The PA Rotation
Exam Review

The PA Rotation Exam Review

Paul Alexander Gonzales, MPAS, PA-C
Physician Assistant
Comprehensive Epilepsy Center
Children's Health
Dallas, Texas

Wolters Kluwer

Philadelphia • Baltimore • New York • London
Buenos Aires • Hong Kong • Sydney • Tokyo

Acquisitions Editor: Matt Hauber
Product Development Editor: Andrew Hall; Andrea Vosburgh
Editorial Coordinator: Tim Rinehart
Marketing Manager: Michael McMahon
Production Project Manager: Linda Van Pelt
Design Coordinator: Holly McLaughlin
Illustration Coordinator: Jennifer Clements
Manufacturing Coordinator: Margie Orzech
Prepress Vendor: TNQ Technologies

9 8 7 6 5 4 3

Printed in the U.S.A.

Library of Congress Cataloging-in-Publication Data

Names: Gonzales, Paul Alexander, author.
Title: The PA rotation exam review / Paul Alexander Gonzales.
Other titles: Physician assistant end of rotation exam review
Description: Philadelphia : Wolters Kluwer, [2019] | Includes bibliographical references and index.
Identifiers: LCCN 2018038939 | ISBN 9781496387271 (paperback)
Subjects: | MESH: Physician Assistants | Internship and Residency | Examination Questions
Classification: LCC R697.P45 | NLM W 18.2 | DDC 610.73/72069–dc23
LC record available at https://lccn.loc.gov/2018038939

shop.lww.com

To my best friend and loyal husband, Conner, who is incredibly patient, loving, and understanding.

To my parents, Fabian and Valerie, who always support me.

To my alma mater, UT Southwestern, and all of the faculty and PA students who have helped perfect this book.

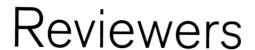

Reviewers

Christine Alexander
Student
University of Texas Southwestern Medical Center
Dallas, Texas

Maria Burk
Student
University of Texas Southwestern Medical Center
Dallas, Texas

Kelsey Devine
Student
University of Texas Southwestern Medical Center
Dallas, Texas

Lauren Esrock
Student
University of Texas Southwestern Medical Center
Dallas, Texas

Mina Fawze
Student
Jefferson College of Health Sciences
Roanoke, Virginia

Dara Goral
Student
University of Texas Southwestern Medical Center Dallas,
Texas

Lindsey Grace Gerke
Student
University of Texas Southwestern Medical Center
Dallas, Texas

Sarah Jane Whinery
Student
University of Texas Southwestern Medical Center
Dallas, Texas

Sarah Lindner
Student
University of Texas Southwestern Medical Center
Dallas, Texas

Elizabeth Lloyd-Davies
Student
University of Texas Southwestern Medical Center
Dallas, Texas

Aaron Longale
Physician Assistant
Interservice Physician Assistant Program
Schererville, Indiana

Allison Loy
Student
Jefferson College of Health Sciences
Roanoke, Virginia

Tanya Michelle Ehart
Student
University of Texas Southwestern Medical Center
Dallas, Texas

Taylor Piatkowski
Student
James Madison University
Harrisonburg, Virginia

Jonathan White
Student
South College
Knoxville, Tennessee

About the Author

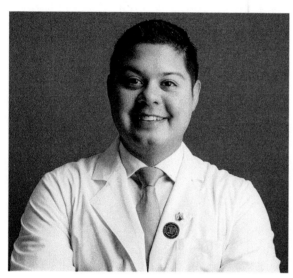

(Photo credit: Omar Ramos Photography.)

Paul Alexander Gonzales studied biomedical engineering as an undergraduate at the University of Texas at Austin and received his Master of Physician Assistant Studies at UT Southwestern Medical Center in December 2016. He began his career in pediatric epilepsy at Children's Health in Dallas, Texas, where he also has elected to precept students. Over the past decade, he has dedicated his life to teaching mathematics and the sciences, eventually leading to other opportunities, including becoming a guest lecturer at a Spark Session for AAPA 2016 and attending both the Future Educator Fellowship and the PAEA™ (Physician Assistant Education Association) Stakeholder Summit in 2016. He was the recipient of the AAPA Student Academy PAragon Student Award in 2015 and is a member of many professional organizations, including the Alpha Eta Society; National Scholastic Honor Society for Allied Health Professionals; Pi Alpha National Honor Society for PAs; the National Hispanic Medical Association; the Hispanic Scholarship Consortium; the American Academy of Physician Assistants; and the Physician Assistant Education Association. He is also a Neal Kocurek Scholar, among many other awards and accolades.

He is best known for the site DoseofPA.blogspot.com (formerly known as "Trust Me, I'm a PA Student"), which contains many free resources available to both pre-PA and PA students. He gained further writing experience volunteering as assistant editor and later senior editor of *First Rounds*, the student section of *PA Professional Magazine*.

In his free time, he is an amateur skier and loves to spend time with his husband, Conner, and their two pugs, Pickles and Pepito.

Preface

Discovering the type of learner you are requires time and effort, and the process is not always straightforward. As learners, as students, we must adapt our learning style to various challenges that come our way. Each day we modify the way we think to recall profound amounts of information, both clinical and nonclinical. That information must be processed and stored in our memory for use in the future.

Through my journey to become a lifelong learner I have encountered many challenges. The world of medicine is vast and even today, as a practicing clinician, there is so much to learn. Pattern recognition, even between seemingly unrelated content, is essential for organizing and retaining such a large volume of knowledge. Developing a method in which you can classify information as you read and learn it can help you to understand and recall it. This method presented in this text is very systematic and may not be for everyone, but I have found that it is extremely useful to study clinical medicine in various formats to improve recollection.

During Physician Assistant (PA) school I discovered that students from previous classes would create study guides to help one another study for examinations in both didactic and clinical education. Contributing study guides and practice questions to this information bank was a helpful study aid for myself and others in my class.

In the PA school I attended, our class was required to take standardized examinations to test our knowledge and skills throughout the "core" clinical rotations. Akin to shelf examinations for medical students, we studied for and took these comprehensive examinations at the end of each rotation.

One of the many challenges of taking these examinations was a lack of expectation. The use of rotation examinations was new at our school, so there were few practice examinations or helpful resources for students. During rotations in my second year of PA school, I decided to create a tabular review for each rotation. After the first few rotations, I realized how helpful they had been and decided to continue creating them. I shared them among my peers and received

positive feedback. I believe these study guides can help all PA students throughout clinical rotations. This is a resource that can tailor your studies, offer a new format for learning the material, and stretch your mind to consider a broader understanding of each disease.

One of the defining features of PA student education is that it is very condensed, requiring us to use our time efficiently. During each 4- to 8-week rotation, we are given a long list of topics to cover—some very narrow and clear-cut and others very broad and vague. Throughout the rotation, we must balance studying for examinations with actively learning how to practice clinical medicine—developing good bedside manner, performing documentation, accessing information you don't know and applying what you do. This pressure is common among medical professionals at every level of training. This book is dedicated to allowing a student to focus more on the latter half, rather than stressing over an examination.

This book can be used not only during clinical rotations but also as a companion text during didactic, when minds are discovering new techniques to study information differently. By no means is this meant to be a book you pick up off the shelf five days before an examination to cram; it is meant to be read during didactic or throughout rotations and can be used as a final review of the topics you struggled with or missed practice questions about.

The book provides a reference at the beginning of each chapter pointing to topics discussed elsewhere in the text to alleviate redundancy. It covers all of the most commonly tested rotations, including Family Medicine, Internal Medicine, Emergency Medicine, Surgery, Pediatrics, Psychiatry, and Obstetrics and Gynecology. It features questions both in print and online to help you tailor your studies to whatever format your examination may be. The organization of the book is as follows: (1) etiology, prevalence, risk factors, and pathophysiology, (2) presentation of signs, symptoms, and associated diagnoses, (3) diagnostic studies and expected results, and (4) clinical therapeutics or intervention, prognosis, and possible prophylaxis or health maintenance. Throughout the text, I try to detail high-yield information by placing topics you should stress in bold. There are also topics listed that may not be on the blueprints but are recommended topics that I feel students should know for real-world clinical practice.

I wish each student the best success, and I hope that this text will serve your every need throughout each of your rotations. This is the exciting beginning of your professional career spent serving a diverse, complex patient population, and there will always be more to learn—even after you become a board-certified physician assistant.

Paul Alexander Gonzales

Contents

Medical Abbreviations

AAA=abdominal aortic aneurysm
AAP = American Academy of Pediatrics
AAT = alpha-1 antitrypsin
Ab = antibody
ABG/VBG = arterial blood gas/venous blood gas
ACEI = angiotensin-converting enzyme inhibitor
ACS = acute coronary syndrome
ADA = American Diabetes Association
ADHF = acute decompensated heart failure
ADL = activity of daily living
AFB = acid-fast bacilli
Ag-EIA = antigen enzyme immunoassay
AICD = automatic implantable cardioverter defibrillator
AMG = urine alpha 1- microglobulin
AMH = anti-Müllerian hormone
AMS = altered mental status
ANA = antinuclear antibody
ANC = absolute neutrophil count
ANCA = antineutrophil cytoplasmic antibody
AP = anteroposterior
aPTT = activated partial thromboplastin time
ARB = angiotensin II receptor blocker
ARDS = acute respiratory distress syndrome
ART = antiretroviral therapy
ASD = atrial septal defect
ATE = arterial thromboembolism
ATG = anti-thyroglobulin antibody
ATLS = advanced trauma life support
ATN = acute tubular necrosis
AV = atrioventricular
AVN = avascular necrosis
BB = beta-blockers
BBB = blood-brain barrier
BDZ = benzodiazepine
B-hCG = beta human chorionic gonadotropin
BID = twice a day
BiPAP = bilevel positive airway pressure
BM = bowel movement
BMP = basic metabolic panel
BPH = benign prostatic hypertrophy

BPM = beats per minute
BSA = body surface area
BUN = blood urea nitrogen
CA = cancer antigen
CAP = coronary artery pressure
CCP = cyclic citrullinated peptide
CF = cystic fibrosis
CFTR = cystic fibrosis transmembrane conductance regulator
CGMP = cyclic guanosine monophosphate
CHF = congestive heart failure
CK-MB =creatine-kinase muscle/brain
CMA = chromosomal microarray analysis
CML = chronic myelogenous leukemia
CMV = cytomegalovirus
CN =cranial nerve
CNS = central nervous system
CoNS = coagulase-negative *Staphylococcus*
COPD = chronic obstructive pulmonary disease
CP = cerebral palsy
CPAP = continuous positive airway pressure
CPR = cardiopulmonary resuscitation
CPS = Child Protective Services
CRAG = cryptococcal antigen assay
CRC = colorectal cancer
CRP = C-reactive protein
CSF = cerebrospinal fluid
CT = computed tomography
CTPA = CT pulmonary angiogram
CVA = cerebrovascular accident
CVD = cardiovascular disease
CVT = cerebral venous thombosis
CXR = chest X-ray
DDAVP = desmopressin acetate
DDx = differential diagosis
DHEA = dehydroepiandrosterone
DI = diabetes insipidus
DIP = distal interphalangeal
DKA = diabetic ketoacidosis

DLCO = diffusing capacity of the lung for carbon monoxide
DMARD = disease-modifying antirheumatic drug
DMSA = dimercaptosuccinic acid
DRE = digital rectal examination
DSM = Diagnostic and Statistical Manual
DTI = direct thrombin inhibitors
DTR = deep tendon reflexes
DVT = deep vein thrombosis
DX = diagnosis
EBV = Epstein–Barr virus
ECI = early childhood intervention
ECT = electroconvulsive therapy
ED = emergency department
EEG = electroencephalogram
EGA = estimated gestational age
EGD = esophagogastroduodenoscopy
ELISA = enzyme-linked immunosorbent assay
EMB = endometrial biopsy
EMG = electromyography
EPS = extrapyramidal symptoms
ESRD = end-stage renal disease
FFP = fresh frozen plasma
FH = family history
FNA = fine needle aspiration
FOBT = fecal occult blood test
FSH = follicle-stimulating hormone
FTA-ABS = fluorescent treponemal antibody
absorption test
FVC = forced vital capacity
GAS = group A streptococcus
GBS = group B streptococcus
GERD = gastroesophageal reflux disease
GFR = glomerular filtration rate
GHD = growth hormone deficiency
GI = gastrointestinal
GMG = generalized myasthenia gravis
GN = glomerulonephritis
GSM = genitourinary syndrome of menopause
GTT = glucose tolerance test
GU = genitourinary
H&H = hemoglobin & hematocrit
HA = headache
HCC = hepatocellular carcinoma
hCG = human chorionic gonadotropin
HD = high dose
HDL = high-density lipoprotein
HIV = human immunodeficiency virus
HLA = human leukocyte antigen
HPA = hypothalamic–pituitary–adrenal
HPF = high-power field
HPV = human papilloma virus
HR = heart rate
HX = history
IABP = intra-aortic balloon pump
IBD = inflammatory bowel disease
IBS = irritable bowel syndrome
ICD = implantable cardioverter defibrillator
ICH = intracranial haemorrhage

ICP = intracranial pressure
ICU = intensive care unit
IDA = iron deficiency anemia
IFG = impaired fasting glycemia
IGF = insulin-like growth factor
ILD = interstitial lung diseases
INO = internuclear ophthalmoplegia
INR = international normalized ratio
IOP = intraocular pressure
IPV = inactivated polio vaccine
ISS = injury severity score
ITP = idiopathic thrombocytopenic purpura
IUGR = intrauterine growth restriction
IVC = inferior vena cava
IVF = in vitro fertilization
IVIG = intravenous immunoglobulin
JRA = juvenile rheumatoid arthritis
JVD = jugular venous distention
LDH = lactate dehydrogenase
LDL = low-density lipoprotein
LFT = liver function test
LOC = loss of consciousness
LP = lumbar puncture
LR = lactated Ringer's solution
LTCF = long-term care facility
LVAD = left ventricular assist device
LVD = left ventricular dysfunction
LVEF = left ventricular ejection fraction
MAOI = monoamine oxidase inhibitor
MC = most common
MCL = medial collateral ligament
MCP = metacarpophalangeal
MDD = major depressive disorder
MEN = multiple endocrine neoplasia
MET = metastasis
MHA-TP = microhemagglutination assay for *Treponema
pallidum* antibodies
MI = myocardial infarction
MIP = maximal inspiratory pressure
MMA = methylmalonic acid
MMR = mumps, measles, rubella
MN = motor neuron
MR = mental retardation
MRA = magnetic resonance angiography
MRCP = magnetic resonance cholangiopancreatography
MRI = magnetic resonance imaging
MSAFP = maternal serum alpha fetoprotein
MTP = metatarsophalangeal
MTX = methotrexate
MVC = motor vehicle crash
NE = norepinephrine
NG = nasogastric
NHL = non-Hodgkin lymphoma
NL = normal
NMJ = neuromuscular junction
NPO = nothing by mouth
NS = normal saline
NT = nuchal translucency

NTG = nitroglycerin
NYHA = New York Heart Association
OAB = overactive bladder
OCD = obsessive-compulsive disorder
OD = right eye
ODD = oppositional defiant disorder
OGL = oral glucose loading
OGTT = oral glucose tolerance test
OMG = ocular myasthenia gravis
OPIDN = organophosphate-induced delayed neuropathy
OR = operating room
OSA = obstructive sleep apnea
PA = physician assistant
PAN = polyarteritis nodosa
p-ANCA = perinuclear anti-neutrophil cytoplasmic antibodies
PCN = penicillin
PCR = polymerase chain reaction
PCWP = pulmonary capillary wedge pressure
PDA = patent ductus arteriosus
PDE = phosphodiesterase
PE = pulmonary embolism
PEA = pulseless electrical activity
PET = positron emission tomography
PHN = postherpetic neuralgia
PHQ = patient health questionnaire
PID = pelvic inflammatory disease
PIP = proximal interphalangeal
PMN = polymorphonuclear
PNA = pneumonia
PND = paroxysmal nocturnal dyspnoea
PPD = purified protein derivative
PPI = proton-pump inhibitor
PR = per rectum
PRTA = percutaneous transluminal renal angioplasty
PSA = prostate-specific antigen
PSC = primary sclerosing cholangitis
PTC = percutaneous transhepatic cholangiography
PTH = parathyroid hormone
PTL = preterm labor
PTT = partial thromboplastin time
PTU = propylthiouracil
PUD = peptic ulcer disease
PVR = pulmonary vascular resistance
QID = four times daily
QOL = quality of life
R/O = rule out
RAT = rapid antigen test
RBC = red blood cell
RCM = restrictive cardiomyopathy
RET = rearranged during transfection
RNS = repetitive nerve stimulation
ROM = range of motion
RPR = rapid plasma reagin
RR = respiratory rate
RSV = respiratory syncytial virus
RT-PCR = reverse transcriptase polymerase chain reaction
RUQ = right upper quadrant

RYGB = Roux-en-Y gastric bypass
SAAG = serum albumin ascites gradient
SAH = subarachnoid hemorrhage
SCC = squamous cell carcinoma
SCD = sequential compression devices
SCFE = slipped capital femoral epiphysis
SCI = spinal cord injury
SGA = small for gestational age
SIADH = syndrome of inappropriate antidiuretic hormone
SIRS = systemic inflammatory response syndrome
SLE = systemic lupus erythematosus
SMA = superior mesenteric artery
SMX = sulfamethoxazole
SNRI = serotonin-norepinephrine reuptake inhibitor
SPN = solitary pulmonary nodule
SQ = subcutaneous
STEMI = ST elevation myocardial infarction
SVT = supraventricular tachycardia
T4 = thyroxine
TB = tuberculosis
TCA = trichloroacetic acid
TFT = thyroid function test
THC = tetrahydrocannabinol
TIA = transient ischemic attack
TIBC = total iron binding capacity
TKA = Takayasu arteritis
TLC = total lung capacity
TMJ = temporomandibular joint
TMP = trimethoprim
tPA = tissue plasminogen activator
TPN = total parenteral nutrition
TPO = thyroperoxidase
TRUS = transrectal ultrasonography
TTP = thrombotic thrombocytopenic purpura
TX = treatment
TZD = thiazolidinedione
U/A = urinalysis
UC = ulcerative colitis
UE = upper extremity
ULN = upper limit of normal
UMN = upper motor neuron
URI = upper respiratory infection
USPSTF = US Preventive Services Task Force
UT = urinary tract
UVA = ultraviolet A
UVB = ultraviolet B
VBG = venous blood gas
VC = vital capacity
VDRL = venereal disease research laboratory
VKA = vitamin K antagonist
VLDL = very-low-density lipoprotein
VO = oxygen consumption
VQ = ventilation/perfusion
VS = vital signs
VTE = venous thromboembolism
VUR = vesicoureteral reflux
VZV = varicella-zoster virus
XRT = external radiation therapy

CHAPTER 1

Cardiology

Refer to Internal Medicine for in-depth coverage of the following topics:

Refer to Appendices for the following topics:

Supplemental material:

CONGESTIVE HEART FAILURE

- Decompensated heart failure: evidence on physical examination or chest radiograph of pulmonary edema, audible third heart sound, or increased JVP
- **Left ventricular failure**: symptoms of low cardiac output and congestion (predominate feature: **SOB**) due to systolic or diastolic dysfunction
- **Right ventricular failure**: symptoms of fluid overload almost always due to left ventricular failure
- Most common cause of systolic heart failure (HF with reduced EF): ischemic cardiomyopathy (CAD with resultant MI and loss of functioning myocardium)
  - Treatment aimed at reducing death and hospitalization
- **Systolic dysfunction**: difficulty with ventricular contraction
- **Diastolic dysfunction** (HF with preserved EF): difficulty with ventricular relaxation; results from hypertension and associated with aging; related to myocardial muscle stiffening and LVH
  - Treatment aimed at improving symptoms and treating comorbidities

Disease	Etiology, Prevalence, Risk Factors	Clinical Symptoms and Signs	Diagnostics	Therapy, Prognosis, and Health Maintenance

Congestive heart failure	MCC: **CAD**, HTN, DM
	LV remodeling: dilation, thinning, mitral valve incompetence, RV remodeling
	75% have preexisting HTN
	MCC of **transudative pleural effusions**
	Mostly >age 65 y
		Most common:
		1. Exertional **dyspnea** (SOB), then with rest
		  • Chronic nonproductive cough, worse in recumbent position
		2. **Fatigue**
		3. Orthopnea (late), night cough, relieved by sitting up or sleeping with additional pillows
		4. Paroxysmal nocturnal dyspnea
		5. Nocturia
		Signs:
		1. Cheyne-Stokes breathing: periodic, cyclic respiration
		2. Edema: ankles, pretibial (cardinal)
		3. **Rales** (crackles)
		4. Additional heart sounds
		S4 = diastolic HF (preserved EF)
		S3 = Systolic HF (reduced EF) with volume overload
		  • Tachycardia, tachypnea
		5. Jugular venous pressure: >8 cm
		6. Cold extremities, cyanosis
		7. Hepatomegaly
		  • Ascites, jaundice, peripheral edema
			For new onset, chronic, or acute decompensation:
			1. Basic labs: CBC, CMP, U/A ± glucose, lipids, TSH
			  • Occult hyperthyroidism or hypothyroidism
			2. **Serum BNP**: increases with age and renal impairment, low in obese
			  • Elevated in HF
			  • Differentiates SOB in HF from noncardiac issues
			3. **12-lead EKG**
			4. CXR: Kerley B lines
			5. Echo: diagnose, evaluate, manage
			  • Most useful, differentiates HF ± preserved LV diastolic function
			6. Other findings: **reduced pulse pressure** and SVR
				Acute management (mnemonic: LMNOP):
				1. Lasix—for diuresis
				2. Morphine—reduces preload
				3. Nitrates (NTG)—reduce preload
				4. O₂
				1. Position
				2. ACE inhibitor + diuretic (unless contraindicated)
				3. CCB in diastolic HF
				4. Poor prognosis factors: chronic kidney disease, diabetes, lower LVEF, severe symptoms, old age
				5. 5-y mortality: 50%

- BNP—elevated when ventricular filling pressures are high (very sensitive); less specific in older patients, women, and patients with COPD
  - NT-pro-BNP <300 pg/mL or BNP <100 pg/mL with a normal EKG makes HF less likely

- Helpful to guide intensity of diuretic use and disease-modifying agents (ACE/BB) for acute setting; less helpful for chronic

When to Refer Versus Admit

Refer	Admit
• New symptoms of HF not explained by obvious cause • Continued symptoms and reduced LVEF (<35%)	• Unexplained new or worsening symptoms or (+) biomarkers indicating acute MI • Hypoxia, fluid overload, pulmonary edema not resolved as outpatient

New York Heart Association Heart Failure Classification

Functional Capacity	Objective Assessment
Class I, <5%	Cardiac disease without **any** limitation of physical activity (ordinary activity **does not** cause fatigue, palpitations, dyspnea, anginal pain).
Class II: moderate activity, 10%-15%	Cardiac disease with **slight** limitation of physical activity (ordinary activity **results in** fatigue, palpitations, dyspnea, anginal pain). *Comfortable at rest.*
Class III, 20%-25%	Cardiac disease with **marked** limitation of physical activity (less than ordinary activity causes fatigue, palpitations, dyspnea, anginal pain). *Comfortable at rest.*
Class IV: symptoms at rest, 35%-40%	Cardiac disease with **inability** to carry on physical activity without discomfort. Symptoms present **even at rest**; if activity undertaken, discomfort increased.
A	No objective evidence of cardiovascular disease. No symptoms and no limitation in ordinary physical activity.
B	Objective evidence of minimal cardiovascular disease. Mild symptoms and slight limitation during ordinary activity. Comfortable at rest.
C	Objective evidence of moderately severe cardiovascular disease. Marked limitation in activity owing to symptoms, even during less-than-ordinary activity. Comfortable only at rest.
D	Objective evidence of severe cardiovascular disease. Severe limitations. Experiences symptoms even while at rest.

HYPERTENSION (EMERGENCIES)

Disease	Clinical Symptoms and Signs	Diagnostics	Therapy, Prognosis, and Health Maintenance
See etiology below	Symptoms: 1. **>140/90 mm Hg** during at least 2 separate visits 2. Mostly asymptomatic with nonspecific headache Signs: 1. BMI and waist circumference 2. BP in both arms, compare radial and femoral pulses 3. Examine for abdominal aortic masses, PMI, murmurs, bruits 4. **Fundoscopic examination** for eye changes	1. **EKG**: LVH with strain 2. CXR 3. Basic labs • CBC, CMP • Toxicology screen • Pregnancy test • TSH • Hgb/Hct: decreased • BUN, creatinine, glucose: elevated • Urinary glucose, protein, sediment: renal disease or DM • U/A: hematuria or proteinuria • Lipid profile	1. Treatment goal: <140/90 **mm Hg** general population, those with diabetes, and those with renal disease[a] • Older than age 60 y: <150/90 **mm Hg**[a] 2. **Lifestyle modification** (first line) • DASH diet • Weight loss • Smoking cessation • Limit ETOH and Na intake 3. Meds • **ACE inhibitors**–for patients with diabetes, renal disease • Thiazide diuretics–AA, check for hypokalemia • CCB • Aldosterone antagonists for refractory HTN, post-MI, HF • α blockers: BPH • Hydralazine: refractory HTN

[a]Follows JNC-8 Guidelines.

	Systolic Pressure (mm Hg)	Diastolic Pressure (mm Hg)
Normal	<120	<80
Prehypertension	120-139 **(120-129)**	80-89 **(<80)**
Stage 1 hypertension	140-159 **(130-139)**	90-99 **(80-89)**
Stage 2 hypertension	>160 **(>140)**	>100 **(>90)**
Urgency	>220	>125
Emergency	>220	>130

As of 2017 ACC/AHA Guidelines.

Metabolic Syndrome

• Consists of (1) truncal obesity, (2) hyperinsulinemia and insulin resistance, (3) hypertriglyceridemia, (4) HTN

• Associated with DM and increased CV complications

	Etiology and Diagnostic Criteria	Treatment
Primary (essential) hypertension: 90%-95%	Multifactorial: • Genetic predisposition (old age, African American) • Environmental (high-salt diet, obesity) • Sympathetic NS activity, abnormal cardiovascular or renal development, imbalance in RAAS, deficit in sodium secretion, abnormal Na-K exchange Exacerbating factors: • Excessive ETOH use, tobacco use • Lack of exercise/sedentary lifestyle • Polycythemia • Use of NSAIDs • Low K+ intake	See above
Secondary HTN: 5%-10%	• Parenchymal disease, **renal artery stenosis**, coarctation of aorta, pheochromocytoma, Cushing syndrome, hyperthyroidism, primary hyperaldosteronism, chronic steroid use, estrogen use, NSAID use, sleep apnea	Treat underlying disease
Hypertensive urgency	• BP that must be reduced within hours • Persistently elevated higher than **220 systolic or 125 diastolic** or accompanied complications **without** end-organ damage	1. Oral agents: **clonidine**, captopril, nifedipine, **labetalol**

(continued)

(continued)

	Etiology and Diagnostic Criteria	Treatment

Hypertensive emergency (malignant hypertension)
Elevated BP with **papilledema** or **retinal hemorrhage**, and either encephalopathy or nephropathy, confusion, left ventricular failure, intravascular coagulation
Difference: HTN emergency always has retinal papilledema and flame-shaped hemorrhages and exudates
	• Elevated BP that must be reduced within 1 h to prevent **progression** of end organ damage or death
	• Persistently elevated higher than **220 systolic**
	• Diastolic pressure **>130 mm Hg**
	Complications:
	• *Encephalopathy, nephropathy*, ICH, aortic dissection, pulmonary edema, unstable angina, MI, **stroke** (most common)
	• Encephalopathy: seizures, visual changes, altered mental status
	• **Fundoscopic examination**: new retinal hemorrhages, exudates, papilledema (Fig. 1-1)
	  • If left untreated → progressive renal failure (hematuria and weight loss)
	• **Hallmark**: fibrinoid necrosis of the arterioles in the kidneys
		<u>Do not reduce BP too rapidly; can cause ischemia:</u>
		1. Sodium nitroprusside
		  • Short acting, titrate minute to minute, constant monitoring
		  • Potential for thiocyanate and cyanide toxicity with prolonged use or if renal/hepatic failure
		2. **Labetalol** (α and β block)
		  • Preferred in acute dissection and ESRD
		  • 10-20 mg bolus, 1 mg/min until desired BP
		Neurologic emergencies:
		• Encephalopathy, stroke, ICH, subarachnoid hemorrhage
		  • Labetalol, nicardipine, esmolol (preferred agents)
		  • Avoid nitroprusside and hydralazine
		  • Reduce MAP 25% over 8 h
		  • For MI: use **NTG or a BB**
		• Aortic dissection: use **nitroprusside** and **BB** (labetalol) and urgent surgery
		• Hydralazine—especially during pregnancy
		• Lower BP within first 24-48 h by 25%
		  • ICU admission
		  • 90% will die after 1-2 y

- Nitroprusside is converted to cyanide in the bloodstream and has the potential to cause **cyanide toxicity**, particularly in the setting of prolonged exposure (infusions lasting several hours), chronic renal insufficiency, and young age. This leads to hypertensive encephalopathy

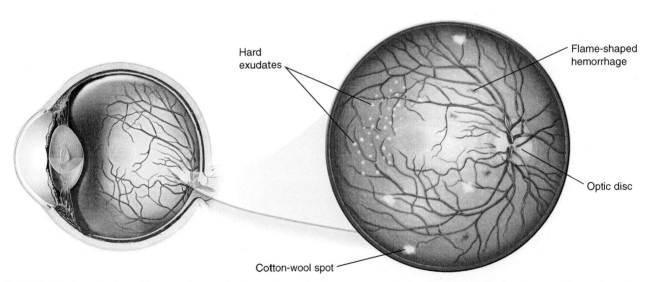

FIGURE 1-1. Complications of hypertension on a funduscopic examination may reveal arteriosclerosis, retinal hemorrhages, cotton wool spots, exudates, and possibly papilledema (leading to blindness). (From Anatomical Chart Co. *Hypertension Anatomical Chart.* Philadelphia: Lippincott Wiliams & Wilkins; 2004.)

ENDOCARDITIS

Disease	Etiology, Prevalence, Risk Factors	Clinical Symptoms and Signs	Diagnostics	Therapy, Prognosis, and Health Maintenance
Endocarditis	MC: Native valve infection (Streptococcus *viridans*, Staphylococcus *aureus*, enterococci) IVDU: • **S. aureus, tricuspid valve** • Prosthetic valve: S. aureus, gram-negative organisms, or fungi → streptococci or staphylococci • Most patients have underlying regurgitant defect providing a nidus • Infection from DIC or bacteremia, especially with procedures	1. Fever 2. Nonspecific SX: **dyspnea, cough, chest pain,** arthralgias, back or flank pain, GI complaints Signs: 1. **Stable murmur** (90%) 2. Palatal, conjunctival, or subungual petechiae (25%), splinter hemorrhages 3. Pallor 4. Splenomegaly Diagnostic signs: 1. **Osler nodes**: painful, violaceous, raised lesions of fingers, toes, feet 2. **Janeway lesions**: painless red lesions of palms/soles 3. **Roth spots**: exudative lesions in retina Associated: Strokes, emboli	1. Three sets of **blood cultures** at least 1 h apart, before starting ABX 2. **Echo**: required to make diagnosis and identify involved valves **(vegetation)**	1. Empiric antibiotics: cover staphylococci, streptococci, and enterococci 2. Native Valve: Vancomycin alone OR + Cefazolin 3. Ill patients w/ HF: **gentamicin** plus • Cefepime • Vancomycin 4. Valve replacement (aortic valve) if refractory or abscess (fungal infection) Prophylaxis: Antibiotic prophylaxis to prevent endocarditis recommended before invasive dental work or surgical procedures: prosthetic valves, previous IE, some congenital heart diseases (transposition, Tetralogy), acquired valve disorders, HCM, cardiac transplant patients with valvulopathy → **amoxicillin** Health maintenance: Anticoagulants not beneficial

Modified Duke Criteria

Must have (1) 2 major, (2) 1 major and 3 minor, (3) 5 minor criteria.

Major	Minor
1. Two positive blood cultures of typical causative microorganism 2. Echo showing new valvular regurgitation	1. Predisposing factor 2. Fever >100.4°F (38°C) 3. Vascular phenomena (embolic disease or pulmonary infarct) 4. Immunologic phenomena: glomerulonephritis, Osler nodes, Roth spots 5. (+) blood culture not meeting major criteria

Endocarditis Prophylaxis

- Prosthetic heart valves or material used for valve repair; repair of congenital heart defect with prosthetic material or device

- History of previous infective endocarditis

- Unrepaired cyanotic congenital heart disease; repaired congenital heart disease with residual defects

- Cardiac transplant with valve regurgitation due to structurally abnormal valve

- Treatment:

  - Amoxicillin 2 g PO 1 hour before procedure (standard), 50 mg/kg in children

  - PCN allergy: clarithromycin or azithromycin 500 mg PO 1-hour pre-op

HYPERLIPIDEMIA

Elevated LDLs increase the risk of CAD; higher HDLs are thought to be protective; elevated triglycerides are also a risk factor for atherosclerosis; severe elevations can cause pancreatitis.

- Recommended screening for patients with no evidence of CVD and **no risk factors** begin **at age 35 years** (USPSTF)

- NCEP recommends screening all adults **at age 20 years** regardless of risk factors

Disease	Etiology, Prevalence, Risk Factors	Clinical Symptoms and Signs	Diagnostics	Therapy, Prognosis, and Health Maintenance
Hyperlipidemia	Genetic: Primary HLD, familial hypercholesterolemia Secondary to DM, ETOH, hypothyroid, obesity, sedentary lifestyle, renal or liver disease, drugs RF: 1. Diabetes (CAD risk equivalent) 2. Smoking 3. Hypertension 4. HDL <40 5. Age (>45 y, men; >55y women) 6. Early CAD in first-degree relatives (<55 y, men; <65 y, women) 7. HIV (CAD risk equivalent)	Most asymptomatic: 1. Eruptive or tendinous xanthomas 2. Two-thirds of all people with **xanthelasmas** affecting eyelids have normal lipid profiles 3. Severe → premature arcus senilis; lipemia retinalis (cream-colored retinal vessels) are seen with TG levels >2000 mg/dL	1. Without RF, order a total cholesterol	1. **Lifestyle changes** (first line): • Reduce total fat intake to 25%-30%, saturated fat <7%, dietary cholesterol <200 mg/d • 30 min of aerobic exercise daily • Increase antioxidants from fruits and vegetables, soluble fiber may reduce LDL • CAD prophylaxis (81 mg aspirin) unless otherwise contraindicated • Smoking cessation 2. Statin therapy Health maintenance: 1. Patients with any evidence of CVD or CAD risk equivalent (DM, HIV) should be screened with fasting complete lipid profile

Pharmacologic Therapy for Hyperlipidemia

	Statins (HMG-CoA Reductase Inhibitors)	Niacin	Bile-Acid Sequestrants (Cholestyramine, Colesevelam, Colestipol)	Fibric Acid Derivatives (Gemfibrozil, Clofibrate)	Fish Oil (Omega-3 Fatty Acids)
MOA	Reduce cholesterol production in the liver and increase ability of liver to remove LDL from blood	Reduces long-term risk of CAD by reducing production of VLDL, lowering LDL, and increasing HDL; may also reduce TG	Bind bile acids in the intestine; resins reduce the incidence of coronary events in middle-aged men; no effect on mortality	Peroxisome proliferator-activated receptor alpha (PPAR-α) agonists—most important meds for lowering of triglyceride levels and raising HDL	
LDL	↓18%-55%	↓5%-25%	↓15%-30%	↓5%-20%	↑2%-5%
Triglycerides	↓7%-30%	↓20%-50%	↓0%-15%	↓25%-50%	↓30%-40%
HDL	↑5%-15%	↑15%-35%	↑3%-5%	↑10%-20%	Increase
Adverse effects	**Myalgias**, mild GI complaints Severe: myositis, liver toxicity, rhabdomyolysis	Prostaglandin-induced **niacin flushing** may be reduced by taking aspirin 30 min prior or a daily NSAID	Constipation, gas	May induce gallstones, hepatitis, myositis	1. Fishy taste after burping 2. Nausea
Monitoring	1. LFTs and creatinine-phosphokinase if myalgias develop 2. Monitor lipids every 6 wk until goals met	1. Baseline LFTs 2. LFTs – every 6-12 wk first year, then every 6 mo 3. Lipid panel 4. Blood sugar (diabetic) or platelets and PT (if on anticoagulants), uric acid (gout)	1. Fasting lipid profile prior to treatment, then 3 mo after initiation, then 6-12 mo thereafter	1. Periodic LFT, CBC, cholesterol in the first year	

• Ezetimibe blocks intestinal absorption of dietary and biliary cholesterol by blocking a cholesterol transport and may be used as monotherapy or in combo with a statin

Lipid Goals for Hyperlipidemia

	LDL		Total Cholesterol			HDL
Optimal	<100	Desirable	<200	Protective	>60
Near optimal	100-129	Borderline high	200-239	Borderline	41-59
Borderline high	130-159	High	>239	At risk	<40
High	160-189				
Very high	>189				

CORONARY VASCULAR DISEASE (CAD/CHD)

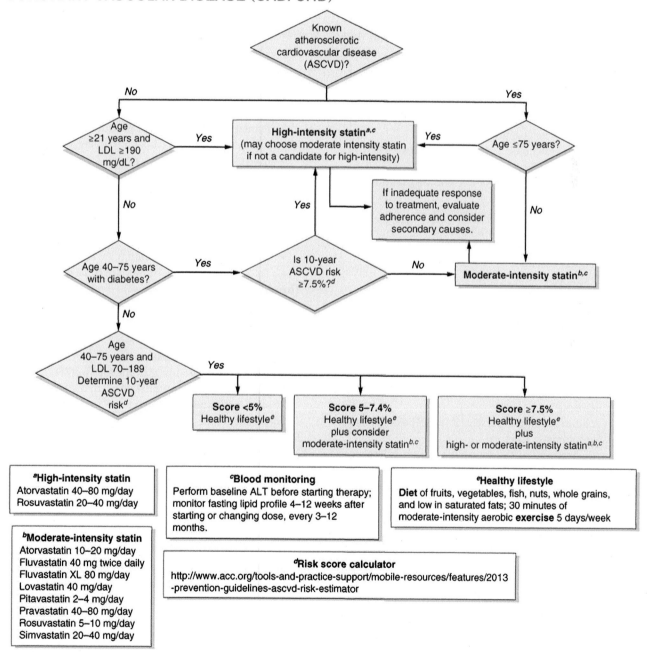

FIGURE 1-2. Recommendations for statin therapy initiation for ASCVD prevention. (From Stone NJ, Robinson JG, Lichtenstein AH, et al. 2013 ACC/AHA guideline on the treatment of blood cholesterol to reduce atherosclerotic cardiovascular risk in adults: a report of the American College of Cardiology/American Heart Association Task Force on Practice Guidelines. *Circulation*. 2014;129[25 suppl 2]:S1-S45.)

- Risk factor modification

Mild	EF: normal Angina: mild Single-vessel disease	**NTG** (SX and prophylaxis) **BB** ± CCB–if refractory
Moderate	EF: normal Angina: moderate 2-vessel disease	± coronary angiography for revascularization (PCI)
Severe	EF: normal Angina: mild 3-vessel disease, *left main* or left anterior descending	Coronary angiography Consider for CABG

- **Smoking cessation**—cuts risk by 50%
- Medical therapy—standard of care is **ASA + BB**
  - **Sublingual NTG** tablets or sublingual isosorbide dinitrate—primary for acute angina
  - **Aspirin**—indicated in all patients with CAD
    - **Decreases morbidity and mortality**, reducing risk of MI due to infarction secondary to emboli
    - Clopidogrel may also be used
    - Inhibits platelet aggregation
  - **β-blockers**—atenolol and metoprolol (first-line choices)
    - Prolong life; first line for chronic angina and treat ischemic symptoms
    - Reduce HR, BP, contractility—lowers O_2 consumption
    - Reduces remodeling post-MI
    - Reduces mortality
  - ACE inhibitors—for patients with heart failure
  - **Morphine** analgesia
    - Venodilation—decreases preload and O_2 demand
  - **Nitrates**—long-acting nitrates (oral, ointment, patch) should include an 8- to 10-hour treatment-free interval to prevent tolerance
    - Dilates coronary arteries—increases supply
    - Venodilation—reduces preload and myocardial O_2 demand
    - Relieves angina and prevents it (taken before exercise)
    - Symptomatic relief
    - AE: headache, orthostatic hypotension, tolerance, syncope
  - CCB—coronary vasodilation and afterload reduction; reduces contractility
    - Secondary treatment when BB or NTG are not fully effective or maximized
    - Can increase mortality because they increase HR
  - **Statins**—stabilize plaques and lower cholesterol (Fig. 1-2)
    - Use atorvastatin 80 mg before discharging
  - If concomitant CHF—use ACE inhibitors and/or diuretics
- Revascularization—does not reduce the risk of MI, but does improve symptoms
  - PCI (also known as coronary **angioplasty**): preferred if contraindications to thrombolytic therapy
    - Coronary angioplasty + balloon and stenting
    - Indications—patients with 1, 2, or 3 vessel diseases

- **Contraindications:** intolerance of long-term antiplatelet therapy or presence of any significant comorbid conditions that severely limit the lifespan of the patient (relative), arteries <1.5 mm diameter (relative), diffuse diseased saphenous vein grafts (relative)
- Restenosis: up to 40% within 6 months!
- CABG
  - Primary method for most institutions
  - Indications: STEMI (though frequently stents are used), cardiogenic shock post-MI, complications with PCI, ventricular arrhythmias, mechanical complications after acute MI, 3-vessel disease with >70% stenosis in each, left main CAD with >50% disease, left ventricular dysfunction
- Antiplatelet therapy
  - Bare metal stents—minimum 4 weeks
  - Drug-eluting stents—minimum of 12 months
- **Thrombolytic therapy (alteplase)**—first-line therapy
  - Patients who present late and PCI contraindicated
  - Administer ASAP up to 24 hours after onset of chest pain, best if given in first 6 hours
  - Indications: ST elevation in 2 contiguous EKG leads with pain onset in 6 hours, refractory to NTG
  - **Contraindications**: trauma (head or CPR), previous stroke, recent invasive surgery/procedure, dissecting aortic aneurysm, active bleeding/diathesis
- Rehabilitation
  - Cardiac rehabilitation—exercise + RF reduction after MI
  - Reduces symptoms and prolongs survival

PERIPHERAL VASCULAR DISEASE OR PERIPHERAL ARTERIAL DISEASE

- In the absence of limb-threatening ischemia, symptoms of PAD tend to remain stable with medical therapy
- Options for revascularization include percutaneous intervention, surgical bypass, or a combination of these, and the choice depends upon the level of obstruction (aortoiliac, femoropopliteal), severity of disease, the patient's risk for the intervention, and the goals for care. Attempt percutaneous revascularization first, reserving surgery for when arterial anatomy is unfavorable.

- Clinical features are useful to help determine if initial thrombolytic therapy (with or without percutaneous intervention) versus surgical revascularization is the most appropriate treatment. These include the following:
  - The presumed etiology (embolus vs thrombus)
  - The location
  - The duration of symptoms
  - The availability of autologous vein for bypass grafting
  - The suitability of the patient for surgery

- As an example, a proximal embolus at the bifurcation of the common femoral artery is an ideal lesion for **embolectomy.** On the other hand, embolus to a distal vessel (eg, to the tibial artery) may be best treated with a thrombolytic agent. The major use of percutaneous transluminal **angioplasty** (PTA) is in the treatment of an underlying lesion after the clot has been lysed with thrombolytic therapy

- **Leriche syndrome** is the triad: (1) claudication, (2) absent or diminished femoral pulses, and (3) erectile dysfunction

Disease	Etiology, Prevalence, Risk Factors	Clinical Symptoms and Signs	Diagnostics	Therapy, Prognosis, and Health Maintenance
Intermittent claudication	Means "limping" Occurs distal to level of stenosis or occlusion Eg, calf pain with walking 10%-35% of people with PAD	1. Reproducible pain in single or multiple muscle groups • Aggravated by sustained exercise • Relieved with rest • Aching, dull pain • Leg pain that occurs after certain walking distance causing patient to stop walking, resolving within 10 min 2. Cramping 3. Numbness, weakness, giving way Physical: 1. **Hair loss** on bilateral lower extremities 2. Thinning of skin 3. Diminished pulses	1. Treadmill testing using **ABIs** at rest and after exercise protocol (confirms) • <0.9 (diagnostic)	**Stop smoking** (first line): 1. Graduated exercise—walk to point of claudication, rest, then continue walking 2. Foot care 3. Control HLD, HTN, weight, DM 4. Avoid extremes of temperature 5. **ASA + ticlopidine** or clopidogrel (symptomatic relief) 6. Cilostazol (PDE inhibitors) Surgery: 1. **Angioplasty** 2. Bypass grafting
Asymptomatic PAD	Screen in patients with: • Abnormal/absent pedal pulses • Age >70 y • Age 50-69 y with HX of smoking or DM	Asymptomatic	1. Ankle-brachial index (ABI) • If <0.90 (diagnostic) • If 0.91-1.3: normal, no further testing • If >1.3: doppler ankle waveforms and toe pressures	1. Preventative treatment: aspirin, lipid lowering, blood pressure control

(continued)

(continued)

Disease	Etiology, Prevalence, Risk Factors	Clinical Symptoms and Signs	Diagnostics	Therapy, Prognosis, and Health Maintenance
PAD (peripheral arterial or vascular disease), or PVD	Occlusive atherosclerotic disease of lower extremities (noncardiac vessels) Sites: **superficial femoral artery (MC)**, popliteal, aortoiliac RF: **smoking**, hyperlipidemia, diabetes mellitus, hypertension Men >40 y, African American MCC: **atherosclerosis** Considered to be a coronary artery disease (CAD) risk equivalent Common in patients with ESRD 20%-50% are asymptomatic and 40%-50% present with atypical leg pain	**1. Pain in one or more lower extremity muscle groups** • Cramping thigh, calf, or buttock pain • Intermittent claudication: Reproduced with exercise and relieved by rest • Worse with elevation (reclining) **2. Rest pain** (continuous): felt over distal metatarsals • **Prominent at night** (wakes patient up from sleep) • **Hangs foot over side of bed** or stands to relieve pain Signs: 1. **Diminished/**absent pulses 2. Muscular atrophy 3. **Hair loss** distal to obstruction 4. **Thick toenails**, decreased skin temperature, localized skin necrosis (toes) 5. Nonhealing, infarction, or gangrene 6. **Pallor** of elevation and rubor of dependency	1. Lipids: hypercholesterolemia >240, hypertriglyceridemia >250 2. **Ankle: brachial index (ABI) testing** • If **<0.90 (diagnostic)** 3. Doppler: reduced or interrupted flow 4. **Arteriography** (gold standard)	1. Prevention of atherosclerosis • Control HLD, HTN, weight, DM 2. Manage primary hyperlipidemia: statins, diet, exercise • Graduated exercise: walk to point of claudication, rest, then continue walking • Foot care 3. Reduce BP 4. **Stop smoking** • Most important Medical intervention: 1. **ASA + ticlopidine** or clopidogrel (symptomatic relief) 2. Cilostazol (PDE inhibitors) Surgery: 1. Angioplasty (preferred) 2. Adjunctive stenting 3. Bypass grafting Prognosis: Stable: 70%-80% Worsening: 10%-20% ALI: 1%-2%
Aortoiliac disease	Inflow disease	1. Buttock or thigh claudication = more disabling	See TASC II classification	1. Percutaneous transluminal angioplasty (PTA) • Iliac artery and stenting 2. Aortoiliac bypass 3. Aortofemoral bypass
Femoropopliteal disease	Disease below inguinal ligament = outflow disease		See TASC II classification	1. Balloon angioplasty/ stenting of femoral or superficial femoral artery 2. Surgical bypass (femoral to above-knee popliteal bypass, femoral to below-knee bypass)

Criteria for Percutaneous Transluminal Angioplasty (Revascularization)	Supportive Care and Risk Factor Modification	

1. Significantly disabled by claudication, resulting in inability to perform normal work or activities important to patient
2. Patient has not had or not predicted to have adequate response to exercise rehabilitation or pharmacologic therapy
3. Characteristics of lesion permit appropriate intervention at low risk with high likelihood of long-term success
4. Patient is able to benefit from improvement in claudication (exercise not limited by another cause—angina, HF, COPD, orthopedic problems)
	1. Cardiovascular risk modification
	  • Antiplatelet therapy: for patients with symptomatic PAD (claudication)
	    • Main indication remains as secondary prevention of CAD and stroke
	    • Aspirin (preferred)
	    • Clopidogrel
	  • Lipid lowering (diet)
	    • Moderate dose of statin, irrespective of baseline LDL (for all patients)
	  • Control of DM and HTN
	    • Blood sugar control with A1C goal <7%, as close to 6% as possible
	    • Hypertension control
	  • Smoking cessation
	    • All patients should be offered pharmacotherapy, behavior modification, referral to smoking cessation program, and counseling
	    • Ask about status of tobacco use at every visit
	    • Cessation favorable alters the progression of PAD
	2. Exercise therapy program (initial treatment for claudication)
	  • Recommended: 30-45 m at least 3 times per week for a minimum of 12 wk
	3. Compression therapy (nonpneumatic calf compression)	

Pharmacologic Therapy	**Referral for Invasive Intervention**	**Invasive Intervention**

For patients who failed risk modification and exercise therapy and revascularization cannot be offered or is declined
1. Therapeutic trial (3-6 mo) of
  • **Cilostazol**: decreases pain with ambulation or increased walking distance
    • Phosphodiesterase inhibitor that suppresses platelet aggregation and is a direct arterial vasodilator
    • Benefits as early as 4 wk after initiation
    • 100 mg BID taken 0.5 h before or 2 h after eating
    • Can be taken safely with aspirin and/or clopidogrel
    • AE: headache, loose/soft stool, diarrhea, dizziness, palpitations
    • Contraindicated: heart failure (all types)
  • Statin therapy
	1. If compliant with risk reduction × 6-12 mo and failed adjunctive pharmacotherapy	1. Percutaneous intervention
		  • Access femoral artery with arterial sheath and pass catheter to guide placement of expandable balloon/stent
		  • Balloon angioplasty
		  • Adjunctive stenting needed if vessel does not remain patent or if dissection progresses
		2. Surgical revascularization
		  • Identify a vessel above and below arterial obstruction onto which you suture a graft to bypass obstruction

- Continued smoking restricts improvements in pain-free walking symptoms that might otherwise be seen with an exercise program

Disease	Etiology, Prevalence, Risk Factors	Clinical Symptoms and Signs	Diagnostics	Therapy, Prognosis, and Health Maintenance
Phlebitis	Inflammation at entry site due to needle or catheter insertion MCC of fever after postop day 3 Most common in lower extremity veins	1. Induration 2. Edema 3. Tenderness Visible signs minimal: redness		Remove catheters at earliest signs Prevention: aseptic technique during insertion, frequent change of tubing (48-72 h), rotation of insertion sites (q 4 d) Use silastic catheters (least reactive) and hypertonic solutions in veins with substantial flow
Suppurative phlebitis	MC bug: **staphylococci** Presence of infected thrombus around indwelling catheter	Local signs of inflammation + pus from venipuncture site High fever	(+) blood cultures	Excise affected vein Extend incision proximally to first open collateral Leave wound open

ANGINA PECTORIS (CHEST PAIN) AND MYOCARDIAL INFARCTION

- **Stress EKG**: performed before, during, and after exercise
  - Confirms angina, evaluates response of therapy, identifies patients with CAD with high risk of ACS
  - 75% sensitive if patient able to get HR to 85% maximum predicted value for age (220−age) → ST depression = ischemia
  - Also (+) if patient experiences chest pain, hypotension, or significant arrhythmias
    - If (+) → send patient for cardiac catheterization
- Stress echo: performed before and immediately after exercise
  - Exercised induced ischemia → wall motion abnormalities (akinesis, dyskinesis) not present at rest
  - More sensitive than stress EKG for ischemia
  - Shows LV size and function, diagnoses valve disease, identifies CAD
  - If (+) → cardiac catheterization
- Reversible areas of ischemia → percutaneous coronary intervention (PCI) or coronary artery bypass graft (CABG)
- Pharmacologic stress test—for patients who cannot exercise
- Holter monitor—detects silent ischemia, evaluates arrhythmias and HR variability, and pacemaker and implantable cardioverter defibrillator (ICD) function
  - Evaluates unexplained syncope and dizziness
- Cardiac catheterization—most accurate method for specific cardiac diagnosis
  - Provides info on hemodynamics, intracardiac pressure, CO, O_2 sat
  - Indications:

- After (+) stress test
- Patient with angina when noninvasive tests are nondiagnostic, angina occurring despite meds, angina soon after MI, diagnostic dilemma
- Severely symptomatic patient needing urgent diagnosis
- Evaluation of valve disease
- **Coronary CT angiography**—definitive test for CAD (gold standard)
  - Most accurate method of identifying presence/severity of CAD
  - Determines whether revascularization is needed
  - Can perform PCI at the same time with balloon or stent
  - Stenosis >70% significant
  - If severe (left main or 3-vessel), refer for CABG

PCI Versus CABG

- Administer aspirin indefinitely and a P2Y12 antagonist for **1 to 3 months** after the implantation of a *bare* metal stent to reduce coronary thrombus formation
- Administer aspirin indefinitely + P2Y12 antagonist for **at least 1 year** after implantation of *drug*-eluting stent
- Defer noncardiac surgery for at least 12 months
- The use of drug-eluting stents that locally deliver antiproliferative drugs can reduce restenosis to less than 10%
  - Delayed endothelial healing puts patient at risk for subacute stent thrombosis
- CABG: anastomosis of one or both of the internal mammary arteries or a radial artery to the coronary artery distal to the obstructive lesion is the preferred procedure; a section of a vein (usually the saphenous) is used to form a connection between the aorta and the coronary artery distal to the obstructive lesion

	PCI (Coronary Angioplasty)	CABG
Indications	• Symptom-limiting angina pectoris, despite medical therapy, accompanied by evidence of ischemia during a stress test • PCI can be used to treat stenoses in native coronary arteries as well as in bypass grafts in patients who have recurrent angina after CABG	• Left main coronary artery stenosis • Ideal candidate is male, <80 y of age, has no other complicating disease, and has troublesome or disabling angina that is not adequately controlled by medical therapy or does not tolerate medical therapy
Benefits	• PCI is more effective than medical therapy for the relief of angina • PCI improves outcomes in patients with unstable angina or when used early in the course of myocardial infarction with and without cardiogenic shock • Less invasive and expensive than CABG, permits savings in initial costs	• The operation is relatively safe, with mortality rates <1% in patients without serious comorbid disease and normal LV function • The survival benefit is greater in patients with abnormal LV function (ejection fraction <50%) • CABG has also been shown to be superior to PCI (including the use of drug-eluting stents) in preventing death, myocardial infarction, and repeat revascularization in patients with diabetes mellitus and multivessel IHD
Contraindications	• Left main coronary artery stenosis	

	PCI (Coronary Angioplasty)	CABG
Prognosis	• Adequate dilation (an increase in luminal diameter >20% to a residual diameter obstruction <50%) with relief of angina, is achieved in >95% of cases • Recurrent stenosis of the dilated vessels occurs in ~20% of cases within 6 mo of PCI with bare metal stents, and angina will recur within 6 mo in 10% of cases • Restenosis is more common in patients with diabetes mellitus, arteries with small caliber, incomplete dilation of the stenosis, long stents, occluded vessels, obstructed vein grafts, dilation of the left anterior descending coronary artery, and stenoses containing thrombi	• Angina is abolished or greatly reduced in ~90% of patients after complete revascularization • Within 3 y, angina recurs in about one-fourth of patients but is rarely severe

Disease	Etiology, Prevalence, Risk Factors	Clinical Symptoms and Signs	Diagnostics	Therapy, Prognosis, and Health Maintenance
Stable angina	Fixed atherosclerotic lesions narrowing major coronary arteries→ **O₂ supply < O₂ demand** = inadequate perfusion Major RF: DM (worst), HLD (high LDL), **HTN (most common)**, smoking, age (M >45 y, W >55 y), family history of premature CAD or MI in first degree relative (M <45 y, W <55 y), low HDL Minor RF: obesity, sedentary, stress, ETOH	1. Chest pain or **substernal pressure** • Lasts <10-15 min • Chest discomfort: **heaviness, pressure, squeezing, tightness**, rarely sharp/stabbing Pain—gradual onset 2. Increased with exertion or emotion 3. **Relieved with rest or NTG** Signs: 1. **Levine sign**—clenched first over sternum and clenched teeth when describing chest pain	1. EKG: normal, Q-waves (prior MI) 2. Cardiac stress test	1. Sublingual NTG → IV NTG 2. **Coronary angiography**—if severely symptomatic despite medical therapy and being considered for PCI, patients with troublesome symptoms difficult to diagnose, angina symptoms in a patient who has survived a cardiac death event and patients with ischemia on noninvasive testings Prognosis: Depends on • LVEF: <50% (increased mortality) • Vessel(s) Involved: left main (poor, ⅔ of heart), 2-3 vessels total (worst)

Acute Coronary Syndrome/Chest Pain (Angina)

- Clopidogrel (Plavix)—reduces incidence of MI in patients with USA compared with ASA alone (9-12 months of therapy)
- LMWH—continue for at least 2 days; PTT not followed
- UFH—PTT 2-2.5× normal if using UFH
- Start patient with **USA or NSTEMI** with **high LDL** on HMG-CoA reductase inhibitor (statin)

Disease	Etiology, Prevalence, Risk Factors	Clinical Symptoms and Signs	Diagnostics	Therapy, Prognosis, and Health Maintenance
Coronary artery vasospasm (Prinzmetal variant)	**Smooth muscle constriction (spasm) of the coronary artery without obstruction** → leads to MI, ventricular arrhythmias, sudden death Known triggers: hyperventilation, cocaine or tobacco use, provocative agents (acetylcholine, ergonovine, histamine, serotonin) Nitric oxide deficiency → increased activity of potent vasoconstrictors and stimulators of smooth muscle proliferation 50-y-old, females	1. **Nonexertional chest pain** similar to unstable angina • Normal exercise tolerance • Pain is **cyclical** (mostly occur in morning hours, no correlation to cardiac workload)	1. EKG: ST segment or T-wave abnormalities 2. Cardiac enzymes: **normal** troponin, CK-MB 3. Check Mg level, CBC, CMP, lipid panel	1. Stress testing with myocardial perfusion imaging or coronary angiography 2. Pharmacotherapy • SL, topical, or IV **nitrates** (initial) • Antiplatelet, thrombolytics, statins, BB 3. Once diagnosis made—**CCB** and long-acting nitrates used for long-term prophylaxis (**amlodipine**)

(continued)

(continued)

Disease	Etiology, Prevalence, Risk Factors	Clinical Symptoms and Signs	Diagnostics	Therapy, Prognosis, and Health Maintenance
Unstable angina (USA)	**O$_2$ demand unchanged** Supply decreased, secondary to low resting coronary flow	1. **Chronic angina**—Increasing in frequency, duration, or intensity of pain Or 2. **New-onset** angina—severe and worsening Or 3. **Angina at rest**	1. <u>EKG</u>: ST segment or T-wave abnormalities 2. Cardiac enzymes: **normal** troponin, CK-MB	1. Admit to unit with continuous cardiac monitoring, establish IV access, **O$_2$**, pain control with **NTG** and **morphine** 2. **ASA**, clopidogrel, **BB** (first line), LMWH 3. Replace electrolytes 4. If response to med therapy → stress test to determine if catheterization/revascularization necessary 5. Reduce RF: stop smoking, weight loss, treat DM/HTN and HLD 6. Heparin Not beneficial: thrombolytics and CCB
NSTEMI	Non-ST elevation myocardial infarction caused by a severely narrowed artery that is not 100% blocked		<u>EKG</u>: pathologic Q waves Cardiac enzymes—**elevated** troponin/CK-MB	
STEMI	ST elevation myocardial infarction caused by 100% blockage of a coronary artery Necrosis of the myocardium (thrombotic occlusion) Asymptomatic in one-third of patients	1. **Chest pain**—intense substernal pressure (crushing or elephant standing on my chest) 2. **Radiation** to neck, jaw, arms, back, **left side** (MC) 3. Similar to angina pectoris—severe, lasts longer 4. Pain does not respond to NTG 5. Epigastric discomfort 6. <u>Others</u>: **SOB, sweating**, weakness, fatigue, **nausea, vomiting**, sense of impending doom, syncope	1. <u>EKG</u>: • Peaked T-waves, early • ST elevation • Q-waves (necrosis), late • T-wave inversion (nonspecific) • ST depression (subendocardial injury) 2. Monitor BP/HR 3. Cardiac enzymes • Troponin I • CK-MB	1. Admit to CCU, establish IV access, O$_2$, NTG/morphine 2. MONA • Morphine • O$_2$ • Nitrates • ASA 3. Plus 4. BB, ACE, heparin, and statins <u>Prognosis:</u> 30% mortality rate
Dressler syndrome	**Post-MI** syndrome Occurs 1-2 wk post-MI	1. Fever 2. Malaise <u>Complications:</u> Pericarditis Pleuritis	1. CBC: leukocytosis	1. **ASA** (first line) 2. Ibuprofen

Disease	Etiology, Prevalence, Risk Factors	Clinical Symptoms and Signs	Diagnostics	Therapy, Prognosis, and Health Maintenance
New papillary rupture (free wall rupture)	Myocardial rupture after AMI Occurs 1 d-3 wk **post-MI** (mostly **3-5 d** after) Common in **older women**, especially those with recurrent post-MI angina, and patients with systemic hypertension	1. Acute-onset **SOB**, chest pain, shock, sweating, unexplained vomiting, cool and clammy skin, syncope 2. Sudden death due to LV free-wall rupture 3. **Pulmonary edema**, CHF, and hypotension following blunt chest trauma Signs: 1. Tachypnea, tachycardia, hypotension 2. Respiratory distress, **diffuse rales** 3. Signs of mitral regurgitation 4. Can also present as post-MI pericarditis (pleuritic chest pain, friction rub)	1. CXR, cardiac catheterization 2. **Echo (TEE, preferred):** LV or RV wall motion abnormality, diffuse or loculated effusion, decreased Doppler flow velocity, mobile echodensity into left atrium during systole, 3. EKG: no changes	1. Early surgical intervention for myocardial rupture: • Mitral valve replacement (definitive) • NPO and bed rest • Inotropes, vasodilators, and diuretics to stabilize patient

Cardiac Biomarkers

	Increases	Return to Normal	Peak	
Troponin	3-5 h	5-14 d	24-48 h	Greater sensitivity/specificity Obtain on admission and q 8 h × 24 h Troponin I—false (+) in CKD
CK-MB	4-8 h	48-72 h	24 h	Greater sensitivity and specificity if measured in 24-36 h (early) of onset SX Measure on admission and q 8 h × 24 h • Use to diagnose reinfarction

Hypertriglyceridemia

Disease	Etiology, Prevalence, Risk Factors	Clinical Symptoms and Signs	Diagnostics	Therapy, Prognosis, and Health Maintenance
Hypertriglyceridemia	Often caused or exacerbated by uncontrolled DM, obesity, sedentary habitus RF: CAD Usually asymptomatic until **TG >1000-2000 mg/dL**	1. GI: midepigastric pain, but can occur in chest or back areas; nausea or vomiting Signs: 1. Tenderness to palpation over midepigastric, RUQ/LUQ 2. Hepatomegaly 3. Respiratory: dyspnea 4. Dermatologic: xanthomas 5. Ophthalmologic: corneal arcus, xanthelasmas 6. Neurologic: memory loss, dementia, depression	1. Decreased pedal pulses or ABI index in the presence of PAD 2. Lipid panel, chylomicron determination, FBG, TSH, U/A, LFTs	1. Lifestyle modification: diet, exercise, weight reduction, smoking cessation, limit alcohol 2. Pharmacotherapy • Fibric acid derivatives (gemfibrozil, fenofibrate) • Niacin • Omega-3 fatty acids • Statins 3. Plasmapheresis in setting of severe hypertriglyceridemia

CHAPTER 2

Pulmonology

Refer to Internal Medicine [icon] for in-depth coverage of the following topics:

Carcinoid Tumor, p 211
Bronchiectasis, p 212
Solitary Pulmonary Nodule, p 212
Sarcoidosis, p 213

Pulmonary Hypertension, p 215
Idiopathic Pulmonary Fibrosis, p 214
Pneumoconiosis, p 214
Cor Pulmonale, p 215

Recommended Supplemental Topics:

Tobacco Use/Dependence, refer to Substance Abuse
    Disorders, p 562

BREATH SOUNDS

Disease	Percussion	Breath Sounds	Adventitia	Special Tests
Normal lung	Resonant	Vesicular Inspiration > expiration	None	F: Normal E: Normal
Chronic bronchitis	Resonant	Vesicular or varied	Crackles, wheezes, rhonchi	F: Normal (or decreased)
CHF	Early: resonant Late: dull	Vesicular	Crackles, wheezes	F: Normal
Pneumonia	**Dull**	Bronchial Inspiration < expiration	Late inspiratory crackles	F: **Increased** E: E → A
Atelectasis	Dull over airless area	Absent	None	F: Absent
Pleural effusion	Dull	**Decreased to absent**	Pleural rub	F: Decreased
Pneumothorax	Hyperresonant or tympanitic over pleural air	Decreased to absent	± Pleural rub	F: Decreased to absent
COPD	Hyperresonant (air trapping)	Decreased or absent	None or "junky" (wheezes, crackles)	F: Decreased
Asthma	Hyperresonant	Decreased or absent (medical emergency)	Expiratory wheeze ± crackles	F: Decreased

- F = tactile fremitus
- E = egophony

Peak expiratory flow—use a peak flow meter

- If <350 L/min, perform PFTs to screen for obstruction

Pulmonary function testing

- FEV_1: amount of air that can be forced out of the lungs in 1 second
  - Airway obstruction diagnosed by: normal/increased TLC with decreased FEV_1
    - $FEV_1/FVC < 0.7$

Disease	FEV$_1$	FVC	FEV$_1$/FVC Ratio	FEF$_{25-75}$	FET	Peak Expiratory Flow
Obstructive	Decreased <80%	**Normal** <80%	Decreased <0.7	Decreased <60%	Increased	Low
Restrictive	Normal or decreased <80%	Decreased <80%	Normal or **increased** ≥0.7	Normal >60%	Normal	Normal
Mixed	Decreased <80%	Decreased <80%	Decreased <0.7	Decreased or normal <60%	Increased or normal	

- Tiffeneau index (FEV$_1$/FVC × 100): % of FVC expired in 1 second
- FET = forced expiratory time
- **Pay attention here:** The important thing to know about how to differentiate an obstructive versus restrictive lung disease is based on their TLC, not the vital capacity, which will be decreased in obstructive lung diseases (this can be misleading)

Disease	TLC	FRC	TV	RV	VC
Obstructive	**Increased**	Increased	N	**Increased**	Decreased
Restrictive	**Decreased**	Decreased	N	Decreased	Decreased

LUNG VOLUME AND CAPACITY (FIG. 2-1)

- **Tidal volume:** volume of air breathed in and out of lungs during quiet breathing
- **Residual volume:** volume of air in the lungs after maximal expiration
- **Inspiratory reserve:** maximum volume inspired after normal end-tidal inspiration (requires you to forcibly inspire after your regular tidal inspiration)
- **Expiratory reserve:** maximum volume expired after resting end tidal expiration (requires you to forcibly exhale after your regular tidal inspiration)
- **Vital capacity:** volume of air expelled from the lungs during a maximum expiration
- **Total lung capacity:** total volume of air in lungs after maximum inspiration
- **Inspiratory capacity:** maximum volume inspired after complete expiration
- **Functional residual capacity:** volume of air in lungs after normal expiration

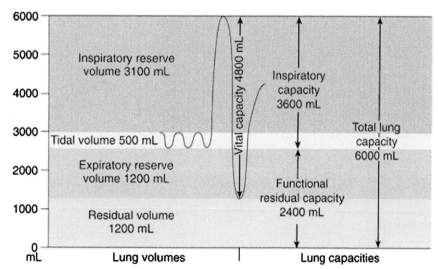

FIGURE 2-1. Lung volume and lung capacity tracings. (From Porth CM, Matfin G. *Pathophysiology: Concepts of Altered Health States*, 8th ed. Philadelphia: Wolters Kluwer Health, 2009, with permission.)

OBSTRUCTIVE VERSUS RESTRICTIVE LUNG DISEASES

- **Obstructive** lung diseases—COPD, asthma, cystic fibrosis, bronchiectasis, and bronchiolar diseases (constrictive bronchiolitis, bronchiolitis obliterans syndrome)

- **Restrictive lung diseases**—interstitial lung diseases (ILD): sarcoidosis, chronic beryllium disease, hypersensitivity pneumonitis, pneumoconiosis, asbestos

Plethysmography Pattern	Feature	DLCO	Likely Dx
Obstructive	Hyperinflation (TLC >120%)	**Decreased**	Emphysema
Obstructive	Hyperinflation	Normal or increased	Asthma
Obstructive	Normal lung volume	Normal	Chronic bronchitis
Restrictive	Low RV	**Decreased**	Scar (sarcoid or fibrosis)
Restrictive	Normal RV	Normal	Neuromuscular disease

- **DLCO** (diffusing capacity of the lung for carbon monoxide) = CO into lungs − CO out of lungs (CO = carbon monoxide)
  - We use carbon monoxide because we can maximize diffusion because of the affinity of Hgb for it → Volume = area/thickness × (P1-P2) × constant

- In emphysema, tissue is destroyed, reducing surface area for diffusion → decreased surface area causes volume to decrease
- In sarcoidosis and fibrosis, lung thickness increases, also driving volume to decrease

Acute/Chronic Bronchitis (Covered Under COPD)

Disease	Etiology, Prevalence, Risk Factors	Clinical Symptoms and Signs	Diagnostics	Therapy, Prognosis, and Health Maintenance
Acute bronchitis	Etiology: viruses (most) Cannot distinguish acute bronchitis from URTI in the first few days	1. **Cough** >5 d (± sputum), lasts 2-3 wk 2. Chest discomfort 3. Shortness of breath 4. ± fever (rare)	1. Labs not indicated, unless pneumonia suspected (HR >100, RR >24, T >38°C, rales, hypoxemia, mental confusion, or systemic illness)→ 1. CXR	1. Antibiotics not recommended—mostly viral 2. Symptomatic-based treatment 1. **NSAIDs**, ASA, tylenol, and/or ipratropium 2. Antibiotics and cough suppressants not indicated • Cough suppressants—codeine-containing cough meds • Bronchodilators (albuterol)

Asthma

1. Characteristics
   - Airway inflammation
   - Airway hyperresponsiveness
   - **Reversible** airflow obstruction

2. May begin at any age

3. **Dyspnea** common when exposed to rapid changes in temperature and humidity

Extrinsic	Intrinsic
• Atopic: produce IgE to environmental triggers (eczema, hay fever) • Become asthmatic at young age	• Not related to atopy or environmental triggers

- PFTs (obstructive): decreased expiratory flow, low FEV_1, and decreased FEV_1/FVC ratio
  - **Increased FEV_1 > 12%** with albuterol

- Decrease in FEV_1 > 20% with methacholine or histamine
- Increase in diffusion capacity of lung for carbon monoxide (DLCO)

General	Signs and Symptoms	Diagnostics	Therapy 1	Therapy 2
Triggers: pollens, house dust, molds, cockroaches, cats, dogs, cold air, viral infections, tobacco smoke, meds (BB, aspirin), exercise	Intermittent: 1. **SOB** 2. **Wheezing** 3. **Chest tightness** 4. **Cough** • Occurs in 30 mins to exposure to triggers • Symptoms worse at night Signs: 1. **Wheezing** (inspiration and expiration) is the most common finding	1. **CXR:** for first time wheezers 2. **PFTs:** required to DX 3. **Spirometry** before and after bronchodilators—increase in **FEV_1 or FVC by 12%**	1. **SABA** (albuterol) for acute attacks • Onset 2-5 min, duration is 4-6 h 2. LABA (salmeterol) for nighttime asthma and exercise-induced asthma 3. Inhaled corticosteroids: moderate to severe asthma • Use regularly to decrease airway hyper-responsiveness and exacerbations	1. Montelukast: prophylaxis for mild exercise-induced asthma and control of mild-moderate • Allows for reduction in steroid and B_2 2. Cromolyn sodium: prophylaxis before exercise 3. Aviod β-blockers in asthmatics
Acute asthma exacerbation	1. Sweating 2. Wheezing 3. Speaking in incomplete sentences 4. **Tachypnea** 5. Paradoxical movement of the abdomen and diaphragm on inspiration 6. Use of accessory muscles	1. Peak expiratory flow: low • Severe <60 2. ABG: **increased A-a** gradient 3. CXR: r/o pneumonia, pneumothorax	1. **Inhaled B_2 agonist via nebulizers** or MDI 2. Corticosteroids: IV or orally 3. IV magnesium: can help prevent bronchospasm	Treatment below: Complications: • Status asthmaticus: does not respond to standard meds • ARDS: respiratory muscle fatigue • Pneumothorax, atelectasis, pneumomediastinum

Monitor **peak flow** (peak expiratory flow rate)—measures airflow obstruction

- Adult normal ranges: 450 to 650 L/min (men) versus 350 to 500 L/min (women)
- Mild >300, moderate to severe 100 to 300, severe <100
- Mild persistent asthma: monitor periodically; increase dose of inhaled steroid if peak flow decreases
- Moderate persistent asthma: daily monitoring required; increase dose of inhaled steroid if peak flow decreases
- Severe persistent: daily monitoring; initiate prednisone if peak flow decreases

Bronchoprovocation test—useful when asthma suspected, but PFTs nondiagnostic

- Measures lung function before and after inhalation of increasing doses of methacholine; hyperresponsive airways → obstruction at low doses

Chest XR—severe asthma reveals hyperinflation

- Only get with severe asthma to r/o pneumonia, pneumothorax, pneumomediastinum, foreign body

Arterial blood gas (ABG)—order if in significant respiratory distress.

- **Hypocarbia** (common) with hypoxemia
- If $Paco_2$ is normal or increased, respiratory failure may ensue—asthmatics have increased respiratory rate, which should cause $Paco_2$ to decrease

Classification of Asthma Severity and Initiating Therapy

Level of severity is determined by the components of severity based on frequency of symptoms, intensity, functional limitations, and the risk of exacerbations. Assessment of impairment is made by events during last 2 to 4 weeks; risk is assessed over the last 12 months. Reassess severity and control of asthma in 2 to 6 weeks; adjust as needed. If no clear benefit in 4 to 6 weeks in children 0 to 4 years of age, consider adjusting therapy or alternate diagnosis.

Stepwise Approach for Managing Asthma in Children and Adults

Components of Control	Impairment						Risk	
	Daytime Symptoms	Nighttime Awakenings <5 y/o → >5 y/o		Interference with Normal Activities	SABA[a] Use for Symptom Control	FEV$_1$ (% Predicted)[b]	Exacerbations Requiring PO Steroids	Stepwise Treatment Approach
Intermittent	≤2 d/wk	None	≤2×/mo	None	≤2 d/wk	>80%	0-1/y	Step 1
Mild persistent	>2 d/wk Not daily	1-2×/mo	3-4×/mo	Minor	<5 y/o: >2 d/wk Not daily >5 y/o: as above, not more than 1×/d	>80%	<5 y/o: ≥2 in 6 mo, wheezing ≥4×/y (lasting >1 d) and risk factors for persistent asthma[c] >5 y/o: ≥2×/y	Step 2
Moderate persistent	Daily	3-4×/mo	>1×/wk Not nightly	Some	Daily	60%-80%	More frequent and intense than above	<5 y/o: Step 3 >5 y/o: Step 3 or Step 3 medium-dose ICS
Severe persistent	Throughout day	>1×/wk	Often, daily	Extremely limited	Several times/d	<60%	More frequent and intense than above	

[a]SABA: short-acting beta-agonist.
[b]Not applicable if <5 years old.
[c]RF for persistent asthma:
FEV$_1$: forced expiratory volume in 1 second.
Adapted from Asthma Care Quick Reference: *Diagnosing and Managing Asthma. Guidelines from the National Asthma Education and Prevention Program Expert Panel Report 3*. Bethesda, MD: U S. Department of Health and Human Services, National Institutes of Health; rev. September 2012. https://www.nhlbi.nih.gov/files/docs/guidelines/asthma_qrg.pdf.

Classification of Asthma Control

	Daytime Symptoms	Nighttime Awakenings ≤11 y/o → ≥12 y/o		Interference with Normal Activities	SABA[a] Use for Symptom Control	FEV$_1$ (% Predicted)[b]	Exacerbations Requiring PO Steroids	Stepwise Treatment Approach
Well controlled	≤2 d/wk	≤1 d/mo	≤2 d/mo	None	≤2 d/wk	>80%	0-1/y	No change FU every 1-6 mo Consider step down if well controlled ≥3 mo
Not well controlled	>2 d/wk or multiple times/d if ≤2 d/wk	≥1-2 d/mo	1-3 d/wk	Some	>2 d/wk	60%-80%	<5: 2-3/y ≥5: ≥2/y	Step up 1 step. Reevaluate in 2-6 wk. If <5, adjust therapy in 4-6 wk if no improvement
Very poorly controlled	Throughout the day	≥1-2 d/wk	≥4 d/wk	Extremely limited	Several times/d	<60%	<5: 3+/y >5: ≥2/y	Consider short course PO steroids. Step up 1-2 steps. Reevaluate in 2 wk

[a]SABA: short-acting beta-agonist.
[b]Not applicable if <5 years old.
Helps to determine adjustments to current medications. The level of control takes into account the severity and the time since the last asthma exacerbation and possible side effects when assessing risk. Always review adherence to medication, inhaler technique, and environmental control before a step-up in treatment. Consider alternative therapies when side effects are experienced, and if an alternate treatment was used, discontinue other treatments and use preferred treatment for that step.
Adapted from Asthma Care Quick Reference: *Diagnosing and Managing Asthma. Guidelines from the National Asthma Education and Prevention Program Expert Panel Report 3*. Bethesda, MD: U.S. Department of Health and Human Services, National Institutes of Health; rev. September 2012. https://www.nhlbi.nih.gov/files/docs/guidelines/asthma_qrg.pdf.

Stepwise Approach to Managing Asthma Long Term

	Intermittent	Persistent				
Alternative therapy		<5: CRM or MLK ≥5: CRM, LTRA, or THE	• <5: *MD*-ICS • ≥5: • *MD*-ICS • LD-ICS + • LABA if ≥5 • LTRA if ≥5 • THE if ≥5 • ZLU if ≥12	MD-ICS+: • LTRA • THE	If ≥5-11: HD-ICS +: • LTRA • THE	If ≥5-11: HD-ICS: • LTRA • THE + OCS
Preferred therapy	SABA as needed[a]	LD-ICS		<5: *MD*-ICS+: • LABA *or* • MLK ≥5: *MD*-ICS+ • LABA if ≥5 • LTRA if ≥5 • THE if ≥5 • ZLU if ≥12	<5: HD-ICS+: • LABA *or* • MLK • ≥5: *HD*-ICS + LABA if ≥5 • ± OMZ if allergic asthma (if ≥12)	<5: HD-ICS +: • LABA *or* • MLK +OCS: ≥5: *HD*-ICS + LABA + OCS ± OMZ if allergic asthma (if ≥12)
	Step 1	**Step 2**	**Step 3**	**Step 4**	**Step 5**	**Step 6**

Note that steps 3 and 4 are the same, except in step 4 you'd use a high-dose ICS rather than a medium-dose. Consult with asthma specialist at step 4+ required. Consider use of SQ allergen immunotherapy (omalizumab) for patients with persistent, allergic asthma.

[a]Up to 3 treatments every 20 minutes as needed. Note: frequent use of SABA (>2 d/wk) may indicate need to go up to the next step in treatment. With viral symptoms, SABA every 4 to 6 hours may be needed up to 24 hours.

CRM, cromolyn; HD-ICS, high-dose ICS; ICS, inhaled corticosteroid (beclomethasone, budesonide, ciclesonide, flunisolide, fluticasone, mometasone). LABA, long-acting beta agonist (salmeterol, formoterol), not for monotherapy; LD-ICS, low-dose ICS; LTRA, leukotriene-receptor antagonist (montelukast, zafirlukast); MD-ICS, medium-dose ICS; MLK, montelukast (Singulair); OCS, oral corticosteroids (methylprednisolone, prednisolone, prednisone); OMZ, omalizumab (anti-IgE); SABA, short-acting beta-agonist; THE, theophylline, a methylxanthine; ZLU, zileuton;.

Adapted from Asthma Care Quick Reference: *Diagnosing and Managing Asthma. Guidelines from the National Asthma Education and Prevention Program Expert Panel Report 3*. Bethesda, MD: U.S. Department of Health and Human Services, National Institutes of Health; rev. September 2012. https://www. nhlbi.nih.gov/files/docs/guidelines/asthma_qrg.pdf.

Chronic Obstructive Pulmonary Disease

- Fourth leading cause of death in the United States
- Coexisting bronchitis and emphysema, rarely one or the other by itself
- Leads to chronic respiratory acidosis with metabolic alkalosis as compensation

- Risk factors and causes
  - **Smoking (tobacco)**
  - α-antitrypsin deficiency—worse with smoking
  - Environmental factors—second-hand smoke
  - Chronic asthma—independent risk factor?

Disease	Etiology, Prevalence, Risk Factors	Clinical Symptoms and Signs	Diagnostics	Therapy, Prognosis, and Health Maintenance
Chronic bronchitis	Excess mucous production narrows airways → productive cough Scarring and inflammation → enlargement of glands → smooth muscle hyperplasia = obstruction	1. Cough 2. Sputum production 3. **Dyspnea** (on exertion or at rest) Signs: 1. **Prolonged forced expiratory time** (takes longer to get all air out) 2. During auscultation: end-expiratory wheezes on forced expiration, decreased breath sounds, inspiratory crackles 3. Tachypnea, tachycardia 4. **Cyanosis** 5. Use of accessory muscles 6. **Hyperresonance** on percussion 7. Signs of cor pulmonale	Clinical diagnosis: chronic cough, productive sputum >3 mo, at least 2 consecutive years 1. **CXR**—low sensitivity; useful in acute exacerbation to r/o pneumonia or pneumothorax • Hyperinflation, flat diaphragm, enlarged retrosternal space • Diminished vascular markings 2. α-antitrypsin levels—FH premature emphysema? 3. ABG—chronic pCO_2 retention, decreased pO_2	See treatment table

(continued)

(continued)

Disease	Etiology, Prevalence, Risk Factors	Clinical Symptoms and Signs	Diagnostics	Therapy, Prognosis, and Health Maintenance

Emphysema
Elastase (protease) excess and overinflation ("pink puffers," barrel chest, pursed lips)
	<u>Types:</u>
	1. **Centrilobular**—most common; seen in smokers; destruction limited to bronchioles (upper lungs)
	2. Panlobular—patients with α-1 antitrypsin deficiency; destruction both proximal and distal acini (lung bases)
	<u>MOA:</u>
	1. Elastase—released from PMNs and macrophages, ingesting lung tissue (normally inhibited by α_1 antitrypsin)
	2. Tobacco smoke—increases PMNs and macrophages, inhibits antitrypsin, and increases oxidative stress on the lung
		1. Productive cough or acute chest tightness
		  • Worse in the morning
		  • Clear to white sputum
		  • 50 y/o typical
		2. Dyspnea (MC)
		  • Presents at 60 y/o
		3. Wheezing
		<u>Signs</u>
		1. Tachypnea
		2. Dyspnea with mild exertion
		3. Cyanosis
		4. JVD
		5. Atrophy of limb musculature
		6. Peripheral Edema
		7. "Barrel Chest" (2:1 anterior: posterior diameter)
		8. Diffuse or focal wheezing
		9. Diminished breath sounds
		10. Hyperresonance to percussion
			Pathologic diagnosis: permanent **enlargement of airspaces distal to terminal bronchioles** due to destruction of alveolar walls
			1. **Decreased DLCO**
			2. **PFTs (spirometry):** diagnostic
			  • $FEV_1/FVC <0.75$
			  • FEV_1 is decreased
			  • Total lung capacity (TLC), residual volume, FRC increased (indicates air trapping)
			3. **Vital capacity decreased**—extra air that does come in is not useful → becomes residual volume (dead space)
			4. CXR (Fig. 2-2)
				See treatment table

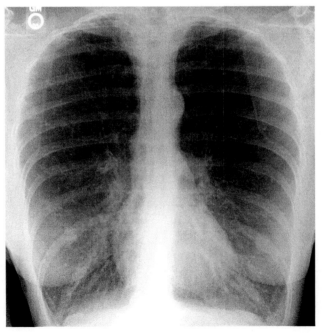

FIGURE 2-2. Severe emphysema seen on chest radiograph. Notice the radiolucency in the upper lobes and the lack of vasculature. (From Webb WR. Chronic obstructive pulmonary disease and empheysema. In Webb WR, Higgins CB, eds. *Thoracic Imaging*. Philadelphia: Wolters Kluwer Health; 2017, with permission.)

Treatment of Chronic Bronchitis Versus Emphysema

Chronic Bronchitis	Emphysema

• **Smoking cessation** (*most important*): smokers have faster decline in FEV_1 (3-4×)
• Inhaled β_2 agonists (**albuterol**): symptomatic relief
  • Long-term agents (salmeterol) for frequent use
• Inhaled **anticholinergics** (**ipratropium** bromide): slower onset of action, lasts longer
• Combination of β-agonist and anticholinergic (helps with adherence to therapy)
• Inhaled **corticosteroids** (*budesonide, fluticasone*): anti-inflammatory; slows decline in FEV_1 over time
• Oxygen therapy: get an ABG to determine need for oxygen; long-standing hypoxemia → pulmonary hypertension and cor pulmonale
• Pulmonary rehabilitation: improves exercise tolerance
• Vaccinations: influenza (annual) and streptococcus pneumoniae every 5-6 y (>65)
• Surgery: lung resection vs transplant
	• **Smoking cessation** and **home O_2** are only interventions shown to lower mortality
	• Give **steroids** and **antibiotics** for acute exacerbations: increased sputum production or change in character or worsening SOB
	• Not responsive to bronchodilators
	• IV methylprednisolone if hospitalized
	• Azithromycin or levofloxacin
	• O_2 > 90%, nasal cannula
	• NPPV: BiPAP or CPAP
	• Can lead to ARDS
	• Criteria for continuous or intermittent long-term O_2:
	  • Pao_2 55 mm Hg
	  • O_2 saturation <88% (pulse oximetry) either at rest or during exercise
	  • Pao_2 55 59 mm Hg + polycythemia or cor pulmonale
	• Look for nocturnal hypoxemia; give CPAP or O_2 as needed

- Clinical monitoring
  - Serial FEV_1 measurements (highest PPV)
  - Pulse oximetry
  - Exercise tolerance testing
- Acute exacerbations
  - Most common causes: infection, noncompliance, cardiac disease
  - Secondary polycythemia (Hct >55% men, 47% women)—response to chronic hypoxemia
  - Pulmonary HTN and cor pulmonale—severe, long-standing COPD

- Mainstay of therapy for stable COPD
  - Inhaled bronchodilators: β-agonists and anticholinergics alone or in combination with inhaled glucocorticoids
  - Administered in metered dose, soft mist, or dry powder inhalers, some via nebulization
- Maintenance therapy—long-acting agents recommended
  - Theophylline—modestly effective, more side effects than inhaled bronchodilators, used for refractory COPD

COPD Staging—Global Initiative for Chronic Obstructive Lung Disease Criteria

GOLD I mild Less symptomatic, low risk (cat A) FEV_1/FVC <0.7 FEV_1 > 50% predicted	No symptoms Cough, sputum Limited exercise capacity: **breathless with strenuous exercise or when walking up slight hill** Infrequent exacerbations 0-1 exacerbations per year	1. SA bronchodilators • **First line: Short-acting anticholinergics and/or β-agonists** prn alone • Second: LAMA or LABA or SABA and SAAC prn • Alt: theophylline	**FEV1 > 80%** predicted
GOLD II moderate More symptomatic, low risk (Cat B) FEV_1/FVC <0.7 FEV_1 > 50% predicted	Significant limitation in exertional capacity: **patient has to walk more slowly than others of same age owing to SOB; must stop to catch breath when walking on level ground at own pace or severe SOB** Limited ADLs 0-1 exacerbations per year	1. SABA prn + pulmonary rehabilitation • First line: **LAMA** or **LABA** • Second: LAMA + LABA • Alt: SABA ± SAAC, theophylline	50% < FEV_1 < 80%

(continued)

(continued)

| GOLD III severe
Less symptomatic, high risk (Cat C)
$FEV_1/FVC <0.7$
$FEV_1 < 50\%$ predicted | SOB, even at rest: **SOB with strenuous exercise or when hurrying on level ground or walking up slight hill**
>2 exacerbations per year or 1 hospitalization | 1. **SABA prn + pulmonary rehabilitation**
• First line: **Combo (LABA + inhaled steroid) OR LAMA**
• Second: LAMA + LABA
• Alt: theophylline, SABA ± SAMA, PDE-4 inhibitor | $30\% < FEV_1 < 50\%$ |
| GOLD IV
Very severe
More symptomatic, high risk (Cat D)
$FEV_1/FVC <0.7$
$FEV_1 < 50\%$ predicted | Frequent, severe exacerbations
>2 exacerbations per year or 1 hospitalization | 1. SABA prn + pulmonary rehabilitation
• First line: **Combo (LABA + inhaled steroid)** or LAMA
• Second: Combo (LABA + inhaled steroid) + LAMA
• Third: Combo (LABA + inhaled steroid) + PDE4-inhibitor
• Fourth: LAMA + LABA
• Fifth: LAMA + PDE4
• Continuous O_2 prn | $FEV_1 < 30\%$ predicted |

Pneumonia (Viral, Bacterial, Fungal, Human Immunodeficiency Virus–Related)

Community Acquired Pneumonia

- Occurs when there is a defect in one of the primary pulmonary defense mechanisms (cough reflex, mucociliary clearance, immune response)
- Urinary Ag for *Streptococcus pneumoniae* helpful screening tool in patients with: leukopenia, asplenia, alcohol use, chronic severe liver disease, pleural effusion, ICU patients
- Urinary *Legionella* Ag helpful screening tool in patients with: active alcohol use, travel previous 2 weeks, pleural effusion, ICU patients
- Extended spectrum β-lactamase species: *Enterobacter, Klebsiella pneumoniae, Escherichia coli*

Disease	Etiology, Prevalence, Risk Factors	Clinical Symptoms and Signs	Diagnostics	Therapy, Prognosis, and Health Maintenance
Community-acquired pneumonia (pneumococcal pneumonia)–**immunocompetent**	<u>MCC</u>: **S. pneumoniae** (²/₃), *Haemophilus influenzae, Mycoplasma pneumoniae, S. aureus, N. meningitidis, M. catarrhalis, K. pneumonia,* other GNR Viruses: Influenza, RSV, adenovirus, parainfluenza virus Occurs outside of the hospital or within 48 h of hospital admission in a patient not residing in a long-term care facility <u>RF</u>: Advanced age, alcoholism, tobacco use, comorbid medical conditions (asthma, COPD) **Most common cause of pulmonary disease in HIV infected patients**	1. Acute or subacute onset of **fever** 2. Gradual onset **cough** with or without sputum production 3. **Shortness of breath** on exertion 4. Others: sweats, chills, rigors, chest discomfort, pleurisy, hemoptysis, fatigue, myalgias, anorexia, headache, abdominal pain <u>Signs</u>: 1. Fever or hypothermia 2. Tachypnea 3. Tachycardia 4. O₂ desaturation 5. Inspiratory crackles and **bronchial** breath sounds 6. Dullness to percussion	<u>Imaging</u>: 1. CXR: patchy airspace opacities to **lobar consolidation with air bronchograms** to diffuse alveolar or interstitial opacities • Not necessary in outpatient because empiric therapy is effective • Recommended if unusual presentation, history, or inpatient • Clearing of opacities can take 6 wk or longer! 2. CT chest • More sensitive and specific <u>Labs</u>: 1. Sputum gram stain and sensitivity • Not sensitive or specific for *S. pneumoniae* 2. Urinary Ag test for *S. pneumoniae* and *Legionella* • As sensitive/specific as gram stain, readily available 3. Rapid Ag test for flu • Sensitive, not specific 4. Pre-antibiotic **sputum and blood cultures** • 2 sticks at separate sites 5. CBC and CMP, LFTs, bilirubin 6. ABG in hypoxemic patients 7. HIV testing in at-risk patients 8. Procalcitonin–released by bacterial toxins and inhibited by viral infections	See later under Treatment of Pneumonia Prophylaxis: 1. Pneumovax 23 2. Prevnar 13 • Ind: age 65+ y and immunocompromised give both, or any chronic illness with increased risk of CAP • Immunocompromised patients at high risk should get single revaccination of 23 6-y after first dose, regardless of age • Immunocompetent and 65+ y get second dose of 23 if first received vaccine 6+ y ago (<65) 3. Influenza • Ind: age 65+, residents of LTCF, pulmonary or CV disease, chronic metabolic disorder, or health care worker
Community-acquired pneumonia–immunocompromised	HIV (ANC < 1000), current or recent exposure to myelo or immunosuppressive medications, or patients taking chronic steroids		1. Sputum induction 2. BAL–r/o PCP pneumonia	
Nosocomial pneumonia	Pathogens: *S. aureus, K. pneumoniae, E. coli, Pseudomonas aeruginosa*	<u>Requires at least 2 of the following</u>: 1. Fever 2. Leukocytosis 3. Purulent sputum	1. CXR: new or progressive parenchymal opacity 2. Blood cultures × 2 3. CBC and CMP 4. Sputum culture and gram stain • Not sensitive or specific 5. ABG, thoracentesis if effusion 6. Procalcitonin	See later under Treatment of Pneumonia

- **Ventilator-associated pneumonia (VAP)**—Develops **more than 48 hours** following endotracheal intubation and mechanical ventilation
  - MC pathogens: *Acinetobacter, Stenotrophomonas maltophilia*
  - Endotracheal aspiration culture—Use sterile suction catheter and fiberoptic bronchoscopy with BAL

- **Hospital-acquired pneumonia (HAP)**—Occurs **more than 48 hours after admission** to hospital or other health care facility and excludes any infection present at time of admission
  - MC pathogens: ***S. aureus*** (MSSA and MRSA), *Pseudomonas*, GNR (ESBL and non-ESBL)

Disease	Etiology, Prevalence, Risk Factors	Clinical Symptoms and Signs	Diagnostics	Therapy, Prognosis, and Health Maintenance

Pneumocystis pneumonia	*Pneumocystis jirovecii*—caused by fungus found in lungs of mammals
	Most common opportunistic infection in HIV/AIDS
		1. **Fever, SOB**, nonproductive **cough**
		2. Examination findings disproportionate to imaging, showing *diffuse interstitial infiltrates*
		3. Fatigue, weakness, weight loss
			1. CXR (definitive): diffuse or **perihilar infiltrates, reticular interstitial** pneumonia or airspace disease that mimics pulmonary edema
			  • 5%-10% normal CXR
			  • Absent pleural effusions (Fig. 2-3)
			2. **Sputum Wright-Giemsa stain or DFA (direct fluorescence Ab)**
			  • Definitive in 50%-80%
			3. **BAL**
			  • Definitive in 95%
			4. **CD4 <200** if AIDS
			5. ABG: hypoxia, hypocapnia, reduced DLCO
			6. LDH: increased, but nonspecific
			7. Serum β-glucan
			  • More sensitive and specific
			8. WBC: low
				1. **Bactrim**, add steroids if Pao$_2$ <70 mm Hg or A-a gradient >35 mm Hg if given in 72 h
				2. Dapsone—if sulfa allergy
				3. All patients with CD4 <200 should undergo prophylaxis (Bactrim)

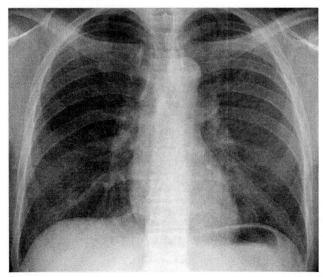

FIGURE 2-3. *P. jirovecii* pneumonia on chest radiograph. Diffuse ground-glass opacity sparing the lung periphery. (From Gotway MB. Pulmonary infections. In Webb WR, Higgins CB, eds. *Thoracic Imaging*. Philadelphia: Wolters Kluwer Health; 2017, with permission.)

Treatment of Pneumonia

Community-Acquired Pneumonia	Pathogens	Previously Healthy Patients with No Recent (90 d) Use of Antibiotics	Patients at Risk for Drug Resistance: Antibiotics in Last 90 d, Age >65 y, Comorbid Illness, Immunosuppression, Exposure to Child in Daycare
Outpatient Duration: 5 d minimum or until patient afebrile × 48-72 h	**S. pneumoniae** M. pneumoniae C. pneumoniae Respiratory viruses: flu	1. Macrolide: **clarithromycin** 500 mg PO BID or azithromycin 500 mg PO first dose, then 250 mg PO daily × 4 d 2. Doxycycline 100 mg PO BID	1. **Respiratory FQ**: Moxifloxacin 400 mg PO daily, levofloxacin 750 mg PO daily 2. Macrolide Plus β lactam (HD amoxicillin 1 g PO TID or augmentin 2 g PO BID)
Smokers		1. Cefdinir	
Inpatient, non-ICU	Pathogens: S. pneumoniae, Legionella, H. influenzae, Enterobacteriaceae, S. aureus, Pseudomonas	First line 1. **Respiratory FQ**: IV levofloxacin 750 mg daily or IV ciprofloxacin 400 mg q 8-12 h	At risk for Pseudomonas 1. IV macrolide plus IV β lactam (HD ampicillin 1-2 g q 4-6 h or Cefotaxime 1-2 g q 4-12 h or Ceftriaxone 1-2 g q 12-24 h)
Hospitalized or ICU patients Duration: 5 d minimum or until patient afebrile × 48-72 h	ICU: S. pneumoniae, Legionella, H. influenzae, Enterobacteriaceae, S. aureus, Pseudomonas	1. Azithromycin or respiratory FQ (moxifloxacin, **levofloxacin**) plus 2. Antipneumococcal β-lactam: **cefotaxime**, ceftriaxone, UNASYN β-lactam allergy: 1. FQ plus 2. Aztreonam 1-2 g q 6-12 h	1. Antipneumococcal and antipseudomonal β-lactam: **Zosyn**, cefepime, imipenem or meropenem plus 2. Ciprofloxacin or **levofloxacin** or 3. Antipneumococcal β-lactam (cefotaxime, ceftriaxone, UNASYN) plus 4. Aminoglycoside (gentamicin, tobramycin, amikacin) plus 5. Azithromycin or respiratory FQ If at risk for MRSA: 1. Add vancomycin or linezolid 600 mg BID
		Low risk for MDR pathogens	High risk for MDR pathogens
Nosocomial pneumonia		One of the following: 1. Ceftriaxone 1-2 g IV q 12-24 h 2. Moxifloxacin 400 mg PO or IV 3. Levofloxacin 750 mg PO or IV 4. Ciprofloxacin 400 mg IV q 8-12 h 5. UNASYN 1.5-3 g IV q 6 h 6. Zosyn 3.375-4 g IV q 6 h 7. Ertapenem 1 g IV daily	One agent from each: 1. Antipseudomonal • Cefepime 1-2 g IV BID or ceftazidime 1-2 g IV q 8 h • Imipenem 0.5-1 g IV q 6-8 h or meropenem 1 g IV q 8 h • Zosyn 3.375-4.5 g IV q 6 h • PCN allergy: aztreonam 1-2 g IV q 6-12 h 2. Second antipseudomonal • Levofloxacin 750 mg IV daily or ciprofloxacin 400 mg IV q 8-12 h • IV gentamicin, tobramycin, amikacin 3. MRSA coverage • IV vancomycin • Linezolid

When to Admit

CURB-65 Score
1. Confusion 2. Uremia 3. Respiratory rate 4. Blood pressure 5. Age >65
<1 = no hospitalization 1-2 = hospitalization (maybe ICU) 3+ = definite ICU admission

Pneumonia Vaccination

- Administer one or the other when pneumococcal vaccination history is incomplete or unknown and indicated
- Other indications for pneumococcal vaccine: sickle cell disease, other hemoglobinopathies, congenital or acquired asplenia/splenic dysfunction/splenectomy, congenital or acquired immunodeficiency, HIV, chronic renal failure, nephrotic syndrome, leukemia, lymphoma, Hodgkin disease, multiple myeloma, solid organ transplant
- No additional dose of PPSV23 indicated for adults vaccinated with PPSV23 at or after age 65 years should not be given during same visit

Have Received	Age 65+ y	Age 19-64 y, Immunocompromised, Functional Asplenia
Both	• If both received <65, give 23 6-12 mo after 13 was received or 5 y after most recent dose of 23	• Give second dose of 23 at least 5 y after first 23
PCV-13	• Give 23 6-12 mo after 13 • When indicated, only a single dose recommended for adults	• Give 23 at least 8 wk after 13 and second dose of 23 at least 5 y after first
PPSV23	• If given 65+, give 13 at least 1 y after 23 was received • If 1+ doses given <65, give 13 at least 1 y after most recent 23	• Give 13 at least 1 y after 23 and second 23 at least 8 wk after 13 and 5 y after first dose of 23 • If 2+ doses of 23, give one dose of 13 after 1 y
Neither	• Give 13 followed by 23 in 6-12 mo	• Give 13 followed by 23 at least 8 wk after 13, then second dose of 23 5 y after first
Give 23 (special population)	• CSF leaks and cochlear implants: give 13 followed by 23 at least 8 wk after 13 is given	• Smoke cigarettes • Nursing home resident or long-term care facility • Chronic heart disease (CHF, not hypertension) • Chronic lung disease (COPD, emphysema, asthma) • Chronic liver disease (cirrhosis), alcoholism • Diabetes

Tuberculosis

Chronic infection that can present as an acute or latent infection

- Only active TB is contagious (cough, sneezing), primary TB not contagious
- Difficult to diagnose in HIV (+)

- PPD will be **negative**
- Atypical CXR findings
- Sputum smears likely negative
- Granuloma formation may not be present
- Patients with (+) PPD have a lifetime risk of 10% for TB, reduced to 1% after 9 months of isoniazid treatment

Disease	Etiology, Prevalence, Risk Factors	Clinical Symptoms and Signs	Diagnostics	Therapy, Prognosis, and Health Maintenance
Tuberculosis	RF: **HIV**, recent immigrants (<5 y), prisoners, health care workers, close contact, alcoholics, diabetic patients, steroid use, blood malignancy, IVDU MC: ***Mycobacterium tuberculosis*** (acid-fast bacilli), slow growing Transmission: inhalation of **aerosolized droplets**	1. Fatigue 2. Weight loss 3. Fever 4. Night sweats 5. Productive cough	1. Sputum stain: acid-fast bacilli on smear • Sputum culture (+) for *M. tuberculosis* 2. PPD 3. CXR: caseating granuloma formation • Pulmonary opacities, most often apical	1. RIPE therapy 2. D/C therapy if transaminases >3-5 × ULN 3. Can spread to vertebral column: Pott disease

Primary TB	Secondary TB (Reactivation)	Extrapulmonary TB
Bacilli inhaled and deposited into lung → ingested by alveolar macrophages Surviving organisms multiply and disseminate via lymphatics and blood **Granulomas** form and "wall off" mycobacteria → remains dormant Insults on immune system reactivates (5%-10%)	Host's immunity weakened (HIV, malignancy, steroids, substance abuse, poor nutrition), gastrectomy, silicosis, diabetes Most oxygenated parts of lung: **apical/posterior** segments	Impaired immunity cannot contain bacteria → disseminates (HIV)

Primary TB	Secondary TB (Reactivation)	Extrapulmonary TB

Asymptomatic:
1. Pleural effusion
2. Can be progressive with incomplete immune response, pulmonary and constitutional symptoms
3. Usually clinically and radiographically silent
	Symptomatic:
	1. Constitutional SX: fever, night sweats, weight loss, malaise (common)
	   • Slowly progressive
	2. **Chronic cough, progressive,** dry → purulent
	   • Cough (MC symptom)
	   • **Blood streaked** (common) → hemoptysis
	Signs:
	1. Chronically ill appearing, malnourished
	2. Posttussive apical rales
		1. Any organ: lymph nodes, pleura, GU tract, spine, intestine, meninges
		2. Miliary TB: hematogenous spread
		   1. Can be due to reactivation or new infection
		   2. HIV (+) patients
		   3. Organomegaly, reticulo-nodular infiltrates, choroidal tubercles in eye

1. High index of suspicion, depending on RF and presentation
2. **CXR**–Small unilateral upper lobe **(apical) infiltrates** with **cavitations**, hilar and paratracheal lymph node enlargement, and segmental atelectasis
   • Pleural effusions (30%-40%), Ghon complex, Ranke complex
   • HIV (immunocompromised): lower lung zone, diffuse, or miliary infiltrates
3. **Sputum studies (sputum AFB)**
   • Definitive diagnosis by **sputum culture**: growth of MTB
   • Obtain **3 morning sputum** specimens–takes 4-8 wk
   • PCR can detect specific mycobacterial DNA (rapid)
4. PPD **(tuberculin skin test, Mantoux test)**–screening to detect previous TB exposure
   • Not for active TB diagnosis, but for latent primary TB
   • If (+), use CXR to r/o active TB
      • Once active infection r/o, **9 mo** of isoniazid initiated
   • Only screen patients with 1+ risk factors, preferred in children <5 y/o
   • If symptomatic or abnormal CXR, order AFB
   • Inject PPD into volar aspect of forearm; measure induration 48-72 h after:
      • (+) if induration >15 mm if no risk factors
      • (+) if induration **>10 mm +** high risk (high prevalence living areas, homeless, immigrants in the last 5 y, prisoners, health care workers, nursing home residents, close contact, alcoholics, diabetic patients)
      • (+) if induration >5 mm + very high risk (HIV, steroid users, organ transplant recipients, contact with active TB patient, CXR with cavitations)
      • Repeat in 1-2 wk if first test negative → second test used for management
5. **Interferon gamma release assay** (QuantiFERON and T-SPOT test): measures interferon gamma release in response to MTB antigens → sensitivity 60%-90%, reduced by HIV (low CD4), specificity 95%
   • Helpful to exclude false positive TST
6. Blood cultures (+) in 50% for MTB if CD4 count <100 (HIV/AIDS)
   • While awaiting definitive diagnosis, err on the side of treating *M. tuberculosis*
7. NAAT-R (nucleic acid amplification testing-resistance) and NAAT-TB to identify rapidly TB and drug resistance

| CXR–signs of healed primary TB:
1. **Ghon complex**–calcified focus with associated lymph node
2. Ranke complex–Ghon complex undergoes fibrosis and calcification | CXR–fibrocavitary apical disease, discrete nodules, pneumonic infiltrates usually in apical or posterior segments of upper lobes or in superior segments of lower lobes | |

Tuberculosis Treatment

| Active TB:
1. Droplet precautions; isolation until sputum negative for AFB
2. **2 m** of treatment with 4 drug RIPE regimen → **4 m** with *INH* and *Rifampin*
   • Once isolate determined to be isoniazid sensitive, ethambutol may be D/C'd
   • If susceptible to isoniazid and rifampin, may continue on 2-drug regimens
   • Treat at least 3 mo past negative cultures for MTB
Pregnant women:
• Should not take pyrazinamide: RIE × 2 mo → isoniazid and rifampin for 7 mo
• Pyridoxine (B₆) 10-25 mg PO daily to prevent peripheral neuropathy
• Breastfeeding *not* contraindicated
Latent (primary) TB: (+) PPD:
1. 9 mo of INH *after* active TB excluded (negative CXR, sputum, or both)
2. Not infectious; no active disease
3. Active TB results in 6% of untreated individuals | Immunocompetent, now seroconverted:
1. INH 300 mg/d × 9 m
   • AE: drug-induced hepatitis
HIV-positive patients:
1. 9 m of **INH**, 2 m of **rifampin** and pyrazinamide, or rifampin × 4 mo
2. Interaction with rifamycin derivatives and PI/NNRTI
3. Pyridoxine (B₆) 50 mg PO daily with isoniazid to rid of CNS/PNS symptoms
4. Rifampin should not be given to patients receiving a boosted protease inhibitor regimen → substitute rifabutin | 1. 9 m of therapy when miliary, meningeal, or bone/joint disease present
2. Surgical drainage and debridement of necrotic bone in skeletal disease
3. Steroid therapy to prevent constrictive pericarditis and neurologic complications |

PULMONARY NEOPLASM (LUNG CANCER)

- Risk factors
  - **Cigarette smoking** (>85%)—Increased risk with increasing pack years
    - Adenocarcinoma—Lowest association of smoking
  - Passive smoke
  - Asbestos—Common in shipbuilding and construction, car mechanics, painting
    - Smoking + asbestos = high risk
  - Radon—High levels in basements
  - COPD—Independent risk factor
- Metastatic disease—**Brain, bone, adrenal glands, liver**

Disease	Etiology, Prevalence, Risk Factors	Clinical Symptoms and Signs	Diagnostics	Therapy, Prognosis, and Health Maintenance
Small cell lung cancer (SCLC)–25%		1. **Recurrent pneumonia** 2. Constitutional SX (advanced disease): **anorexia, weight loss, weakness, cough** Associated: 1. **Superior vena cava syndrome** (SCLC): obstruction of SVC by mediastinal tumor, facial fullness, facial and arm edema, dilated veins over anterior chest, arms, face; JVD 2. Phrenic nerve palsy–hemidiaphragmatic paralysis 3. Recurrent laryngeal nerve palsy–hoarseness 4. **Horner syndrome**: invasion of cervical sympathetic chain by apical tumor → unilateral facial anhidrosis (no sweating), ptosis, miosis 5. Malignant pleural effusion 6. **Eaton-Lambert syndrome** (most common in SCLC): similar to myasthenia gravis (proximal muscle weakness/fatigue, diminished DTRs, paresthesias (lower extremity) 7. Digital clubbing	1. **CXR** most important for DX, but not used for screening 2. **CT chest** with IV contrast (use to stage) 3. **Tissue biopsy**–determine histologic type (definitive) 4. Cytologic examination of sputum–DX central tumors, not peripheral lesions 5. Fiberoptic bronchoscope–DX central tumors, not peripheral lesions 6. PET scan 7. Transthoracic needle biopsy–suspicious masses, highly accurate for peripheral lesions 8. Mediastinoscopy–advanced disease	1. Limited: **chemo + radiation** 2. Extensive: **chemo only** → if responsive, radiation therapy Prognosis: 1. Limited: **10%-13%** 5-y survival 2. Extensive: 1%-3% 5-y survival Staging: 1. Limited–confined to CHEST + supraclavicular nodes (not cervical or axillary) 2. Extensive–outside chest and supraclavicular nodes
Non–small cell lung cancer (NSCLC)–75%	Etiology: **squamous cell carcinoma**, adenocarcinoma, large cell carcinoma, bronchoalveolar cell carcinoma	1. Airway involvement (SCC) = cough, hemoptysis, obstruction, wheezing 2. **Pancoast syndrome** (SCC): superior sulcus tumor → shoulder pain, radiates down arm; pain and upper extremity weakness due to brachial plexus invasion, Horner syndrome (60% of time) Associated: Paraneoplastic syndromes • SIADH: with SCC • Ectopic ACTH–SCC • PTH-like secretion–SCC • Hypertrophic pulmonary osteoarthropathy–adenocarcinoma and SCC	Diagnostics as above: 1. CXR shows pleural effusion (LP for malignant cells) • Always perform a biopsy for intrathoracic lymphadenopathy	1. **Surgery**–best option • If metastatic outside chest, not a candidate • May recur after surgery 2. **Radiation**–important adjunct to surgery • Chemotherapy–uncertain benefit Staging: • Primary TNM system

Lung Cancer Screening

- The USPSTF recommends annual screening for lung cancer with low-dose computed tomography (LDCT) in adults aged 55 to 80 years who have a 30 pack-year smoking history and currently smoke or have quit within the past 15 years.

- Screening should be discontinued once a person has not smoked for 15 years or develops a health problem that substantially limits life expectancy or the ability or willingness to have curative lung surgery

SLEEP DISORDERS

Obesity-hypoventilation (Pickwickian) syndrome—condition in which severely overweight people fail to breathe rapidly or deeply enough, resulting in **low blood O_2** and **high CO_2 levels**.

- May result in OSA (periods of frequent absence of breathing for short periods of time) resulting in partial awakenings at night and sleepiness during the day

- This may lead to eventual heart failure symptoms, such as leg swelling

- Clinical features: **obesity (BMI > 30)**, hypoxemia during sleep, and hypercapnia resulting from hypoventilation

- TX: **weight loss** and **continuous positive airway pressure** (CPAP)

Disease	Etiology, Prevalence, Risk Factors	Clinical Symptoms and Signs	Diagnostics	Therapy, Prognosis, and Health Maintenance

Obstructive sleep apnea (90%)	Loss of pharyngeal muscle tone leads to collapse during inspiration
	RF: micrognathia, macroglossia, obesity, tonsillar hypertrophy, hypothyroidism, smoking
	Aggravators: ingestion of ETOH or sedatives before sleeping, nasal obstruction (eg, cold)
	Most middle-age, obese men
		1. HX of loud snoring
		  • Witnessed cyclical snoring, restlessness, thrashing of extremities during sleep
		2. Apnea—cessation of breathing
		3. Interrupted sleep and excessive daytime sleepiness
		4. Fatigue
		5. Personality changes, poor judgment, memory impairment, inability to concentrate
		6. Other: depression, hypertension, headaches worse in AM, impotence
		Signs:
		1. Appears sleepy
		2. Narrow oropharynx, excessive soft tissue folds, large tonsils, pendulous uvula, large tongue
		3. Deviated nasal septum
		4. "Bull neck" appearance
			1. **Polysomnography** (definitive)
			  • **5+ episodes** of apnea, hypopnea, or respiratory-related arousals per hour (high AHI) during sleep
			2. CBC: erythrocytosis
			3. TFTs: r/o hypothyroidism
			4. ABG $CO_2 > 45$ mm Hg
				1. **Weight loss**, avoid hypnotic meds
				2. CPAP (curative)
				  • Only 75% use after 1 y
				3. If $O_2 < 90\%$, switch to BiPAP (higher pressure during inspiration, lower pressure during expiration)
				4. If both ineffective, add O_2 therapy
				5. UPPP—works in 50%
				6. **Tracheostomy**–definitive treatment

(Obesity) hypoventilation syndrome (10%)	Alveolar hypoventilation results from blunted ventilatory drive and increased mechanical load imposed by obesity → voluntary hyperventilation returns the P_{CO_2} and P_{O_2} toward normal values Rise of CO_2 by 10 mm Hg after sleep compared to awake measurements and overnight drops in O_2 levels *without* apnea or hypopnea		1. **Polysomnography** (required): EEG, EKG, pulse oximetry 2. Screen for **TSH** (hypothyroid) and **CBC** (polycythemia) 3. CXR or CT scan, spirometry performed Complications: cor pulmonale (33%)	1. **Weight loss**: improves hypercapnia and hypoxemia 2. NPPV 3. Acetazolamide, theophylline, medroxyprogesterone acetate • Reduces bicarbonate levels 4. Treat underlying OSA

TOBACCO USE/DEPENDENCE

1 pack of cigarettes = 20 cigarettes
1 carton = 10 packs = 200 cigarettes

First-Line Therapies Approved for Use by the FDA for Smoking Cessation

Drug Name	Bupropion (Zyban)	Nicotine Gum (Nicorette)	Nicotine Patch (NicoDerm CQ, Nicotrol)	Varenicline (Chantix)
Class	Norepinephrine/dopamine Reuptake inhibitor (NDRI)	Nicotinic cholinergic receptor agonist		Partial cholinergic receptor agonist
Route	PO	PO	Transdermal	PO
Onset of action	1-2 wk			
Half-life	21 h			
Excretion	Mostly urine			
MOA	Blocks the reuptake of dopamine and norepinephrine, enhancing their respective neurotransmission	**Agonist to nicotinic receptors** at autonomic ganglia, adrenal medulla, neuromuscular junctions, and the brain		1. Bind with high affinity $\alpha_4\beta_2$ nicotinic acetylcholine receptors on dopamine neurons, preventing nicotine from exerting action 2. Reduces craving 3. **Agonist at receptors** inducing nicotine effects
Contraindications/precautions	HX seizure disorder HX eating disorder Undergoing abrupt D/C of ETOH or sedatives (benzos, AEDs) Use of MAOIs within 14 d Linezolid or IV methylene blue	None	None	Cardiovascular disease (CHF) Mood disorders
Boxed warning	Suicidality (especially in first 1-2 mo)			Suicide, psychosis
Adverse effects	Insomnia Headache Dry mouth Constipation Nausea/vomiting, weight loss	Mouth soreness or ulcers Dyspepsia (if chewed too rapidly): nausea, vomiting, abdominal pain, constipation, hiccups Headache Excess salivation Sore jaw	Insomnia Local skin reaction	Nausea, vomiting Headache Vivid dreams Constipation
Required monitoring	Kidney/liver function Behavioral changes Body weight Blood pressure	None	None	Kidney function Behavioral changes

Drug Name	Bupropion (Zyban)	Nicotine Gum (Nicorette)	Nicotine Patch (NicoDerm CQ, Nicotrol)	Varenicline (Chantix)
Clinical pearls	150 mg q AM × 3 d, then 150 mg BID (begin 1-2 wk before cessation) Prescription only *Most effective when combined with behavioral therapies Not approved for pediatric patients	Use up to 12 wk (3 mo) 1-24 CG/d: 2 mg 25+ CG/d: 4 mg Up to 24 pieces/d *Chew at least 1 piece every 1-2 h while awake "Chew and park": chew/bite down q 30 min and place in buccal mucosa *Adjunct therapy *Avoid acidic beverages (coffee, sodas) OTC only	Wear for 4 wk, then 2 wk, then 2 wk, then 8 wk OTC only	12 or 24 wk 0.5 mg daily × 3 d, then 0.5 mg BID × 4 d, then 1 mg PO BID Prescription only Give s/e at least 2 wk to resolve May impair capacity to drive *Only take with bupropion

Second-Line Therapies Approved for Use by the FDA for Smoking Cessation

Drug Name	Clonidine (Catapres)	Nortriptyline
Class	Centrally acting α_2 adrenergic agonist	Tricyclic antidepressant
Route	PO	PO
Onset of action	N/A	N/A
Half-life	12-16 h	30 h
Excretion	Urine	Urine, mostly
MOA	Stimulates α_2 receptors in the brain, effectively decreasing peripheral vascular resistance, lowering blood pressure By binding to presynaptic α_2 receptors in the brain, it decreases presynaptic calcium levels, inhibiting the release of **norepinephrine**	Inhibits the reuptake of **norepinephrine** more than **serotonin**
Contraindications/ precautions	Rebound hypertension if discontinued abruptly	Risk of arrhythmia Do not use in acute recovery phase after MI
Boxed warning		
Adverse effects	Dry mouth Drowsiness Dizziness, **hypotension** **Sedation**, dizziness Headache	Sedation Dry mouth Constipation Increased appetite Blurred vision Tinnitus
Required monitoring	None	None
Clinical pearls	0.15-0.75 mg/d × 3-10 wk Gradually taper if D/C Prescription only	75-100 mg/d × 12 wk Prescription only

CHAPTER **3**

Gastrointestinal System and Nutrition

Supplemental Resources :

Cancer of the Esophagus, Liver, Stomach, Pancreas, and Gallbladder, p 218

Diverticular Disease, p 216

Celiac Disease, p 220

Hemochromatosis, see Hematology, p 285

Achalasia, see Family Medicine, p 66

LIVER FUNCTION TESTS

- **ALT** is more sensitive than **AST** for liver damage
  - ALT primarily found in the *liver* and AST found in many tissues (skeletal muscle, heart, kidney, brain)
  - Most common causes of elevated aminotransferases: alcohol, hepatitis C virus, hemochromatosis, and hepatitis B virus
- **Alkaline-phosphatase:** nonspecific to the liver (bone, intestine, placenta), elevated with obstruction to bile flow (cholestasis) in any part of biliary tree
  - If levels very high (10× increase): think extrahepatic biliary tract, obstruction, or intrahepatic cholestasis (PBC, drug-induced cirrhosis)
  - If levels are elevated—measure GGT (liver only)
    - **GGT** elevated—strongly suggests hepatic origin
- Bilirubin—rarely exceeds 20 mg/dL with any cause. The highest bilirubin levels are observed in cirrhosis, especially with accompanying hepatic failure (eg, hepatorenal syndrome). If extrahepatic obstruction is present, the serum bilirubin level will rise to about 15 mg/dL, but the kidneys compensate by excreting excess bilirubin, resulting in bilirubinuria. In hepatic failure this mechanism is lost, which explains why the highest serum bilirubin levels are seen in advanced cirrhotic liver disease with hepatorenal syndrome.
- **Albumin**—decreased in *chronic* liver disease, nephrotic syndrome, malnutrition, and inflammatory states (burns, sepsis, trauma)
- **Prothrombin time (PT)**—liver synthesizes clotting factors I, **II**, V, **VII, IX, X,** XII, and XIII, the function of which is reflected by PT

- Not prolonged until most of liver's synthetic capacity is lost, which corresponds to <u>advanced</u> liver disease
- The prothrombin time and partial thromboplastin time are usually both normal in acute viral hepatitis. However, in a patient with acute viral hepatitis, a prolonged prothrombin time and an international normalized ratio (INR) greater than 1.8 may be the harbinger of submassive necrosis of the liver and impending liver failure
- The prothrombin time and partial thromboplastin time are prolonged in chronic liver disease and cirrhosis
- The prothrombin time may be prolonged in patients with prolonged obstructive jaundice because of failure to absorb vitamin K
- Cholestatic LFTs: markedly elevated alkaline phosphatase and GGT
- Hepatocellular necrosis or inflammation: NL or slightly elevated alk-phos; markedly elevated AST/ALT
- If AST/ALT are:
  - Mildly elevated (low hundreds): chronic viral hepatitis or acute ETOH hepatitis
  - Moderately elevated (high hundreds-thousands): acute viral hepatitis
  - Severely elevated (>10 000): extensive hepatic necrosis (APAP toxicity, severe viral hepatitis, ischemia, shock liver)
- Note: LFTs are often NL or can be low in patients with cirrhosis (no active cell necrosis) or metastatic liver disease → number of healthy functioning hepatocytes is reduced

Type of Disorder	Direct Bilirubin	AST/ALT Ratio	GGT	Alk-Phos	PT/INR	Albumin
Acute hepatocellular necrosis	↑	↑>10-fold AST ~ ALT	NL/↑	NL/↑	↑	NL/↓(late)
Chronic hepatocellular necrosis	↑	↑1- to 5-fold AST ~ ALT	NL/↑	NL/↑	NL/↑ (late)	NL/↓(late)
Alcoholic liver disease	↑	AST = ALT 2- to 3-fold	↑	NL/↑	NL/↑	NL/↓
Cirrhosis	NL to ↑	AST:ALT > 1-2-fold	↑	↑	↑	↓
Obstruction/cholestasis	↑	5- to 10-fold ↑ AST ~ ALT	↑	↑↑↑↑	NL	NL

ANAL FISSURE AND FISTULA (FIG. 3-2)

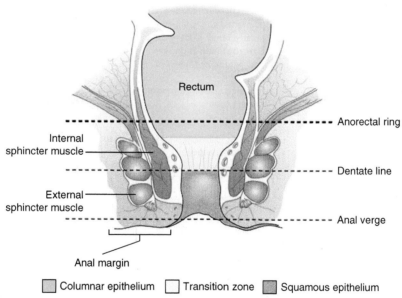

Columnar epithelium   Transition zone   Squamous epithelium

FIGURE 3-1. Dentate line. The anorectal ring extends about 4 cm to the anal verge, which compromises the entire anal canal. The dentate line divides the upper canal from the lower canal, which is lined by columnar epithelium and squamous epithelium. (From Jiang Y, Beddy DJ, Nelson H, Kachnic LA, Ajani JA. Cancer of the anal region. In: DeVita VT, Lawrence TS, Rosenberg SA, et al, eds. *DeVita, Hellman, and Rosenberg's Cancer: Principles and Practice of Oncology*. Philadelphia: Wolters Kluwer Health; 2012, with permission.)

Disease	Etiology, Prevalence, Risk Factors	Clinical Symptoms and Signs	Diagnostics	Therapy, Prognosis, and Health Maintenance
Anal fissure Irritation caused by trauma to anal canal results in increased resting pressure of internal sphincter → ischemia in region of fissure and poor healing of injury	More common in 30-50s, M = F Primary: local trauma, passage of hard stool, prolonged diarrhea, anal sex, vaginal delivery Secondary: previous anal surgical procedures; IBD (**Crohn disease**), granulomatous disease (TB, sarcoidosis), malignancy (squamous cell anal cancer, leukemia), HIV, syphilis, chlamydia MC site: **posterior** anal midline, *below or distal to the dentate line* Chronic = more than 6 wk (40% of patients develop)	Acute: 1. **Tearing pain with defecation** • May avoid using bathroom 2. Perianal **pruritus** and/or skin irritation 3. **Bright red bleeding** (on toilet paper) Signs: 1. **Superficial** laceration (paper cut–like) Chronic: 1. Anal spasm 2. High anal pressure Signs: 1. Laceration has raised edges exposing the white, horizontally oriented fibers of internal anal sphincter muscle fibers at base 2. **External skin tags** (sentinel pile) at distal end of fissure 3. **Hypertrophied** anal **papillae** at proximal end	1. Endoscopy—if patient has rectal bleeding beyond 2 mo of treatment 2. Sigmoidoscopy in patients <50 with no FH of colon cancer 3. Colonoscopy if suspicion for Crohn disease	Acute: Heals in 6 wk 1. Dietary fiber and water intake 2. **Sitz baths**, topical anesthetics, and vasodilator (nifedipine, NTG) • Stool softeners or laxative Failed therapy/chronic: • Fails conservative; requires aggressive approach 1. **Botulinum toxin A injection** 2. Lateral sphincterotomy (gold standard): last resort; may result in fecal incontinence Prevention: 1. Proper anal hygiene: keep dry and wipe with soft cotton or moistened cloth 2. High-fiber diet, adequate fluids, avoid straining during defecation 3. Avoid trauma to anus 4. Prompt treatment of diarrhea
Anorectal fistulas (fistula-in-ano): • 10% associated with IBD, tuberculosis, malignancy, radiation • Communication of abscess cavity with an identifiable internal opening within the anal canal, most commonly located at the dentate line where the anal glands enter the anal canal (Fig. 3-1)	Arise through obstruction of anal crypts or glands **Intersphincteric** (70%), transsphincteric (23%), extrasphincteric (5%), suprasphincteric (2%) 40% are (+) for intestinal bacteria Male (2×) > female MCC: Anorectal abscess	1. Nonhealing anorectal abscess following drainage or **chronic purulent drainage** and pustule-like **firm mass** in perianal or buttock area 2. Intermittent **rectal pain** • Worse with defecation, sitting, and activity 3. Malodorous perianal drainage 4. Pruritus Signs: 1. Excoriation and inflammation of perianal skin 2. Inflamed, tender, draining external opening	1. All require **anoscopy** with diluted hydrogen peroxide to look for internal opening 2. Imaging (not required): endosonography, fistulography, CT, or MRI–air or contrast material within fistula 3. Drain with Mallenkot catheter, then fistulagram to search for an occult fistula tract 4. Parks classification system (see Fig. 3-3)	Simple: 1. **Fistulotomy** with probing (preferred) • Decreased risk of incontinence and recurrence, shorter healing time 2. Simple ligation of the internal fistula tract (LIFT) procedure 3. Fistulectomy • Larger wound, prolonged healing time, higher risk of incontinence Complex: 1. Seton • Vessel loop or silk tie placed through fistula tract • Reduces risk of incontinence in cases where poor wound healing expected • Can be initial temporary intervention or for complex fistulas who fail initial therapy 2. Treatment as above

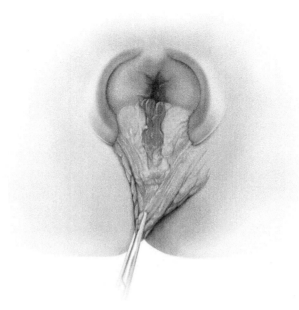

FIGURE 3-2. Anal fissure. (From Albo D. Surgical management of anal fissures. In: Albo D, ed. *Operative Techniques in Colon and Rectal Surgery.* Philadelphia: Wolters Kluwer Health; 2016, with permission.)

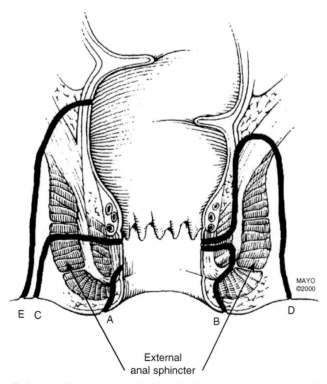

FIGURE 3-3. Parks classification system. **A,** Superficial fistula. **B,** Intersphincteric. **C,** Transphincteric. **D,** Suprasphincteric. **E,** Extrasphincteric. (From Michelassi F, Nanadakumar G, Katdare MB, Fichera A, Hurst RD. Surgical treatment of Crohn's disease. In: Fischer JF, Bland KI, Callery MP, et al, eds. *Fischer's Mastery of Surgery.* Philadelphia: Wolters Kluwer Health; 2019, with permission.)

HEMORRHOIDS (FIGS. 3-4 AND 3-5A)

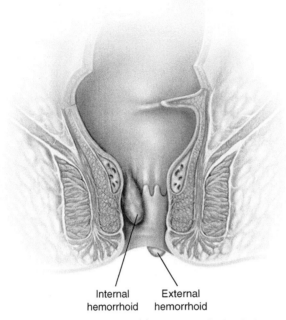

Internal   External
hemorrhoid   hemorrhoid

FIGURE 3-4. Internal and external hemorrhoids. (From Bidhan D. Surgical management of hemorrhoids. In: Albo D, ed. *Operative Techniques in Colon and Rectal Surgery.* Philadelphia: Wolters Kluwer Health; 2016, with permission.)

Disease	Etiology, Prevalence, Risk Factors	Clinical Symptoms and Signs	Diagnostics	Therapy, Prognosis, and Health Maintenance
Hemorrhoids	Varicose veins of anus and rectum Risk factor: Constipation/straining, pregnancy, portal HTN, obesity, prolonged sitting or standing, anal intercourse	1. **Hematochezia–rectal bleeding** (BRBPR) • Painless • Associated with bowel movement 2. Perianal pruritus 3. Fecal soilage 4. Rectal prolapse	1. Anoscopy–if BRBPR or suspected thrombosis	1. Conservative: • Sitz bath • Apply ice packs to anal area • Bed rest • Stool softeners • High fiber/fluid diet • Topical steroids Complications: Iron deficiency anemia (chronic)
External	Dilated veins arising from *inferior* hemorrhoidal plexus **distal to dentate line** (sensate area)	Asymptomatic unless thrombosed→ 1. Sudden, **painful** swelling 2. Lasts several days, then subside		1. Conservative management (above) 2. **Rubber band ligation** • If protrudes with defecation, enlargement, or intermittent <u>bleeding</u> • For stages I, II, or III nonresponsive 3. Closed **hemorrhoidectomy**–for permanently prolapsed • Stage III or IV with chronic bleeding or stage II that is acutely thrombosed • External do not require surgical management, unless thrombosed or large and symptomatic
Internal	Dilated submucosal veins of *superior* rectal plexus; **above dentate line** (insensate area) Thrombosed: increased with defecation and sitting; **tender, swollen, bluish ovoid mass**	1. **Painless** rectal bleeding 2. Bulging perianal mass with straining 3. Present when they prolapse • Mild fecal incontinence • Mucous discharge • Wetness • Sensation of fullness Signs: 1. Bulging purplish-blue Refer to Fig. 3-5 for Prolapsed hemorrhoids		

Disease	Etiology, Prevalence, Risk Factors	Clinical Symptoms and Signs	Diagnostics	Therapy, Prognosis, and Health Maintenance
Thrombosed (Fig. 3-5B)	More common with external hemorrhoids	1. Acute severe perianal pain • **Painful** defecation 2. BRBPR 3. Anal pruritus <u>Signs</u>: 1. Palpable perianal mass (purplish hue) 2. Perianal swelling 3. Acutely tender	1. Anoscopy Thrombosed external hemorrhoid	1. Conservative management unless persistent or present within 72 h from onset of pain 2. **Surgery** recommended (definitive) <u>Complications</u>: Internal hemorrhoids can become prolapsed, strangulated, and develop gangrenous changes

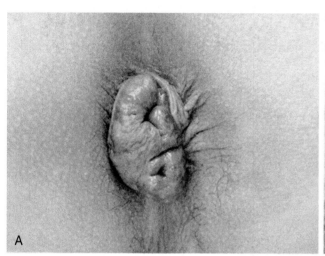 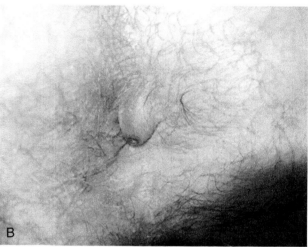

FIGURE 3-5. A, Prolapsed internal hemorrhoid. **B,** Thrombosed hemorrhoid. (From Burney RE. Thrombosed hemorrhoids. In: Dimick JB, Upchurch GB, Sonnenday CJ, eds. *Clinical Scenarios in Surgery*. Philadelphia: Wolters Kluwer Health; 2013, with permission.)

Treatment of Hemorrhoids

External hemorrhoids **Low-grade internal hemorrhoids** 1. Grade I hemorrhoids are visualized on anoscopy and may bulge into the lumen but do not prolapse below the dentate line 2. Grade II hemorrhoids prolapse out of the anal canal with defecation or with straining but reduce spontaneously	<u>Conservative</u>: 1. Dietary changes (fiber, water)—treats bleeding • Psyllium or methylcellulose 2. Topical venoactive agents: hydroxyethylrutoside 3. Local analgesics: hydrocortisone/lidocaine 4. Itching or irritation: hydrocortisone suppository, warm sitz baths, or steroid cream BID • Not recommended >1 wk <u>If conservative management fails or bleeding internal hemorrhoids</u>: 1. Nonsurgical office-based procedures (rubber band ligation)—fewer complications and pain 2. Surgery—more effective for recurrence or bleeding external hemorrhoids
Painful thrombosed external hemorrhoids Medium-grade internal hemorrhoids Grade III hemorrhoids prolapse out of the anal canal with defecation or straining and require manual reduction	1. Rubber band ligation (initial) • Contraindications: coagulopathies, anticoagulants (warfarin), antiplatelets (Plavix) • Aspirin is okay 2. Sclerotherapy: for symptomatic internal hemorrhoids: phenol 5% in vegetable oil • Indications: Grades I-II bleeding internal or patients on anticoagulants 3. Surgery recommended (<u>definitive</u>)
Grade IV hemorrhoids are irreducible and may strangulate	1. **Requires** *definitive* surgical treatment: • Surgical excision • Hemorrhoidectomy

COLORECTAL CANCER OR COLORECTAL CARCINOMA

- Pattern of spread
  - Direct extension—circumferentially, then through bowel wall

- Hematogenous—portal circulation to **liver** (liver is the most common site of distant spread), lumbar/vertebral veins to LUNGS
- Lymphatic—regionally
- Transperitoneal and intraluminal

Disease	Etiology, Prevalence, Risk Factors	Clinical Symptoms and Signs	Diagnostics	Therapy, Prognosis, and Health Maintenance
Colorectal cancer Most arise from adenomas (endoluminal **adenocarcinomas** arising from the mucosa)	Premalignant, but most do not develop into cancer Malignancy: **Villous** > tubular adenomas Larger the size and greater the number = higher risk of cancer CRC is the most common cause of **large bowel** OBST in adults RF: **Age** (>50 y), adenomatous polyps (premalignant), personal history of CRC or adenomatous polyps, IBD (**ulcerative colitis** > Crohn disease), family history (first degree with CRC), dietary (high fat, low fiber), major polyposis syndromes (see below)	1. **Abdominal pain:** due to obstruction or peritoneal dissemination 2. **Change in bowel habit** 3. **Weight loss** 4. **Blood in stool (hematochezia)** • Asymptomatic • Unexplained iron deficiency anemia • Mostly in advanced states: melena or hematochezia Right-sided tumors: Obstruction unusual because of large luminal diameter • Occult blood stool, IDA, and **melena** • No change in bowel habits • Triad of anemia, weakness, and RLQ mass Left-sided tumors: Smaller lumen, obstruction common • **Change in bowel habits**: alternating constipation/diarrhea, *narrowing of stools* ("pencil") • Hematochezia (common)	See Screening Guidelines	1. **Surgery**–Only curative treatment • CEA levels before surgery 2. Adjuvant therapy: chemo + radiation 3. Follow up with: • Stool guaiac • Annual CT of abdomen/pelvis and CXR up to 5 y • Colonoscopy at 1 y, then q 3 y • CEA levels every 3-6 mo • Very high CEA = possible liver involvement 90% of recurrences are within 3 y after surgery
Familial adenomatous polyposis (FAP)	**Autosomal dominant**–hundreds of adenomatous polyps in colon (duodenum in 90%) 20-30s Risks: Colon cancer, follicular or papillary thyroid cancer, gastric carcinoma, medulloblastoma, duodenal ampullary carcinoma	1. **>100 cumulative colorectal adenomas** or HX of adenomas in combination with extracolonic features (duodenal or ampullary adenomas, desmoid tumors, papillary thyroid cancer, congenital hypertrophy of the retinal pigment epithelium, epidermal cysts, osteomas) Complications: Iron deficiency anemia	1. Endoscopy starting at age 25-30 y • Random sampling of fundic gland polyps • Diagnosed with 10 or more colorectal adenomas	1. Prophylactic **colectomy** recommended • Indications: large (>1 cm) or high-grade dysplasia • Annual endoscopy of rectum, ileostomy eval every 1-3 y 2. Screen thyroid annually (TST, U/S) Surveillance: • Stage 0-1: q 4 y • Stage 2: q 2-3 y • Stage 3: q 6-12 m • Stage 4: surgery Risk of CRC **100%** by 30s-40s
Peutz-Jeghers	Single or multiple hamartomas that may be scattered: 78%, small bowel; 60%, colon; 30% stomach Hamartomas–very low malignant potential (unlike adenomas)	Pigmented spots around lips, oral mucosa, face, genitalia, palmar surface		Increased incidence in various carcinomas (stomach, ovary, breast, cervix, testicle, lung) Complications: intussusception or GI bleed

Colorectal Cancer Screening Guidelines

	CDC Recommendations		Average Risk
Colorectal cancer	1. Begin at age 50 y, continue until age 75 y • **FOBT** every year • Do not screen adults >85 y • Start 10 y younger than age of diagnosis of youngest affected relative 2. **Flexible sigmoidoscopy**: every 5 y combined with FOBT every 3 y 3. **Colonoscopy**: every 10 y • Colonoscopy every 5 y for patients with single first-degree relative diagnosed with CRC or advanced adenoma	For screening purposes, patients with 1 first-degree relative diagnosed with colorectal cancer or advanced adenoma at age 60 y or older are considered at average risk For patients with a single first-degree relative diagnosed with colorectal cancer or advanced adenoma before age 60 y, or those with 2 first-degree relatives with colorectal cancer or advanced adenomas; the guideline recommends colonoscopy every 5 y, beginning at age 40 y or at 10 y younger than the age at diagnosis of the youngest affected relative	Patients are considered at average risk if all answers to initial screening questions are "no" • Have you ever had CRC or an adenomatous polyp? • Have you had inflammatory bowel disease? • Have you received abdominal radiation for childhood cancer? • Have any family members had CRC or an adenomatous polyp? If so, were they first-degree relatives and what age was it diagnosed?

- The highest familial risk is in people with **multiple first-degree relatives** or relatives who have developed **colorectal cancer at a relatively young age** (eg, younger than 50 years)
  - Risk for colorectal cancer is greater for relatives of patients with colon, as compared to rectal, cancer

- Patients who have a family member with an adenomatous colonic polyp may also be at increased risk for adenoma or colorectal cancer

---

CRC Screening Methods

- FOBT—poor sensitivity/specificity
- Digital rectal examination—only 10% are palpable
- **Colonoscopy**—most sensitive and specific test
  - Perform if FOBT (+) or any other test is positive
  - Diagnostic and therapeutic—biopsy + polypectomy
- Flexible sigmoidoscopy—can reach area where 50%-70% of tumors occur
- Barium enema—evaluates entire colon, complementary to flex-sig, abnormal findings require colonoscopy
- **Carcinoembryonic antigen (CEA)**—not useful for screening; useful for **baseline and recurrence surveillance**
  - Prognostic significance—if >5 ng/mL, worse prognosis
- CT chest/abdomen/pelvis and physical (ascites, HSM, lymphadenopathy)—clinical staging

PEPTIC ULCER DISEASE

Disease	Etiology, Prevalence, Risk Factors	Clinical Symptoms and Signs	Diagnostics	Therapy, Prognosis, and Health Maintenance
Peptic ulcer disease	Causes: • *Helicobacter pylori* infection • NSAIDs • Acid hypersecretory states (Zollinger-Ellison syndrome) Other causes: • Smoking (2×) • ETOH and coffee • Emotional stress • Dietary factors	1. Epigastric pain: • Aching or *gnawing* in nature • Nocturnal symptoms • Effect of <u>food</u> on symptoms variable 2. Nausea/vomiting 3. Early satiety 4. Weight loss	1. **Endoscopy**: required to DX gastric ulcers to r/o malignancy, duodenal do not require, can biopsy for *H. pylori* • Use of IV PPI to prevent rebleeding 2. Barium swallow 3. *H. pylori* antigen • Antibodies to *H. pylori* can remain elevated for months-years after infection gone • False-negatives with PPI, Pepto, antibiotics 4. Biopsy (gold standard) 5. Urease detection via urea breath test 6. Serum gastrin measurement: if considering Zollinger-Ellison syndrome	See treatment table <u>Complications</u>: GI bleed

Peptic Ulcer Disease Treatment

Supportive
- D/C aspirin/NSAIDs, no alcohol, stop smoking and decrease emotional stress, avoid eating before bedtime, decrease coffee intake

Acid suppression
- H$_2$ (accelerate healing), **PPI** (most effective), antacids (adjunctive/symptomatic relief)
- Eradicate *H. pylori* with 3-4 drug therapy (**amoxicillin and clarithromycin and PPI**) or clarithromycin and flagyl
  - Alternative: Pepto Bismol, tetracycline, flagyl, PPI

Cryoprotection
- Sucralfate: facilitates ulcer healing → for pregnant women
- Misoprostol: reduces risk for ulcer formation with NSAID use

Surgical intervention
1. Truncal vagotomy and antrectomy
   - Indications: hemorrhage, perforation, obstruction, failure of medical management

Duodenal Versus Peptic (Gastric) Ulcer

Duodenal: 70%-90% *H. pylori*	Gastric: 60%-70% *H. pylori*
Cause: Increase in offensive factors (higher rates of basal and stimulated gastric acid secretion) RF: **NSAIDs**	Cause: Decrease in defensive factors (gastric acid level normal/low unless ulcer is pyloric) RF: **smoking**
Low malignancy potential Younger patients <40 y Type O blood Relieved with eating, **nocturnal pain more common**	High malignancy potential Older patients >40 y Type A blood Eating can make pain worse → anorexia, weight loss

GASTRITIS

Disease	Etiology, Prevalence, Risk Factors	Clinical Symptoms and Signs	Diagnostics	Therapy, Prognosis, and Health Maintenance
Acute gastritis: inflammation of the gastric mucosa	1. **NSAIDs**, aspirin, *H. pylori* infection 2. Alcohol, heavy cigarette smoking, caffeine 3. Extreme physiologic stress (shock, sepsis, burns)	1. Asymptomatic or epigastric pain: relationship b/w eating and pain not consistent (aggravated or relieved) 2. **Dyspepsia** (belching, bloating, distention, heartburn) 3. **Abdominal pain**	1. **Upper GI endoscopy with biopsy** (first line) 2. Urea breath test to detect *H. pylori* 3. *H. pylori* antigen	1. Stop NSAIDs, empiric therapy with acid suppression 2. 4-8 wk of PPI • If no response, consider upper GI endoscopy and ultrasound, test for *H. pylori* infection • If *H. pylori* (+)–treat with antibiotics
Chronic gastritis	MCC: *H. pylori*	1. Most asymptomatic: epigastric pain similar to PUD 2. Nausea, vomiting, anorexia–rare		1. Triple therapy (PPI + 2 antibiotics) for 2 wk or quadruple therapy (PPI, Pepto, and 2 antibiotics) for 1 wk

GASTROENTERITIS

Disease	Etiology, Prevalence, Risk Factors	Clinical Symptoms and Signs	Diagnostics	Therapy, Prognosis, and Health Maintenance
Acute viral gastroenteritis	Causes: rotavirus, **Norwalk virus**, enterovirus Duration: 48-72 h, SX may linger up to 1 wk Transmission: Fecal-oral Most common cause of acute diarrhea	1. Myalgias, malaise, possible low-grade fever 2. Headache 3. Watery diarrhea 4. Abdominal pain 5. **Nausea and vomiting**	1. Fecal leukocytes: none 2. Hypokalemia and metabolic acidosis	1. Supportive look for similar illness in family members

Disease	Etiology, Prevalence, Risk Factors	Clinical Symptoms and Signs	Diagnostics	Therapy, Prognosis, and Health Maintenance

Traveler's diarrhea	<u>Cause:</u>
	Food/water contaminated with fecal matter
	<u>Etiology:</u>
	ETEC, *Campylobacter, Salmonella, Shigella*
	<u>RF:</u>
	Travel destination
	Occurs in first 2 wk of travel, lasts 4 d without treatment
		<u>Defined as:</u> 3+ unformed stools in 24 h with at least one of the following:
		1. Fever
		2. Nausea
		3. Vomiting
		4. Abdominal cramps
		5. Tenesmus
		6. Bloody stools
		<u>Complications:</u>
		Dehydration (MC), Guillain-Barre, Reiter syndrome
			<u>Clinical DX:</u>
			1. Fecal leukocytes
			2. *Clostridium difficile* toxin
			3. Test 3 stool samples for ova and parasites
			4. Bacterial stool culture
			5. FOBT
				1. Empiric treatment with **ciprofloxacin** 500 mg BID × 1-3 d and loperamide (if older than 2 y)
				  • Campylobacter and Shigella: FQ
				  • FQ-resistant, children, pregnant: **azithromycin**
				  • Complications from treatment: *C. difficile* colitis
				2. Bismuth-subsalicylate is 60% effective
				  • Not recommended for patients taking anticoagulants or other salicylates
				  • AE: black tongue, dark stools, tinnitus, Reye syndrome in children
				<u>Prophylaxis:</u>
				1. Prophylaxis with FQ is 90% effective

Salmonella	Duration: resolves in 1 wk Transmission: most commonly **food or water** (poultry and eggs), **fecal-oral route** Incubation: 5 d to 2 wk for enteric fever (typhoid)	1. Inflammatory diarrhea (small volume) 2. Nausea and vomiting 3. SX *appear* **24-48 h after** ingesting food *Salmonella typhi*–presents as constipation Possible fever	1. Fecal leukocytes: yes 2. *C. difficile* toxin and culture 3. Test 3 stool samples for ova and parasites 4. Bacterial stool culture 5. Hypokalemia and metabolic acidosis	1. Ciprofloxacin • No treatment except in immunocompromised or enteric fever (*S. typhi*)
Shigella	Duration: resolves in 1 wk (4-5 d) Transmission: **fecal-oral route** more common than food More common in developing countries, children <5 y and their caregivers (especially people who work in nurseries or nursing homes)	1. Abdominal pain 2. Inflammatory diarrhea (small volume) 3. Frequent, mucous and bloody stool 4. Nausea, vomiting (less common) 5. **Tenesmus:** feeling of constantly needing to pass stools 6. Possible fever	1. **Fecal leukocytes:** (+) 2. *C. difficile* toxin and culture 3. Test 3 stool samples for ova and parasites 4. Bacterial stool culture 5. Hypokalemia and metabolic acidosis Produces the largest quantity of fecal leukocytes than any other cause of gastroenteritis	1. **TMP/SMX** (Bactrim)
Enterohemorrhagic *E. coli* (EHEC), also referred to by *E. coli* O157:H7 or Shiga-toxin producing *E. coli* (STEC)	Consumption of **under-cooked ground beef** Shiga-like toxin	1. Onset: 12-60 h 2. Duration: 5-10 d 3. Watery, *voluminous*, nonbloody diarrhea with nausea and vomiting→ 4. Dysentery (bloody)	1. No fecal leukocytes	1. **Antibiotics not recommended**, except in severe disease <u>Complication:</u> Hemolytic uremic syndrome (AKI, thrombocytopenia, hemolytic anemia)
Enteroinvasive *E. coli* (EIEC)	<u>Source:</u> Food	1. Onset: 5-15 d 2. Duration: 1-5 d 3. Cramping, watery diarrhea	1. Fecal leukocytes (+)	1. Pepto-Bismol, Imodium 2. Hydration

(continued)

(continued)

Disease	Etiology, Prevalence, Risk Factors	Clinical Symptoms and Signs	Diagnostics	Therapy, Prognosis, and Health Maintenance
Cholera	Acute diarrheal disease that can result in profound, rapidly progressive dehydration and death Protein **enterotoxin** produced by organism as it colonizes small intestine Consumption of contaminated, locally harvested **shellfish**	1. Onset: 24-48 h after consumption 2. Watery diarrhea "**rice water stool**" is due to action of cholera toxin <u>Signs:</u> 1. "Fishy odor"		1. Tetracycline, **fluoroquinolones**, or macrolide 2. Oral rehydration

ACUTE AND CHRONIC PANCREATITIS

Disease	Etiology, Prevalence, Risk Factors	Clinical Symptoms and Signs	Diagnostics	Therapy, Prognosis, and Health Maintenance
Acute pancreatitis	Inflammation of pancreas from prematurely activated enzymes → pancreatic autodigestion <u>Causes:</u> **ETOH (40%), gallstones (40%)**, post-ERCP, viral infection, drugs, scorpion stings, pancreatic cancer, **hypertriglyceridemia**, hypercalcemia, uremia Blunt trauma (MCC in children)	<u>Mild (most common):</u> 1. **Abdominal pain, epigastric, radiates to back** (50%), steady, dull, and severe • Worse when supine and after meals 2. Nausea, vomiting, anorexia <u>Signs:</u> 1. Low grade fever, tachycardia, hypotension, leukocytosis 2. Epigastric tenderness, abdominal distention 3. Decreased/absent bowel sounds 4. Hemorrhagic pancreatitis: Gray Turner sign (flank), Cullen sign (periumbilical), Fox sign (inguinal ligament)	1. Serum amylase (MC)–nonspecific, absence does not r/o, 5xULN, normal 48-72 h after 2. **Serum lipase**–more specific (3xULN) 3. LFTs–possible gallstone pancreatitis 4. **Hyperglycemia**, hypoxemia, leukocytosis 5. *Ranson criteria:* glucose, calcium, hematocrit, BUN, ABG, LDH, AST, WBC 6. KUB–r/o perforation 7. Abdominal U/S–identifies cause 8. **CT scan** (confirmatory)–most accurate 9. ERCP–severe with obstruction	1. Mild–**bowel rest (NPO), IVF, replete electrolytes, pain control** (fentanyl, meperidine) 2. Severe–high mortality; ICU admit • Enteral nutrition in first 72 h through NJ tube Recurrence high in ETOH related <u>Complications:</u> • Pancreatic necrosis • Pancreatic pseudocyst
Chronic pancreatitis	Persistent, continued inflammation of pancreas → fibrosis and alteration of ducts = *irreversible* <u>Causes:</u> **Chronic ETOH-ism** <u>Other causes:</u> hereditary, tropical, idiopathic	Severe epigastric pain, recurrent or persistent • **Nausea and vomiting** • Aggravated by drinking or eating • Radiates to back • **Weight loss** due to malabsorption, ETOH, diabetes • **Steatorrhea** due to malabsorption	1. **CT scan** (first)–calcifications, normal does not r/o 2. KUB–pancreatic calcifications (95% specific) 3. **ERCP** (gold standard): "chain of lakes" 4. Serum amylase and lipase not elevated, other labs not helpful 5. Stool elastase–most sensitive and specific for pancreatic insufficiency (steatorrhea secondary to malabsorption): low	1. Pain meds, NPO, pancreatic enzymes and H$_2$ blockers, insulin, ETOH abstinence 2. Frequent, small-volume, low-fat meals 3. Surgery–**pancreaticojejunostomy** or pancreatic resection (Whipple syndrome) <u>Complications</u> • **Narcotic addiction (most common)** • DM–loss of islets of Langerhans <u>Malabsorption:</u> Late manifestation • Pseudocyst • CBD obstruction • B$_{12}$ malabsorption • Effusions • Pancreatic carcinoma

• Pancreatic enzymes—inhibit CCK release, decreasing pancreatic secretions after meals

• H$_2$ blockers—inhibit gastric acid secretion, preventing degradation of enzyme supplements by gastric acid

INFLAMMATORY BOWEL DISEASE: ULCERATIVE COLITIS VERSUS CROHN DISEASE

- Sulfasalazine—metabolized by bacteria to 5-ASA (active metabolite) and sulfapyridine (causes side effects)
- **Tenesmus** (rectal dry heaves)

Disease	Etiology, Prevalence, Risk Factors	Clinical Symptoms and Signs	Diagnostics	Therapy, Prognosis, and Health Maintenance
Ulcerative colitis	Chronic inflammation of the colon or rectal mucosa Any age MC: **Rectum** and left colon Smoking is protective Mucosal and submucosal involvement only	1. Gradual or **abrupt onset** of LLQ **abdominal pain** 2. **Tenesmus** (most common) 3. **Hematochezia** (bloody diarrhea) **and pus-filled diarrhea** 4. Bowel movements frequent, but small 5. **Fever**, anorexia, **weight loss** (severe disease) Extraintestinal SX: Scleritis and episcleritis, **primary sclerosing cholangitis**, erythema nodosum and pyoderma gangrenosum, ankylosing spondylitis	Anemia, increased ESR and low serum albumin ANCA (+) in 60%-70% KUB: colonic dilation 1. Stool cultures for *C. difficile*, OandP 2. Fecal leukocytes–WBC present in UC, ischemic colitis, and infectious diarrhea 3. **Colonoscopy**–assess extent and complications, no skip lesions • Avoid in acute disease owing to risk of perforation or toxic megacolon 4. Sigmoidoscopy–rectal pseudopolyps, diffuse ulcerations and bleeding	1. **Topical or PO sulfasalazine** (mesalamine, 5-ASA)–more effective in UC; good for maintenance therapy 2. 5-ASA enema–proctitis and distal colitis 3. Steroids–acute exacerbations 4. Immunosuppression–prevent relapses, not for acute attacks 5. **Proctocolectomy**– considered curative; indications are severe disease, toxic megacolon, obstruction, severe hemorrhage, fulminant exacerbation, evidence or risk of colon cancer, growth failure (FTT), systemic complications Complications: IDA, hemorrhage, electrolyte imbalance, strictures, colon cancer, sclerosing cholangitis (PSC), cholangiocarcinoma, toxic megacolon (leading cause of death), growth retardation, narcotic abuse, depression
Crohn disease	Chronic inflammatory diseases affecting any part of the GI tract (**mouth-anus**), but MC small bowel (terminal ileum) Unpredictable flares and remissions Chronic granulomatous inflammation, transmural inflammation that can lead to fistulization, submucosal inflammation leading to bowel lumen narrowing MC: **Terminal ileum** and **cecum** (40%) <40 y/o	**Gradual onset:** 1. Diarrhea (nonbloody), abdominal cramps 2. Malabsorption, **weight loss** (common) 3. **Abdominal pain** (RLQ), nausea, vomiting 4. Fever, malaise 5. Extraintestinal manifestations (15%-20%): uveitis, arthritis, erythema nodosum, **aphthous oral ulcers**, cholelithiasis, nephrolithiasis Complications: **Fistula, abscess**, luminal strictures, noncaseating granulomas, **transmural thickening** and inflammation (full-thickness, "wall to wall"), "fat creeping" onto antimesenteric border of small bowel	1. Abdominal CT: inflammation throughout the bowel wall at ileocecal junction, mesenteric fat wrapping (fat creeping) 2. Upper GI with small bowel follow-through: narrowing of terminal ileum or fistulas 3. Endoscopy (sigmoid or **colonoscopy**) with biopsy–aphthous ulcers, **cobblestone appearance**, pseudopolyps, patchy **skip lesions** with discontinuous involvement • Rectal sparing	1. Sulfasalazine (**mesalamine, 5-ASA**) for maintenance 2. **Prednisone**–acute exacerbations 3. Metronidazole–if not responsive to ASA, or perianal disease, fistula or fissure 4. Immunosuppression (azathioprine, 6-mercaptopurine) 5. Bile acid sequestrants (cholestyramine, colestipol) Not antidiarrheals: 1. Surgery–for complications of Crohn disease, **SBO** (MC), fitsulae, disabling disease, perforation, **abscess**; noncurative 2. IV nutrition Health maintenance: 1. Supplement with B$_{12}$, folate, and vitamin D 2. Smoking cessation Prognosis: 1. Effectiveness of treatment decreases with advancing disease; recurrence common after surgery

(continued)

(continued)

Disease	Etiology, Prevalence, Risk Factors	Clinical Symptoms and Signs	Diagnostics	Therapy, Prognosis, and Health Maintenance

Ischemic colitis	Insufficient blood supply to a segment or entire colon, resulting in ischemic necrosis from superficial to full-thickness transmural necrosis
	RF:
	Old age, atherosclerosis
	Most common form of intestinal ischemia
		1. Acute-onset, mild, crampy abdominal pain
		2. Passage of blood mixed with stool within 24 h
		  • Minimal blood loss
		3. Urge to defecate
		4. Possible anorexia, nausea, vomiting
		Signs:
		1. Tenderness over the affected area
			Leukocytosis, metabolic acidosis, elevated lactate:
			1. Abdominal radiograph: generalized bowel distention and air-filled bowel loops
			2. Barium enema: thumbprinting (nonspecific), longitudinal ulcers
			3. CT w/ contrast: segmental circumferential wall thickening
			4. **Colonoscopy** (*definitive*)
			  • Early: petechial hemorrhage with interspersed pale edematous mucosa
			  • **Late: segmental erythema with or without ulcerations** and bleeding
			  • Colon single stripe sign: single longitudinal ulcerated or inflamed colon strip
				1. IV fluids, stabilize hemodynamically, bowel rest, avoid vasoconstrictive drugs
				2. Empiric antibiotics
				3. 20% require surgery owing to peritonitis or deterioration despite supportive therapy: bowel resection with colostomy
				Prognosis:
				1. 20% develop peritonitis

Extraintestinal Manifestations of IBD

	Crohn Disease	Both	Ulcerative Colitis
Eye (5%)	Episcleritis–parallels bowel disease activity	Scleritis Anterior uveitis–independent course	
Skin (10%)	**Erythema nodosum**–parallels bowel disease Oral aphthous ulcers		**Pyoderma gangrenosum**; parallels bowel disease in 50%
Ortho		Arthritis–most common EM of IBD Osteoporosis Migratory monoarticular–parallels bowel disease (coincides with acute exacerbations of colitis) Sacroiliitis–does not parallel disease	**Ankylosing spondylitis** (30% greater than general population)
Heme		Idiopathic thrombocytopenic purpura Vitamin B_{12} deficiency (pernicious anemia) Thromboembolic-hypercoagulable state–can lead to DVT, PE, or CVA	
GI/renal	Gallstones (ileal involvement) Kidney stones		**Primary sclerosing cholangitis** (5%); not parallel to bowel disease, not prevented by colectomy
Respiratory		Bronchiectasis, ILD, BOOP (bronchiolitis obliterans with organizing pneumonia), sarcoidosis, pulmonary infiltrates with eosinophilia (PIE) syndrome, serositis, pulmonary embolism	

APPENDICITIS

Disease	Etiology, Prevalence, Risk Factors	Clinical Symptoms and Signs	Diagnostics	Therapy, Prognosis, and Health Maintenance
Acute appendicitis	1. Lumen **obstructed by hyperplasia of lymphoid tissue** (60%), fecalith (35%), foreign body 2. Obstruction → stasis → bacterial growth and inflammation 3. Distention = ischemia, infarction, necrosis Peak incidence: mid-20s	1. Abdominal pain—begins in epigastrium → umbilicus → RLQ 2. **Anorexia (always present)** 3. Nausea, vomiting (follow pain) 4. **McBurney point:** RLQ tenderness 5. Rebound tenderness, guarding, diminished bowel sounds 6. Low-grade fever 7. **Rovsing sign:** LLQ deep palpation → RLQ referred pain 8. Psoas sign: LQ pain with hip flexed against resistance or hip extension while lying on L-side 9. Obturator sign: LQ pain when hip and knee flexed and hip internal rotated, patient supine	1. **Clinical DX** CBC—neutrophilia (supportive) 2. Imaging if atypical presentation • CT scan: lowers false (+) rates • U/S	1. Appendectomy (lap) 2. IVF, antibiotics, NPO • See Preoperative for antibiotics 3. Pain management

GASTROINTESTINAL BLEED

Disease	Etiology, Prevalence, Risk Factors	Clinical Symptoms and Signs	Diagnostics	Therapy, Prognosis, and Health Maintenance
Upper GI bleed	Bleeding that originates proximal to ligament of Treitz Consider: Peptic ulceration, esophageal varices or gastric bleeding from portal hypertension, gastritis, AVM, tumor, Mallory-Weiss tear RF: Use of NSAIDs, aspirin, anticoagulants, antiplatelets; alcohol abuse; previous GI bleed; liver disease; coagulopathy	1. **Hematemesis:** vomiting of blood or coffee ground emesis 2. **Melena:** black, tarry stools 3. Hematochezia: can be seen with massive upper GI bleeds Signs: 1. Orthostatic hypotension 2. Tachycardia 3. Rectal examination 4. Abdominal tenderness, guarding	1. Obtain type and screen, Hgb, platelet count, coagulation studies, liver enzymes, albumin, BUN/Cr 2. NG lavage to check for intragastric blood (+) lavage is *confirmatory* 3. Endoscopy once stabilized (80% confirmed) • Give erythromycin before examination if likely to have large amount of blood in stomach • Antibiotics prophylactically for known cirrhotics	1. Supportive care: • NPO • IV access • Oxygen • IV Fluids of isotonic crystalloid • Transfuse for: hemodynamic instability despite fluids, Hgb <9 in high-risk patients (elderly, CAD), Hgb <7 in low-risk patients 2. Treat with IV PPI until confirmation of cause of bleeding 3. Consult GI and interventional radiology or surgery 4. Treat underlying cause 5. Surgery—duodenotomy or gastroduodenotomy, ligation of bleeding
Lower GI bleed	Bleeding from site distal to ligament of Treitz Consider: **Diverticulosis (MC)**, angiodysplasia, colitis (infectious, ischemic, inflammatory bowel disease), colon cancer, anorectal disorders, proctitis	1. **Hematochezia** (BRBPR): passage of maroon or bright red blood or clots per rectum 2. Melena: seen with GI bleeding from the right colon (or small intestine) 3. Orthostatic hypotension or shock	1. CBC, serum chemistry, liver tests, coagulation studies 2. Monitor Hgb every 2-8 h, depending on severity 3. Automated BP, O_2, and EKG monitoring 4. Colonoscopy—only once upper GI bleed ruled out 5. CT or mesenteric angiography—require active bleeding to identify source	1. Supportive care • O_2 • IV access • Fluid and blood resuscitation • Management of coagulopathies, antiplatelets and anticoagulants

- Most common cause of rectal bleeding in patients <50 y: hemorrhoids
- High-risk features for upper GI bleed: hemodynamic instability (systolic <100 mm Hg or HR >100 BPM, Hgb <10 g/L, active bleeding during endoscopy, large ulcer size (>1-3 cm), ulcer location (high lesser gastric curvature or posterior duodenal bulb)
- High-risk features for lower GI bleed: hemodynamic instability (hypotension, tachycardia, orthostasis, syncope), persistent bleeding, comorbid illness, advanced age, history of bleeding from the same cause, current aspirin use, prolonged PT, nontender abdomen, anemia, elevated BUN, abnormal WBC count

BOWEL OBSTRUCTION

Disease	Etiology, Prevalence, Risk Factors	Clinical Symptoms and Signs	Diagnostics	Therapy, Prognosis, and Health Maintenance
SBO (small bowel obstruction)	<u>MCC:</u> **Adhesions or hernias,** cancer, IBD, volvulus, intussusception	1. Abdominal pain 2. Distention 3. Vomiting of partially digested food 4. Obstipation <u>Signs:</u> 1. Dehydration + electrolyte imbalance 2. High-pitched bowel sounds, come in rushes → silent bowls	1. KUB: air-fluid levels, multiple dilated bowel loops	1. NPO, nasogastric suction, IV fluids, monitoring Partial obstruction in hemo-stable patient → IV hydration and NG decompression 2. Pain management
LBO (large bowel obstruction)	<u>MCC:</u> **Cancer,** strictures, hernias, volvulus, fecal impaction	1. Distention and pain 2. Complete strangulation of bowel tissue → infarction, necrosis, peritonitis → death <u>Signs:</u> 1. Febrile, tachycardia → shock 2. Dehydration + electrolyte imbalance	1. KUB: air-fluid levels, multiple dilated bowel loops	1. NPO, nasogastric suction, IV fluids, monitoring 2. Pain management Urgent surgery when mechanical obstruction expected

Volvulus	Twisting of any portion of bowel on itself, commonly in **sigmoid or cecum** of bowel
	Sigmoid volvulus: most common form (8% of all obstructions)
	Most common in elderly (>50 y) with a history of chronic constipation
		1. **Cramping** abdominal pain (LLQ) and **distention**
		2. Nausea, vomiting (late), obstipation
		3. Failure to pass flatus or stool
		<u>Signs:</u>
		1. **Abdominal tympany**
		2. Tachycardia
		3. Fever
		4. Severe pain if ischemic
		  • Ischemia → gangrene, peritonitis, sepsis
			1. Abdominal radiograph: **colonic distention**
			  • Inverted U-shaped appearance of distended sigmoid loop
			  • **Loss of haustra**
			  • **Coffee bean sign** at midline crease corresponding to mesenteric root in a greatly distended sigmoid
			  • Sigmoid = bowel loop points to RUQ
			  • Cecal = bowel loop points toward LUQ (dilated cecum comes to rest in LUQ)
			2. Barium Enema
			  • Bird's-beak or bird-of-prey sign
			3. CT Abd/Pelvis
			  • Whirl pattern
				1. Emergent endoscopic decompression to avoid ischemic injury
				  • Laparoscopic **derotation** or laparotomy ± bowel resection
				  • Derotation and decompression by barium enema or with rectal tube, colonoscope, or sigmoidoscope if no signs of ischemia or perforation
				2. Surgical evaluation if fails to resolve quickly

DISEASES OF THE GALLBLADDER AND BILIARY TRACT (FIG. 3-6)

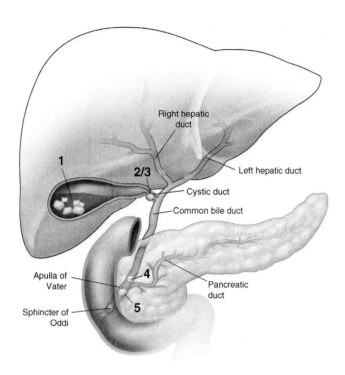

FIGURE 3-6. The biliary tree disorders. (*1*) Cholelithiasis—gallstones located in the gallbladder, but not causing obstruction. (*2*) Biliary colic—occurs after a fatty meal in which the gallbladder contracts and pushes stones into the cystic duct; when the duct relaxes, the stone retreats back into the gallbladder causing visceral pain. (*3*) Cholecystitis—obstruction of the cystic duct resulting in acute inflammation of the gallbladder wall. (*4*) Choledocholithiasis—gallstones located in the common bile duct. (*5*) Ascending cholangitis—gallstones located in the ampulla of Vater.

Disease	Etiology, Prevalence, Risk Factors	Clinical Symptoms and Signs	Diagnostics	Therapy, Prognosis, and Health Maintenance
Cholestasis	Blockage of bile flow (intra- or extrahepatic) with increase in conjugated bilirubin levels	1. Jaundice, gray stool, dark urine 2. Pruritus (bile salt deposition in skin) 3. Skin xanthomas 4. Malabsorption of fats and fat-soluble vitamins	1. **Alkaline phosphatase: high** 2. Serum cholesterol: high (impaired secretion) 3. DX with serum levels of conjugated and unconjugated bilirubin	
Biliary colic		1. RUQ or epigastric pain • May not have an obvious relationship to food intake	Cholestatic labs: total and direct bilirubin levels, alkaline-phosphatase elevated	

(continued)

(continued)

Disease	Etiology, Prevalence, Risk Factors	Clinical Symptoms and Signs	Diagnostics	Therapy, Prognosis, and Health Maintenance
Cholelithiasis (Fig. 3-6, _1_)	Stones in the _gallbladder_, pain secondary to contraction of gall against obstructed cystic duct 3 types: • Cholesterol (yellow to green): obesity, DM, HLD, multiple gestation, OCP use, Crohn disease, ileal resection, old age, Native American, cirrhosis, CF • Pigment stones (black): **hemolysis** (SS, thalassemia, spherocytosis, artificial heart valve), **alcoholic cirrhosis** • Pigment stones (brown): found in bile ducts; due to biliary tract infection • Mixed stones—cholesterol + pigment	Asymptomatic (most) SX only last few hours 1. Biliary colic—RUQ pain or epigastric 2. Pain after eating and at night 3. **_Boas sign_**—referred right subscapular pain	1. **RUQ ultrasound**—high sensitivity and specificity if >2 mm 2. CT scan and MRI	Asymptomatic—**No treatment necessary** 1. Elective cholecystectomy for recurrent bouts Complications: Cholecystitis Choledocholithiasis Gallstone ileus Malignancy
Acute cholecystitis (Fig. 3-6, _2_)	Obstruction of cystic duct (_not infection_) induces acute inflammation of gallbladder wall	1. **Pain** lasts days, **RUQ** or epigastrium, may radiate to R shoulder or scapula 2. **Nausea, vomiting,** anorexia 3. Pruritus, clay-colored stools, dark urine Signs: 1. RUQ tenderness, rebound in RUQ 2. **Murphy sign**—inspiratory arrest during deep palpation 3. Hypoactive bowel sounds 4. Low-grade **fever, leukocytosis** 5. Jaundice	1. **RUQ ultrasound** (first line)—thickened gallbladder wall, bile sludge, pericholecystic fluid, distended gall, stones (Fig. 3-7) 2. Radionuclide scan (**HIDA**)—when u/s inconclusive; if normal, r/o acalculous cholecystitis (+) HIDA means gall not visualized, if not visualized in 4 h, A.C. diagnosed 3. CT scan—alternative, more sensitive for perforation, abscess, pancreatitis Labs: 1. Elevated ALK-P and GGT 2. Elevated _conjugated_ bilirubin	1. Admit patient 2. **IV fluids, bowel rest (NPO), IV antibiotics, analgesics,** correct electrolytes 3. **Cholecystectomy** (first 24-48 h), timing depends on severity Prognosis: 1. 70% recurrence if left untreated
Acalculous cholecystitis	Acute cholecystitis without stones obstructing the cystic duct Common in critically ill (ICU patients) with TPN, chronically debilitated, trauma or burn patients Associated: Dehydration, ischemia, burns, severe trauma, post-op state	Same as acute cholecystitis, except _without_ stones 1. RUQ pain 2. Fever 3. Nausea, vomiting Signs: (+) Murphy sign	Diagnosis difficult owing to comorbid conditions: 1. Ultrasound: bile sludge	1. **Emergent cholecystectomy** 2. Percutaneous drainage of gall with cholecystectomy (if too ill) 3. Antibiotics

Disease	Etiology, Prevalence, Risk Factors	Clinical Symptoms and Signs	Diagnostics	Therapy, Prognosis, and Health Maintenance
Choledocholithiasis (Fig. 3-6, 4)	Stones in common bile duct (CBD) <u>Primary</u>: Originate in CBD <u>Secondary</u>: Originate in gall, pass into CBD	<u>Asymptomatic for years</u>: 1. RUQ or epigastric pain • May not have an obvious relationship to food intake 2. Jaundice	1. RUQ U/S (first line): not sensitive (ranges from 20%-90%) • Dilated common bile duct 2. **ERCP** (gold standard): diagnostic and therapeutic 3. PTC–alternative <u>Labs</u>: 1. Total and direct bilirubin levels, ALK-P elevated	1. **ERCP with sphincterotomy** and **stone extraction with stent placement** 2. Lap-choledocholithotomy <u>Complications</u>: **Cholangitis** Obstructive jaundice **Acute pancreatitis** Biliary colic Biliary cirrhosis
Cholangitis	Infection of biliary tract secondary to obstruction, leading to biliary stasis and bacterial overgrowth Choledocholithiasis (60% of cases)	***Charcot Triad*** (50%-70%): 1. RUQ pain 2. Jaundice 3. Fever ***Reynold Pentad:*** 1. RUQ pain, jaundice, fever 2. Plus 3. Septic shock: *hypotension* 4. AMS–coma, disorientation	1. RUQ U/S (first) 2. CBC, bilirubin (high): leukocytosis, mildly elevated AST/ALT 3. PTC or **ERCP** (definitive), but not for use in acute cases	1. Blood cultures, IV fluids, IV antibiotics, decompress CBD when stable 2. Closely monitor BP, hemodynamics, and UOP 3. Must be afebrile 48 h for ERCP/PTC 4. **Decompression via PTC (cath) or ERCP (sphincterotomy)** or T-tube insertion (laparotomy) 5. Potential life threatening, emergent treatment <u>Complications</u>: **Hepatic abscess** (life threatening)
Ascending cholangitis (Fig. 3-6, 5)	Due to gallstone in ampulla of Vader, leading to infection of biliary tract			
Primary sclerosing cholangitis (PSC)	Chronic idiopathic, progressive disease of intrahepatic and/or extrahepatic bile ducts characterized by thickening of duct walls and narrowing of lumens → cirrhosis, portal HTN, and liver failure In essence, this is progressive inflammation, fibrosis, and stricturing of the biliary tree likely triggered by an immunologically mediated bile duct injury Strong association with **ulcerative colitis** (50%-70%)	1. Insidious onset 2. Chronic cholestasis–***progressive jaundice, itching*** 3. Other: fatigue, malaise, weight loss	1. **ERCP** and PTC–diagnostic of bead-like stricturing and dilatation of intrahepatic and extrahepatic ducts 2. LFTs–cholestasis	1. **Liver transplant** 2. Cholestyramine–symptomatic relief of itching

(continued)

(continued)

Disease	Etiology, Prevalence, Risk Factors	Clinical Symptoms and Signs	Diagnostics	Therapy, Prognosis, and Health Maintenance

Primary biliary cirrhosis	Chronic, progressive cholestatic disease with destruction of intrahepatic bile ducts with portal inflammation and scarring
	Autoimmune, middle aged-women (40-60s)
	Immune-mediated bile duct injury leading to chronic cholestasis and secondary inflammation and scarring
		1. Asymptomatic (no pain)–50%-60%
		2. Symptomatic
		  • **Fatigue**
		  • **Itching**
		  • Signs and symptoms of jaundice
		Signs:
		1. Skin findings: hyperpigmentation, excoriations, xanthelasmas, jaundice
		2. Jaundice
		3. Hepatosplenomegaly
		4. Spider nevi, temporal and proximal limb muscle wasting
		5. Ascites, edema
		6. Kayser-Fleischer rings
			1. LFTs–**Elevated alkaline-phosphatase**
			2. (+) **AMA** (antimitochondrial antibodies, 90%-95%) → liver biopsy
			3. High cholesterol, LDL, IgM
			4. **Liver biopsy** (*confirms* DX)
			5. Abdominal U/S or CT to r/o obstruction
				1. Symptomatic:
				  • **Cholestyramine** (itching)
				  • **Calcium, bisphosphonates, vitamin D** (osteoporosis)
				2. Ursodeoxycholic acid–slows progression
				3. Liver transplant (curative)

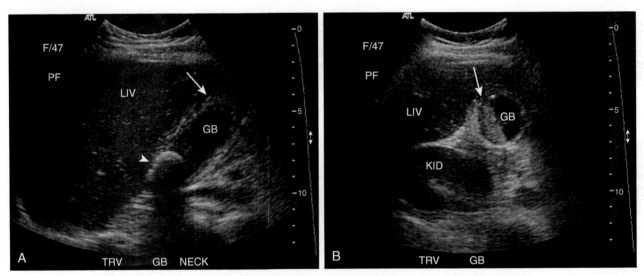

FIGURE 3-7. Acute cholecystitis. **A,** Dilated gallbladder with a large shadowing stone and thickened wall. Arrowhead refers to the large shadowing stone, the arrow refers to a dilated gallbladder with a thickened gallbladder wall. **B,** Hyperechoic sludge. Sonographic Murphy sign, wall thickening >3 mm, dilated gallbladder, affected stone, and pericholecystic fluid are all hallmarks of acute cholecystitis. Arrow refers to hyperechoic sludge. (From Vachha BA, Tsai LL, Lee KS, Camacho MA. Diagnostic imaging in acute care surgery. In: Britt LD, Peitzman AB, Barie PS, Jurkovich GJ, eds. *Acute Care Surgery.* Philadelphia: Wolters Kluwer Health; 2012, with permission.)

JAUNDICE

- Conjugated (direct) bilirubin is water soluble and excreted in the urine

Disease	Etiology, Prevalence, Risk Factors	Clinical Symptoms and Signs	Diagnostics	Therapy, Prognosis, and Health Maintenance
Jaundice (Fig. 3-8)	Refers to the yellowish discoloration of the skin, sclera, and mucous membranes resulting from the deposition of bilirubin in tissues; this indicates that the serum bilirubin is likely **3 mg/dL or higher** If the examiner suspects scleral icterus, a second site to examine is underneath the tongue	1. Yellow discoloration of skin or eyes 2. Weight loss 3. Fever, chills 4. Abdominal pain 5. Flu-like symptoms 6. Itching Associated signs: 1. Scleral icterus 2. Pallor 3. Abdominal mass 4. Palpable gall 5. Oliguria 6. Pruritus 7. Spider angioma 8. Muscle wasting 9. Ecchymosis or petechiae 10. Parotid enlargement 11. Palmar erythema 12. Gynecomastia 13. Dupuytren contracture 14. HSM 15. ± **Ascites** 16. Testicular atrophy 17. Bruising	1. Urinary bilirubin–indicates that conjugated hyperbilirubinemia present • Confirm with serum total and direct bilirubin 2. CBC, LFTs, GGT, alkaline-phosphatase, hepatitis panel 3. **Abdominal ultrasound** (preferred) or CT abdomen 4. Liver biopsy (definitive)	1. Treat underlying cause Prognosis: 1. If post-op, should clear by 3 wk

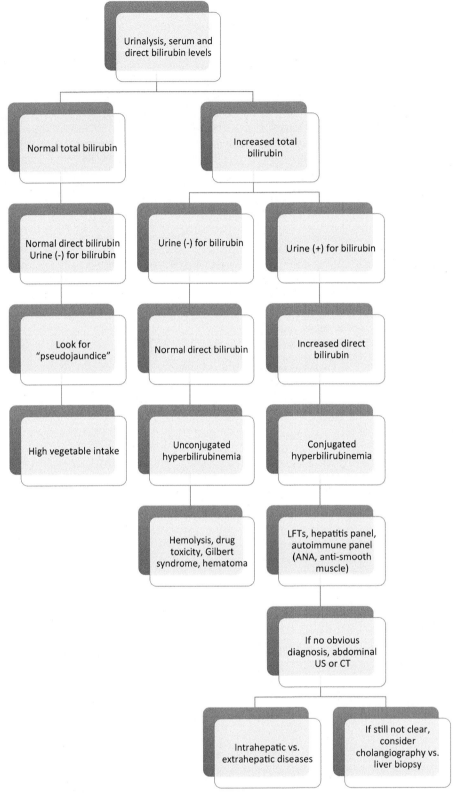

FIGURE 3-8. Systematic approach to the adult patient with jaundice.

Differential Diagnosis of Prehepatic Jaundice

Comes from breakdown of RBCs and ineffective erythropoiesis

Unconjugated (Indirect) Bilirubin	Conjugated (Direct) Bilirubin
1. Hemolysis • Hereditary spherocytosis • Glucose-6-phosphate dehydrogenase Deficiency: 1. Hematoma	1. Alcohol 2. Infectious hepatitis 3. Drug reaction 4. Autoimmune disorders

Differential Diagnosis of Intrahepatic Jaundice

Unconjugated (Indirect) Bilirubin	Conjugated (Direct) Bilirubin
1. Gilbert syndrome	1. Hepatocellular disease—hepatitis, chronic alcohol use, autoimmune disorders 2. Drugs: OCPs, Tylenol, Thorazine, estrogenic or anabolic steroids 3. Pregnancy 4. Parenteral nutrition 5. Sarcoidosis 6. Primary biliary cirrhosis 7. Primary sclerosing cholangitis

Differential Diagnosis of Posthepatic Jaundice

Conjugated (Direct) Bilirubin
1. Cholelithiasis (MC)   2. Cholecystitis or cholangitis   3. Pancreatitis   4. Malignancy

Differential Diagnosis of Extrahepatic Jaundice

Conjugated (Direct) Bilirubin
Intrinsic to ductal system: 1. Gallstones   2. Surgical strictures   3. Infection (CMV, *Cryptosporidium*)   4. Cholangiocarcinoma   5. Intrahepatic malignancy   Extrinsic to ductal system: 1. Extrahepatic malignancy (pancreas, lymphoma)   2. Pancreatitis

CIRRHOSIS (FIG. 3-9)

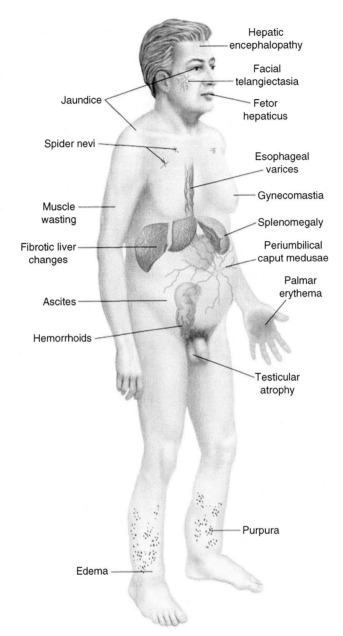

FIGURE 3-9. Common findings in a cirrhosis patient. (From Norris T. *Porth's Pathophysiology: Concepts of Altered Health States*. 11th ed. Philadelphia: Wolters Kluwer Health; 2019.)

- Chronic liver disease characterized by fibrosis, disruption of the liver architecture, and widespread nodules in the liver
- Irreversible when advanced
- Distortion of liver anatomy causes
  - Portal HTN: decreased blood flow through the liver → hypertension in portal circulation; causes ascites, peripheral edema, splenomegaly, varicosity of veins
  - Hepatocellular failure → decreases albumin synthesis and clotting factor synthesis
- Child-Pugh scores: estimates hepatic reserve in liver failure; measures disease severity
  - A = mild, C = most severe

- Most common cause is alcoholic liver disease
- Second most common cause: chronic hepatitis B and C infections
- Chronic liver disease
  - Ascites, varices, hemorrhoids
  - Gynecomastia, testicular atrophy
  - Palmar erythema, spider angiomas
  - Caput medusae
- Monitoring: periodic lab values **q 3 to 4 months** (CBC, renal function, electrolytes, LFT, coagulation panel), perform endoscopy for varices, CT-guided biopsy for HCC

Disease	Etiology, Prevalence, Risk Factors	Clinical Symptoms and Signs	Diagnostics	Therapy, Prognosis, and Health Maintenance
Esophageal variceal rupture	Dilated submucosal veins Occurs in 50% of patients with cirrhosis	1. Preceding retching or dyspepsia Signs: 1. Hypovolemia: hypotension, tachycardia	1. Upper endoscopy– once hemodynamically stable	1. Spontaneously stops in 50% 2. See treatment table Complications: Upper GI bleed (30%) Poor prognosis RF: Size of varices, presence at endoscopy of red wale markings (longitudinal dilated venules on varix surface), severe liver disease (Child Pugh score), active alcohol abuse
Portal HTN		Ascites Peripheral edema Splenomegaly Varicosities	Paracentesis	Treat complications Transjugular intrahepatic portosystemic shunt (**TIPS**) to lower portal pressure
Ascites: accumulation of fluid in peritoneal cavity due to portal HTN (increased hydrostatic pressure) and hypoalbuminemia (reduced oncotic pressure)	Most common complication of **cirrhosis**	Abdominal distention, shifting fluid dullness, fluid wave	Abdominal ultrasound **Diagnostic paracentesis** for new-onset, worsening, or suspected SBP Examine: • Cell count, ascites albumin, gram stain, culture to r/o SBP • MC site: **posterior anal midline, *below* or *distal* to the dentate line** • Measure serum ascites albumin gradient • If >1.1 = portal HTN • If <1.1 = portal HTN unlikely	**Salt restriction** and diuretics (furosemide, spironolactone) Bed rest Paracentesis if tense ascites, SOB, or early satiety
Hepatic encephalopathy	Cause: **ammonia** accumulates and reaches the brain Precipitants: alkalosis, hypokalemia (*diuretics*), *sedating drugs* (narcotics, sleep meds), GI bleed, systemic infection, *hypovolemia*	Decreased mental function, confusion, poor concentration, stupor, or coma **Asterixis** (flapping tremor)–have patient extend and dorsiflex hands Rigidity, hyperreflexia *Fetor hepaticus*: musty breath odor		**Lactulose**–prevents absorption of ammonia Neomycin (antibiotic): kills bowel flora Diet: **limit protein** to 30-40 g/d
Hepatorenal syndrome: Progressive renal failure in ESLD, secondary to renal hypoperfusion from vasoconstriction	Precipitated by: **infection, diuretics**	Azotemia–elevated BUN Oliguria–low urine output Hypotension	Low urine sodium (<10 mEq/L) Hyponatremia	Liver transplant (only cure) Poor prognosis "Functional renal failure"
Spontaneous bacterial peritonitis (SBP): infected ascitic fluid (20%)	Cause: **E. coli (MC)**, *Klebsiella*, *S. pneumoniae* Patients with ascites with abdominal pain, fever, vomiting, rebound tenderness → Sepsis		Paracentesis: **WBC >500, PMN >250** (+) ascites culture	Broad spectrum ABX Clinical improvement in 24-48 h → repeat paracentesis in 2-3 d High recurrence rate in first year (70%)

(continued)

(continued)

Disease	Etiology, Prevalence, Risk Factors	Clinical Symptoms and Signs	Diagnostics	Therapy, Prognosis, and Health Maintenance
Hyperestrinism	Spider angiomas—dilated cutaneous arterioles with central red spot and reddish extension that radiate outward like a spider's web Palmar erythema Gynecomastia and testicular atrophy			
Coagulopathy: secondary to synthesis of clotting factors			**Prolonged PT** PTT prolonged in severe disease Vitamin K ineffective (cannot be used by diseased liver)	Fresh frozen plasma
Hepatocellular carcinoma (HCC)	10%-25% of patients with cirrhosis			

Treatment of Esophageal Varices

A. First-line measures	1. Rapid infusion of fluids/blood products
	2. FFP or platelets
	  • Many patients have underlying coagulopathy, especially if INR >1.8-2.0 or PL count <50k
	3. Prophylactic IV ABX
	  • Target gram negatives
	  • Norfloxacin, ceftriaxone
	4. Somatostatin, Octreotide

B. Second-line measures	1. Sclerotherapy ≪ **band ligation** • Band ligation not recommended for small varices, but is preferred for medium/large varices at high risk for bleeding over β-blockers 2. IV vitamin K, for abnormal PT 3. Lactulose for encephalopathy

C. Third-line measures	1. Balloon tube tamponade
	  • Initially controls active bleeds in 60%-90%
	  • Complications: esophageal/oral ulcers, perforation, aspiration, airway obstruction
	  • Only in patients with bleeding that cannot be controlled pharmacologically or endoscopically, until decompression is available
	2. TIPS: expandable wire mesh stent passed over catheter into jugular vein through liver parenchyma creating a portosystemic shunt from portal vein to hepatic vein
	  • Controls acute hemorrhage in 90% of active bleeds
	  • Only for patients that cannot be controlled with pharmacologic or endoscopic therapy
	3. Emergency portosystemic shunt surgery

D. Prophylaxis	1. **Combination BB** (nadolol, propranolol) plus **variceal band ligation**
	2. TIPS ≫ endoscopic sclerotherapy or band ligation
	  • Higher incidence of encephalopathy, stenosis, and thrombosis of stents
	  • Reserved for patients with 2+ episodes of variceal bleeding who have failed endoscopic or pharmacologic therapies, recurrent bleeding from gastric varices or portal hypertensive gastropathy, and noncompliance with other therapies
	3. Portosystemic shunts
	  • Higher incidence of encephalopathy
	4. Liver transplant

E. Rescreening	1. For patients without varices on screening endoscopy, repeat endoscopy in 3 y 2. Higher risk of bleeding if: varices >5 mm, varices with red wale markings, or Child-Turcotte-Pugh class B or C cirrhosis

INFECTIOUS DIARRHEA, GIARDIASIS, AND OTHER PARASITIC INFECTIONS

Disease	Etiology, Prevalence, Risk Factors	Clinical Symptoms and Signs	Diagnostics	Therapy, Prognosis, and Health Maintenance
Cryptosporidiosis	Origin: *Cryptosporidium* spp. (spore-forming protozoa) Transmission: Fecal-oral	1. Watery diarrhea	1. Stool sample: oocytes	1. **Supportive**
Amebiasis	Origin: *Entamoeba histolytica* (protozoa) Transmission: Fecal-oral, contaminated water/food, anal-oral	1. Bloody diarrhea 2. Tenesmus 3. Abdominal pain Associated: ±**liver abscess**	1. Stool sample—trophozoites	1. **Iodoquinol** or paromomycin 2. Flagyl for liver abscess
Giardiasis	Origin: *Giardia lamblia* (protozoa) Transmission: Fecal-oral, food/water, person-to-person (anal-oral sex) Incubation: **1-3 wk** "Foul smelling diarrhea"	1. Acute profuse **fatty** (nonbloody) **diarrhea** • Chronic diarrhea with cramps • Nausea • Malaise • Anorexia • **Flatulence** • Bloating 2. HX: daycare, **recent camping trip,** watery diarrhea, chronic infection causing weight loss	1. Stool sample—cysts or trophozoites	1. Supportive Care 2. Antibiotics • **Tinidazole (first line)** • For patients >3 y/o • Nitazoxanide • For patients 12 m-3 y • Flagyl (Metronidazole) 250-750 mg PO TID • for <12 mo Health Maintenance: 1. Symptoms resolve in 5-7 d, no need to repeat stool exam 2. Remove from at-risk settings until asymptomatic x 48 h
Roundworms: ascariasis	Origin: *Ascaris lumbricoides* (nematodes) Transmission: Ingestion of human feces (water/food)	1. Asymptomatic 2. Symptomatic • Postprandial abdominal pain • Vomiting Associated: Bowel, pancreatic duct, or common bile duct obstruction—if heavy worm burden	1. Stool sample—eggs or adult worms	1. Albendazole, **mebendazole**, pyrantel pamoate
Hookworm	Origin: *Ancylostoma duodenale* or *Necator americanus* Transmission: Larvae invade skin, travel to lung, cough, and swallow, reside in the intestine	1. Asymptomatic 2. Symptomatic • Cough Signs: 1. Malabsorption—weight loss Associated: Eosinophilia, anemia	1. Stool sample—see adult worms	1. **Mebendazole** or pyrantel pamoate
Pinworm	Origin: **Enterobius vermicularis** Transmission: Fecal-oral (anus-hand-mouth), children	1. Perianal pruritus, worse at night	1. "Tape test" on anus—eggs on tape	1. **Mebendazole** or pyrantel pamoate
Tapeworm	Origin: *Taenia saginata* (beef), *T. solium* (pork), *Diphyllobothrium latum* (fish) Transmission: raw or undercooked meat	1. Asymptomatic 2. Symptomatic • Nausea • Abdominal pain • Weight loss Associated: B_{12} deficiency (if due to fish)	1. Tape test for *D. latum* (fish) 2. Stool sample: eggs	1. Praziquantel; vitamin B_{12} if deficient
Schistosomiasis	Origin: *Schistosoma mansoni, S. haematobium, S. japonicum* Transmission: Penetration of skin (contaminated freshwater) → lungs → portal vein → venules of mesenteric, bladder, ureters	1. Dermatitis • Localized erythema • Pruritic maculopapular rash 2. Within 2-8 wk: • acute fever, myalgias, malaise • abdominal pain • Hepatosplenomegaly • HA, cough, +/- bloody diarrhea, lymphadenopathy	1. Eggs in urine or feces	1. Praziquantel

ESOPHAGEAL HIATAL HERNIA AND MALLORY-WEISS TEAR

- During forceful vomiting, the marked increase in intra-abdominal pressure is transmitted to the esophagus, potentially leading to one of two conditions

- If the tear is mucosal and at the gastroesophageal junction → Mallory-Weiss syndrome
- If the tear is transmural (causing perforation) → Boerhaave syndrome

Disease	Etiology, Prevalence, Risk Factors	Clinical Symptoms and Signs	Diagnostics	Therapy, Prognosis, and Health Maintenance
Sliding (type 1) hernia	**>90%** GE junction and stomach herniate into thorax through esophageal hiatus <u>Associated:</u> GERD	1. Asymptomatic 2. Heartburn 3. Chest pain 4. Dysphagia	1. Barium upper GI series 2. Upper endoscopy	1. Antacids, small meals, elevation of head after meals • 15% require surgery <u>Complications:</u> **GERD**, reflux esophagitis (risk of Barrett esophagus/cancer), aspiration
Paraesophageal (type 2) hernia	<5% Stomach herniates into thorax through esophageal hiatus, but GE junction does not	• Can become **strangulated** • Enlarge with time • Does not cause GERD		1. Elective surgery <u>Complications:</u> Obstruction, hemorrhage, incarceration, strangulation (life threatening)
Mallory-Weiss syndrome	Mucosal tear at (or just below) the GE junction as a result of forceful vomiting or retching Example—binge drinking alcoholics	1. Occurs after repeated episodes of vomiting 2. **Hematemesis** (always) • Painful	1. **Upper endoscopy** (diagnosis)	1. Surgery or angiographic embolization <u>Prognosis:</u> 1. Most **resolve spontaneously** (90%)
Boerhaave syndrome	Transmural ruptured esophagus due to vomiting	1. Retrosternal chest pain 2. Odynophagia 3. Fever, hypotension, tachypnea 4. Hamman's sign: mediastinal crackling	1. **Gastrografin swallow**—water-soluble contrast preferred over barium when perforated suspected	1. Surgery for thoracic perforations 2. Antibiotics for cervical perforation

GASTROESOPHAGEAL REFLUX DISEASE

Disease	Etiology, Prevalence, Risk Factors	Clinical Symptoms and Signs	Diagnostics	Therapy, Prognosis, and Health Maintenance
Gastroesophageal reflux disease (GERD)	• Inappropriate relaxation of LES (decreased tone) • Retrograde flow of stomach contents into esophagus • Decreased esophageal motility • Gastric outlet obstruction • **Hiatal hernia** (common) <u>Dietary RF:</u> ETOH, tobacco, chocolate, high-fat foods, coffee Prevalence increases with age <u>Complications:</u> • **Barrett esophagus** (*squamous epithelium replaced with columnar*) → adenocarcinoma, get EGD • Dental erosion, gingivitis • Laryngitis, pharyngitis • Recurrent pneumonia • Peptic stricture: dysphagia, dilation with EGD • Erosive esophagitis—long-term PPI therapy	• **Heartburn, dyspepsia**—retrosternal pain, burning shortly after eating, worse with lying down after meals, *mimics cardiac chest pain* • Regurgitation • Waterbrash (reflex salivary hypersecretion) • Cough—due to aspiration of refluxed material • Hoarseness, sore throat, feeling a lump in the throat • Early satiety, postprandial nausea, vomiting	1. Upper GI series (**barium contrast study**)—identifies complications, but does not DX; good for chronic GERD 2. **Endoscopy (EGD)** with biopsy: if refractory to TX, dysphagia, odynophagia, GI bleed 3. **24-h pH monitor** (gold standard) 4. Manometry (if motility d/o suspected)	1. **Diet changes**—avoid fatty food, orange juice, coffee, ETOH, chocolate, large meals before bed; sleep with trunk of body elevated • Stop smoking • Antacids—after meals and at bedtime 2. Phase II: add H_2 blocker 3. Phase III: switch to PPI 4. Phase IV: Add promotility (metoclopramide or Reglan, bethanechol) 5. Phase V: H_2 + promotility + PPI 6. Phase VI: antireflux surgery for intractable cases, aspiration, other complications

IRRITABLE BOWEL SYNDROME

Disease	Etiology, Prevalence, Risk Factors	Clinical Symptoms and Signs	Diagnostics	Therapy, Prognosis, and Health Maintenance

Irritable bowel syndrome	• Change in consistency and frequency of stool **without** abnormal findings on colonoscopy
	• Abnormal resting activity of GI tract
	• **Sigmoid colon** most common location
	• Exacerbations with **stress** or menses
	• Women > men, begins during early to mid adulthood
	• Psychiatric symptoms precede bowel symptoms, worse with stress and irritants in intestinal lumen
		1. SX present at **LEAST 3 mo**
		2. Change in **frequency or consistency of stool**: diarrhea, constipation (or alternating)
		3. **Cramping abdominal pain**
		  • Relieved by defecation
		  • Worse with food intake
		4. **Dyspepsia** (common)
		5. Bloating or feeling of abdominal distention
		  • Associated with accumulation of gas, associated spasm of smooth muscle
		  • Postprandial urgency common
		6. Urinary frequency and urgency (common in women)
		Signs:
		1. Tender, palpable sigmoid colon
		2. Hyperresonance on percussion of abdomen
			All labs normal, no mucosal lesions: CBC, renal panel, FOBT, O&P, sed rate, ± flex sig
			1. Clinical DX–**diagnosis of exclusion**
			2. **Colonoscopy**, barium enema, ultrasound, or CT
			3. Endoscopy in patients with persistent symptoms, weight loss/anorexia, bleeding or history of other GI
				1. Diarrhea–diphenoxylate or **loperamide** (Imodium)
				2. Constipation–**Colace, psyllium**, cisapride
				3. Tegaserod maleate (Zelnorm) is a serotonin agonist introduced for the treatment of IBS
				4. Rifaximin (Xifaxan)–antibiotic approved for IBS-D
				Health maintenance:
				1. Avoid dairy products and excessive caffeine
				Comorbid:
				Depression, anxiety, somatization

ESOPHAGITIS AND ESOPHAGEAL STRICTURES

Disease	Etiology, Prevalence, Risk Factors	Clinical Symptoms and Signs	Diagnostics	Therapy, Prognosis, and Health Maintenance
Infectious	• Immunosuppressed patients with AIDS, solid organ transplants, leukemia, and lymphoma • MC pathogens: **Candida albicans**, herpes simplex, CMV	1. Odynophagia, dysphagia, substernal chest pain 2. **Oral thrush** (75%) 3. CMV infection at other sites (colon, retina) 4. Oral ulcers (herpes labialis)	1. Endoscopy with biopsy and brushings	Empiric: 1. *Candida*: fluconazole 14-21 d 2. CMV: Ganciclovir 3-6 wk 3. AIDS–HAART 4. Herpetic: symptomatic TX unless immunocompromised, then acyclovir × 2-3 wk
Pill induced	Most common: alendronate, clindamycin, doxycycline, iron, **NSAIDs**, KCl tablets, quinidine, tetracycline, bactrim, vitamin C, zidovudine	1. **Odynophagia** 2. **Dysphagia** 3. Severe retrosternal chest pain	1. Endoscopy: one or several discrete; shallow or deep ulcers	Prevention: 1. Take with 4 ounce water and remain upright for 30 mins after
Eosinophilic	HX: food allergies, asthma, atopic dermatitis	1. Dysphagia 2. Impaction (food being stuck at lower end of esophagus)	1. Upper endoscopy 2. Biopsy: eosinophil inflammation, stacked circular rings, strictures, linear furrows	1. Topical steroids (budesonide)
Radiation	Radiosensitizing drugs: Doxorubicin, bleomycin, cyclophosphamide, cisplatin	1. Dysphagia 2. Odynophagia lasting weeks-months after therapy		1. Radiation exposure of 5000 cGy associated with increased risk for stricture→ 2. Supportive therapy 3. Dilation
Corrosive	Ingestion of alkali or acid from attempted suicide			1. Steroids

(continued)

Disease	Etiology, Prevalence, Risk Factors	Clinical Symptoms and Signs	Diagnostics	Therapy, Prognosis, and Health Maintenance
Esophageal stricture	1. Narrowing of esophageal lumen through inflammation, fibrosis, neoplasia 2. Direct invasion or lymph node enlargement 3. Disruption of peristalsis or lower esophageal sphincter function Causes: Mostly sequelae of long-term **gastroesophageal reflux induced esophagitis** (70%-80%) Originate at *squamocolumnar junction* MC: Old white men	1. **Heartburn**–absence does not rule out 2. **Dysphagia**–progressive with *solid foods* (first, most common) → *liquids* 3. **Odynophagia** 4. Food impaction 5. Weight loss 6. Chest pain Atypical: 1. Chronic cough 2. Asthma secondary to aspiration	1. Barium swallow–location, length, and diameter, irregularity 2. Manometry–measures LES pressure, increased 3. CT scan–used for staging 4. **EGD**–use to confirm, r/o malignancy, biopsy, and cytology, more sensitive than barium • Edema, cellular infiltration, basal cell hyperplasia, increased type III collagen deposition 5. CXR	1. Mechanical dilation 2. Lifestyle modifications, weight loss, small meals, correct poor dentition, avoid NSAIDs/ASA 3. PPI > H$_2$ blockers 30% require repeat dilation in 1 y Poor prognostic factors: Lack of heart burn and significant weight loss Complications: 8. Bleeding, bacteremia
Zenker diverticulum	Older patients Outpouching of the posterior pharyngeal wall immediately above the upper esophageal sphincter in an area of weakness between the 2 parts of the inferior posterior constrictor Stores undigested food and pushes on lumen of esophagus	1. **Dysphagia** with solids (98%) 2. **Halitosis** (fetor ex ore) 3. **Regurgitation of undigested food** hours after eating • Globus sensation • Coughing after eating 4. Unexplained weight loss 5. Borborygmi in the neck	1. Barium swallow–outpouching just above the cricopharyngeus muscle 2. Manometry–indicated if contrast study suggests achalasia or motility disorder	1. Requires treatment only if symptomatic–cricopharyngeus myotomy 2. No intervention if small (<2 cm) • Botulinum toxin for temporary relief Complications: Aspiration and pneumonia

CONSTIPATION

- **Obstipation:** severe or complete constipation

Disease	Etiology, Prevalence, Risk Factors	Clinical Symptoms and Signs	Diagnostics	Therapy, Prognosis, and Health Maintenance
Bowel obstruction	Paralytic ileus or mechanical obstruction		1. XR: air-fluid levels with dilated loops of bowel	
Mechanical **(intestinal) obstruction**	Postoperative adhesions or internal (mesenteric) ischemia	1. Short period of normal intestinal function before obstructive symptoms 2. Cramping 3. **Abdominal distension** Signs: 1. **High-pitched hyperactive bowel sounds** 2. Visible peristalsis 3. Minimal tenderness	1. XR: air fluid levels in loops of small bowel	1. **NG suction** for several days 2. Invasive hemodynamic monitoring if cardiac, pulmonary, or renal disease 3. If no resolution in 24-48 h or peritoneal signs, laparotomy • Antibiotics for surgery
Small bowel intussusception	10% in pediatric cases Occurs during first 2 wk postop Most ileoileal or jejunoileal	Atypical symptom complex 1. Vomiting 2. Abdominal distention 3. Abdominal pain	1. Abdominal **ultrasound:** target/bull's eye/coiled spring sign 2. CT scan: target lesion representing layers of intussuscepted segment	1. **Barium/air enema:** diagnostic + therapeutic 2. NPO, IVF, NG, ABX 3. Manual reduction or resection with primary anastomosis
Ileus	Ileus that persists for more than 3 d following surgery is termed postoperative adynamic ileus or paralytic ileus Hypomotility of the gastrointestinal tract in the absence of mechanical bowel obstruction	Signs: 1. Absent bowel sounds	1. **CT scan with gastrografin**–must exclude mechanical obstruction	1. Physiologic ileus spontaneously resolves within 2-3 d, after sigmoid motility returns to normal 2. D/C opiates

Disease	Etiology, Prevalence, Risk Factors	Clinical Symptoms and Signs	Diagnostics	Therapy, Prognosis, and Health Maintenance
Gastroparesis	<u>MCC:</u> **Diabetes** <u>Other causes:</u> Anorexia, bulimia, scleroderma, Ehlers-Danlos, abdominal surgery Female	1. Chronic nausea 2. *Vomiting* 3. Abdominal pain 4. Feeling of fullness after eating small amounts <u>Others:</u> Palpitations, heartburn, bloating, decreased appetite, GERD	1. KUB, manometry, gastric emptying scan	1. Low-fiber and low-residue diets, restrict fat intake, smaller meals spaced 2-3 h apart 2. **Metoclopramide** (Reglan)–D_2 receptor antagonist increases contractility and resting tone in GI tract

DIARRHEA

Disease	Etiology, Prevalence, Risk Factors	Clinical Symptoms and Signs	Diagnostics	Therapy, Prognosis, and Health Maintenance
Pseudomembranous colitis	*C. difficile* Occurs secondary to **treatment with antibiotics** Mostly elderly hospitalized patients Relies on secretion of toxins A (enterotoxin) and B (cytotoxin) Occurs after use of broad spectrum penicillins, cephalosporins, and FQ Disruption of normal colonic flora	1. Mild **watery foul-smelling diarrhea** (>3 but <20 stools/d) 2. **Fever** (30%-50%), but lack of fever does not rule it out 3. Abdominal pain 4. Generalized constitutional symptoms	1. **PCR identification** of *C. difficile* toxin or *C. difficile* toxin gene in stool–if patient has clinically significant diarrhea • Toxin B is clinically important 2. Culture from stool sample or rectal swab–for patients with ileus and suspected *C. difficile* infection • Most sensitive method, but cannot distinguish toxin-producing strains from nontoxin-producing 3. Radiograph: severe inflammation of inner lining of bowel 4. CBC: **Leukocytosis**	1. IV metronidazole OR 2. PO vancomycin (this is the only use for oral vancomycin) <u>Prevention</u> • Strict hand washing • Enteric precautions • Minimize antibiotic use <u>Complications:</u> Bowel perforation, toxic megacolon

ACUTE AND CHRONIC HEPATITIS: INFLAMMATION OF THE LIVER

- Hepatitis B: associated with *polyarteritis nodosa (PAN)*
- Hepatitis C: associated with cryoglobulinemia
- Hepatitis C—most common cause of liver transplantation in the United States
- If transaminases are markedly elevated (>500), think acute viral hepatitis, shock liver, or drug-induced hepatitis

Disease	Etiology, Prevalence, Risk Factors	Clinical Symptoms and Signs	Diagnostics	Therapy, Prognosis, and Health Maintenance
Acute hepatitis A	• Cause: foodborne (RNA) hepatovirus (in Picornavirus family) associated with **contaminated seafood** • Foreign travel • Daycare • RF: poor sanitation, crowding, exposure of food, water, milk, **shellfish** <u>Transmission:</u> **Fecal-oral** Incubation: 30 d Major cause of acute hepatitis	<u>Prodromal phase:</u> • 2-6 wk of **flu-like symptoms** • Low grade fever • Nausea/vomiting (frequent) • Constipation, diarrhea • Fatigue • Myalgias, malaise • Arthralgia • Upper respiratory SX • Anorexia <u>Icteric phase:</u> • Hepatic compromise (bilirubinemia) • Jaundice, after 5-10 d • Icterus • Abdominal pain: RUQ or epigastrium, worse with exertion <u>Signs:</u> 1. Hepatomegaly (>50%) 2. Splenomegaly (15%)	1. Labs • WBC: NL to low • U/A: proteinuria, bilirubinuria • AST/ALT: very high • ALK-P: high (late), **marked cholestasis** • Anti-HAV: (+) (early) 2. IgM/IgG anti-HAV (+), IgM peaks in first week, disappearing by 3-6 mo • Diagnoses acute hepatitis A • IgG rises 1 mo after onset, persists for years, indicates previous exposure, noninfection, and immunity	1. Supportive therapy • Avoid ETOH, hepatotoxic agents, and strenuous exercise • Recovery in 3 mo <u>Prophylaxis:</u> 1. Handwash after bowel movements 2. **Unvaccinated exposure advised to get postexposure prophylaxis** • Single dose of HAV vaccine or IG • Vaccine for age 1-40, IG for immunocompromised or chronic liver disease <u>Prognosis:</u> • No chronic carrier state • Low mortality rate <u>When to Admit:</u> 1. Encephalopathy 2. INR > 1.6 3. Unable to maintain hydration 4. Complications: acute cholecystitis

(continued)

(continued)

Family Medicine

Disease	Etiology, Prevalence, Risk Factors	Clinical Symptoms and Signs	Diagnostics	Therapy, Prognosis, and Health Maintenance
Acute hepatitis B	Hepadnavirus with a double-stranded DNA genome, inner core protein, and outer surface coat; 8 genotypes (A-H) Transmission: Blood products, infected blood, sexual contact Incubation: 6W-6M Prevalent in: **MSM, IVDA** DNA virus (hepadnavirus) Natural immunity not possible—risk of reactivation Age of exposure is important	1. Insidious onset of signs and symptoms • Low grade fever • Similar to Hep A • Subsides in 2-3 wk 2. Defervescence: jaundice and bradycardia Complications: **Cryoglobulinemia** (polyarteritis nodosa, membranoproliferative glomerulonephritis, renal, skin, joint), **cirrhosis, HCC, superinfection with HDV**	1. Labs • AST/ALT–1000-5000 (high) • No cholestasis • PT: prolonged 2. Hepatitis serology **HBsAg: +** (first evidence of infection) HBc IgM: + (diagnostic for acute Hep B, persists 3-6 mo) HBe Ag: may or may not be + HBV DNA: parallels HBeAg Anti-HBs: signals recovery, noninfection, or immunity • Treat anyone (+) with elevated enzymes • Anyone with viral load >2000, normal AST/ALT, but fibrosis on biopsy	1. Refer to hepatologist—risk of reactivation 2. Postexposure • HBIG within 7 d, followed by HB vaccine • Newborn infants of HBsAg (+) moms 3. Antiviral therapy • Interferon α or lamivudine • Tenofovir if pregnant (third trimester) Prophylaxis: 1. Supportive • **Vaccinate**: infants, children, adults at risk (including <60 y/o with DM); standard is 10-20 µg repeated again at 1 and 6 mo • Safe sex precautions • Clean contaminated utensils, bedding, clothing Screening: 1. Recommended in high-risk groups: previous incarceration or STD, MSM, IVDU Prognosis: 1. 0.1%-1% mortality 2. Most recover in 3-6 mo 3. HBV infected are at high risk for *cirrhosis and HCC* (25%-40%), M > F • **Biannual HCC screen** for carriers and chronic infection: **AFP** and **US** every 6 mo When to refer: 1. Acute hepatitis requiring liver biopsy for diagnosis Admit: 1. Same as Hep A
Chronic hepatitis B	Characterized by elevated aminotransferase levels for 6+ mo Develops in 1%-2% of healthy adults, but in 90% of neonates and infants		1. Hepatitis serology HBc IgM: – **HBsAg: +** (persistent 6+ mo) HBc IgM: – (appears during flares of inactive chronic Hep B) HBe Ag: ±(beyond 3 mo increases likelihood of chronic) Anti-HBe: +(follows disappearance of HBeAg) HBV DNA: parallels HBeAg (can be high in chronic) Anti-HBs: signals recovery, noninfection or immunity	1. Treatment as above Prophylaxis: 1. Vaccination against HBV

Disease	Etiology, Prevalence, Risk Factors	Clinical Symptoms and Signs	Diagnostics	Therapy, Prognosis, and Health Maintenance
Acute hepatitis C	Prevalence: **IVDA (50%)**, military service, cocaine use RF: Body piercings, tattoos, hemodialysis, **MSM** (multiple sex partners, HIV coinfection, unprotected receptive anal intercourse with ejaculation, sex while on meth) MC: Genotype 1 (of 7 identified) Incubation: 6-7 wk Single-stranded RNA (flavivirus) Increases the hepatotoxicity of antiretroviral therapy	1. Mild, usually asymptomatic • Jaundice 2. Complications: cryoglobulinemia, membranoproliferative glomerulonephritis, **lichen planus,** autoimmune thyroiditis, lymphocytic sialadenitis, IPF, sporadic porphyria cutanea tarda, monoclonal gammopathies	1. Labs • Waxing and waning AST/ALT elevations 2. Hepatitis serology 3. Anti-HCV: (+) 4. Enzyme immunoassay (EIA): diagnoses HCV • Moderate sensitivity in early course and low specificity if high GGT 5. **HCV RNA assay:** confirmatory	1. Antivirals: • **Interferon** α × 6-24 wk • Reserved for patients whose RNA levels do not clear after 3 mo untreated • ± ribavirin • Newer, more expensive agents: Solvadi, Harvoni, Daklinza, Viekira Pak Prophylaxis: 1. Safe sex precautions Health maintenance: 1. Vaccinate against HAV and HBV Prognosis: 1. 85%-90% of acute infections develop into chronic infections 2. 20%-30% increased risk of non-Hodgkin lymphoma 3. Clears in 3-6 mo 4. Mortality: <1%
Chronic hepatitis C	Develops in 85% of acute cases HIV infection leads to increased risk of acute liver failure and rapid progression of chronic Hep C to cirrhosis			1. Treatment as above Prognosis: 1. 30% develop cirrhosis 2. 3%-5% will develop HCC
Hepatitis D (delta agent)	"Passenger virus": requires the outer envelope of HBs-Ag for replication Can only be transmitted as coinfection with HBV or superinfection in a chronic HBV carrier Defective RNA virus Mediterranean countries (nonpercutaneous) United States/Europe (blood)	1. Acute HDV + acute HBV = similar in severity to acute HBV alone 2. Chronic HBV + superinfection HDV = worse short-term prognosis • Fulminant hepatitis → cirrhosis	1. Anti-HDV (+)	1. Treat HBV infection as above Prognosis: 1. 3× risk of HCC

(continued)

(continued)

Disease	Etiology, Prevalence, Risk Factors	Clinical Symptoms and Signs	Diagnostics	Therapy, Prognosis, and Health Maintenance
Hepatitis E (non-A, non-B)	**RF:** Consumption of **undercooked pork** or wild boar, pets in home, consuming undercooked organ meats Herpesviridae family India, Pakistan, southeast Asia, parts of Africa Transmission: Fecal-oral	Same presentation as HAV, but markers are negative Extrahepatic manifestations: Arthritis, pancreatitis, monoclonal gammopathy, thrombocytopenia, Guillain-Barre, peripheral neuropathy	1. Serologies IgM Anti-HEV (+) HEV RNA (+)	1. Antiviral • PO ribavirin × 3 mo 2. Public hygiene

Hepatitis Serologies

Marker	Acute Infection	Chronic Infection (Actively Replicating)	Resolution	Chronic Infection (Inactive)	Postimmunization
Anti-HAV IgM	+	N/A	–	N/A	–
Anti-HAV IgG	–	N/A	+	N/A	+
Anti-HCV	+	+	+	+	
HBsAg	+	+	–	+	–
Anti-HBs	–	–	+	–	+
Anti-HBc IgM	+	–	–	–	–
Anti-HBc Total**	+	+	+	+	–
HBeAg	+	+	–	–	–
Anti-HBe	–	–	+	+	–

** Anti-Hepatitis B core total antibodies.

- HBsAg is (+) if actively infected or chronically infected
- HBeAg is (+) if active <u>acute</u> or chronic infection
- Antibodies
  - HBs = (+) if resolved or *immunized*
  - HBe = (+) if resolved or inactive chronic infection
  - HBc IgM = (+) only in <u>active</u> acute infection
  - HBc total = (+) if virus has ever been active inside the body
- If resolving an active infection—these 2 antigens disappear and 2 antibodies appear
  - HBeAg disappears, HBe-Ab appears
  - HBsAg disappears, HBs-Ab appears
- How to distinguish if someone is vaccinated versus recovered? If they are vaccinated, they will have a (−) anti-HBc total, and the only (+) serology will be HBsAb, whereas an immune/recovered patient will show positive HBc total Ab (+) in addition to HBsAb and anti-HBe

Disease	Etiology, Prevalence, Risk Factors	Clinical Symptoms and Signs	Diagnostics	Therapy, Prognosis, and Health Maintenance
Achalasia	Idiopathic motility disorder resulting in loss of peristalsis in the distal two-thirds of the esophagus and impaired relaxation of the lower esophageal sphincter	1. Slowly progressive dysphagia 2. Episodic regurgitation 3. Chest pain	1. Barium esophagography (nonconfirmatory) • Esophageal dilation • Loss of esophageal peristalsis • Poor esophageal emptying • Smooth, symmetric "birds beak" tapering of distal esophagus 2. Esophageal manometry (confirmatory)	1. Calcium channel blockers, nitrates, botulinum toxin 2. Surgery (endoscopic dilatation or resection) <u>Health maintenance:</u> 1. Increased risk of esophageal squamous cell carcinoma

CHAPTER 4

Orthopedics and Rheumatology

Refer to Appendices for the Following Topics:

Acute and Chronic Low Back Pain, see Appendix G: Fractures, Dislocations, and Tears, p 734

Bursitis/Tendinitis, see Appendix G: Fractures, Dislocations, and Tears, p 735

Sprains/Strains, see Appendix G: Fractures, Dislocations, and Tears, p 733

Recommended Topics:

Mallet Finger, see Appendix G: Fractures, Dislocations, and Tears, p 716

Osteomyelitis, see Appendix G: Fractures, Dislocations, and Tears, p 709

Ankylosing Spondylitis, see Appendix G: Fractures, Dislocations, and Tears, p 734

ACUTE AND CHRONIC LOW BACK PAIN

Disease	Etiology, Prevalence, Risk Factors	Clinical Symptoms and Signs	Diagnostics	Therapy, Prognosis, and Health Maintenance
Costochondritis	Tietze syndrome: <40 y, M = F; much less common than costochondritis Age >40 y, mostly F	1. Anterior chest pain • Sudden or gradual • Sharply localized or radiates to arms or shoulders • Worse with sneezing, cough, deep inspiration, or twisting • Brief and darting • Persistent dull ache 2. Reproduced with palpation <u>Tietze syndrome:</u> 1. 1+ joints are **swollen**, red, and tender	1. Radiograph 2. Bone scan 3. Vitamin D level 4. Biopsy	1. Analgesics, anti-inflammatories 2. Local steroid injections

BURSITIS/TENDINITIS

Reactive Arthritis

• **Reiter syndrome**—most patients **do not** have the classic findings, so term reactive arthritis is used

  • Classic triad: **arthritis**, **urethritis**, ocular inflammation (conjunctivitis or anterior **uveitis**): "can't see" (uveitis), "can't pee" (urethritis), "can't climb a tree" (arthritis)

• Patient can develop reactive arthritis after non-gonococcal urethritis or after enteric infections with *Salmonella*, *Shigella flexneri*, *Campylobacter jejuni*, or *Yersinia enterocolitica*

Disease	Etiology, Prevalence, Risk Factors	Clinical Symptoms and Signs	Diagnostics	Therapy, Prognosis, and Health Maintenance
Reactive arthritis	HLA-B27 (+) patients Asymmetric inflammatory oligoarthritis of the lower extremities (upper less common); preceded by an infectious process that is remote from the site (1-4 wk prior); usually after urogenital or enteric infections Sterile inflammatory process	1. Evidence of **infection** (GI or GU) 1-4 wk before onset of symptoms → **_Campylobacter infection_** 2. **Asymmetric arthritis**: new joints may be involved sequentially over days (joints are painful, with effusions and lack of mobility) • Joint pain may persist or recur over a long-term period 3. Conjunctivitis 4. Urethritis 5. Mucocutaneous lesions 6. **Constitutional SX**: fatigue, malaise, weight loss, fever are common	1. Synovial fluid for analysis (r/o infection or crystals)	1. **NSAIDs** (first line) 2. If no response → • Sulfasalazine Or • Azathioprine

OSTEOARTHRITIS (FIG. 4-1)

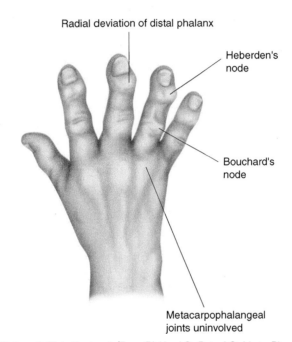

Radial deviation of distal phalanx

Heberden's node

Bouchard's node

Metacarpophalangeal joints uninvolved

FIGURE 4-1. Osteoarthritis in the hand. (From Bickley LS. *Bates' Guide to Physical Examination and History Taking.* 10th ed. Philadelphia: Lippincott Williams & Wilkins; 2009.)

	Osteoarthritis	Rheumatoid Arthritis	Gouty Arthritis
Onset	Insidious	Insidious	Sudden
Common locations	Weight-bearing joints (knees, **hips, lumbar/cervical spine**), hands	Hands (*PIP, MCP*), **wrists**, ankles, knees	**Great toe**, ankles, knees, **elbows**
Presence of inflammation	No	Yes	Yes
Radiographic changes	Narrowed joint space, **osteophytes**, subchondral sclerosis, subchondral cysts	Narrowed joint space, bony erosions	**Punched-out erosions** with overhanging rim of cortical bone
Laboratory findings	None	High ESR, RF, anemia	Crystals
Other features	• No systemic findings • **Bouchard nodes** and **Heberden nodes** in hands	• Systemic findings: extra-articular manifestations common • Ulnar deviation, swan neck and boutonniere deformity	• Tophi • Nephrolithiasis

	Osteoarthritis	Rheumatoid Arthritis	Gouty Arthritis
Treatments	1. Tylenol—prn 3-4 times daily if no inflammation 2. NSAIDs—prn for mild inflammation • Topicals if CI to oral agents 3. Intra-articular steroids—for persistent symptoms despite oral and topical NSAIDs • Repeat q 3 mo 4. **Intra-articular hyaluronic acid**—for patients with OA of knee nonresponsive to APAP or NSAIDs, nor relief from intra-articular steroids I	See treatment table	1. Avoid secondary causes of hyperuricemia • Meds that increase uric acid (thiazide, loop diuretics) • Obesity • **Alcohol intake** • **Dietary purines** (seafood/red meat) 2. Acute gout • Bed rest; early ambulation • See treatment table

GOUT

- Hyperuricemia—hallmark of disease
- MOA is multifactorial
  - Increased production of uric acid
    - Hypoxanthine-guanine phosphoribosyltransferase deficiency (eg, in Lesch-Nyhan syndrome)
    - Phosphoribosyl pyrophosphate synthetase overactivity
    - Increased cell turnover with chemotherapy, chronic hemolysis, and hematologic malignancies
  - Decreased excretion of uric acid (**90%**)
    - Renal disease
    - NSAIDs/diuretics
    - Acidosis
- Inflammation
  - PMNs play a key role in acute inflammation
  - Uric acid crystals collect in synovial fluid as extracellular fluid becomes saturated
  - IgGs coat monosodium urate crystals, which are phagocytosed by PMNs, leading to the release of inflammatory mediators and proteolytic enzymes from the PMNs, which then result in inflammation

Disease	Etiology, Prevalence, Risk Factors	Clinical Symptoms and Signs	Diagnostics	Therapy, Prognosis, and Health Maintenance
Gout	Inflammatory monoarticular arthritis caused by the crystallization of monosodium urate in joints Precipitants: **cold temperature, dehydration, stress** (emotional or physical), **excessive alcohol intake,** starvation 90% are men >30 y, women unaffected until menopause	See presentation table, later	1. Joint aspiration and synovial fluid analysis • **Needle-shaped and negatively birefringent urate** crystals 2. Gram stain and culture—r/o septic arthritis 3. Serum uric acid—not helpful 4. XR: punched out erosions with overhanging rim of cortical bone	See treatment table, later
Pseudogout (calcium pyrophosphate)	RF: Increases with age and **OA** of joints (elderly with DJD), **hemochromatosis, hyperparathyroidism, hypothyroidism,** Bartter syndrome	1. Most common joints affected—**knee and wrist** • Classically monoarticular, but can be polyarticular	1. Joint aspiration • Weakly **positively birefringent, rod-shaped, and rhomboidal crystals** 2. XR—chondrocalcinosis (cartilage calcification)	1. Treat underlying disorder 2. Symptomatic management: NSAIDs, colchicine, intraarticular steroids 3. Total joint replacement if symptoms debilitating

Presentation of Gout

Four Stages

1. Asymptomatic hyperuricemia–increased serum uric acid level in the absence of clinical findings; presents without SX for 10-20 y
2. Acute gouty arthritis–peak onset 40-60 y/o
   - Initial attack usually involves one joint of lower extremity
     - **Sudden onset exquisite pain**–may be unable to tolerate bed sheet on joint; pain awakens patient up from sleep
     - Most often big toe–**first MT joint** (*podagra*); ankles and knees
   - Pain and cellulitic changes–redness, swelling, tenderness, warmth
   - ± fever
   - Desquamation of overlying skin
3. Intercritical gout–asymptomatic period after the initial attack; 60% recur within 1 y
   - 75% likelihood of second attack in 2 y
   - Attacks become polyarticular and increase in severity
4. Chronic tophaceous gout–occurs in people with **poorly controlled gout for >10-20 y**
   - Tophi–aggregations of urate crystals surrounded by giant cells in an inflammatory reaction
   - Seen only after several attacks of acute gout; noted after average of 10 y following first attack
   - Cause deformity and destruction of hard and soft tissue
   - Common locations–extensor surfaces of forearms, elbows, knees, Achilles tendon, pinna of external ear

Treatment of Gout

1. Asymptomatic hyperuricemia–do not treat
2. Avoid secondary causes of hyperuricemia
   - Meds that increase uric acid (thiazide, loop diuretics)
   - Obesity
   - **Alcohol intake**
   - **Dietary purines** (*seafood*/red meat)
3. Acute gout
   - Bed rest; early ambulation
   - **NSAIDs** (indomethacin)
   - Colchicine–alternative for patients who cannot take NSAIDs or do not respond
     - AE: nausea, vomiting, abdominal cramps, severe diarrhea
     - CI: renal insufficiency, cytopenia
   - Steroids (PO prednisone) 7-10 d: if does not respond or intolerant of NSAID/colchicine, intra-articular injections
4. Prophylaxis
   - Must have **2-3 attacks** before initiating prophylactic therapy
   - NSAIDs (indomethacin) × 3-6 mo→
   - Uricosuric drugs (probenecid, sulfinpyrazone)–increase renal excretion; only for patients with normal kidney function (undersecretion)
   - Allopurinol–24-h urine uric acid >800 mg/d; watch for rash or SJS; not for acute cases (overproduction)

1. If untreated, acute gouty attack lasts 7-10 d and then resolves
   - Severe episodes may last longer
2. Complications
   - Nephrolithiasis (1%)
   - Degenerative arthritis (15%)
3. **Avoid aspirin** (makes it worse) and **tylenol** (no anti-inflammatory properties)

RHEUMATOID ARTHRITIS (FIG. 4-2)

Inflammatory autoimmune disease involving the synovium of joints, which can cause damage to cartilage and bone

- Osteophytes are not present in RA as they are in OA; because the entire synovium is involved, the changes more significant and extensive
- Can involve every joint in the body *except* DIP joints
- Poor prognostic risk factors: high RF titers, subcutaneous nodules, erosive arthritis, autoantibodies to RF
- If (+) RF and/or ACPA—at high-risk of developing erosive joint damage

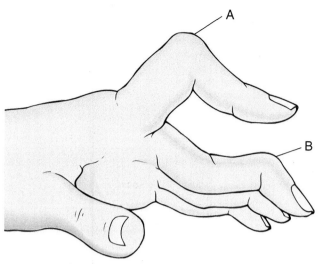

FIGURE 4-2. Rheumatoid arthritis. Boutonniere deformity (*A*) and swan neck deformity (*B*). (From Young VB, Kormos WA, Chick DA. *Blueprints Medicine.* 6th ed. Philadelphia: Wolters Kluwer Health; 2016.)

<u>Age</u>: 20-40 y
F > M (3:1)
<u>Etiology</u>: uncertain, may be due to viral infection or genetic predisposition

1. Inflammatory polyarthritis (joint swelling)
   • Pain on motion of joints with tenderness
   • Joints of hands (**PIP, MCP**) and **wrists,** knees, ankles, elbows, hips, shoulders
2. Hand deformities
   • Ulnar deviation of the MCP joints
     • *Boutonniere deformities* of the PIP joints (PIP flexed, DIP hyperextended)
     • *Swan-neck deformities* of PIP joints (PIP hyperextended, MCP flexed, DIP flexed)
3. Constitutional symptoms (prominent)
   • **Morning stiffness** (all patients) with improvement later in the day; symmetric involvement
   • Low-grade fever, weight loss
   • Fatigue (prominent)
4. Cervical spine involvement at C1-C2 (subluxation and instability)
   • Instability of cervical spine, seen in 30%-40%
5. Cardiac involvement: pericarditis, pericardial effusion, conduction involvement, valvular competence
6. Pulmonary involvement: usually pleural effusions; interstitial fibrosis may occur
7. Ocular involvement: episcleritis or scleritis
8. Soft tissue swelling

<u>Labs:</u>
1. **Rheumatoid factor**–high titers associated with severe disease, nonspecific (80%); higher = more severe, but rarely change with disease activity
2. **Anticitrullinated peptide/** protein antibodies (ACPA): 50%-75% sensitive, 90% specific
   • ESR/CRP: elevated
3. Normocytic normochromic anemia
<u>XR:</u>
1. Loss of juxtaarticular bone mass (periarticular osteoporosis) near fingers
2. **Narrowing of joint** space (late)
3. **Bony erosions** at margins
4. Synovial joint fluid analysis

Extraarticular Manifestations

Skin	• Skin becomes thin and atrophic and bruises easily • Vasculitic changes/ulcerations involving fingers, nail folds • **Subcutaneous rheumatoid nodules** (elbows, sacrum, occiput)–pathognomonic for RA • Nearly always in seropositive patients
Lungs	• **Pleural effusions** (very common)–pleural fluid has **low glucose** and complement • Pulmonary fibrosis (restrictive on PFTs with honeycombing on CXR) • Rheumatic nodules in lungs can cavitate or become infected
Heart	• Rheumatoid nodules leading to conduction disturbances • **Pericarditis** (40%) • Pericardial effusion
Eyes	• Scleritis • Scleromalacia (softening) → can perforate → blindness • Dry eyes and mucous membranes → Sjögren xerostomia
Nervous system	• Mononeuritic multiplex–infarction of nerve trunk • Patient cannot move arm or leg → systemic vasculitis

(continued)

(continued)

Felty syndrome	• Triad: RA, neutropenia, and splenomegaly • Also, anemia, thrombocytopenia, and lymphadenopathy • Associated with high titers of RF and extraarticular disease • Increased susceptibility to infection • Late in disease process
Blood	• **Anemia of chronic disease**: mild, normocytic, normochromic anemia • Thrombocytosis
Vasculitis	• Microvascular vasculitis → mesenteric vasculitis, PAN, or other syndromes
Juvenile RA	• Begins before 18 y of age • Extraarticular manifestations: **Still disease** or arthritis

Rheumatoid Arthritis Treatments

- Goal: prevent/halt destruction and enter remission with least toxicity

Preventative acute therapy	• Exercise—maintain ROM and strength
	• **NSAIDs**—pain control • Steroids (low dose)—refractory to NSAIDs, short term

Primary	• Disease-modifying antirheumatic drugs (**DMARDs**)
	  • Reduce morbidity and mortality (30%)
	  • Initiate early (at diagnosis)
	  • Slow onset (6+ wk)
	• First-line agents
	  • **Methotrexate**—best initial DMARD; 80% respond
	    • AE: GI upset, oral ulcers (stomatitis), mild alopecia, bone marrow suppression, ***hepatocellular injury***, idiosyncratic interstitial pneumonitis → **pulmonary fibrosis**
	    • Monitor LFTs and renal function, supplement with folate
	  • Leflunomide—alternative; same efficacy as MTX
	  • Hydroxychloroquine—alternative; requires biannual eye examinations (risk of retinopathy)
	  • Sulfasalazine—alternative
	  • Anti-TNF inhibiting agents—etanercept, infliximab; secondary, if refractory

Severe	• Surgery
	  • Synovectomy (arthroscopic)—decreases joint pain/swelling, won't improve ROM
	  • Joint replacement—for severe cases

Synovial Joint Fluid Analysis

Condition	Appearance	WBC/mm³	PMNs	Other
Normal	Clear	<200	<25%	
Noninflammatory arthritis (OA/trauma)	Clear, yellow ±red if traumatic	<2000 Mild WBC	<25%	RBCs for trauma
Inflammatory (RA, gout, pseudogout, Reiter syndrome)	**Cloudy yellow**	**>5000 Moderate-severe WBC**	**50%-70% Moderate PMNs**	• Positively birefringent crystals with pseudogout • Negatively birefringent crystals with gout
Septic arthritis (bacteria, TB)	Turbid, purulent	>50 000 Extreme WBC counts	>70% Greatest percentage of PMNs	Synovial fluid culture (+) for bacterial arthritis, except gonococcal

SYSTEMIC LUPUS ERYTHEMATOSUS

An autoimmune disorder leading to inflammation and tissue damage involving multiple organ systems

- Genetic, environmental, and hormonal factors involved
- Autoantibody production, deposition of immune complexes, complement activation, and tissue destruction/vasculitis

- Types
- Spontaneous
- Discoid lupus (skin lesions, no systemic disease): **erythematous raised patches** with adherent keratotic scaling; present on the face, neck, and scalp
- Drug-induced lupus
- ANA-negative lupus

- Arthritis, Raynaud phenomenon, subacute cutaneous lupus
- Serology: Ro (anti-SS-A) antibody (+), ANA negative
- Risk of neonatal lupus in infants of affected mothers: skin lesions, cardiac abnormalities (AV block, transposition of great vessels), valvular/septal defects
- Clinical course
  - Chronic disease with exacerbations and remissions
  - Malar rash, joint pain, and fatigue (Fig. 4-3)

	Presentation	Diagnostic Studies
Systemic lupus erythematosus	1. Constitutional SX: **fatigue**, **malaise**, **fever**, weight loss 2. Skin: *butterfly **rash*** over cheeks and bridge of nose (1/3), *photosensitivity*, *discoid lesions*, *oral and nasopharyngeal ulcers*, alopecia, Raynaud phenomenon (20%) 3. MS: **joint pain** (90%), ***arthritis*** (symmetric), arthralgias, myalgia ± myositis 4. Cardiac: *pericarditis*, endocarditis, myocarditis 5. Lung: ***pleuritis***, pleural effusion, pneumonitis 6. Heme: ***hemolytic anemia*** or reticulocytosis of chronic disease, *leukopenia, lymphopenia, thrombocytopenia* 7. Renal: *proteinuria >0.5 g/d, cellular casts*, GN, azotemia, pyuria, uremia, HTN 8. Immune: impaired response due to autoantibodies to lymphocytes, abnormal T cell function, and immunosuppressive meds 9. GI: nausea, vomiting, dyspepsia, dysphagia, PUD 10. CNS: *seizures, psychosis*, depression, headaches, TIA, CVA 11. Other: conjunctivitis, Sjogren syndrome	1. (+) **ANA screening**: sensitive, not specific 2. **Anti-ds DNA**: 100% specific, correlates with dz 3. **Anti-Sm Ab**: 55%-100% very specific, not sensitive; does not correlate with disease extent 4. **Antiphospholipid Ab**: 33% specific 5. Anti-ss DNA (70%) 6. Antihistone Abs (70%) in 100% of drug-induced lupus (Ro 9SS-A) and La (SS-B) • Also, positive in other diseases such as: Sjögren syndrome 7. False (+) with syphilis 8. Complement: decreased 9. CBC, BUN/Cr, U/A, serum electrolytes 10. Anticardiolipin and lupus anticoagulant

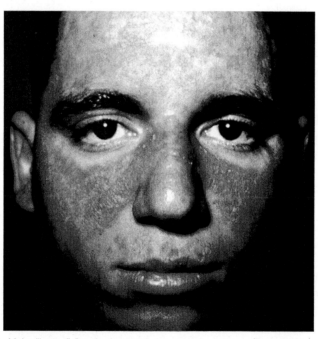

FIGURE 4-3. Malar "butterfly" rash of systemic lupus erythematosus. (From McConnell TH. *The Nature of Disease: Pathology for the Health Professions.* 2nd ed. Philadelphia: Wolters Kluwer Health; 2014.)

Treatment for Lupus

• Treatment: • Avoid sun exposure • NSAIDs if less severe • Local or systemic **corticosteroids** • Systemic **steroids** for severe manifestations • Best long-term therapy: antimalarials **(hydroxychloroquine)** with annual eye examination • Cytotoxic agents (cyclophosphamide)–for active GN	Monitoring: 1. BUN/Cr–renal disease 2. Blood pressure–HTN	**Prevalence:** **Women of childbearing age (90%), African American** Prognosis: More severe in children Appears in late childhood or adolescence

OSTEOPOROSIS

Disease	Etiology, Prevalence, Risk Factors	Clinical Symptoms and Signs	Diagnostics	Therapy, Prognosis, and Health Maintenance
Osteoporosis Systemic skeletal disorder characterized by low bone mass, deterioration of bone tissue, increased fragility of bone, and susceptibility to fracture	More women who fracture are osteopenic > osteoporotic RF: 1. Lifestyle (increased caffeine, **smoking**, ETOH, lack of exercise, low calcium intake) 2. Hormonal (menopause estrogen deficiency, eating disorder) 3. Genetic (FH, cystic fibrosis, Ehlers-Danlos) 4. Endocrine (hyper-PT, hyperthyroid) 5. Medical (SLE, lymphoma) 6. Medications (steroids, chemotherapy, thyroid hormone) 7. Vitamin D deficiency 8. Advanced age Age: 50 y+, white F (2-3 risk of M)	Asymptomatic: 1. 1+ fracture • Most common sites: vertebral body, proximal femur, distal forearm/wrist	1. **DEXA scan** to measure BMD • Dual energy radiograph absorptiometry (DXA) • **T score:** ≥-2.5 • Decreased by 1-point increases the risk of fracture 2- to 3-fold • Only apply WHO T score criteria to postmenopausal women 2. Imaging of vertebra: FRAX: • Fracture Risk Algorithm • Therapy indicated for patients with 10-y probability of hip fracture 3% or higher or major osteoporosis-related fracture of >20% Treat if: • BMD −2.5 or less (spine/hip) with no RF • HX of spine/hip fracture • FRAX: over 3%, T-score less than −1	1. **Bisphosphonates**: Alendronate, BMD prior and repeated biennially 2. Calcitonin 3. Estrogens (± progestogen) 4. PTH 5. Raloxifene 6. Denosumab Prophylaxis: 1. Ovarian estrogen and estrogen administered postmenopausally 2. Calcium: **1200 mg/d** Vitamin D: 800-1200 IU/d 3. Counseling: balanced diet, avoid alcohol, quit smoking, regular exercise, calcium and vitamin D 4. Reduce risk of falls 5. **Avoid smoking/ETOH** 6. Most severe in women with early oophorectomy or premature ovarian failure, gonadal dysgenesis Health Maintenance: 1. Recheck bone mineral density 1-2 y after starting bisphosphonate therapy
Osteopenia: low bone mass			T score: −1.0 and −2.5 SD	

- T score: number of standard deviations above or below the mean BMD for sex-matched young normal controls
- Z score: compares patient with an age- and sex-matched population
- Measurement of bone mineral density (BMD) recommended for:
  - Postmenopausal patients younger than 65 years who have 1+ risk factor for osteoporosis (other than white postmenopausal female)
  - All women 65+ years regardless of risk factors
  - Postmenopausal women who present with fractures
  - Women considering therapy for osteoporosis if testing would facilitate decision
- Women who have been on HRT for extensive periods
- Women who have been on treatment to monitor treatment effect
- Women considering discontinuation of treatment

Fibromyalgia

Chronic nonprogressive course waxing and waning in severity

- Must rule out: myofascial syndromes, rheumatoid disease, polymyalgia rheumatica, ankylosing spondylitis, spondyloarthropathy, chronic fatigue syndrome, Lyme disease, hypothyroidism, polymyositis, depression, and somatization disorder, and hypertrophic osteoarthropathy

Disease	Etiology, Prevalence, Risk Factors	Clinical Symptoms and Signs	Diagnostics	Therapy, Prognosis, and Health Maintenance
Fibromyalgia	Adult women Etiology: unknown, somatization not a proven cause	1. **Stiffness**, body aches, fatigue 2. Pain is constant and aching, aggravated by weather, stress, sleep deprivation, cold temperature (worse in AM) 3. Pain better with rest, warmth, and mild exercise 4. Sleep patterns disrupted and sleep unrefreshing 5. **Anxiety and depression** common	1. Diagnosis: **multiple trigger points** (tender to palpation) • Symmetrical • 18 characteristic locations have been identified (occiput, neck, shoulder, ribs, elbows, buttocks, knees) 2. Widespread pain including **axial pain for at least 3 mo** 3. Pain in at **least 11** of the 18 possible tender point sites	1. Advise patient to stay active and productive 2. Meds not very effective • SSRI and **TCAs**, avoid narcotics 3. CBT, exercise, psychiatric evaluation

GANGLION CYSTS (FIG. 4-4)

Disease	Etiology, Prevalence, Risk Factors	Clinical Symptoms and Signs	Diagnostics	Therapy, Prognosis, and Health Maintenance
Ganglion cysts	Benign soft-tissue mass	1. Soft, nontender, transilluminating mass 2. Usually on dorsum of hand or wrist		1. **Surgical excision** (definitive)—recommended if cyst causes pain, disruption of function, or cosmetic distress

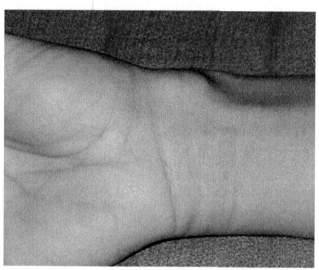

FIGURE 4-4. Volar wrist ganglion cyst. (From Wiesel SW. *Operative Techniques in Orthopaedic Surgery.* Lippincott Williams & Wilkins; 2011.)

PLANTAR FASCIITIS (FIG. 4-5)

Disease	Etiology, Prevalence, Risk Factors	Clinical Symptoms and Signs	Diagnostics	Therapy, Prognosis, and Health Maintenance
Plantar fasciitis	Common in runners and overweight patients Caused by microscopic tears in plantar fascia at calcaneal origin	1. Patients will complain of pain with first few steps in AM and heel pain at night Signs: 1. Pain at calcaneal origin 2. Inflexible Achilles tendon	1. Plain XR normal, but may reveal calcaneal fracture or bone spur 2. MRI: calcifications of plantar fascia	1. Conservative treatment × 6-12 mo • Physical therapy for stretching plantar fascia and Achilles tendon • Heel pads • Arch supports • Massage of area with tennis ball 2. Steroid injections used with caution owing to risk of rupture of plantar fascia 3. Surgery for extreme cases

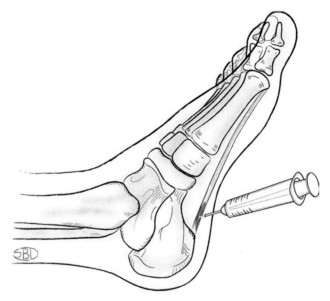

FIGURE 4-5. Treatment for plantar fasciitis. Injection occurs at the insertion of the plantar fascia along the base of the calcaneus, the most common site of pain. (From Simon RR, Ross C, Bowman SH, Wakim PE. *Cook County Manual of Emergency Procedures.* Philadelphia: Lippincott Williams & Wilkins, a Wolters Kluwer business; 2012.)

OVERUSE SYNDROME

The result of repetitive stresses and microtrauma outpacing the body's ability to heal

Hip Myofascial Syndromes

Disease	Etiology, Prevalence, Risk Factors	Clinical Symptoms and Signs	Diagnostics	Therapy, Prognosis, and Health Maintenance
External snapping hip syndrome (posterior lateral hip pain, coxa saltans)	Young women Occurs with activities such as dancing or stair climbing	1. Snapping sound heard and popping sensation felt as IT band slips over greater trochanter 2. Snap heard with hip flexion and extension	1. MRI	
Fascia lata syndrome (lateral thigh pain)	Unilateral enlargement of the tensor fascia lata	1. Pain to palpation and trigger points 2. Pain in anterior groin 3. Point tenderness over anterior iliac crest	1. Ultrasound	

Knee Myofascial Syndromes

- **Q-angle**: measured at the junction of a line drawn from the central patella to the tibial tubercle and the line of the femur
  - Normal: 15°
  - Increased angle increases risk for patellar subluxation (females tend to have large Q angle, increasing their risk)
- Patellar grind test—press patella away from femoral condyles while asking patient to contract quadriceps (Figs. 4-6 and 4-7)

Disease	Etiology, Prevalence, Risk Factors	Clinical Symptoms and Signs	Diagnostics	Therapy, Prognosis, and Health Maintenance
Patellofemoral syndrome (runner's knee or anterior knee pain, "moviegoer syndrome")	Major cause of anterior knee pain 3 causes: focal trauma, overuse, and abnormal patellar tracking (weak quads) More common in females owing to the presence of increased Q angle (>20°)	1. Anterior knee pain–gradual onset, nonradiating, unilateral 2. Worse with prolonged flexion of the knee (air flights or movie theater) 3. Occurs with ADLs: walking, stair climbing <u>Signs:</u> 1. Crepitus to palpation 2. Patellar grind test (+ if sudden patellar pain and relaxation of the muscle)	1. XR–limited use	1. Physical therapy and strengthening 2. Brace support of knee
Iliotibial band syndrome (lateral knee pain)	Most common in distance runners or cyclists Bursa underlying band becomes irritated	Pain reproduced after consistently reaching certain mileage during running or other physical exertion <u>Signs:</u> Localized tenderness to palpation over lateral epicondyles		1. Rest, decrease distance in training 2. Change shoes to reduce stress on structures 3. Stretching exercises 4. Steroid injections
Patellar tendinitis (jumper's knee, anterior superior knee pain) (Fig. 4-7)	Microtears of the patellar ligament Caused by jumping, running (uphill), squatting, cutting maneuvers, standing from sitting position, walking	1. Focal pain at inferior pole of patella or proximal tendon 2. Improves with activity early in course or can have discomfort at rest		1. Rest 2. NSAIDs 3. Cryotherapy 4. Ultrasound-guided intratendinous injection of platelet-rich plasma 5. No steroid injections (contraindicated)
Popliteal (Baker) cyst, posteroinferior knee pain (Fig. 4-6)	Distention of a local bursa, communicating with the knee; herniation of the synovial membrane through the posterior joint capsule	1. Posterior knee pain or stiffness 2. Swelling/mass in popliteal fossa	1. Ultrasound 2. Arthrography or MRI for complete evaluation	1. Excision for relief

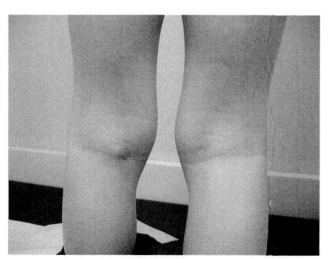

FIGURE 4-6. Popliteal (Baker) cyst. (From Waldman SD. *Comprehensive Atlas of Ultrasound-Guided Pain Management Injection Techniques.* Philadelphia: Lippincott Williams & Wilkins, a Wolters Kluwer business; 2014.)

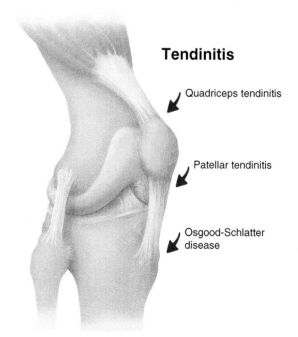

Tendinitis

Quadriceps tendinitis

Patellar tendinitis

Osgood-Schlatter disease

FIGURE 4-7. Types of tendinitis affecting the knee. (From Anatomical Chart Company. *Hip and Knee Inflammations.* Philadelphia: Wolters Kluwer; 2000.)

CHAPTER 5

Head, Ear, Eyes, Nose, and Throat

Recommended Supplemental Topics:

HEAD

Acute and Chronic Sinusitis (Rhinosinusitis)

- Sinusitis—inflammation of the area near the osteomeatal complex

- Rhinitis—inflammation of the nasal mucosa

Disease	Etiology, Prevalence, Risk Factors	Clinical Symptoms and Signs	Diagnostics	Therapy, Prognosis, and Health Maintenance

Acute sinusitis	Mostly viral
	MCC:
	S. pneumoniae,
	  H. influenzae,
	  Moraxella
	  catarrhalis
	Cofactor:
	Air pollution (tobacco
	  smoke), nasal
	  polyps, pregnancy,
	  rhinitis medica-
	  mentosa, oral
	  antihypertensives,
	  anti-osteoporosis
	  agents or HRT
	  sprays, mucociliary
	  dysfunction
		1. Follows URI
		2. Up to **4 wk**, 2 or more major signs and symptoms, 1 major and 2+ minor
		3. Nasal purulence on exam
		4. Rapid onset
		Major:
		1. **Facial pain, pressure**, or fullness
		2. **Nasal obstruction or blockage, nasal**, or **postnasal discharge**
		3. Purulence
		4. Hyposmia/anosmia
		5. **Fever** (acute only)
		Minor:
		1. Headaches
		2. Halitosis
		3. Fatigue
		4. Dental pain
		5. Cough
		6. Ear pain, pressure, or fullness
		Signs:
		1. **Tenderness to palpation over affected sinus**
		2. Nasal purulence or postnasal discharge
		3. Transillumination–decreased light transmission
			Clinical DX:
			1. Routine radiographs not recommended, but useful if unclear presentation
			2. Nasal endoscopy–for patients who do not respond to therapy
			3. CT ≫ MRI
				1. Supportive care
				• **NSAIDs** (for pain)
				• Hydration with oral fluid intake
				• **Nasal saline sprays**
				• **Steam**
				• Mucolytic: guaifenesin (Mucinex, Robitussin)
				Oral decongestant:
				• Pseudoephedrine (Sudafed)
				• Topical nasal vasoconstrictors–phenylephrine (Neo-Synephrine) or oxymetazoline (Afrin)
				• Intranasal steroids
				
				2. Oral antibiotics × 7-14 d, for fever, facial pain, or swelling
				• **Amoxicillin** (first line)
				• Amoxicillin/clavulanic acid (Augmentin)
				• PCN allergy–macrolides, **Bactrim**, or doxycicline
				• Fluoroquinolones
				• Third-generation cephalosporin
				3. Consider bacterial if symptoms worsen after 5 d, persist 10+ d, or out of proportion to viral infections

Subacute		4-12 wk; same as above Complications: orbital cellulitis, osteomyelitis, cavernous sinus thrombosis		
Chronic	MCC: S. aureus	12+ wk; same as above		
Recurrent cute		4+ episodes of acute disease per year, lasting 7+ d		

EARS

Labyrinthitis, Tinnitus, Meniere Disease, Tympanic Membrane Perforation

Disease	Etiology, Prevalence, Risk Factors	Clinical Symptoms and Signs	Diagnostics	Therapy, Prognosis, and Health Maintenance
Meniere disease (endolymphatic hydrops)	Excessive endolymph fluid in cochlea overstimulates hairs causing vertigo and sudden hearing loss with aural fullness Unknown etiology	1. **Sudden**, recurrent **vertigo** (lasting minutes to hours), lower range hearing loss 2. **Tinnitus** 3. One-sided aural pain, pressure, and/or fullness (unilateral) 4. **Hearing loss (low frequency)** 5. Nausea, vomiting Signs: 1. Nystagmus on impaired side	1. Audiometry at time of attack 2. Caloric testing	1. **Low-sodium, high-water diet** 2. **Diuretics** (acetazolamide) 3. Intratympanic gentamicin 4. Referral to ENT Health maintenance: 1. Avoid alcohol, caffeine, and tobacco

(continued)

(continued)

Disease	Etiology, Prevalence, Risk Factors	Clinical Symptoms and Signs	Diagnostics	Therapy, Prognosis, and Health Maintenance
Acoustic neuroma (vestibular schwannoma)	Intracranial benign tumor affecting CN VIII Bilateral acoustic neuromas, associated with **neurofibromatosis type II**	1. **Unilateral, progressive** sensorineural hearing loss (may also be acute) 2. **Unsteadiness** 3. **Vertigo** (continuous, late): vestibular deficit compensated centrally as it develops 4. **Tinnitus** 5. Impaired speech discrimination 6. Headache Signs: 1. Decreased corneal reflex sensitivity 2. Diplopia 3. Facial weakness	1. Head impulse test: deficient response when head rotated toward affected side 2. **MRI**: densely enhancing lesions, enlarging the internal auditory canal, and extending into the cerebellopontine angle 3. Lumbar puncture–elevated protein	1. Asymptomatic • Serial MRIs 2. Surgery or SRS for larger lesions Complication: loss of corneal reflex from trigeminal involvement
Labyrinthitis	Unknown etiology Likely viral, head injury, stress or allergy related	1. Acute severe vertigo, lasting several *days to a week* • Improves over a few weeks, but hearing loss may or may not resolve • Imbalance 2. Hearing loss 3. Nausea or vomiting Signs: 1. Severe nystagmus		1. Antibiotics for fever or signs of infection 2. Vestibular suppressants for acute symptoms • Diazepam • Meclizine 3. Symptoms regress after 3-6 wk
Tinnitus		1. Ringing in the ears	1. Comprehensive audiologic examination for unilateral persistent tinnitus or associated hearing impairment 2. Imaging for unilateral tinnitus, pulsatile tinnitus, asymmetric hearing loss, or focal neuro deficits	1. Hearing aids for tinnitus with hearing loss 2. CBT or sound therapy for persistent, bothersome tinnitus
Tympanic membrane perforation (barotrauma/ TM perforation)	1. **MCC: infection** (AOM) 2. Trauma (barotrauma, direct impact, explosion)	Most asymptomatic: 1. Audible **whistling** sounds during sneezing and nose blowing 2. **Decreased hearing** 3. Increased tendency of ear infection during colds and with water immersion Signs: 1. **Copious** sanguineous purulent drainage 2. Painless, if no overlying infection or cholesteatoma	Clinical DX: Tympanometry	1. Most self-resolve and asymptomatic, not requiring treatment • No treatment for nonswimming patients with minimal hearing loss and no history of recurrent ear infection • If only hearing loss: treat with hearing aid 2. Systemic antibiotics: Bactrim, amoxicillin 3. Trichloroacetic acid (10% solution) to cauterize edges of TMP 4. Surgical repair of TM as well as ossicular chain • Fat plug tympanoplasty • Tympanoplasty under sedation Health maintenance: 1. Avoid water exposure to ear 2. Avoid eardrops containing gentamicin, neomycin sulfate, or tobramycin

Drugs that cause vertigo (MALES-TIP)

- Methanol, alcohol, lithium, ethylene glycol, sedative hypnotics/solvents

- Thiamine depletion/carbamazepine (Tegretol), isopropanol, PCP/phenytoin (Dilantin)

Otitis Externa, Otitis Media, Cholesteatoma (Figs. 5-1–5-2)

Disease	Etiology, Prevalence, Risk Factors	Clinical Symptoms and Signs	Diagnostics	Therapy, Prognosis, and Health Maintenance
Otitis externa–bacterial	AKA "swimmer's ear" RF: Water exposure, trauma (scratching or cleaning), exfoliative skin conditions (psoriasis, eczema) MC bugs: *Pseudomonas*, proteus, fungi	1. Ear pain (especially with the movement of tragus or auricle or eating) Signs: 1. Redness/swelling of ear canal and purulent exudate 2. Foul smelling 3. Pre- or postauricular LAD	1. Tuning fork: BC > AC	1. Antibiotic otic drops and avoid further moisture or ear injury • Aminoglycosides: neomycin, polymyxin • **Fluoroquinolone**: ofloxacin (Floxin otic) 2. ±topical steroid Complications: In diabetic or immunocompromised patients–*malignant otitis externa* may develop (requires hospitalization with IV antibiotics) , periauricular cellulitis, cranial nerve palsies
Otitis externa–fungal (mycotic otitis externa)	MC pathology: *Aspergillus niger* (black), *A. flavus* (yellow), or *A. fumigatus* (gray) *Candida albicans* (white)	1. Pruritus 2. Weeping, pain, hearing loss, aural fullness Signs: 1. Swollen 2. Hyphae ± spores 3. Moist/wet appearance		1. Hygiene, clean 2. Topical antifungal powder + 3. Antifungal otic drops: acetic acid, Vosol 4. Prophylaxis: 1:1 ethanol (ETOH)/white vinegar in each ear after showering
Acute otitis media	Viral URI → eustachian tube dysfunction or blockage, buildup of fluid/mucus, anatomic deformities, or edema In infants and children (**S. pneumoniae,** *Haemophilus influenzae, Moraxella catarrhalis, Streptococcus pyogenes)* Adults–mostly viral (45%-70%)	1. Fever 2. Ear pain (otalgia)–supine or leaning forward 3. Ear pressure or fullness 4. Hearing impairment Otoscopic examination: 1. Tympanic membrane redness (erythema) 2. Pneumotoscopy–limited mobility 3. Bulging and/or rupture of tympanic membrane, leading to otorrhea and abrupt decrease in pain, pre- or postauricular LAD	1. Tuning fork: BC > AC 2. Tympanometry	1. Watchful waiting for older children without severe pain or fever 2. **HD amoxicillin** (first line) 80-90 mg/kg/d × 10-14 d • Ceftriaxone • Resistant cases: cefaclor or augmentin • Recurrent: *tympanostomy*, tympanocentesis, myringotomy Complications: Mastoiditis, facial nerve paralysis (Bell's palsy), central venous sinus thrombosis, short- or long-term hearing loss, speech delay, bacterial meningitis, intracranial abscess, TM perforation
Chronic otitis media	Repeated episodes of AOM, trauma or cholesteatoma MC bugs: *Pseudomonas,* **S. aureus**, Proteus, anaerobes	1. Perforated tympanic membrane and chronic clear discharge with or without pain 2. Tympanic membrane and/or ossicular damage can result in conductive hearing loss		1. Removal of infected debris, avoidance of water exposure, topical antibiotic drops • Ciprofloxacin and dexamethasone (CIPRODEX) 2. Surgery is definitive (tympanic membrane repair or reconstruction) 3. Tympanostomy tubes indicated for: chronic otitis media and its complications, recurrent AOM, and antibiotic failure in children • Made of silicon or Teflon, fall out spontaneously after 2-5 y

(continued)

(continued)

Disease	Etiology, Prevalence, Risk Factors	Clinical Symptoms and Signs	Diagnostics	Therapy, Prognosis, and Health Maintenance

Serous otitis media	Effusion without infection Retention of transudate fluid in the middle ear	HX:
		Recent viral URTI, sinus infection, flare of allergies, flying while congested, recent AOM, adenoid hypertrophy, nasopharyngeal mass
		1. Fullness, pressure
		2. Hearing loss
		3. *Popping/gurgling* after a yawn or blowing nose
		4. Dizziness or swimming sensation
		5. Unilateral or bilateral
		Signs:
		1. Retracted TM
		2. Amber- or "Coca Cola"–colored fluid
		3. Displacement of cone of light
		4. Air bubbles behind TM
			1. Pneumatic otoscopy reveals decreased movement of TM
			2. Tuning fork: BC > AC
				1. Resolves slowly (up to 12 wk)
				2. Follow up q 4-6
				  • Nasal steroid sprays
				  • Short course of PO steroids
				3. Consider tympanostomy after 3 mo
				Health maintenance:
				1. Avoid decongestants, antihistamines, antibiotics

Cholesteatoma	Chronic negative pressure thins the TM and retracts, adhering the TM to the middle ear → squamous epithelium forms inside and expands	HX of AOM or previous surgery: 1. Worsening hearing loss 2. Chronic discharge, fullness 3. **Not painful** Signs: 1. Pearly white mass 2. Squamous debris 3. Discharge 4. Conductive hearing loss	1. Weber test: lateralization to affected ear 2. Rinne test–bone > air conduction on affected side	1. Progressive, may lead to permanent hearing loss if left untreated

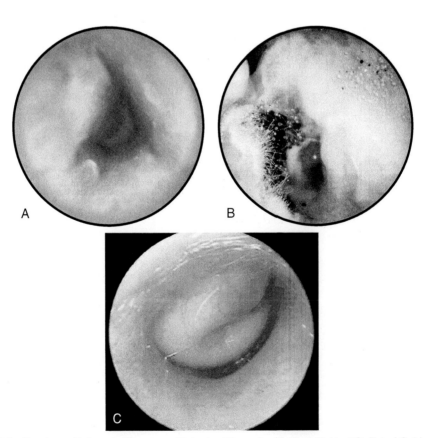

FIGURE 5-1. A, Bacterial otitis externa. **B**, Fungal otitis externa. **C**, Acute otitis media. (**A**, From Bickley LS. *Bates' Guide to Physical Examination and History Taking.* 8th ed. Philadelphia: Lippincott Williams & Wilkins; 2002. **B**, From Chung EK. *Visual Diagnosis and Treatment in Pediatrics.* 3rd ed. Philadelphia: Wolters Kluwer; 2015. **C**, From Johnson JT, Rosen CA, et al. *Bailey's Head & Neck Surgery: Otolaryngology.* 5th ed. Philadelphia: Lippincott Williams & Wilkins, a Wolters Kluwer business; 2014.)

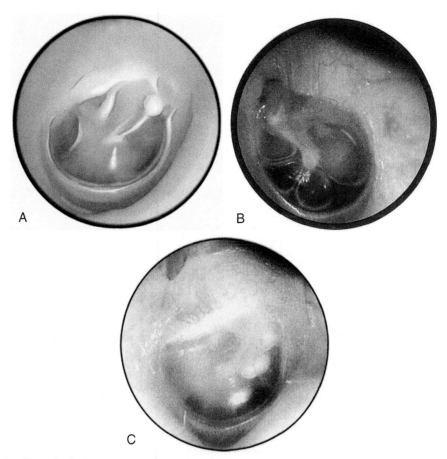

FIGURE 5-2. A, Chronic otitis media. **B**, Serous otitis media. **C**, Cholesteatoma. (**A**, From Jensen S. *Nursing Health Assessmet: A Best Practice Approach.* 2nd ed. Philadelphia: Wolters Kluwer; 2015. **B**, From Bickley LS. *Bates' Guide to Physical Examination and History Taking.* 8th ed. Lippincott Williams & Wilkins; 2002. **C**, From Chung EK. *Visual Diagnosis and Treatment in Pediatrics.* 2nd ed. Philadelphia: Wolters Kluwer; 2011.)

EYES

Blepharitis, Conjunctivitis, Dacryocystitis, Hordeolum

- Meibomian gland: sebaceous glands found within the tarsal plates of the eyelid and express oily layer of tear film responsible for preventing tear evaporation, reducing surface tension of tear layer, and aggregating tears over the corneal surface

Disease	Etiology, Prevalence, Risk Factors	Clinical Symptoms and Signs	Diagnostics	Therapy, Prognosis, and Health Maintenance

Blepharitis (Fig. 5-3A)	Chronic conjunctival and lid margin inflammation
	Causes: Seborrhea, staph or strep infection, dysfunction of the Meibomian glands
	Posterior blepharitis—more common, inflammation of inner eyelid at level of Meibomian gland (also known as Meibomian gland dysfunction)
		1. Rims are red, eyelashes adhere
		2. Dandruff-like deposits (scurf) and fibrous scales (collarettes)
		3. Clear to red conjunctiva
		4. Possible thick, cloudy discharge
		5. Gritty or burning sensation
		6. Excessive tearing
		7. Itchy eyelids
		8. Light sensitivity
		Signs:
		1. Greasy appearance of lid margin with scaling around the base of the lashes
			1. Slit lamp exam	1. **Warm compresses**
				  • 5-10 min, 2-4 times per day
				2. Lid massage to empty glands and improve secretion
				3. Lid washing
				  • Lid scrubs using diluted baby shampoo on cotton-tipped swabs
				4. Topical antibiotics if suspected infection
				  • Azithromycin 1%, erythromycin, bacitracin
				5. Oral antibiotics
				  • Azithromycin, doxycycline, tetracycline
				6. Associated—rosacea, seborrheic dermatitis

(continued)

(continued)

Disease	Etiology, Prevalence, Risk Factors	Clinical Symptoms and Signs	Diagnostics	Therapy, Prognosis, and Health Maintenance
Bacterial conjunctivitis (Fig. 5-3B)	Associated: steroid or OTC eye drops, contact lens wearers, age, sexual activity, immunodeficiency MC: *S. pneumoniae*, *S. aureus*, *Hemophilus aegyptius*, *Moraxella catarrhalis* Transmission: Direct contact or fomites; autoinoculation Rare: *Chlamydia trachomatis*, *Neisseria gonorrhoeae* Transmission: Direct contact, fomites, nonchlorinated swimming pools, sexual contact, vaginal delivery	1. Segmental or diffuse injection, **purulent discharge**, "mattering" or lid margin 2. Difficulty prying open lids after awakening Signs: 1. No preauricular lymphadenopathy 2. Yellow-green discharge from eyes 3. Bilateral conjunctival injection		Self-limiting, but secondary keratitis may develop 1. Topical **sulfonamide**, gentamicin, tobramycin, norfloxacin, or trimethoprim polymyxin B sulfate 2. Good handwashing 3. Avoid contaminated pillows, makeup, and towels to prevent reinfection
Viral conjunctivitis (pinkeye) (Fig. 5-3C)	Most common: Adenovirus 3, 8, or 19 Highly contagious Transmission: Direct contact, **swimming pools** MC: Midsummer to early fall Benign	Associated symptoms: recent URTI, no resolution with eye drops 1. Unilateral or bilateral erythema of the conjunctiva 2. Ipsilateral **preauricular lymphadenopathy** 3. Epiphora—excessive watery discharge (tearing) Signs: 1. Hyperemia 2. Chemosis 3. Follicular conjunctival injection 4. Subconjunctival hemorrhage		1. Eye lavage with normal saline × 7-14 d • Vasoconstrictor antihistamine drops • **Ophthalmic sulfonamide drops** 2. Supportive (cold compress, lubricants—artificial tears), hand hygiene Prognosis: 1. Self-limiting (2-4 wk)
Seasonal allergic	Occurs year-round, usually symptom free in the winter	HX of rhinitis (runny nose) 1. Itchy eyes 2. Clear, watery discharge Signs: 1. Conjunctival injection 2. Chemosis 3. Eyelid edema		1. Supportive therapy: cool compresses 2. Topical histamine H1 receptor antagonists
Hordeolum (Fig. 5-3D)	Acute development of a small, mildly painful nodule or pustule within a gland in upper or lower eyelid MC bug: **S. aureus** Not contagious Inflammation of Meibomian gland (internal) with pustular formation; deep **Glands of Zeis** (external, **stye**) infection at eyelid margin, points outward	1. Acute onset, redness and pain 2. Edema of involved eyelid 3. Occurs on upper or lower eyelid Palpable indurated area on eyelid with central purulence and surrounding erythema		Spontaneously resolves 1. Warm compress several times daily × 2 d 2. Topical antibiotics for secondary infection 3. I&D if no resolution

Disease	Etiology, Prevalence, Risk Factors	Clinical Symptoms and Signs	Diagnostics	Therapy, Prognosis, and Health Maintenance
Chalazion (Fig. 5-3E)	Obstruction of Meibomian gland (granuloma) or internal posterior hordeolum Secondary to chronic inflammation of internal hordeolum	1. *Painless*, nontender, noninflamed swelling (nodule) 2. Develops *over weeks* (chronic), minimal irritation 3. White or gray 4. May become itchy 5. Eyelid may become red	Deep indurated lesion from palpebral margin	1. **Hot compress** 2. Referral to ophthalmologist for elective excision • Oral doxycycline or tetracycline
Dacryocystitis (Fig. 5-4A)	Inflammation of the lacrimal gland caused by obstruction Acute: ***S. aureus* and β-hemolytic strep**, *S. epidermidis*, *Candida* <u>Chronic:</u> *Candida albicans*, anaerobic streptococci, *S. epidermidis*	1. Painful erythema over the tear duct at nasal side of eye • Swelling, tenderness 2. Tearing and/or purulent drainage		1. Hot compress 2. Antibiotics If an abscess forms → zI&D required If recurrent → dacryocystorhinostomy or dacryocystectomy
Dacryostenosis (Fig. 5-4B)	Common in newborn (first month) when duct does not open	1. Epiphora from affected eye from birth 2. Morning crusting and heavy matting		Resolves by 9 mo of age 2. Hot compress, massage 3. Surgical probe
Dacryoadenitis (Fig. 5-4C)	Acute inflammation of the lacrimal gland seen in sterile inflammatory disease Mostly due to gram-positive bacteria <u>MC virus:</u> EBV	1. Abrupt onset of swelling of upper eyelids, laterally	Bilateral dacryoadenitis seen in mumps	

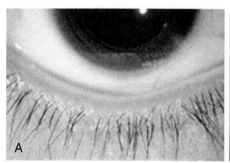
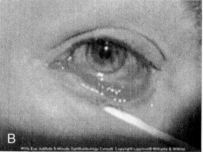
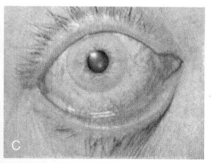
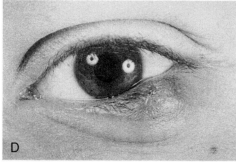
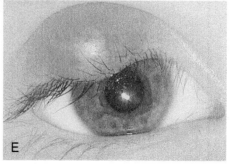

FIGURE 5-3. **A**, Blepharitis. **B**, Bacterial conjunctivitis. **C**, Viral conjunctivitis. **D**, Hordeolum. **E**, Chalazion. (**A-C**, From Wolters Kluwer Health Library. **D**, From Goodheart HP. *Goodheart's Photoguide of Common Skin Disorders: Diagnosis and Management.* 2nd ed. Philadelphia: Lippincott Williams & Wilkins; 2003. **E**, From Nurse's 5-Minute Clinical Consult. *Diseases.* Philadelphia: Lippincott Williams & Wilkins, a Wolters Kluwer business; 2007.)

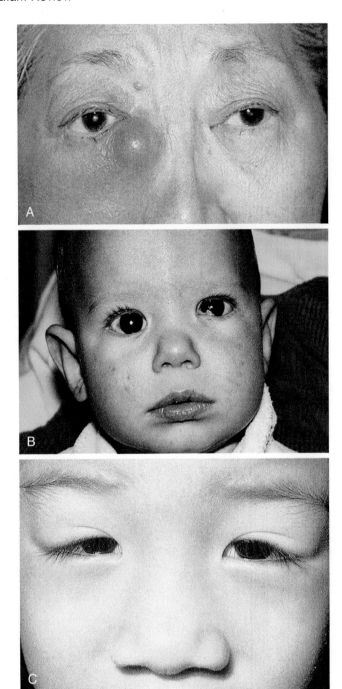

FIGURE 5-4. A, Dacryocystitis. **B,** Dacryostenosis. **C,** Dacryoadenitis. (**A,** From Chern KC, Saidel MA. *Ophthalmology Review Manual.* 2nd ed. Lippincott Williams & Wilkins, a Wolters Kluwer business; 2012. **B,** From Shaw KN, Bachur RG. *Fleisher & Ludwig's Textbook of Pediatric Emergency Medicine.* 7th ed. Philadelphia: Wolters Kluwer; 2016. **C,** From Gold DH, Weingeist TA. *Color Atlas of the Eye ini Systemic Disease.* Philadelphia: Lippincott Williams and Wilkins; 2001.)

Ectropion, Entropion (Fig. 5-5A and B)

Disease	Etiology, Prevalence, Risk Factors
Ectropion	Outward turning of eyelid
Entropion	Inward turning of eyelid

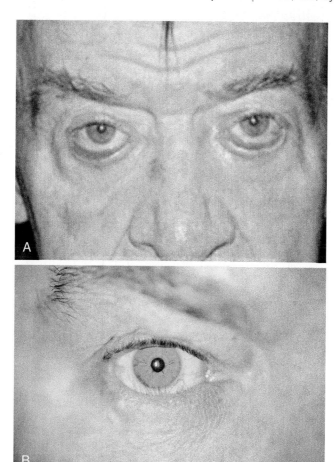

FIGURE 5-5. **A**, Ectropion. **B**, Entropion. (**A**, From Wolters Kluwer Health Library. **B**, From Penne RB. *Wills Eye Institute Color Atlas & Synopsis of Clinical Ophthalmology: Oculoplastics.* 2nd ed. Philadelphia: Lippincott Williams & Wilkins, a Wolters Kluwer business; 2012.)

Corneal Abrasion and Corneal Ulcer

Disease	Etiology, Prevalence, Risk Factors	Clinical Symptoms and Signs	Diagnostics	Therapy, Prognosis, and Health Maintenance
Corneal abrasion (Fig. 5-6A)	MC etiology: contact lenses Other causes: Fingernail, eyelash, small foreign body	1. Eye pain and foreign body sensation 2. Photophobia 3. Tearing, injection 4. Blepharospasm 5. Blurred vision Signs: 1. Multiple vertical linear abrasions (*ice rink sign*) under upper eyelid suggests foreign body 2. Record visual acuity before examining or treating	1. Slit-lamp examination or fluorescein stain–epithelial defect but clear cornea	1. Topical anesthetic to confirm diagnosis only 2. Saline irrigation to loosen debris 3. Antibiotic ointment (gentamicin or sulfacetamide), Tylenol for pain 4. Patching no longer than 24 h for large abrasions (5-10 mm) 5. Daily follow-up and referral
Corneal ulcer	MC bugs: **Pseudomonas**, *Staph, Strep*, HSV, *Acanthamoeba* Etiology: Contact lenses, especially if wearing underwater; trauma, poor lid apposition	1. Eye pain 2. Photophobia 3. Discharge–tearing 4. Decreased vision 5. Foreign-body sensation Signs: 1. Circumcorneal injection 2. Watery to purulent discharge	1. Stains and cultures ASAP • Slit-lamp examination: dense corneal infiltrate with overlying epithelial defect Dendritic lesion = herpes keratitis	1. **Immediate ophthalmology consult** 2. Intensive topical antibiotics • Fluoroquinolone • Cephalosporin or vancomycin ± aminoglycoside **Steroids and eye-patching contraindicated** • Discontinue lens wearing, discard opened lens and solutions, sterilize lens equipment

(continued)

Disease	Etiology, Prevalence, Risk Factors	Clinical Symptoms and Signs	Diagnostics	Therapy, Prognosis, and Health Maintenance
Acute iritis (anterior uveitis) (Fig. 5-6B)		1. Eye or periorbital pain 2. Headaches Signs: 1. Hypopyon 2. Irregular pupil 3. Consensual photophobia 4. Floaters 5. Dilated ciliary vessels (injection or flush)	1. Slit lamp examination: "cells and flare" in anterior chamber 2. Keratic precipitates (KP) on posterior surface of cornea	Refer to ophthalmology or rheumatology 1. Steroid and dilating drops
Herpes keratitis (Fig. 5-6C)	Etiology: HSV-1	1. Painful eye 2. Blurred vision 3. Tearing 4. Photophobia Signs: 1. Conjunctivitis 2. Hutchinson sign: herpetic lesion on tip of nose	1. Slit-lamp examination: dendritic ulcer (branch-like) lesion	1. Most spontaneously resolve in 3 wk

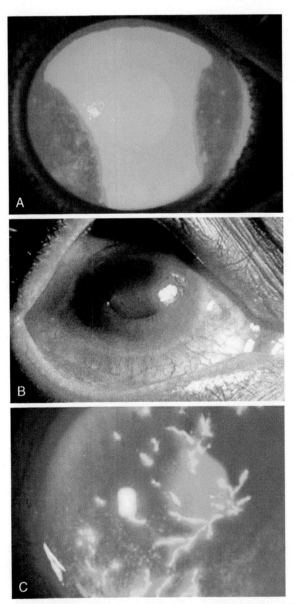

FIGURE 5-6. A, Corneal abrasion. **B,** Acute iritis. **C,** Herpes keratitis. (**A,** From Miller MG, Berry DC. *Emergency Response Management for Athletic Trainers.* 2nd ed. Philadelphia: Wolters Kluwer; 2016. **B,** From McDonagh D. *FIMS Sports Medicine Manual: Event Planning and Emergency Care.* Philadelphia: Lippincott Williams & Wilkins, a Wolters Kluwer business; 2012. **C,** From Rapuano CJ. *Wills Eye Institute Color Atlas & Synopsis of Clinical Ophthalmology: Cornea.* 2nd ed. Philadelphia: Lippincott Williams & Wilkins, a Wolters Kluwer business; 2012.)

Glaucoma (Fig. 5-7)

Disease	Etiology, Prevalence, Risk Factors	Clinical Symptoms and Signs	Diagnostics	Therapy, Prognosis, and Health Maintenance
Glaucoma		Increased IOP with optic nerve damage	1. Visual field testing, ophthalmoscopy, gonioscopy (determines cause), tonometry to measure IOP Normal IOP: 10-21 mm Hg	
Acute (angle closure or closed angle) "Halos around lights"	Peripheral iris blocks outflow of aqueous humor from the anterior chamber into the canal of Schlemm, associated papillary dilation RF: Elderly, Asians, hyperopes	1. Sudden **dull or severe eye pain** (bilateral), worse in dark rooms 2. Blurry vision, decreased visual acuity 3. Frontal headache 4. Tearing 5. GI: **nausea, vomiting** 6. Sweating Physical examination: 1. Conjunctival hyperemia with ciliary flush 2. **Cloudy,** "steamy" **or** "stippled" **(hazy) cornea** 3. **Mid-position or mid-dilated and nonreactive pupil**	1. Penlight test—hold laterally and direct nasally; will project a shadow on nasal side of iris with narrow anterior chamber 2. **Tonometry**—Markedly increased IOP (>50) 3. Cornea is edematous 4. Pupil dilated and nonreactive	1. Refer immediately 2. First-line **topical** agents decrease aqueous humor production • **β-Blockers** (timolol, betaxolol, levobunolol) • α-Antagonists (brimonidine, apraclonidine) • Prostaglandin analogues (latanoprost) 3. Topical miotic: pilocarpine ineffective with severe or prolonged high IOP 4. Adjunct cycloplegic agents • **IV acetazolamide** • Osmotic diuretics: **IV mannitol**, glycerol, isosorbide 5. Laser iridotomy (*definitive*) or incisional peripheral iridectomy done by an ophthalmologist Do not administer mydriatics to these patients
Chronic (primary open angle)	More common than acute RF: **Age 40+, African Americans**, and patients with FH of glaucoma or **diabetes** MCC: Outflow obstruction through trabecular meshwork	1. **Gradual loss of peripheral vision** 2. Painless	1. Increased IOP, defects in peripheral visual field, increased cup-to-disc ratio	1. Refer immediately 2. Topical meds (β-blocker, α-agonist, carbonic anhydrase inhibitor) to decrease production 3. Prostaglandin analogue, cholinergics, or epinephrine to increase outflow 4. Laser or surgical treatment

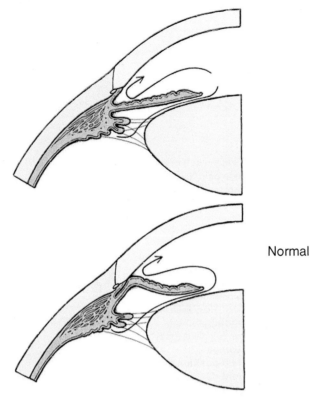

Normal

FIGURE 5-7. Glaucoma. *Top*, A normal angle between the iris and cornea exists where aqueous humor drains, but the eye's drainage canals become clogged over time and excess fluid cannot drain appropriately in open angle glaucoma. The iris blocks the canal, limiting flow of aqueous humor from the anterior chamber in angle-closure glaucoma. (From Ford FM. *Roach's Introductory Clinical Pharmacology.* 11th ed. Philadelphia: Wolters Kluwer; 2018.)

- Note: elevated IOP without optic nerve damage is called ocular hypertension

Hyphema, Papilledema, Pterygium

Disease	Etiology, Prevalence, Risk Factors	Clinical Symptoms and Signs	Diagnostics	Therapy, Prognosis, and Health Maintenance
Hyphema (Fig. 5-8A)	Blood in the anterior chamber resulting from a rupture of one or more iris stromal vessels Most common in children (70%) <u>RF:</u> Sickle cell disease or trait, African American, aspirin use			1. Rest, elevation of head 2. Topical steroids <u>Health maintenance:</u> 1. Avoid ASA and NSAIDs <u>Complications:</u> 4 S's 1. **S**taining of the cornea 2. **S**ynechiae (iris adheres to cornea or lens) 3. **S**econdary rebleed on days 2-5 4. **S**ignificantly increased IOP <u>Prognosis:</u> 1. Poor prognostic factors—hyphema in greater $\frac{1}{3}$ of anterior chamber, treatment after 24 h, high IOP, prior low visual acuity

Disease	Etiology, Prevalence, Risk Factors	Clinical Symptoms and Signs	Diagnostics	Therapy, Prognosis, and Health Maintenance
Papilledema (Fig. 5-8B) Bilateral edema of the head of the optic nerve due to increased intracranial pressure → disc margins are blurred, cup is diminished or absent, nerve head is elevated with vascular congestion, flame-shaped hemorrhages are seen on or adjacent to nerve head	Increased intracranial pressure that causes optic disc swelling Causes: **Malignant hypertension**, hemorrhagic stroke, acute subdural hematoma, pseudotumor cerebri	Asymptomatic or: 1. Transient visual alterations (*seconds*) 2. **Bilateral** 3. Develops over hours to weeks	1. Disc appears swollen, margins blurred, obliteration of the vessels 2. ICP: increased	1. Treat underlying cause
Optic neuritis (Fig. 5-8C) Optic nerve swelling causes destruction of myelin sheath	MCC: Multiple sclerosis	1. **Pain** with movement of the affected eye • Precedes visual loss 2. Sudden **unilateral central** vision loss • Blurry or "foggy" vision 3. Central scotoma and change in color perception Signs: 1. No chemosis or conjunctival injection 2. APD present 3. Fundoscopic examination: swollen, edematous optic disc (papillitis)	1. ICP—normal 2. Red desaturation test—have patient look with one eye at a dark red object and then test other eye to see if object looks same color → affected eye will see red object as pink or light red	1. IV or PO steroids 2. Consult neurology and ophthalmology
Pterygium (Fig. 5-8D)	"Surfer's eye" Commonly grows from the nasal side of the conjunctiva Small, raised, conjunctival nodule at the temporal or nasal limbus that encroaches on the corneal surface	1. Slowly growing thickening of bulbar conjunctiva 2. Unilateral or bilateral 3. Interferes with vision if it reaches the cornea		1. Excision (if interference with vision) Recurrence is common, may be more aggressive

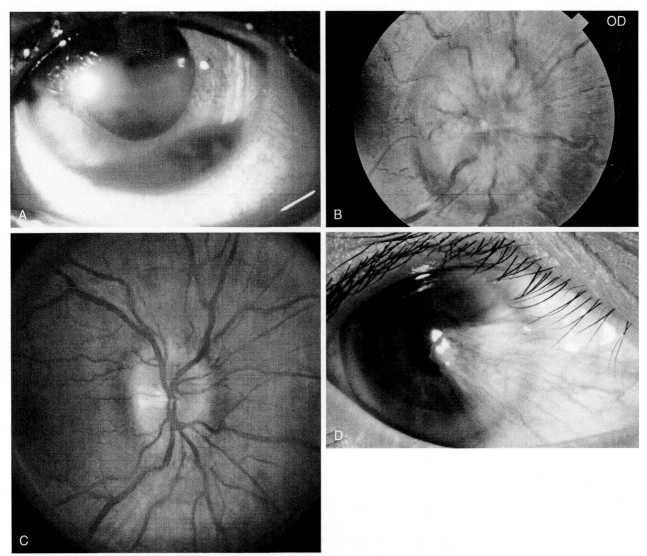

FIGURE 5-8. **A**, Hyphema. **B**, Papilledema. **C**, Optic neuritis. **D**, Pterygium. (**A**, From Rhee DJ. *Wills Eye Institute Color Atlas & Synopsis of Clinical Ophthalmology: Glaucoma.* 2nd ed. Lippincott Williams & Wilkins, a Wolters Kluwer business; 2012. **B**, From Joynt RJ. *Baker and Joynt's Clinical Neurology 2004.* Lippincott Williams & Wilkins; 2004. **C**, From Miller NR, Subramanian PS, Patel VR. *Walsh and Hoyt's Clinical Neuro-Ophthalmology: The Essentials.* 3rd ed. Philadelphia: Wolters Kluwer; 2015. **D**, From Rapuano CJ. *Wills Eye Institute Color Atlas & Synopsis of Clinical Ophthalmology: Cornea.* 2nd ed. Philadelphia: Lippincott Williams & Wilkins, a Wolters Kluwer business; 2012.)

Retinopathy

Disease	Etiology, Prevalence, Risk Factors	Clinical Symptoms and Signs	Therapy, Prognosis, and Health Maintenance
Retinopathy	Systemic disorders, including diabetes, hypertension, preeclampsia-eclampsia, blood dyscrasias, and HIV disease may affect the retina		
Diabetic *proliferative* retinopathy (Fig. 5-9A)	Prolonged **hyperglycemia** <u>causes</u>: 1. Basement membrane thickening 2. Decreased pericytes (hyperproliferation) 3. Microaneurysms 4. Neovascularization Leading cause of blindness in adults	1. **Neovascularization** breaks through ILM (inner limiting membrane) leading to tractional retinal detachment 2. **Vitreous hemorrhage**	1. If diabetic, get yearly dilated ophthalmoscopic examinations 2. Optimize glucose control 3. Regulate blood pressure 4. Laser photocoagulation 5. Vitrectomy
Nonproliferative retinopathy (Fig. 5-9B)		1. Microaneurysms 2. Hard exudates 3. Retinal hemorrhage 4. Venous dilation	

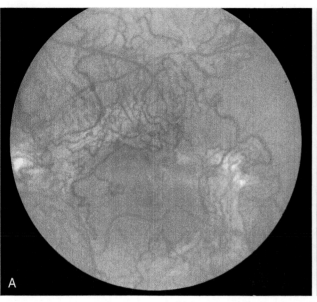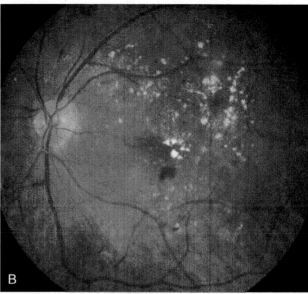

FIGURE 5-9. A, Diabetic proliferative retinopathy. **B,** Nonproliferative retinopathy. (**A,** From Grossman S, Porth CM. *Porth's Pathophysiology: Concepts of Altered Health States.* 9th ed. Wolters Kluwer Health; 2014. **B,** From Gerstenblith AT, Rabinowitz MP. *The Wills Eye Manual Office and Emergency Room Diagnosis and Treatment of Eye Disease.* 6th ed. Philadelphia: Lippincott Williams & Wilkins, a Wolters Kluwer business; 2012.)

Retinal Detachment, Retinal Vascular Occlusion, Macular Degeneration

Disease	Etiology, Prevalence, Risk Factors	Clinical Symptoms and Signs	Diagnostics	Therapy, Prognosis, and Health Maintenance
Retinal detachment (Fig. 5-10A)	Separation of the retina from the pigmented epithelial layer causing the detached tissue to appear as a flap in the vitreous humor Can occur spontaneously or secondary to trauma or extreme myopia	"**Curtain of darkness**" with peripheral flashes or spider webs and floaters 1. Preceding posterior vitreous detachment: *photopsia* (**flashes of light**), **floaters**, feeling of heaviness in eye → followed by 2. **Acute onset, painless vision loss** • Peripheral to central vision loss 3. Blurred or blackened (Fig. 5-10B) vision (over several <u>hours</u>) → partial or complete monocular blindness <u>Physical examination:</u> 1. Relative APD	Gray detached retina flapping in vitreous humor	1. **Emergent ophthalmology consult** • Remain supine with head turned to side of retinal detachment 2. Laser surgery or cryosurgery <u>Prognosis:</u> 1. 80% recover with no recurrence with intervention 2. 15% require retreatment 3. 5% will never reattach
Central retinal artery occlusion (*cherry-red spot*, ischemic retina) (Fig. 5-11A)	Flow through CRA occluded <u>Associated:</u> ***Atherosclerotic*** thrombosis, embolus, giant cell arteritis	1. **Sudden**, painless **unilateral** vision loss <u>Physical examination:</u> • ***Pale-gray retina***, APD, cherry dot	Funduscopy: arteriolar narrowing, separation of arterial flow (box-carring), retinal edema, perifoveal atrophy (cherry red spot), ganglionic death leads to optic atrophy and pale retina	1. **Emergent ophthalmologic consult** (decrease IOP; arterial dilation, paracentesis) 2. Workup and management of atherosclerotic disease Irreversible damage to retina after 90 min • Poor prognosis

(continued)

(continued)

Disease	Etiology, Prevalence, Risk Factors	Clinical Symptoms and Signs	Diagnostics	Therapy, Prognosis, and Health Maintenance
Central retinal vein occlusion (*blood and thunder fundus*) (Fig. 5-11B)	50+ MC associated: HTN, POAG Occurs secondary to **thrombotic** event	1. **Sudden**, painless **unilateral** vision loss 2. Blurred vision or complete visual loss Exam: 1. Retinal hemorrhages in all quadrants 2. Edema of optic disc	Funduscopy: dilated veins, macular edema, cotton wool spot, massive superficial/deep hemorrhage with vitreous involvement	1. Spontaneously resolves over time 2. Workup for thrombosis
Age-related macular degeneration (ARMD) (Fig. 5-12A)	RF: *Long history of **smoking**,* metabolic syndrome, family history, female, white, **age 50+** Other causes: drugs (chloroquine, phenothiazine) Leading cause of irreversible central vision loss	1. Insidious onset 2. **Gradual** loss of ***central vision*** clarity • Metamorphopsia: wavy or distorted vision, measured with Amsler grid (Fig. 5-12B)	1. **Drusen formation**, mottling, serous leaks, hemorrhages on retina	No effective treatment: 1. Laser therapy 2. **Anti-VEGF intravitreal injections** of monoclonal antibody drugs: slows progression 3. Vitamins and antioxidants slow progression
Senile (age-related) cataract (Fig. 5-13)	Leading cause of blindness in world Opacity of lens of the eye that causes partial or total blindness MCC: Age-related nuclear sclerosis Other RF besides age: Smoking (2×), ETOH, **sunlight exposure,** low education, malnutrition, physical inactivity, metabolic syndrome, diabetes, steroid use, statin use	1. Painless, progressive loss of vision 2. Bilateral, asymmetrical field of vision 3. Difficulty driving at night, reading road signs, or reading fine print Signs: 1. Funduscopic examination: darkening of red reflex, obscured ocular fundus		1. Nonurgent referral to ophthalmologist 2. Conservative–change in glasses prescription 3. Surgery • Indications: if symptoms interfere with ability to perform ADLs; no criteria based on level of visual acuity • No advantage to removing sooner • Extracapsular cataract extraction vs. phacoemulsification

- Blindness: Internationally defined as the inability to count fingers at 10 feet; this converts to 10/200 on Snellen notation. This means that at 10 feet you can see what a normal person would see at 200 feet. In the United States, 20/200 is considered legal blindness.

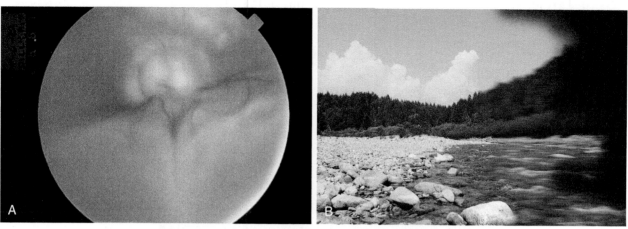

FIGURE 5-10. **A**, Retinal detachment. **B**, Its visual effect. (**A**, From Nelson LB, Olitsky SE. *Harley's Pediatric Ophthalmology*. 6th ed. Philadelphia: Wolters Kluwer; 2014. **B**, From Cosby KS, Kendall JL. *Practical Guide to Emergency Ultrasound*. 2nd ed. Philadelphia: Wolters Kluwer; 2014.)

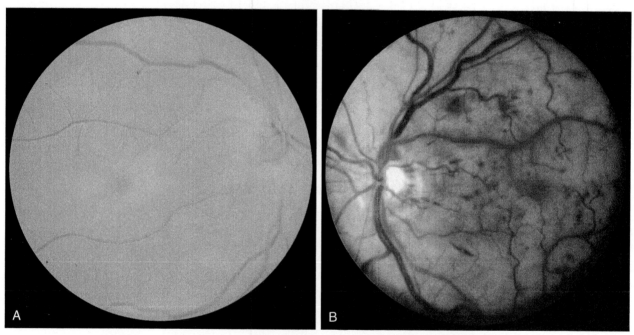

FIGURE 5-11. **A**, Central retinal artery occlusion. **B**, Central retinal vein occlusion. (**A**, From Stoller JK, Nielsen C, Buccola J, Brateau A. *The Cleveland Clinic Foundation Intensive Review of Internal Medicine*. 6th ed. Philadelphia: Wolters Kluwer Health; 2014. **B**, From Fineman MS, Ho AC. *Wills Eye Institute Color Atlas & Synopsis of Clinical Ophthalmology: Retina*. 2nd ed. Philadelphia: Lippincott Williams & Wilkins, a Wolters Kluwer business; 2012.)

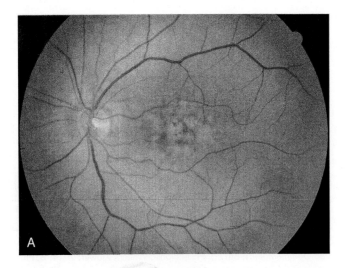

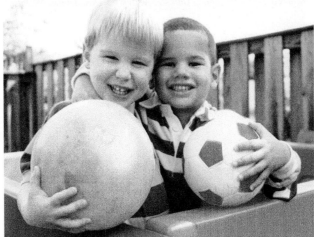

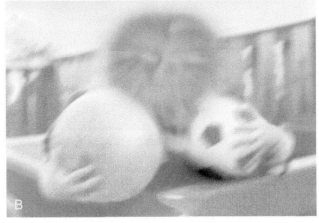

FIGURE 5-12. **A**, Acute related macular degeneration. **B**, Its visual effect. (**A**, From King M, Lipsky M. *Step-Up to Geriatrics*. Philadelphia: Wolters Kluwer; 2017. **B**, From Timby BK, Smith NE. *Introductory Medical-Surgical Nursing*. 11th ed. Philadelphia: Wolters Kluwer Health; 2014.)

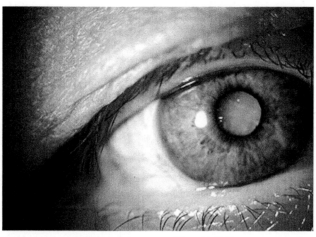

FIGURE 5-13. Senile, age-related cataract. (From UpToDate. www.uptodate.com.)

NOSE

Allergic Rhinitis/Nasal Congestion

Disease	Etiology, Prevalence, Risk Factors	Clinical Symptoms and Signs	Diagnostics	Therapy, Prognosis, and Health Maintenance
Allergic rhinitis	IgE-mediated reactivity to airborne antigens (pollen, molds, danders, dust) RF: Family history, atopic triad Atopic triad: Asthma, eczema, allergic rhinitis	Symptoms similar to common cold 1. Allergic shiners (blue discoloration below eyes) 2. Rhinorrhea 3. Itchy, watery eyes 4. Sneezing 5. Nasal congestion 6. Dry cough Signs: 1. Pale, boggy, bluish mucosa 2. Horizontal nasal crease from habitual rubbing of nose 3. Clear and watery discharge	Clinical DX	1. Avoid known allergens and use antihistamines 2. Cromolyn sodium 3. Nasal or systemic corticosteroids 4. Nasal saline drops or washes 5. Immunotherapy
Vasomotor rhinitis	Rhinorrhea caused by increased secretion of mucus from the nasal mucosa	1. Bogginess of the nasal mucosa + stuffiness and rhinorrhea 2. Symptoms disappear quickly 3. Worse with changes in temperature or humidity, odors, or alcohol, or results from neurologic imbalance	Clinical DX	1. Avoid irritants or precipitants
Rhinitis medicamentosa	Overuse of decongestant drugs containing oxymetazoline or phenylephrine	1. Rebound congestion promoting increased use of decongestant drug 2. Severe congestion and pain 3. Minimal discharge	Clinical DX	1. Discontinue decongestants

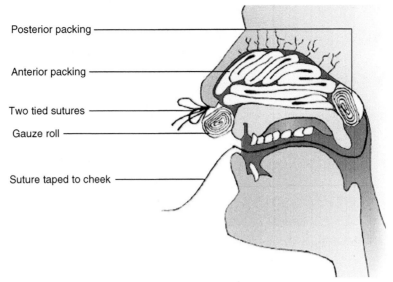

Posterior packing

Anterior packing

Two tied sutures

Gauze roll

Suture taped to cheek

FIGURE 5-14. Nasal packing. When nasal packing is administered, families and staff should be mindful of the patient's vital signs, watching for signs of shortness of breath, hypoxia, tachycardia, or restlessness. The patient's head of bed should be elevated allowing them to breathe through the mouth and oxygen should be given if needed. Flashlights, scissors, and hemostats should be kept nearby in case the cheek suture needs to be cut or the catheter needs to be deflated. The pack should be removed if signs of airway obstruction or respiratory distress ensue. Lastly, avoid tension on the cheek suture. Remind the patient not to blow their nose for 48 hours after packing is removed. (From *Lippincott's Nursing Advisor 2013*. Philadelphia: Wolters Kluwer; 2013.)

Epistaxis

- Local trauma is the most common cause, followed by facial trauma, foreign bodies, sinus infections, and prolonged inhalation of dry air (low humidity), medications (antihistamines, corticosteroids)

- Children typically present owing to local irritation or recent URI

Disease	Etiology, Prevalence, Risk Factors	Clinical Symptoms and Signs	Diagnostics	Therapy, Prognosis, and Health Maintenance
Anterior epistaxis	Anterior—**Kiesselbach plexus,** also known as Little area (most common) RF: Nose picking, dry nasal mucosa, HTN, cocaine use, alcohol use More than 90% of bleeds	1. Typically unilateral and easily visualized	Clinical DX	1. **Direct pressure** at site of bleeding • Sit, leaning forward • Compress nares 15 min 2. If continued, identify site (anterior vs posterior) 3. Topical cocaine used as anesthetic and vasoconstrictor, or other topical decongestants (oxymetazoline) and anesthetics (lidocaine) 4. Electrocautery or silver nitrate can be used with visible bleeding source 5. Anterior packing (Fig. 5-14)
Posterior epistaxis	Posterior—less common (5%) occurring in Woodruff plexus RF: HTN, atherosclerosis	1. Typically bilateral or from the posterior pharynx 2. If placement of anterior pack does not stop bleeding and bleeding noted in posterior pharynx	Clinical DX	1. Posterior packing is difficult and high risk of complications 2. Consult with inpatient monitoring • Balloon catheter 3. Nasal arterial supply ligation Prognosis: 1. Greater risk of airway compromise, aspiration of blood, and more difficult to control bleeding
Nasal polyps (Fig. 5-15)	Associated: allergic rhinitis, history of nasal polyps and asthma	1. Pale, boggy masses on the nasal mucosa 2. Chronic congestion 3. Decreased sense of smell		1. 3-mo course of topical nasal corticosteroid (first line) for small polyps 2. Oral steroids with 6-d taper to reduce size 3. Surgical removal Note: aspirin contraindicated—possibility of severe bronchospasm (Samter triad)

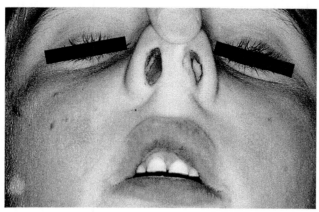

FIGURE 5-15. Nasal polyps. (From Fleisher GR, Ludwig S, Baskin MN. *Atlas of Pediatric Emergency Medicine.* Lippincott Williams & Wilkins; 2004.)

THROAT

Pharyngitis and Tonsillitis

Disease	Etiology, Prevalence, Risk Factors	Clinical Symptoms and Signs	Diagnostics	Therapy, Prognosis, and Health Maintenance
Acute (*Strep*) pharyngitis and tonsillitis (Fig. 5-16A)	Group A B-hemolytic streptococci (GABHS)—treat to prevent complications Viral ≫ bacterial	1. **Rapid onset high fever (>38°C or 100.4°F)** 2. **Sore throat** 3. **Lack of cough** 4. Not-suggestive of strep pharyngitis: coryza, hoarseness, cough Signs: • Beefy-red uvula • Tender anterior cervical adenopathy • Palatal petechiae • Gray furry tongue 4. **Pharyngotonsillar (white) exudate** Centor criteria: Presence of 1-4 suggests GABHS	1. If 3/4 criteria met → **rapid streptococcal test** sensitivity >90% 2. If negative → throat culture (confirms, gold standard)	1. **IM penicillin** (if compliance unlikely) 2. Oral penicillin or cefuroxime 3. PCN allergy: macrolide (erythromycin) Complications: scarlet fever, glomerulonephritis, abscess formation
Exudative pharyngitis (Fig. 5-16B)				

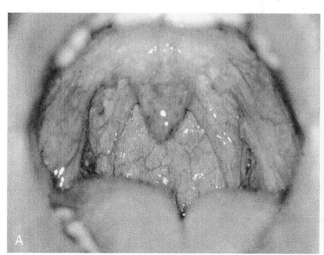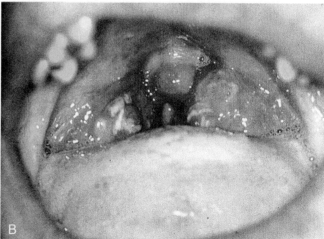

FIGURE 5-16. **A**, Streptococcal pharyngitis. **B**, Exudative pharyngitis. (From Bickley LS. *Bates' Guide to Physical Examination and History Taking.* 8th ed. Lippincott Williams & Wilkins; 2002.)

Peritonsillar Abscess, Aphthous Ulcers, and Laryngitis

Disease	Etiology, Prevalence, Risk Factors	Clinical Symptoms and Signs	Diagnostics	Therapy, Prognosis, and Health Maintenance
Peritonsillar abscess/ cellulitis (quinsy) (Fig. 5-17A)	Penetration of infection through tonsillar capsule	1. Sore throat 2. Pain with swallowing (odynophagia) 3. Trismus—spasm of jaw muscles 4. Deviation of soft palate or uvula 5. **Muffled** "hot potato" **voice** Signs: 1. Deviation of the soft palate 2. Asymmetric rise of the uvula (*abscess*) 3. Erythematous and edematous tonsil	1. Neck CT	1. **Needle aspiration**, incision, and drainage ± antibiotics • IV amoxicillin, Unasyn, and clindamycin • Less severe: oral antibiotics 7-10 d 2. Tonsillectomy (10%)
Aphthous ulcers (canker sores, ulcerative stomatitis) (Fig. 5-17B)	Unclear etiology May be associated with HHV-6	1. Single or multiple painful, round ulcers with yellow-gray centers and red halos • Occur on nonkeratinized mucosa (buccal or labia) • Usually recurrent		1. OTC topical anesthetics 2. Nonspecific, topical therapies (**steroids**) provide symptomatic relief 3. 1-wk oral prednisone taper can be helpful 4. Cimetidine (maintenance) in recurrent cases
Laryngitis	**Viral** ≫ Bacterial Bacteria: *M. cat, H. flu*	Follows a URI: 1. Hoarseness (hallmark) 2. Cough 3. Absence of pain or sore throat		1. Supportive therapy • Vocal rest and avoidance of singing or shouting 2. If bacterial → erythromycin, cefuroxime, or augmentin for cough or hoarseness 3. Oral or IM steroids for faster recovery but requires vocal fold evaluation Complications: Vocal fold hemorrhage, polyp or cyst formation

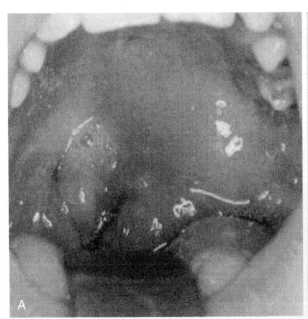
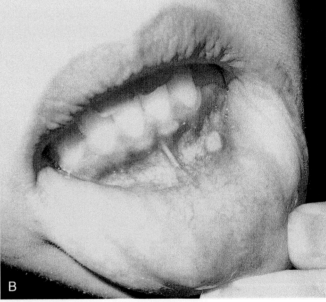

FIGURE 5-17. **A**, Peritonsillar abscess. **B**, Aphthous ulcers. (**A**, From Jensen S. *Nursing Health Assessmet: A Best Practice Approach.* 2nd ed. Philadelphia: Wolters Kluwer; 2015. **B**, Image provided by Stedman's.)

Tonsillectomy Indications

- Tonsillar hypertrophy with sleep disordered breathing
- Recurrent throat infections for

- ≥7 episodes of recurrent throat infection in last year
- ≥5 episodes per year in last 2 years
- ≥3 episodes per year in last 3 years

Parotitis, Sialadenitis

Disease	Etiology, Prevalence, Risk Factors	Clinical Symptoms and Signs	Diagnostics	Therapy, Prognosis, and Health Maintenance
Parotitis	**Viral** (parainfluenza)	1. Unilateral or bilateral	1. Elevated amylase	
Mumps parotitis (Fig. 5-18)	Develops in 70%-90% of symptomatic infections within 24 h of prodromal symptom onset, but can begin as long as 1 wk after First most common complication/manifestation of mumps MCC: **Paramyxovirus,** but also caused by influenza, parainfluenza, coxsackie virus, echovirus, HIV MC: Children <15 Transmission: Airborne droplets	Prodrome of low-grade fever, malaise, myalgia, arthralgias, headache, anorexia 1. Acute onset unilateral or **bilateral swelling** of the parotid or other **salivary glands** lasting >2 d (average: 1-5 d) 2. Tenderness and obliteration of space between earlobe and angle of mandible 3. Patient reports earache and difficulty swallowing, eating, or talking Signs: 1. Gland is tense, painful 2. Erythema and warmth are absent 3. No pus expressed from Stensen duct Associated: Epididymo-orchitis (15%-30%)	Clinical DX: 1. CT scan	1. Supportive care: self-limiting manifestation, without risk of death or long-term sequelae Complications: 1. Recurrent sialadenitis 2. Mastitis, pancreatitis, aseptic meningitis, sensorineural hearing loss, myocarditis, polyarthritis, hemolytic anemia, thrombocytopenia Health maintenance: 1. Contagious for 9 d after onset of parotid swelling 2. Children should not attend school for 9 d after onset of swelling

Suppurative parotitis	Newborns and debilitated elderly
	Bacterial infection of the parotid gland in patients with compromised salivary flow
	Caused by retrograde flow of oral bacteria into salivary ducts and parenchyma
	MCC:
	S. aureus
	RF:
	Recent anesthesia, dehydration, prematurity, advanced age, sialolithiasis, oral cancer, salivary duct strictures, tracheostomy, ductal foreign bodies; medications; chronic illness (HIV, Sjogren syndrome, depression, hypothyroidism, diabetes, renal or hepatic failure, hyperuricemia, anorexia, bulimia, cystic fibrosis)
		1. Rapid onset—Swollen parotid gland
		2. Tenderness and erythema
		3. Usually unilateral
		4. Drainage of purulent material from Stensen duct
		5. Fever
		Signs:
		1. Gland is tense, painful
		2. Erythema and warmth are present
		3. Pus expressed from Stensen duct
		4. Fever
		5. Trismus
			Clinical DX:
			1. Culture discharge
			2. CBC—leukocytosis
				1. Hydration with fluids
				2. Massage and apply heat to affected gland
				3. Stimulate salivation with sialogogues (lemon drops)
				4. Discontinue drugs that cause dry mouth
				5. PO antibiotics if they can tolerate liquids and no signs of systemic illness or trismus
				  • Augmentin
				  • Clindamycin
				  • Cephalexin with Flagyl
				6. IV antibiotics
				  • Nafcillin
				  • Unasyn
				  • Vancomycin + Flagyl
				7. Neonates
				  • Gentamicin + Antistaphylococcal antibiotics

(continued)

(continued)

Disease	Etiology, Prevalence, Risk Factors	Clinical Symptoms and Signs	Diagnostics	Therapy, Prognosis, and Health Maintenance
Malignant otitis externa	Consider in patients with persistent otitis externa despite 2-3 wk of topical antibiotics	1. Severe otalgia (90%) 2. Edema of the external auditory canal with otorrhea (70%) <u>Signs of infected ear:</u> 1. Erythema, edema 2. **Parotitis** 3. Trismus (involvement of TMJ or masseter muscle) 4. CN VII involvement	<u>Clinical Diagnosis:</u> 1. WBC—within normal ranges 2. ESR/CRP—elevated, nondiagnostic and nonspecific 3. **Contrast CT head** or MRI (either will confirm)	1. Use imipenem in children 2. In adults, use an • Aminoglycoside plus • Antipseudomonal penicillin or cephalosporin or quinolone *Note: IV Ciprofloxacin has replaced combo therapy of aminoglycosides with third generation cephalosporins
Sialadenitis	Affects the parotid or submandibular gland Occurs with dehydration or chronic illness (Sjogren syndrome), ductal obstruction <u>MC bug:</u> S. aureus	1. Acute swelling of the gland 2. Increased pain and swelling with eating 3. Tenderness and erythema of the duct opening 4. Pus will drain with massage	1. Ultrasound or CT scan to diagnose	1. IV antibiotics: Nafcillin 2. Hydration, warm compresses, sialagogues (lemon drops), massage gland 3. Oral antibiotics for less severe cases 4. Resolves in 2-3 wk <u>Complications:</u> Abscess formation, ductal stricture, stone, tumor
Suppurative sialadenitis	Acute, severe, potentially life-threatening	1. No pus will drain from Stensen papilla		Do not respond to rehydration or IV antibiotics 1. Incision and drainage required
Sialolithiasis	Development of calcium carbonate and calcium phosphate stone (sialolith) in a stagnant salivary duct Can occur at any age Mostly men, 30-60 y Most in submandibular gland (80%) Mimics parotitis	1. Pain, swelling • Colicky • Worse with meals 2. Tenderness 3. Typically unilateral <u>Signs:</u> Firm gland palpated	<u>Clinical DX:</u> Intraoral XR—radiopaque calculi	1. Outpatient therapy • PO analgesics • Antibiotics if concurrent infection • Massage • Sialagogues (lemon drops) <u>Complications:</u> Recurrent or persistent duct obstruction, strictures, infection, gland atrophy

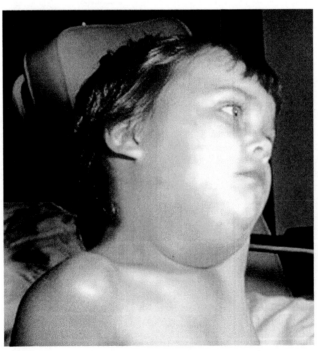

FIGURE 5-18. Mumps parotitis. (From Knipe DM, Howley PM. *Fields Virology.* 6th ed. Philadelphia: Wolters Kluwer; 2014.)

CHAPTER 6
Obstetrics and Gynecology

Refer to Section V 🔍 for In-depth Coverage of the Following Topics:

Recommended Supplemental Topics:

PELVIC INFLAMMATORY DISEASE

Disease	Etiology, Prevalence, Risk Factors	Clinical Symptoms and Signs	Diagnostics	Therapy, Prognosis, and Health Maintenance
Pelvic inflammatory disease (acute *salpingitis*)	Infection that ascends from the cervix or vagina to involve the endometrium and/or fallopian tubes <u>MCC:</u> ***N. gonorrhoeae***, *Chlamydia trachomatis*, genital mycoplasmas *(Mycoplasma hominis, Ureaplasma urealyticum, Mycoplasma genitalium)* <u>RF:</u> Presence of endocervical infection, bacterial vaginosis, history of salpingitis (PID), or recent vaginal douching, recent insertion of IUD, D&C or C-section	1. **Mucopurulent malodorous vaginal discharge** (cervicitis) 2. Midline abdominal pain 3. Abnormal vaginal bleeding *Progresses→* 4. **Bilateral lower abdominal and pelvic pain** • Dull, aching • May be absent • *Abnormal uterine bleeding* coincides with pain (40%) • Duration <3 wk 5. **Nausea, vomiting** 6. Urethritis (20%): dysuria 7. Proctitis: anorectal pain, tenesmus, rectal discharge, or bleeding 8. Fever >38°C (33%) <u>Signs:</u> 1. Speculum examination: yellow endocervical discharge, easily induced bleeding 2. Bimanual examination: • **Uterine or adnexal tenderness and swelling** 50%) • **Cervical motion tenderness:** by stretching the adnexae 3. Rebound, guarding Abdominal tenderness (if peritonitis develops)	1. Labs • ESR elevated >15 mm/h (75%) • Leukocytosis (60%) • Serum B-hCG • NAATs: r/o GC/CT • Gram stain and culture of endocervical secretions 2. Ultrasound: enlarged fallopian tubes with fluid in cul-de-sac <u>Rule:</u> If cultures (+), r/o by laparoscopy or endometrial biopsy 3. Laparoscopy: last line to r/o acute appendicitis, ectopic pregnancy, corpus luteum bleeding, and ovarian tumor (do if unilateral pain or mass) • Other indications: absence of lower genital tract infection, missed period, (+) pregnancy test, failed response to therapy 4. Endometrial biopsy–r/o endometritis Complications/sequelae: Tubo-ovarian abscess, infertility, ectopic pregnancy, chronic pelvic pain, recurrent salpingitis	1. Outpatient • IM **ceftriaxone** 250 mg once + PO **doxycycline** 100 mg BID × 14 d ± PO flagyl 500 mg BID × 14 d 2. Inpatient • Consider hospitalization if: • Diagnosis uncertain, ectopic and appendicitis cannot be r/o • Patient pregnant • Pelvic abscess suspected • Severely ill or nausea and vomiting preclude outpatient management • HIV positive • Unable to follow or tolerate outpatient regimen • Failed to respond to outpatient therapy • **Doxycycline + IV cefotetan or cefoxitin** × 48 h until condition improves, then PO doxycycline 100 mg BID × 14 d • **Clindamycin + gentamicin daily**, if normal renal function, ×48 h until condition improves, then PO doxycycline 100 mg BID × 14 d

BREAST MASS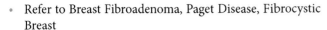

- Refer to Breast Fibroadenoma, Paget Disease, Fibrocystic Breast

MENOPAUSE

- **Menopause (natural):** 12 months of amenorrhea with no obvious pathological cause
  - Oocytes responsive to gonadotropins disappear from the ovary
  - The few remaining oocytes do not respond to gonadotropins
- **Induced (artificial) menopause:** Permanent cessation of menstruation after bilateral oophorectomy or ablation of ovarian function (chemotherapy, radiation)
  - Used as treatment for endometriosis, estrogen-sensitive neoplasms of the breast and endometrium (rarely)
- **Perimenopause/menopause transition:** Menstrual cycle and hormonal changes that occur a few years before and 12 months after the final menstrual period resulting from natural menopause
- **Premature menopause (spontaneous premature ovarian failure):** Menopause reached at or before age 40
- The early rise of FSH in menopause is related to **inhibin** (polypeptide synthesized and secreted by granulosa cells), which causes negative feedback on FSH release by pituitary → as oocyte number decreases, inhibin levels decrease resulting in elevated FSH
  - Note: during the menopausal transition, high FSH stimulates follicles to secrete estradiol (2-3 times higher than normal)

Changes in Hormone Metabolism

- In postmenopausal women, there is a reduction of circulating androstenedione to approximately 50% of the concentration found in young women, reflecting the absence of follicular activity
- The level of testosterone found in postmenopausal women is only minimally lower than that found in premenopausal women before oophorectomy and is distinctly higher than the level observed in ovariectomized young women
- Levels of the adrenal androgens dehydroepiandrosterone (DHEA) and dehydroepiandrosterone sulfate (DHEAS) are reduced by 60% and 80%, respectively, with age
- A decrease of **estradiol** occurs up to 1 year after the last menstrual period
  - Although both estrone and testosterone are converted in peripheral tissues to estradiol, it is conversion from estrone that accounts for most estradiol in older women (adrenal gland is major source)
  - Last hormonal change associated with loss of ovarian function
- In young women, the major source of **progesterone** is the ovarian corpus luteum after ovulation. During the follicular phase of the cycle, progesterone levels are low. With ovulation the levels rise greatly, reflecting the secretory activity of the corpus luteum. Because postmenopausal ovaries do not contain functional follicles, ovulation does not occur and progesterone levels remain low
  - Dexamethasone suppresses level, ACTH increases level, hCG has no effect
- Gonadotropins: With menopause, both LH and FSH levels rise substantially, with FSH usually higher than LH

Disease	Etiology, Prevalence, Risk Factors	Clinical Symptoms and Signs	Diagnostics	Therapy, Prognosis, and Health Maintenance
Menopause	**Average age:** 51.3 y Range: 44-56 RF (early menopause): genetics, **smoking**, cancer therapies Consider in differential: Pregnancy and hypothyroidism, premature ovarian failure (if <35 y) Most common symptom: hot flash or flush	Early menopause: 1. **Menstrual irregularity** (more frequent) 2. Vasomotor symptoms: hot flashes, night sweats, 3. Sleep disturbances 4. Irritability, mood disturbances 5. Vaginal dryness → dyspareunia Vulvovaginal atrophy/**GSM** (intermediate): 1. Vaginal atrophy, loss of urogenital integrity, loss of skin elasticity Late menopause: 1. Osteoporosis 2. CVD 3. Macular degeneration 4. Periodontal disease 5. Decreased hearing, balance, skin integrity 6. Alzheimer disease, memory, and cognition	DX: **1 y of no periods** (amenorrhea) after age 40 with no pathological cause 1. **FSH: elevated** (21-100 mU/mL) • Elevated during early follicular phase, decrease during follicular maturation 2. **Estradiol <20 pg/mL, low** • Establishes diagnosis of menopause • Determines ovarian status of patient 3. Progesterone levels: same as younger women • No clinical use in postmenopausal women 4. AMH, Inhibin B: low 5. LH: elevated, but not necessary to measure	1. Estrogens • Used to treat hot flashes • Woman with **intact uterus** should **not** use estrogen alone because of increased risk of endometrial cancer 2. Progestins • Hot flashes • Increased risk of breast cancer 3. SSRI and SNRIs • Caution use with Tamoxifen 4. Black cohosh 5. HRT−severe menopausal symptoms (hot flashes, night sweats, vaginal dryness) • "Smallest dose for shortest possible time and annual reviews of the decision to take hormones" • HRT should not be used to prevent cardiovascular disease owing to slight increased risk of breast cancer, MI, CVD, DVT • Hormone therapy effect on lipid profile: HDL and *TG levels increase*, LDL levels decrease

CHAPTER 7

Neurology

Supplemental Resources:
Intracranial Tumors 📟, p 243

DIZZINESS AND VERTIGO

- **Dizziness**—describes a variety of sensations (vertigo, light-headedness, faintness, imbalance)
  - Vascular disorders cause presyncopal dizziness due to cardiac dysrhythmia, orthostatic hypotension, medication effects
  - Vestibular causes (vertigo or imbalance) can be due to peripheral lesions affecting labyrinths or vestibular nerves
  - Ask the D's: Diplopia, Dysarthria, Dysphagia, Dysphonia, Dysmetria, Dysesthesia, Drop Attacks
  - Deafness (transient and bilateral hearing loss is bad; abrupt onset unilateral loss may be bad or benign)
  - Dyspnea (SOB)
- **Vertigo**—when dizziness describes a sense of spinning or other motion (specifically, the illusion of self or environmental motion)

- Can be physiologic, occurring during or after sustained head rotation, or pathologic (vestibular dysfunction)—implies asymmetry of vestibular inputs from the 2 labyrinths or their central pathways
- Light-headedness—commonly refers to presyncopal sensations due to brain hypoperfusion; also refers to disequilibrium and imbalance
- Approach to the patient
  - Delineate nature—unilateral vs. bilateral, acute vs. chronic or progressive
  - Focus on the history—is this the first attack? Duration of this episode or prior episodes? Provoking factors? Accompanying symptoms?
  - Common causes of dizziness

Lasts Seconds	Lasts Minutes	Lasts Hours
• Benign paroxysmal positional vertigo (BPPV) • Orthostatic hypotension • Provoked by changes in head or body position	• Transient ischemic attacks of the posterior circulation • Migraine	• Vestibular migraine • Meniere disease

- Symptoms that accompany vertigo distinguish peripheral vestibular lesions from central causes

Peripheral Vertigo	Central Vertigo
• Unilateral hearing loss and aural symptoms (ear pain, pressure, fullness)	• Causes bilateral hearing loss, unless lesion lies near root entry zone of auditory nerve • Double vision, numbness, limb ataxia: brainstem or cerebellar lesion

- Examination
  - Neurologic examination—focus on assessment of eye movements, vestibular function, and hearing
    - Peripheral eye movement disorders (cranial neuropathies, eye muscle weakness) are different in 2 eyes
    - Check pursuit: ability to follow smoothly moving target

- Saccades: ability to look back and forth accurately between 2 targets
  - Poor pursuit or inaccurate saccades indicates central pathology (cerebellum)
- Spontaneous nystagmus: involuntary back and forth movement of eyes
  - Cerebellar (central) lesions
    - Vertical nystagmus with downward fast phases (downbeat)

- Horizontal nystagmus that changes direction with gaze (gaze-evoked)
- Peripheral lesions
  - Unidirectional horizontal nystagmus—use Frenzel eyeglasses to aid detection
- Head impulse test—examines vestibuloocular reflex (VOR) with 20° rapid head rotations
  - Patient fixates on target, head rotated to right or left
  - If deficient, rotation is followed by a catch-up saccade in opposite direction
  - Identifies both unilateral and bilateral vestibular hypofunction
- Dix-Hallpike maneuver—begin in sitting position with patient's head turned 45°; hold back of head and lower patient into supine position with head extended backward 20° while watching eyes
  - Posterior canal BPPV—transient upbeating torsional nystagmus
  - If no nystagmus after 15 to 20 seconds → raise patient to sitting, repeat with head turned to other side
- Ancillary testing
  - Audiometry if vestibular disorder suspected
    - Unilateral sensorineural hearing loss = peripheral (vestibular schwannoma)
    - Low frequency hearing loss = Meniere disease
  - Electronystagmography or videonystagmography
  - Caloric testing assesses response of 2 horizontal semicircular canals
  - Neuroimaging if central vestibular disorder suspected: MRI with gadolinium to r/o schwannoma

Disease	Etiology, Prevalence, Risk Factors	Clinical Symptoms and Signs	Diagnostics	Therapy, Prognosis, and Health Maintenance

Vertigo	Sensation of movement (spinning, tumbling, or falling) in the absence of actual movement or an overresponse to movement
	Central etiology: multiple sclerosis, brain tumor, head injury, medications
		1. Duration and presence of hearing loss or nystagmus
		2. Peripheral vertigo—sudden onset, intermittent, nausea/vomiting, tinnitus, hearing loss, nystagmus (horizontal with rotary component)
		3. Central vertigo—gradual onset, continuous, nausea or vomiting, vertical nystagmus, **no auditory symptoms**; motor, sensory, or cerebellar deficits
			1. **Dix-Hallpike maneuver**–nonfatigable nystagmus = central cause
			2. Audiometry, caloric stimulation, ENG, MRI, evoked potentials
				Peripheral–
				1. Vestibular suppressants help with acute symptoms
				  • Diazepam (Valium)
				  • Meclizine
				  • Less helpful for chronic dizziness
				2. Epley maneuver
				Central–treat the source
				1. Deep head-hanging maneuver

Acute prolonged vertigo (*vestibular neuritis*)	Owing to sudden asymmetry of inputs from 2 labyrinths or in central connections, stimulating continuous rotation of the head Central (cerebellar, brainstem infarct, hemorrhage) can be life-threatening Peripheral–affects vestibular nerve or labyrinth	1. Sudden, unilateral vertigo • **Persists even when head remains still** 2. Nausea, vomiting 3. Oscillopsia–motion of the visual scene 4. Imbalance 5. Central symptoms: diplopia, weakness, numbness, dysarthria	1. Head impulse test	Spontaneously resolves 1. Steroids within 3 d of symptom onset 2. Antivirals nonbeneficial unless herpes zoster oticus (Ramsay Hunt syndrome) suspected 3. Vestibular suppressant medications for acute symptoms 4. Resume normal activity ASAP and directed vestibular rehab
Benign paroxysmal positional vertigo (BPPV)	Common cause of recurrent vertigo Caused by free-floating otoconia (calcium carbonate crystals) dislodged from utricular macula and moved to semicircular (posterior) canal	1. Brief episodes (**<1 min**), last 15-20 s • Provoked by changes in head position relative to gravity (lying down, rolling over in bed, rising from supine position, extending head to look upward) Posterior canal BPPV: **Upward, torsional nystagmus** Horizontal canal BPPV: Horizontal nystagmus when lying ear down Superior (anterior) BPPV: Rare	1. **(+) Dix-Hallpike maneuver** produces delayed fatigable nystagmus 2. Posterior canal BPPV: **Epley maneuver**	1. Dix-Hallpike maneuver (quickly turn patient's head 90° while supine) 2. Avoid using meclizine or similar medicines

Disease	Etiology, Prevalence, Risk Factors	Clinical Symptoms and Signs	Diagnostics	Therapy, Prognosis, and Health Maintenance
Psychosomatic dizziness or vertigo	Phobic postural vertigo, psychophysiologic vertigo, or chronic subjective dizziness HX: Previous vestibular disorder (neuritis)	Somatic manifestation of psychiatric condition (major depression, anxiety, panic disorder) 1. Chronic (months) dizziness and disequilibrium 2. Increased sensitivity to self-motion and visual motion (movies) 3. Worse with complex visual environments (supermarket)	1. Neurologic examination and vestibular testing: normal	1. SSRIs and cognitive behavioral therapy 2. Vestibular rehabilitation therapy Comorbidity: **anxiety**, autonomic symptoms

Disease	Etiology, Prevalence, Risk Factors	Clinical Symptoms and Signs	Diagnostics	Therapy, Prognosis, and Health Maintenance
Meniere disease (endolymphatic hydrops)	Excessive endolymph fluid in cochlea overstimulates hairs causing vertigo and sudden hearing loss with aural fullness Unknown etiology **Triad:** Vertigo, hearing loss, tinnitus	1. Sudden, recurrent **vertigo** (lasting *minutes to hours*), lower-range hearing loss 2. **Tinnitus** 3. One-sided aural "fullness" pain, or pressure **(unilateral)** 4. **Hearing loss** (low frequency), sensorineural 5. Nausea, vomiting Signs: Nystagmus on impaired side	1. Audiometry at time of attack 2. Caloric testing	1. Symptomatic treatment: meclizine, dimenhydrinate (Dramamine), prochlorperazine (Compazine), promethazine (Phenergan) 2. Valium in refractory cases Management: 1. **Low-sodium, high-water diet** 2. **Diuretics:** (acetazolamide), hydrochlorothiazide 3. Intratympanic gentamicin 4. Referral to ENT Avoid alcohol, caffeine, and tobacco
Acoustic neuroma (*vestibular schwannoma*)	Intracranial benign tumor affecting CN VIII Bilateral acoustic neuromas, associated with **neurofibromatosis type II** "Progressive vertigo"	1. **Unilateral, progressive** sensorineural *hearing loss* (may also be acute) 2. *Unsteadiness* 3. *Vertigo* (continuous, late): vestibular deficit compensated centrally as it develops 4. **Tinnitus** 5. Impaired speech discrimination 6. Headache Signs: 1. Decreased corneal reflex sensitivity 2. Diplopia 3. Facial weakness or numbness	1. Head impulse test: deficient response when head rotated toward affected side 2. **MRI:** densely enhancing lesions, enlarging the internal auditory canal and extending into the cerebellopontine angle 3. Lumbar puncture: elevated protein	1. Asymptomatic • Serial MRIs 2. Surgery or SRS for larger lesions Complication: Loss of corneal reflex from trigeminal involvement

SYNCOPE

Loss of consciousness/postural tone secondary to acute decrease in cerebral blood flow; rapid recovery of consciousness without resuscitation.

- 20% of patients who present with "syncope" have a primary diagnosis of mood, anxiety, or substance abuse disorder, the most common being panic disorder
- Differential

- Seizure disorder
- Cardiac—sudden, no prodromal symptoms (face hits floor)
  - Arrhythmias (sick sinus syndrome, v-tach, AV block, rapid SVT)
  - Obstruction of blood flow (aortic stenosis, HCM, mitral valve prolapse)
  - Massive MI

- **Vasovagal syncope** ("neurocardiogenic, simple faints, vasodepressor"): paradoxical withdrawal of sympathetic stimulation and enhanced parasympathetic stimulation
  - Most common cause (50%)
  - Emotional stress, pain, fear, extreme fatigue, claustrophobic situations
  - Premonitory SX: pallor, sweating, light-headed, nausea, dimming of vision, roaring in ears
  - First episode usually >40
  - **Tilt-table study** to reproduce symptoms
  - Treatment: supine posture, elevate legs, β-blockers
- Orthostatic hypotension: ganglionic blocking agents, diabetes, old age, prolonged by bed rest; defect in vasomotor reflexes
  - Posture is main cause, sudden standing or prolonged standing
  - (+) tilt table test
  - Premonitory symptoms: light-headed, nausea, etc
  - Treat with increased sodium and fluids, fludrocortisone
- Severe cerebrovascular disease—rare
  - TIA involving vertebrobasilar circulation
- Noncardiogenic causes: hypoglycemia, hyperventilation, hypersensitivity (wearing tight collar or turning head), mechanical reduction of venous return (Valsalva or postmicturition), meds (BB, NTG, antiarrhythmics)
- Evaluation—r/o life-threatening causes (MI, hemorrhage, arrhythmias)
  - History: events before, during, and after, check meds, witness reports
  - Physical: orthostatics, postictal mental status, murmurs, carotid pulses, apply pressure to carotid sinus (reflex bradycardia and hypotension)
  - **EKG**—for all patients
  - CBC, CMP
  - 24-hour ambulatory EKG (Holter)
  - Tilt-table testing
  - CT or EEG—if seizure suspected
  - Echo—if evidence of structural heart disease or abnormal EKG
  - Electrophysiologic studies

- Serum Prolactin—though it may not differentiate between syncope or seizures, measurement after an event may rule out nonepileptic psychogenic events if performed within 10 to 20 minutes after an event; will be elevated after syncope or seizures

SEIZURE DISORDERS

Seizure

A sudden abnormally highly synchronous discharge of electrical activity, or a chronic disorder of recurrent, idiopathic seizures are not reproduced by a secondary cause.

- In seizures, duration of unconsciousness tends to be longer than in syncope (momentary)
- Causes: 4 M's and 4 I's
  - Metabolic and electrolyte disturbances—**hyponatremia**, water intoxication, **hypoglycemia** and hyperglycemia, hypocalcemia, uremia, thyroid storm, hyperthermia
    - Hyponatremia (<120), hypernatremia (>155), hyperosmolarity (>310), hypocalcemia (<7), hypoglycemia (<30)
  - Mass lesions—brain mets, primary brain tumors, hemorrhage
  - Missing drugs
    - Noncompliance with anticonvulsants (most common reason)
    - Acute withdrawal from **alcohol**, benzos, barbituates
  - Miscellaneous
    - Pseudoseizures—psychiatric in origin
    - Eclampsia
    - Hypertensive encephalopathy
    - Childhood febrile seizures
  - Intoxication—**cocaine**, lithium
  - Infection—septic shock, bacterial or viral meningitis, brain abscess
  - Ischemia—embolic stroke, TIA (common in elderly), syncope
  - Increased ICP due to trauma

Disease	Etiology, Prevalence, Risk Factors	Clinical Symptoms and Signs	Diagnostics	Therapy, Prognosis, and Health Maintenance
Epilepsy (seizure disorder)	Chronic disorder: condition with recurrent seizures not produced directly by a secondary cause *Nocturnal epilepsy*: seizures that occur exclusively during sleep *Catamenial epilepsy*: seizures that occur around menses or ovulation **Triggers** (lower seizure threshold): Sleep deprivation, emotional stressors, medications, infection, alcohol Causes: Childhood (perinatal injury, infection, genetic factors), and age (stroke, tumor, dementia)	1. Diagnosis requires 2+ separate seizures that are unprovoked	1. If *known epileptic* → check anticonvulsant levels 2. If *first seizure* →CBC, CMP (LFTs), blood glucose, renal function tests, serum calcium, urinalysis 3. **EEG**: most helpful diagnostic test, abnormal pattern is not diagnostic alone 4. **CT scan** of head: r/o structural lesions 5. **MRI of brain** with and without gadolinium: more sensitive than CT for structural changes 6. **LP/blood cultures** if febrile 7. **Pregnancy test**— before initiating anticonvulsants!!! 8. **Serum prolactin** levels rise abruptly in the postictal state only in true epilepsy	1. ABCs first, secure airway and roll patient to side 2. *Known epileptics* • Check for noncompliance of anticonvulsant, check levels • If persistent with monotherapy, increase dose of first anticonvulsant until signs of toxicity appear → add second drug if seizures uncontrolled If controlled → continue regimen × 2 y, then taper 3. *First seizure* • **EEG** with neurology consult • If normal EEG, recurrence low (15%) compared with abnormal EEG (41%) • Do not treat most patients with single seizure • Start antiepileptics only if EEG abnormal, MRI abnormal or status epilepticus Associated: Comorbid depression (50%)

Partial Seizures (70%)

Begins in one part of brain (single lobe) and produces symptoms referable to region of cortex involved.

- Seizure itself is referred to as the ictus and the period of time during which the seizure occurs is called the *ictal phase*
- The time after the seizure until the patient is fully recovered is called the *postictal phase*
- The time between seizures (which can be years) is referred to as the *interictal phase*
- **Clonic** (rhythmic jerking) or **tonic** (stiffening) movements
- Reflex seizures: precipitated by specific stimulus (touch, musical tune, particular movement, reading, stroboscopic lights, certain complex visual images)

Disease	Clinical Symptoms and Signs	Diagnostics	Therapy, Prognosis, and Health Maintenance
Simple partial seizure (*focal*), or aura	1. Consciousness *intact* (not impaired) 2. Seizure—*localized*, but may evolve • May be described as a *sensation*, autonomic function (nausea, epigastric sensation), abnormal thought (fear, deja vu), or involuntary movement • Patient can interact normally with environment except for limitations imposed by seizure itself on localized brain functions 3. May involve transient *unilateral* **clonic-tonic** movement Occurs in about 60% of patients with partial epilepsy	**EEG**	1. **Phenytoin and carbamazepine** 2. Alternatives—phenobarbital, depakote, primidone

(continued)

(continued)

Disease	Clinical Symptoms and Signs	Diagnostics	Therapy, Prognosis, and Health Maintenance

Complex partial	1. Consciousness *impaired*—consciousness spans from minimal to complete unresponsiveness
	2. Preceding **aura**
	3. **Ictal manifestations** (ictus lasts 1-3 min)
	  • Eyes usually open during ictus (indicating awake)
	  • **Automatisms**: purposeless, involuntary, repetitive movements (lip smacking, chewing)
	  • Epigastric sensation or vague cephalic sensation (most common)
	  • **Olfactory and gustatory hallucinations**
	  • Deja vu, odd thinking
	  • Visual changes: micropsia, macropsia
	  • Fear, pleasure, anger, dreamy sensation
	  • Voices, music
	  • Speech arrest, aphasia
	  • Absence-like symptoms
	  • Contralateral eye deviation
	  • Contralateral arm extension, fencing posture
	  • Contralateral clonic movements of face, fingers, hand, foot
	4. **Postictal confusion**
	  • Typically, some fatigue and ipsilateral headache
	  • Lasts few minutes to hours
		EEG	1. **Trileptal**
			2. Lamictal
			3. Phenytoin and carbamazepine

Generalized Seizure

Loss of consciousness; disruption of electrical activity in entire brain.

- **Secondarily generalized** convulsive seizures—a focal onset seizure that spreads throughout the brain

Disease	Clinical Symptoms and Signs	Diagnostics	Therapy, Prognosis, and Health Maintenance

Generalized tonic clonic (**grand mal**, *convulsion, generalized tonic-clonic, major-motor seizure)*	1. Eyes open and "roll to back of head"
	  • Begins with **sudden LOC**, "falls to ground"
	2. Apnea: Breathing does not occur
	3. *Tonic* phase: extensor posturing lasting 20-60 s
	  • Rigid trunk and limb extension occurs
	  • Bilaterally symmetric and without focal onset
	4. *Clonic* phase: progressively longer periods of inhibition manifesting as a clonic phase lasting up to 60 s
	5. *Postictal* phase: Transient deep stupor, followed by **15-30 min** of lethargy, and confusion → headache, muscle soreness, mental dulling, lack of energy, mood changes (hours-days)
	6. **Urinary incontinence**, fecal (rare)
	7. Vomiting
	The arm contralateral to the seizure focus may extend first while the ipsilateral arm is flexed at the elbow (*figure 4 sign*) with a loud "*tonic cry*" heard at the onset of a convulsion as air is forcibly expelled through the contracted vocal cords
	Signs:
	1. Cyanosis
	2. Foaming at the mouth
	3. Tongue biting (oral trauma)
	4. Hypoxemia
		1. Lactic acidosis, elevated catecholamine levels, increased serum CK, prolactin, corticotropin, and cortisol
		2. EEG: generalized high amplitude, rapid spiking
			1. Roll patient onto side to allow saliva to drool from mouth, decreasing likelihood of aspiration
			Treatment:
			1. Levetiracetam (Keppra), topiramate (Topamax), zonisamide (Zonegran)
			2. **Phenytoin and carbamazepine**
			3. Alternatives—phenobarbital, depakote, primidone
			Complications:
			Oral trauma, vertebral compression, fractures, shoulder dislocation, aspiration pneumonia, sudden death (rare) due to asphyxiation, edema, or cardiac arrhythmia

Disease	Clinical Symptoms and Signs	Diagnostics	Therapy, Prognosis, and Health Maintenance
Absence (**petitmal**) School-aged children, resolves with age	1. Disengage from current activity and "stare into space"–then returns to activity • Patient looks "absent minded" during episodes which are confused with "daydreaming" • Minor clonic activity (eye blinks, head nodding, 45%) 2. Brief (lasts **few seconds**), but quite frequent (up to 100 times/d) 3. Impairment of consciousness 4. No loss of postural tone and **no postictal confusion** Signs: Loss of neck tone	EEG: 3/s **spike and slow wave** activity (2.5 Hz or less)	1. **Ethosuximide** 2. Valproic acid (Depakote) 3. Zonegran (Zonisamide)
Myoclonic seizures	1. Rapid, recurrent, brief muscle jerks of the face or hands → massive bilateral spasms simultaneously affecting head, limbs, and trunk 2. Occur bilaterally 3. Synchronously or asynchronously 4. May occur shortly after waking up, but can occur at any time	**EEG**	1. Keppra 2. Depakote

Disease	Etiology, Prevalence, Risk Factors	Clinical Symptoms and Signs	Diagnostics	Therapy, Prognosis, and Health Maintenance
Status epilepticus	Causes: noncompliance, alcohol withdrawal, intracranial infection, neoplasm, metabolic disorder, drug overdose	1. Prolonged, sustained unconsciousness with persistent convulsive activity in seizing patient lasting **longer** than **30 min**[a] Or 2. **2 or more** sequential seizures without full recovery of consciousness between seizures	1. EEG 2. Consider MRI	1. Step 1: make diagnosis • Establish an airway, monitor O_2, give O_2 if needed • Check CMP, Ca, Mg, Phos • CBC, UTox, troponin, AED levels, glucose 2. Step 2 (6-10 min) • If hypoglycemic, give 100 mg IV thiamine and **50 mL 50% dextrose** IV, **0.1 mg/kg IV lorazepam** (no more than 2 mg/min), repeat if persistent • May give rectally 3. Step 3: IV fosphenytoin 20 mg PE/kg, no faster than 150 mg PE/min or **IV phenytoin 20 mg/ kg IV** no faster than 50 mg/min • Monitor HR and BP • May give add. 10 mg/kg fosphenytoin or phenytoin (total 30 mg/kg) • Phenytoin level 2 hours after (goal ~20) 4. Step 4 (31-50 min) • Intubation • IV phenobarbital 20 mg/kg slow push 5. Resistant: IV phenobarbital Mortality: 20%

[a]Note: although by definition, status is longer than 30 min, most patients are treated after 5 min of convulsive seizures.

STROKES: TRANSIENT ISCHEMIC ATTACK AND CEREBROVASCULAR ACCIDENT (CVA)

- Evolving stroke: worsening
- Completed stroke: maximal deficit has occurred
- *Duration of symptoms* is the determining difference between TIA and CVA
- Transient Ischemic Attacks (TIA)
  - Neurologic deficit that lasts few mins to <24 hours (N: 30 minutes)
  - Symptoms transient because reperfusion occurs owing to collateral circulation or breaking up of embolus
  - **Blockage in blood flow does not last long enough to cause permanent infarction**

- Clinical pearls
  - Triptans are contraindicated in patients with coronary artery disease or peripheral vascular disease and should be avoided in all patients with an increased risk for stroke
  - Contraindications to thrombolytic therapy: previous hemorrhagic stroke, stroke within 1 year, a known intracranial neoplasm, active internal bleeding, suspected aortic dissection. Relative contraindications: severe uncontrolled hypertension, use of anticoagulation, active peptic ulcer disease.
  - **Hypertension** is the most common and most important stroke risk factor (Fig. 7-1)

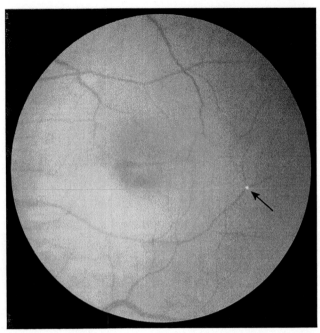

FIGURE 7-1. Amaurosis fugax, a Hollenhorst (cholesterol) plaque causing temporary occlusion of the retinal artery. (From Fineman MS, Ho AC. *Wills Eye Hospital Color Atlas & Synopsis of Clinical Ophthalmology: Retina.* 3rd ed. Philadelphia: Wolters Kluwer; 2018.)

Disease	Etiology, Prevalence, Risk Factors	Clinical Symptoms and Signs	Diagnostics	Therapy, Prognosis, and Health Maintenance
Ischemic stroke (85%) <u>Causes in young patients:</u> OCP use, hypercoaguable states (pregnancy, malignancy, vWF, antiphospholipid antibody syndrome), vasoconstrictive drug use (cocaine, amphetamines), polycythemia vera, sickle cell	<u>RF:</u> **Age** and **HTN,** smoking, DM, hyperlipidemia, **atrial fibrillation** (*cardioembolic*), family history of CAD, family history of stroke, previous stroke/TIA, carotid bruits, drugs (sympathomimetics, OCPs, cocaine)	<u>Clinical manifestations:</u> See below	1. **CT *without* contrast of head**—differentiates ischemic from hemorrhagic (first line), may have to wait 2448 h to see infarct 2. MRI of brain—more sensitive than CT and identifies all infarcts earlier than CT, not preferred in emergent setting 3. EKG—acute MI or A-fib may be cause of embolic strokes 4. Carotid duplex scan—determines degree of stenosis 5. MRA—definitive test for stenosis of vessels of head/neck and for aneurysms	*Acute*—supportive treatment (airway protection, O_2, IV fluids) 1. C-A-B 2. *Gradual* BP control • Preferred: **IV labetalol 20 mg** • Do not give antihypertensives unless • SBP >200, DBP >120, or MAP >130 mm Hg • Acute MI, aortic dissection, severe HF, hypertensive encephalopathy • Receiving thrombolytic therapy <u>Prevention:</u> • Control RF: HTN, DM, smoking, cholesterol, obesity • Aspirin • Carotid endarterectomy • Prevention of lacunar strokes: control HTN <u>Stable:</u> 1. **t-PA therapy** • If administered within first **3** h of onset, improved outcome at 3 mo • Do not initiate if: >3 h, uncontrolled HTN, bleeding disorder or anticoagulated, history of recent trauma or surgery • Do not give aspirin for first 24 h if t-PA given, perform frequent neuro checks, carefully monitor BP 2. **Aspirin** is best if given within 24 h of symptom onset • If within 3 h—give thrombolytics • If *after 3 h*—give aspirin, and if patient allergic, give clopidogrel (Plavix) → ticlopidine 3. Anticoagulants (heparin/warfarin) have not been proven to have efficacy in acute stroke 4. Assess patient's ability to protect airway, keep NPO, elevate HOB to 30°

Disease	Etiology, Prevalence, Risk Factors	Clinical Symptoms and Signs	Diagnostics	Therapy, Prognosis, and Health Maintenance
Embolic stroke	Most common type MC location: Heart (due to embolization of mural thrombus in patient with **atrial fibrillation**), internal carotid, aorta, paradoxical	1. Onset of symptoms very rapid (seconds), and deficits are maximal initially 2. Clinical features depend on artery occluded 3. **MCA most commonly affected**: • Contralateral hemiparesis (weakness) • Hemi-sensory loss • Hyperreflexia • Aphasia (90% left) • Apraxia		Prognosis: 1. High risk of restroke in subsequent months • Risk is ~10% per year • 30% 5-y risk of restroke
Thrombotic stroke	Atherosclerotic lesions in large arteries of neck or medium-sized arteries of brain (MCA)	1. Onset may be rapid or stepwise 2. Patient **awakens from sleep** with neurologic deficits		
Lacunar stroke (internal capsule, pons, thalamus) Causes 20% of all strokes; usually affects subcortical structures	*Narrowing* of large arterial lumen due to **thickening of vessel wall** (*not* by thrombosis) RF: History of chronic **HTN** and DM Affected arteries: MCA, circle of Willis, basilar and vertebral arteries	*Hemiparesis*–weakness of entire left or right side 1. **Internal capsule**: pure **motor** hemiparesis 2. Pons: dysarthria, clumsy hand 3. **Thalamus**: Pure **sensory** deficit	Focal features and usually contralateral pure motor or pure sensory deficits	Prevention of lacunar strokes: control HTN
Transient ischemic attack	Brief episode of neurologic dysfunction caused by focal brain or retinal ischemia Blockage in flow does not last long enough to cause permanent infarction Retinal artery (MCA) → amaurosis fugax	1. Sudden onset neurologic deficit 2. Lasts **minutes to <1 h** (N: 15-30 min) 3. Reversal of symptoms within 24 h	1. Carotid doppler ultrasound 2. MRA of neck	1. Hospital admission for new onset and recurrent TIA, unless confident diagnosis of cause of event can be made 2. **Antiplatelet therapy**: Aspirin ± dipyridamole OR clopidogrel Note: If high risk → warfarin should be used RF for recurrent stroke, average 5% risk per year
Amaurosis fugax	Etiology: **Atherosclerosis** (emboli to the ophthalmic artery), carotid stenosis	"Fleeting blindness" or "curtain coming down" vertically into field of vision 1. Painless, transient 2. *Unilateral* (monocular) vision loss 3. Seconds of a *graying out* of vision in one eye	Retinoscopy: refractile arterial lesions (**Hollenhorst plaques**, cholesterol crystals) (Fig. 7-1)	Prognosis: 1. Annual risk of stroke is 1%-2%

(continued)

(continued)

Disease	Etiology, Prevalence, Risk Factors	Clinical Symptoms and Signs	Diagnostics	Therapy, Prognosis, and Health Maintenance
Carotid stenosis	Extracranial internal carotid artery stenosis >80% ± symptoms of ischemia *Asymptomatic*–refers to presence of narrowing of the ICA in individuals without a history of recent ipsilateral ischemic stroke or TIA *Symptomatic*–refers to neurologic symptoms caused by TIA or ischemic stroke in the carotid artery territory and ipsilateral to significant carotid atherosclerotic pathology	Symptoms of *ischemia:* 1. Partial and complete blindness in one eye and absent pupillary light response 2. Contralateral homonymous hemianopsia, hemiparesis, hemisensory loss 3. Left hemisphere– Aphasia 4. Right hemisphere–left visuospatial neglect, constructional apraxia, dysprosody 5. Unilateral limb shaking, transient loss of monocular vision upon exposure to bright light 6. Does not cause vertigo, light-headedness, or syncope Signs: 1. Carotid bruit 2. Funduscopic examination: arterial occlusion or ischemic damage to retina	1. **Cerebral angiography** (gold standard) • Permits use of entire carotid system, provides info about tandem atherosclerotic disease, plaque morphology, and collateral circulation • Identifies people who would benefit from endarterectomy (CEA) 2. **Carotid duplex ultrasound** • Noninvasive, but hairline residual lumens can be missed and can overestimate degree of stenosis 3. **Magnetic resonance angiography (MRA) neck** • Less accurate for detecting moderate stenosis, more expensive, time-consuming, patient must lie still, renal insufficiency can be an issue 4. CT angiography (CTA) • Impaired renal function is a relative contraindication since contrast bolus must be given (DM/CHF)	See treatment of asymptomatic and symptomatic CAS below

Treatment of Carotid Stenosis

Asymptomatic Bruits
1. Start daily **antiplatelet therapy**, statin therapy, manage diabetes, treat hypertension, and healthy lifestyle (limit ETOH consumption, weight control, aerobic physical activity, Mediterranean diet)
2. **Carotid endarterectomy (CEA): >80% stenosis**, recurrent TIAs on medical therapy (preferred)
   • If patient has life expectancy of >5 y
3. Duplex ultrasonography–repeat annually to assess progression or regression of disease and response to therapeutic intervention if stenosis >50%
4. Carotid artery stenting (CAS) only for high risk patients
   • Unlikely to benefit if: severe comorbidity, prior ipsilateral stroke, total occlusion of ICA

Symptomatic Bruits–manifested as recent TIA or ischemic stroke and ipsilateral CAS
1. *Anticoagulation (Warfarin)*
2. Carotid endarterectomy (CEA) indicated for:
   • Severe stenosis (70%-99%) → CEA recommended
   • Mod stenosis (50%-69%) → CEA recommended
   • Mild stenosis (<50%) → no indication for CEA or carotid angioplasty with stenting
   • Consider age: If >70, CEA may be associated with better outcome compared with CAS; for younger patients, CAS = CEA in terms of periprocedural complications
3. CAS is indicated as an alternative to CEA for symptomatic patients at average or low risk of complications when diameter of lumen of ICA is reduced by >70% by noninvasive imaging, or >50% by catheter angiography, or >50% by noninvasive imaging with corroboration
High risk: progression of asymptomatic CAS, detection of embolism, plaque burden and morphology, reduced cerebrovascular reserve, silent embolic infarcts

Brain Perfusion Territories (Fig. 7-2)

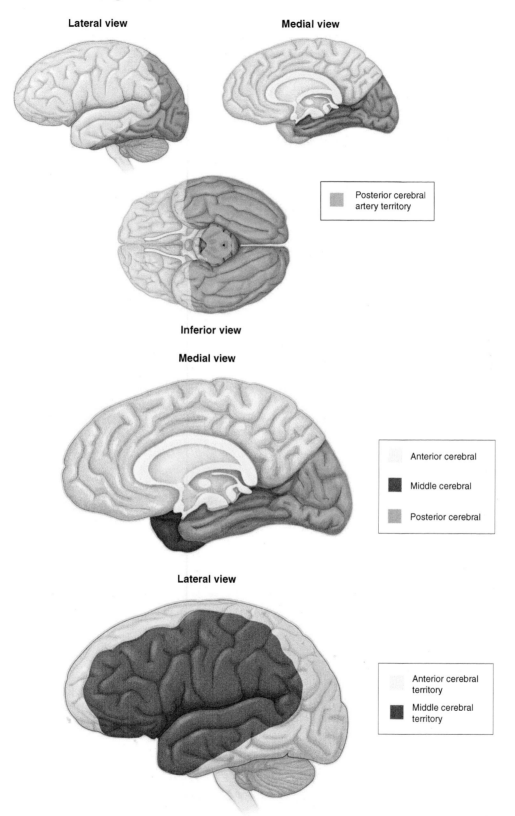

FIGURE 7-2. Brain perfusion territories.

Deficits Seen in Ischemic Strokes (Fig. 7-3)

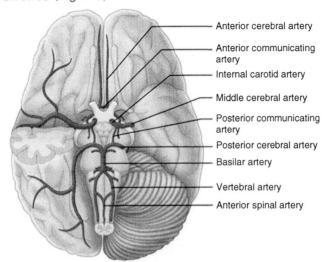

FIGURE 7-3. The circle of Willis and adjacent circulation. (From Morton PG, Fontaine DK. *Critical Care Nursing: A Holistic Approach.* 10th ed. Philadelphia: Wolters Kluwer Health; 2013.)

Distribution	Location and/or Type of Deficiency
Anterior cerebral artery (ACA)	1. **Contralateral** lower extremity **hemiparesis** and hemisensory loss (leg > arm) 2. Abulia (especially if bilateral)–inability to make decisions
Middle cerebral artery (MCA)	1. **Aphasia** (if dominant hemisphere involved)–90% LEFT 2. Agnosia (nondominant)–inability to process sensory information 3. Apraxia, contralateral body neglect, confusion (if nondominant hemisphere involved) 4. *Contralateral* **hemiparesis** and hemisensory loss 5. Homonymous hemianopsia (variable)
Internal carotid artery (ICA)	1. Ipsilateral blindness (variable) 2. MCA syndrome
Vertebral or PICA (posterior inferior cerebellar artery)	1. Ipsilateral: hemiataxia, nystagmus, facial sensory loss, Horner syndrome 2. Contralateral loss of temperature or painful sensation 3. Dysphagia
Basilar artery	1. Quadriparesis 2. Dysarthria 3. Dysphagia 4. Diplopia 5. Somnolence 6. Amnesia
Posterior cerebral artery	1. Contralateral homonymous hemianopsia 2. Amnesia 3. Sensory loss
Lacunar (internal capsule, pons, thalamus)	1. **Internal capsule**: pure **motor** hemiparesis 2. Pons: dysarthria, clumsy hand 3. **Thalamus**: pure **sensory** deficit

- Cocaine use is one of the main causes of stroke in the young
- Common sites of SAH
  - Junction of anterior communicating artery and anterior cerebral artery
  - Junction of posterior communicating artery and internal carotid
  - Bifurcation of the MCA

CHADS2 Scoring

The presence of congestive cardiac failure (C), hypertension (H), age >75 years (A), and diabetes (D) each scores one point, and a history of prior stroke or TIA (S) scores 2 points. A CHADS score of 2 or more is associated with an annual risk of stroke of over 4%.

- International recommendations: aspirin 325 mg/d for those with a CHADS score of 0

- For those with a CHADS2 score of 1: aspirin or warfarin may be used depending on patient preference.
- Patients with a CHADS2 score of 2 or more: anticoagulated, unless there is a specific contraindication
- Patients with bacterial endocarditis should not receive warfarin because of the risk of cerebral hemorrhage from septic embolization
- CHADS2 scoring is used specifically for people with atrial fibrillation

ALZHEIMER'S DISEASE

- Pathology:
  - Sensile plaques—focal collections of dilated, tortuous neuritic processes surrounding a central amyloid core (amyloid β-protein)
  - Neurofibrillary tangles: bundles of neurofilaments in cytoplasm of neurons, neuronal degeneration

- Early stages—mild forgetfulness, impaired ability to learn new material, poor performance at work, poor concentration, changes in personality, impaired judgment (inappropriate humor)
- Intermediate—memory is progressively impaired; aware of condition, yet denial present; visuospatial disturbances are common (getting lost in familiar place and difficulty following directions), repeat questions over and over
- Late—assistance needed for ADLs, difficulty remembering names of relatives/friends or major aspects of lives, paranoid delusions (victim of theft) and hallucinations common
- Advanced—complete debilitation and dependence on others, incontinence, forgets own name
- Death—secondary to infection or other complications of debilitated state

Disease	Etiology, Prevalence, Risk Factors	Clinical Symptoms and Signs	Diagnostics	Therapy, Prognosis, and Health Maintenance
Alzheimer's disease	66% of all cases of dementia (most common form of dementia) 60-70 y old, mostly 85 or older (50%) Decreased acetylcholine synthesis, impaired cortical cholinergic function	1. Begins *insidiously* and *progresses* at steady rate 2. Progressive memory loss 3. Cognitive deficits: disorientation, language difficulties, inability to perform complex motor functions, inattention, visual misperception, poor problem solving, inappropriate social behavior, hallucinations 4. Intellectual decline in 2+ areas of cognition documented by MMSE or similar scale 5. Formal neuropsychological testing to confirm diagnosis	Clinical DX: 1. CT or MRI: diffuse **cortical atrophy with enlargement of ventricles** 2. Pathology: intracellular neurofibrillary tangles and extracellular neuritic plaques 3. CBC, CMP, heavy metal, calcium, glucose, TSH, B_{12}, renal, LFT, drug/ETOH levels	No treatment found to have significant effects 1. Cholinesterase inhibitors: **donepezil**, rivastigmine, galantamine 2. Memantine (NMDA-receptor antagonist): mod-severe 3. Ginkgo, lecithin 4. Vitamin E Avoid anticholinergics Onset to death: 5-10 y

ESSENTIAL TREMOR, PARKINSON'S DISEASE

- Parkinson disease is an imbalance in the dopaminergic and cholinergic systems of the basal ganglia and striatal region
  - Treatment directed at enhancing dopamine's effect or inhibiting acetylcholine

Disease	Etiology, Prevalence, Risk Factors	Clinical Symptoms and Signs	Diagnostics	Therapy, Prognosis, and Health Maintenance
Essential tremor	Familial (**autosomal dominant**)	1. Worse with certain postures (eg, arms outstretched) or certain tasks (handwriting), drinking from a cup or use of utensils 2. Head tremor, vocal tremulousness 3. **Improved with alcohol**		1. **Propranolol** (first line) 2. Primidone 3. Alprazolam 4. Small amounts of alcohol 5. Gabapentin, Topiramate, or Nimodipine 6. Drug resistant cases - Deep brain stimulation

(continued)

(continued)

Disease	Etiology, Prevalence, Risk Factors	Clinical Symptoms and Signs	Diagnostics	Therapy, Prognosis, and Health Maintenance
Parkinson's disease	Loss of dopamine containing neurons located in substantia nigra and locus ceruleus _Age onset:_ After 50 y Meds that cause parkinsonism: neuroleptics (chlorpromazine, metoclopramide, reserpine)	1. *Pill-rolling* **tremor at rest** (worse with emotional stress), goes away when performing routine tasks 2. **Bradykinesia**–slowness of voluntary movements 3. Rigidity (**cogwheel rigidity**)–refers to rachet-like jerking, examined by testing tone in one limb while patient clenches the opposite fist 4. Poor postural reflexes; difficulty initiating first step and walking with small **shuffling steps**; stooped posture 5. Masked (expressionless) facies; decreased blinking 6. Dysarthria and dysphagia, micrographia (small handwriting) 7. Impairment of cognitive function (dementia) 8. Autonomic dysfunction can lead to orthostatic hypotension, constipation, increased sweating, and oily skin 9. Personality changes present in early stages • Patients become withdrawn, apathetic, and dependent on others • Depression common and can be significant 10. Follows progressive course → significant disability within 5-10 y Clinical DX		1. No cure–goals are to delay disease progression and relieve symptoms 2. **Carbidopa-levodopa (Sinemet)**–drug of choice for treating Parkinsonian symptoms; most effective • Dyskinesias (involuntary, choreic movements) after 5-7 y of treatment • Nausea/vomiting, anorexia, HTN, hallucinations • "On-off" phenomenon: fluctuations in symptoms due to dose-response relationships 3. **Dopamine receptor agonists** (bromocriptine, *pramipexole*)–first to initiate • May control symptoms and delay need for levodopa • Used for sudden episodes of hesitancy or immobility ("freezing") 4. **Selegiline**–inhibits monoamine oxidase B activity (increases dopamine pathway), reducing metabolism of levodopa; adjunctive therapy 5. Amantadine (antiviral)–mild or early disease 6. Anticholinergics–helpful for tremor • trihexyphenidyl and **benztropine** 7. Amitriptyline–anticholinergic and antidepressant 8. Surgery (deep brain stimulation)–for refractory cases, severe disease before age 40

BELL'S PALSY

Disease	Etiology, Prevalence, Risk Factors	Clinical Symptoms and Signs	Diagnostics	Therapy, Prognosis, and Health Maintenance
Bell's palsy: hemifacial weakness/paralysis of muscles innervated by CN VII due to swelling of cranial nerve	Uncertain cause, possibly viral (herpes simplex)	1. URI preceding event 2. Acute onset **unilateral facial weakness/ paralysis**, both upper and lower parts of face affected • Mastoid pain • Decreased tearing • **Cannot raise eyebrow on affected side** 3. Weak orbicularis oculis muscle (**unable to close eye**) on affected side 4. Dysgeusia (impairment of taste) or ageusia (loss of taste) _Signs:_ 1. Check external ear canal for rash or vesicles to r/o Ramsay Hunt syndrome (herpes zoster oticus) 2. Hyperacusis (tuning fork)	<u>Clinical DX:</u> 1. Consider Lyme disease (do not use steroids) 2. EMG testing if paresis fails to resolve in 10 d	1. Usually no treatment required 2. Short course of **prednisone** and **acyclovir** 3. Wear eye patch to prevent corneal abrasion 4. Surgical decompression of CN VII 5. Prognosis good: 80%-90% recover fully within 6 wk-3 mo

- Aberrant reinnervation
  - Synkinesis: abnormal contraction of facial muscles while smiling or closing eyes
  - Crocodile tears: eye tearing with salivation or eating

DELIRIUM AND DEMENTIA

Delirium

Acute period of cognitive dysfunction due to a medical disturbance or condition.

- Elderly very prone
- Causes include those of coma (SMASHED) plus (P. DIMM WIT)
  - P = postoperative state (pain meds)
  - D = dehydration
  - I = infection (sepsis, meningitis, encephalitis, UTI)
  - M = Meds (TCAs, steroids, anticholinergics, hallucinogens, cocaine)
  - M = Metals (heavy metal exposure)
  - W = Withdrawal state (ETOH, benzos)
  - I = inflammation, fever
  - T = trauma, burns
- SMASHED
  - Structural brain pathology: stroke, subdural or epidural hematoma, tumor, hydrocephalus, herniation, abscess
  - Meningitis, mental illness
  - Alcohol, acidosis

- Seizures (postictal), substrate deficiency (thiamine)
- Hypercapnia, hyperglycemia; hyponatremia, hypoglycemia, hypoxia, hypotension, hypothermia
- Endocrine (Addisonian crisis, thyrotoxicosis, hypothyroidism); encephalitis, encephalopathy
- Drugs (opiates, barbiturates, benzos)

Dementia

Progressive deterioration of intellectual function, typically characterized by preservation of consciousness.

- The most important risk factor for dementia: age
- Reversible causes: hypothyroidism, neurosyphilis, Vitamin B_{12}/folate/thiamine deficiency, medications, hydrocephalus, depression, subdural hematoma
- Patient history—ask about nature of onset, specific deficits, physical symptoms, comorbid conditions, review all meds, FH/SH
- Physical—focus on a thorough neurologic examination and MSE, gait analysis
- Labs and imaging—CBC, chemistry, TSH, B12/folate, VDRL, HIV, CT scan or MRI of head
- Treatment
  - Avoid and/or monitor doses of meds with adverse cognitive effects (steroids, opioids, sedative hypnotics, anxiolytics, anticholinergics, lithium)
  - Treat/control: HTN, diabetes, depression, visual and hearing impairment
  - Pharmacologic therapy: vitamin E, tacrine, **donepezil**

Disease	Etiology, Prevalence, Risk Factors	Clinical Symptoms and Signs	Diagnostics	Therapy, Prognosis, and Health Maintenance
Delirium	**"Waxing and waning,"** rapid onset **"Sundowning"** = worse at night	1. *Rapid* deterioration in mental status (hours-days), a fluctuating level of awareness, disorientation, abnormal vitals 2. May be accompanied by acute abnormalities of perception, such as **visual hallucinations** 3. May not necessarily be agitated, but may have slow, blunted responsiveness 4. Tremor sometimes (asterixis)	1. Mental status examination (MMSE) 2. Labs (chemistry, B_{12}/folate) 3. LP in febrile, delirious patient (cerebral edema)	Almost always reversible 1. Treat underlying cause 2. **Haloperidol** for agitation/psychosis 3. Supportive
Dementia	RF: Increasing age	1. *Insidious*, progressive 2. Preserved consciousness 3. Rarely hallucinations present 4. No tremor unless due to Parkinson disease		Typically irreversible

(continued)

(continued)

Disease	Etiology, Prevalence, Risk Factors	Clinical Symptoms and Signs	Diagnostics	Therapy, Prognosis, and Health Maintenance
Vascular dementia	Multi-infarct, stepwise decline due to series of infarcts Men > women	Forgetfulness in absence of depression and inattentiveness 1. Cortical—speech difficulty, trouble performing routine tasks, sensory interpretation difficulty, confusion, amnesia, executive dysfunction 2. Subcortical symptoms: gait problems, urinary difficulties, motor deficits, personality changes		1. Control HTN and metabolic disorders 2. Same as Alzheimer disease
Frontotemporal dementia		1. Frontal lobe symptoms: behavioral SX (euphoria, apathy, disinhibition) and Compulsive disorders 2. Primitive reflexes (frontal release signs): palmomental, palmar grasp, rooting reflexes	MRI: frontal or anterior temporal lobe atrophy PET: frontal and/or anterior temporal hypometabolism	Supportive care SSRIs for depression
Lewy-body dementia	Features of Alzheimer and Parkinson diseases, but progression more rapid than in Alzheimer disease	1. **Visual hallucinations** predominate, extrapyramidal features and fluctuating mental status 2. Sensitive to adverse effects of neuroleptics (make worse)		1. Neuroleptics for hallucinations and psychosis 2. Cholinesterase inhibitors: **donepezil**, rivastigmine, galantamine 3. Selegiline—slows progression

HEADACHES (CLUSTER, MIGRAINE, TENSION)

- Caused by *vasodilation* of blood vessels
- Sensitization: refers to the process in which neurons become increasingly responsive to nociceptive and non-nociceptive stimulation → responsible for clinical symptoms of migraine, including throbbing quality, worsening with cough, bending, sudden head movements, hyperalgesia, and allodynia.
- **Status migrainosus**: debilitating migraine attack lasting for >72 hours.

- Visual aura in migraine: bilateral homonymous scotoma; bright, flashing, crescent shaped images with jagged edges appear on a page, obscuring the underlying print, lasts 10-20 minutes.
- Indications for preventive treatment: frequent or long-lasting migraines, migraine attacks that cause significant disability or decreased QOL, contraindication to acute treatment, failure of acute therapy, serious adverse effects of acute therapy, risk of medication overuse headache, menstrual migraine.

Disease	Etiology, Prevalence, Risk Factors	Clinical Symptoms and Signs	Diagnostics	Therapy, Prognosis, and Health Maintenance
Migraines	12% of general population Women > men <u>MC:</u> 3039 (+) family history <u>Precipitating factors:</u> Emotional stress, hormones (women), not eating, weather, sleep disturbance, odors, neck pain, lights, alcohol, smoke, sleeping late, heat, food, exercise, sexual activity <u>Comorbidities:</u> Sleep disturbances (insomnia)	1. Recurrent attacks, over hours to days 2. 4 phases • Prodrome (60%, 24-48 h prior): euphoria, depression, irritability, food cravings, constipation, neck stiffness, increased yawning • Aura (25%): see below • Headache: **Unilateral**, throbbing, **pulsatile**, increasing **(gradual)** intensity over 4-72 h → nausea ± vomiting, photophobia, phonophobia; **better with lying down in dark, quiet room**, osmophobia, cutaneous allodynia • Postdrome: pain with sudden head movement in location of antecedent headache; patient may feel drained or exhausted	<u>Clinical DX:</u> 1. Neuroimaging unnecessary in most **Indications:** **First/worst headache**, recent significant change in pattern, frequency, or severity of headaches, new or unexplained neurologic signs/sx, headache always on same side, unresponsive to treatment, onset **after age 50**, onset with cancer or HIV, or associated sx (fever, stiff neck, papilledema, cognitive impairment, personality change) 2. **Head CT** (with and without contrast) 3. **MRI**–r/o lesions or CSF leak 4. MRA and MRV–r/o arteriovenous lesions	See treatment table <u>Complications:</u> Status migrainosus, persistent aura without infarction, migrainous infarction, migraine aura-triggered seizure

(continued)

(continued)

Disease	Etiology, Prevalence, Risk Factors	Clinical Symptoms and Signs	Diagnostics	Therapy, Prognosis, and Health Maintenance
Migraines with aura "classic migraine"	Autosomal dominant with incomplete penetrance <u>Causes:</u> Serotonin depletion?	1. Aura • Does not always precede headache • Gradual development, but can be acute (<5 min) • No longer than **1 h** • Positive and negative features • Completely reversible 2. **Positive symptoms:** visual (bright lines, shapes, objects), auditory (tinnitus, noises, music), somatosensory (burning, pain, paresthesia), or motor (jerking, repetitive rhythmic movements) • Paresthesias may affect the buccal mucosa and half of the tongue, can mimic ischemic events 3. Negative Symptoms: **Loss of vision**, hearing, feeling, or ability to move a part of the body	<u>ICHD-3 Criteria:</u> 1. At least **2 attacks** 2. Fully reversible aura • Visual, sensory, speech and/or language, motor, brainstem, retinal 3. Characteristics, at least 2: • 1 aura spreads gradually over >5 min, and 2+ symptoms occur in succession • Each aura lasts 5-60 min • At least 1 aura is unilateral • Aura followed by headache within 60 min 4. No other better ICHD-3 diagnosis	1. Acute migraines • Mild-mod: NSAIDs, Tylenol, antiemetics • Mod-severe: PO Triptan or Sumatriptan-Naproxen, SQ Sumatriptan, nasal Sumatriptan and Zolmitriptan • **DHE** (5-HT1) agonist: highly effective • **Sumatriptan** (5-HT1 agonist): rapid and effective, 1-2 times/wk 2. Prophylaxis: • Avoid precipitants • TCAs and **propranolol** (most effective) *Do not use BB as initial therapy in patients >60 and in smokers • Verapamil (Calan), depakote, methysergide (Deseril) 3. Emergent migraines: • Sumatriptan 6 mg SQ • **Metoclopramide 10 mg IV**, prochlorperazine 10 mg IV or IM, or chlorpromazine 0.1-1 mg/kg IV • DHE 1 mg IV with metoclopramide 10 mg IV • Ketorolac 30 mg IV or 60 mg IM
Migraines without aura "common migraine"	Most common type (75%)	1. Prodromal phase (30%) • Excitation or inhibition of CNS: elation, excitability, increased appetite or craving for foods, depression, irritability, sleepiness, fatigue 2. **Severe, throbbing, unilateral headache** • Lasts 4-72 h • Generalized over entire head, lasting for days • Aggravated by coughing, physical activity, or bending down • "Throbbing, dull, achy" 3. **Nausea, vomiting** (90%), photophobia, increased sense of smell	ICHD-3 criteria: 1. At least **5 attacks** 2. Lasting 4-72 h (untreated or treated) 3. Characteristics: • Unilateral • Pulsating • Intensity: mod/severe • Aggravation or avoiding physical activity (walking/stairs) 4. At least one of: • Nausea, vomiting, both • Photo/phonophobia 5. No other better ICHD-3 diagnosis	
Menstrual migraines (catamenial migraine)		1. Occurs 2 d before menstruation and last day of menses, estrogen withdrawal 2. May also have migraine at other times during the month		1. NSAIDs 2. Estrogen supplementation

Disease	Etiology, Prevalence, Risk Factors	Clinical Symptoms and Signs	Diagnostics	Therapy, Prognosis, and Health Maintenance
Chronic migraines		1. Headache occurring 15 or more days/month for more than 3 mo 2. Features of migraine on at least 8 d/mo		
Tension-type headaches (stress, muscle contraction, psychogenic, or psychomyogenic)	Unknown cause, but originally named for suspected cause (excessive *stress or tension* leading to muscle contraction) Women > men Precipitants: anxiety, depression, stress Most prevalent headache in general population and second most prevalent disorder in the world	1. **Bilateral** 2. Pain—steady, aching, "vise-like" and encircles entire head (tight **band-like**), generalized but most intense around neck or back of head • Mild to moderate intensity • Nonthrobbing • Descriptors: dull, pressure, head fullness, head feels large, like a tight cap, band-like, or like a heavy weight on my head or shoulders 3. Characteristics: **Pressure or** "tightness" in posterior neck muscles, which waxes and wanes 4. Lasts 30 min to 7 d Signs: 1. Patient may remain active or may need to rest 2. Increased pericranial muscle tenderness	1. CT/MRI, blood work, and spinal fluid analysis—normal ICHD-3 criteria: 1. At least **10 episodes** of headache, lasting 30 min to 7 d each • At least 2 of: • Bilateral • Pressing or tightening (nonpulsating) • Mild or moderate • Not aggravated by routine activity • Neither: • No nausea or vomiting • No more photo or phonophobia	1. Mild/mod: **NSAIDs** (ibuprofen, ketoprofen, naproxen, diclofenac), Tylenol, aspirin 2. Severe: triptans, nonpharmacologic treatments (ice, heat, massage, rest, biofeedback) 3. Failure: Emergent setting: 1. Metoclopramide + diphenhydramine 2. IM ketorolac 60 mg 3. IV chlorpromazine Pregnancy: 1. Butalbital with Tylenol (also used with ulcers or renal failure)
Cluster headaches	Rare Middle-aged men Chronic cigarette smokers (85%) 1. **Episodic (90%)**—last 2-3 mo, with remissions of months to years 2. Chronic cluster headaches (10%)—last 1-2 y, headaches do not remit	1. Always **unilateral** • Excruciating orbital, supraorbital, or temporal pain ("**behind the eye**") • Deep, burning, searing, or stabbing pain • Occurs up to 8 times/d, short lived 2. Associated: **Ipsilateral lacrimation, facial flushing, nasal stuffiness/ discharge** 3. Begins few hours after patient goes to bed, **lasts 15 min to 3 h**, awakens from sleep (daytime cluster headaches occur) 4. Occur nightly 2-3 mo, then disappear 5. Worse with alcohol and sleep Signs: 1. Pallor, diaphoresis 2. Horner syndrome 3. Restlessness, agitation 4. Focal neurologic symptoms (rare) 5. Sensitivity to alcohol	ICHD-3 Criteria: 1. At least 5 attacks 2. Characteristics: • Severe unilateral orbital, supraorbital, and/or temporal pain lasting 15-180 min when untreated 3. Either or both: • Ipsilateral to headache: conjunctival injection or lacrimation, nasal congestion or rhinorrhea, eyelid edema, forehead or facial sweating or flushing, sensation of fullness in ear, miosis or ptosis • Restlessness or agitation 4. Attacks occur between once every other day and 8/d for more than half the time when disorder is active 5. No other better ICHD-3 diagnosis	1. Acute attacks • 100% **O₂ inhalation** (first) via nonrebreathing facial mask at flow rate 12 L/min in sitting, upright position × 15 min • SQ triptans: **sumatriptan** (Imitrex) 6 mg • Intranasal triptans 2. Prophylaxis (2+ mon) • Most responsive to **verapamil 80 mg TID** • Ergotamine, **methysergide, lithium**, steroids • Resolution of headaches within 1 wk

CHAPTER 8

Dermatology

DERMATITIS (ECZEMA, SEBORRHEA), NUMMULAR ECZEMA

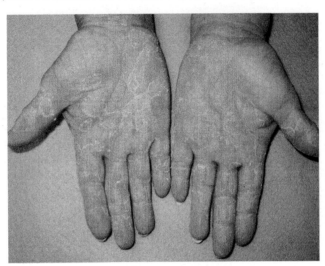

FIGURE 8-1. Irritant contact dermatitis; likely caused by latex gloves. Tympanogram showing perforation of the tympanic membrane. (Image provided by Stedman's.)

Disease	Etiology, Prevalence, Risk Factors	Clinical Symptoms and Signs	Diagnostics	Therapy, Prognosis, and Health Maintenance
Contact	**Irritant:** nonimmune modulated skin irritation caused by skin injury, direct cytotoxic effects, or cutaneous inflammation from contact with irritant **Allergic:** *Type IV, T-cell mediated, delayed hypersensitivity* reaction from foreign substance Most common: Poison ivy, nickel, fragrances	1. Not painful, but **red** and itchy 2. Onset after contact with irritant or allergen 3. Distribution patterns from irritant or allergen Signs: 1. **Scaly** occurring on thin areas of skin (flexural surfaces, eyelids, face, anogenital region) 2. Acute = erythema, vesicles, and bullae 3. Chronic = lichenification with cracks and fissures	1. Determine if problem resolves with removal of substance	1. Localized = mid- or high-potency topical steroids (triamcinolone 0.1%/triamcinolone acetonide (Kenalog) or clobetasol 0.05%) If >20% of BSA, systemic steroids recommended with resolution in 12-24 h • 5-7 d of prednisone 0.5-1 mg/kg/d

Irritant (Fig. 8-1)	**Allergic**
Usually occurs on hands Burning, itching, painful Dry and fissured Less distinct borders	Usually exposed areas of skin (hands most common) Itching (predominant symptom) Vesicles or bullae—redness and scaling with relatively well-demarcated visible borders

Seborrheic Dermatitis

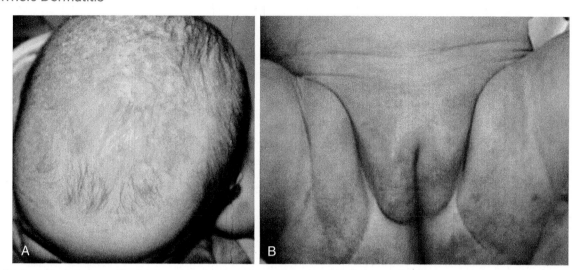

FIGURE 8-2. Seborrheic dermatitis. **A,** Infant with seborrheic dermatitis on the scalp. **B,** Infant with seborrheic dermatitis in diaper area, which is not found to be bright red and is without satellite lesions. (From Shaw KN, Bachur RG. *Fleisher & Ludwig's Textbook of Pediatric Emergency Medicine.* 7th ed. Philadelphia: Wolters Kluwer; 2016.)

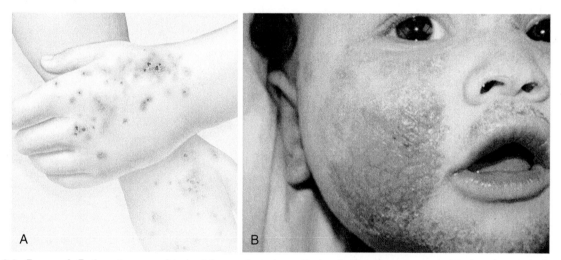

FIGURE 8-3. Eczema. **A,** Erythematous, excoriated patches, and papules on the hands; **B,** erythematous, excoriated patches on the face. (**A,** From Anatomical Chart Company. *Understanding Allergies.* Philadelphia: Wolters Kluwer; 2006. **B,** From White AJ. *The Washington Manual of Pediatrics.* 2nd ed. Philadelphia: Wolters Kluwer; 2016.)

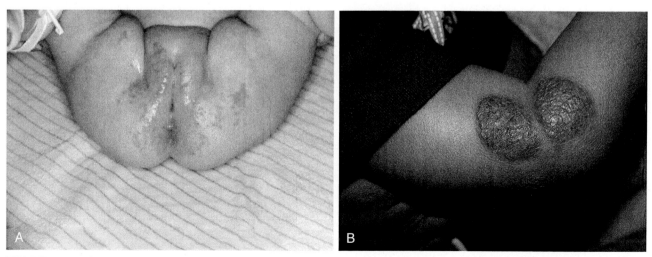

FIGURE 8-4. **A,** Mucocutaneous candidiasis. Erythematous patches in the genital area with surrounding satellite macules. **B,** Nummular eczema. Round, eczematous patches on the arm. (**A,** From Chung EK. *Visual Diagnosis and Treatment in Pediatrics.* 3rd ed. Philadelphia: Wolters Kluwer; 2015. **B,** From White AJ. *The Washington Manual of Pediatrics.* 2nd ed. Philadelphia: Wolters Kluwer; 2016.)

Disease	Etiology, Prevalence, Risk Factors	Clinical Symptoms and Signs	Diagnostics	Therapy, Prognosis, and Health Maintenance
Seborrhea (Fig. 8-2)	Malassezia yeast Immunocompromised at risk—HIV Bimodal: 2-12 mo, adolescence/early adulthood M > F	1. Scaling erythema, itching • Most common—scalp, face, chest, back, axilla, groin Infants: 1. Thick white or yellow greasy scale on scalp (benign) Adults: 1. Flaky, greasy, erythematous patches on scalp, nasolabial folds, ears, eyebrows, anterior chest, or upper back	1. Mainly clinical DX, but biopsy may reveal parakeratosis in epidermis, plugged follicular ostia, and spongiosis	1. **Topical ketoconazole/ Nizoral 2%, daily** (mainstay) • <u>AE</u>: Irritation, itching, xeroderma 2. Antifungal shampoo (long-term): • **Selenium sulfide** twice/ wk AE: alopecia, hair discoloration, irritation 3. Zinc pyrithione twice/wk, irritation 4. Topical steroids (betamethasone valerate 0.12% foam) AE: hypopigmentation, itching, atrophy, stinging 5. Calcineurin inhibitors second line, short term Infants—resolves spontaneously
Atopic **(eczema)** (Fig. 8-3)	More susceptible to skin infections, *S. aureus* (most common) Associated **allergic triad**: asthma, allergic rhinitis, atopic dermatitis	Onset before age 2, 10% diagnosed after age 5 <u>Acute phase</u>: vesicular, weeping, crusting eruption <u>Subacute</u>: dry, scaly, red papules and plaques <u>Chronic</u>: Excoriations and lichenification of skin, Xerosis, hyperpigmentation Flexural lichenification in adults: anterior and lateral neck, eyelids, forehead, face, wrists, dorsa of feet, hands Facial and EXTENSOR involvement in children and infants	<u>Clinical DX</u>: Complications: 1. Secondary bacterial infections—pustules and crusts	1. Moisturizers or **emollients** (mainstay): Cetaphil or Eucerin • Ointments: Aquaphor, petroleum jelly 2. Bathing—removes scale, crust, irritants, allergens • Limit use of nonsoap cleansers (hypoallergenic, no fragrance) 3. **Topical steroids** (first line)—flare ups 4. Topical calcineurin inhibitors—second line mod-severe (pimecrolimus 1%/Elidel or tacrolimus 0.03%) 5. Antibiotics to reduce flare ups 6. UV phototherapy for severe or refractory
Mucocutaneous candidiasis (Fig. 8-4A)	Associated: oral thrush and vitiligo Begins in infancy or during first 2 decades of life	1. Diffuse eruption over trunk, thorax, and extremities • Face, scalp, hands, nails 2. Pruritus, worse in genitocrural folds, anal region, axillae, hands/feet Signs: 1. Rash that begins as individual vesicles → large confluent areas 2. Satellite lesions 3. Erythema and maceration Complications: bacterial sepsis	1. Wet mount, scrapings, or smears • Taken from skin, nails, oral or vaginal mucosa • KOH prep, gram stain, or methylene blue	1. Topical antifungal • Clotrimazole, miconazole, ketoconazole, nystatin 2. For onychomycosis use itraconazole (Sporanox)
Nummular eczema (Fig. 8-4B)		One or several coin-shaped plaques on extremities, typically on backs of hands		

DYSHIDROSIS (FIG. 8-5)

Disease	Etiology, Prevalence, Risk Factors	Clinical Symptoms and Signs	Diagnostics	Therapy, Prognosis, and Health Maintenance
Dyshidrosis (pompholyx)		Occurs on lateral digits (hands) Clear, deep-seated erythematous **"tapioca pudding" vesicles** ± scaling	History/clinical DX	1. Topical steroids and emollients

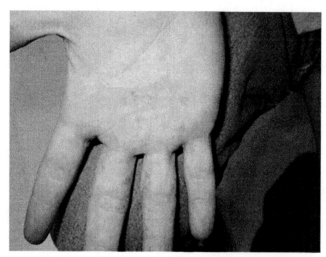

FIGURE 8-5. Dyshidrosis. Intensely pruritic vesicles and erosions on the palm and digits. (From Werner R. *A Massage Therapist's Guide to Pathology*. 5th ed. Philadelphia: Wolters Kluwer Health; 2013.)

LICHEN SIMPLEX CHRONICUS (FIG. 8-6)

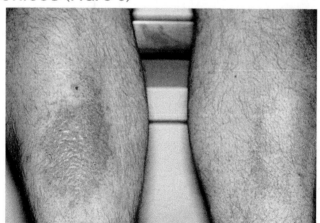

FIGURE 8-6. Lichen simplex chronicus. Lichenified plaques and excoriations on the bilateral shins. (From Goodheart HP, MD. *Goodheart's Photoguide of Common Skin Disorders*. 2nd ed. Philadelphia: Lippincott Williams & Wilkins; 2003.)

Disease	Etiology, Prevalence, Risk Factors	Clinical Symptoms and Signs	Diagnostics	Therapy, Prognosis, and Health Maintenance
Lichen simplex chronicus	<u>MC:</u> Adults, possible in children	1. **Eczematous** eruption caused by habitual scratching of single localized area 2. One or more plaques with lichenification in an area that is easily scratched		1. **High potency topical steroids** (first line) for all forms: Clobetasol <u>Health maintenance:</u> Avoid scratching and picking at skin

LICHEN PLANUS (FIG. 8-7)

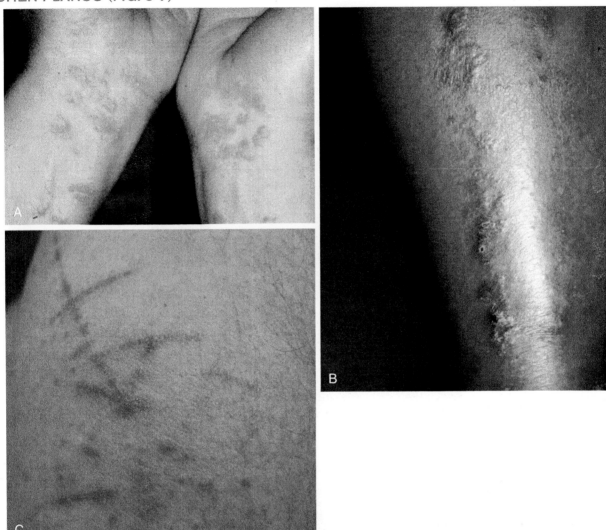

FIGURE 8-7. Lichen planus. **A**, Erythematous flat-topped, polygonal, pruritic papules, and patches on the volar surfaces of the wrists. **B**, Purple, flat-topped lesions of lichen planus on the lower leg. **C**, Koebnerized lesions of lichen planus from scratching. (**A**, From DeLong L, Burkhart NW. *General and Oral Pathology for the Dental Hygienist*. 2nd ed. Philadelphia: Wolters Kluwer Health; 2013. **B**, From Goodheart HP, Gonzalez ME. *Goodheart's Photoguide to Common Pediatric and Adult Skin Disorders*. 4th ed. Philadelphia: Wolters Kluwer; 2016. **C**, Image provided by Stedman's.)

Disease	Etiology, Prevalence, Risk Factors	Clinical Symptoms and Signs	Diagnostics	Therapy, Prognosis, and Health Maintenance

Lichen planus	Chronic, inflammatory autoimmune disease
	Most common in peri-menopausal women, **30-60 y/o**
	Commonly associated with **hepatitis C**
		1. Acute onset, affects **flexor surfaces of wrists**, forearms, legs
		  • Generalized eruption occurs after 1 wk with maximal spreading after 2-16 wk
		2. **6 P's: p**lanar (flat topped), **p**urple, **p**olygonal, **p**ruritic (itchy), **p**apules, **p**laques
		3. **Pruritus** (common)
		Signs:
		1. Koebner phenomenon—follow lines of trauma
		2. Covered by lacy, reticular, white lines (**Wickham striae**)
		3. Postinflammatory hyperpigmentation as skin lesions clear, especially with darker skin
			Clinical DX:
			4 mm punch biopsy helpful and required for atypical cases
				1. **High-potency topical steroids** (first line) for all forms: Clobetasol
				  • Oral antihistamines (hydroxyzine/Vistaril) for itching
				  • Intralesional triamcinolone acetonide (Kenalog) 5-10 mL for hypertrophic lesions
				2. Topical calcineurin inhibitors (tacrolimus or pimecrolimus) for vulvovaginal lichen planus
				3. 3-6 wk of oral prednisone for severe, widespread cases
				Prognosis:
				1. Most self-limited: **resolves spontaneously within 1-2 y**, although recurrence is common
				Health maintenance:
				Screen for hepatitis C

PITYRIASIS ROSEA (FIG. 8-8)

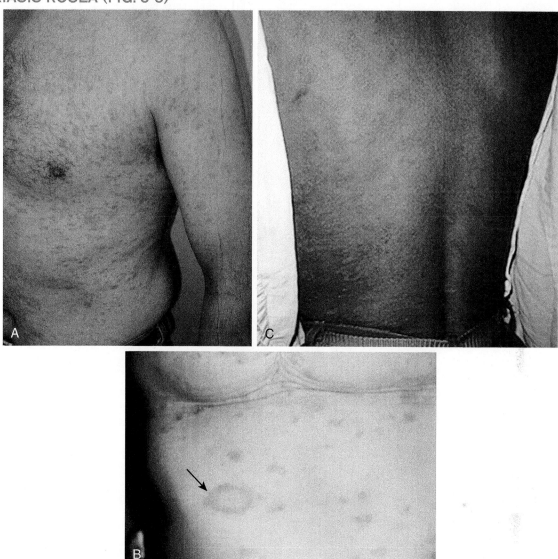

FIGURE 8-8. Pityriasis rosea. **A**, Pink macules and patches distributed along the skin tension lines of the trunk and arm. **B**, Salmon-colored herald patch with fine collarette scale on the abdomen. **C**, Purple patches of pityriasis rosea on a darker skinned individual. Note the distribution down the back in a "Christmas tree" pattern. (**A**, Image provided by Stedman's. **B**, From Porth CM. *Essentials of Pathophysiology*. 4th ed. Philadelphia: Wolters Kluwer; 2015. **C**, From Arndt KA, Hsu JTS, Alam M, et al. *Manual of Dermatologic Therapeutics*. 8th ed. Philadelphia: Wolters Kluwer; 2014.)

Disease	Etiology, Prevalence, Risk Factors	Clinical Symptoms and Signs	Diagnostics	Therapy, Prognosis, and Health Maintenance
Pityriasis rosea	Children and young adults Related to herpes type 7 **Not contagious** Common on trunk, upper arms, and thighs	1. Begins with herald patch 2. Pruritus 3. Progression to generalized rash in 1-3 wk 1. Multiple salmon-pink oval papules, Scattered symmetrically 2. **Christmas-tree–like distribution** over the neck, trunk and proximal extremities 3. Annular plaques with collarette scale		1. Self-limiting (reassurance) in 6-8 wk without treatment 2. Antihistamines for itching

PSORIASIS (FIG. 8-9)

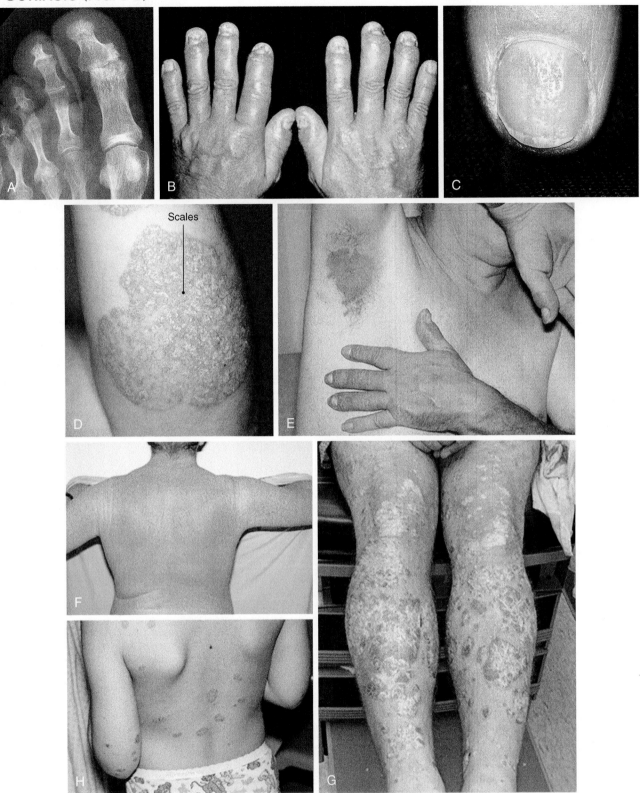

Scales

FIGURE 8-9. **A,** Psoriatic arthritis. Radiograph showing pencil in cup deformity of the second distal interphalangeal joint. **B,** Psoriatic onycho-dystrophy with nail plate **thickening** and breakage. **C,** Nail pitting showing multiple pinprick indentations of the nail. **D,** Plaque psoriasis. One large, erythematous psoriatic plaque with overlying silvery scale. **E,** Inverse psoriasis. Erythematous plaque with overlying scale on the right axilla. **F,** Erythrodermic psoriasis showing wide spread, confluent erythema. **G,** Pustular psoriasis showing scattered erythematous papules and plaques with scattered, coalescing pustules on the lower legs. **H,** Guttate psoriasis showing small erythematous papules and plaques with overlying scale on the back of a child. (**A,** From Berquist TH. *Imaging of the Foot and Ankle.* 3rd ed. Wolters Kluwer; 2011. **B,** From Huang JJ, Gaudio PA. *Ocular Inflammatory Disease and Uveitis Manual: Diagnosis and Treatment.* Philadelphia: Lippincott Williams & Wilkins, a Wolters Kluwer Business; 2010. **C,** From Goodheart HP, Gonzalez ME. *Goodheart's Photoguide to Common Pediatric and Adult Skin Disorders.* 4th ed. Philadelphia: Wolters Kluwer; 2016. **D,** From *Wound, Ostomy and Continence Nurses Society: Core Curriculum: Wound Management.* Philadelphia: Wolters Kluwer; 2016. **E,** From Nicol NH. *Dermatologic Nursing Essentials: A Core Curriculum.* 3rd ed. Philadelphia: Wolters Kluwer; 2016. **F,** From Werner R. *A Massage Therapist's Guide to Pathology.* 5th ed. Philadelphia: Wolters Kluwer Health; 2013. **G,** From Council ML, Sheinbein DM, Cornelius LA. *The Washington Manual of Dermatology Diagnostics.* Philadelphia: Wolters Kluwer; 2016. **H,** From Werner R. *A Massage Therapist's Guide to Pathology.* 5th ed. Philadelphia: Wolters Kluwer Health; 2013.)

Disease	Etiology, Prevalence, Risk Factors	Clinical Symptoms and Signs	Diagnostics	Therapy, Prognosis, and Health Maintenance

Psoriasis	Etiology: genetic and environmental factors
	Immune-mediated disease
	Most common form: plaque psoriasis
	RF:
	Direct skin trauma (Koebner phenom), strep infection, stress, smoking, obesity, and alcohol use
		1. Distinctive red, scaling patches and papules that coalesce to form round-to-oval plaques on extensor surfaces
		2. Itchy and sometimes painful
		3. Associated comorbidities: cardiovascular disease, lymphoma, **depression**
			1. Clinical DX
			2. Biopsy rarely needed to confirm DX
				1. Potent **topical steroids**
				  • **Topical vitamin D** (calcipotriene/Dovonex, Calcitriol/Vectical)
				  • **Tazarotene** (Tazorac) for mild psoriasis
				  • Calcineurin inhibitors, such as tacrolimus (Protopic) or pimecrolimus (Elidel)
				2. PO biologics for severe psoriasis
				3. TNF inhibitors for psoriatic arthritis

Psoriatic arthritis	• Seronegative • Develops 12 y after onset of skin lesions • 6%-42% prevalence • Severity not related to skin disease	1. Nail pitting 2. Splinter hemorrhages 3. "Oil staining" 4. Yellow-gray or silvery-white nails	1. Pencil and cup deformity	
Psoriatic onychodystrophy (nail pitting)	Occurs in 80%-90% over lifetime	1. Fingernails > toenails 2. Pitting, subungual hyperkeratosis, onycholysis		1. Treatment resistant
Plaque psoriasis	90% of psoriasis	1. Well-defined round or oval plaques that differ in size and coalesce 2. Occur on extensor surfaces of arms, legs, scalp, buttocks, trunk		
Inverse psoriasis	Heat, trauma, infection contribute to development	1. Less scaly than plaque form, occurs in skin folds, such as flexor surfaces and perineal, inframammary, axillary, inguinal and intergluteal areas		
Erythrodermic psoriasis		1. Widespread generalized erythema 2. Systemic symptoms may develop from long-standing psoriasis or appear abruptly in patients with mild versions		
Pustular psoriasis		1. Pustules on palms/feet, without plaque formation 2. Severe acute form can be life-threatening		
Guttate psoriasis	More common <30 y/o 2% of all cases	1. Located on trunk 2. 1-10 mm pink papules with fine scale 3. Presents several weeks after **group A β-hemolytic streptococcal** infection		

- Classification criteria for psoriatic arthritis
  - Established inflammatory articular disease PLUS
  - 3 or more

DRUG ERUPTIONS, ERYTHEMA MULTIFORME, STEVENS-JOHNSON SYNDROME, TOXIC EPIDERMAL NECROLYSIS, BULLOUS PEMPHIGOID, URTICARIA

Disease	Etiology, Prevalence, Risk Factors	Clinical Symptoms and Signs	Diagnostics	Therapy, Prognosis, and Health Maintenance

Erythema multiforme (Fig. 8-10)	Delayed-type hypersensitivity reaction to infection or drugs
	Adults 20-40 y/o
	Infectious causes:
	HSV-1 or 2, M. pneumoniae, fungal
	Meds:
	Barbiturates, hydantoins, NSAIDs, penicillin, phenothiazines, sulfonamides
		1. Acute onset, mild to no prodromal symptoms
		2. Polymorphous eruption of macules, papules, and characteristic "**target or iris lesions**" without scale = round shape, 3 concentric zones
		  • Appear days after onset
		3. Itching or burning at site
		Signs:
		1. Sharply demarcated red or pink macules → papular → plaques
		2. Central portion becomes darker red, brown, dusky, or purpuric
		3. Crusting or blistering of center
		4. Symmetrically distributed
		5. Spreads distal to proximal
		6. **Minimal mucous membrane involvement**
			<10% of body surface area	1. Treat existing infection or discontinue drug
				  • Mild = no TX
				  • Recurrent = continuous acyclovir
				Prognosis:
				1. Resolves spontaneously in 3-5 wk without sequelae
				2. May recur

Stevens-Johnson syndrome (SJS) (Fig. 8-11)	Most often caused by medication MC: Sulfonamides (TMP-SMX), allopurinol, antipsychotics, antiseizure medications	1. No typical target lesions 2. Flat atypical targets, confluent purpuric macules on face and trunk 3. Severe mucosal erosions at one or more sites	**<10%** of body surface area	1. Stop medication immediately and transfer patient to burn center

Toxic epidermal necrolysis (TEN) (Fig. 8-12)	Causes:
	NSAIDs, antibiotics (ampicillin), anticonvulsants (carbamazepine), sulfonamides (TMP-SMX), allopurinol, phenytoin
		1. Fever
		2. Mucocutaneous lesions
		3. Necrosis and sloughing of epidermis
		  • **Diffuse**, macular rash with indistinct margins and central purpuric region followed by eventual formation of vesicles and bullae as epidermal necrosis develops over days
		  • Start on face and spread inferiorly to trunk and lower extremity
		4. No typical target lesions
		5. Flat atypical target lesions
		6. Begins with severe mucosal erosions and progresses to **diffuse, generalized detachment of epidermis**
			DX criteria:
			>30% of body surface area
			1. Nikolsky sign (+): sloughing of superficial skin layers with gentle pressure
			2. Must have erythema and sloughing of mucosal surfaces including: conjunctiva, oral cavity, and vagina (2 or more)
			1. Biopsy: full-thickness involvement of dermis
				1. Prednisolone

Disease	Etiology, Prevalence, Risk Factors	Clinical Symptoms and Signs	Diagnostics	Therapy, Prognosis, and Health Maintenance
Bullous pemphigoid (Fig. 8-13)	IgG antibody complexes deposit between the epidermis and dermis causing formation of fluid-filled bullae **Autoimmune** skin disorder with subepidermal blistering Mostly elderly, onset 60-80, men = women *S. aureus* <u>Scenario:</u> Elderly patient who takes multiple medications	1. **Large, tense bullae**, but may begin as an urticarial eruption, filled with clear fluid or hemorrhagic 2. Discrete lesions arise on axilla, medial thigh, groin, abdomen, flexor arms, and lower legs 3. **Itchy**, <u>not</u> painful 4. Tense, not easy to rupture Lesions start as urticarial eruption, developing into bullae over weeks to months No scar formation after, but milia appear at sites of previously involved skin	1. **Nikolsky sign (-):** sloughing of superficial skin layers with gentle pressure 2. Skin biopsy required for DX: subepidermal separation and intact epidermis	1. **Oral prednisone**, alone or in combo with steroid-sparing Azathioprine, mycophenolate mofetil or a tetracycline Self-limiting, months to years
Urticaria (hives) (Fig. 8-14)	Vascular reaction of the skin marked by the transient appearance of smooth, slightly elevated papules or plaques (wheals) that are erythematous and often severely itchy <u>Etiology:</u> 1. Drugs: NSAID, aspirin, opiates, succinylcholine, antibiotics (polymyxin, ciprofloxacin, rifampin, vancomycin, β-lactams 2. Radiocontrast media IgE triggers the release of histamine from mast cells	1. Rapid onset, pruritic erythematous wheals • Lack of epidermal change • Intense itching • Presence of advancing edge and receding edge 2. Life-threatening angioedema 3. Features of anaphylaxis: hypotension, respiratory distress, stridor, GI distress, swallowing difficulty, joint swelling, or pain	1. RAST (radioallergosorbent assay test)	1. Second-generation H1 antagonists: **Cetirizine, loratadine, fexofenadine (first line)** 2. H2 antagonists: use in combo with second generation H1s • Famotidine, ranitidine 3. First generation H1 antagonists: diphenhydramine, hydroxyzine, chlorpheniramine • Drowsiness, anticholinergic, cognitive defects 4. 0.3-0.5 mg IM epinephrine for laryngeal angioedema <u>Prognosis:</u> 1. Most self-limited and short duration <u>Health maintenance:</u> 1. Avoid exposure to antigen

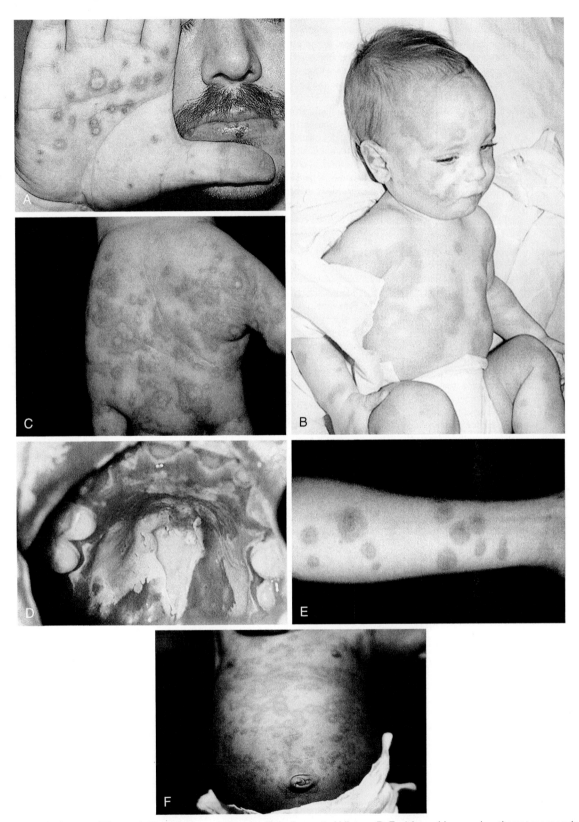

FIGURE 8-10. Erythema multiforme. **A**, Target lesions of the palm. Note the central blisters. **B**, Evolving, widespread erythematous macules and target lesions on the head, trunk, and limbs of an infant. **C**, Target lesions and erythematous macules of the palm. **D**, Ulceration, hemorrhage, and erosion of the oral mucosa in a patient with erythema multiforme. **E**, Target lesions on the forearm. Notice the dusky red center and surrounding erythema and pallor. **F**, Target lesions of the trunk in an infant with a dark skin tone. (**A**, From Bobonich MA, Nolen ME. *Dermatology for Advanced Practice Clinicians*. Philadelphia: Wolters Kluwer; 2015. **B**, From *Lippincott's Nursing Advisor 2014*. Philadelphia: Wolters Kluwer; 2014. **C**, From White AJ. *The Washington Manual of Pediatrics*. 2nd ed. Philadelphia: Wolters Kluwer; 2016. **D**, From Langlais RP, Miller CS, Gehrig JS. *Color Atlas of Common Oral Diseases*. 5th ed. Philadelphia: Wolters Kluwer; 2017. **E**, From McConnell TH. *The Nature of Disease: Pathology for the Health Professions*. 2nd ed. Philadelphia: Wolters Kluwer Health; 2014. **F**, From Ricci SS, Kyle T, Carman S. *Maternity and Pediatric Nursing*. 3rd ed. Philadelphia: Wolters Kluwer; 2017.)

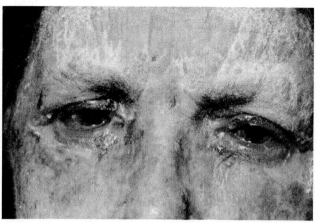

FIGURE 8-11. Stevens-Johnson syndrome in a woman with erosion of the conjunctivae. (From Rapuano CJ. *Wills Eye Institute Color Atlas & Synopsis of Clinical Ophthalmology: Cornea.* 2nd ed. Philadelphia: Lippincott Williams & Wilkins, a Wolters Kluwer business; 2012.)

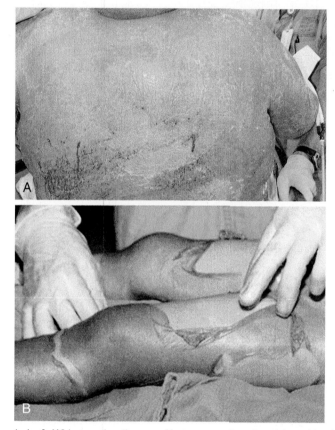

FIGURE 8-12. Toxic epidermal necrolysis. **A,** Widespread erythema and large areas of erosion of the epidermis on the back. **B,** Denuded epidermis on the legs of a child. (**A,** From McConnell TH. *The Nature of Disease: Pathology for the Health Professions.* 2nd ed. Philadelphia: Wolters Kluwer Health; 2014. **B,** From Lawrence PF. *Essentials of General Surgery.* 5th ed. Philadelphia: Lippincott Williams & Wilkins, a Wolters Kluwer business; 2013.)

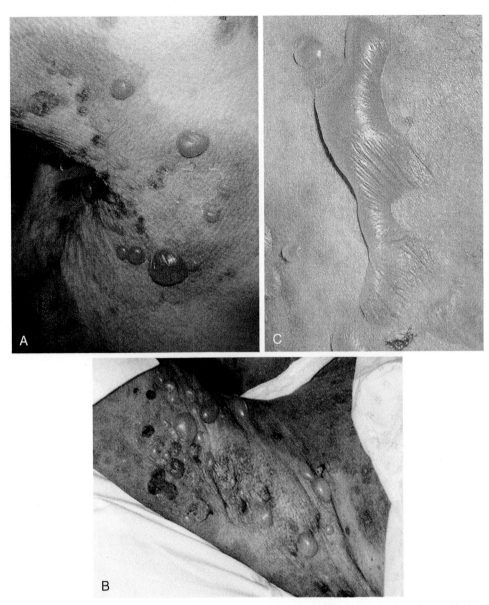

FIGURE 8-13. Bullous pemphigoid. **A,** Erythematous patches and bullae on the trunk. **B,** Hyperpigmented patches and bullae on the axilla. **C,** Large, tense bulla with surrounding erythema. (**A,** From Edward S, Yung A. *Essential Dermatopathology*. Philadelphia: Wolters Kluwer Health; 2012. **B,** From Wound, Ostomy and Continence Nurses Society. *Core Curriculum: Wound Management*. Philadelphia: Wolters Kluwer; 2016. **C,** From Ayala C, Spellberg B. *Boards and Wards for USMLE Steps 2 & 3*. 5th ed. Philadelphia: Wolters Kluwer Health; 2013.)

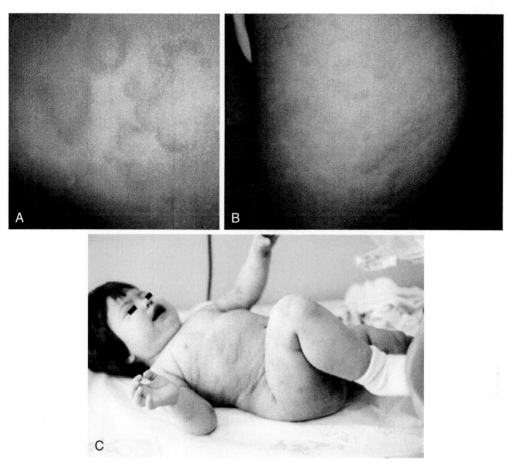

FIGURE 8-14. Urticaria/hives. **A**, Well-circumscribed, raised, erythematous plaques with central pallor. **B**. Erythematous wheals on the hip and buttocks. **C**, Generalized hives with erythematous wheals and plaques on a toddler. (**A**, From Elder DE, Elenitsas R, Rubin AI, et al. *Atlas and Synopsis of Lever's Histopathology of the Skin*. 3rd ed. Philadelphia: Lippincott Williams & Wilkins, a Wolters Kluwer business; 2013. **B**, From Council ML, Sheinbein DM, Cornelius LA. *The Washington Manual of Dermatology Diagnostics*. Philadelphia: Wolters Kluwer; 2016. **C**, From Salimpour RR, Salimpour P, Salimpour P. *Photographic Atlas of Pediatric Disorders and Diagnosis*. Philadelphia: Wolters Kluwer Health; 2014.)

ACTINIC KERATOSIS AND SEBORRHEIC KERATOSIS (FIG. 8-15)

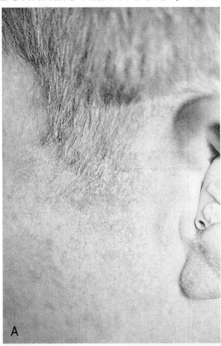

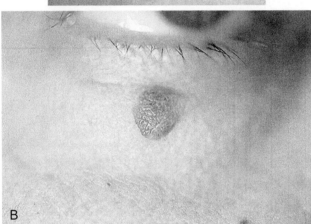

FIGURE 8-15. **A**, Actinic keratosis. **B**, Seborrheic keratosis. (**A**, From Bickley LS. *Bates' Guide to Physical Examination and History Taking*. 8th ed. Lippincott Williams & Wilkins; 2002. **B**, From Penne RB. *Wills Eye Institute Color Atlas & Synopsis of Clinical Ophthalmology: Oculoplastics*. 2nd ed. Philadelphia: Lippincott Williams & Wilkins, a Wolters Kluwer business; 2012.)

Disease	Etiology, Prevalence, Risk Factors	Clinical Symptoms and Signs	Diagnostics	Therapy, Prognosis, and Health Maintenance
Actinic keratosis (Fig. 8-15A)	RF: sun-exposed areas (head, neck) Considered premalignant (of SCC)	1. 3-6 mm in size 2. Rough texture (like sandpaper), red, scaly plaques 3. Formation of yellow adherent crust	1. Biopsy recommended to exclude SCC	1. Cryotherapy 2. Curettage ± electro-cautery, shave excision 3. Topical 5-FU or imiquimod 4. Photodynamic therapy
Seborrheic keratosis (Fig. 8-15B)	Age 40+ Benign Hereditary—autosomal dominant No association with sunlight	1. Usually multiple, located on all body surfaces *except* palms and soles Signs: 1. Well-circumscribed border, stuck-on or waxy (velvety) appearance 2. Tan-brown—black color	1. Dermoscopy—keratin pseudocyst Tend to get darker the longer they've been present	1. Cryotherapy 2. Curette, electrocautery, shave removal

LICE/SCABIES

Disease	Etiology, Prevalence, Risk Factors	Clinical Symptoms and Signs	Diagnostics	Therapy, Prognosis, and Health Maintenance
Lice (Fig. 8-16)	<u>Head:</u> <u>Pediculus humanis capitis or</u> <u>Pediculus capitis</u> <u>Genital:</u> Phthirus pubis <u>Transmission:</u> Sexual contact, clothing, towels	1. SEVERE Itching of scalp, body, or groin <u>Signs:</u> 1. Live lice and nits attached to hair on exam	1. DX—requires observation of live lice • Most commonly found behind ears and on back of neck	1. **Permethrin cream 1% shampoo (Elimite)** • Apply neck down and wash off after several hours • Combs, clothes, bed linens washed thoroughly
Scabies (Fig. 8-17)	Mites tunnel into skin, lay eggs, depositing feces (scybala), causing delayed type IV hypersensitivity reaction Highly contagious via skin-skin contact, towels, bed linens, or clothes Caused by skin mite *Sarcoptes scabiei var hominis*	1. Burrows and typical distribution on hands, feet, waist, axilla, or groin = linear marks 2. **SEVERE ITCHING, especially at night** <u>Signs:</u> 1. Erythematous papules on wrists, between fingers, and in genital area 2. Excoriation 3. Characteristic burrows on hands, wrists, and ankles, and in genital region	<u>DX:</u> 1. History of itching 2. Rash in typical distribution 3. History of itching in close contacts <u>Definitive DX:</u> 1. Finding mites, eggs, fecal pellets 2. Skin scraping from nonexcoriated burrows, papules, or vesicles	1. **Overnight therapy with permethrin 5% (elimite)** • Apply neck down (under nails), around genitals, and in cleft of buttocks, leave cream on overnight 8-10 h and wash off next morning • Causes paralysis of mite (nerve cell membrane) 2. Treat close contacts simultaneously 3. No longer contagious after one treatment, although itching may continue for weeks as dead mites are shed • Topical steroids and oral antihistamines for itching 4. Wash bedding in hot water and dry on heat

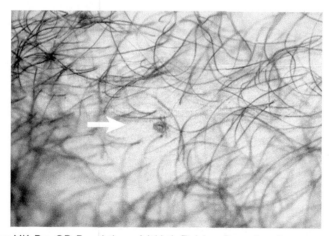

FIGURE 8-16. Lice. (From Anderson MK, Parr GP. *Foundations of Athletic Training: Prevention, Assessment, and Management.* 5th ed. Philadelphia: Wolters Kluwer; 2013.)

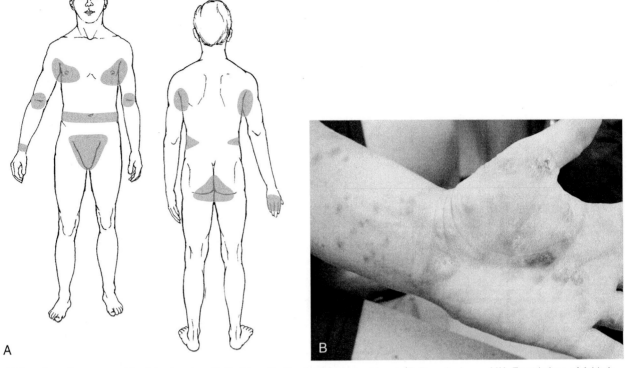

FIGURE 8-17. **A**, Common scabies infection sites. **B**, Scabies affecting the forearm and hand. (**B**, From Anderson MK. *Foundations of Athletic Training: Prevention, Assessment, and Management.* 6th ed. Philadelphia: Wolters Kluwer; 2017.)

ROSACEA (FIG. 8-18)

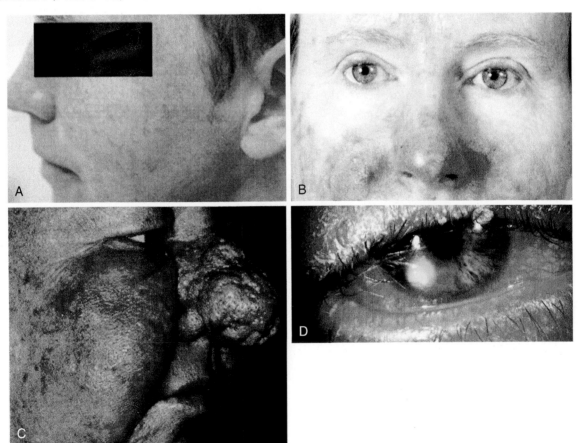

FIGURE 8-18. **A**, Erythematotelangiectatic rosacea. **B**, Papulopustular and ocular rosacea. **C**, Phymatous rosacea. **D**, Ocular rosacea. (**A**, From Council ML, Sheinbein DM, Cornelius LA. *The Washington Manual of Dermatology Diagnostics.* Philadelphia: Wolters Kluwer; 2016. **B**, From Porth CM. *Essentials of Pathophysiology.* 4th ed. Philadelphia: Wolters Kluwer; 2015. **C**, From Hannon RA, Porth CM. *Porth Pathophysiology: Concepts of Altered Health States.* 2nd ed. Philadelphia: Wolters Kluwer; 2016. **D**, From Rapuano CJ. *Wills Eye Institute Color Atlas & Synopsis of Clinical Ophthalmology: Cornea.* 2nd ed. Philadelphia: Lippincott Williams & Wilkins, a Wolters Kluwer business; 2012.)

Disease	Etiology, Prevalence, Risk Factors	Clinical Symptoms and Signs	Diagnostics	Therapy, Prognosis, and Health Maintenance
Rosacea	Common, chronic, progressive dermatosis MC: white F Avoid sun exposure, emotional stress, hot weather, wind, strenuous exercise, alcohol consumption, hot baths, cold weather, spicy food, humidity, indoor heat, hot beverages	1. Central facial **erythema** 2. Symmetric flushing 3. Stinging sensation 4. Inflammatory lesions 5. **Telangiectasias** 6. Phymatous changes Signs: 1. Erythematous, edematous eruptions of papules and pustules on forehead, cheeks, nose, and eyes 2. **NO COMEDONES**		1. Emollients, moisturizers, and fragrance and soap-free cleansers (Fig. 8-19) • Broad-spectrum sunscreen with zinc oxide • Avoid astringents 2. **Topical metronidazole** (Metrogel) first line 3. Topical + oral tetracycline, doxycycline, or minocycline for mod-severe disease
Erythematotelangiectatic rosacea			Persistent erythema of central face, prolonged flushing, telangiectasias, burning/stinging, ocular may coexist	Most difficult to treat
Papulopustular rosacea			Persistent central erythema with small papules and pinpoint pustules, burning/stinging, sparing of periocular and perioral areas, resembles acne vulgaris WITHOUT comedones ± facial edema	Easiest to treat
Phymatous rosacea	More common in men		Marked skin thickening and irregular nodularities of nose, chin, ears, forehead, or eyelid Rhinophyma	
Ocular rosacea			Watery, bloodshot eyes Dry eye, foreign body sensation, irritation, photophobia	

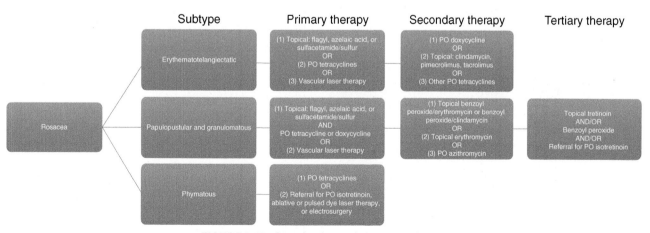

FIGURE 8-19. Stepwise therapy for rosacea subtypes.

ACNE VULGARIS (FIG. 8-20)

- Four factors responsible
  - Increased sebum production
  - Hyperkeratinization of the follicle
- Colonization by *Propionibacterium acnes* (anaerobe)
- Inflammatory reaction

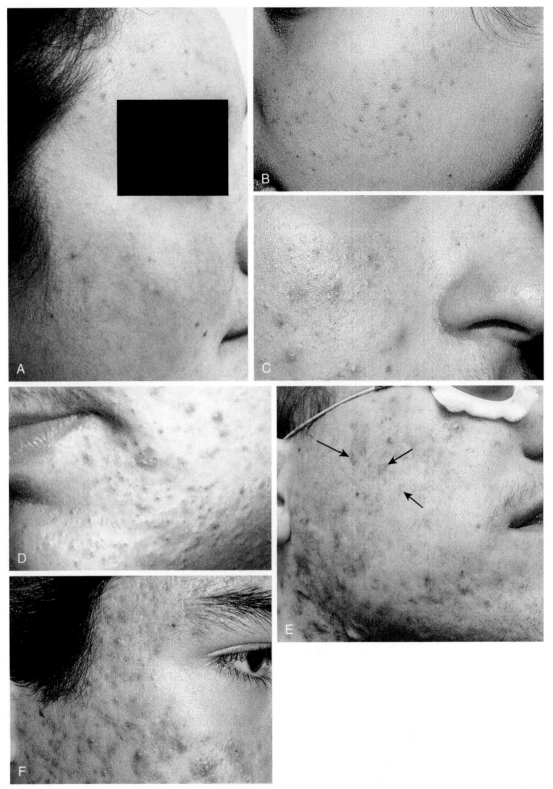

FIGURE 8-20. Acne. Mild acne examples in (**A** and **B**); mostly blackheads and an occasional papule or pustule. **C** and **D**, Moderate acne examples. Seen here are multiple blackheads and whiteheads alongside pustules and papules. **E** and **F**, Severe recalcitrant acne examples. Note the nodules, cysts, and/or pits in both photos. (**A**, From Goroll AH, Mulley AG. *Primary Care Medicine: Office Evaluation and Management of the Adult Patient.* 7th ed. Philadelphia: Wolters Kluwer; 2014. **B**, From Goodheart HP. *Goodheart's Photoguide of Common Skin Disorders: Diagnosis and Management.* 2nd ed. Philadelphia: Lippincott Williams & Wilkins; 2003. **C**, From Jensen S. *Nursing health assessment.* Philadelphia: Lippincott Williams & Wilkins; 2010. **D**, From James WD. Acne. *N Engl J Med.* 2005;352:1464. Copyright © 2005. Massachusetts Medical Society. **E**, From Krakowski AC, Shumake PR. *The Scar Book: Formation, Mitigation, Rehabilitation, and Prevention.* Philadelphia: Wolters Kluwer, 2017. **F**, From Burkhart C, Morrell D, Goldsmith LA, et al. *Essential Pediatric Dermatology.* Philadelphia: Lippincott Williams & Wilkins; 2009.)

- Occur on the face, neck, chest, back
- Adding benzoyl peroxide to antibiotic therapy prevents risk of bacterial resistance
- After treatment goals reached, oral antibiotics should be replaced with topical retinoids for maintenance therapy

Noninflammatory	Inflammatory
Open (blackheads) Closed (whiteheads)	Papules, pustules, nodules

1. Topical retinoids–monotherapy
  • Adapalene (Differin)
  • Tazarotene (Tazorac)
  • Tretinoin (Retin-A)
    • AE: redness, peeling, dryness, itching, stinging
	1. Topical retinoids + topical antibiotics for mild-mod acne
	  • Clindamycin and erythromycin: AE: redness, peeling, dryness, itching, stinging, oiliness
	  • With benzoyl peroxide–AE: dry skin, redness
	  • Salicylic acid–AE: dryness, irritation
	2. Oral antibiotics for mod to severe acne
	  • Tetracycline and erythromycin
	  • AAD recommends Minocycline
	    • AE: vestibular dysfunction, photophobia, hepatotoxicity, lupus-like reaction, pseudo-tumor cerebri
	  • With benzoyl peroxide

Disease	Etiology, Prevalence, Risk Factors	Clinical Symptoms and Signs	Diagnostics	Therapy, Prognosis, and Health Maintenance
Acne vulgaris	Most common skin disorder in the United States MC: P. acnes More prevalent in adolescents and more severe in males Pathology: plugged follicles, retained sebum, bacterial overgrowth, release of fatty acids	Noninflammatory: 1. Open comedones = blackheads 2. Closed comedones = whiteheads, flesh colored Inflammatory: • Erythematous papules, pustules, nodules or cysts • Size: 1-5 mm	1. Testosterone, FSH, LH, DHE-5 levels (not necessary for DX)	See treatment table (Fig. 8-21)
Mild acne		1. Noninflammatory acne (comedones) 2. Inflammatory acne (papules + pustules)	Papular and comedonal acne	*Noninflammatory:* 1. **Topical retinoids**–prevent comedones, reduce existing ones, and target inflammation (**first line** and *maintenance*) 2. **Benzoyl peroxide**–bactericidal that does not lead to resistance 3. Salicylic acid or azelaic acid *Inflammatory acne:* 1. Topical Tretinoin 2. Topical benzoyl peroxide 3. Topical antibiotic • Erythromycin or clindamycin

Moderate acne		1. *Nodular* acne: nodules or cysts
		2. Hyperpigmentation
		3. Scarring
			Mixed inflammatory and comedonal with inflammatory papules and pustules, erythematous macules and open comedones	1. **Oral** antibiotics–effective as monotherapy, but better when combined with retinoids
				  • Tetracyclines
				  • Erythromycin, doxycycline, minocycline, Bactrim, clindamycin
				Topical retinoid
				2. Topical benzoyl peroxide

Severe recalcitrant acne		1. Nodular or cystic acne
		2. Inflammatory acne (papules + pustules)
			Erythematous violaceous macules and papules, pustules, nodules, and scarring	1. **Oral isotretinoin**, must be member of iPLEDGE program
				  • AE: dry eyes/nose/lips, epistaxis, joint pains, mood swings, suicidal thoughts
				  • Premature closure of long bones, visual changes, elevated LFTs, leukopenia, ***triglyceridemia***, teratogenicity 0.5-1 mg/kg per day × 20 wk
				2. Cumulative dose of 120 mg/kg
				3. Oral antibiotic topical retinoid benzoylperoxide

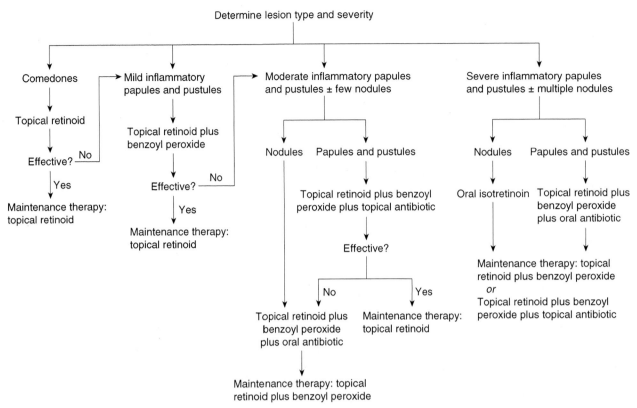

FIGURE 8-21. Acne stepwise therapy. (Redrawn from Titus S, Hodge J. Diagnosis and treatment of acne. *Am Fam Physician* 2012;86[8]:734-740.)

SPIDER BITES (FIG. 8-22)

- Appropriate and timely tetanus prophylaxis for all
- Antivenin recommended for significant latrodectism (widow)
- Wound cleansing and conservative debridement for brown recluse
- Referral to ophthalmologist for ophthalmia nodosa caused by embedded tarantula hairs

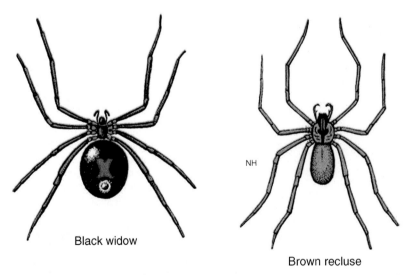

Black widow

Brown recluse

FIGURE 8-22. A, Black widow. **B,** Brown recluse. (From Miller MG, Berry DC. *Emergency Response Management for Athletic Trainers.* 2nd ed. Philadelphia: Wolters Kluwer; 2016.)

Disease	Etiology, Prevalence, Risk Factors	Clinical Symptoms and Signs	Therapy, Prognosis, and Health Maintenance
Black widow	Latrodectus species Massive presynaptic release of most neu-rotransmitters (AcH, NE, Dopamine, glutamate)	Moderately to severely painful bite, no surrounding inflammation Muscle spasms and rigidity starting at bite site within 30 min-2 h • Spreads proximally to abdomen and face • Rebound tenderness mimicking acute appendicitis	Resolve over 2-3 d Death rarely occurs
Brown recluse	Loxosceles species Local cytotoxicity with subsequent ulcerating dermonecrosis	Occur early in morning, painless Delayed reaction (3-7 d) Systemic symptoms: arthralgias, fever, chills, maculopapular rash, nausea, vomiting Progress to ulcerating dermonecrosis at bite site	Most necrotizing ulcers heal over 1-8 wk 10%-15% scar
Tarantula		Contain urticating hairs on dorsal abdomens, which can be flicked off by thousands, irritating and incapacitating aggressors • Penetrate skin causing foreign body keratoconjunctivitis or ophthalmia nodosa	Refer to ophthalmologist if suspected eye injury (slit lamp examination)

BASAL CELL CARCINOMA (FIG. 8-23)

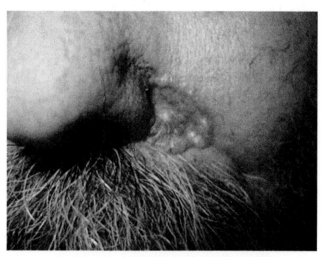

FIGURE 8-23. Basal cell carcinoma of the nose. Note the red, scaly plaque with a raised pearly white border. (From Werner R. *A Massage Therapist's Guide to Pathology.* 5th ed. Philadelphia: Wolters Kluwer Health; 2013.

Disease	Etiology, Prevalence, Risk Factors	Clinical Symptoms and Signs	Diagnostics	Therapy, Prognosis, and Health Maintenance
Basal cell carcinoma	Most common cutaneous neoplasm 85% occur on head or neck <u>RF:</u> Fair skin, **sun exposure**, male gender	Signs: 1. Firm, round, and pearly or waxy papule or nodule on the head or neck (**PEARLY PINK PAPULES**) 2. Margin telangiectasia ("**rolled border**") 3. Fragile~bleed and scab	1. Shave biopsy for nod-ular or thick superficial BCC 2. Scoop shave or punch biopsy for sclerosing or flat superficial BCC	1. Curettage, cryotherapy, ***Excision*, Mohs** (gold standard) 2. Imiquimod, 5% FU 3. Photodynamic/radiation

KAPOSI SARCOMA (FIG. 8-24)

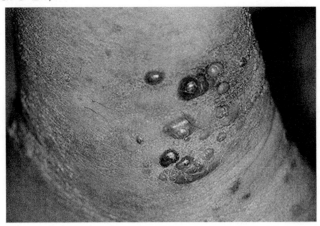

FIGURE 8-24. Kaposi sarcoma. (From Schwartz RA, Micali G, Nasca MR, et al. Kaposi sarcoma: a continuing conundrum. *J Am Acad Dermatol.* 2008;59:179–206.)

Disease	Etiology, Prevalence, Risk Factors	Clinical Symptoms and Signs	Diagnostics	Therapy, Prognosis, and Health Maintenance
Kaposi sarcoma	Typically seen in HIV or AIDS patients	1. Lesions anywhere: eyelids, conjunctiva, pinnae, palate, toe webs Signs: 1. Purplish, nonblanching papules or nodules		1. Resolves with effective ART

MELANOMA (FIG. 8-25)

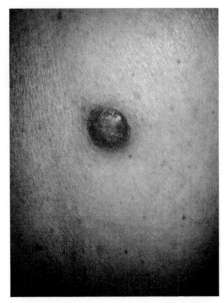

FIGURE 8-25. Nodular melanoma. (From Nicol NH. *Dermatologic Nursing Essentials: A Core Curriculum.* 3rd ed. Philadelphia: Wolters Kluwer; 2016, courtesy of Grace Chung.)

Family Medicine

Disease	Etiology, Prevalence, Risk Factors	Clinical Symptoms and Signs	Diagnostics	Therapy, Prognosis, and Health Maintenance
Melanoma	<u>MC:</u> Cancer among 25-29 y/o Number one cause of death due to skin cancer <u>RF:</u> Fair complexion, sun exposure, family history, xeroderma pigmentosum, old age, lots of moles, dysplastic nevus syndrome, giant congenital nevi <u>Most common types:</u> Superficial spreading melanoma (70%); flat macule or slightly raised discolored plaque with irregular borders, on trunk in men and legs in women	1. Asymmetry 2. Border–irregular 3. Color variation–brown, tan, black ± red, white, blue 4. **Diameter >6 mm** 5. Evolving–size, shape, symptoms (itching, tenderness), surface (bleeding), shades of color Changing mole on back → itching, bleeding	1. **Excision biopsy** (standard) • Shave and punch are less accurate 2. Lymph node dissection	1. **Complete full-skin depth excision** using margins determined by Breslow depth <u>Breslow depth:</u> Tumor thickness from granular layer of epidermis to point of deepest invasion 5-mm: in-situ lesions 1-2 cm: invasive lesions Most important indicator of prognosis: depth of invasion

ALOPECIA (FIG. 8-26 TO 8-29)

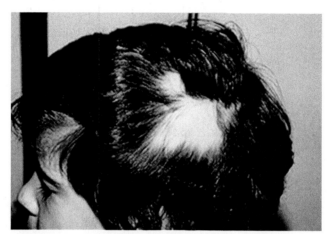

FIGURE 8-26. Alopecia areata. (From Goodheart HP. *Goodheart's Photoguide of Common Skin Disorders.* 2nd ed. Philadelphia, PA: Lippincott Williams & Wilkins; 2003.)

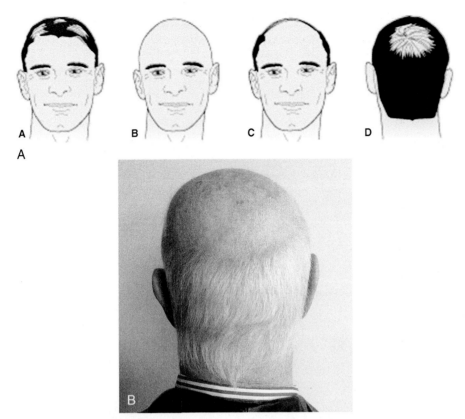

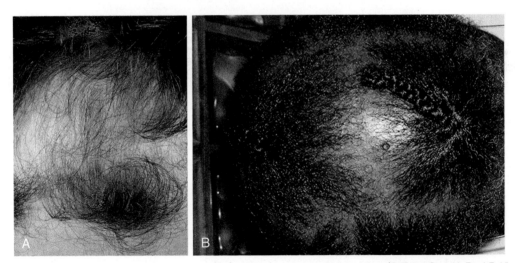

FIGURE 8-27. **A** and **B**, Androgenic alopecia hair loss patterns. (**A**, From Timby BK, Smith NE. *Introductory Medical-Surgical Nursing.* 10th ed. Philadelphia: Wolters Kluwer; 2010. **B**, From Council ML, Sheinbein DM, Cornelius LA. *The Washington Manual of Dermatology Diagnostics.* Philadelphia: Wolters Kluwer; 2016.)

FIGURE 8-28. **A**, Telogen effluvium with nonuniform hair loss. **B**, Traction alopecia from hair-braiding. (**A**, From Craft N, Fox LP. *VisualDx: Essential Adult Dermatology.* Philadelphia: Wolters Kluwer Health; 2011. **B**, From Hall BJ, Hall JC. *Sauer's Manual of Skin Diseases.* 11th ed. Philadelphia: Wolters Kluwer; 2018.)

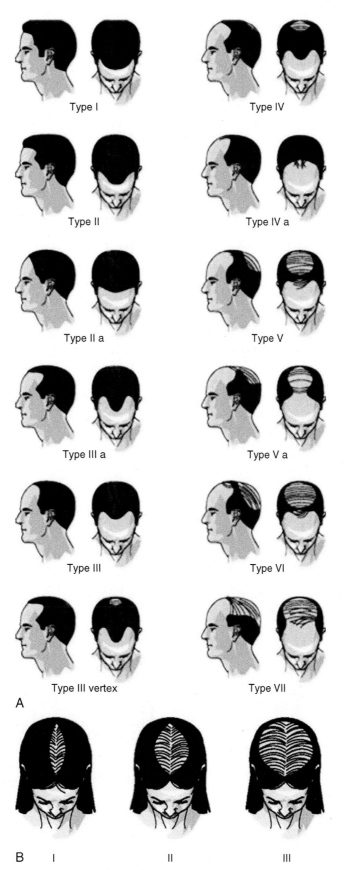

FIGURE 8-29. A, Norwood-Hamilton classification of male androgenetic alopecia. **B,** Ludwig classification of female androgenetic alopecia. (From Schalock PC, Hsu JTS, Arndt KA. *Lippincott's Primary Care Dermatology*. Philadelphia: Lippincott Williams & Wilkins, a Wolters Kluwer business; 2011.)

Disease	Etiology, Prevalence, Risk Factors	Clinical Symptoms and Signs	Diagnostics	Therapy, Prognosis, and Health Maintenance
Alopecia areata	Autoimmune	Oval shaped, well-circumscribed hair loss		Clobetasol
Androgenic alopecia (male pattern)		Top of head		Topical minoxidil
Telogen effluvium		1. Diffuse, extensive hair loss or thinning 2. Occurs after stress, illness, or meds (chemo), radiation 3. No evidence of scaling		Self-limiting
Traction alopecia	Tight hairstyle (braids)			

PARONYCHIA (FIG. 8-30)

Inflammation of the folds of tissue surrounding the nail of a toe or finger.

- Acute = direct or indirect trauma to cuticle or nail fold → pathogens inoculate the nail, resulting in infection
    - Avoid nail trauma, biting, picking, and manipulation, and finger sucking
    - Keep affected areas clean and dry
- Chronic = multifactorial inflammatory reaction of the proximal nail fold to irritants and allergens, cuticle separates from the nail plate leaving the region between the proximal nail fold and nail plate vulnerable to infection by bacteria/fungus

- Apply moisturizing lotion after hand washing
- Avoid chronic prolonged exposure after hand washing
- Avoid finger sucking
- Keep nails short
- Use rubber gloves, preferably with inner cotton glove or cotton liners
- Recommendations
    - Avoid trimming of cuticles or using cuticle removers
    - Improve glycemic control in patients with diabetes
    - Provide adequate patient education

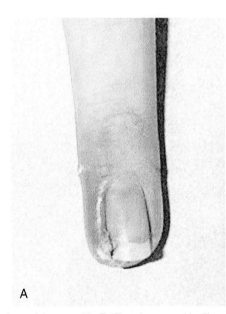
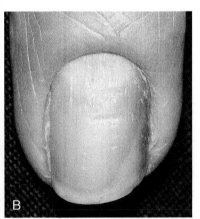

FIGURE 8-30. **A**, Acute bacterial paronychia. **B**, Chronic paronychia—illustrating Beau lines as well as swelling of the proximal nail fold, nail plate dystrophy, and cuticle loss. (**A**, From Schalock PC, Hsu JTS, Arndt KA. *Lippincott's Primary Care Dermatology*. Philadelphia: Lippincott Williams & Wilkins, a Wolters Kluwer business; 2011. **B**, From Goodheart HP, MD. *Goodheart's Photoguide of Common Skin Disorders*, 2nd ed. Philadelphia: Lippincott Williams & Wilkins; 2003.)

Disease	Etiology, Prevalence, Risk Factors	Clinical Symptoms and Signs	Diagnostics	Therapy, Prognosis, and Health Maintenance
Acute paronychia	<u>MC causative agent:</u> *S. aureus* Others: *S. pyogenes*, *Pseudomonas pyocyanea*, *Proteus vulgaris*	1. Rapid onset of erythema, edema, and discomfort or tenderness of proximal and lateral nail folds 2. 2-5 d after trauma 3. Drainage of pus when nailfold compressed <u>Signs:</u> 1. Swelling 2. Erythema 3. Discharge	1. History of minor trauma and physical exam	1. Warm compresses, soak in Burow solution (aluminum acetate or vinegar) • Tylenol or NSAIDs 2. <u>Topical</u> antibiotics with or without steroids • Mupirocin (bactroban), Neosporin • Betamethasone (Diprolene) 3. Oral antibiotics 4. Surgical I&D
Chronic paronychia	Chronic inflammation of the proximal paronychia More common in **children** <u>RF:</u> Diabetes and chronic use of systemic retinoids or protease inhibitors	1. HX of continuous immersion of hands in water, contact with soap, detergents, or other chemicals 2. Similar to acute paronychia: erythema, tenderness, swelling of proximal nail fold 3. Retraction of proximal nail fold 4. **Absence of adjacent cuticle** <u>Signs:</u> 1. Nail plate thickened and discolored with pronounced **Beau lines** (inflammation of matrix) and nail loss 2. Cross-striations of the nail 3. ± pus below nail fold	1. History and physical examination, present for at least *6 wk* at time of DX 2. *Strep, Staph,* or *Candida* on smear/culture	Avoid exposure to contact irritants 1. *Topical* antifungal and steroid • Use emollient lotions

CONDYLOMA ACUMINATUM (FIG. 8-31)

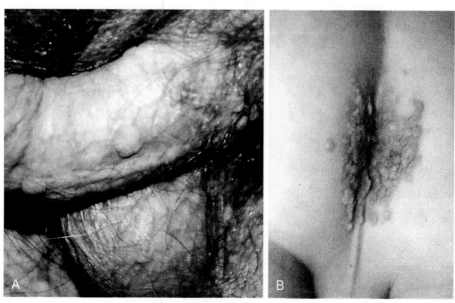

FIGURE 8-31. Condyloma acuminatum of the (**A**) penis and (**B**) anus. (From Nicol NH. *Dermatologic Nursing Essentials: A Core Curriculum.* 3rd ed. Philadelphia: Wolters Kluwer; 2016, courtesy of Charles E. Lewis, MD.)

Disease	Etiology, Prevalence, Risk Factors	Clinical Symptoms and Signs	Diagnostics	Therapy, Prognosis, and Health Maintenance
Condyloma acuminatum (external genital warts)	HPV type 6, 11, 16, 18, 31 External genitalia, perineum, perianal, inguinal fold F: 20-24 M: 25-29 RF: Early intercourse, numerous partners, unprotected sex	1. Soft, rather than hard 2. Hyperkeratotic, exophytic 3. Sessile papules or large confluent plaques		1. Cryotherapy 2. Imiquimod or podophyllin 3. Laser and electrocautery 4. Scissors or shave debulking Vaccine: • Gardasil: quadrivalent against 6, 11, 16, 18 for M/F age 9-26 • Cervarix: bivalent against 16, 18 for F 10-25

EXANTHEMS (FIG. 8-32 AND 8-33)

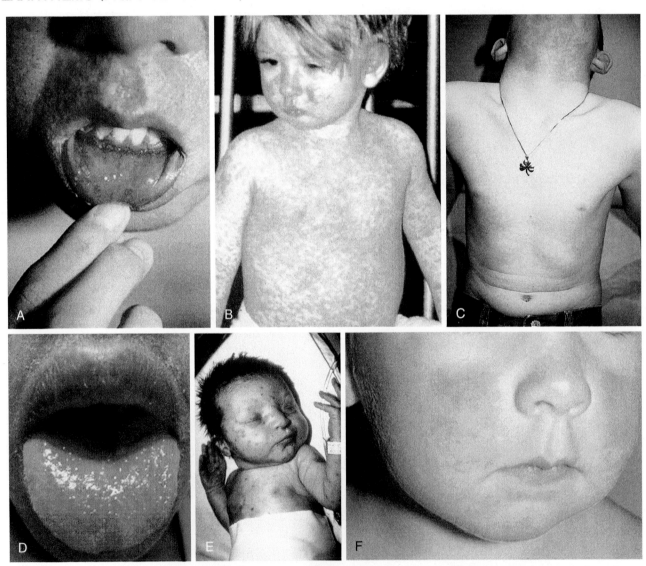

FIGURE 8-32. **A,** Measles (rubeola), illustrating Koplik spots that appear 2 to 3 days after onset of symptoms. **B,** The blotchy rash of measles (rubeola). **C,** The rash of scarletina. **D,** The strawberry tongue characteristic of scarletina. **E,** The characteristic rash of rubella. **F,** The characteristic rash of erythema infectiosum, illustrating a slapped cheek appearance. (**A,** From Mallory SB, Bree A, Chern P. *Illustrated Manual of Pediatric Dermatology.* New York: Taylor and Francis Publishing; 2005. **B,** From Anderson MK, Parr GP. *Foundations of Athletic Training: Prevention, Assessment, and Management.* 5th ed. Philadelphia: Wolters Kluwer; 2013. **C,** From Ricci SS, Kyle T. *Maternity and Pediatric Nursing.* Philadelphia: Wolters Kluwer; 2009. **D,** From Sherman S, Cico SJ, Nordquist E, et al. *Atlas of Clinical Emergency Medicine.* Philadelphia: Wolters Kluwer; 2016. **E,** Photo courtesy of Centers for Disease Control and Prevention. **F,** From Burkhart C, Morrell DS. *VisualDx: Essential Pediatric Dermatology.* Philadelphia: Lippincott Williams & Wilkins, a Wolters Kluwer business; 2010.)

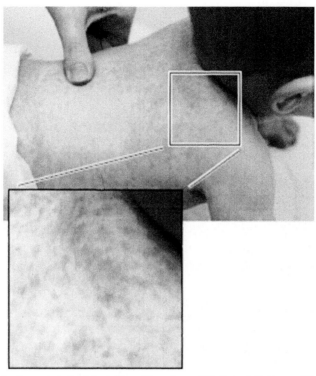

FIGURE 8-33. The characteristic rash of roseola in the infant. (From Cornelissen CN, Fisher BD, Harvey RA. *Lippincott's Illustrated Reviews: Microbiology.* 3rd ed. Philadelphia: Lippincott Williams & Wilkins, a Wolters Kluwer business; 2013.)

Disease	Etiology, Prevalence, Risk Factors	Clinical Symptoms and Signs	Diagnostics	Therapy, Prognosis, and Health Maintenance

First disease: **measles** (rubeola) hard measles, 14-d measles, measles virus	Incubation: 2 wk Measles virus	Prodromal: malaise and anorexia
		1. **High fever** (up to 105°F) and **lethargy**
		  • Lasts 4-7 d
		Triad: 3 C's
		2. **Cough**
		3. **Coryza** (runny nose, nasal congestion)
		4. **Conjunctivitis**
		5. Rash on day 3
		Signs:
		1. **Koplik spots**: bluish gray specks or "grains of sand" on red base on buccal mucosa
		  • Appear 1-2 d before rash, last 3-5 d
		2. Blanching, erythematous macules and papules on face at hairline, sides of neck, and behind ears
		  • Coalesce into patches and plaques on trunk and extremities (palms/soles)
		    • Lasts 5-7 d
			Clinical DX:
			1. Measles IgM titer
			  • Obtain on third day of rash up to 1 mo
			2. Measles IgG titer
			  • 4× rise between acute and convalescent
			3. Viral culture from throat and nasal swab
			4. RT-PCR
				1. Ibuprofen (Motrin)
				2. Fluids
				3. Vitamin A supplementation
				Complications:
				1. Pneumonia
				2. Otitis media
				3. Encephalitis

(continued)

(continued)

Disease	Etiology, Prevalence, Risk Factors	Clinical Symptoms and Signs	Diagnostics	Therapy, Prognosis, and Health Maintenance
Second disease: Scarletina	**S. pyogenes,** group A strep Incubation: 12 h-7 d Transmission: **respiratory droplets** Common in over-crowded places (schools), children age 1-10 y	1. **Fever**, abdominal pain, headache, sore throat, and rhinorrhea 2. **Rash** 12-48 h after onset of fever • Erythematous patches below ears, on neck, chest, and axilla • Dry, *rough texture of fine sandpaper*; blanchable • Disseminates to flexural areas (axillae, popliteal fossa, inguinal folds) 3. **Pastia lines**: confluent petechiae in skin creases, neck, antecubital, axilla, groin Signs: 1. Enlarged **anterior cervical lymph nodes** or swollen tonsils 2. Mucous membranes—bright red, scattered petechiae and red papular lesions on soft palate 3. *Strawberry tongue*—tongue heavily coated with white membrane with edematous red papillae (day 1-2) 4. Day 4-5: shiny red tongue with prominent papillae	1. **Clinical DX** 2. CBC: leukocytosis with left shift 3. Throat or nasal culture or rapid strep test 4. Antistreptolysin titer	1. Calamine lotion 2. Tylenol 3. **Amoxicillin**, or Macrolide Prognosis: 1. Desquamation begins 7-10zd after resolution of rash with flakes peeling from face Complications: Rheumatic fever, septicemia, vasculitis, hepatitis, otitis media, pneumonia, osteomyelitis, glomerulonephritis
Third disease: Rubella "Blueberry muffin baby," *German measles*, 3-d measles	*Rubella virus* Incubation: 2-3 wk Prodromal phase absent in children Transmission: droplet Incubation period: 14-19 d RNA virus: Rubivirus	1. Mild URI (may not be present in child) 2. Low grade fever (no systemic symptoms) 3. Macular rash on day 1 (face), fades by 3 d Face → trunk → limbs 4. **Arthralgia** Signs: 1. **Postauricular**, postcervical, and **occipital nodes** • Tender, generalized	Clinical DX	1. Ibuprofen (Motrin) 2. Fluids Health maintenance: 1. Contagious for 7 d after onset of rash—isolate from work, school, or other public places Complications: **PDA**, pulmonary artery stenosis, aortic stenosis, ventricular defects, thrombocytopenic purpura with purple macular lesions, cataracts, retinopathy, sensorineural deafness
Fifth disease: Erythema infectiosum (slapped cheek syndrome)	*Parvovirus B19* Incubation: 4-14 d Transmission: Aerosolized respiratory droplets, mother to fetus	1. Mild URI (last 2-3 d): headache, sore throat, itching, coryza, abdominal pain, arthralgias • Infectious period 2. Low-grade fever 3. 1 wk later • **Slapped cheek** • Nasal, perioral, and periorbital sparing • Fades over 2-4 d • **Lacy reticular rash** on proximal extremities (usually arms and extensor surfaces) and trunk • Palms, soles spared • Occurs 1-4 d later • Clearing and recurrence for weeks to months Complications: Arthritis, anemia, and fetal hydrops	Clinical DX	1. Ibuprofen (Motrin) 2. Fluids Health maintenance: 1. Not infectious, may attend school or childcare
Sixth disease: Roseola exanthem subitum, sudden rash, 3-d fever	*HHV 6B or 7* Incubation: 5-15 d MC: 9-12 mo old	1. **High fever** for 3-4 d ± febrile seizure 2. After 3 d, rapid defervescence, **rash occurs** (small pink blanchable rash) • Mild, pink, morbilliform rash • Nagayama spots: red papules on soft palate and base of uvula	1. CBC, U/A, blood cultures, CSF examination 2. Roseola IgM	1. Ibuprofen (Motrin) 2. Fluids Complications: 1. Febrile seizures (15%)

MOLLUSCUM CONTAGIOSUM (FIG. 8-34)

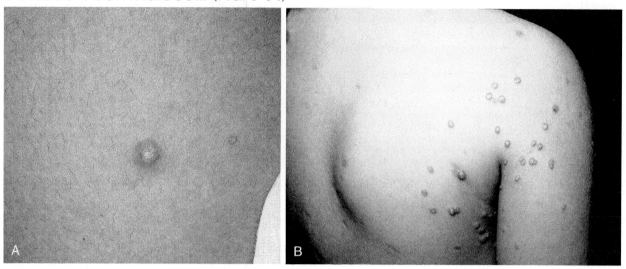

FIGURE 8-34. A and **B**, Molluscum contagiosum. (**A,** From Fleisher GR, MD, Ludwig S, MD, Baskin MN, MD. *Atlas of Pediatric Emergency Medicine.* Philadelphia: Lippincott Williams & Wilkins; 2004. **B,** From Hall BJ, Hall JC. *Sauer's Manual of Skin Diseases.* 11th ed. Philadelphia: Wolters Kluwer; 2018.)

Disease	Etiology, Prevalence, Risk Factors	Clinical Symptoms and Signs	Diagnostics	Therapy, Prognosis, and Health Maintenance
Molluscum contagiosum	Trunk, face, extremities, genitalia <u>MC:</u> Children with atopy, immunosuppressed, wrestlers Highly contagious via skin-skin contact Common in sexually active adults and children (r/o child abuse) Caused by **poxvirus**	1. Itching <u>Signs:</u> 1. Discrete 2-5-mm diameter flesh-colored, dome-shaped macules or papules with central umbilication 2. Pruritus 3. Koebnerize		1. Topical keratolytic (**cantharidin**) 2. Cryotherapy 3. Curettage <u>Prognosis:</u> 1. Persists up to 6 mo, but spontaneously regresses with time

Verrucae (Fig. 8-35)

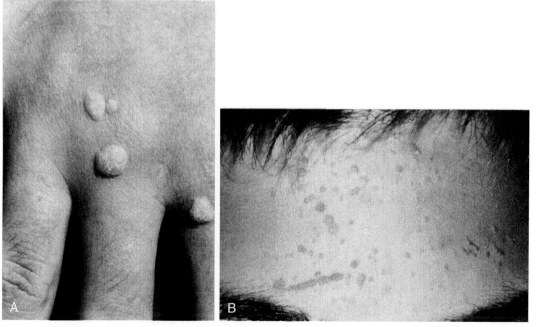

FIGURE 8-35. A, Verruca vulgaris. **B,** Verruca planae affecting the forehead. (From Elder DE, Elenitsas R, Rubin AI, et al. *Atlas and Synopsis of Lever's Histopathology of the Skin.* 3rd ed. Philadelphia: Lippincott Williams & Wilkins, a Wolters Kluwer business; 2013.)

Disease	Etiology, Prevalence, Risk Factors	Clinical Symptoms and Signs	Therapy, Prognosis, and Health Maintenance
Verruca vulgaris (common wart)	HPV—infects basal keratinocytes of cutaneous and mucosal epithelium Type 2 or 4 Skin-skin contact or contaminated surfaces/objects <u>MC:</u> Fingers, dorsal hands, knees, elbows	<u>Signs:</u> 1. Hyperkeratotic, exophytic, dome-shaped papules or nodules • Well circumscribed • Flesh-colored 2. Black punctate dots 3. May koebnerize	1. Cryotherapy • Freeze 30 s, 2 times • Blister, color change, pain, scar, nail dystrophy 2. Salicylic acid • Applied and changed every 1-2 d under occlusion
Verruca planae (flat warts)	HPV Type 3 or 10 Dorsal hands, arms, face (exposed areas)	Skin colored or pink Smooth surfaced, slightly elevated, flat-topped papules	1. Cryotherapy not recommended for face 2. Refer to dermatology
Palmoplantar verruca	HPV Type 1	Thick, endophytic papules Mosaic warts—coalesce into large plaques Painful with ambulation	Observe—spontaneously resolve at 2 y (75%)

CELLULITIS AND ERYSIPELAS

Disease	Etiology, Prevalence, Risk Factors	Clinical Symptoms and Signs	Diagnostics	Therapy, Prognosis, and Health Maintenance
Cellulitis (Fig. 8-36A)	80% caused by **S. aureus** or GABHS Cat or dog bite: *Pasteurella multocida* <u>MRSA RF:</u> Antibiotics, prolonged hospitalization, surgical site infection, ICU, hemodialysis Usually lower leg Deeper than erysipelas, ill-defined border Acute infection of the skin involving the dermis and subcutaneous tissues	HX: break in skin from trauma, bite, or dermatosis (tinea pedis, stasis dermatitis) 1. **Erythema, warmth, tenderness, pain, edema** • Margins indistinct • Bulla formation to necrosis • Extensive epidermal sloughing and superficial erosion • Spreading, erythematous, nonfluctuant tender plaque 2. **Firm, tender induration** 3. **Usually NO fluctuance** 4. ± fever (26%), crepitus 5. Streaks of lymphangitis	1. Aspiration—if fluctuance in area of erythema • Culture for antibiotic susceptibility 2. Blood cultures if febrile <u>DX:</u> 1. Rubor (red) 2. Calor (warm) 3. Tumor (swollen) 4. Dolor (pain)	1. <u>Outpatient nonpurulent:</u> treat for group A strep • PCN: Oxacillin, nafcillin, **dicloxacillin × 7-10 d** • Cefazolin, Cephalexin • PCN allergy: Clindamycin 2. <u>Outpatient purulent:</u> treat for MRSA • Clindamycin, **Bactrim**, FQ, tetracyclines (doxycycline, minocycline) 3. <u>Inpatient</u> • Hospitalize patients who are immunocompromised (HIV, transplant, chronic renal or liver disease, on prednisone, uncontrolled DM) • IV antibiotics until signs of infection improve, then oral antibiotics × 2 wk • IV Nafcillin 2 g q 4 h • **Cefazolin** 1 g IV q 8 h • Vancomycin 1 g IV BID

Disease	Etiology, Prevalence, Risk Factors	Clinical Symptoms and Signs	Diagnostics	Therapy, Prognosis, and Health Maintenance
Erysipelas (Fig. 8-36B)	Superficial cellulitis with dermal-lymphatic involvement (edema) Group A *Strep* Most common on lower extremities and face Predisposing factors: lymphatic obstruction (after radical mastectomy), local trauma, abscess, fungal infection, diabetes, alcoholism	1. Prodromal SX: **chills, high fever**, headache, vomiting, joint pain • Follows bacterial pharyngitis or trauma 2. Presents with pain, superficial (bright red) **"fiery" erythema** 3. Plaque-like edema with a sharply **demarcated area with slowly advancing margin** • Described as peau d'orange • **"Streaking"** lymphatic involvement 4. Plaques may develop overlying blisters (bullae)	High WBC (>20k)	1. **Penicillin VK IM** 2. Erythromycin for PCN allergy High rate of recurrence <u>Complications:</u> Sepsis, local spread to SQ tissue, necrotizing fasciitis

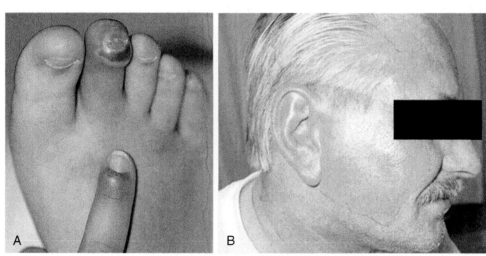

FIGURE 8-36. A, Cellulitis of the toe. **B**, Characteristic rash of erysipelas. (**A**, From Engleberg NC, DiRita V, Dermody TS. *Schaechter's Mechanisms of Microbial Disease.* 5th ed. Philadelphia: Lippincott Williams & Wilkins, a Wolters Kluwer business; 2013. **B**, From Werner R. *A Massage Therapist's Guide to Pathology.* 5th ed. Philadelphia: Wolters Kluwer Health; 2013.)

IMPETIGO

Disease	Etiology, Prevalence, Risk Factors	Clinical Symptoms and Signs	Diagnostics	Therapy, Prognosis, and Health Maintenance
Impetigo	Strep and/or staphylococci Most commonly affects children 2-5 y/o Highly contagious Most common areas: exposed skin of face (nares, perioral area) and extremities	Superficial skin infection that begins as: 1. Vesicles with thin, fragile roof	Clinical DX	Resolves within 2-3 wk without scarring 1. Topical antibiotics: **mupirocin** 2. Oral antibiotics for large bullae: Augmentin, dicloxacillin, cephalexin, clindamycin, doxycycline, Bactrim, macrolides <u>Complications (rare):</u> 1. Poststrep GN (most serious)

Impetigo Contagiosa

Nonbullous (70%) (Fig. 8-37A) Cause: *S. aureus* or *S. pyogenes*	Bullous (30%) (Fig. 8-37B) Cause: *S. aureus*
Honey-colored crusts on face and extremities Primarily affects skin Secondarily affects insect bites, eczema, or herpetic lesions	Honey-colored crusts on face and extremities Primarily affects skin Secondarily affects insect bites, eczema, or herpetic lesions

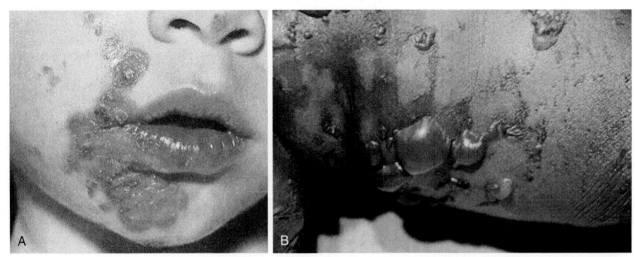

FIGURE 8-37. **A**, Nonbullous impetigo. **B**, Bullous impetigo. (**A**, From Kronenberger J, Durham LS, Woodson D. *Lippincott Williams & Wilkins' Comprehensive Medical Assisting.* 4th ed. Philadelphia: Wolters Kluwer; 2012. **B**, From Stocker JT, Dehner LP, Husain AN. *Stocker & Dehner's Pediatric Pathology.* 3rd ed. Philadelphia: Wolters Kluwer; 2011.)

ACANTHOSIS NIGRICANS (FIG. 8-38)

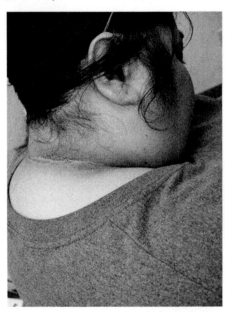

FIGURE 8-38. Acanthosis nigricans. (From DeLong L, Burkhart NW. *General and Oral Pathology for the Dental Hygienist.* 2nd ed. Philadelphia: Wolters Kluwer Health; 2013, courtesy of Dr. Frank Varon.)

Disease	Etiology, Prevalence, Risk Factors	Clinical Symptoms and Signs	Diagnostics	Therapy, Prognosis, and Health Maintenance
Acanthosis nigricans (AN)	Hyperkeratosis and epidermal papillomatosis; increased melanin in basal layer of epidermis Most cases benign, can be acquired or inherited MC in Native American, African American, or Hispanic patients Associated: Type 2 **diabetes** and **obesity** (insulin resistance), polycystic ovarian syndrome, gastric cancers (MCC malignant AN), drug reactions	1. Velvety to verrucous hyperpigmented plaques in intertriginous areas Signs: 1. Thick, velvety hyperpigmented plaques and accentuated skin lines • Gray-brown color 2. Located on the **neck, axilla**, groin, or inframammary folds 3. Acrochordons (skin tags) may be present around affected areas 4. Typically symmetrically distributed	Clinical DX: 1. Labs: fasting blood sugar, LDL, HgbA1C 2. r/o PCOS in females 3. Skin biopsy (definitive)	1. Treat underlying cause 2. Topical retinoids and vitamin D analogues Health maintenance: 1. Discourage excessive scrubbing of the affected skin, which results in lichenification and hyperpigmentation Prognosis: 1. In isolation, no physical adverse consequences in the long term 2. Subject to sequelae of associated underlying medical disorders

Disease	Etiology, Prevalence, Risk Factors	Clinical Symptoms and Signs	Diagnostics	Therapy, Prognosis, and Health Maintenance
Malignant AN	Occurs in older, nonobese patients Associated: gastric or lung cancer	1. Recent unintentional weight loss 2. Extensive or rapidly progressive AN 3. Mucous membrane involvement 4. Prominent palm or sole involvement 5. No other identifiable cause Signs: 1. Cachexia 2. Cutaneous plaques in unusual locations (oral cavity, palms, soles) 3. Multiple skin tags, seborrheic keratoses 4. Tripe palm (acanthosis palmaris): velvety thickening of palms	Clinical DX	1. Definitive treatment of underlying malignancy

HIDRADENITIS SUPPURATIVA

Disease	Etiology, Prevalence, Risk Factors	Clinical Symptoms and Signs	Diagnostics	Therapy, Prognosis, and Health Maintenance
Hidradenitis suppurativa (acne inversa or Verneuil disease) (Fig. 8-39)	"Tombstone comedone" Chronic follicular occlusive disease <1%-4% prevalence Onset: Puberty to age 40 (mean: 20-30s) F > M RF: Genetic, mechanical stress on skin, obesity, **smoking**, hormonal factors 40% have (+) FH, autosomal dominant	1. Recurrent inflamed nodules and abscesses or draining sinus tracts and bands of severe scar formation • Affects the intertriginous areas: **axillae** (MC), groin, perianal, perineal, inframammary, buttocks, scrotum, vulva, chest, scalp 2. Pain 3. Malodorous 4. Drainage Signs: 1. Solitary, painful, deep-seated inflamed nodule in intertriginous area 2. Open comedones; double-headed open comedones ± closed 3. Dense fibrotic bands or indurated, thick, scarred plaques Associated: Acne vulgaris	Clinical DX: 1. Skin biopsy—not required, but definitive 2. Culture—r/o infection 3. Hurley staging system • Stage 1: abscess formation without sinus tracts or scarring • Stage 2: recurrent abscesses with sinus tracts and scarring • Stage 3: diffuse involvement of interconnected sinus tracts and abscesses	I&D **only** for tense abscess for immediate relief of pain; not effective for definitive management 1. Dietary and behavioral modifications • Skin hygiene, smoking cessation, elimination of dairy products, weight loss • Psychological support 2. Topical and systemic medications • Stage 1: daily topical clindamycin, punch debridement, intralesional steroids • Stage 2: PO doxycycline • Stage 3: adalimumab, infliximab, acitretin 3. Surgery • Stage 4: unroof nodules and sinus tracts • Stage 5: wide excision Prognosis: 1. Increased risk for metabolic syndrome, diabetes, dyslipidemia, hyperglycemia, cardiovascular associated death, etc. Complications: Strictures and contractures, lymphatic obstruction, lymphedema of limbs and genitalia, malaise, depression, suicide, infections complications (abscess, osteomyelitis), arthritis, **squamous cell carcinoma**, anemia, hypoproteinemia, amyloidosis

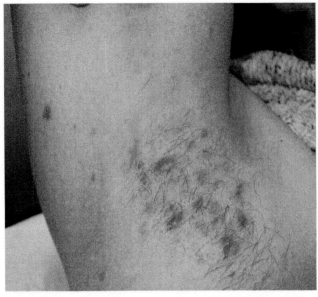

FIGURE 8-39. Hidradenitis suppurativa. (Image provided by Stedman's.)

LIPOMAS/EPITHELIAL INCLUSION CYSTS

Disease	Etiology, Prevalence, Risk Factors	Clinical Symptoms and Signs	Diagnostics	Therapy, Prognosis, and Health Maintenance
Lipomas (Fig. 8-40)	Solitary or multiple (familial) Consist of mature fat cells enclosed by a thin fibrous capsule Can occur anywhere on the body Most common benign soft tissue neoplasms Can be familial (familial multiple lipomatosis)	1. Soft, painless, subcutaneous nodules 2. 1->10 cm, most frequently on trunk or upper extremities Signs: 1. Subcutaneous nodules few cm in diameter 2. Located on trunk or proximal extremities 3. Soft, mobile, no epidermal skin change 4. ± tenderness	Clinical DX: 1. Biopsy if: • SX of pain or restriction of movement • Rapidly enlarging • Firm rather than soft	1. Surgical excision (elective) • AE: scarring, seroma, hematoma 2. Liposuction Prognosis: Recurrence not common
Epithelial inclusion cysts (sebaceous cysts, epidermoid cysts) (Fig. 8-41)	Benign Cyst wall consists of stratified squamous epithelium and is filled with laminated layers of keratinous material Most common cutaneous cyst Can occur anywhere on the body Sterile, do not require oral antibiotics	1. Skin colored dermal nodules with visible central punctum Signs: 1. Discrete cyst or nodule filled with nasty smelling white material with overlying punctum 2. Compressible, mobile	Clinical DX: Culture drained contents	1. Resolve spontaneously if inflamed, uninfected • May recur 2. Incision and drainage—if fluctuant • If inflamed: IL steroid 3. Excision—for when non-inflamed only 4. Antibiotics pending culture results—MRSA Prognosis: Recurrence is common

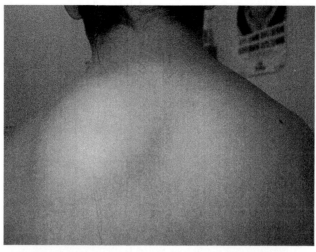

FIGURE 8-40. Lipomas of the back. (Image provided by Stedman's.)

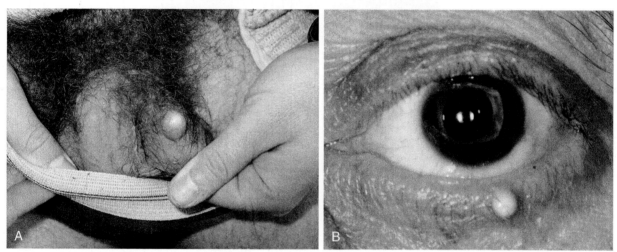

FIGURE 8-41. **A** and **B**, Epithelial inclusion cysts. (**A**, Image provided by Stedman's. **B**, From Shields JA, Shields CL. *Eyelid, Conjunctival, and Orbital Tumors: An Atlas and Textbook*. 3rd ed. Philadelphia: Wolters Kluwer; 2016.)

Disease	Etiology, Prevalence, Risk Factors	Clinical Symptoms and Signs	Diagnostics	Therapy, Prognosis, and Health Maintenance
Melasma (Chloasma) "mask of pregnancy"	Acquired hyperpigmentation of the skin affecting the sun exposed areas of the face MC: F with darker complexion living in areas of intense UV radiation exposure Occurs in 15%-50% of pregnant F F > M RF: Darker skin, UV radiation, pregnancy, OCPs, genetic predisposition, cosmetic use, thyroid dysfunction, AEDs	1. Irregularly shaped, hyperpigmented macules on face Signs: 1. Hyperpigmented macules in sun exposed areas 2. Colors: light-brown to dark-brown or ash/blue 3. Confluent and symmetrically distributed	Clinical DX: 1. Wood lamp: enhancement of epidermal melasma 2. Tissue biopsy—increased melanin deposition in all layers of epidermis on Fontana-Masson stain	1. Photoprotection • Sun avoidance • Wear wide brimmed hats • Broad spectrum sunscreen 2. Topical skin-lightening agents (mainstay) • Hydroquinone • Azelaic acid • Mequinol • Kojic acid 3. Topical retinoids • Tretinoin • Teratogenic Prognosis: 1. Regresses within 1 y after delivery in pregnant women Grading: Melasma area and severity index (MASI)

MELASMA (FIG. 8-42)

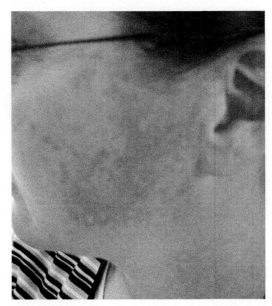

FIGURE 8-42. Melasma (cholasma), the mask of pregnancy. (From Jensen S. *Nursing Health Assessmet: A Best Practice Approach.* 2nd ed. Philadelphia: Wolters Kluwer; 2015.)

PILONIDAL DISEASE (FIG. 8-43)

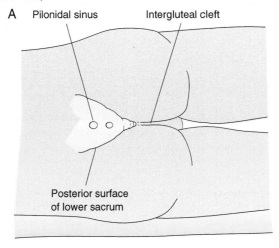

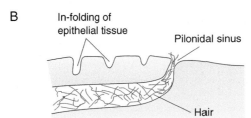

FIGURE 8-43. The pilonidal sinus and intergluteal (natal) cleft extending from below the sacrum to the perineum, ending just superior to the anus **(A)** where the skin is prominently affected by pilonidal cysts **(B)**. (From Smeltzer SC, Bare BG. *Brunner & Suddarth's Textbook of Medical-Surgical Nursing.* 9th ed. Philadelphia: Lippincott Williams & Wilkins; 2000.)

- Acquired infection of the skin and subcutaneous tissue near natal cleft of buttocks

- These cavities are not true cysts as they lack an epithelial lining

- Median age is 19 for women, 21 for men (men 2-4× as likely to be affected)

- RF: overweight/obese, local trauma/irritation, sedentary lifestyle or prolonged sitting, deep natal cleft, family history

Disease	Etiology, Prevalence, Risk Factors	Clinical Symptoms and Signs	Diagnostics	Therapy, Prognosis, and Health Maintenance
Pilonidal cyst or abscess	Fluid-filled sac found above the crease where the buttocks come together (natal cleft)	Asymptomatic or: 1. Redness 2. Sudden onset, mild to severe pain in intergluteal region 3. Swelling 4. Discomfort with sitting, bending, situps 5. Drainage—fluid, blood, pus Signs: 1. Asymptomatic—one or more primary pores (pits) in natal cleft 2. Symptomatic—tender mass or sinus draining (mucus, pus, blood) 3. Hair protruding from sinus opening	Clinical DX: 1. No imaging 2. CBC—leukocytosis	Acute 1. Incision and drainage under local anesthesia • Incision lateral to midline or over maximal fluctuance 2. Debridement within sinus 3. Pack wound with gauze • Wounds heal by secondary intention Definitive/chronic: 1. Surgical excision of all sinus tracts • Excision (mainstay) • Primary closure: faster wound healing, sooner return to work • Delayed closure: lower recurrence rate Antibiotics: 1. Limited, use if cellulitis develops 2. First gen cephalosporin (cefazolin) + flagyl Prognosis: 1. Recurrence ranges: 20%-55% 2. Cure rate: 45%

PRESSURE ULCERS (FIG. 8-44)

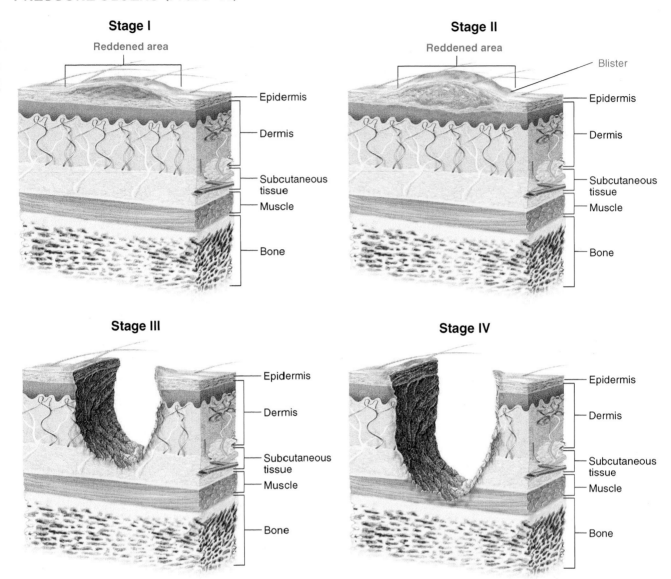

FIGURE 8-44. Pressure or decubitus ulcer staging system. (From Werner R. *A Massage Therapist's Guide to Pathology: Critical Thinking and Practical Application.* 6th ed. Philadelphia: Wolters Kluwer; 2016; assets provided by Anatomical Chart Company.)

- The stage is determined on initial assessment by noting the deepest layer of tissue involved. The ulcer is not restaged unless deeper layers of tissue become exposed. The most commonly used staging system is the **National Pressure Ulcer Advisory Panel's (NPUAP) classification system** describing 4 stages of pressure ulcers
- Each grade of pressure ulceration was defined by the anatomic limit of soft tissue damage that could be observed

- Assessment of ulcer status should be performed **weekly** and whenever a significant change is noted in the wound; assessment should not be confused with monitoring the ulcer at each dressing change
- At a minimum, the ulcer should be assessed for location, depth and stage, size, and wound bed description such as necrotic tissue, exudate, wound edges for undermining and tunneling, and presence or absence of granulation and epithelialization

Disease	Etiology, Prevalence, Risk Factors	Clinical Symptoms and Signs	Diagnostics	Therapy, Prognosis, and Health Maintenance
Pressure or decubitus ulcers (bedsores) Occur over bony prominences—sacrum, ischial tuberosities, trochanters, and heels most often	Result from necrosis of tissue that becomes ischemic and ulcerates, caused by prolonged pressure from the weight of the patient RF: **Immobilization**, PAD, dementia, incontinence, malnutrition, altered sensation or response to pain and discomfort Occurs within first 2 wk of hospitalization (first 5 d in critical care) MC pathogen: *P. aeruginosa, Providencia*	1. Blanchable erythema (first sign)—discoloration of patch of flat, nonraised area of skin >1 cm • Varies from pink to bright red or purple/blue-gray in dark skin 2. Edema 3. Increased temperature of area	Risk assessment on admission and at periodic intervals thereafter (48 h) • Norton scale: lower scores = lower function, high risk for ulcer • Braden scale for predicting pressure sore risk	1. Reposition every 2 h 2. Debridement of necrotic tissue, adequate wound cleansing, and application of topical therapy 3. Reassess every 4-wk postdischarge Complications: Septicemia (most severe), wound infection, cellulitis, osteomyelitis
	Skin color	Temperature	Texture	
Stage 1	Nonblanching erythema Dark-red to purple or cyanotic Dark-skinned: purple or gray, changes in texture, with induration, orange peel appearance	Cool compared with healthy tissue	Indurated	1. Reversible, although tissue takes 1-3 wk to return to normal 2. Cover with transparent film for protection
Stage 2: epidermis disrupted with subepidermal blisters, crusts, or scaling	Superficial, early: indistinct margins, red, shiny base; may be surrounded by erythema Chronic, deep ulcer: begins at bony prominence; dusky red wound base, does not bleed easily, surrounded by blanchable or nonblanchable erythema or deepening of normal skin tone	Warm	Indurated	1. May resolve in 2-4 wk if treated • Dressing that maintains moist environment • Avoid wet-to-dry dressings • Use semiocclusive (transparent film) or occlusive (hydrocolloids or hydrogels) so that necrotic tissue is digested by enzymes present in the wound base
Stage 3: full thickness loss of skin extending into subcutaneous tissue, but not through fascia	Eschar formation			1. Debridement of necrotic tissue 2. Coverage with dressings 3. Treat underlying infection, if present
Stage 4: full thickness loss of skin extending into muscle, bone, joints, tendons	Severe tissue necrosis present, osteomyelitis, pathologic fractures, sinus tracts present			

- Undermining, or pocketing, and tunneling may be present with large necrotic cavity
- Eschar formation may be result of larger vessel damage below skin from shearing; formation of an acellular dehydrated compressed area of necrosis, usually surrounded by outer rind of blanchable erythema → indicates full thickness loss of skin
- Pressure ulcer healing is accelerated during the initial 3 months after development

Forms of Debridement

Surgical or sharp	Extensive necrosis or need to obtain clean wound bed quickly • Removes thick, adherent, or large amounts of nonviable tissue and when advancing cellulitis or signs of sepsis present	• Most rapid form • Requires high level of competency in sharp tool skills and must meet licensure requirements • Considered nonselective, as viable and necrotic tissue both removed	Use of scalpel, scissors, or sharp instruments to remove nonviable tissue
Mechanical	Removes viable and nonviable tissue using hydrosurgery or whirlpool debridement	• Increased time and labor for application/removal of dressing • Not specific, but fast results • Painful and can harm viable tissue • Use cautiously: can traumatize new granulation and epithelial tissue	1. Use of wet-to-dry dressings, whirlpool, lavage, or wound irrigation 2. Hydrosurgery or wound cleansing 3. Ultrasound debridement
Autolytic	Moistens necrotic tissue, allowing degradation by host enzymes Long-term care or home care environments	• More conservative than sharp debridement, but more effective than mechanical • Must cleanse wound before • Selectively removes only the necrotic tissue, protects healthy tissues	1. Process of using body's own mechanisms to remove nonviable tissue 2. Maintaining moist environment allows collection of fluid at site 3. Enzymes within wound digest necrotic tissue
Enzymatic	Use of **collagenase**, papain-urea, papain-urea with chlorophyllin to remove necrotic tissue Long-term care or home care environments	• More conservative than sharp debridement • Faster than autolysis • Frequent dressing changes required	1. Apply a concentrated, commercially prepared enzyme to the surface of necrotic tissue 2. Aggressively degrades necrosis by digesting devitalized tissue
Biosurgical	Selective microdebridement using species of larvae (*Lucilia sericata*, *Phaenicia sericata*, and *Lucilia cuprina*)	• Targets only necrotic tissue	1. Application of maggots (*Phaenicia sericata*) to wound at density of 5-8/cm²

- Use of antiseptic and antimicrobial solutions for cleansing *clean* pressure ulcers is not indicated based on in vitro studies of the toxicity of topical wound cleansers.
- Use of antiseptic and antimicrobial solutions for cleansing pressure ulcers with *necrotic* debris should be employed thoughtfully with attention to the solution chosen, the characteristics of the microorganisms present in the wound, and duration of use
- Moist wound healing allows wounds to re-epithelialize up to 40% faster than wounds left open to air
- Use hydrocolloid dressings for Stage II to IV pressure ulcers
- There is some evidence supporting use of negative pressure wound therapy (NPWT) in large Stage III and IV nonhealing pressure ulcers with poor granulation tissue or excess exudate.
- Clinicians should institute systemic antibiotics for patients exhibiting signs and symptoms of systemic infection such as *sepsis* or *cellulitis* with associated fever and an elevated white blood cell count. Systemic antibiotics should also be initiated for osteomyelitis or for the prevention of bacterial endocarditis in persons with valvular heart disease and who require debridement of a pressure ulcer.

- Examples of systemic antibiotics: Ampicillin–sulbactam, imipenem, meropenem, ticarcillin–clavulanate, piperacillin–tazobactam, and a combination of clindamycin or metronidazole with ciprofloxacin, levofloxacin, or an aminoglycoside are appropriate choices for initial antibiotic therapy
- The most effective strategy for preventing infection and dealing with existing infection is adequate debridement of necrotic tissue
- Topical antibiotics are most appropriate for Stage III or IV ulcers when there is evidence of local infection such as erythema surrounding the wound, failure to improve with adequate treatment, or friable granulation tissue → silver sulfadiazine
  - Do not use hydrogen peroxide or iodine on clean pressure ulcers → toxic to fibroblasts, impair wound healing

VITILIGO (FIG. 8-45)

- Poliosis: decrease or absence of melanin or color in head hair, eyebrows, and/or eyelashes

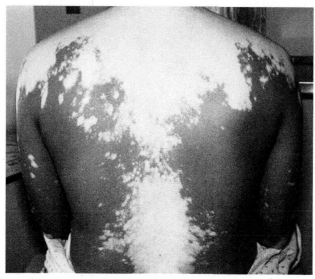

FIGURE 8-45. Vitiligo. (From *Lippincott's Nursing Advisor 2014.* Philadelphia: Wolters Kluwer; 2014.)

Disease	Etiology, Prevalence, Risk Factors	Clinical Symptoms and Signs	Diagnostics	Therapy, Prognosis, and Health Maintenance
Vitiligo	A complete loss of melanin pigment in the epidermis and absence of melanocytes, with occasional lymphocytes at advancing border Unknown cause, likely hereditary <u>Nonsegmental (MC):</u> No increase in size of existing lesions, absence of new lesions in previous 3-6 mo <u>Subtypes:</u> Generalized, acral, acrofacial, or universal	1. Asymptomatic depigmented macules without inflammation 2. Preceded by: severe sunburn, pregnancy, skin trauma, and/or emotional stress 3. Occurs anywhere: mostly face, area around orifices, genitals, or hands 4. Poliosis 5. Premature graying of scalp hair <u>Signs:</u> 1. Well demarcated, discrete, uniformly white or depigmented macules with convex borders surrounded by normal skin 2. Absence of inflammation or textural changes <u>Associated:</u> Alopecia areata, psoriasis, IBD, DM type I, rheumatoid arthritis, linea morphea, myasthenia gravis, discoid and systemic Lupus, Sjögren syndrome, autoimmune hypothyroidism, pernicious anemia, Addison disease	1. **Wood lamp examination** (diagnostic): appears bright blue with white fluorescence, sharply demarcated 2. Dermoscopy: residual perifollicular pigmentation or telangiectasia 3. Skin biopsy—not routine (definitive)	1. Topical steroids and photochemotherapy <u>Health maintenance:</u> 1. Screen for thyroid disease: TSH, anti-TPO, antithyroglobulin antibodies 2. ANA if (+) family hx of autoimmune disease, prior to phototherapy 3. Serial photography to mark progression <u>Prognosis:</u> 1. Progresses slowly over years, unless FH of nonsegmental vitiligo, longer duration of disease, koebnerization, and mucosal involvement 2. Flare ups common, separated by stable periods (no change in 12 mo)

Treatment of Vitiligo

Rapidly Progressive Disease	<10% TBSA Localized	<10% TBSA Disseminated Multiple Anatomic Sites	<10% TBSA Segmental	10%-40% TBSA or >40% TBSA Stable Nonsegmental
1. Low dose PO prednisone 5-10 mg/d (children), 10-20 mg/d (adults) × 2 wk max 2. With or without concomitant narrowband UVB phototherapy 2-3 times/wk	1. Mild to high potency topical steroids (first line) 2. High potency and mid-potency topical steroids • Betamethasone dipropionate, mometasone furoate, clobetasol propionate 3. Topical calcineurin inhibitors: tacrolimus and pimecrolimus, for face or high risk of skin atrophy 4. Unresponsive to above: phototherapy twice weekly Monitor for side effects: skin atrophy, telangiectasias, hypertrichosis, acneiform eruptions	1. NB-UVB phototherapy	1. Topical steroids 2. Calcineurin inhibitors 3. Targeted phototherapy 4. NB-UVB phototherapy for extensive disease affecting multiple dermatomes 5. Autologous grafting	1. NB-UVB phototherapy 2-3 times per wk × 9-12 mo

FOLLICULITIS (FIG. 8-46)

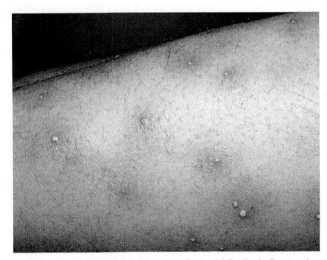

FIGURE 8-46. Bacterial folliculitis. (From Burkhart C, Morrell DS. *VisualDx: Essential Pediatric Dermatology*. Philadelphia: Lippincott Williams & Wilkins, a Wolters Kluwer business; 2010.)

Disease	Etiology, Prevalence, Risk Factors	Clinical Symptoms and Signs	Diagnostics	Therapy, Prognosis, and Health Maintenance
Bacterial folliculitis Inflammation of the superficial or deep portion of the hair follicle	Bacterial: **S. aureus (MCC, MC on scalp and face)** and *P. aeruginosa* ("hot tub," occurs on trunk and buttocks) <u>RF:</u> Male sex, nasal carriage of *S. aureus,* hyperhidrosis, occlusion of hair follicles, underlying skin disease (eczema), prolonged application of steroids, long-term oral antibiotics for acne, shaving against direction of hair growth, exposure to heated swimming pools or hot tubs (appears 8-48 h after) Occurs on any hair-bearing surface Fungal: Malassezia (Pityrosporum), Dermatophyte (Trichophyton), *Candida albicans* <u>Viral:</u> Herpesvirus, poxvirus (molluscum contagiosum virus)	1. Itching (MC symptom) 2. Painful pustules <u>Signs:</u> 1. Follicular pustules 2. Follicular erythematous papules on hair-bearing skin 3. Nodules	<u>Clinical DX:</u> 1. Gram stain and culture (confirms) 2. Skin biopsy—rarely needed	1. Most mild cases resolve spontaneously 2. Treat if: numerous papules/pustules, involvement of 1+ body area, or folliculitis that does not spontaneously resolve after several weeks • Topical mupirocin, clindamycin (first line) • 7-10 d course of PO dicloxacillin, cephalexin • If MRSA suspected: 7-10 d course of PO Bactrim DS, clindamycin, or doxycycline • *Pseudomonas* suspected: ciprofloxacin, ampicillin, or Bactrim DS × 14 d • Recalcitrant disease: Isotretinoin 0.5-1 mg/kg/d × 4-5 mo <u>Health maintenance:</u> 1. Avoid predisposing factors (occlusive clothing, hyperhidrosis) 2. 5-d course of topical mupirocin ointment in nares and daily chlorhexidine body washes with daily washing of personal items (towels, clothing) 3. Benzoyl peroxide washes and bleach baths 4. Avoid contaminated water and chlorinate pools and hot tubs properly

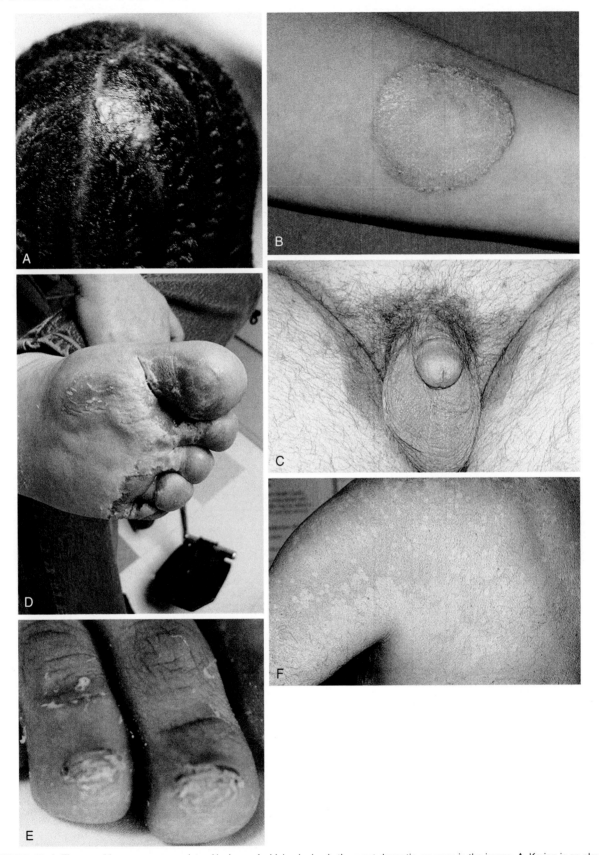
DERMATOPHYTE (TINEA) INFECTIONS: TINEA INFECTIONS, TINEA VERSICOLOR, ONYCHOMYCOSIS (FIG. 8-47)

FIGURE 8-47. A, Tinea capitis may cause a variety of lesions, of which a kerion is the most dramatic, as seen in the image. A, Kerion is an elevated, exudative, boggy, lesion covered by matted hair. **B**, Tinea corporis. **C**, Tinea cruris. **D**, Tinea pedis. **E**, Tinea unguium. **F**, Tinea versicolor. (**A**, From Fleisher GR, MD, Ludwig S, MD, Baskin MN, MD. *Atlas of Pediatric Emergency Medicine*. Philadelphia: Lippincott Williams & Wilkins, 2004. **B** and **C**, From Goodheart HP, MD. *Goodheart's Photoguide of Common Skin Disorders*. 2nd ed. Philadelphia: Lippincott Williams & Wilkins; 2003. **D**, From Council ML, Sheinbein DM, Cornelius LA. *The Washington Manual of Dermatology Diagnostics*. Philadelphia: Wolters Kluwer; 2016. **E**, From Salimpour RR, Salimpour P, Salimpour P. *Photographic Atlas of Pediatric Disorders and Diagnosis*. Philadelphia: Wolters Kluwer Health; 2014. **F**, From Goodheart HP. *Goodheart's Photoguide of Common Skin Disorders*. 2nd ed. Philadelphia: Lippincott Williams & Wilkins; 2003.)

Disease	Etiology, Prevalence, Risk Factors	Clinical Symptoms and Signs	Diagnostics	Therapy, Prognosis, and Health Maintenance
Tinea capitis (scalp)	MC: Trichophyton tonsurans Most common in African American children, age 3-9 y Classic "ringworm" pattern	1. Scalp or body 2. **Leading edge** (active border), scaly red, and slightly elevated with central clearing 3. Vesicles appear at active border when inflammation is intense 4. Scaling of the scalp or circumscribed alopecia with broken hair at scalp Signs: 1. Cervical and suboccipital **adenopathy** 2. Alopecia 3. Itching 4. Scaling	Clinical DX: 1. **KOH Prep**—more sensitive than culture 2. Fungal culture, takes 2-6 wk 3. Histologic tissue exam	1. **Oral antifungals** (griseofulvin/grifulvin 20 mg/kg/d × 8 wk) • AE: nausea, vomiting, photosensitivity 2. Oral terbinafine (Lamisil) 62.5 mg/d × 4 wk • Not effective for *Microsporum* species • Short duration, less expensive • Liver toxicity, baseline AST/ALT 3. Oral ketoconazole 4. **Selenium sulfide 2.5% shampoo** 2-3 times/wk, leave on for at least 5 min
Tinea corporis (body)	MC: *Trichophyton rubrum*	1. Annular patch or plaque with advancing, raised, scaling border and central clearing	Clinical DX: 1. KOH prep Culture not required	1. Topical antifungals-Fungicidal allylamines (terbinafine and butenafine)
Tinea cruris (groin)	MC: *T. rubrum, Trichophyton mentagrophytes, Epidermophyton floccosum* Adolescent and young adult men, postpubertal females who are overweight or wearing tight jeans/pantyhose Usually occurs with tinea pedis	1. Lesion border is usually active with pustules or vesicles 2. Background rash is red to reddish-brown, symmetric macule with fairly well-demarcated borders 3. Spares the scrotum 4. Itchy		1. Topical antifungals • Fungicidal allylamines (terbinafine and butenafine) applied daily × 2 wk
Tinea pedis (athlete's foot)	MC: *T. rubrum* Predisposing factors: exposure to a moist environment and maceration of the skin	1. White macerated area between the toes, although more diffuse dry scaling can occur (mocassin type) 2. Another pattern is inflammatory vesiculobullous eruption occurring on the soles 3. Does not spare intertriginous areas		1. Topical antifungals • Fungicidal allylamines (terbinafine and butenafine) 2. Oral steroids—if severe
Tinea unguium (**onycho-mycosis**)	Mostly caused by dermatophytes: **Trichophyton**, *Candida* Infection of the finger or toenails Subset of onychomycosis RF: Associated tinea pedis, improperly fitting shoes, diabetes	1. Discomfort in walking 2. Pain 3. Limitation of activities	1. Clean with 70% isopropyl alcohol, then collect samples of subungual debris and 8-10 nail clippings 2. Place on microscope with **KOH** 10%-20% solution, leave for 5 min before viewing → identification of hyphae or pseudohyphae • If negative → **periodic acid-Schiff (PAS) staining** to <u>confirm</u> infection	1. **Oral terbinafine** AE: • Sensory loss (taste, smell, hearing) • Diarrhea, rash, headache • 250 mg PO once daily × 6 wk (fingernails) or 12 wk (toenails) • Baseline LFTs, CBC and LFT if used >6 wk 2. Itraconazole 3. Fluconazole
Tinea (pityriasis) versicolor	MC: **Malassezia** *furfur* Superficial fungal infection caused by several *Malassezia* species Affects young adults and adolescents	1. Worse with hot/humid weather, excessive sweating, skin oils Signs: 1. Well-demarcated hyper- or hypo-pigmented lesions affecting the trunk 2. Light, dark, or pink/tan	1. KOH: "Spaghetti and meatballs"	1. Topical imidazoles (antifungals) 2. Selenium sulfide 2%, zinc pyrithione, or ketoconazole shampoo Prognosis: 1. Recurs annually in summer

CHAPTER **9**

Urology and Renal

Recommended Supplemental Topics:

Balanitis Xerotica Obliterans (Penile Lichen Sclerosis), p 183

Chronic Kidney Disease, p 237

Testicular Torsion, p 241

HERNIAS (FIG. 9-1)

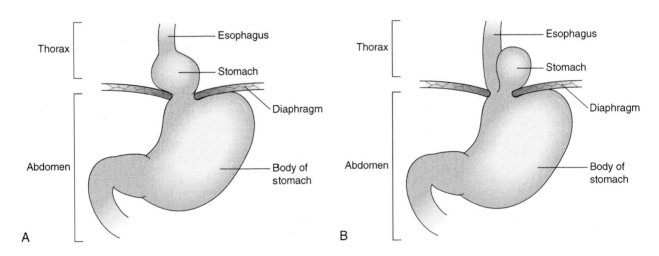

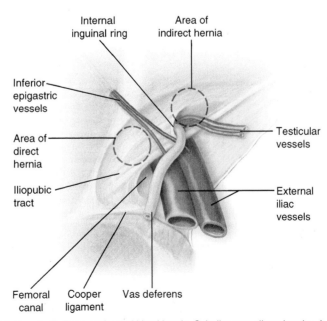

FIGURE 9-1. Hernia. **A**, Sliding hiatal hernia. **B**, Paraesophageal hiatal hernia. **C**, Indirect vs. direct hernias. Left side (anterior view). (**A** and **B**, From Porth C. *Essentials of Pathophysiology: Concepts of Altered States*. Philadelphia: Wolters Kluwer Health; 2014. **C**, From Jones D, ed. *Master Techniques in Surgery: Hernia*. Philadelphia: Wolters Kluwer Health; 2013.)

Disease	Etiology, Prevalence, Risk Factors	Clinical Symptoms and Signs	Diagnostics	Therapy, Prognosis, and Health Maintenance
Indirect inguinal hernia	• Obliteration of the **processus vaginalis** (peritoneal extension accompanying the testis in its descent into the scrotum) fails to occur • Hernial sac passes through internal inguinal ring, a defect in the transversalis fascia halfway between the ASIS and pubic tubercle • Sac located anteromedially to spermatic cord • Descends into the scrotum	1. Asymptomatic 2. Lump or swelling in groin with sudden pain and bulge that occurs while lifting or straining 3. "Dragging" sensation, radiation of pain into the scrotum 4. With enlargement → discomfort, aching pain, must lie down to reduce	1. Mass that may or may not be reducible 2. Examine patient both supine and standing, with cough and strain 3. Ask patient to cough/strain while finger directed laterally and upward into inguinal canal → protrudes against tip of finger 4. Tissue must be felt protruding the inguinal canal during coughing in order for diagnosis • Posterior wall of inguinal canal is firm and resistant	1. All symptomatic groin hernias should be repaired if patient can tolerate **surgery** • Especially painful or tender hernias • Repair may be deferred if hernia reduces with gentle manipulation and no evidence of strangulation (gangrenous tissue) 2. Nonsurgical management: truss • Use if patient refuses operative repair or when absolute contraindications to operation • Fit to provide adequate external compression over defect • Take off at night at put on in AM before arising • Does not preclude later repair of hernia Health maintenance: 1. Sedentary workers return to work in few days after surgery, no heavy manual labor 4-6 wk Prognosis: 1. Recurrence rate after hernia repair: 4%
Direct inguinal hernia	• A weakness or defect in the transversalis fascia • Funicular type more likely to become incarcerated because it has distinct borders		1. Appears as symmetric, circular swelling at external ring with standing and straining 2. Ask patient to cough/strain while finger directed laterally and upward into inguinal canal → protrudes against side of finger • Bulges forward through Hesselbach triangle 3. Disappears when lying supine • Posterior wall of inguinal canal is relaxed or absent	
Hiatal hernia Congenital or acquired Acquired may be nontraumatic (common) or traumatic Nontraumatic 1. Sliding hiatal hernia 2. Paraesophageal hiatal hernia	A portion of the stomach herniates through the diaphragmatic esophageal hiatus RF: Pregnancy, obesity, ascites, muscle weakening	Most asymptomatic, discovered incidentally 1. **GERD symptoms**–reflux or worsening reflux 2. Pain radiates to chest, not back Physical examination: 1. No palpable mass	1. **Upper GI series (barium swallow):** outpouching of barium at lower end of esophagus, wide hiatus, free reflux of barium • Distinguishes sliding from paraesophageal 2. **Upper GI endoscopy (EGD):** diagnoses hiatal hernia, diagnosis complications, good for biopsy of suspicious areas	1. Lifestyle modification 2. **PPI therapy** 3. Surgical treatment—remove hernial sac and close wide hiatus—only necessary if refractory to PPI • Nissen fundoplication, Belsey fundoplication, hill repair Complications: • Intermittent bleeding from esophagitis, erosions, discrete ulcers, or IDA • Incarcerated hernia (rare) • Barrett esophagus • Tumor
Femoral hernia	Acquired protrusion of a peritoneal sac through the femoral ring • Passes beneath the iliopubic tract and inguinal ligament into upper thigh Predisposing factor: Small empty space between lacunar ligament medially and femoral vein laterally	1. Bulge near groin or thigh		Prognosis: 1. **Highest incidence of strangulation and incarceration** ≫ inguinal hernias

(continued)

(continued)

Disease	Etiology, Prevalence, Risk Factors	Clinical Symptoms and Signs	Diagnostics	Therapy, Prognosis, and Health Maintenance
Umbilical hernias (adults) (Fig. 9-2A)	Owing to gradual yielding of the cicatricial tissue closing the ring F > M <u>RF:</u> Multiple pregnancies with prolonged labor, ascites, obesity, large intra-abdominal tumors	1. Increasing in size • Usually contain omentum, but small and large bowel may be present 2. Sharp pain on coughing or straining • Large hernias produce dragging or aching sensation		1. Observation 2. Requires emergency repair if strangulated or incarcerated • Neck is usually narrow compared with size of herniated mass → incarceration and strangulation common • Mesh = lowest recurrence rate, use for all but smallest • Control significant ascites preop: medically or TIPS • Correct fluid and electrolyte imbalances RF for high complication and recurrence: large size, old age, debility of patient, obesity, intra-abdominal disease
Epigastric hernia	Protrudes through linea alba above level of umbilicus 3%-5% of population have M > F, ages 20-50 y/o	1. Painless, found on routine examination 2. Symptomatic–varies • Mild epigastric pain and tenderness • Deep, burning epigastric pain with radiation to back or lower abdominal quadrants 3. Abdominal bloating, nausea, vomiting 4. SX occur after large meal and may be relieved by reclining <u>Signs:</u> 1. Palpable–diagnose with maneuvers that increase intra-abdominal pressure	1. Ultrasound 2. CT 3. XR	1. Most repaired • Smaller masses (only fat) prone to incarceration and strangulation, tender • Mesh for large hernias Recurrence rate: 10%-20% (high)
Incisional (ventral) hernia (Fig. 9-2B)	10% of operations	1. Asymptomatic 2. S/Sx of small bowel obstruction		1. Small–early repair due to obstruction • If unwilling or poor surgical risk → elastic binder 2. Large–may be left if asymptomatic, less likely to incarcerate • Considered large if fascial edges cannot be approximated without tension • Mesh > primary suture repair, even if small • Recurrence rate increases with each subsequent reoperation • Factors that increase recurrence: wound infection, abdominal aneurysms, smoking, poor nutrition

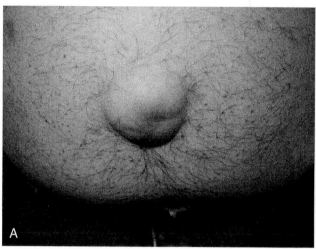
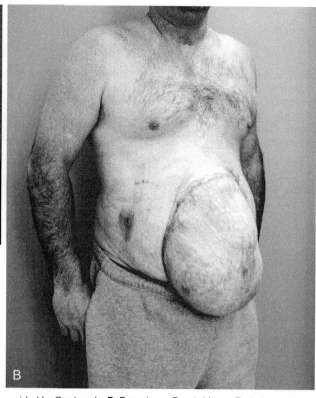

FIGURE 9-2. A, Umbilical hernia. **B**, Incisional/ventral hernia. (**A**, Image provided by Stedman's. **B**, From Jones D, ed. *Master Techniques in Surgery: Hernia*. Philadelphia: Wolters Kluwer Health; 2013.)

URINARY TRACT INFECTION (CYSTITIS) AND PYELONEPHRITIS, URETHRITIS

- Urinary tract infection: denotes symptomatic disease
- Cystitis: symptomatic infection of the bladder
- Pyelonephritis: symptomatic infection of the kidneys (renal parenchyma) without inflammatory mass or abscess

Disease	Etiology, Prevalence, Risk Factors	Clinical Symptoms and Signs	Diagnostics	Therapy, Prognosis, and Health Maintenance
Uncomplicated urinary tract infection: cystitis in immunocompetent nonpregnant women (**healthy patients**) w/o underlying structural or neurologic disease	RF: Recent use of a diaphragm with spermicide, frequent sexual intercourse, and a history of UTI are independent risk factors for acute cystitis MCC: ***E. coli* (80%)**, *Proteus, Klebsiella, S. saprophyticus* In healthy postmenopausal women, sexual activity, diabetes mellitus, and incontinence are risk factors for UTI	1. **Dysuria, urgency**, frequency 2. Hematuria Signs: 1. Change in urine color/odor 2. **Suprapubic pain** 3. Fever (absent)	1. Urine dipstick: nitrite, leukocyte esterase 2. U/A: **pyuria, bacteriuria** ± hematuria ± nitrites 3. CBC: **leukocytosis** 4. Urine culture (clean-catch midstream or straight cath): only get if **symptomatic** • >10 ^ 5 CFU/mL (F) • >10 ^ 3 CFU/mL M or cath patients • →takes 24 h to obtain results 5. Blood cultures: obtain in febrile Pts; consider in complicated UTI	1. Nitrofurantoin (Macrobid) 100 mg × 5 d 2. **Bactrim DS PO × 3 d**

(continued)

(continued)

Disease	Etiology, Prevalence, Risk Factors	Clinical Symptoms and Signs	Diagnostics	Therapy, Prognosis, and Health Maintenance
Complicated urinary tract infection Infection in patient with structural or functional abnormality that would reduce the efficacy of antibiotic therapy	MCC: **E. coli (30%)**, enterococci, PsA, *Staphylococcus epidermidis* Catheter associated: yeast (30%), E. coli (25%) Complicated: children, men, nosocomial or nursing home acquired, kidney allograft, **pregnancy**, immunosuppression RF: DM, sickle cell disease, BPH, recurrent UTI, indwelling catheter, neurogenic bladder, polycystic kidney disease	Same as uncomplicated UTI	1. Urine culture (clean-catch midstream or straight cath): only get if **symptomatic** • >10 ^ 5 CFU/mL	1. **Fluoroquinolone** OR • Bactrim PO × 7-14 d 2. Pregnant: • Nitrofurantoin • Ampicillin • cephalosporins
Recurrent UTI	Relapse: Recurrence of UTI within 2 wk of treatment caused by same organism Reinfection: Recurrent UTI caused by different bacteria; more common than relapse	1. 2 uncomplicated UTI in 6 mo OR 3+ uncomplicated UTIs in previous year	1. Urine culture (clean-catch midstream or straight cath)	1. Empiric treatment 2. Repeat culture in 1-2 wk
Urethritis (nongonococcal)	Inflammation of the urethra caused by infectious or noninfectious causes (trauma, foreign body) MC: M, age 20-24, African American **C. trachomatis**, *Ureaplasma urealyticum, Trichomonas. vaginalis, Mycoplasma genitalium*, HSV	1. **Urethral discharge** 2. Dysuria • Both, usually without frequency of urination 3. Urethral itching Signs: 1. Proximal to distal "milking" of urethra	1. **NAAT**s of first voided urine • Recommended for screening asymptomatic at-risk men and testing symptomatic men 2. **Gram stain** of anterior urethral specimen: >5 WBC 3. Urinalysis w/ culture: (+) leuk-esterase 4. Prostate examination, to r/o bacterial prostatitis and cystitis	1. If no gonococci • azithromycin or doxycycline 2. If gonococci detected • Treat for both Neisseria and Chlamydia (CTX 125 mg IM × 1, Doxy 100 mg PO BID × 7 d or Azithro 1 g PO × 1 3. Recurrency • Flagyl or tinidazole 4. Plus azithromycin
Asymptomatic bacteriuria	Pregnant: asymptomatic bacteriuria at 12-16 wk ASB is common among **elderly** and **catheterized** patients	1. No signs or symptoms referable to UTI	1. Urine culture: >10^5 CFU/mL except in catheter associated disease (>10^2) • Get cultures if pregnant and treat	No treatment unless pregnant, invasive urologic procedure, neutropenic patients and renal transplant patients 1. Antibiotics × 3 d Indications not to treat: 1. Nonpregnant or premenopausal women 2. Diabetic patients 3. Indwelling urethral catheters 4. Spinal cord injury 5. Elderly

Disease	Etiology, Prevalence, Risk Factors	Clinical Symptoms and Signs	Diagnostics	Therapy, Prognosis, and Health Maintenance

Pyelonephritis	RF: sexual intercourse, a new sexual partner, a UTI in the previous 12 mo, a maternal history of UTI, diabetes, and incontinence **E. coli** (most common)	1. Cystitis: **dysuria, urgency, frequency**
		2. Fever + chills
		3. Nausea, vomiting, diarrhea
		Signs:
		1. **Flank** or back pain,
		2. CVA Tenderness
			1. U/A: **pyuria, bacteriuria, WBC casts** ± hematuria ± nitrites
			2. CBC: leukocytosis, left shift
			3. Urine culture (clean-catch midstream or straight cath): only get if symptomatic
			  • >10^5 CFU/mL (women)
			  • >10^3 CFU/mL men or cath patients
			4. Blood cultures: obtain in febrile patients; consider in complicated UTI
			5. Abdominal CT: r/o abscess in patients with pyelo who fail to defervesce after 72 h
			6. Urologic w/u (renal U/S, abd CT, VCUG): recurrent UTI in men
				1. First-line: fluoroquinolones
				  • ciprofloxacin PO 500 mg BID ± initial IV 400 mg load

Treatment of Pyelonephritis

Outpatient	Inpatient	Pregnant	Men
1. **FQ × 7 d** **Or** 2. **Bactrim DO × 14 d**	1. **IV 1-g CTX** Or 2. **Amp/Sulbactam** Or 3. Aminoglycoside × 14 d (change to PO if clinically improved and afebrile 24-48 h)	1. IV B-lactam (**ampicillin**) +/– 2. Aminoglycoside (**gentamicin**) × 14 d→ Increased risk of pyelonephritis, PTB, low birth weight, and perinatal mortality, if untreated	1. FQ or bactrim × 7-14 d

GLOMERULONEPHRITIS

Caused by immune-mediated mechanisms, metabolic or hemodynamic disturbances

Nephrotic Syndrome	Nephritic Syndrome
• Abnormal glomerular permeability = increased filtration of macromolecules • Many causes—**membranous GN** (MCC), diabetes, SLE, drugs, infection • Minimal change disease (children, MCC) • Associated: 30% have DM, amyloidosis, or SLE	• Inflammation of glomeruli due to any of the causes of GN • Causes: **poststreptococcal GN** (MCC), Berger disease, hepatitis C, SLE

1. Hypercoagulable state
2. **Hypoalbuminemia** (urinary loss)
3. **Hyperlipidemia, fatty casts** in urine (**lipiduria**)
  • Hypercholesterolemia, hypertriglyceridemia: decreased plasma oncotic pressure stimulates hepatic lipoprotein synthesis
4. **Proteinuria** >3.5 g/24 h
  • Can also calculate protein-to-creatinine ratio on random urine specimen
5. **Edema (peripheral):** periorbital edema in AM and pedal edema
	1. **Asymptomatic gross hematuria (30%-50%)**
	  • Smoke, tea, or coca cola colored
	2. Mild **proteinuria**, <3.5 g/24 h
	Advanced findings
	1. Hypertension
	2. AKI: Oliguria, azotemia
	3. Edema (generalized)

1. U/A: **oval fat bodies** 2. 24-hour urine collection 3. Renal biopsy (required for diagnosis) • Contraindications: bleeding diathesis, small kidneys, severe uncontrolled HTN, multiple bilateral cysts, hydronephrosis, active renal infection, uncooperative patient	1. U/A: Dysmorphic RBC ± RBC casts, pyuria 2. C3 and CH50 (total complement) decreased in first 2 wk 3. (+) ASO titer (streptozyme test) 4. Renal biopsy (not usually performed): only if late or without clear history of prior strep infection

(continued)

Nephrotic Syndrome	Nephritic Syndrome

1. ACE inhibitors for HTN: lower intraglomerular pressure → decrease protein excretion
  • Decrease GFR and cause hyperkalemia, measure SCr, potassium
2. Sodium restriction (2 g/d): reduces peripheral edema and ascites
  • Loop diuretics
3. Steroids and cytotoxic agents
4. **Statin** for hyperlipidemia
5. **Anticoagulation** for hypoalbuminemia
  • Heparin followed by warfarin as long as nephrotic (esp in membranous nephropathy)
	1. Steroids and cytotoxic agents: Methylprednisolone
	2. **Loop diuretics** and *sodium/H_2O restriction* for edema
	  • IV Furosemide 1 mg/kg, max 40 mg
	3. ACE inhibitors for HTN encephalopathy
	  • Oral nifedipine or IV nicardipine

1. **Increased risk of VTE:** DVT/PE and renal vein thrombosis (membranous nephropathy) 2. Increased risk of infection: pneumonia	

- Diagnosis
  - Urinalysis (hematuria, proteinuria, RBC casts)
  - Blood tests: renal function tests
  - Needle biopsy of kidney

Primary Glomerular Disorders

Minimal change disease	• Most common GN of children • Associations: Hodgkin and non-Hodgkin lymphoma • Proteinuria, edema, hypoalbuminemia, hyperlipidemia, HTN • Hematuria • Fusion of foot processes on electron microscopy • Good prognosis TX: steroids 4-8 wk
Membranous GN	• Usually presents with nephrotic syndrome; thick glomerular capillary walls • Primary idiopathic, secondary due to infection (Hep-C, Hep-B, syphilis, malaria), drugs (gold, captopril), or SLE • Prognosis is fair, remission common, renal failure (33%) TX: **steroids**, but won't change survival
IgA nephropathy (Berger disease)	• Asymptomatic recurrent hematuria/mild proteinuria common • Most common cause of **glomerular hematuria** • **Gross hematuria after URI** (or exercise) common • Renal function normal • Electron microscopy: Mesangial deposition of IgA and C3 • Prognosis good, preserved renal function TX: **Steroids** for unstable disease

Secondary Glomerular Disorders

Diabetic nephropathy	• Most common cause of ESRD • HX: type 1 DM, male, African American, (+) family history • Albuminuria (micro or macro) • End organ issues: retinopathy or CVD • Elevated SCr • Annual screening for albuminuria, strict glycemic control, ACE/ARB, low sat/protein diet
Membranoproliferative GN	• Usually due to **Hep-C infection** • Commonly associated with cryoglobulinemia • Poor prognosis, renal failure (50%), TX rarely effective
Poststreptococcal GN	• **Most common cause** of nephritic syndrome • Occurs after infection with group A β-hemolytic streptococcal infection of URT (impetigo), develops 10-14 d after • Primarily children (+) ASO titer U/A: **RBC casts, dysmorphic** RBCs • Features: hematuria, edema, HTN, *low complement* and proteinuria
Goodpasture GN	• Classic triad of proliferative GN (crescentic), pulmonary hemorrhage, and IgG antiglomerular basement membrane antibody • Features: rapidly progressive renal failure, hemoptysis, cough, dyspnea • Lung disease before kidney disease (days-weeks) • Renal biopsy: linear immunofluorescence • TX: **plasmapheresis** to remove circulating anti-IgG antibodies, cyclophosphamide, and steroids

NEPHROLITHIASIS (RENAL CALCULI) (FIG. 9-3)

- Most clinically important inhibitor of calcium-containing stones is urine citrate

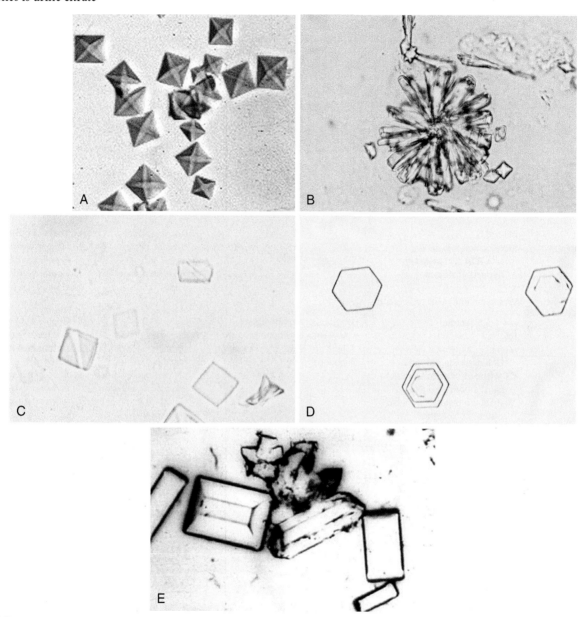

FIGURE 9-3. **A**, Calcium oxalate. **B**, Calcium phosphate. **C**, Uric acid. Calcium phosphate. **D**, Cystine stones. Calcium phosphate. **E**, Struvite. (**A**, From Bergin J. *Medicine Recall*. Philadelphia: Wolters Kluwer Health; 2007. **B-D**, From Mundt L, Shanahan K. *Graff's Textbook of Urinalaysis*. Philadelphia: Wolters Kluwer Health; 2016. **E**, From Leehey DJ, Moinuddin I. *Handbook of Nephrology*. Philadelphia: Wolters Kluwer Health; 2014.)

Disease	Etiology, Prevalence, Risk Factors	Clinical Symptoms and Signs	Diagnostics	Therapy, Prognosis, and Health Maintenance
Nephrolithiasis (renal calculi)	MC types of stones: calcium oxalate (75%), calcium phosphate, uric acid, struvite, cystine M > F <u>RF:</u> Family history (2×), hyper-calciuria, weight gain, low urine output (2×), sweet beverages, working in a hot environment, dietary (animal protein, oxalate, sodium, sucrose, fructose)	1. Unilateral flank pain • Radiates anteriorly (upper ureter) or ipsilateral testicle or labium (lower ureter) 2. Nausea, vomiting 3. Painless gross hematuria (90%) <u>Signs:</u> 1. CVAT	1. CMP 2. U/A with culture 3. KUB (initial test) • Cannot see cystine or uric acid 4. **Helical CT without contrast** (highly sensitive)	1. Treat colic pain • **NSAIDs** (Ketorolac or Toradol) • PO fluids (maintain euvolemia) • α blockers 2. Extracorporeal shockwave lithotripsy • For stones **>6 mm** up to 2 cm, intractable pain • Ureteral stent or percutaneous nephrolithotomy 50% recur in 10 y

Type of Stone	Etiology/Imaging/Description	Factors that Increase Stone Formation	Factors that Decrease Stone Formation	Treatment
Calcium oxalate	No influence by pH XR: Visible on abdominal radiograph Bipyramidal and biconcave ovals	1. Increased serum calcium 2. Increased urine oxalate 3. Increased urine uric acid 4. Decreased urine citrate	1. Avoid high dose vitamin C 2. Avoid foods with oxalate: spinach, rhubarb, potatoes 3. Avoid alkali foods (fruits, vegetables) and supplement with **potassium citrate**, sodium bicarbonate 4. Decrease sucrose, fructose, Na intake (<2.5 g/d) 5. Decrease urine calcium and urine oxalate, and increased urine citrate	1. Dietary calcium restriction not beneficial 2. High dose **thiazide diuretic** 3. Allopurinol
Calcium phosphate	pH > 6.5 More common in patient with **RTA** and **primary hyperthyroidism** XR: Visible on abdominal radiograph		1. Decrease urine calcium, urine phosphate, and pH 2. Increased urine citrate	1. **Thiazide diuretics** with Na restriction 2. Potassium citrate—increases urine citrate
Uric acid	pH < 5.5 (**acidic**) RF: Metabolic syndrome (obesity, DM, dyslipidemia), gout **CT without contrast:** "radiolucent" stones "Flat square plates," "rhombic plates" or "rosettes"	HX: gout, chemotherapy of leukemia or lymphoma with high cell destruction releases purines → hyperuricemia	1. pH goal: 6-7 2. Decrease purine containing foods 3. **Increase urine pH** and decrease uric acid excretion (alkalinize the urine!) 4. Increase alkaline foods (fruits, vegetables), reduce acidic foods (animal flesh)	1. Supplement with bicarbonate or **potassium citrate (Bicitra)** 2. Allopurinol (xanthine oxidase inhibitor) or febuxostat
Cystine stones	Cystinuria is **autosomal recessive**—defect in renal transport of amino acids **CT without contrast:** "radiolucent" stones "stop signs" "benzene rings" "hexagon shaped"		1. Increase cystine solubility 2. Maintain high urine volume	1. **Tiopronin** and penicillamine—binds cysteine 2. Alkalinize the urine—**potassium citrate**
Struvite (infection stones, triple-phosphate stones, Mg-NH_3-PO_4)	Upper UT infected with urease-producing bacteria: ***Proteus mirabilis***, *K. pneumoniae*, Providencia → hydrolyze urea → **increase urine pH > 8** Staghorn calculi: grow quickly and fill renal pelvis KUB: "Staghorn calculi" **"Coffin lids"** or "rectangular prisms"	HX: **recurrent UTIs** due to urease-producing orgs (Proteus, Klebsiella, Serratia, Enterobacter) **Alkaline pH** + calcium crystal nidus + urease producing bacteria RF: Women 50+, neurogenic bladder, h/o stones, medullary sponge kidney (MSK)	1. Prevent UTIs for prophylaxis	1. Requires complete removal by **urologist** 2. Acetohydroxamic acid—urease inhibitor

BENIGN PROSTATIC HYPERPLASIA (FORMERLY HYPERTROPHY), PROSTATITIS

Disease	Etiology, Prevalence, Risk Factors	Clinical Symptoms and Signs	Diagnostics	Therapy, Prognosis, and Health Maintenance
Benign prostatic hyperplasia (formerly Hypertrophy) (BPH) Bladder outlet obstruction	70+ (10%-30%) Associated: DM, cold/sinus medications, OSA, insomnia, hematuria Occurs in the **TRANSITION** zone	1. Obstructive (prostate): **decreased force of stream**, hesitancy, post-void dribbling, sensation of incomplete emptying 2. Irritative (bladder): dysuria, **frequency, urgency** 3. Nocturia Manifestations: UTI, hematuria, renal insufficiency, retention, LUTS (lower urinary tract symptoms)	1. **Urinalysis:** r/o infection, hematuria 2. PSA: if 10+ life expectancy 3. Renal U/S: if renal insufficiency 4. Other testing • Urodynamics • Uroflowmetry • Postvoid residual-urine	First line: 1. Reassurance 2. Lifestyle modification • decrease fluid intake before bed • decrease caffeine/ETOH • time-void 3. **α blockers:** most effective with severe BPH and HTN 4. **5-α reductase** inhibitors (finasteride, dutasteride): larger prostates 5. PDE-5 inhibitors 6. Saw palmetto 7. **Surgery: TURP** if: Interfere with QOL, acute retention, recurrent UTI or hematuria, Azotemia, bladder stones Complications: Acute urinary retention
Acute prostatitis	Rare, class I "sick" Most community acquired, others occur after catheterization and cystoscopy or after transrectal prostate biopsy **Gram-negative organisms: E. coli,** *Klebsiella, Proteus, Enterobacter, Staph* Peak: 20-40 y/o	1. Acute onset of **pelvic pain** • Perineal, sacral, or suprapubic pain 2. Irritative **UTI symptoms:** Frequency, urgency, dysuria 3. Obstructive: straining, hesitancy, poor or interrupted stream, incomplete emptying 4. Systemic febrile illness: **Fever**/chills, malaise, nausea, vomiting Signs: 1. Toxic, febrile 2. Sepsis: Tachycardia, hypotension 3. Tachypnea 4. Suprapubic pain	1. U/A + culture: large WBC, (+) culture 2. Postvoid residual 3. CBC: **elevated WBC** 4. DRE: tender, enlarged "boggy" **prostate** • **Prostatic massage contraindicated!** 5. In cases of treatment failure, transrectal ultrasonography of the prostate may detect prostate calculi or abscess 6. CBC and blood cultures if toxic of sepsis suspected	1. Outpatient • FQ (ciprofloxacin) 750 mg BID or • **Bactrim BID** × 4-6 wk 2. Inpatient: systemically ill or unable to voluntarily urinate, unable to tolerate PO intake, or RF for resistance • IV **ampicillin** 1 g q 12 h + **gentamicin** 1 mg/kg q8h 3. Noncontrast pelvic CT if fever persists >36 h after antibiotics
Chronic prostatitis Persistent infection of prostate lasting 3+ mo	5%-15% of men develop over lifetime More common M 40-70 y/o Causes: BPH, stones, or foreign body within urinary tract, bladder cancer, prostatic abscess, enterovesical fistula MCC: *E. coli*	1. **Recurrent or relapsing UTI, urethritis, or epididymitis** • Asymptomatic between episodes 2. Localized pain in **lower back, perineal, testicular** region • Dull 3. Irritative: frequency, urgency, dysuria 4. No fever Signs: 1. Do not appear ill 2. Afebrile	1. U/A and culture: WBC (+) and **culture (+)** or negative 2. **2-glass pre- and post-prostatic massage test** 3. DRE: prostate enlarged and nontender	1. Fluoroquinolone • **Ciprofloxacin** 500 mg BID • Levofloxacin 500 mg daily 2. Bactrim DS 160/800 mg BID

GONORRHEA AND CHLAMYDIA

Disease	Etiology, Prevalence, Risk Factors	Clinical Symptoms and Signs	Diagnostics	Therapy, Prognosis, and Health Maintenance
Chlamydia	Most common bacterial STD • Most coinfected with gonorrhea (40% F, 20% M) • Incubation: 1-3 wk RF: Lack of condom use, lower socioeconomic status, living in an urban area, having multiple sex partners Most common in F: 15-19, then **20-24 (75%)** Independent risk factor for **cervical cancer**	Mostly asymptomatic Men: **dysuria**, *purulent urethral* **discharge**, **itching**, scrotal pain and swelling, fever Women: *purulent urethral dis-charge*, intermenstrual or **post-coital bleeding**, **dysuria** Signs: 1. Mucopurulent discharge from cervical os 2. Friable cervix	1. **NAAT** (nucleic acid amplification tests)—most sensitive 2. **Wet mount**: leukor-rhea (>10 WBC/hpf) 3. Culture, enzyme immunoassay, PCR • No serologic testing • Screen sexually active females for chlamydia, even if asymptomatic	1. **1 g Azithromycin** PO × 1 or doxycycline (100 mg BID × 7 d) 2. Treat all partners Pregnant women: **Azithromycin 1 g** × 1 or amoxicil-lin 500 mg TID × 7 d • Complications: preterm labor, chorioamnionitis, endometritis, transmission to infant Complications: Men—epididymitis, proctitis, prostatitis Women: PID, salpingitis, tubo-ovar-ian abscess, ectopic pregnancy, Fitz-Hugh Curtis syndrome, **infertility**
Gonorrhea	• ***N. gonorrhoeae*** (gram-negative, intra-cellular diplococci) • Transmission: sexual or neonatal • Coinfection with chlamydia (30%)	• Asymptomatic in women, symp-tomatic in men • Check: pharynx, conjunctiva, and rectum M: 10% symptomatic, contagious • Urethral discharge, dysuria, erythema, edema, frequency in urination F: most asymptomatic or few symptoms • Cervicitis or **urethritis** (purulent discharge, dysuria, intermenstrual bleeding) Disseminated (1%-2%), F • Fever, arthralgias, tenosynovitis (hands and feet) • Migratory polyarthritis/**septic arthritis,** endocarditis, meningitis • Skin rash (distal extremities)	1. **NAAT** (nucleic acid amplification tests)—most sensitive 2. **Gram stain** of urethral discharge: leukocytes 3. **Cultures (all)**: men from urethra, women from endocervix 4. Test for syphilis and HIV 5. Obtain blood cul-tures for dissemi-nated disease	Treat empirically because cultures take 1-2 d 1. **Ceftriaxone** (250 mg IM × 1), also protects against syphilis, but can use cefixime, ciprofloxa-cin or ofloxacin 2. **Add azithromycin** PO × 1 or doxycycline (PO × 7 d) to cover chlamydia • If disseminated: hospitalize and IV or IM Ceftriaxone × 7 d Complications: PID, infertility with chronic pelvic pain, epididymitis, prostati-tis, salpingitis, tubo-ovarian abscess, Fitz-Hugh-Curtis syn-drome (perihepatitis, bleeding, dyspareunia), disseminated gonococcal infection

EPIDIDYMITIS, ORCHITIS, BALANITIS

Disease	Etiology, Prevalence, Risk Factors	Clinical Symptoms and Signs	Diagnostics	Therapy, Prognosis, and Health Maintenance
Epididymitis Inflammation or infection of the epididy-mis → can spread to entire testicle (epididymo-or-chitis)	<35: Gonorrhea or chlamydia >35: *E. coli* h/o: UTI, urethritis, discharge, sex-ual activity, foley catheterization Most common cause of scrotal pain in adults	1. Gradual **unilateral pain** and swelling of scrotum • Dull ache, swelling of scrotum, tender testicle • Indolent onset (hours-days) • **Radiation to ipsilateral inguinal canal (flank)** 2. Symptoms of cystitis: frequency, urgency, hematuria, **dysuria** 3. **Fever**, chills 4. Symptoms of urethritis: urethral discharge and pain at the tip of the penis Signs: 1. Mass palpable 2. Erythema of scrotal skin 3. **Prehn sign (+)**: pain relief with elevation of scrotum 4. (+) Cremasteric reflex 5. Tachycardia	1. Doppler ultrasound: **increased blood flow** 2. CRP and ESR: elevated r/o torsion, which is more acute and not associated with fever	1. Rest, scrotal elevation, ice packs, NSAIDs 2. <35: **ceftriaxone** and **doxycycline** or azithromycin 3. >35: ciprofloxacin and **Bactrim**

Disease	Etiology, Prevalence, Risk Factors	Clinical Symptoms and Signs	Diagnostics	Therapy, Prognosis, and Health Maintenance
Orchitis	Inflammation from epididymis spreads to adjacent testicle	1. Abrupt onset of testicular pain Signs: 1. Testicular swelling and tenderness 2. Cremasteric reflex (+)	History, physical, UA Doppler ultrasound: Testicular masses or swollen testicles with hyperechoic and hypervascular areas	1. Supportive: NSAIDs, scrotal support 2. Antibiotics: ciprofloxacin, doxycycline, rocephin
Viral orchitis	Occurs most commonly after mumps, but may be caused by viral or bacterial infection	7-10 d after mumps, as parotitis resolves→ 1. Painful, tender unilateral scrotal swelling→ 2. Resolves and testicles may atrophy		1. Supportive: NSAIDs, scrotal support 2. Resolves spontaneously after 3-10 d
Balanitis xerotica obliterans (penile lichen sclerosis) (Fig. 9-4)	Occurs in males of all ages, average 42 y/o Squamous cell carcinoma (4%-6%) Precancerous	1. Phimosis, painful erections, or obstructive voiding, itching, pain, bleeding • Initial complaint of urinary retention 2. Hypopigmented lesion with skin similar to crinkled paper or cellophane • Affects glans penis and prepuce • Bullae, erosions, atrophy	1. Biopsy—if SCC suspected	1. Moderate to ultrapotent fluorinated **topical steroids** 2. Surgery for persistent disease or history of SCC • Circumcision of glans and prepuce 3. PO retinoids

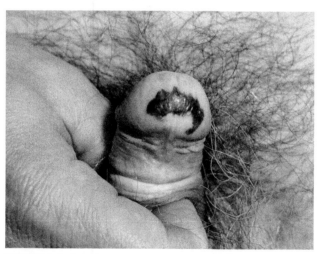

FIGURE 9-4. Balanitis xerotica obliterans. (From Craft N, Fox LP, Goldsmith LA, et al. *VisualDx: Essential Adult Dermatology.* Philadelphia: Wolters Kluwer Health; 2011.)

TESTICULAR CANCER (FIG. 9-5)

Testicular Self-Examination

Disease	Etiology, Prevalence, Risk Factors	Clinical Symptoms and Signs	Diagnostics	Therapy, Prognosis, and Health Maintenance
Testicular carcinoma	MC type: seminoma Most common in M 20-35 RF: History of **cryptorchidism** or Klinefelter syndrome	1. **Painless enlarging testicular mass**, lump, or firmness 2. Gynecomastia Signs: 1. Scrotal enlargement	1. **Ultrasound** (first line) 2. Tumor markers: *AFP*: increased in embryonal tumors (80%), but chorio and seminoma never have elevated AFP 3. *β-hCG*: always elevated in choriocarcinoma 4. CT chest/abd/pelvis and CXR for staging	1. Surgery, radiation, or chemotherapy offered • Orchiectomy • Nonseminomatous: 2 rounds of chemotherapy • Seminoma: external beam radiation Relatively high cure rate for cancer Most common site of spread: retroperitoneal lymph nodes Complications: scrotal hematoma

(continued)

(continued)

Disease	Etiology, Prevalence, Risk Factors	Clinical Symptoms and Signs	Diagnostics	Therapy, Prognosis, and Health Maintenance
Germ cell tumors (95%)	Most common 20-40 Mostly **seminomas** (35%)– slow growth and late invasion Nonseminomatous (65%) • Embryonal carcinoma = highly malignant, hemorrhage, necrosis, mets to abdominal lymphatics and lungs • Choriocarcinoma = most aggressive, mets occur by diagnosis • Teratoma = rarely metastasize • Yolk sac carcinoma = rare in men, usually younger boys		1. If testicular cancer suspected, remove testicle surgically to confirm diagnosis (orchiectomy) → CT of chest, abdomen, pelvis for staging 2. B-hCG and AFP measurement before and after orchiectomy for comparison with pre-op	• Seminomas (95% curable) • Most radiosensitive, inguinal orchiectomy and radiation • Nonseminomatous: orchiectomy + retroperitoneal lymph node dissection ± chemotherapy

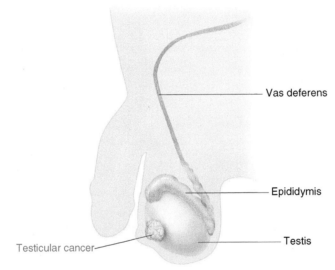

Vas deferens

Epididymis

Testis

Testicular cancer

FIGURE 9-5. Testicular carcinoma. (Anatomical Chart Co.)

CHAPTER **10**

Endocrinology

Refer to Internal Medicine 🩺 for in-depth coverage of the following topics:

Diabetes Mellitus, p 231

Adrenal Insufficiency, see Addison's Disease and Secondary Adrenal Insufficiency, p 228

Cushing Disease, p 234

Hyperthyroidism, p 226

Hypothyroidism, p 227

Recommended Supplemental Resources:

Pituitary Adenoma, see Internal Medicine 🩺 p 233

Thyroid Cancer, see Internal Medicine 🩺 p 232

Diabetic Ketoacidosis, see Emergency Medicine ⛑ p 432

Pheochromocytoma, see Internal Medicine 🩺 p 229

Paget Disease of the Bone, p 233

CHAPTER 11

Psychiatry and Behavioral Medicine

Refer to Psychiatry [icon] for in-depth coverage of the following topics:

Recommended Supplemental Topics:

The fifth edition of the American Psychiatric Association's *Diagnostic and Statistical Manual (DSM-5)* utilizes specific criteria with which to objectively assess symptoms, rather than purely discrete diagnostic categories. For example, personality dimensions are more prominent than they were in *DSM-IV*. Nonetheless, the diagnosis is still based on a solid history and examination. **All of the following are currently updated with DSM-V criteria.**

INSOMNIA DISORDER (DYSSOMNIAS)

- Electroencephalographs show two distinct states of sleep, both of which are normal
  - Rapid Eye Movement (REM) sleep, also known as "dream sleep," D-state sleep, paradoxic sleep
  - Non-REM (NREM) sleep, also called S-stage sleep, divided into stages 1 to 4
    - Stages 3 and 4 are called "delta sleep"

- Sleep has 4 ro 5 REM periods throughout the night accounting for 25% of the total night's sleep (1.5-2 hours)
- The first REM period occurs 80-120 minutes after onset of sleep and lasts 10 minutes; later REM periods are longer (15-40 minutes) and occur mostly in the last several hours of sleep.
- Most stage-4 sleep (deepest) occurs in the first several hours
- As you age, the percentage of REM sleep does not change, however, stages 3 and 4 of sleep decrease in duration. This leads to early bedtimes and daytime naps and is a result of insomnia complaints in older patients.
- Any persistent sleep disorder that is not attributed to another condition (depression, mania, alcohol abuse, heavy smoking, uremia, asthma, thyroid disorders, nocturia, pain, delirium, respiratory distress syndromes) should be evaluated by a sleep medicine specialist

Disease	Etiology, Prevalence, Risk Factors	Clinical Symptoms and Signs	Diagnostics	Therapy, Prognosis, and Health Maintenance
Insomnia	Contributing factors: stress, caffeine, physical discomfort, daytime napping, early bedtimes	1. Difficulty getting to sleep or staying asleep 2. Intermittent wakefulness during night 3. Early morning awakening 4. Combinations of any of above	Clinical diagnosis	1. Cognitive-behavioral therapy (CBT) • Indications: Primary insomnia 2. Pharmacologic therapy • Indications: grief reaction

Psychological Treatment of Insomnia	Pharmacologic Treatment of Insomnia

1. Good sleep hygiene
 • Go to bed only when sleepy
 • Use the bed and bedroom for sleeping and sex only
 • If still awake after 20 min, leave the room and pursue a restful activity (bath, meditation), return only when sleepy
 • Get up at the same time every morning regardless of the amount of sleep during the night
 • Discontinue caffeine and nicotine, at least in the evening if not completely
 • Daily exercise regimen
 • Avoid alcohol—disrupts continuity of sleep
 • Limit fluids in evenings
 • Learn and practice relaxation techniques
 • Establish bedtime rituals and routine for going to sleep
2. CBT as effective as zolpidem (Ambien) with benefits sustained 1 y after treatment
	1. Benzodiazepines
	 • Lorazepam (0.5 mg PO QHS)
	 • Temazepam (7.5-15 mg PO QHS)
	 • Flurazepam (HL > 48 h)—can cause ataxia, cognitive slowing, falls, and somnolence in elderly
	2. Nonbenzo hypnotics:
	 • Zolpidem (5-10 mg PO QHS)—good for long term use
	   • AE: amnestic episodes if used on daily basis
	 • Zaleplon (5-10 mg PO QHS)—good for long term use
	 • Eszopiclone (2-3 mg PO QHS)
	3. Antihistamines—no dependency, but anticholinergic effects (confusion, urinary retention in elderly)
	 • Diphenhydramine 25 mg PO QHS
	 • Hydroxyzine 25 mg PO QHS
	4. Atypical antidepressants—non–habit-forming, lower doses than antidepressants
	 • Trazodone 25-150 mg PO QHS
	   • AE: priapism
	5. Melatonin receptor agonist—helps with sleep onset, no abuse potential
	 • Ramelteon 8 mg PO QHS
	6. Dual orexin receptor antagonists (DORAs)—approved in 2014 to initiate and maintain sleep
	 • Suvorexant
	   • AE: worsens preexisting depression

BIPOLAR AND RELATED DISORDERS

Disease	Etiology, Prevalence, Risk Factors	Clinical Symptoms and Signs	Diagnostics	Therapy, Prognosis, and Health Maintenance
Intimate partner violence (IPV)	Abusive behavior (physical, sexual, emotional) by a person in an intimate relationship with the victim F > M to be victims Goal of abuser: Gain control over victim RF: Young (<35), pregnant; being single, divorced or separated; ETOH or drug abuse in victim or partner, smoking, low economic status	1. Explanation of injuries that do not fit with examination findings 2. Frequent visits to ED 3. Somatic complaints: headache, abdominal pain, fatigue Signs: 1. Vague during history 2. Minimal eye contact 3. Abuser in room answers all questions or declines to leave room 4. Injuries to central area of body, forearms 5. Bruises in various stages of healing	Screening tools: 1. HITS (Hurt, Insult, Threaten, Screamed at tool) 2. WAST (Women Abuse Screening Tool) 3. PVS (Partner Violence Screen) 4. AAS (Abuse Assessment Screen) 5. WEB (Women's Experience with Battering) scale	1. Most important: Speak with patient alone 2. Document all history and findings carefully 3. USPSTF recommends screening women of childbearing age for IPV including domestic violence and refer women who screen (+) to intervention services Interventions: leave abusive situation ensuring a safe place to go, counseling to assess risk of danger, create plan for safety

CHAPTER 12
Urgent Care

Refer to Family Medicine 👪 for in-depth coverage of the following topics:

Acute Abdomen, refer to Acute Appendicitis, Acute Pancreatitis, Peritonitis, SBO, LBO, Volvulus on GI, p 189

Cardiac Failure, see Heart Failure on Cardiology, p 1

Myocardial Infarction, see Cardiology, p 12

Hypertensive Crisis, see Hypertension on Cardiology, p 3

Refer to Internal Medicine 💉 for in-depth coverage of the following topics:

Deteriorating Mental Status/Unconscious Patient, refer to Neurology—Coma, p 249

Acute Abdomen, refer to Ischemic Bowel Disease: Toxic Megacolon, Acute Mesenteric Ischemia on GI, p 257

Cardiac Arrest, see Critical Care, p 257

Refer to Emergency Medicine ✳ for in-depth coverage of the following topics:

Acute Respiratory Distress/Failure, see Pulmonology, p 396

Pulmonary Embolism, see Pulmonology, p 395

Pneumothorax, see Pulmonology, p 397

Refer to Pediatrics 🧍 for in-depth coverage of the following topics:

Burns, see Dermatology, p 293

Recommended Supplemental Topics:

Fractures/Dislocations, see Appendix G: Fractures, Dislocations, and Tears, p 709

Sprains/Strains, see Appendix G: Fractures, Dislocations, and Tears, p 733

Supracondylar Fracture, see Appendix G: Fractures, Dislocations, and Tears, p 713

Lisfranc Fracture, see Appendix G: Fractures, Dislocations, and Tears, p 722

ALLERGIC REACTION/ANAPHYLAXIS

Disease	Etiology, Prevalence, Risk Factors	Clinical Symptoms and Signs	Therapy, Prognosis, and Health Maintenance
Allergic reaction (Fig. 12-1)	Nonimmunologic reaction to food are more common than true food allergies Food allergy is due to abnormal immunologic response following exposure (ingestion) of food Non-IGE mediated allergy isolated to GI tract and/or skin manifestations	1. More subacute and/or chronic 2. Vomiting and diarrhea 3. Itching and/or burning <u>Signs:</u> 1. Vesicular eruption—symmetrical on extensor surfaces of elbows, knees, buttocks, sacrum, face, neck, trunk, and occasionally within the mouth	1. Stop the transfusion if medication related 2. Treat with antihistamines

Disease	Etiology, Prevalence, Risk Factors	Clinical Symptoms and Signs	Therapy, Prognosis, and Health Maintenance

Anaphylactic reaction (anaphylaxis)	Potentially life threatening, generalized allergic reaction that is rapid in onset and may cause death
	<u>Prevalence:</u>
	<2%
	Immunologic mechanism involving **immunoglobulin E (IgE)**
	<u>MCC in children:</u>
	Foods
	<u>MCC in adults:</u>
	Insect stings and medications
	<u>RF:</u>
	1. Asthma
	2. Cardiovascular disease
	3. Respiratory disease (COPD, ILD, pneumonia)
	4. Acute infection (URI, fever), emotional stress, exercise, disruption of routine, premenstrual status
		1. Severe reaction with difficulty breathing
		2. LOC
		3. Flushing
		4. Swollen lips, tongue, or uvula
		5. Nasal discharge or congestion
		6. Change in voice quality
		7. Sensation of choking or throat closure
		8. Shortness of breath
		9. Cough
		10. Nausea, vomiting, diarrhea, crampy abdominal pain
		<u>Signs:</u>
		1. Generalized hives
		2. Pruritus
		3. Periorbital edema
		4. Conjunctival swelling
		5. Wheezing
		6. Stridor
		7. Hypotonia (collapse), syncope
		8. Incontinence
		9. Dizziness
		10. Tachycardia
		11. Hypotension
			1. General
			  • Airway, breathing, circulation
			  • Place in recumbent position
			  • 8-10 L/min O$_2$
			  • NS rapid bolus
			  • Albuterol
			2. Immediate administration of 1 mg/mL IM epinephrine to mid-outer thigh
			  • Repeat every 5-15 min as needed
			  • There are NO absolute contraindications
			  • AE: anxiety, restlessness, headache, dizziness, palpitations, pallor, tremor
			  • Okay for pregnancy
			3. Adjunctive
			  • Diphenhydramine 25-50 mg IV
			  • Ranitidine 50 mg IV
			  • Methylprednisolone 125 mg IV
			4. If refractory
			  • Epinephrine IV 0.1 mcg/kg/min

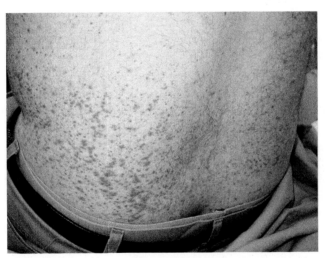

FIGURE 12-1. Allergic reaction. (Image provided by Stedman's.)

Diagnostic Criterion for Anaphylaxis

Criterion 1	Acute onset of illness (minutes to several hours) involving the skin, mucosal tissue, or both and at least one of the following • Respiratory compromise (dyspnea, wheezing or bronchospasm, stridor, reduced peak expiratory flow, hypoxemia) • Reduced blood pressure or associated symptoms/signs of organ hypoperfusion (hypotonia/syncope, incontinence)
Criterion 2	**Two or more** of the following that occur rapidly (seconds to several hours) after exposure likely to **an allergen** • Involvement of skin-mucosal tissue (hives, itching, flushing; swollen lips, tongue, or uvula) • Respiratory compromise as above • Reduced BP or associated symptoms • Persistent GI symptoms (abdominal cramping, vomiting)

Criterion 3	**Reduced BP** after exposure to **known allergen** for that patient (minutes to several hours). Eg, hypotension/shock from insect sting
	1. Reduced BP in adults: systolic <90 mm Hg or greater than 30% decrease from baseline
	2. Infants and children: low systolic BP for age or greater than 30% decrease from baseline
	  • <70 mm Hg from 1 mo-1 y
	  • Less than (70 mm Hg + [twice age]) from 1-10 y/o
	  • Less than 90 mm Hg from 11-17 y/o

BURNS ⚕, ACUTE ABDOMEN⚕

- The "rule of nines" is a crude but quick and effective method of estimating burn size. In adults, the anterior and posterior trunk each account for 18%, each lower extremity is 18%, each upper extremity is 9%, and the head is 9%. In children younger than 3 years, the head accounts for a larger relative surface area and should be taken into account when estimating burn size

- Follow American Burn Association criteria for transfer of a patient to a regional burn center
  - Partial thickness burns >10% BSA
  - Burns involving the face, hands, feet, genitalia, perineum, major joints
  - Third degree burns in any age
  - Electrical burns, including lightning injury
  - Chemical burns
  - Inhalation injury
  - Burn injury in patients with preexisting medical disorders
  - Patients with burns and trauma in which burn is greatest risk
  - Burned children without qualified personnel for care of children in hospital

- Patients who require social, emotional or rehabilitative intervention

- The **zone of coagulation** is the most severely burned portion and is typically in the center of the wound; likely needs excision and grafting

- Peripheral to that is a **zone of stasis**, with variable degrees of vasoconstriction and resultant ischemia, much like a second-degree burn

- The last area of a burn is called the **zone of hyperemia**, which will heal with minimal or no scarring and is most like a superficial or first-degree burn.

- Appropriate resuscitation and wound care may help prevent conversion to a deeper wound, but infection or suboptimal perfusion may result in an increase in burn depth

- Burn wounds evolve over the 48 to 72 hours after injury

- One of the most effective ways to determine burn depth is full-thickness biopsy, but this has several limitations; not only is the procedure painful and potentially scarring, but accurate interpretation of the histopathology requires a specialized pathologist and may have slow turnaround times

- Prognosis is directly related to the extent of injury both size and depth

THIRD TRIMESTER BLEEDING: ABRUPTIO PLACENTAE AND PLACENTA PREVIA

Disease	Etiology, Prevalence, Risk Factors	Clinical Symptoms and Signs	Diagnostics	Therapy, Prognosis, and Health Maintenance
Placenta previa	Placenta implants over the internal cervical os Most common abnormality of placental implantation RF: **A**dvanced Maternal Age **M**ultiparity, multiple gestation **P**rior previa C-section, D&C Smoking	1. **Painless** vaginal bleeding • Light spotting to profuse hemorrhage • Latter half of pregnancy, occasional contractions Signs: 1. Uterus: rarely tender 2. Breech/transverse lie common, lie often abnormal or head high and tachycardic 3. Consequences: PPH, required c-section, placenta accreta, increta, or percreta, abruption, and growth restriction	1. If DX in first or second trimester, repeat ultrasound 2. U/S: TAUS or **TVUS: placenta low** 3. CBC, coags 4. Type and screen 5. Fetal HR monitoring 6. Do not perform digital examination—can cause severe hemorrhage	1. Hospitalization for extended evaluation (initial) 2. If 37+ wk with continued bleeding, delivery is indicated 3. <36 wk expectant management Asymptomatic/mild (preterm <37 wk): close observation, steroids Mature fetus ± contractions/labor: base on fetal testing, document lung maturity, schedule 36-38 wk Delivery regardless of gestational age: severe fetal status, life threatening hemorrhage, bleeding after 34 wk
Placental abruption	Premature separation of the placenta from its implantation site before delivery Vascular RF: pre-eclampsia, chronic **HTN**, smoking, cocaine, thrombophilia Maternal-fetal RF: prior abruption, **AMA, multiparity**, multifetal gestation, **prior uterine surgery**, polyhydramnios, fibroid, PPROM	1. Painful vaginal bleeding • Common, severe, constant with exacerbations • Bleeding: absent or dark 2. **Uterine tenderness** 3. Frequent contractions Signs: 1. **Uterine tenderness,** • Tender, **"woody"** 2. *Fetal distress* 3. Shock: tachycardia, hypotension 4. Cervix: dilation from labor	Clinical DX: 1. U/S: exclude previa 2. CBC, coags, fibrinogen, type and screen, BUN/Cr 3. Tocodynamometry Fetal HR monitoring 4. Monitor urine output/blood Profound coagulopathy and acute hypovolemia from blood loss	1. **Immediate delivery** due to high risk of fetal death 2. Preterm/no distress (34-37): induce labor 3. Term/no distress: vaginal delivery 4. Fetal distress: emergent CS regardless of age 5. Fetal demise: vaginal delivery, induction; D&E if second trimester Complications: Life-threatening PPH and increased need for emergent hysterectomy

(continued)

(continued)

Disease	Etiology, Prevalence, Risk Factors	Clinical Symptoms and Signs	Diagnostics	Therapy, Prognosis, and Health Maintenance
Invasive placenta	Abnormally adherent placenta that has invaded the uterus—does not separate after delivery and bleeding can be torrential RF: **Prior uterine scar** (invasive placenta or c-section, placenta previa), AMA, multiparity	Suspect in patients with 1 or more prior cesarean deliveries and an anterior placenta previa	Ultrasound: intraplacental lacunae, bridging vessels into the bladder, loss of the retroplacental clear space	1. Emergent **hysterectomy** 2. Transfusion

Further classified depending on depth of invasion

1. **Placenta accrete**—limited to endometrium (*accreta adheres* to myometrium)

2. Placenta increta—extends into myometrium (*increta invades* the myometrium)

3. Placenta percreta—invades beyond the uterine serosa (possibly bladder), *percreta penetrates*

BITES/STINGS

- Appropriate and timely tetanus prophylaxis for all
- Antivenin recommended for significant latrodectism (widow)
- Wound cleansing and conservative debridement for brown recluse
- Referral to ophthalmologist for ophthalmia nodosa caused by embedded tarantula hairs

Disease	Etiology, Prevalence, Risk Factors	Clinical Symptoms and Signs	Therapy, Prognosis, and Health Maintenance
Black widow	Latrodectus species Massive presynaptic release of most neurotransmitters (AcH, NE, Dopamine, glutamate)	Moderately to severely painful bite, no surrounding inflammation Muscle spasms and rigidity starting at bite site within 30 min to 2 h • Spreads proximally to abdomen and face • Rebound tenderness mimicking acute appendicitis	Resolve over 2-3 d Death rarely occurs
Brown recluse	Loxosceles species Local cytotoxicity with subsequent ulcerating dermonecrosis	Occur early in morning, painless Delayed reaction (3-7 d) Systemic symptoms: arthralgias, fever, chills, maculopapular rash, nausea, vomiting Progress to ulcerating dermonecrosis at bite site	Most necrotizing ulcers heal over 1-8 wk 10%-15% scar
Tarantula		• Contain urticating hairs on dorsal abdomens, which can be flicked off by thousands, irritating and incapacitating aggressors • Penetrate skin causing foreign body keratoconjunctivitis or ophthalmia nodosa	Refer to ophthalmologist if suspected eye injury (slit lamp examination)

FOREIGN BODY ASPIRATION

Disease	Etiology, Prevalence, Risk Factors	Clinical Symptoms and Signs	Diagnostics	Therapy, Prognosis, and Health Maintenance
Foreign body aspiration	Aspiration of gastric contents, inert material, toxic material, or poorly chewed food Degree of injury depends on substance	1. Choking and coughing 2. Wheezing or hemoptysis Complications: Asphyxia, pneumonia, acute gastric aspiration	1. CXR: regional hyperinflation caused by check valve effect Cultures if postobstructive pneumonia suspected	1. Heimlich maneuver 2. Bronchoscopy—diagnostic and therapeutic

INGESTING HARMFUL SUBSTANCES (POISONINGS)

- History
  - What, when, how?
  - Obtain offending agent if possible
- Physical
  - Breath odors, check skin for dryness, sweating, discoloration and fever
  - Pupillary size and lacrimation
  - Vomiting or excessive salivation
- Neurologic changes: ataxia, tremor, agitation, convulsion, coma
- Tachycardia, tachypnea or dysrhythmias (TCAs)
- Labs
  - Anion and osmolar gaps (ETOH causes anion gap, methanol causes osmolar gap)
  - Initial and ongoing EKG
  - Standard emergency dept toxin panels (toxicology screen), then order specifics for diuretics, ethylene glycol, lithium, aromatic hydrocarbons, cyanide

Disease	Etiology, Prevalence, Risk Factors	Clinical Symptoms and Signs	Diagnostics	Therapy, Prognosis, and Health Maintenance
Hydrocarbons (benzene, petroleum distillates, gasoline)		Mucosal irritation Vomiting, bloody diarrhea Cyanosis, respiratory distress Fever, tachycardia	CXR Urinalysis EKG	Avoid emetics and lavage Oxygen with mist Antibiotics if pneumonia develops
Bases (Clorox, Drano)		Irritated mucous membranes Stomach perforation, hepatotoxicity Respiratory distress secondary to edematous epiglottis	EGD to determine degree of damage to larynx, esophagus, stomach	Small amounts of water (diluent) Avoid vomiting Supportive care
Acetaminophen (Tylenol)	Especially in depressed patients Acetaminophen converted to free radicals → liver necrosis (occurs in hypoxic area around central veins, called zone III)	Hepatic failure: elevated LFTs	Monitor APA plasma concentration (nomogram) LFTs–nonemergent	1. Gastric lavage–only works in first hour 2. Charcoal–prevents enterohepatic recirculation, but only works <2 h of ingestion 3. **N-Acetylcysteine** (antidote): increases glutathione levels, which acts as a neutralizer of free radicals 4. 4-h APAP levels to determine response to therapy
Aspirin (salicylates)		Vomiting Hyperpnea, pulmonary edema Fever Encephalopathy, convulsions, coma Renal failure	Check serum salicylate level Look for metabolic acidosis and hypokalemia High or reduced serum glucose	Induce emesis Charcoal to bind drug Correct dehydration with IVF Hemodialysis
Organophosphates (chlorthion, diazinon)		Salivation, lacrimation Sweating Urination, diarrhea Pulmonary congestion Twitching, convulsions, coma Miosis	Measure red cell cholinesterase levels Blood glucose levels	ABCs Decontamination of skin Atropine + pralidoxime
Iron		Intestinal bleeding Impaired coagulation Shock, coma Red urine	Blood indices Metabolic panel: Acidosis UOP Type and screen LFTs	Evoke emesis Gastric lavage Whole-bowel irrigation Desferoxamine Dialysis
Mercury	Overconsumption of fish	**Diarrhea**, constricted visual fields, peripheral neuropathy, hyperhidrosis (**sweating**) Renal failure Tachycardia, hypertension		**Chelating agents** (succimer, dimercaprol, penicillamine)

(continued)

(continued)

Disease	Etiology, Prevalence, Risk Factors	Clinical Symptoms and Signs	Diagnostics	Therapy, Prognosis, and Health Maintenance
Lead	Ingestion of lead-based paint, working with batteries or working with lead-based casting materials	Neuropathy and renal failure		**Chelating agents** (succimer, dimercaprol)
Arsenic	Pesticides or contaminated ground water	Severe headaches, abdominal pain, diarrhea, delirium, convulsions, and **breath that smells like garlic**		**Chelating agents** (succimer, dimercaprol)
Carbon monoxide	House fires and automobile exhaust ingestion	Headache, cherry-red skin Lactic acidosis due to hypoxia		100% O$_2$
Cyanide	House fires Cyanide–produced from combustion of furniture materials	Coma, seizures Heart dysfunction Metabolic acidosis and breath that smells like **bitter almonds**		TX: amyl nitrite and thiosulfate

ORBITAL CELLULITIS

Disease	Etiology, Prevalence, Risk Factors	Clinical Symptoms and Signs	Diagnostics	Therapy, Prognosis, and Health Maintenance
Orbital cellulitis (Fig. 12-2)	More common in children Median age: 7-12 y Associated: sinusitis Causes: dental infection, facial infection, infection of globe or eyelids or lacrimal system, trauma MC bugs: *S. pneumoniae, S. aureus, H. flu,* gram-negative bacteria, MRSA	1. Ptosis, eyelid edema, exophthalmos, purulent discharge, conjunctivitis 2. Fever 3. Restricted ROM of eyes, sluggish pupillary response 4. Edema and erythema of lids	1. CBC, blood cultures, cultures of any drainage– high WBC 2. CT scan: broad infiltration of orbital soft tissue	Medical emergency requiring hospitalization 1. IV antibiotics • Broad spectrum until fever subsides, then 2-3 wk of PO • Nafcillin and Flagyl, or clindamycin, 2nd or 3rd generation cephalosporin, and fluoroquinolones 2. Surgical I&D If MRSA suspected, vancomycin

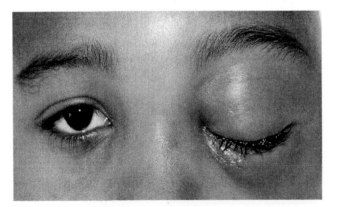

FIGURE 12-2. Orbital cellulitis. (From Chung EK. *Visual Diagnosis and Treatment in Pediatrics.* Philadelphia: Wolters Kluwer; 2015.)

CHAPTER 13

Hematology

Refer to Internal Medicine ⚕ **for in-depth coverage of the following topics:**

Anemia, see Iron Deficiency Anemia, Thalassemia, Vitamin B12 and Folic Acid Deficiency Anemia, Sickle Cell Anemia, and Hemolytic Anemias, p 275

Leukemia, see Acute and Chronic Leukemia, p 280

Thrombocytopenia, see ITP and TTP, p 284

Clotting Disorders, see DIC, vWF Disease, and Hemophilia, p 282

Lymphomas, p 281

Recommended Supplemental Material:

Immune Thrombocytopenia, p 284 ⚕

von Willebrand Disease, p 283 ⚕

Blood Cell Morphology and Life Cycle, p 274 ⚕

Vitamin K Deficiency, see below, p 193

VITAMIN K DEFICIENCY

- SNOT factors = Seven, Nine, 10, Two

Disease	Etiology, Prevalence, Risk Factors	Clinical Symptoms and Signs	Diagnostics	Therapy, Prognosis, and Health Maintenance
Vitamin K deficiency	Rare Sources: Liver, green leafy vegetables, broccoli, peas, green beans, soybeans Occurs from deficient intake of vitamin K, malabsorption, or decreased intestinal production by bacteria (from chemotherapy or antibiotics) Vitamin K plays a role in activity of coagulation factors II, VII, IX, and X	Soft tissue ecchymosis, hematomas, and mucosal bleeding	1. PT: prolonged, corrects upon mixing 2. Clotting factors are low: VII, IX, X, II (SNOT)	1. **Vitamin K$_1$ (phytonadione)** via IV or PO route • 5-10 mg/d PO • 1 mg/d IV over 30 min

POLYCYTHEMIA VERA

- Increased production of basophils and mast cells → itching after hot shower from histamine release

Disease	Etiology, Prevalence, Risk Factors	Clinical Symptoms and Signs	Diagnostics	Therapy, Prognosis, and Health Maintenance
Polycythemia vera (primary polycythemia)	Onset 50-70 y Clonal stem disorder with excessive proliferation of erythroid, myeloid, and megakaryocytic progenitor cells Spent phase—extramedullary hematopoiesis in liver and spleen with normocytic anemia	1. **Elevated Hgb/Hct** (>20 g/dL/>60%) 2. Full body itching with use of warm water 3. **Hypertension** 4. Intermittent **headache, fullness of face/head**, dizziness 5. Impaired vision 6. Chest pain 7. Claudication Signs: 1. **Splenomegaly** (75%) 2. Hepatomegaly (30%) 3. Plethora or ruddy complexion	1. CBC: hyperviscosity, high total blood volume • **High RBC count** • Red cell mass: increased • Hgb/Hct >50 • Thrombosis • Leukocytosis 2. Low serum EPO 3. Elevated B$_{12}$ 4. Hyperuricemia 5. **Bone marrow biopsy** (confirmatory)	1. **Phlebotomy** • Goal: Hct <45% • Frequent, may cause IDA 2. **Low-dose aspirin** 3. Hydroxyurea Median survival: 9-14 y

CHAPTER **14**

Infectious Disease

Refer to Internal Medicine 🩺 **for in-depth coverage of the following topics:**

Mononucleosis, p 271
Lyme Disease, p 268
Human Immunodeficiency Virus, p 259

Influenza, p 272
Meningitis, see Neurology, p 247

Refer to Family Medicine 👥 **for in-depth coverage of the following topics:**

Salmonellosis and Shigellosis, see GI for FM, p 43

PRACTICE QUESTIONS

1. A 42-year-old woman with a history of rheumatic fever as a child undergoes a mitral valve replacement with a bovine bioprosthetic valve. She is anticoagulated post-operatively and discharged home on warfarin. What is the recommended anticoagulation goal?
   A. INR 1.0 to 2.0 indefinitely
   B. INR 2.0 to 3.0 indefinitely
   C. INR 2.5 to 3.5 indefinitely
   D. INR 2.0 to 3.0 for 3 months after insertion

2. A 21-year-old G1P0 woman at 18 weeks' gestation is found to have a low-lying placenta abutting, but not covering, the internal os on routine sonogram. What is the most appropriate management?
   A. This is a normal finding. Continue routine prenatal care
   B. Repeat the ultrasound at 32 weeks
   C. Follow up with serial ultrasounds every 4 weeks
   D. Admit to the hospital for observation

3. A 13-year-old girl presents to the clinic for concern about heavy menses. She had her first period 3 months ago and during each menstrual cycle the bleeding has been so heavy she has had to change her pad 3 to 4 times per day. Upon reviewing her history, the physician assistant discovers that the patient has experienced easy bruising for several years, and on multiple occasions has had a nosebleed that lasted longer than 10 minutes before resolving. She denies history of bleeding gums, spontaneous bleeding, or bleeding into joints. Physical examination is normal without evidence of petechiae or purpura. A trial of which medication is indicated in this patient?

   A. Desmopressin (DDAVP)
   B. Factor VIII
   C. Vitamin K
   D. Fresh frozen plasma

4. A 65-year-old woman presents to her primary care provider because she noticed a bump under the skin on her left upper arm. It is not itchy or painful and not really bothersome, but she wants to have it looked at for her own peace of mind. On physical examination, you find a soft, mobile, 2 cm subcutaneous ovoid nodule with no clinically visible epidermal changes. What is the most likely diagnosis?
   A. Epidermoid cyst
   B. Ganglion cyst
   C. Pyogenic granuloma
   D. Lipoma

5. A 69-year-old woman with history of atrial fibrillation on chronic warfarin therapy presents with a nosebleed. The epistaxis began four hours ago and has not resolved with holding pressure. The patient denies lightheadedness, fatigue, or loss of consciousness. Vital signs are all normal. You observe brisk bleeding from both nares. You place temporary anterior nasal packing to examine the patient but are unable to identify the bleeding source and the patient continues to bleed. What is the most appropriate clinical intervention?
   A. Continue to hold pressure. The bleeding should resolve on its own.
   B. Administer vitamin K
   C. Electrical cautery of bleeding source
   D. Place a balloon catheter

6. A 60-year-old man presents for anal pain for the past 3 days. He describes a tearing pain when he defecates and is scared to use the bathroom. He also admits perianal pruritus and minimal bright red streaking on the toilet paper when he wipes. On physical examination, you note a skin tag lateral to the anal sphincter. What is the first-line therapy for this patient given the most likely diagnosis?

A. Sitz baths

B. Botulinum toxin injection

C. Placement of a seton

D. Sclerotherapy

7. A 75-year-old woman sees her physician assistant because she is scared she is having a stroke. Two hours ago, she suddenly lost her vision in her right eye, which she described as if, "someone pulled a shade down over my eye." The blindness lasted less than 10 minutes, then returned to normal. She reports severe headaches for the past 2 days over the right temple, worse if she touches her scalp or brushes her hair. Upon further questioning he also admits fatigue and loss of appetite, as well as a low-grade fever of 100.1°F. What is the best initial treatment?

A. Prednisone 45 mg daily

B. Alteplase 0.9 mg/kg, 10% given as a bolus followed by a 60-minute infusion

C. Warfarin 5 mg titrated to an INR between 2.0 and 3.0

D. Cephalexin 500 mg BID for 7 days

8. Which of the following is not commonly associated with lobar pneumonia?

A. Increased tactile fremitus

B. Hyperresonance to percussion

C. Bronchial breath sounds

D. Coarse rales

E. Egophony

9. A 25-year-old male presents to his PCP complaining of dizziness. He reports that earlier this morning he felt like he was going to pass out. Upon further questioning he also admits that his heart felt like it was racing and his chest felt heavy. An EKG in the office shows a shorted PR interval, wide QRS complex, and a delta wave in leads V1 to V4. What is the most likely diagnosis?

A. Wolff-Parkinson-White syndrome

B. Myocardial infarction

C. Hypertrophic cardiomyopathy

D. Second-degree heart block, Mobitz I

10. A 59-year-old Asian man with a 20-pack year smoking history who immigrated to the US 30 years ago presents with gradual onset of solid food dysphagia. He describes a sensation of food "sticking" in his throat when he tries to swallow. He denies pain with swallowing, acid reflux, or regurgitation of undigested food. Which of the following would you be most worried about in this patient?

A. Achalasia

B. Zenker diverticulum

C. Schatzki ring

D. Squamous cell carcinoma

11. A 36-year-old obese man with type 2 diabetes would like to lose weight. Which class of medication would NOT be a good choice for this patient?

A. Biguanide

B. GLP-1 receptor agonist

C. SGLT-2 inhibitor

D. Sulfonylurea

12. A 19-year-old woman presents for her annual physical. On breast examination, you note a 2-cm solid, firm, well-defined, mobile mass in the left breast. What is the initial work up for this lesion?

A. Ultrasound

B. Mammogram

C. Biopsy

D. Surgical excision

13. What is the mechanism of action of Zyban as used for smoking cessation?

A. Weak inhibitor of norepinephrine and dopamine uptake to reduce cravings and withdrawal symptoms

B. Partial nicotinic receptor agonist, allowing it to stimulate dopamine activity but to a lesser degree than nicotine

C. Increase synaptic concentration of serotonin and/or norepinephrine in the central nervous system

D. Nicotine replacement to be substituted for tobacco-containing products

14. A 72-year-old man presents for painless vision loss. He describes his vision as hazy. The problem started 2 years ago when he had to get new reading glasses, but it continues to worsen. He admits difficulty driving at night because his vision is fuzzy. On examination, the red reflex is diminished and visual acuity is 20/50 on the right, 20/70 on the left. What is the most likely diagnosis?

A. Nuclear cataract

B. Retinal detachment

C. Age-related macular degeneration (ARMD)

D. Open angle glaucoma

15. A 35-year-old man with no significant past medical history presents complaining of chest pain that is worse when he takes a deep breath. He reports 2 weeks ago he thinks he had the flu but thought he could ride it out. The patient is febrile and tachycardic. Physical examination reveals an S3 gallop without murmur or rub, with decreased breath sounds over the lower lobes bilaterally, and mild lower extremity edema. EKG shows sinus tachycardia but is otherwise normal. WBC is 13.7 and ESR, CRP and troponin I levels are all elevated. What is the most likely cause of this patient's problem?

A. Coxsackievirus B

B. *Cytomegalovirus*

C. *S. pneumoniae*

D. Occlusion to the right coronary artery

16. A 49-year-old woman with a 25 pack-year smoking history presents with shortness of breath. She says her symptoms started abruptly this morning while she was mowing her lawn. The dyspnea is constant and does not improve with rest. She also complains of chest pain, worse when she takes a deep breath, and also says she has been coughing a lot throughout the day. On physical examination she is tachycardic and tachypneic and you hear decreased breath sounds diffusely on the right. You also note redness and swelling of her right calf and the patient complains of tenderness when you palpate the area. Which of the following is the test of choice to confirm the suspected diagnosis?

A. Chest radiograph

B. D-dimer

C. CT pulmonary angiography

D. Ventilation/perfusion scan

17. A 58-year-old man with history of hypertension, hyperlipidemia, diabetes mellitus, myocardial infarction 6 years ago s/p revascularization, and a 40 pack/y smoking history, presents for cramping pain in his calves that worsens with exercise and improves with rest. Physical examination reveals diminished DP and PT pulses, loss of hair over his shins, and thickened toenails. He is already taking aspirin, clopidogrel, atorvastatin, lisinopril, metformin, and liraglutide. He has made changes to his diet and exercise routines and has stopped smoking. What additional medication could you consider adding to provide additional symptom relief?

A. Cilostazol (Pletaal)

B. Warfarin (Coumadin)

C. Diltiazem (Cardizem)

D. Gabapentin (Neurontin)

18. A 22-year-old woman who recently emigrated from Bulgaria presents with fatigue. You order labs, which show hemoglobin of 10.2, MCV of 110, and hypersegmented neutrophils. Her vitamin B_{12} level is normal. You diagnose her with megaloblastic anemia secondary to folate deficiency. In addition to starting her on a folic acid supplement, which food can you recommend that is high in folic acid?

A. Beans/lentils

B. Red meat

C. Cheese

D. Oatmeal

19. A 21-year-old woman presents requesting treatment for her asthma. She can't remember what medications she has used in the past because she ran out several months ago and never got them refilled. She reports wheezing on a daily basis and usually wakes up in the middle of the night coughing about 1 to 2 times per week. She is concerned because she feels her asthma is interfering with her daily life. In the office, her FEV_1 is 76% predicted. How would you classify the severity of this patient's asthma?

A. Mild intermittent

B. Mild persistent

C. Moderate persistent

D. Severe persistent

20. A 56-year-old data analyst presents to his PCP for numbness and tingling in his thumb and first finger of his right hand and right wrist that worsens at night. He has tried using a wrist splint for the past couple weeks, which has helped some but he still wakes at night with symptoms. What is the next step in management?

A. Glucocorticoid injection with continued use of nocturnal wrist splinting

B. Glucocorticoid injection alone

C. Start oral prednisone

D. Refer for surgery

21. Which of the following seen on ophthalmoscopic examination supports the diagnosis of age-related macular degeneration (AMD)?

A. Soft drusen

B. Cotton wool spots

C. AV nicking

D. Roth spot

22. What is the most common cause of thyrotoxicosis?

A. Grave disease

B. Hashimoto thyroiditis

C. De Quervain thyroiditis

D. Follicular thyroid cancer

23. A 61-year-old man with a history of type 2 diabetes presents with lower abdominal pain with associated dysuria and urinary frequency. Physical examination reveals normal genitalia. On DRE there is mild prostate tenderness, but the prostate is smooth and not enlarged. PSA is 3.5 and urine dipstick is positive for leukocyte esterase and nitrates. The physician assistant also notes that the patient had positive urine leukocytes and nitrates at his last physical, but he was asymptomatic at that time and did not pursue further workup. What is the most likely diagnosis?

A. Chronic bacterial prostatitis

B. Benign prostatic hyperplasia (formerly Hypertrophy)

C. Bladder cancer

D. Hydronephrosis

24. A 27-year-old man suffers from chronic, progressive pain in his back, neck, and sacroiliac joints that is worse at night and improves with exercise. Lateral spine radiographs show squaring of the vertebral bodies, and he has already been counseled on the hyperkyphosis and postural abnormalities he may face down the road. In addition to the condition described, from which other medical problem is this patient most likely to suffer?

    A. Ulcerative colitis

    B. Gout

    C. Autoimmune hepatitis

    D. Dermatomyositis

25. A 46-year-old man with a BMI of 32 presents for routine physical examination. His blood work reveals total cholesterol of 220, LDL of 146, HDL of 35, and triglycerides of 140. What is the first-line therapy that you should prescribe for this patient?

    A. Lifestyle modification

    B. Pravastatin 10 mg daily

    C. Atorvastatin 40 mg daily

    D. Metformin 500 mg BID

ANSWERS

1. Health Maintenance: Mitral Regurgitation. Answer D. Bioprosthetic valves in the mitral position require anticoagulation with a goal of 2.0 to 3.0 for 3 months after insertion. A, An INR of 1.0 to 2.0 is subtherapeutic. B, Mechanical aortic valves require INR of 2.0 to 3.0 long term. C, Mechanical mitral valves require INR of 2.5 to 3.5 long term.

2. Clinical Therapeutics: Placenta Previa. Answer B. For pregnancies >16 weeks, the placental location is considered normal if the edge is ≥2 cm from the internal os. If the edge is <2 cm from, but not covering, the internal os the placenta is labeled as low-lying. If the edge covers the internal os, the placenta is labeled as previa. For either low-lying or previa, appropriate management is to follow up with ultrasonography for placental location at 32 weeks' gestation, as the majority of placenta previa identified early in pregnancy go on to resolve with advancing gestational age. A, A low lying placenta is a normal finding of pregnancy in early gestation, but not typically in pregnancies >16 weeks. C, Follow up with a serial ultrasound is not appropriate and (D) there is no life threatening indication for hospitalization.

3. Diagnosis: von Willebrand Disease. Answer A. The mild bleeding this patient describes is consistent with von Willebrand disease (vWD). Desmopressin is an analog of antidiuretic hormone that promotes the release of von Willebrand factor. B, Factor VIII is the treatment for Hemophilia A, which is usually only seen in boys and would have presented much earlier in life with more severe bleeding. C, Vitamin K works to reverse the effects of warfarin, which is not applicable here. Fresh frozen plasma is not indicated as prophylaxis for vWD. D, A trial of desmopressin is recommended in all type 1 and most type 2 vWD patients.

4. Diagnosis: Lipoma. Answer D. Lipomas are the most common benign soft-tissue neoplasms that can occur anywhere on the body but are most commonly found on the trunk and upper extremities. They present as soft, painless masses ranging from 1 to 10 cm in size. The diagnosis of lipoma is clinical. Other causes should be considered if the mass is firm rather than soft, rapidly enlarging, or causing symptoms such as pain or restriction of movement. A, Epidermoid cysts, also called epidermal or epidermal inclusion cysts, present as skin-colored dermal nodules with a central punctum that can range from a few millimeters to several centimeters. Epidermoid cysts can be infected or sterile, and in either case can develop inflammation. As they get larger they are more likely to become erythematous, fluctuant, and painful. B, Ganglion cysts are fluid-filled sacs overlying a joint or tendon sheath that arise from a herniation of the connection tissue. Ninety percent of ganglion cysts are found in the dorsal or volar wrist. C, Pyogenic granuloma is a benign vascular tumor characterize by rapid growth and a friable surface that bleeds profusely after minor trauma.

5. Clinical Intervention: Posterior Epistaxis. Answer D. The brisk bleeding despite proper packing as well as the inability to identify a bleeding source on examination strongly suggest a posterior bleeding source. Acute management of posterior epistaxis includes posterior nasal packing, preferably with a balloon catheter, though Foley catheter and cotton packing can also be used if no balloon catheter is available. A, It is already clear from the history that conservative measures have not worked to stop the bleeding, so continuing to hold pressure for the bleed to spontaneously resolve is inappropriate. B, Vitamin K administration is appropriate in warfarin-treated individuals experiencing serious or life-threatening bleeding, which this patient is not. Vitamin K would also take several hours to work and thus would not treat the acute problem and would only put her at an increased stroke risk by dropping her INR. C, Electrical or chemical cautery is the treatment of choice in anterior bleed if the bleeding source can be identified.

6. Clinical Therapeutics: Anal Fissure. Answer A. In addition to recommending the patient increase his dietary fiber and water intake, sitz baths are the first-line therapy for treatment of acute anal fissures. B, Botulinum toxin A injection can be considered for the treatment of chronic anal fissures or in patients who have failed conservative therapy. C, Setons can be used in the treatment of complex anorectal fistulas. D, Sclerotherapy is a second-line treatment for symptomatic internal hemorrhoids.

7. Clinical Therapeutics: Giant Cell Arteritis (temporal arteritis). Answer A. This patient demonstrates the classic signs and symptoms of giant cell arteritis (GCA). High-dose glucocorticoids, such as prednisone 40 to 60 mg/d, is the well-established standard of care for GCA and has been shown to improve or resolve symptoms and decrease the risk of vascular complications. C, The addition of warfarin to glucocorticoids and low-dose aspirin for the treatment of GCA in patients without contraindications to anticoagulation has been proposed, but there is very little evidence to support its use. B, Alteplase, or tPA, if given within 4.5 hours of onset, has been shown to improve functional outcomes after ischemic stroke, but has no role in the treatment of GCA. D, Antibiotics also have no role in the treatment of GCA.

8. Scientific Concepts: Pneumonia. Answer B. In a patient with pneumonia you can expect to find dullness to percussion, not hyperresonance. Hyperresonance is associated with overinflated lungs, such as with asthma or COPD, or with a large pneumothorax. A, Increased tactile fremitus, (C) bronchial breath sounds, (D) coarse rales, and (E) egophony are all expected findings in lobar pneumonia.

9. Clinical Intervention: Wolf-Parkinson-White Syndrome. Answer A. Wolff-Parkinson-White (WPW) syndrome classically presents on EKG with a short PR interval (less than 0.12 seconds) and slurred upstroke of the QRS complex termed delta wave. WPW is often asymptomatic, but some patients may develop an arrhythmia (atrial fibrillation with rapid ventricular response) and symptoms may include palpitations, lightheadedness and/or dizziness, syncope or presyncope, chest pain, sudden cardiac death. B, Myocardial infarction, (C) hypertrophic cardiomyopathy, and (D) Mobitz I second-degree heart block do not result in delta waves.

10. Diagnosis: Squamous Cell Carcinoma. Answer D. Squamous cell carcinoma commonly presents with solid food dysphagia and weight loss. Early symptoms are nonspecific, but patients may describe a transient "sticking" of food in their throat and/or retrosternal discomfort. While adenocarcinoma is more common in patients with a history of gastroesophageal reflux disease (GERD) and Barrett esophagus, squamous cell carcinoma is associated with tobacco and alcohol use and is reported at a higher frequency in northern Iran and central Asia. Not only does this diagnosis best fit the history, it is also the most worrisome of the listed diagnoses and needs to be ruled out. A, Achalasia typically presents with dysphagia with solids and/or liquids and regurgitation of undigested food. B, Zenker diverticula usually occur in adults older than 60 years, often >75 years, and presents with transient dysphagia, halitosis, gurgling in the throat, and/or regurgitation of food into the mouth. C, Schatzki ring is a narrowing of the mucosa at the squamocolumnar junction and is almost always associated with a hiatal hernia.

11. Clinical Therapeutics: Type 2 Diabetes. Answer D. Sulfonylureas work by stimulating insulin release from pancreatic beta cells. Common side effects include weight gain and hypoglycemia. A, Biguanides (metformin), (B) GLP-1 receptor agonists, and (C) SGLT-2 inhibitors all promote varying degrees of weight loss.

12. Diagnostic Studies: Fibroadenoma. Answer A. The physical examination findings are consistent with a fibroadenoma, which can be confirmed with ultrasound. B, Mammogram should not be used as an initial diagnostic test in women younger than 30 years as their breasts are hypersensitive to radiation exposure. C, Biopsy and/or (D) complete removal may be indicated if the ultrasound reveals suspicious features but are not indicated for initial management.

13. Scientific Concepts: Smoking Cessation. Answer A. Bupropion (Zyban) is a dopamine/norepinephrine-reuptake inhibitor than can be used as an antidepressant, smoking cessation aid, and off label to assist with weight loss. Zyban, specifically, is marketed as a smoking cessation aid. B, Varenicline (Chantix) is a partial nicotine agonist. C, Nortriptyline (Pamelor)is a tricyclic antidepressant that increases serotonin and/or norepinephrine. D, Nicotine replacement therapy is also frequently used as a smoking cessation aid and is available in several forms including patch, gum, lozenge, and nasal spray.

14. Diagnosis: Cataract. Answer A. Cataracts should be suspected in anyone who presents with a complaint of painless, progressive decline in vision. Cataracts typically occur in patients over 60 and common complaints include problems with night driving, reading road signs, or difficulty with fine print. Frequently, a patient with cataracts will also experience a myopic shift that increases nearsightedness. B, Retinal detachment usually presents with a sudden onset of floaters and/or monocular decreased visual fields. C. ARMD will also present as gradual vision loss, such as difficulty reading or driving, but is also characterized by scotomas, distorted vision and eventually loss of central vision. D, Open angle glaucoma is generally asymptomatic and diagnosed on eye examination. Visual acuity is typically preserved, but late manifestations may include visual field loss ("tunnel vision").

15. Scientific Concepts: Myocarditis. Answer A. This patient has myocarditis, which is most commonly associated with a viral infection such as coxsackie B. B, While *Cytomegalovirus* can cause myocarditis, it is much less common than coxsackievirus, especially in an immunocompetent host. C, *S. pneumoniae* is the most common cause of bacterial pericarditis, not myocarditis. D, Myocardial infarction caused by occlusion of the right coronary artery would not present with fever or leukocytosis, and would be accompanied by EKG changes in leads II, III, and aVF.

16. Diagnostic Studies: Pulmonary Embolism. Answer C. In patients with a high suspicion of pulmonary embolism, CTPA is the imaging modality of choice because of its high sensitivity and specificity. A, A chest radiograph is not helpful in the diagnosis of pulmonary embolism. B, An elevated D-dimer alone is insufficient to make a diagnosis of pulmonary embolism but is useful in ruling out PE in patients thought to be at intermediate risk. D, In patients with a contraindication to CTPA (pregnancy, contrast allergy, renal insufficiency), alternate imaging such as a V/Q scan may be used.

17. Clinical Therapeutics: Peripheral Arterial Disease. Answer A. Cilostazol is a phosphodiesterase inhibitor that can be used in the treatment of peripheral arterial disease with intermittent claudication. B, Warfarin, (C) diltiazem, and (D) gabapentin are not indicated in the treatment of PAD.

18. Health Maintenance: B_{12} Deficiency. Answer A. Beans and lentils are rich in folic acid. Other foods with high folic acid content include leafy green vegetables, citrus fruits, and fortified breads and cereals. B, Red meat is high in saturated fat and protein. C, Cheese is high in fat, protein, calcium, vitamin A and B_{12}, riboflavin, zinc, and phosphorus. D, Oatmeal is high in fiber, protein, and some antioxidants; none of the latter are rich in folic acid.

19. Diagnosis: Asthma. Answer C. In patients 12 years of age and older, moderate persistent asthma is characterized by daily symptoms, nighttime awakenings >1 times per week but not nightly, FEV_1 of 60% to 80% of predicted, and some limitation or interference with normal activity. A, Mild intermittent describes daytime symptoms <2 days per week, nighttime awakenings <2 times per month, and FEV_1 >80% predicted, with no interference with normal activity. B, Mild persistent describes daytime symptoms >2 days per week but not daily, nighttime awakenings 3 to 4 times per month, and FEV_1 >80% predicted with minor interference with normal activity. D, Severe persistent describes continuous daytime symptoms throughout the day, nighttime awakenings nearly every night, and FEV_1 <60% predicted with extreme limitation of normal activity.

20. Clinical Intervention: Carpal Tunnel Syndrome. Answer A. Carpal tunnel syndrome classically presents with pain or paresthesia in the median nerve territory, worse at night and often waking patients from sleep. Symptoms are exacerbated by activities that involve flexion or extension of the wrist, such as typing, driving, or holding a phone. First-line treatment includes nocturnal wrist splinting. B, For patients who remain symptomatic after a month, it is recommended to add a single injection of methylprednisolone, as addition of a second treatment modality is more effective than a single therapy. C, The addition of oral glucocorticoids is an option in patients who decline injection therapy, but not preferred due to the negative effects of prolonged steroid use. D, Surgical decompression is recommended for most patients with severe median nerve injury only after electrodiagnostic studies.

21. Diagnosis: Age Related Macular Degeneration. Answer A. Drusen are bright yellow spots usually concentrated in the macula caused by deposits of extracellular material. While hard drusen are a normal consequence of aging, soft drusen develop in people with ARMD and are associated with vision loss. B, There are numerous etiologies for cotton wool spots, including ischemic, embolic, infectious, traumatic, autoimmune, and other causes, but they are most commonly caused by systemic hypertension or diabetes mellitus. Cotton wool spots are not a sign of ARMD. C, Arteriovenous, or AV, nicking is seen in systemic hypertension. D, Roth spots are associated with infective endocarditis.

22. Scientific Concepts: Thyrotoxicosis. Answer A. Thyrotoxicosis is synonymous with hyperthyroidism. Grave disease is the most common cause of thyrotoxicosis. Other common causes include toxic adenoma, toxic multinodular goiter, and excess exogenous thyroid hormone. B, Hashimoto thyroiditis causes hypothyroidism, not hyperthyroidism. C, De Quervain thyroiditis, commonly referred to as subacute thyroiditis, is a viral or postviral syndrome that causes a transient hyperthyroidism followed by euthyroidism or hypothyroidism, and eventually restoration of euthyroid state. It is an uncommon cause of thyrotoxicosis. D, Follicular thyroid cancer is rarely functional, though it may result in functional metastases.

23. History and Physical: Prostatitis. Answer A. The presentation of chronic bacterial prostatitis can be subtle, as men as often asymptomatic and may only have incidentally noted persistent or recurrent bacteriuria. Symptoms may include recurrent urinary tract infection with irritative voiding symptoms, repeated isolation of the same organism from the urine, and/or pain in the perineum, lower abdomen, testicles, or penis. Rectal examination may reveal prostatic hypertrophy, tenderness, edema, or nodularity, but is frequently normal. B, In benign prostatic hyperplasia (formerly hypertrophy), patients typically present with both obstructive and irritative symptoms and nocturia. C, Bladder cancer typically presents with gross hematuria, irritative symptoms, and obstructive symptoms if near the urethra or bladder neck and flank pain. The patient often has a history of smoking. D, Hydronephrosis typically presents with sudden or new onset hypertension, difficulty voiding, severe steady pain that radiates to the lower abdomen or testicles.

24. Scientific Concepts: Ankylosing Spondylitis. Answer A. This patient suffers from ankylosing spondylitis. Approximately 5% to 10% of patients with ankylosing spondylitis go on to develop overt inflammatory bowel disease. B, Gout, (C) hepatitis, and (D) dermatomyositis are not associated with ankylosing spondylitis.

25. Clinical Therapeutics: Hyperlipidemia. Answer A. The first-line treatment for hyperlipidemia is lifestyle modification, including aerobic exercise and adopting a diet lower in saturated fats. This is particularly useful in overweight patients with high LDL cholesterol. B, Pravastatin and (C) atorvastatin are statins that would be indicated for patient with an ASCVD risk score of 5% or greater. Factors that are used to determine ASCVD include gender, age, total cholesterol, HDL cholesterol, blood pressure, history of diabetes or smoking, and whether or not the patient has been treated for hypertension, with statin therapy or aspirin therapy. D, Metformin would be indicated for a patient with type II diabetes, not necessarily in a patient with hyperlipidemia.

CHAPTER 15

Cardiovascular

Refer to Family Medicine [icon] for in-depth coverage of the following topics:

Hypertension, p 3
Endocarditis, p 5
Hyperlipidemia, p 5
Peripheral Vascular Disease, p 8
Coronary Vascular Disease, p 7
Myocardial Infarction/Angina (Chest Pain), p 12
Cardiomyopathy, p 205

Refer to Appendices for the following topics:

Heart Murmurs, including Aortic Regurgitation, p 674
Cardiac Arrhythmias/Conduction Disorders, including Atrial Fibrillation, Ventricular Tachycardia, Sinus Sick Syndrome, see Appendix A, p 659
Valvular Heart Disease, including Coarctation of the Aorta, p 681

Recommended Supplemental Material:

Cerebral Vascular Accident, see Neurology [icon], p 111

CONGESTIVE HEART FAILURE

- Decompensated heart failure—Evidence on physical exam or chest x-ray of pulmonary edema, audible third heart sound, or increased JVP

- **Left ventricular failure**—Symptoms of low cardiac output and congestion (predominate feature: **SOB**) due to systolic or diastolic dysfunction

- **Right ventricular failure**—Symptoms of fluid overload almost always due to left ventricular failure

- Most common cause of systolic heart failure (HF with reduced EF)—Ischemic cardiomyopathy (CAD with resultant MI and loss of functioning myocardium)

  - Treatment aimed at reducing death and hospitalization

- **Systolic dysfunction**—Difficulty with ventricular contraction

- **Diastolic dysfunction** (HF with preserved EF)—Difficulty with ventricular relaxation; results from hypertension and associated with aging; related to myocardial muscle stiffening and LVH

- Treatment aimed at improving symptoms and treating comorbidities

Disease	Etiology, Prevalence, Risk Factors	Clinical Symptoms and Signs	Diagnostics	Therapy, Prognosis, and Health Maintenance
Congestive heart failure	MCC: **CAD**, HTN, DM LV remodeling: dilation, thinning, mitral valve incompetence, RV remodeling 75% have pre-existing HTN MCC of *transudative pleural effusions* Mostly > age 65	1. Most common: Exertional **dyspnea** (SOB), then with rest • Chronic nonproductive cough, worse in recumbent position 2. **Fatigue** 3. Orthopnea (late), night cough, relieved by sitting up or sleeping with additional pillows 4. Paroxysmal Nocturnal Dyspnea 5. Nocturia Signs: 1. Cheyne-Stokes breathing: periodic, cyclic respiration 2. Edema: ankles, pretibial (cardinal) 3. **Rales** (crackles) 4. Additional heart sounds S4 = diastolic HF (preserved EF) **S3** = systolic HF (reduced EF) with volume overload • Tachycardia, tachypnea 5. Jugular venous pressure: >8 cm 6. Cold extremities, cyanosis 7. Hepatomegaly • Ascites, Jaundice, Peripheral edema	For new onset, chronic, or acute decompensation: 1. Basic labs: CBC, CMP, U/A +/− glucose, lipids, TSH • Occult hyperthyroidism or hypothyroidism 2. **Serum BNP**: increases with age and renal impairment, low in obese • Elevated in HF • Differentiates SOB in HF from noncardiac issues 3. **12-lead EKG** 4. CXR: Kerley B lines 5. Echo: diagnose, evaluate, manage • Most useful, differentiates HF +/− preserved LV diastolic function 6. Other findings: **Reduced pulse pressure** and SVR	Acute management (mnemonic: LMNOP): 1. Lasix—for diuresis 2. Morphine—reduces preload 3. Nitrates (NTG)—reduces preload 4. O₂ 5. Position 1. ACE inhibitor + diuretic (unless contraindicated) 2. CCB in diastolic HF Poor prognosis factors: chronic kidney disease, diabetes, lower LVEF, severe symptoms, old age 5-y mortality: 50%
Refractory HF		1. Rapid or repetitive recurrences of symptoms 2. Symptoms at rest or on minimal exertion that require repeated or prolonged hospitalizations		

- BNP—Elevated when ventricular filling pressures are high (very sensitive), less specific in older patients, women, and patients with COPD
  - NT-proBNP <300 pg/mL or BNP <100 pg/mL with a normal EKG makes HF less likely

- Helpful to guide intensity of diuretic use and disease modifying agents (ACE/BB) for acute setting, less helpful for chronic

Therapies for Refractory or Decompensated HF

IV (+) inotropic agent and/or vasodilator	1. Dobutamine, milrinone, nitroprusside, NTG, and nesiritide—improve hemodynamic and symptoms • Milrinone has inotropic and vasodilator activity
Swan Ganz catheters	1. Used to monitor CVP, pulmonary artery and capillary wedge pressure, CO, systemic and pulmonary vascular resistance
Extracorporeal ultrafiltration	1. Removes intravascular fluid → compensatory movement of fluid from the interstitial compartment 2. Relieves pulmonary and peripheral edema and improves NYHA class 3. Restores responsiveness to loop diuretics and decreases proinflammatory cytokine levels

Mechanical circulatory support	1. Intra-aortic balloon pump (IABP) • Most commonly used, long record of success, simple design, easily and rapidly inserted, least expensive, does not require constant monitoring • Best for short term use 2. Cardiopulmonary assistive devices • Provides full cardiopulmonary support analogous to bypass during cardiac surgery, but has limited use outside cardiac catheter lab 3. Left ventricular assist devices (LVAD) • Intermediate LVADs provide temporary support until cardiac transplant is available not designed for chronic, permanent support, but are used in chronic HF patients with poor long-term prognosis who are not transplant candidates (due to age, ESRD, or COPD) • Long-term LVADs are used as a bridge to transplant and are approved as a permanent therapy in patients who are not candidates for transplant; also implanted in patients who have failed all other pharmacologic therapies 4. **Cardiac transplantation (definitive)–**improves survival and QOL in select patients with severe HF • Survival at 1-3 y is 85%-79%, respectively • VO$_2$max is a good objective predictor of survival and is used to determine when a patient should be placed on waiting list • Criteria • **History of repeated hospitalizations for HF** • **Escalation in intensity of medical therapy** • **Reproducible VO$_2$max <14 mL/kg/min is relative indication, while <10 mL/kg is stronger indication** • Others: Refractory cardiogenic shock, dependence on IV inotropes to maintain adequate organ perfusion, severe symptoms of ischemia not amenable to revascularization or recurrent unstable angina, recurrent symptomatic ventricular arrhythmias refractory to all therapy

When to Refer versus Admit

Refer	Admit
• New symptoms of HF not explained by obvious cause • Continued symptoms and reduced LVEF (<35%)	• Unexplained new or worsening symptoms or (+) biomarkers indicating acute MI • Hypoxia, fluid overload, pulmonary edema not resolved as outpatient

New York Heart Association (NYHA) Heart Failure Classification

Functional Capacity	Objective Assessment
Class I: <5%	Cardiac disease without **any** limitation of physical activity (ordinary activity **does not** cause fatigue, palpitations, dyspnea, anginal pain)
Class II: Moderate activity, 10%-15%	Cardiac disease with **slight** limitation of physical activity (ordinary activity **results in** fatigue, palpitations, dyspnea, anginal pain). *Comfortable at rest.*
Class III: 20%-25%	Cardiac disease with **marked** limitation of physical activity (less than ordinary activity causes fatigue, palpitations, dyspnea, anginal pain). *Comfortable at rest.*
Class IV: Symptoms at rest, 35%-40%	Cardiac disease with **inability** to carry on physical activity without discomfort. Symptoms present **even at rest**; if activity undertaken, discomfort increased.
A	No objective evidence of cardiovascular disease. No symptoms and no limitation in ordinary physical activity.
B	Objective evidence of minimal cardiovascular disease. Mild symptoms and slight limitation during ordinary activity. Comfortable at rest.
C	Objective evidence of moderately severe cardiovascular disease. Marked limitation in activity due to symptoms, even during less-than-ordinary activity. Comfortable only at rest.
D	Objective evidence of severe cardiovascular disease. Severe limitations. Experiences symptoms even at rest.

MYOCARDITIS

Inflammation of the myocardium, with many possible causes.

Disease	Etiology, Prevalence, Risk Factors	Clinical Symptoms and Signs	Diagnostics	Therapy, Prognosis, and Health Maintenance

Myocarditis	Viruses:
	• **Coxsackie A virus**, Parvovirus 19, HHV-6
	• Bacteria: group A strep, Lyme disease, *Mycoplasma*
	  • Lupus
	  • Meds (sulfonamides)
	  • Idiopathic
	• Classic: **young M**
		Asymptomatic OR
		Viral prodrome
		1. **Fatigue, fever** malaise, myalgias
		2. **Heart failure SX**
		  • Dyspnea at rest
		  • Exercise intolerance
		  • Syncope
		Signs:
		1. Tachypnea, tachycardia
		2. Hepatomegaly
		3. S3 +/– S4
		4. Hypotension, decreased pulses, AMS
		Complications:
		Pericarditis, CHF, toxic mega-colon, arrhythmias, death
			1. Elevated cardiac enzymes
			  • CK-MB, Troponin
			2. ESR: high
			3. **Endomyocardial biopsy** (definitive, gold standard): infiltrations of lymphocytes with myocardial tissue necrosis
			Imaging:
			1. CXR: cardiomegaly
			2. EKG: sinus tachycardia
			3. Echo: ventricular dysfunction
				1. **Supportive**
				  • Diuretics (ACE inhibitor)
				  • Inotropic drugs: dopamine, dobuta-mine, milrinone)
				Treat underlying cause and any complications

PERICARDITIS

Disease	Etiology, Prevalence, Risk Factors	Clinical Symptoms and Signs	Diagnostics	Therapy, Prognosis, and Health Maintenance

Acute pericarditis	Most commonly **idio-pathic** (90%) or due to viral infection (**Coxsackie virus**), **lupus**
	MC in men <50 y/o
	Post-viral illness
	1-2 wk after MI (*Dressler's syndrome*)
	Renal failure (uremia)
		1. **Pleuritic** substernal radiating chest pain
		  • Sharp, worse with deep inspiration
		2. **Positional**-relieved: By sitting upright and leaning forward
		  • Worse: with lying supine, coughing, swallowing
		Signs:
		1. Pericardial **friction rub** (spe-cific, not always present):
		  • Heard during end expi-ration, patient sitting up, leaning forward
		  • Intermittent, scratching high pitched sound
			1. **Leukocytosis** → get blood and pericardial fluid cultures
			2. EKG: **Diffuse ST ele-vation** and PR depres-sion in precordial leads
			3. Echo: normal (r/o tamponade) (Fig. 15-1A-C)
				1. **NSAIDs** or aspirin
				2. Colchicine
				3. Steroids if refractory
				4. Antibiotic therapy if infectious
				Prognosis:
				1. Most recover in 1-3 wk

Pericardial effusion	Secondary to peri-carditis, uremia, or cardiac trauma
	Restrictive pressure on the heart
		1. Painful or painless
		2. Cough and dyspnea
		3. Atypical chest discomfort
		4. Dizziness (low BP)
		5. Palpitations
		Signs:
		1. Peripheral edema
		2. **Distant heart sounds**
		Complications:
		As effusion increases, CO and BP decrease, falling to critical levels (tamponade)
			1. CXR or echo: determines extent of effusion or calcification
			  • Increased pericardial fluid
			  • Cardiomegaly
			2. EKG: nonspecific T wave changes, low QRS voltage (**alternans**)
				1. **Pericardiocentesis** to relieve fluid accumulation
				2. Recurrent → surgery with a pericardial window

Cardiac tamponade	Fluid compromises cardiac filling and impairs cardiac output	Signs: 1. **Beck's triad:** biphasic scratching sound (muffled heart sounds), hypotension, JVD 2. **Tachycardia, Tachypnea** 3. **Kussmaul's sign** 4. **Pulsus paradoxus**	1. Echo: increased peri-cardial fluid, **diastolic collapse of cardiac chambers** 2. **Narrow pulse pressure**	1. **Pericardiocentesis**

Disease	Etiology, Prevalence, Risk Factors	Clinical Symptoms and Signs	Diagnostics	Therapy, Prognosis, and Health Maintenance

Constrictive pericarditis	Fibrotic, calcified pericardium limiting filling of the ventricles during diastole	1. **Dyspnea** (most common)
		2. R-sided HF SX
		  • Peripheral edema
		  • Elevated JVP
		  • Hepatic congestion, nausea, vomiting
		Signs:
		1. Pulsus paradoxus
		2. Kussmaul's sign
		3. **Pericardial knock**
		4. Hepatojugular reflux
			1. Echo: pericardial thickening and calcification	1. **Pericardiectomy**

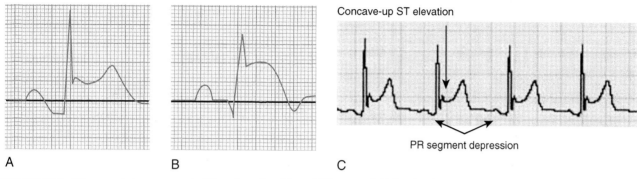

FIGURE 15-1. ST-segment changes seen in **(A)** acute pericarditis and **(B)** myocardial infarction. In myocardial infarctions, you'll more commonly find ST elevation and T wave abnormalities, such as T wave inversion (which is nonspecific). **C,** Acute pericarditis. Demonstration of the diffuse ST elevation commonly seen on EKG in pericarditis. PR depression may also be seen in precordial leads. (From Morton PG, Fontaine DK. *Critical Care Nursing: A Holistic Approach.* Philadelphia: Wolters Kluwer Health; 2018.)

- **Pulsus paradoxus**: >10 mm drop in systolic blood pressure with inspiration; pulses disappear with inspiration as well
- **Kussmaul's sign**: increased JVP with inspiration
- **Pericardial knock**: high pitched third heart sound from sudden cessation of ventricular filling in early diastole due to a thick inelastic pericardium
- **Electrical alternans**: alteration of QRS complex height on EKG due to movement of the heart within the pericardial sac

- **Beck's triad**: JVD, hypotension, muffled heart sounds
- When Is Pericardiocentesis Indicated?
  - Life-threatening hemodynamic changes in patient with suspected cardiac tamponade
  - Nonemergent: to aspirate pericardial fluid in hemodynamically stable patients for diagnostic, palliative, or prophylactic reasons
  - No absolute contraindications exist

CARDIOMYOPATHIES

Dilated Cardiomyopathy (Fig. 15-2)

Normal

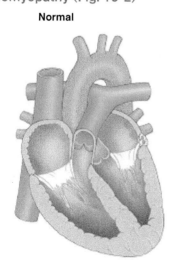

Dilated

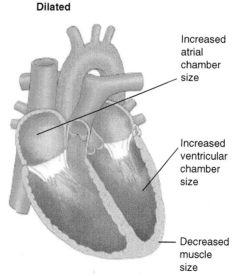

Increased atrial chamber size

Increased ventricular chamber size

Decreased muscle size

FIGURE 15-2. Dilated cardiomyopathy includes findings such as increased left ventricular chamber size, as well as decreased ventricular wall and septum. This leaves the heart weaker and does not allow for blood to be pumped effectively to the body. (From Timby BK, Smith NE. *Introductory Medical-Surgical Nursing.* 11th ed. Philadelphia: Wolters Kluwer; 2013.)

Disease	Etiology, Prevalence, Risk Factors	Clinical Symptoms and Signs	Diagnostics	Therapy, Prognosis, and Health Maintenance

Dilated cardiomy-opathy (DCM)	• **Most common type** (95%) and associated with reduced strength of ventricular con-traction, resulting in dilation of left ventricle
	• Most **idiopathic** (50%), age 20-60 y
	• **CAD with prior MI** is com-mon cause
	• **Genetic abnormalities**
	  • Excessive ETOH
	  • Postpartum
	  • Doxorubicin
	  • Endocrinopathy
	  • Myocarditis
		1. **Dyspnea** (MC)
		2. Fatigue
		3. SX of L and R-HF
		Signs:
		1. **S3 gallop**
		2. Pulmonary crackles (rales)
		3. Increased JVP
		Complications:
		• Arrhythmias
		• Sudden death
		• Embolic events (10%)
			1. EKG: nonspecific ST and T wave changes, conduction abnormalities, ventricular ectopy
			2. CXR: **cardiomegaly**, pulmonary congestion
			3. Echo:
			• **LV dilation** and dysfunction
			• High diastolic pressures
			• Low cardiac output
			• **Decreased ejection fraction**
			• **Regional or global LV hypokinesis**
				1. CHF supportive therapy
				• ACE inhibitor
				• Diuretics
				• β blockers
				• Na restriction
				2. Digoxin, vasodilators
				3. ICD if EF <30%-35%
				4. Cardiac transplant
				5. Poor prognosis—most die within 5 y
				Health Maintenance:
				1. **Abstinence from ETOH**

Hypertrophic Cardiomyopathy

Massive hypertrophy (of the septum), small left ventricle, systolic anterior mitral motion, and diastolic dysfunction.

- Conditions, positions, and maneuvers that reduce LVED (decreased preload and afterload) worsen the outflow obstruction, intensifying the murmur

- Valsalva—decreases preload
- Moving from squatting to standing, nitrates—decreases preload
- Vasodilators—decrease afterload

Disease	Etiology, Prevalence, Risk Factors	Clinical Symptoms and Signs	Diagnostics	Therapy, Prognosis, and Health Maintenance
Hypertrophic cardio myopathy (HCM) (Fig. 15-3)	Asian descent, elderly (distinct form) Most: **autosomal dominant trait** Stiff, hypertrophied ventricle with elevated diastolic filling pres-sures (diastolic dysfunction) Secondary HCM: Due to longstanding HTN or aortic stenosis (not true HCM)	1. **Dyspnea** (90%) 2. **Angina pectoris** (75%) 3. Syncope and arrhythmias common • Palpitations, dizziness 4. Sudden cardiac death (<30, 2 %-3%) Signs: 1. Sustained PMI or triple apical impulse 2. **Loud S4** gallop 3. Variable systolic murmur 4. **Bisferious pulse** (carotid pulse with two upstrokes) 5. Jugular venous pulse with-out prominent "a" wave 6. Harsh systolic, **crescendo-decrescendo** murmur heard at LUSB • Better with: **squatting, lying** down or straight leg raise; sustained handgrip • Worse with: exercise, **valsalva, standing** (decrease preload and afterload)	1. CXR: unremarkable 2. EKG: nonspecific ST and T wave changes, septal Q waves, **LVH** 3. **Echo** • Asymmetric septal hypertrophy (>15 mm) • Systolic anterior motion of mitral valve • Small left ventricle • Diastolic dysfunction	1. **Beta blockers (first line)** or CCB; disopyramide for negative inotropic effects • Increases ventricular diastolic filling time • *Caution*: use of digoxin (increases contractility), nitrates, & diuretics (decrease volume) 2. Surgery (myomectomy) • Resection of hypertro-phied septum • For severe, refractory pts 3. Alcohol septal ablation • Ethanol destroys extra myocardial tissue 4. Dual chamber pacing, implantable defibrillator, mitral valve replacement Health maintenance: 1. **Avoid extreme exertion or strenuous exercise** 2. Avoid dehydration

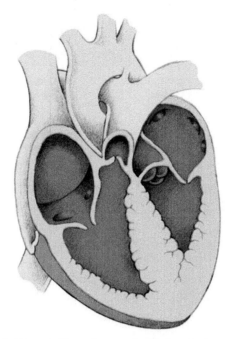

FIGURE 15-3. Hypertrophic cardiomyopathy. Findings include a stiff, enlarged septum, resulting in a small left ventricle. In effect, this increases diastolic filling pressures. (From *Lippincott's Nursing Advisor 2011. Philadelphia: Wolters Kluwer Health; 2012.*)

Restrictive Cardiomyopathy

Results from fibrosis or infiltration of the ventricular wall.

Disease	Etiology, Prevalence, Risk Factors	Clinical Symptoms and Signs	Diagnostics	Therapy, Prognosis, and Health Maintenance

Restrictive cardio myopathy (RCM)	Infiltration of the myocardium → impaired diastolic ventricular filling due to decreased ventricular compliance
	MCC:
	Collagen defect diseases (amyloidosis, radiation, post-op changes, DM, endomyocardial fibrosis)
		1. MC: **Dyspnea**
		2. Decreased exercise tolerance
		3. Advanced: **right**-sided congestive HF symptoms
		  • Peripheral edema
		  • Hepatic congestion (anorexia, nausea, vomiting)
		Signs:
		1. Pulmonary hypertension
		2. HSM, RUQ tenderness, hepatojugular reflex
		3. JVD
		4. Kussmaul's sign
		5. S3
			1. CXR: mild to mod enlarged cardiac silhouette
			  • Enlarged atria
			2. EKG: **low volt changes**
			3. Echo
			  • **Ventricules not dilated** with normal wall thickness
			  • Marked dilation of both atria
			  • **Diastolic dysfunction** with normal systolic function
			  • High pulmonary capillary wedge pressure
			4. Endomyocardial biopsy (gold standard)
				• **Diuretics and vasodilators**, cautiously
				• Treat underlying d/o
				  1. Hemochromatosis–phlebotomy and deferoxamine
				  2. Sarcoidosis–glucocorticoids
				  3. Amyloidosis–no TX
				  4. Systolic dysfunction–digoxin

RHEUMATIC FEVER AND RHEUMATIC HEART DISEASE

Disease	Etiology, Prevalence, Risk Factors	Clinical Symptoms and Signs	Diagnostics	Therapy, Prognosis, and Health Maintenance

Acute rheumatic fever	Supporting RF: previous (+) throat culture or RAT (66%), elevated or rising strep antibody titer
	Complications:
	Mitral stenosis
		Major criteria:
		1. Polyarthritis
		2. Carditis
		3. Chorea
		4. Erythema marginatum
		  • Red patches with central clearing
		5. Subcutaneous nodules
		Minor criteria:
		1. Fever (>39)
		2. Arthralgia
		3. Elevated CRP or ESR
		4. Prolonged PR interval (mitral regurgitation)
			1. Throat culture or RAT
			2. **ASO titer**: establishes recent strep infection (>320 = +)
			DX criteria:
			1. **2 Major**
			OR
			2. **1 major + 2 minor**
			+ Supporting evidence
			Exceptions: chorea or indolent carditis with normal anti strep antibody levels
				1. **PO Aspirin** (50-100 mg/kg/d) QID for 2-4 wk, then taper 4-6 wk
				2. **1.2 million U benzathine penicillin IM** or 10 days PO penicillin
				  • Erythromycin if PCN allergy
				3. **Prednisone** 2 mg/kg/d BID for 2-4 wk
				4. Prophylaxis: **Benzathine penicillin G** (first line) q 4 wk, erythromycin (PCN allergy)

ARTERIAL OR VENOUS ULCER DISEASE (VASCULAR DISEASE)

Disease	Etiology, Prevalence, Risk Factors	Clinical Symptoms and Signs	Diagnostics	Therapy, Prognosis, and Health Maintenance

Chronic Venous Insufficiency (Venous Stasis)
Mostly due to valvular dysfunction - leads to loss of compartmentalization of veins, leading to distention and increased pressure → transmitted to microvasculature → basement membrane thickening, increased capillary elongation, skin changes
	Varicose veins, postphlebitic syndrome
	Age 30-40 y, F
	Aggravating factors:
	Pregnancy, increased blood volume, increased cardiac output or venocaval pressure, progesterone
	F > M
	RF:
	Family history, DVT, female, estrogen increase, age, obesity, prolonged standing
	2% of general population
		1. **Heaviness** or aching of leg (**lower extremity edema**)
		  • *Worse with prolonged standing and relieved by walking*
		  • **Relief with elevation**
		2. Edema worse **at end of day and with standing**
		  • Shoes feel tight in evening
		  • Night cramps
		3. Itching 2/2 irritation
		Signs:
		1. **Hyper pigmentation**
		2. **Distal edema**
		3. Erythema, dry tight skin
		4. Ulceration (severe)
		Complications:
		50% have varicose veins, fibrosis, atrophy
			1. **Duplex ultrasound** to assess valve closure
			  • NL: 0.5-1 s
			    <0.5 s (diagnostic)
			2. See CEAP Categorization for classification
			(Fig. 15-4A)
				Conservative Methods:
				For at least 3 mo
				1. **Graduated compression hose** (first line)
				2. Compression for open ulcer
				Vein ablation therapies:
				  • Indications: vein hemorrhage superficial thrombophlebitis
				  • Contra: pregnant, DVT, mod to severe PAD, joint disease
				1. **Injection sclerotherapy (initial)**
				  • For telangiectasias (CEAP cat 1), reticular veins, small varicose veins
				2. Vein ligation/excision
				  • For CEAP cat 2 (>3 mm)
				3. Thermal ablation
				4. Venous reconstruction

Varicose veins	"Blow out" of incompetent veins 10%-30% of general population MC in F	1. Enlarged, tortuous superficial leg veins • Seen best with standing 2. Painful and itchy	1. Tourniquet test: applied to leg that has been elevated; release after patient stands and veins fill instantly (Fig. 15-4B)	1. **Injection sclerotherapy** with prolonged compression 2. Vascular surgery: ligation, remove saphenous veins 3. Endoscopic subfascial dissection of perforating veins

Disease	Etiology, Prevalence, Risk Factors	Clinical Symptoms and Signs	Diagnostics	Therapy, Prognosis, and Health Maintenance
Eczematous (stasis) dermatitis		1. Inflammatory plaques, scaly, and crusted erosions 2. Pigmentation with stippled hemorrhage 3. Dermal sclerosis 4. Excoriations from scratching	1. Culture for MSSA (Fig. 15-4C)	1. Topical steroids (short term) 2. Topical antibiotics (mupirocin)
Venous ulcers	Prevalence: 1% Occur on medial lower calf, single or multiple, **medial** > lateral over malleolus RF: Diabetes, PAD	1. Irregularly shaped, sharply defined, shallow with sloping border 2. Painful (mild) 3. Occurs over medial and lateral malleolar area, posterior calf Signs: 1. Irregular margins, pink or red base that may be covered with yellow fibrinous tissue, exudate common 2. Warm 3. Pulses and sensation intact 4. Erythema, brown-blue hyperpigmentation; edema, dry skin, varicose veins	(Fig. 15-4D)	1. Correct underlying risk factors 2. Corrective surgery +/− elastic stockings daily 3. Distribute weight in special shoes
Arterial Ulcer	Associated with PAD Occur on lower leg (pretibial, supramalleolar, toes)	1. Severe pain at night • Worse when legs elevated • Over toe joints, malleoli (bony prominence), anterior shin, base of heel, pressure points Signs: 1. Punched out, with sharply demarcated irregular borders • Base dry and often pale or necrotic 2. Tissue slough at base (see tendon) 3. Pulses absent 4. Warm or cool 5. Shiny, taut, loss of hair 6. Dependent rubor of leg and foot, pale with elevation	(Fig. 15-4E)	1. Endarterectomy or bypass surgery to correct arterial flow
Gangrene	Dry gangrene common with PAD	1. Dry: hard, dry texture occurring in the distal aspects of toes and fingers with clear demarcation between viable and black, necrotic tissue 2. Wet: moist appearance, gross swelling, blistering	(Fig. 15-4F)	1. Dry−revascularize first (vascular bypass or angioplasty) 2. Wet−debride immediately

• The ABI is the ratio of the ankle systolic blood pressure divided by the brachial systolic pressure detected with a Doppler probe

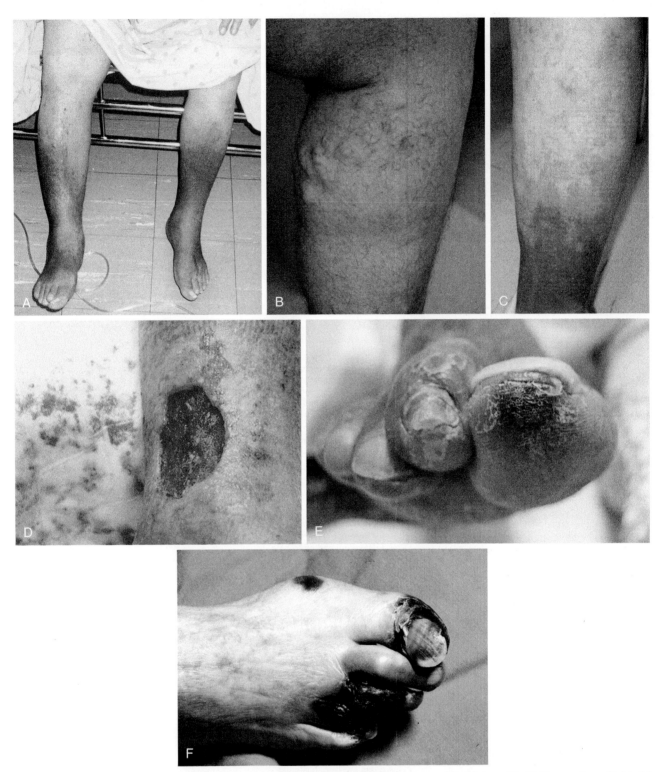

FIGURE 15-4. A, Chronic venous insufficiency (venous stasis). **B**, Varicose veins. **C**, Eczematous (stasis) dermatitis. **D**, Venous ulcers. **E**, Arterial ulcer. **F**, Gangrene. (**A**, Dale Berg and Katherine Worzala, *Atlas of Adult Physical Diagnosis*. Philadelphia: Lippincott Williams & Wilkins, 2006. **B**, Image provided by Stedman's. **C**, Image provided by Stedman's. **D**, From Sussman C, Bates-Jensen B. *Wound Care: A Collaborative Practice Manual for Health Professionals*. Philadelphia; Wolters Kluwer Health; 2012. **E**, From Nicol N. *Dermatologic Nursing Essentials*. Philadelphia: Wolters Kluwer Health; 2016. **F**, From McGreer MA, Carter PJ. *Lippincott's Textbook for Personal Support Workers: A Humanistic Approach to Caregiving*. Philadelphia: Wolters Kluwer Health; 2011.)

CHAPTER 16
Pulmonology

Refer to Family Medicine [icon] for in-depth coverage of the following topics:

Breath Sounds, p 16
Acute/Chronic Bronchitis, p 18
Asthma, p 18
Chronic Obstructive Pulmonary Disease, p 21

Pneumonia, p 24
Pulmonary Neoplasm, p 30
Hypoventilation Syndrome, p 31

Recommended Supplemental Topics:

Pleural Effusion, refer to Emergency Medicine [icon],
   p 391

CARCINOID TUMOR

- Originate from neuroendocrine cells and secrete **serotonin**
- Most begin in the small bowel and appendix
- When it spreads to the liver, patients become symptomatic because the carcinoid is no longer able to be metabolized
- After spreading to the liver, it will then spread to the heart and lung (right heart valve)

Disease	Etiology, Prevalence, Risk Factors	Clinical Symptoms and Signs	Diagnostics	Therapy, Prognosis, and Health Maintenance

Carcinoid tumor	Tryptophan is converted from vitamin B$_3$ (niacin) to serotonin by tumor = niacin deficiency
	MC site:
	Appendix, but can be found in a variety of locations (small bowel, rectum, bronchus, kidney, pancreas)
	M = F, <60 y/o
		1. Cough
		2. Hemoptysis
		3. Focal Wheezing
		4. Recurrent pneumonia
		5. Pellagra
		  • Dermatitis
		  • Dementia
		  • Diarrhea
			1. Fiberoptic bronchoscopy: pink or purple tumor in a central airway
			2. CT scan–to localize and follow growth
			3. Octreotide Scintigraphy
				1. Surgical excision, if symptomatic
				2. Resistant to radiation and chemotherapy
				Complications:
				Bleeding, airway obstruction
				Prognosis:
				Favorable

Carcinoid syndrome (10%)	Excess serotonin secretion Flushing and wheezing is result of serotonin overproduction	1. Cutaneous **flushing** 2. **Diarrhea** 3. Sweating 4. **Wheezing** 5. Abdominal pain 6. Heart valve dysfunction (murmurs) 7. Weight loss Signs: 1. Hypotension	1. Urinalysis: elevated serotonergic precursors (5-HIAA)	1. Surgical resection: of tumor 2. Octreotide for tumors that are metastatic to the liver Risk factors of mets increased with size–ileal tumors have greatest likelihood

BRONCHIECTASIS

Permanent, abnormal dilation and destruction of the bronchial walls; cilia damaged; onset in childhood (usually).

Disease	Etiology, Prevalence, Risk Factors	Clinical Symptoms and Signs	Diagnostics	Therapy, Prognosis, and Health Maintenance
Bronchiectasis	Causes: **Cystic fibrosis** (most common, 50%), infection, immunodeficiency, airway obstruction Infection with airway obstruction or impaired defense/drainage precipitates disease	1. Chronic cough with large amounts of mucopurulent, **foul smelling sputum** 2. Dyspnea (SOB) 3. Hemoptysis—mild, self-limited 4. Recurrent or persistent pneumonia +/− weight loss Signs: 1. Crackles at the lung bases	1. **High resolution CT** (gold standard) 2. PFTs (obstructive pattern) 3. CXR (abnormal, nonspecific) Other labs: CBC (anemia)	1. Antibiotics—acute exacerbations 2. Bronchial hygiene—fluids, chest physiotherapy, inhaled bronchodilators

SOLITARY PULMONARY NODULE

Disease	Etiology, Prevalence, Risk Factors	Clinical Symptoms and Signs	Diagnostics	Therapy, Prognosis, and Health Maintenance
Solitary pulmonary nodule (SPN)	Single, isolated, less than 3 cm, well-circumscribed nodule or "coin lesion" with no associated mediastinal or hilar lymph node involvement (determines if malignant) RF for malignancy: Age 30+, smokers, more cigarettes per day, prior malignancy	1. Asymptomatic • Incidental on CXR	1. **Review old imaging studies** • Compare with prior studies, estimate doubling time 2. **CT chest**—for any suspicious SPN 3. Flexible bronchoscopy—central lesions 4. Transthoracic fine needle biopsy (FNA)—determines if malignant 5. PET scan	See treatment based on probability of malignancy below Prognosis—significant risk of malignancy (10%-68%)
Hamartoma	<5% of SPNs Benign neoplasm of tissue growing in a disorganized manner			

Determinants of Malignancy and Treatment

Benign	Malignant
• Young (<50) • Size: small (<1 cm) • Borders: smooth, discrete • Calcification: dense, central, or laminated calcification • CXR: stable for >2 y	• Older age (**>50**) • Size: large (>2 cm), thick walls (>16 mm) • Borders: irregular • Calcification: *eccentric, asymmetric* • **Change in size: enlarging** • Currently smoking • Lobular appearance • CT findings: peripheral halo, spiculated margins
Follow every **3 mo**	Biopsy and resect

Probability of Malignancy

This probability helps to determine whether to recommend biopsy versus surgical excision in light of each patient's unique clinical scenario.

Probability	Examples	Treatment
Low probability (<5%) of malignancy	Age <30, lesions stable more than 2 y, characteristics suggestive of benign calcification	1. Watchful waiting 2. Serial CT scans or CXRs 3. 3D High Res CT

Intermediate probability (5%-60%) of malignancy		1. Diagnostic biopsy: TTNA (50%-97% yield) vs. bronchoscopy (10%-80% yield) depending on location of lesion
		2. PET Scan
		  • Positive: increases likelihood of cancer
		  • Negative: excludes cancer in most cases
		3. VATS

High probability (>60%) of malignancy		1. Staging → resection 2. Biopsy NOT indicated

INTERSTITIAL LUNG DISEASES (DIFFUSE PARENCHYMAL LUNG DISEASE)

Inflammatory process involving the alveolar wall (resulting in widespread fibroelastic proliferation and collagen deposition) that can lead to **irreversible fibrosis, distortion** of lung architecture, and **impaired** gas exchange.

- History: medications (chemotherapy, gold, amiodarone, penicillamine, nitrofurantoin)
  - Previous jobs: asbestos (electrical or building insulation), beryllium, coal, silicone
- Symptoms: **dyspnea** (first with exertion → rest)
  - Cough (nonproductive)
  - Fatigue

- Signs: **rales at the bases** (common), **digital clubbing** (IPF), signs of pulmonary HTN and cyanosis in advanced disease
- Diagnosis: CXR (reticular, reticulonodular, ground glass, honeycombing)
  - **High resolution CT**: shows extent of fibrosis better
  - PFTs (restrictive): increased FEV1/FVC, lung volumes low, FEV1 and FVC are low but FVC lower
  - O_2 desaturation with exercise
  - Bronchoalveolar lavage (culture/cytology): controversial, variable results
  - **Tissue biopsy**: definitive diagnosis
  - Urinalysis: if signs of glomerular injury (Goodpasture's syndrome and Wegener's granulomatosis)

Interstitial Lung Diseases Associated with Granulomas

Disease	Etiology, Prevalence, Risk Factors	Clinical Symptoms and Signs	Diagnostics	Therapy, Prognosis, and Health Maintenance

Sarcoidosis	Chronic systemic granulomatous disease characterized by noncaseating granulomas, often involving multiple organ systems; lungs most involved
	Etiology:
	Unknown
	Most often occurs in African Americans, especially in F
	75% of cases occur when <40
		1. Constitutional SX: **malaise, fever**, anorexia, **weight loss**
		2. Lungs: Dry cough, **dyspnea on exertion**
		3. Musk (25%-50%): **arthralgias**, arthritis, bone lesions
		4. Skin (25%): **erythema nodosum**
		5. Eyes (25%): **anterior uveitis** (75%), posterior uveitis (25%), conjunctivitis
		6. Heart (5%): arrhythmias, heart block, sudden death
		7. Nervous (5%): CN VII (Bell's palsy), optic nerve dysfunction, papilledema, peripheral neuropathy
			1. CXR: **bilateral hilar adenopathy** (hallmark, nonspecific, 50%)
			2. Serum angiotensin-converting enzyme (**ACE**): elevated (50%-80%, not sens/spec)
			3. **Hypercalciuria, hypercalcemia** (common)
			4. PFTs:
			  • Decreased VC/TLC
			  • Decreased DLCO
			  • Increased FEV1/FVC ratio
			5. Definitive DX: **transbronchial biopsy**—must see noncaseating granulomas (not diagnostic by itself)
				Most resolve spontaneously in 2 y, no treatment
				1. **Systemic (PO) steroids**: if symptomatic, active lung disease, PFT deterioration, conduction disturbances, severe skin or eye involvement
				2. Methotrexate—if refractory
				Prognosis:
				1. Good for most patients

Sarcoidosis Staging

- **Honeycombing**: scarred shrunken lung; air space dilated, fibrous scarring in interstitium; associated with a poor prognosis.

Stage 1	Stage 2	Stage 3	Stage 4
Bilateral hilar adenopathy WITHOUT Parenchymal infiltrates	Hilar adenopathy WITH Parenchymal infiltrates	NO hilar adenopathy + *Diffuse* parenchymal infiltrates	Pulmonary fibrosis with honeycombing + Fibrocystic parenchymal changes

IDIOPATHIC PULMONARY FIBROSIS (IDIOPATHIC FIBROSING INTERSTITIAL PNEUMONIA)

Disease	Etiology, Prevalence, Risk Factors	Clinical Symptoms and Signs	Diagnostics	Therapy, Prognosis, and Health Maintenance
Idiopathic pulmonary fibrosis (idiopathic fibrosing interstitial pneumonia)	Etiology: unknown, more common in **male smokers**	• Gradual onset of progressive dyspnea, nonproductive cough • Constitutional symptoms • Clubbing • Inspiratory crackles	CT: progressive fibrosis over several years CXR: Diffuse patchy fibrosis with pleural based honeycombing or *ground glass*; may be normal PFTs: Restrictive pattern, decreased lung volume with NL to increased FEV1/FVC ratio Exclude other cause of ILD	• **No effective treatment** • >70% do not respond and experience gradual respiratory failure • Supplemental O_2, steroids with or without cyclophosphamide, lung transplant Prognosis: Variable, but mean survival is 3-7 y after first DX

PNEUMOCONIOSIS (ENVIRONMENTAL LUNG DISEASE)

Accumulation of dust in the lungs, and the tissue reaction to its presence.

- eg, silica, beryllium, asbestos, coal dust, graphite, carbon black, aluminum, talc

Disease	Etiology, Prevalence, Risk Factors	Clinical Symptoms and Signs	Diagnostics	Therapy, Prognosis, and Health Maintenance
Coal worker's	Inhalation of coal dust (carbon + silica), nodular opacities at upper lung fields Coal mining	1. Simple: no respiratory disability 2. Complicated: fibrosis (restrictive lung disease)	1. FEV1: decreased 2. (+) ANA, nonspecific	1. Progressive massive fibrosis
Asbestosis	Diffuse interstitial fibrosis caused by inhalation of asbestos fibers (**lower lobes**) Insulation, demolition, construction >90% have lung involvement Highest incidence in north American black F and North European whites	1. Insidious development (>15-20 y) post-exposure 2. Nonspecific ILD findings	Clinical DX, HX of exposure to asbestos: 1. CXR: pleural plaques, hazy infiltrates, and bilateral linear opacities 2. Biopsy: asbestos bodies	1. No specific treatment 2. **Stop smoking** Prognosis: 1. Increased risk of **bronchogenic carcinoma** (smoking synergistic) and **malignant mesothelioma**
Silicosis	Localized and nodular peribronchial fibrosis (**upper lobes**) Sources: Mining, stone cutting, glass manufacturing	1. Exertional dyspnea (MC) 2. Cough with sputum production Signs: Restrictive pulmonary function findings	1. CXR: "**egg shell calcification** of enlarged hilar lymph nodes"	1. Removal from exposure to silica Prognosis: Increased risk of tuberculosis, progressive fibrosis
Berylliosis	High technology fields: Aerospace, nuclear power, ceramics, foundries, tool and die manufacturing	Acute: Diffuse pneumonitis by massive exposure to beryllium Chronic: Similar to sarcoidosis with granulomas, skin lesions, and hypercalcemia	1. Beryllium lymphocyte proliferation test	1. **Chronic glucocorticoid therapy** for both acute/chronic 2. **Glucocorticoid therapy** for both acute/chronic

PULMONARY HYPERTENSION

Mean **pulmonary arterial pressure greater than 25 mm Hg** at rest or 30 mm Hg during exercise.

- Passive type—resistance to pulmonary venous drainage
  - Eg, **mitral stenosis**, LVHF, atrial myxoma, pulmonary veno-occlusive disease
- Hyperkinetic—high pulmonary blood flow (L to R shunts)
  - Eg, VSD, ASD, PDA
- Obstructive type—resistance to flow through large pulmonary arteries
  - Eg, PE, pulmonary artery stenosis
- Obliterative type—resistance to flow through small pulmonary vessels (arterioles) due to parenchymal inflammation leading to fibrosis
  - Eg, **primary pulmonary hypertension**, collagen vascular disease, CREST syndrome
- Vasoconstrictive type—resistance to flow due to hypoxia-induced vasoconstriction
  - Eg, chronic hypoxemia, COPD, OSA
- Increased intrathoracic pressure—transmitted to pulmonary vasculature
  - Eg, mechanical vent with PEEP, COPD
- Increased blood viscosity—polycythemia vera

Primary Pulmonary Hypertension (PPH) and Cor Pulmonale

Disease	Etiology, Prevalence, Risk Factors	Clinical Symptoms and Signs	Diagnostics	Therapy, Prognosis, and Health Maintenance
Primary pulmonary hypertension (PPH)	Young or middle-aged F Cause: Unknown Abnormal increase in pulmonary arterial resistance → thickening of pulmonary arterial walls Pulmonary HTN in absence of disease of heart or lung; DX of exclusion	• **Dyspnea on exertion** • **Fatigue** • **Chest pain** (exertional) • Syncope (exertional) in 50% Signs: • Loud pulmonic P2 sound, subtle lift of sternum • **JVD**, hepatomegaly, **ascites, peripheral edema**	DX of exclusion: 1. EKG: **right ventricular hypertrophy**, right axis deviation and right atrial abnormality 2. Echo: **dilated pulmonary artery**, dilation and hypertrophy of RA/RV, abnormal movement of IV septum 3. **Right heart cath** (gold standard): increased PA pressure 4. CXR: clear lungs, enlarged RV, central pulm arteries, "**peripheral pruning** of large pulmonary arteries" 5. PFTs: restrictive 6. ABGs, serology 7. V/Q scan: PE vs. PPH	1. **IV prostacyclins** (epoprostenol) and CCB: lower pulm vasc resistance 2. Anticoagulation with Warfarin (goal: 2.0) due to venous stasis, physical inactivity, risk of thrombosis 3. Lung transplant Prognosis: Poor, mean survival 2-3 y from DX
Cor pulmonale	Right ventricular hypertrophy with eventual RV failure, resulting from pulmonary HTN, secondary to pulmonary disease Most commonly secondary to **COPD** Other causes: Recurrent PE, ILD, asthma, CF, OSA, pneumoconiosis	1. Decreased exercise tolerance (**DOE**) Signs: • Parasternal lift • Cyanosis • Clubbing • JVD, hepatomegaly, ascites, peripheral edema • Polycythemia (if COPD present)	1. CXR: **enlarged RA, RV**, and **pulm-arteries** 2. EKG: right axis deviation, **P-pulmonale** (peaked P waves), right ventrical hypertrophy	1. Treat underlying pulmonary disorder 2. Use **diuretic** therapy cautiously, patient may be preload dependent 3. Apply continuous **long-term O₂** therapy if hypoxic 4. Digoxin—if coexistent LV failure

CHAPTER **17**

Gastrointestinal System and Nutrition

Refer to Family Medicine [icon] for in-depth coverage of the following topics:

DIVERTICULAR DISEASE

- A diverticulum is a sac-like protrusion of the colonic wall
- Diverticulosis—most common cause of bright red blood per rectum in patients 65+

Disease	Etiology, Prevalence, Risk Factors	Clinical Symptoms and Signs	Diagnostics	Therapy, Prognosis, and Health Maintenance
Diverticulosis	<u>MOA:</u> Increased luminal pressure <u>RF:</u> low fiber diet, (+) family history Prevalence—increased age (>60) MC location in **US—sigmoid** colon The presence of diverticula: constipation leads to expulsion of diverticula in sigmoid colon	<u>History of constipation:</u> Asymptomatic—discovered incidentally, only 20% symptomatic 1. LLQ discomfort, bloating, constipation, diarrhea 2. **Lower GI bleeding**	<u>KUB:</u> r/o free air CT if patient does not respond to therapy 1. **Barium enema**– avoid during acute episode, leads to perforation and peritonitis 2. Colonoscopy (avoid during acute episodes)	1. **High-fiber diet (bran)** to bulk up stool 2. **Psyllium** <u>Complications:</u> • **Painless rectal bleeding** (40%) with sudden-onset large volume hematochezia; spontaneously resolves → if continuous or recurrent go to surgery • Diverticulitis (15%-25%)

Disease	Etiology, Prevalence, Risk Factors	Clinical Symptoms and Signs	Diagnostics	Therapy, Prognosis, and Health Maintenance
Acute diverticulitis	Acute diverticulitis is defined as inflammation and/or infection of a diverticulum Feces impacted in diverticulum = erosion + microperfusion Mean age: 63 Gram negative rods and anaerobes: *E. coli, B. fragilis*	1. **Sudden onset abdominal pain** in **LLQ** or suprapubic region • Constant over several days • 50% w/previous episode 2. Nausea, vomiting 3. Constipation (50%), diarrhea (25%-30%) 4. +/– **Fever** Signs: 1. Painful mass on rectal exam	1. Abdominal CT with contrast: **localized bowel wall thickening** (>4 mm), increase soft tissue density in pericolonic fat, colonic diverticula 2. FOBT (+) 3. CBC: leukocytosis 4. Avoid colonoscopy and barium enemas during acute episodes	Uncomplicated: See Treatment below Complicated: See Treatment below Complications: • Diverticular **abscess** • Colovesical fistula • Bowel obstruction • **Perforation**

Treatment of Diverticulitis

Outpatient	Prophylaxis	Inpatient
1. **PO antibiotics** × 7-10 d • **Ciprofloxacin + Flagyl** • Bactrim + Flagyl • Augmentin 2. Consume clear liquids only until reassessed after 2-3 d 3. Repeat imaging not necessary if clinically improved	1. Do **not** need to avoid nuts, seeds, popcorn 2. High fiber diet	Uncomplicated 1. IVF (LR or NS), pain meds (morphine, Tylenol, hydromorphone), NPO (bowel rest) or clear liquid diet 2. IV antibiotics until abdominal pain resolves (3-5 d) → PO antibiotics × 10-14 d • **Flagyl PLUS** • Cefazolin, cefuroxime, ceftriaxone, cefotaxime, **ciprofloxacin**, levofloxacin • OR single-agent: ertapenem, piperacillin/tazobactam (Zosyn) 3. Repeat imaging–r/o abscess, perforation 4. After 6 wk–pt needs colonoscopy to r/o colon cancer Complicated or recurrent SX 1. Bowel resection

- Criteria for admission: immunosuppression, high fever (>102.5°F/39°C), leukocytosis, severe abdominal pain, advanced age, comorbidities, PO intolerance, failed outpatient treatment, noncompliance or unreliability, lack of support system

Disease	Etiology, Prevalence, Risk Factors	Clinical Symptoms and Signs	Diagnostics	Therapy, Prognosis, and Health Maintenance
Meckel diverticulum	Most common congenital abnormality of the small intestine Incomplete obliteration of the vitelline duct (omphalomesenteric duct)	Most asymptomatic 1. Hematochezia (most common)–**painless rectal bleeding** 2. Abdominal pain (**periumbilical**) that radiates to RLQ 3. **Iron deficiency anemia** and megaloblastic anemia	1. Technetium-99m **(Meckel) scintiscan**: uptake by heterotopic gastric mucosa	1. IV crystalloid fluids, NPO status, NG decompression 2. Excision of the diverticulum along with adjacent ileal segment Complications: Adhesive intestinal obstruction

ESOPHAGEAL VARICES

Disease	Etiology, Prevalence, Risk Factors	Clinical Symptoms and Signs	Diagnostics	Therapy, Prognosis, and Health Maintenance
Esophageal (90%) or gastric varices, including rectal hemorrhoids and caput medusae		1. Massive hematemesis 2. Melena 3. Exacerbation of hepatic encephalopathy	1. **Upper GI endoscopy** (once stabilized) for diagnosis and treat hemorrhage	1. Hemodynamic stabilization 2. IV antibiotic prophylaxis 3. **Nonselective β-blocker** for long term therapy: propranolol 4. Active bleed: **IV octreotide** → 5. Sclerotherapy or *ligation* High mortality rate

CANCER (ESOPHAGUS, HEPATIC, STOMACH, GALLBLADDER)

- The most common malignant liver tumors are **hepatocellular carcinomas** and **cholangiocarcinomas**
- The most common benign liver tumor is the hemangioma
- Gastric Cancer Mets—**VISK-shelf** (superior to inferior)
  - Virchow's Node—metastasis to the supraclavicular FOSSA NODES
  - Irish's Node—metastasis to LEFT AXILLARY ADENOPATHY
  - Sister Mary Joseph's node—metastasis to the periumbilical LYMPH NODE
  - Krukenberg's tumor—metastasis to OVARY
  - Blumer's **shelf**—metastasis to the RECTUM (pelvic-cul-de-sac); palpable

Disease	Etiology, Prevalence, Risk Factors	Clinical Symptoms and Signs	Diagnostics	Therapy, Prognosis, and Health Maintenance
Esophageal cancer	1. **SCC**–African American M, upper thoracic and midthoracic esophagus • RF: alcohol and smoking 2. Adenocarcinoma–white men; distal ⅓ of esophagus/GE junction • RF: GERD and Barrett's esophagus	1. **Dysphagia** (most common; solids first, then liquids) 2. **Weight loss** 3. Anorexia 4. Odynophagia–pain with swallowing (late finding) 5. Hematemesis, hoarseness 6. Aspiration pneumonia 7. Tracheoesophageal or bronchoesophageal fistula 8. Chest pain	1. **Barium swallow** 2. **Upper endoscopy with biopsy** and brush cytology (required) 3. Transesophageal ultrasound–depth 4. CT scan of chest/abdomen, CXR, and bone scan	1. Palliative care 2. Surgery 3. Chemotherapy with radiation Poor prognosis: 5-y survival rate is 5%-15% for both types
Barrett's esophagus	Complication of long standing acid reflux–**columnar** metaplasia of the **squamous** epithelium Typical patient: Middle aged (55) White M with chronic GERD Prolonged stated of untreated GERD → adenocarcinoma	1. ⅔ have longstanding heartburn 2. **Odynophagia** (concerning) +/– Virchow node (left supraclavicular LAD)	1. 24-h pH monitor: severe reflux and reduced LES pressure 2. **EGD** (first line) with biopsy → can screen in patients 50+ with >5 y history of GERD	1. Periodic endoscopic surveillance with intensive biopsy at 3-mo intervals 2. Endoscopic ablation 3. Surgical resection 4. PPI and H2 Increased risk of developing adenocarcinoma
Gastric cancer Ulcerative carcinoma–ulcer through all layers Polypoid carcinoma–solid mass projects into stomach *Superficial spreading*–best prognosis *Linitis plastic*–through all layers, poor prognosis	Most **adenocarcinomas** Rare in U.S. RF: **H. pylori infection** (3-6×), **pernicious anemia** (3×), severe atrophic gastritis, gastric dysplasia, adenomatous gastric polyps, post-antrectomy (15-20 y), blood type A, high intake of preserved foods (high salt, nitrates, nitrites)	1. **Abdominal pain** 2. Unexplained **weight loss** 3. Reduced appetite, anorexia, dyspepsia, early satiety 4. Nausea, vomiting, anemia, melena Signs: 1. Acanthosis nigricans–hyperpigmented, velvety, thickening of the skin occurring in the skin folds, such as the groin, axilla, neck, and intra-mammary folds	1. **FOBT**–Guaiac (+) stool 2. **Endoscopy** with multiple biopsies (most accurate) 3. Barium upper GI series 4. Abdominal CT for staging	1. Surgical **resection** with wide (>5 cm) margins: total or subtotal gastrectomy or extended lymph node dissection 2. Chemotherapy
Gastric lymphoma	Type of non-Hodgkin's arising in stomach	Similar to adenocarcinoma of stomach: abdominal pain, weight loss, anorexia Complications: Bleeding, obstruction, perforation	1. **EGD** with biopsy	Same as above

Disease	Etiology, Prevalence, Risk Factors	Clinical Symptoms and Signs	Diagnostics	Therapy, Prognosis, and Health Maintenance

Hepatocellular carcinoma (HCC), also known as malignant hepatoma	>80% of primary liver cancers
	Most common type:
	non-fibrolamellar, associated with Hep B/C and cirrhosis, unresectable with short survival time
	Fibrolamellar: not associated with Hep B/C or cirrhosis, resectable, long survival time; seen in younger age
	RF:
	Cirrhosis (ETOH, Hep B/C), chemical carcinogens, AAT deficiency, hemochromatosis, Wilson's disease, schistosomiasis, hepatic adenoma, smoking, glycogen storage disease (type 1)
		1. Abdominal pain (**painful hepatomegaly**), *palpable* liver mass
		2. **Weight loss, anorexia**, fatigue
		3. Signs/SX of chronic liver disease–portal HTN, ascites, jaundice
		4. Paraneoplastic syndromes–high RBC/platelet, calcium, cholesterol
		  • Hypoglycemia
		  • Carcinoid syndrome
		  • Pulmonary osteodystrophy
			1. **Liver biopsy** (req)
			2. Labs: Hep B and C serology, LFTs, coags
			3. Imaging: U/S, CT chest/abdomen/pelvis, MRI or MRA if surgery is an option
			4. **A-1-FP tumor marker**: high in 40%-70% of pts
				Liver resection and/or liver transplant
				Survival/prognosis:
				1. If unresectable: less than 1 y
				2. If resectable: 25% 5-y prognosis

Pancreatic cancer	Most common in **elderly** patients (>60), African Americans Anatomic location: pancreatic **head** (75%), body (20%), tail (5%-10%) RF: **Smoking**, high fat diets, age >45, male gender, chronic pancreatitis, diabetes, heavy alcohol use, exposure to chemicals, first degree relative Most adenocarcinomas (50%) involving **head of pancreas**	1. **Abdominal pain:** vague and dull ache, epigastric, may radiate to back 2. **Painless jaundice:** most common with carcinoma of the head 3. **Weight loss**; anorexia 4. Recent onset glucose intolerance, but diabetes is mild 5. Depression, weakness, fatigue Signs: 1. **Trousseau's sign:** Migratory thrombophlebitis (10%) 2. **Courvoisier's sign:** painless palpable gall in 30%	1. **CT scan** (preferred): pancreatic mass, pancreatic and hepatic metastases, vascular involvement 2. **ERCP**–most sensitive (confirms diagnosis); obtain sample for biopsy 3. MRCP–noninvasive, visualize hepatic and biliary structures, no tissue sampling Tumor markers: 1. **CA 19-9** (more sens/spec) 2. CEA	1. Surgical resection with pancreatico-duodenectomy (Whipple's procedure) 2. Chemotherapy: 5-FU and gemcitabine 3. If unresectable–ERCP or PTC with stent placement 4. Most treatment is **palliative care** because of metastases Prognosis: 5-y survival rate is 10%
Carcinoma of the gallbladder	Most **adenocarcinomas**, occur in elderly RF: Cholecystoenteric fistula, porcelain gallbladder	Associated gallstones 1. Nonspecific SX, suggest extrahepatic bile duct obstruction: jaundice, biliary colic, weight loss, anorexia, RUQ mass Signs: 1. Palpable gallbladder		Cholecystectomy vs. radical cholecystectomy depending on depth of invasion Prognosis: 90% die within 1 y
Cholangio-carcinoma	Tumor of intrahepatic or extrahepatic bile ducts Most **adenocarcinomas** Mean age: 70s Regions affected: **proximal 1/3** of CBD (MC, Klatskin's tumor, poor prognosis), distal extrahepatic (best prognosis), intrahepatic RF: **PSC** (major), UC, choledochal cysts, *Clonorchis sinensis* (liver fluke)	1. Obstructive jaundice–dark urine, clay stool, itching 2. Weight loss	1. Cholangiography–PTC or ERCP for DX and resectability	1. Stent placement for Klatskin's tumor (most nonresectable) 2. Chemotherapy, biliary drainage) Prognosis: <1 y after diagnosis

(continued)

(continued)

Disease	Etiology, Prevalence, Risk Factors	Clinical Symptoms and Signs	Diagnostics	Therapy, Prognosis, and Health Maintenance
Carcinoid tumors and syndrome	Originate from neuroen-docrine cells, secrete serotonin MC site: **appendix**	Syndrome (10%): 1. Cutaneous flushing 2. Diarrhea 3. Sweating 4. Wheezing 5. Abdominal pain 6. Heart valve dysfunction	1. **Bronchoscopy:** pink or purple central lesion, well-vascular-ized, pedunculated, or sessile 2. CT and octreotide scintigraphy localize the disease and moni-tor growth	1. Surgical resection 2. Octreotide for symptoms Metastasis risk increased with size

CELIAC DISEASE

Disease	Etiology, Prevalence, Risk Factors	Clinical Symptoms and Signs	Diagnostics	Therapy, Prognosis, and Health Maintenance
Celiac sprue	Autoimmune disease caused by transglu-taminase antibodies after being exposed to gluten → reacts with small intestine causing villus atrophy Hypersensitivity to gluten caused by autoanti-bodies that attack the intestinal villi	1. **Diarrhea**, weight loss 2. Abdominal distention, **bloating** 3. **Infertility** in women Signs: 1. **Dermatitis herpeti-formis** (10%): vesicular rash found on extensor surfaces of arms and legs	1. (+) **anti-endomy-sial antibodies** OR anti-transglutaminase antibodies 2. **Biopsy in proximal small bowel:** Villus atrophy and blunting in the small bowel 3. **Iron deficiency anemia** (poor iron absorption) 4. **Megaloblastic ane-mia** (poor folic acid/B_{12} absorption)	1. Gluten free diet Prognosis: 1. Increased risk of cirrhosis

CHAPTER 18

Orthopedics and Rheumatology

Refer to Family Medicine ⚕ **for in-depth coverage of the following topics:**

Recommended Topics:

POLYARTERITIS NODOSA (PAN)

- Vasculitis of medium-sized vessels involving the nervous system and GI tract
- Pathophysiology: PMN invasion of all layers and fibrinoid necrosis plus resulting intimal proliferation lead to reduced luminal area, which results in ischemia, infarction, and aneurysms
- No pulmonary involvement! Distinguishes this from Wegener's granulomatosis

Disease	Etiology, Prevalence, Risk Factors	Clinical Symptoms and Signs	Diagnostics	Therapy, Prognosis, and Health Maintenance
Polyarteritis nodosa (PAN)	Associated: **hepatitis B**, HIV, drug reactions	1. Early symptoms are **constitutional symptoms** (fever, weakness, weight loss, myalgias, and arthralgias) 2. **Abdominal pain** (bowel angina) 3. **HTN** Signs: 1. Mononeuritic multiplex 2. Livedo reticularis (Fig. 18-1)	1. **Biopsy** of involved tissue or mesenteric angiography 2. ESR: high 3. +/− p-ANCA 4. Test for FOBT	1. **Corticosteroids** • If severe, add cyclophosphamide Prognosis: Poor, but improved to limited extent with treatment

POLYMYOSITIS

Condition does not involve the skin.

- Dermatomyositis—when polymyositis is associated with a skin rash
- Hypothesis: genetically susceptible individual + environmental trigger
- Pathologic changes
  - Dermatomyositis—humoral immune mechanisms
  - Polymyositis and inclusion body—cell-mediated process

Disease	Etiology, Prevalence, Risk Factors	Clinical Symptoms and Signs	Diagnostics	Therapy, Prognosis, and Health Maintenance

Polymyositis	Females	1. Symmetrical **proximal *muscle weakness***, develops subacutely over weeks or months
		• Earliest and most severely affected muscles: neck flexors, shoulder girdle, and pelvic girdle
		• **Myalgias** (33%)
		• **Dysphagia** (30%)
		2. Dermatomyositis (Fig. 18-2)
		• *Heliotrope rash* (butterfly): eyes, bridge of nose, cheeks
		• *Gottron's papules*: papular, red, scaly lesions over knuckles (MCP, PIP, DIP)
		• *V-sign*: rash on face, neck, and anterior chest
		• *Shawl sign*: rash on shoulders, upper back, elbows, and knees
		• Periungual erythema with telangiectasias
		• Subcutaneous calcifications (children)
		• Associated findings
		  • **Arthralgias** (common)
		  • CHF and conduction defects
		  • Interstitial lung disease
		3. Dermatomyositis only
		• Vasculitis of GI tract, kidneys, lungs, eyes (children)
		• **Increased malignancy risk** in adults (lung, breast, ovary, GI tract, myeloproliferative disorders)
			DX criteria:
			1. If 2 of first 4 → possible
			2. If 3 of first 4 → probable
			3. If all 4 → definite
			• Symmetric ***proximal muscle weakness***
			• Elevation in serum creatinine phosphokinase
			• **EMG** findings of a myopathy
			• **Biopsy** evidence of myositis
			• Characteristic rash
			Labs:
			• **CK elevated**, corresponds to degree of necrosis/severity
			• LDH, aldolase, AST/ALT elevated
			• (+) ANA in 50%
			• Anti-synthetase antibodies (***anti-Jo-1***): abrupt onset fever, cracked hands, Raynaud's, pulmonary fibrosis, arthritis → does not respond well
			• Anti-signal recognition particle: cardiac manifestations and worst prognosis
			• **EMG**: abnormal in 90%
			• **Muscle biopsy**: inflammation and muscle fiber FIBROSIS
			• Dermato: perivascular and perimysial
			• Poly and IBM: **endomysial**
				1. **Steroids** (initial) until symptomatic improvement, then taper up to 2 y
				2. Immunosuppressants: methotrexate, cyclophosphamide, chlorambucil
				3. Physical therapy

- *Inclusion body myositis* - affects males more often, absence of autoantibodies; distal muscle involvement and relatively low creatine kinase (CK); poor prognosis

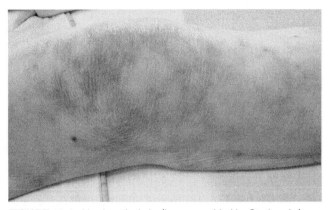

FIGURE 18-1. Livedo reticularis. (Image provided by Stedman's.)

POLYMYALGIA RHEUMATICA

- 10% develop temporal arteritis, whereas 40% to 50% of people with temporal arteritis have coexisting polymyalgia rheumatica

Disease	Etiology, Prevalence, Risk Factors	Clinical Symptoms and Signs	Diagnostics	Therapy, Prognosis, and Health Maintenance

Polymyalgia rheumatica	Elderly (mean: 70), more common in F HLA-DR4 allele	1. **Hip and shoulder muscle *pain*** (bilateral): abrupt stiffness in shoulder and hip regions after long period of inactivity
		2. **Constitutional symptoms**: malaise, fever, depression, weight loss, fatigue
		3. **Joint swelling**: up to 20% have synovitis in knees, wrists, or hand joints (tenosynovitis and synovitis around shoulder may lead to rotator cuff tendinitis or adhesive capsulitis)
		4. Signs/SX of **temporal arteritis**
			Clinical DX
			1. ESR: elevated
			  • >50, but can be >100
			  • Correlates with disease activity
				1. **Corticosteroids**
				  • Responds in 1-7 d
				  • Taper after 4-6 wk
				  • Most people stop steroids in 1-2 y
				Self-limited: 1-2 y
				Few patients have symptoms for up to 10 y

SYSTEMIC SCLEROSIS (SCLERODERMA)

Chronic connective tissue disorder that can lead to widespread fibrosis.

- Cytokines stimulate fibroblasts, causing abnormally *high quantity* of collagen deposition, which causes the problem associated with the disease
- Lupus glomerulonephritis (GN, present at diagnosis): most common finding

Disease	Etiology, Prevalence, Risk Factors	Clinical Symptoms and Signs	Diagnostics	Therapy, Prognosis, and Health Maintenance

Scleroderma	F, age 35-50 (Fig. 18-3)	1. **Raynaud's phenomenon**
		  • Cutaneous fibrosis: **sclerodactyly** (claw-like appearance), can lead to contractures disability, and disfigurement
		2. **GI**: most patients, dysphagia/reflux from esophageal motility, delayed gastric emptying, constipation/diarrhea, abdominal distention, prolonged reflux can lead to strictures
		3. Lungs: most common cause of death; **interstitial fibrosis** +/− pulm HTN
		4. Cardiac: pericardial effusion, myocardial involvement, arrhythmias
		5. Renal: renal crisis (malignant HTN) with diffuse disease
			1. All have elevated ANAs
			2. **Anticentromere Ab:** very specific for LIMITED (CREST syndrome)
			3. **Anti-topoisomerase I** (Anti-Scl-70) Ab: very specific for DIFFUSE
			Barium swallow (esophageal dysmotility) and PFTs
				1. No effective cure
				2. Treat SX:
				  • **NSAIDs** for musculoskeletal pains
				  • **H2 blockers** or PPI for reflux
				3. Raynaud's—avoid cold and smoking, keep hands warm, use CCB if severe
				4. Treat pulmonary and renal complications if present

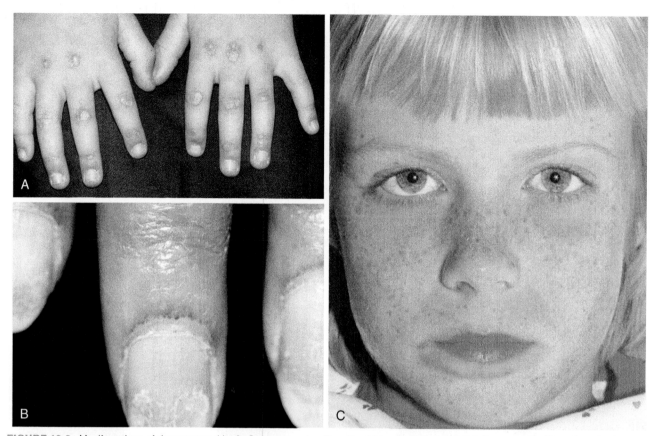

FIGURE 18-2. Manifestations of dermatomyositis. **A**, Gottron papules, **B**, nailbed telangiectasias, and **C**, heliotrope rash. (From Coombs C. *Oski's Pediatric Certification and Recertifications Board Review.* Philadelphia: Wolters Kluwer Health; 2011.)

Diffuse versus Limited Disease

Diffuse	Limited
Widespread skin involvement	Skin involvement limited to distal extremities (face, neck), sparing the trunk
Rapid onset	Delayed onset—skin involvement slowly after onset of long-history of Raynaud's phenomenon
Significant visceral involvement (ie, fibrosis of internal organs)—lung, heart, GI tract, kidneys	Visceral involvement (late)—pulmonary HTN and ischemic vascular disease Minimal constitutional SX
Associated with ANAs, absence of centromere Ab	Anticentromere Ab (most patients)
Poor prognosis—10-y survival is 40%-65%	Better prognosis, normal life span unless severe pulm HTN
• Peripheral edema (hands/legs), polyarthritis, fatigue, weakness, carpal tunnel syndrome • Renal failure can occur • **Interstitial lung disease** (more common)	**CREST syndrome:** • **C**alcinosis of the digits • **R**aynaud phenomenon • **E**sophageal motility disorder • **S**clerodactyly of fingers • **T**elangiectasias (over digits, under nails)

SJÖGREN SYNDROME

Disease	Etiology, Prevalence, Risk Factors	Clinical Symptoms and Signs	Diagnostics	Therapy, Prognosis, and Health Maintenance
Sjögren syndrome	Autoimmune disease most commonly seen in women Lymphocytes infiltrate and destroy the lacrimal and salivary glands 20% with scleroderma have Sjögren syndrome	Primary: 1. **Dry eyes and dry mouth** • Burning, redness, blurred vision (Fig. 18-4) 2. Arthralgias, arthritis, fatigue 3. **Extraglandular manifestations**: chronic arthritis, interstitial nephritis, vasculitis Secondary: 1. Dry eyes and mouth 2. Another connective tissue disease (RA, scleroderma, SLE, polymyositis)	1. ANA (+) in 95%, RF (+) in 50%-75% 2. **Anti-Ro (SS-A)** in 55%, La (SS-B) Ab in 40% 3. Nonspecific: high ESR, normocytic and normochromic anemia, leukopenia 4. Schirmer test: filter paper inserted into eye to measure lacrimal gland output 5. Salivary gland biopsy (lip/parotid): most accurate, not needed for dx	1. Pilocarpine or Cevimeline • Increases oral/ocular secretions 2. Artificial tears 3. Good oral hygiene 4. NSAIDs, steroids Increased risk of *non-Hodgkin lymphoma* (most common cause of death)

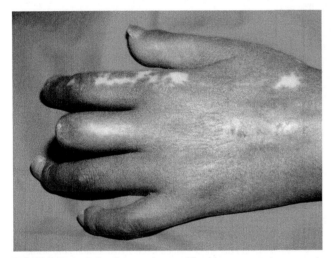

FIGURE 18-3. Scleroderma stigmata. Distal bone resorption caused the third digit to be shortened in this patient. (From Goodheart HP, MD. *Goodheart's Photoguide of Common Skin Disorders*, 2nd Edition. Philadelphia: Lippincott Williams & Wilkins; 2003.)

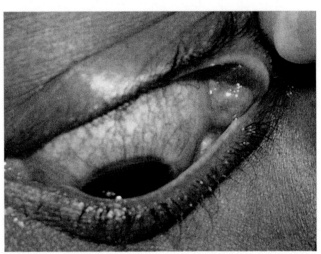

FIGURE 18-4. Sjögren syndrome ocular manifestations. Chronic dry eyes, also known as keratitis sicca or keratoconjunctivitis sicca, can lead to scarring or infection of the eyes. Blepharitis, or inflammation of the eyelid, may also be seen. (From Jensen S. *Nursing Health Assessment: A Best Practice Approach*. Philadelphia: Wolters Kluwer Health; 2011.)

Internal Medicine

CHAPTER 19

Endocrinology

Recommended Supplemental Resources:

HYPERTHYROIDISM/ THYROIDITIS, HYPOTHYROIDISM, HYPOPARATHYROIDISM, HYPERPARATHYROIDISM

- T4 is converted to T3 by deiodination outside of the thyroid

- T3 is more biologically active than T4

- Most of T4 (and T3) is reversibly bound to TBG and is inactive—it is highly bound to protein, especially albumin, and can cause hypoalbuminemia when too elevated

- Factors that increase TBG (and total T4): pregnancy, liver disease, OCPs and ASA

Disease	Etiology, Prevalence, Risk Factors	Clinical Symptoms and Signs	Diagnostics	Therapy, Prognosis, and Health Maintenance
Hyper-parathyroidism	Primary: One or more glands produce inappropriate PTH relative to calcium MCC: **Parathyroid adenoma** Secondary: High PTH and low or NL calcium MCC: **Chronic renal failure**, vitamin D deficiency, renal hypercalciuria Most found incidentally by hypercalcemia on routine lab testing Most F >50	Most asymptomatic 1. Stones: **nephrolithiasis**, frequent urination 2. Bones: body aches and pains 　• **Osteitis fibrosa cystica** (brown tumors)—predisposes to fracture 　• **Weakness** 3. Groans **Abdominal pain, constipation**, nausea, vomiting, anorexia 4. Psychiatric overtones: **depression**, *fatigue*, anorexia, sleep disturbance, **anxiety**, lethargy Signs: 1. **Hypertensive** 2. **Decreased DTRs**	Serum calcium: **high (hypercalcemia)** Serum phosphate: low (**hypophosphatemia**) 1. Serum PTH (first line): **high** 　• Total and ionized calcium: high 　• Albumin: low 　• Urine cAMP: high 　• Hypercalciuria 2. X-ray: subperiosteal bone resorption, osteopenia	1. If serum calcium >12 mg/dL 　• IV fluid resuscitation 2. Otherwise, follow up Primary: 1. β-blockers, K-phosphate supplementation, dietary calcium restriction 2. Bisphosphonates 3. Calcimimetic agents: cinacalcet 4. Parathyroidectomy (definitive) Secondary: 1. 400 IU vitamin D (calcitriol) daily for vitamin D deficiency 　• Annual calcium and Cr measurements 　• Annual KUB for stones 　• DEXA: every 2-3 y 2. PO calcium, dietary phosphorous restriction for renal failure

(continued)

(continued)

Disease	Etiology, Prevalence, Risk Factors	Clinical Symptoms and Signs	Diagnostics	Therapy, Prognosis, and Health Maintenance
Hypo-parathyroidism	MCC: Head and neck surgery—**thyroidectomy**, parathyroidectomy; nonsurgical is rare	1. **Numbness and tingling**—fingers, toes, tip of nose 2. Tetany: **hyperactive DTRs** 3. Rickets, osteomalacia 4. Cataracts Signs: 1. Chvostek sign (tap facial nerve, contraction of muscles) 2. Trousseau sign (carpal spasms with inflating BP cuff higher than systolic BP × 3 min)	EKG: **QT prolongation** PTH: low Low serum calcium: Hypocalcemia High serum phosphate Low urine calcium NL alkaline phosphatase	1. Mild to moderate: **PO calcium supplements** 2. Vitamin D (calcitriol) • Goal: 8-8.5 • Too high can cause kidney stones 3. Severe: IV calcium gluconate
Hyper-thyroidism (thyrotoxicosis)	Associated: atrial fibrillation Subclinical hyperthyroidism = low TSH, normal T3/T4	1. Anxiety, nervousness, insomnia, irritability 2. Palpitations 3. Weight loss 4. Heat intolerance, Sweating 5. Diarrhea, increased frequency 6. Oligomenorrhea 7. Tremor, hyperactivity, tremulousness Signs: 1. Moist skin 2. **Tachycardia** 3. **Hyperreflexive** 4. Flushed, diaphoretic skin 5. Wide pulse pressure	Primary hyperthyroidism: 1. **Thyroid function tests (TFTs)** TSH: low Total T3: high Free T4: high 2. **Autoantibody tests** • Anti-thyroid peroxidase Ab • TS-immunoglobulin 3. **Scintigraphy (thyroid scan with I-123)**—if etiology unclear after initial labs	1. Symptomatic relief A. **Propranolol** (relieves tachycardia, tremor, sweating, anxiety) • Contraindicated in pregnancy 2. Anti-thyroid medications • Methimazole • Contraindicated in pregnancy • Potent, long acting • Propylthiouracil (PTU) • Recommended in pregnancy and thyroid storm 3. RAI (I-131) therapy • Not for children <5 or severe ophthalmopathy • Contraindication: Pregnancy, breast feeding, lactation 4. Thyroidectomy • Indicated in pregnancy if treatment with PTU unsuccessful • Large goiters, severe ophthalmopathy • Noncompliant or intolerant to antithyroids • Refractory amiodarone induced
Graves' disease (diffuse toxic goiter)–80%	Metabolically active gland **Most common cause of hyperthyroidism** Mostly younger women with other autoimmune conditions **Autoimmune**; thyroid stimulating IgG antibody binds TSH receptors on surface of thyroid cells triggering synthesis of excess thyroid hormone	1. ***Pretibial myxedema*** 2. Exophthalmos: periorbital edema, diplopia, or proptosis 3. Thyroid bruit 4. Diffusely enlarged, symmetric, ***nontender*** gland	1. Measurement of thyroid antibodies • Anti-TPO: high • TSI: high 2. Scintigraphy: ***diffuse uptake***	1. Antithyroid Meds as above • May experience remission for 12-18 mo • Titrate every 4 wk until normalized 2. **Radioactive iodine (I-131) preferred** 3. Saline eye drops and tight-fitting sunglasses 4. High-dose steroids with orbital decompression surgery and ocular radiation therapy for severe exophthalmos

Internal Medicine

Disease	Etiology, Prevalence, Risk Factors	Clinical Symptoms and Signs	Diagnostics	Therapy, Prognosis, and Health Maintenance
Multinodular toxic goiter (Plummer disease)–15%	Hyperfunctioning areas that produce high T4 and T3 levels, decreasing TSH → rest of thyroid doesn't function (atrophy with low TSH) MC: Elderly F	Multinodular, bumpy, **irregular, asymmetric**	1. Measurement of thyroid antibodies • Anti-TPO: low or absent 2. Scintigraphy: *patchy* uptake	1. Symptomatic relief A. **Propranolol** (relieves tachycardia, tremor, sweating, anxiety) • Contraindicated in pregnancy 2. Anti-thyroid medications 3. *Radioactive iodine* therapy (preferred)
Toxic adenoma–2%		Single nodule with atrophic gland	1. Measurement of thyroid antibodies • Anti-TPO: low or absent 2. Scintigraphy: very low RAI uptake	
Thyroid storm	Rare, life-threatening complication of thyrotoxicosis Acute exacerbation of hyperthyroidism Precipitating factors: Infection, DKA, stress (trauma, surgery, illness, labor)	1. Marked fever 2. Agitation, psychosis 3. Confusion 4. Nausea, vomiting, diarrhea Signs: Tachycardia		1. Supportive therapy 2. Antithyroid agents • PTU q 2 h • Iodine 3. • β-blockers: HR control • Dexamethasone: generates peripheral T3 from T4, adrenal support High mortality–20%
Hypothyroidism	1. Primary: failure of thyroid to produce sufficient T3 (95%) • Iatrogenic–prior treatment of hyperthyroidism (lithium, thyroidectomy, iodine therapy) • Hashimoto's thyroiditis 2. Secondary: hypothyroidism due to pituitary disease (TSH deficiency), low TSH/free T4 3. Tertiary: due to hypothalamic disease (TRH deficiency), low TSH/free T4 Associated: Carpal tunnel syndrome	1. **Constipation** 2. **Fatigue**, lethargy, **weakness** 3. Weight gain (10-30 lb) 4. **Depression** 5. Menorrhagia 6. Cold intolerance 7. Cramps (Charley horses) 8. Slow mentation, inability to concentrate, dull expression 9. Muscle weakness, arthralgias 10. Hoarseness Signs: 1. Dry, rough skin, coarse hair 2. Palpable enlarged thyroid, 3. Brittle nails 4. Puffy face and eyelids 5. Yellowing of skin (carotenemia) 6. **Decreased DTRs**	1. Thyroid function tests Primary–**high TSH** (most sensitive) Secondary–low TSH Tertiary–low TSH Free T4–**low** in clinically overt 2. Antibody Testing 3. CBC: **Normocytic anemia (MC)**	1. **Levothyroxine** (T4) → effects in 2-4 wk → Monitor TSH and clinical state periodically

Goiter

Disease	Etiology, Prevalence, Risk Factors	Clinical Symptoms and Signs	Diagnostics	Therapy, Prognosis, and Health Maintenance
Subacute (granulomatous) thyroiditis (hypothyroidism)	Gland is releasing preformed thyroid hormone Follows *viral illness*, assoc. HLA-B35	1. Prodromal phase (weeks): fever, flu-like illness 2. Transient **hyperthyroidism** (leak of T3/T4 from inflamed gland) → euthyroid → **hypothyroid** 3. *Painful*, **tender**, enlarged goiter, symmetric	1. TSH: low (secondary to increased T4/T3) 2. High ESR 3. RAI uptake scan–low uptake	1. Self-limited • NSAIDs and ASA, steroids for refractory pain
Hashimoto's thyroiditis (chronic lymphocytic) (hypothyroidism)	MCC: Autoimmune thyroid disorder, and **most common cause of hypothyroidism** MC in F Genetics (+) FH common Slow decline in thyroid function	1. Puffiness of face and eyelids: Periorbital myxedema 2. Thinning of outer halves of eyebrows 3. *Goiter* (MC feature): hard, nonpainful, nontender, multi nodular, irregular, asymmetric	1. **Anti-peroxidase antibodies** (90% +) 2. Anti-thyroglobulin Ab (50% +) 3. **Anti-microsomal antibodies:** high 4. Irregular I-131 on thyroid scan (not required to DX)	1. Levothyroxine (T4)
Myxedema coma	Rare condition Precipitating factors: cold exposure, infection, trauma, narcotics	1. Depressed state of consciousness 2. Profound *hypothermia* 3. Respiratory depression		1. Supportive therapy for BP and breathing 2. **IV thyroxine** 3. **IV hydrocortisone** High mortality rate: 50%-75%

ADDISON'S DISEASE

Disease	Etiology, Prevalence, Risk Factors	Clinical Symptoms and Signs	Diagnostics	Therapy, Prognosis, and Health Maintenance
Primary adrenal insufficiency (**Addison disease**) "Chronic adrenocortical insufficiency"	Adrenal gland does not produce cortisol, aldosterone, or sex hormones (retain no sodium) Primary adrenal failure from **autoimmune adrenalitis**	1. **Hyperpigmentation** due to increased ACTH, MSH (POMC) 2. GI: Anorexia, **abdominal pain, nausea, vomiting**, weight loss 3. **Lethargy**, confusion, psychosis 4. Weakness, malaise 5. Postural hypotension, dizziness 6. Salt craving Signs: *Hypotension* (orthostasis)	1. Electrolytes • Serum Na: low (**hyponatremia**) • Serum K+: high (**hyperkalemia**) • Hypercalcemia • **Hypoglycemia** • Elevated SCr 2. Serum cortisol: low 3. Serum **ACTH: high** Low aldosterone and high renin 4. Standard ACTH test or **Cosyntropin test** (definitive) • Cortisol will *not* elevate sufficiently	1. **Daily oral steroids** • Hydrocortisone, prednisone 2. **Daily fludrocortisone** (mineralocorticoid)
Secondary adrenal insufficiency	**Long-term steroid therapy**—most common cause overall Dysfunction of the hypothalamic-pituitary component of HPA axis: only steroid and androgen deficiency present	HX: prior use of oral steroids–shuts down adrenal axis and causes acute adrenal crisis when stopped 1. Weakness, malaise 2. Postural hypotension 3. Lethargy, confusion, psychosis Signs: Alabaster pale skin	1. Electrolytes • Hyponatremia • Hyperkalemia • **Hypoglycemia** 2. Serum cortisol: low 3. Serum **ACTH: low** • NL aldosterone and renin 4. ACTH test • Cortisol will not respond at all	1. Only daily steroid required

Disease	Etiology, Prevalence, Risk Factors	Clinical Symptoms and Signs	Diagnostics	Therapy, Prognosis, and Health Maintenance
Addisonian (adrenal) crisis	Hypotension refractory to IV fluids or acutely ill patients with chronic steroid use (moon facies, buffalo hump) Any stress (eg, trauma, infection, surgery) can precipitate adrenal crisis	1. Fatigue, anorexia, generalized aches, weakness, lethargy, abdominal pain, nausea, vomiting 2. **Shock**–refractory to fluids or vasopressors Signs: Severe hypotension (**orthostasis**)	1. Electrolytes • Serum Na: low (*hyponatremia*) • Serum K: high (*hyperkalemia*) • Hypercalcemia • **Hypoglycemia** • Elevated SCr • Metabolic acidosis 2. Acute renal failure 3. **Cortisol**: low (<3 ug/dL) 4. **ACTH stimulation test or Cosyntropin** test–cortisol will not elevate sufficiently	1. IV *hydrocortisone* **100 mg q 8 h** 2. Fludrocortisone 0.05-0.2 mg/d for mineralocorticoid support 3. IV fluids (several liters of normal saline with 5% dextrose), and a search for the underlying condition that precipitated the crisis 4. Monitor fluid intake and output, and serum K+ levels frequently
Primary aldosteronism (Conn syndrome)	Benign **adenoma of the adrenal cortex** (makes aldosterone, retain sodium)	1. Patient on no medications with hypertension	1. Electrolytes–**Hypokalemia (unprovoked)** • Hypernatremia	
Cushing syndrome (hypercortisolism)	Excessive exogenous cortisol Most common cause: **iatrogenic** due to prescribed prednisone (steroids), androgen excess absent (exogenous steroids suppress production by adrenals) Second most common cause: 1. ACTH-secreting **adenoma** (also known as Cushing disease) → bilateral adrenal hyperplasia (androgen excess common)	1. Purple striae, buffalo hump, central obesity 2. "Moon" facies, lanugo hair, acne, easy bruising 3. **Proximal muscle weakness** and wasting, osteoporosis, AVN of femoral head 4. Headache 5. Depression, mania Signs: 1. Hypertension 2. **Diabetes** (decreased glucose tolerance) 3. **Menstrual irregularity, infertility** (hypogonadism) 4. Cushing disease only: masculinization (androgen excess)	1. **HD dexamethasone suppression test** • Decrease by 50% 2. Midnight serum cortisol, late night salivary cortisol 3. Urinary free cortisol 4. CT or MRI Sustained elevated cortisol: Hypercortisolism Hypokalemia Hyperglycemia Glucosuria	If iatrogenic → taper steroids 1. If ACTH-secreting pituitary adenoma → transsphenoidal resection of tumor 2. Adrenal adenoma → pituitary radiation, medical adrenalectomy 3. Bilateral adrenalectomy Ectopic ACTH production (**2/3 SCC from lungs**)

PHEOCHROMOCYTOMA

Disease	Etiology, Prevalence, Risk Factors	Clinical Symptoms and Signs	Diagnostics	Therapy, Prognosis, and Health Maintenance
Pheochromocytoma	Rare tumors that produce, store, and secrete catecholamines from the adrenal medulla (90%) Arise from chromaffin cells (adrenal medulla) or from sympathetic ganglia (extrarenal) Pheochromocytoma is associated with MEN 2A and MEN 2B, von Recklinghausen neurofibromatosis, von Hippel–Lindau disease	1. Paroxysms of **headache** 2. Profuse **sweating**, *palpitations* 3. Weight loss 4. *Feelings of warmth* along with **episodic** (later sustained) **hypertension**, sometimes severe • Feeling of impending doom Signs: **Tachycardia**	1. **24-h urine metanephrines** Plasma metanephrines > urine metanephrines 2. CT or MRI 3. Other: **glucosuria**, hyperlipidemia, hypokalemia, hypercalcemia	Give clonidine if equivocal results 1. Tumor resection with ligation of venous drainage (**laparoscopic adrenalectomy**) • α blockers: **phenoxybenzamine** × 10-14 d prior to surgery to control BP and replete intravascular volume • β-blockers: propranolol 2-3 d prior to surgery to control HR Fatal if left undiagnosed and treated

- Rule of TENS for pheochromocytoma
  - 10% are familial, 10% are bilateral (suspect MEN type II)
  - 10% are malignant, 10% are multiple
  - 10% occur in children, 10% are extra-adrenal (malignant)
  - The most common site is **organ of Zuckerkandl** (at aortic bifurcation)

DIABETES

- Water restriction test: restricting water intake raises the plasma osmolality → progressive elevation in ADH release → retention of water → increases urine osmolality (in normal individuals)

- Must measure urine volume and osmolarity every hour and plasma sodium concentration and osmolality every 2 hours
- No drinking 2 to 3 hours before test
- Continue until urine osmolality reaches normal value (above 600) indicating that ADH release and effect are intact
- Once plasma osmolality reaches 295 to 300 mOsmol/kg (N: 275 to 290) or plasma sodium 145 meq/L or higher, the effect of endogenous ADH of kidney is maximal; thus, administering DDAVP (desmopressin) will not further elevate urine osmolality unless endogenous ADH release is impaired (ie, unless patient has central DI)
- Unless inappropriately dilute urine present in setting of serum hyperosmolarity → attempt a fluid deprivation test

Diabetes Insipidus

Disease	Etiology, Prevalence, Risk Factors	Clinical Symptoms and Signs	Diagnostics	Therapy, Prognosis, and Health Maintenance
Primary polydipsia (Psychogenic, water intoxication): secondary insufficiency of ADH due to physiologic inhibition of ADH secretion by excess water intake	Middle aged women, patients with psychiatric illness, carbamazepine, thiazide diuretics	1. Polyuria–appropriate response to increased H_2O intake • Gradual	1. Plasma Na^+ concentration: low (<137), **hyponatremia** 2. Plasma osmolality: 255-280 (NL) 3. Urine osmolality: low	1. Do not treat with antidiuretics–eliminating polyuria does not eliminate urge to drink 2. Patient education
Diabetes insipidus Excretion of a large volume of dilute urine (osmolality <250 mOsmol/kg)		1. **Polyuria**: urinary frequency, enuresis 2. **Nocturia**–may disturb sleep and cause daytime fatigue or somnolence 3. **Polydipsia**–increase in fluid intake	1. Plasma sodium concentration: high (>142), **hypernatremia** (only occurs if patient has thirst defect or no access to water) 2. 24-h urine collection: >50 mL/kg/d Urine osmolality: low (<300) 3. **Water restriction test** (confirmatory)–differentiates central diabetes insipidus from primary polydipsia 4. Administer exogenous ADH once plasma osmolarity reaches 295-300 or plasma sodium 145+ • Increase of >50% indicates pituitary DI	
Central diabetes insipidus (neurohypophyseal, neurogenic): deficient secretion of ADH resulting in variable degree of polyuria *"The sodium is high, in central DI"*	*Idiopathic* (50%), possibly autoimmune injury to ADH producing cells, but also, pituitary surgery, trauma, hypoxia, or ischemia **Most common type**	1. **Polyuria** (5-10 L in 24 h) • Abrupt • Excretion of dilute colorless urine 2. Polydipsia 3. Nocturia	1. Plasma sodium concentration: high (**Hypernatremia**) Plasma osmolality: 280-310 (high) 2. Urine osmolality: <150 mOsm/L (low), low specific gravity 3. **Water restriction and desmopressin test**: *increase in urine osmolality by >300* 4. ADH: *low* (takes forever to get results)	1. **Desmopressin** (DDAVP) • Acts at V2 receptors to increase urine concentration and decrease urine flow • Via nasal spray, PO, or injection 2. **Chlorpropamide**– increases ADH secretion and enhances effect of ADH (retain H_2O)

Disease	Etiology, Prevalence, Risk Factors	Clinical Symptoms and Signs	Diagnostics	Therapy, Prognosis, and Health Maintenance

Nephrogenic diabetes insipidus
Normal ADH secretion, but varying renal resistance to water-retaining effect
	Children: X-linked
	Acquired from drug exposure: **chronic lithium use**, amphotericin B, metabolic conditions (hypercalcemia, hypokalemia), or renal damage
		1. Polyuria
		  • Gradual
		2. Nocturia
			1. Plasma sodium concentration: high (*hypernatremia*)
			  • Plasma osmolality: 280-310 (high)
			2. Urine osmolality: low
			3. **Water restriction and desmopressin test:** will not increase urine osmolality
			4. ADH: *NL to high*
				1. High dose of DDAVP
				2. **Thiazide diuretics:** +/− amiloride with **low sodium diet** and indomethacin
				  • AE: hypokalemia, gastric irritation

Diabetes Mellitus (Types I and II)

Disease	Etiology, Prevalence, Risk Factors	Clinical Symptoms and Signs	Diagnostics	Therapy, Prognosis, and Health Maintenance
Type I	Onset: Slow in adults, **rapid in children** **Autoimmune, Finland/ Sardinia (by Italy) children** **Type 1A:** immune mediated, HLA associated, White, no family history, Autoantibody (+) **Type 1B:** idiopathic, AA/Asian, autoantibody (−), family history	3 Ps: 1. **P**olyuria 2. **P**olydipsia 3. **P**olyphagia 4. **W**eight loss 5. **I**nfection 6. **N**octuria 7. Blurry vision	1. Autoimmune markers (90% +) 2. GAD65 autoantibodies 3. Islet cell autoantibodies 4. Insulin autoantibodies 5. C-peptide (low)—no active insulin in body	Insulin pen Vial and−basal + bolus with carbohydrate counting Check glucose at LEAST 4 × daily

Type II	Insulin resistance: hyperinsulinemic at first, then hypoinsulinemic
	Insulin resistance does not change—**insulin SECRETION** changes
	B-cell decline is gradual
	Deficiency of amylin
	Deficiency of GLP-1: stops glucagon, satiety, increases insulin release
	Postprandial glucose increases over time−not making insulin to control
	Genetics−first degree relative
	Age
	Obesity
		Blurred vision
		3 Ps: **P**olyuria, **p**olydipsia, **p**olyphagia
		WIN: **W**eight loss
		Infection (frequent): UTI, yeast infection, fungal
		Nocturia
		Acanthosis nigricans: hyperpigmented, **velvety** plaques of body folds
		Ketonuria and weight loss (rare)
		Other:
		Fatigue, pruritus, recurrent candidal vaginitis, chronic skin infections, blurred vision, poor wound healing
			American Diabetes Association (ADA)
			1. Random glucose >200 mg/dL (with symptoms)
			2. Fasting >126 mg/dL (2+ occasions)
			3. **HbA1C > 6.5%**
			  • Used to monitor control
			4. OGTT if fasting levels 100-125 mg/dL
			Diabetic dyslipidemia: high triglycerides, low HDL, altered LDL
				1. Primary efforts: diet, exercise, weight loss
				  • Diet: High protein, low fat, no artificial sweetener, low cholesterol
				  • Exercise 150 min/wk
				  • 5%-7% weight loss
				2. Metformin
				Pre-diabetes:
				HbA1C goal: 6%-6.5%
				FBS goal: 100-124
				Post-prandial (1-2 h after meals): <180
				Monitor/treat any CV risk factors
				Screen for diabetes **annually**

- **Dawn phenomenon:** increased resistance to insulin in the early morning due to counter-regulatory hormones
  - Increase overnight basal insulin, exercise, metformin, TZD
- **Somogyi phenomenon:** rebound fasting hyperglycemia following undetected hypoglycemia overnight
  - Excessive hunger, weight gain, worsening hyperglycemia
  - Decrease overnight basal insulin or eat a snack at bedtime

Screening Adults for Diabetes

- All adults overweight (**BMI >25 or >23** in Asian Americans) with risk factors
  - Physical inactivity, first degree relatives with DM, high risk race/ethnicity

- Women who delivered >9 lb. baby or diagnosed with GDM
- Hypertension (>140/90 or on HTN therapy)
- HDL <35 mg/dL +/− triglycerides >250 mg/dL
- Women with PCOS
- A1C >5.7%, IGT or IFG on previous testing
- Other clinical conditions showing insulin resistance (acanthosis nigricans, severely obese)
- History of CVD
- All patients at age 45, especially if overweight or obese
- If normal results, repeat every 3 years at minimum

	HbA1C (%)	Fasting Glucose (mg/dL)	75 g Oral Glucose Tolerance Test (mg/dL)	Treatment
Normal	≤5.7	≤99	≤139	Weight loss, diet counseling, physical activity, monitor/treat CV risk factors, screen at least every 3 y
Pre-diabetes	5.7-6.4	100-125	140-199	Lifestyle changes + Screen annually
Diabetes	≥6.5	≥126	≥200	Lifestyle changes + Screen annually + Metformin

THYROID

- FNA Biopsy Results
  - Cold = hypofunctioning (decreased accumulation of radioactive iodine) → lobectomy
  - Warm = normal functioning
  - Hot = hyperfunctioning (increased accumulation of radioactive iodine)

- **Thyroglobulin (Tg):** Thyroglobulin is a protein produced by *thyroid cells* (both normal and cancerous cells)
  - After removal of the thyroid gland, Thyroglobulin can be used as a "cancer marker." Its number should be as low as possible, termed "undetectable."
  - After surgery and RAI, it may take months or years for the Tg number to come down to zero or undetectable
  - A positive Tg test indicates that thyroid cells, either normal or cancerous, are still present in your body

Thyroid Nodules

Disease	Etiology, Prevalence, Risk Factors	Clinical Symptoms and Signs	Diagnostics	Therapy, Prognosis, and Health Maintenance
Thyroid nodules	Cancer found in 4%-10% of investigated nodules	1. Fixed nodule without movement on swallowing • Firm, irregular 2. HX of radiation therapy to neck or family history 3. Rapid progression 4. Obstructive symptoms: vocal cord paralysis, dysphagia, odynophagia Signs: 1. Must be >1 cm to be palpable on exam	1. Thyroid tests (TTs) • TSH • T3, T4 • Serum calcitonin: high 2. Thyroid ultrasound • Only differentiates solid vs. cystic 3. **Fine needle aspiration biopsy** (initial) • Even if clinically and chemically euthyroid, if <u>palpable or >1.5 cm</u> • Only reliable test that differentiates benign vs. malignant • Reliable for all cancers, except follicular • If indeterminate → RAI uptake	Benign—observe 1 y, f/u with U/S 1. Radioactive iodine therapy • Prefer if <40 y and reliable for lifetime T4 (levothyroxine) • For overactive thyroid without risk of subsequent cancer, leukemia, or other malignancy 2. Thyroidectomy • Cold nodules

Thyroid Cancer

Disease	Etiology, Prevalence, Risk Factors	Clinical Symptoms and Signs	Diagnostics	Therapy, Prognosis, and Health Maintenance
Thyroid cancer	F > M (3:1)			
Differentiated papillary thyroid carcinoma	Most common type (80%-90%) Least aggressive, slow growth and spread RF: HX of radiation to head/neck Papillary cancers are characterized histologically by **psammoma bodies**	1. Typically found incidentally on exam • Thyroid nodule	TSH: normal T3, T4: normal 1. Thyroid ultrasound—differentiates solid vs. cystic 2. **Fine needle aspiration (FNA)**—required for diagnosis • Histo: *Psammoma bodies* (laminated calcified bodies) 3. RAI uptake: (+) uptake	1. **Total thyroidectomy** with limited cervical lymph node removal • Complications: vocal cord paralysis, hypoparathyroidism (Hypocalcemia), hypothyroidism 2. Postoperative radioactive iodine ablation therapy Spreads via lymphatics in neck, metastasizes to cervical lymph nodes

Disease	Etiology, Prevalence, Risk Factors	Clinical Symptoms and Signs	Diagnostics	Therapy, Prognosis, and Health Maintenance

Medullary thyroid carcinoma	Neuroendocrine tumor of the parafollicular or C cells of the thyroid gland
	3%-5% of thyroid carcinomas
	Associated with familial syndromes in about one third of the cases (MEN 2A or 2B)
		1. Dysphagia
		2. Hoarseness
		3. Diarrhea
		4. Facial flushing
		Signs:
		1. Palpable solitary thyroid nodule (MC presentation) in upper portion of thyroid lobe
		2. Cervical lymph nodes palpable
			1. Ultrasound of neck: hypoechoic microcalcifications
			2. Labs
			  • Calcitonin: elevated
			  • CEA
			3. FNA biopsy (diagnostic)
			4. Genetic testing for germline RET mutations
				1. Total thyroidectomy most commonly recommended
				2. Thyroxine therapy started immediately post-op to maintain euthyroidism
				Health maintenance:
				1. Measure serum calcitonin and CEA 2-3 mo after surgery to r/o residual disease
				  • If undetectable, measure levels twice yearly × 2 y, then annually if stable
				2. Neck ultrasound 6-12 mo post-op

PAGET DISEASE OF THE BONE (OSTEITIS DEFORMANS)

Disease	Etiology, Prevalence, Risk Factors	Clinical Symptoms and Signs	Diagnostics	Therapy, Prognosis, and Health Maintenance

Paget disease of the bone (osteitis deformans)	Most common symptom: bone pain
	Age 60+, M = F, rare before age 40
	Viral:
	Paramyxovirus (measles, RSV, canine distemper virus)
	Genetic: familial (15%-30% have FH)
	Localized disorder of accelerated bone remodeling
		1. Asymptomatic (70%-90%)
		2. Bone pain: pelvis, lumbar spine, skull, proximal femur
		  • Mild to severe, not related to physical activity
		3. Periarticular pain (50%): hip, knee, spine
		4. Neuro SX: nonspecific headaches, deafness
		Signs:
		1. Mixed conductive and sensory hearing loss
		2. Frontal bossing of forehead or maxilla
		Complications:
		Chalk stick fractures (10%-40% nonunion, femur), osteosarcoma, chondrosarcoma, fibrosarcoma, nephrolithiasis, gout
			1. **Elevated Alk-phos** (first sign, most useful)
			  • 90% of affected pts
			2. NL LFTs, hyperuricemia, **hypercalcemia**, hypercalciuria
			3. XR: areas of lysis, sclerotic areas, cortical thickening
			  • Bowing of weight bearing bone (femur, tibia, humerus, ulna)
			4. **Total body bone scan** with technetium-labeled bisphosphonate (most sensitive)
			5. Histology: increased number and size of osteoclasts and nuclei
				1. Bone pain—aspirin, Tylenol, NSAIDs
				2. **Bisphosphonates** and calcitonin
				  • Bisphosphonates are more effective in controlling the increased remodeling rates
				3. Check alk-phos annually and perform XRs when change in symptoms
				In pagetic lesions, the primary abnormality is in the osteoclast

PITUITARY ADENOMA, CUSHING'S DISEASE, ACROMEGALY

Disease	Etiology, Prevalence, Risk Factors	Clinical Symptoms and Signs	Diagnostics	Therapy, Prognosis, and Health Maintenance
Pituitary adenoma	Tumors arising in the anterior pituitary → compresses pituitary, then optic chiasm → cavernous sinus → third ventricle, temporal lobes, posterior fossa **60%-70% are prolactin secreting**, 10%-15% growth hormone, small amount ACTH	1. Headaches (50%) 2. Complete or partial **bitemporal hemianopia** 3. Oculomotor palsy Complications: Diabetes insipidus, somnolence, CSF rhinorrhea, seizures	1. MRI with gadolinium	1. Transsphenoidal surgery or stereotactic radiosurgery

(continued)

(continued)

Disease	Etiology, Prevalence, Risk Factors	Clinical Symptoms and Signs	Diagnostics	Therapy, Prognosis, and Health Maintenance
Amenorrhea-galactorrhea syndrome (**prolactinoma**)	Manifests during child-bearing years	1. HX: patient quit taking OCPs and menstrual cycle did not re-establish itself (amenorrhea) 2. Galactorrhea	1. Serum prolactin: increased (>100 ng/mL)	1. Dopamine agonist: Bromocriptine • Inhibits prolactin 2. Transphenoidal surgery with radiation therapy 15% recur after 1 year
Cushing disease	Excessive secretion of ACTH → adrenal hyperplasia Cushing's syndrome: refers to *effects* of cortisol excess from a number of sources, one of which can be an adenoma of the pituitary gland	1. Truncal obesity 2. Hypertension 3. Proximal muscle weakness 4. Amenorrhea 5. Hirsutism 6. Abdominal striae 7. Hyperglycemia 8. Osteoporosis 9. Mental disorder	1. **Increased plasma cortisol** • Not suppressed by small dose dexamethasone, but are suppressed by high doses 2. **High ACTH** 3. Increased free urinary cortisol	
Acromegaly	Broadening of skeleton **due to excess GH** AFTER epiphyseal closure MCC: 10% of acromegaly is caused by a **GH secreting pituitary adenoma** MCC of death: **Cardiovascular disease** Prior to puberty, oversecretion of GH leads to gigantism	Growth promotion: 1. Soft tissue and skeletal overgrowth 2. Coarse facial features 3. **Abnormally large hands/feet** 4. Organomegaly 5. Arthralgias 6. *Prognathism*: Enlarged jaw Metabolic Disturbances: 1. *Diabetes* 2. Hyperhidrosis—sweaty palms Parasellar manifestations: 1. *Headache* 2. **Bitemporal hemianopsia** 3. Cavernous sinus compression 4. Sphenoid sinus invasion 5. **HTN and OSA** Complications: *Hypertrophic CM*	1. GH: elevated (0.10 ng/mL) IGF-1 (Somatomedin C): very high 2. OGTT: glucose load fails to suppress GH; confirms if IGF-1 NL 3. MRI 4. Random GH level is not useful	1. **Octreotide** (somatostatin analog) and Bromocriptine 2. **Transsphenoidal surgery** (first line) 3. Radiation therapy

CHAPTER 20

Urology and Renal

Refer to Family Medicine 👥 **for in-depth coverage of the following topics:**

Recommended Supplemental Topics:

Internal Medicine

PROSTATE CANCER

Disease	Etiology, Prevalence, Risk Factors	Clinical Symptoms and Signs	Diagnostics	Therapy, Prognosis, and Health Maintenance
Prostate cancer	Second most common cancer in men worldwide 95% **adenocarcinomas** RF: **Age 65+** (most important), African American, high fat diet, (+) family history, exposure to herbicides and pesticides	Early—asymptomatic Cancer begins in the **PERIPHERY** and moves centrally Late—obstructive symptoms (**difficulty voiding, dysuria, increased urinary frequency**) Late late—bone pain from mets (most common vertebral bodies, pelvis, and long bones in legs), weight loss	1. **DRE**—hard, nodular, irregular If indurated, asymmetric, or nodularity → biopsy, especially if >45 • When palpable, 60%-70% have spread beyond prostate • Transrectal ultrasonography (**TRUS**) with biopsy regardless of PSA level 2. PSA—not cancer specific (elevated in BPH, old age, prostatitis) • Age adjustment • PSA velocity • Quantify free and **protein bound forms** (cancer) • PSA density 3. TRUS with biopsy • Indicated if • PSA>10 ng/dL (50% chance of cancer) • PSA velocity >0.75/y • Abnormal DRE	1. Localized disease—**radical prostatectomy** or watchful waiting in older men who are asymptomatic Complications: Erectile dysfunction and urinary incontinence 2. Locally invasive—**radiation therapy + androgen deprivation** Metastatic disease: 1. Orchiectomy (remove testes) 2. Antiandrogens 3. LH agonists (leuprolide) 4. GnRH antagonists—degarelix

ACUTE RENAL FAILURE

Disease	Etiology, Prevalence, Risk Factors	Clinical Symptoms and Signs	Diagnostics	Therapy, Prognosis, and Health Maintenance
Acute kidney injury (AKI)	Abrupt, typically reversible decline in GFR, usually **within 48 h** Most commonly due to **acute tubular necrosis (ATN)** Because creatinine is filtered and secreted, changes lag behind and underestimate the decline in GFR. By the time the serum creatinine rises, the GFR has fallen significantly	1. Reduction in kidney function defined as: • Absolute **INCREASE** in SCr level of **more than or equal to 0.3 mg/dL** • Percent INCREASE in SCr >=50% (1.5× baseline) • **DECREASE** in urine output (less than 0.5 mL/kg/h) of 6+ h (about 210 mL/h for 70 kg male) Signs: 1. JVD 2. Orthostatics 3. Periorbital edema, pedal edema 4. Rash, thick skin, mucus ulcers 5. Fever 6. **Pleural rub**, crackles 7. S3 8. Prostate masses 9. Bladder distention Associated: Arthritis, foot drop	Initial management: 1. Serum electrolytes (K+, bicarbonate), serum phosphate, serum calcium, and albumin 2. Serum uric acid, magnesium 3. CBC If obstruction suspected 1. **U/S**: • Prerenal: no obstruction, no evidence of intrarenal causes or acute renal failure • Intrinsic: kidney disease or normal, no obstruction • Postrenal: hydronephrosis	1. Rule out reversible causes • hypotension • volume depletion • obstruction • hyperkalemia • volume overload 2. Identify cause and determine complications that require immediate action 3. If not responsive to therapies, consider urgent dialysis

Complications of AKI

- Volume overload, hyperkalemia, metabolic acidosis, hypocalcemia, hyperphosphatemia

- In severe cases: mental status changes, hyperuricemia, hypermagnesemia

Internal Medicine

Complication	Management	
Volume Imbalance	**Depletion** Eg, vomiting, diarrhea	**Overload** Eg, Sepsis patient receiving aggressive IV fluids
	1. IV fluid therapy (fluid challenge)–r/o prerenal failure • Crystalloids (isotonic saline–preferred for initial therapy • Avoid K^+ containing solutions (lactated Ringer's) • If not responsive, unlikely prerenal disease, more likely ATN or other intrinsic AKI	1. Diuretics trial • Loop: 40-80 mg furosemide, if unresponsive in 30 min, double dose • Thiazide diuretics alone or in combination with Loops 2. Dialysis initiation–see indications below
Hyperkalemia (serum potassium >5.5 mEq/L) or rapidly increasing serum potassium Eg, Rhabdomyolysis and tumor lysis syndrome patients	1. Conservative therapy: discontinue ACE inhibitor or ARB, IV fluid repletion, and/or low K^+ diet 2. Dialysis 3. Immediate therapy if EKG changes or peripheral neuromuscular abnormalities are present–see Appendix	
Signs of uremia (pericarditis, unexplained decline in mental status)	1. Treat symptomatically	
Severe metabolic acidosis (pH < 7.1)	1. Dialysis and/or bicarbonate administration 2. Treat reversible causes of metabolic acidosis	

Etiology of AKI

Pre-Renal (Volume Depletion)	Intrinsic Renal	Post-Renal

• **Renal**: diuretics, osmotic diuresis, Addison's
• **Extrarenal**: vomiting, diarrhea, skin loss
• Other: hypotension, CHF, **cirrhosis**, arrhythmia, intrarenal vasoconstriction, hypercalcemia, hepatorenal syndrome, abdominal compartment syndrome
• **Drugs**: contrast, NSAIDs, cyclosporine, tacrolimus, ACE/ARB, Ampho-B
	• **Vascular**: renal infarction, RAS, renal vein thrombosis, malignant hypertension, atheroemboli, scleroderma
	• **Tubular**
	  • **Ischemic**: prolonged renal state, sepsis, **hypotension**
	  • **Nephrotoxic**: aminoglycosides, MTX, cisplatin, myoglobin, hemoglobin
	• **Glomerular**: acute GN, vasculitis, TTP/HUS
	• **Interstitium**: penicillin, cephalosporins, FQ, NSAIDs, phenytoin, PPI, tumors (leukemia, lymphoma)
		Obstruction: BPH, neurogenic bladder, ureteral obstruction (calculi, tumors, clots), extraureteral (tumors, retroperitoneal fibrosis)

- FE_{Na}: amount of sodium filtered by the kidneys that is not reabsorbed (NL: <1%)
- If on diuretics, check FE_{Urea} (fractional excretion of urea); diuretics increase FE_{Na} when patients have pre-renal failure
- In glomerulonephritis—kidneys reabsorb sodium avidly, leading to low urinary sodium and FE_{Na}

Type of AKI	U/A	UNa	FE_{Na}	FE_{Urea}	BUN: Cr
Pre-renal	**High specific gravity** Hyaline casts/NL	<20	<1%	<35%	>20:1
Intrarenal ATN	Low specific gravity Muddy brown casts	>40	>1%	>50%	<20:1
Vascular d/o	Hematuria	>20	~		
GN	Hematuria, proteinuria Dysmorphic RBC, RBC casts	<20	<1%		
Interstitial nephritis (AIN)	Hematuria, proteinuria WBC, WBC casts Eosinophils	>20	>1%		
Post-renal	Hematuria or NL WBC, granular casts Isothenuria: urine = serum osmolality	>20	~		>20:1

Treatment for AKI

Prerenal	Intrinsic	Postrenal

• Hydrate in depleted states
• Diuresis in overloaded states
• Dobutamine—improves forward flow
• Treat causes: hypotension, nephrotoxins
	• CBC, ESR
	• Steroids or immunosuppressants
	• Consider nephrology consult/kidney biopsy
	• Treat causes, eliminate toxins
		• Relieve obstruction
		• Foley catheter (if BPH)
		• Percutaneous nephrostomy
		• Remove any tumors
		   • *Order CT (no contrast) if cause not evident*
		   • *Consider urology consult*

Common Criteria for Initiating Dialysis

- **A**cidosis—metabolic acidosis, refractory to therapy
- **E**lectrolytes: **Hyperkalemia** (most common) unresponsive to conservative measures, severe hypophosphatemia—give calcium gluconate, D5W, insulin, bicarbonate, kayexalate
- **I**ngestion: salicylates or ethylene glycol
- **O**verload: volume overload (pulmonary edema), persistent extracellular volume expansion despite diuretics
- **U**remic symptoms: confusion, pericarditis, seizures, bleeding diathesis, intractable N/V

CHRONIC RENAL FAILURE

- Progressive loss of nephron and GFR loss → compensatory glomerular hyperfiltration

Disease	Etiology, Prevalence, Risk Factors	Clinical Symptoms and Signs	Diagnostics	Therapy, Prognosis, and Health Maintenance

Chronic renal failure (chronic kidney disease)	Renal failure or insufficiency (stages 2-5)
	<u>RF</u>:
	Diabetes,
	  hypertension
	Independent risk factor for cardiovascular disease
		1. Abnormally elevated SCr for 3+ months
		2. Abnormal **GFR <60 mL/min for 3+ months**
		3. Persistent proteinuria or abnormalities on renal imaging, even if GFR normal
			1. U/A, spot urine sample for albumin or protein:Cr ratio, SCr level
			  • Broad waxy casts
			2. GFR estimation
			3. **Anemia,** hyponatremia, **hyperkalemia, hyperphosphatemia, hypocalcemia,** hypermagnesemia, hyperuricemia
			4. **Metabolic acidosis** with high anion gap
			5. Renal ultrasound: symmetrically small echogenic kidneys (<8.5 cm)
				1. Prevention:
				  • Aggressive glucose and BP control, low salt diet
				  • Target: <130/80
				  • Avoid nephrotoxic agents
				  • Dose adjust meds
				  • Refer for stage 3+ (GFR <30)
				  • ACE/ARBs
				2. Diet and Medication
				  • Protein restriction to 0.6-0.8 g/kg/day
				  • Sodium: 2 g/d
				  • K+ restriction if hyperkalemic
				  • Phosph: 800-1000 mg/d
				3. Kidney transplant with dailysis
				  • CKD stage 5 (GFR 5-10 mL/min)
				<u>Prognosis</u>:
				1. 80% with CKD die, from CVD mostly before getting dialysis

(continued)

(continued)

Disease	Etiology, Prevalence, Risk Factors	Clinical Symptoms and Signs	Diagnostics	Therapy, Prognosis, and Health Maintenance
Uremic syndrome	The buildup of metabolic waste products or uremic toxins	1. General malaise, weakness, fatigue 2. Insomnia, restlessness 3. Inability to concentrate, memory impairment, irritability 4. Nausea, vomiting, hiccups 5. Anorexia 6. Metallic taste in mouth, epistaxis 7. Paresthesias 8. Generalized itching without rash 9. Decreased libido 10. Menstrual irregularities 11. Nocturia, ED Signs: 1. Slow appearing, chronically ill 2. Pallor, ecchymoses, excoriations, edema, xerosis, pale conjunctiva 3. Urinous breath 4. Twitching 5. **Hypertension** (MC finding), cardiomegaly, friction rub 6. Rales, pleural effusion 7. Stupor, asterixis, myoclonus, peripheral neuropathy Complications: Pericarditis, hypoglycemia	1. GFR <10-15/min 2. BUN: SCr	1. Dietary changes • Low salt (2-3 g/d) • Loop diuretics, thiazides if GFR <30 • Reduce water intake (1.5 L/d) • Low K⁺ diet (40-60 mEq/d) • Phosphorous restriction • Avoid blood transfusion, salt substitute, and NSAIDs

Signs of Uremia

Skin	• Paleness, hyperpigmentation • Ecchymosis, hematoma • Pruritus • Skin necrosis (calciphylaxis) • Bullous lesions
Cardiovascular	• Volume overload, systemic **hypertension** (most common complication) • Accelerated atherosclerosis and ischemic heart disease • Left ventricular hypertrophy • Heart failure • Rhythm disturbances • Uremic pericarditis
Neurologic	• Cerebral vascular accidents • Encephalopathy • Seizures • Peripheral and autonomic neuropathy
Gastrointestinal	• Anorexia, nausea, vomiting, malnutrition • Uremic fetor • Inflammatory/ulcerative lesions • GI bleed
Hematologic	• Anemia • Increased infections • Bleeding diathesis (platelet dysfunction)
Bone	• Renal osteodystrophy • Growth retardation (children) • Muscle weakness
Endocrine	• Sexual dysfunction • Infertility (women) • Glucose intolerance (women) • Hyperlipidemia
Labs	• Hyponatremia (excessive water intake), hypocalcemia • Hyperkalemia, hypermagnesemia, hyperuricemia • Metabolic acidosis

Internal Medicine

Indications for Dialysis

- Uremic symptoms: pericarditis, encephalopathy, GI complications (anorexia, nausea, vomiting), azotemia
- GFR <10 mL/min/1.73 m^2
- Fluid overload unresponsive to diuresis
- Refractory hyperkalemia

Types of Dialysis

Hemodialysis (HD)	• Acquired through an AV fistula (preferred) or prosthetic graft; comes with high risk of infection, thrombosis, and aneurysm • Treatment three times per week, lasting 3-5 h each session
Peritoneal dialysis (PD)	• Peritoneal membrane is the "dialyzer" while dialysate is instilled into the peritoneal cavity through indwelling catheter • Water/solutes move across capillary bed between visceral/parietal layers into the dialysate; dialysate is drained and fresh dialysate instilled creating an exchange • Most common complication: peritonitis (nausea, vomiting, abdominal pain, diarrhea or constipation, fever)

ACUTE INTERSTITIAL NEPHRITIS, NEPHRITIS

Disease	Etiology, Prevalence, Risk Factors	Clinical Symptoms and Signs	Diagnostics	Therapy, Prognosis, and Health Maintenance
Acute interstitial nephritis (AIN)	Inflammation involving the interstitium (surrounds glomeruli and tubules), 10%-15% of AKI Causes: **Acute allergic reaction to meds** (PCN, cephalosporin, sulfa drugs, diuretics, anticoagulants, allopurinol, PPI), infection (Streptococcus, Legionella pneumophila), sarcoidosis, SLE, Sjogren's	1. AKI with associated symptoms (weight gain, edema, oliguria, dry mucous membranes, *hypotension, tachycardia*, decreased turgor) 2. Recent infection or **start of new medication** 3. General *aches and pains* 4. **Rash, fever, eosinophilia** 5. (+/−) Pyuria, hematuria	1. Renal function tests (high BUN/Cr) 2. Urinalysis: **eosinophils**, mild proteinuria	1. Remove offending agent 2. **Steroids** 3. Treat infection if present

POLYCYSTIC KIDNEY DISEASE (PKD)

Disease	Etiology, Prevalence, Risk Factors	Clinical Symptoms and Signs	Diagnostics	Therapy, Prognosis, and Health Maintenance
Polycystic kidney disease (PKD)	Family history (75%); **autosomal dominant** Most common GENETIC cause of CKD ESRD develops in 50% of patients	1. **Microscopic or gross hematuria** 2. **Abdominal or flank pain** 3. **Resistant hypertension** (50%) Signs: 1. Palpable abdominal mass 2. **Palpable** kidneys on exam Associated: Kidney stones, Infection	1. **Ultrasound** CONFIRMATORY: multiple cysts 2. CT and MRI alternatives	1. No curative therapy 2. Drain cysts if symptomatic 3. Treat infection with antibiotics 4. Control HTN Complications: **Intracerebral berry aneurysm**, infection of renal cysts, renal failure (late), kidney stones, mitral valve prolapse, cysts in other organs, hernias, diverticula

HYDRONEPHROSIS

Refers to the distention of the renal calyces and pelvis of one or both kidneys by urine → not a disease, but a *physical* result of urinary blockage that may occur at the level of the KUB or urethra.

- Bilateral hydronephrosis—caused by blockage of urine flow occurring at or <u>below</u> the level of the bladder or urethra

- Unilateral hydronephrosis—caused by blockage to urine flow occurring <u>above</u> the level of the bladder

- Urinary obstruction causes a rise in ureteral pressure leading to declines in GFR, tubular function (sodium, K$^+$ transport, or urine concentration), and renal blood flow

Disease	Etiology, Prevalence, Risk Factors	Clinical Symptoms and Signs	Diagnostics	Therapy, Prognosis, and Health Maintenance
Hydronephrosis	MCC of congenital bilateral hydronephrosis: posterior urethral valves (males) MC acquired causes: pelvic tumors, renal calculi, urethral stricture Common in pregnancy	1. Sudden or **new onset HTN** 2. **Severe, steady pain**, radiates down to lower abdomen, testicles, or labia 3. Disturbed excretory function or **difficulty voiding**: oliguria, anuria (complete obstruction) vs. polyuria, nocturia (partial obstruction) 4. Dysuria with UTI Signs: 1. Fever 2. Distention of kidney or bladder 3. DRE: enlarged prostate or rectal/pelvic mass 4. Pelvic exam: enlarged uterus or pelvic mass	1. U/A: hematuria, pyuria, proteinuria, or bacteriuria 2. BUN/Cr: Azotemia due to impaired excretion of Na, urea, and H_2O 3. Urodynamic testing for neurogenic bladder 4. **Ultrasound imaging**: sensitive and specific (90%) if no diuresis occurs with cath • IV urogram and/or CT scan: for intraabdominal and retroperitoneal causes • MR pyelography: detects obstruction • VCUG if VUR, bladder neck or urethral obstruction expected	1. **Bladder catheterization**: if diuresis occurs, the obstruction is below the bladder neck • **Frequent voiding** or **catheterization** 2. Antibiotics 3-4 wk +/− percutaneous nephrostomy 3. Anticholinergics (oxybutynin, tolterodine) for neurogenic bladder 4. VUR • Surgical repair (ureteral reimplantation or ureteroneocystostomy)

ERECTILE DYSFUNCTION

Disease	Etiology, Prevalence, Risk Factors	Clinical Symptoms and Signs	Diagnostics	Therapy, Prognosis, and Health Maintenance
Erectile dysfunction	M **40-70 y/o** CVD risk factors: **Smokers**, HTN, DM **2× risk of heart attack** Cannot dilate cavernosal artery (smooth muscle relaxation) OR venous leakage	The consistent or recurrent inability of a man to attain and/or maintain an erection for sexual performance	Clinical DX	1. **PDE-5 inhibitors**: accumulate cGMP 2. Vacuum constriction device 3. Intracavernosal injection 4. Transurethral system: Alprostadil 5. Penile prosthesis

HYDROCELE, VARICOCELE, TESTICULAR TORSION

Disease	Etiology, Prevalence, Risk Factors	Clinical Symptoms and Signs	Diagnostics	Therapy, Prognosis, and Health Maintenance
Hydrocele	Accumulation of fluid in tunica vaginalis Recurs with drainage	1. Painless, fluctuates in size 2. Smaller in morning, increases size while upright	1. U/S: r/o testicular cancer **(transilluminates)**	1. Watch/wait: small, scrotal support 2. Hydrocelectomy: painful or large
Varicocele	Left-sided (90%) May be infertile Left spermatic vein enters left renal vein Right spermatic vein enters IVC Majority not associated with fertility	Asymptomatic (adolescent males): 1. Vague testicular pain Signs: 1. **"bag of worms"** → decompresses while supine	1. U/S	1. **NSAIDs** 2. Scrotal support 3. Rarely surgery

Disease	Etiology, Prevalence, Risk Factors	Clinical Symptoms and Signs	Diagnostics	Therapy, Prognosis, and Health Maintenance
Testicular torsion	Twisting of spermatic cord leading to arterial occlusion and venous outflow obstruction → ischemia → testicular infarction Adolescent male patients Most: **12-18 y/o**	1. Acute severe **unilateral** testicular pain • Worse with physical activity • Radiates into lower abdomen 2. **Nausea and vomiting** 3. **Absent** dysuria or bladder symptoms Signs: 1. **Absent (–) cremasteric reflex** on affected side, affected testis higher than opposite 2. Swollen and tender scrotum, **elevated high-riding testicle** 3. Bilateral "bell clapper" deformity, horizontal orientation 4. Prehn's sign (–): lift up testicle, no relief	1. Color doppler U/S: **reduced flow** 2. Definitive: scrotal exploration	1. **Manual detorsion**: rotate caudal to cranial and medial to lateral 2. Immediate surgical detorsion and **orchiopexy** to the scrotum (bilateral) SURGICAL EMERGENCY If delayed >6 h → infarction, may not be salvageable → infertility 3. Orchiectomy if nonviable testicle found

BLADDER CANCER, RENAL CELL CARCINOMA

Disease	Etiology, Prevalence, Risk Factors	Clinical Symptoms and Signs	Diagnostics	Therapy, Prognosis, and Health Maintenance
Bladder carcinoma	White males, age 65-75 y/o RF: **Smoking** (2-4×), chronic cyclophosphamide, **Schistosoma haematobium exposure** Protective—vitamin A supplements >95% are transitional cell in origin Most tumors are superficial (75%-85%) MC sites of hematogenous spread: Lung, bone, liver, brain	1. Gross **hematuria** (80%-90%) 2. Irritative symptoms: dysuria, frequency 3. Obstructive symptoms if near urethra or bladder neck Signs: 1. Flank pain	1. U/A and culture–r/o infection 2. Urine cytology • Highly specific, low sensitivity 3. CT scan of pelvis or MR urogram or IV pyelogram 4. **Cystoscopy with biopsy**, histology (required for diagnosis) • Bladder barbotage for cytology 5. Selective catheterization and visualization of upper tracts if cytology (+)	1. Nonmuscle invasive disease • **Complete endoscopic resection** (transurethral surgery) for solitary papillary lesions • Add intravesical therapy for CIS and recurrent disease • Monitor every 3 mo 2. Muscle-invasive disease • **Radical cystectomy** (standard) and removal of pelvic lymph nodes, including prostate, seminal vesicles, and urethra • Impotence
Renal cell carcinoma	**M (2×) > F** 85% of primary renal cancers in adults Cause: Unknown RF: **Smoking**, phenacetin analgesics, adult polycystic kidney disease, chronic dialysis, exposure to heavy metals, hypertension	1. **Hematuria** (most common, 70%) 2. Abdominal or **flank pain** (50%) 3. **Abdominal** (flank) **mass** (40%) 4. Weight loss, fever 5. Paraneoplastic syndromes: polycythemia, hypercalcemia, HTN, Cushing's syndrome, feminization, or masculinization	1. Renal ultrasound 2. **Abdominal CT** with and without contrast: optimal test for DX and staging	1. **Radical nephrectomy** (remove kidney and adrenal gland) for stages I-IV Metastasis—liver, lung, brain, bone

RENAL VASCULAR DISEASE

Renal artery stenosis causes decreased blood flow to JGA → RAAS system becomes activated leading to HTN.

• Most common cause of **secondary HTN**

• Indications for renal artery stenting: Hypertension in patients who are intolerant of medications, or have a unilateral small kidney, or have resistant (>3 classes of medications at maximum dose) or accelerated hypertension with a significant stenosis

Disease	Etiology, Prevalence, Risk Factors	Clinical Symptoms and Signs	Diagnostics	Therapy, Prognosis, and Health Maintenance
(Renovascular hypertension) renal artery stenosis	<u>MCC</u> (67%): **atherosclerosis** (elderly men, smoking, high cholesterol) 1%-2% of patients with hypertension Cause in most young individuals is fibromuscular dysplasia	1. **HTN**—sudden onset without family history, age <20 or >50, severe and refractory to 3+ drugs <u>Signs:</u> 1. Abdominal bruit (RUQ, LUQ, epigastrium) in 50%-80% of patients 2. Atherosclerotic disease of aorta or peripheral arteries 3. Pulmonary edema with increase in blood pressure	1. **Hypokalemia** 2. Decreased renal function 3. Abrupt increase in serum creatinine after use of ACE inhibitors 1. **Renal arteriogram** (gold standard, definitive), but contrast is nephrotoxic 2. MRA: high sensitivity and specificity, can be used in renal failure • For medium to low suspicion 3. Duplex Doppler ultrasonography of renal arteries and contrast enhanced CT scan	1. Revascularization with **percutaneous transluminal renal angioplasty** (PRTA) initial treatment 2. Surgery (bypass) 3. ACEI or CCB may be tried alone or in combo
Fibromuscular dysplasia (of renal artery)	F <50, bilateral 50% 10%-15% of renal artery stenosis	<u>Signs:</u> Abdominal bruit (RUQ, LUQ, epigastrium); common with **fibromuscular dysplasia**	1. Doppler ultrasound, CT angiography, or MRA—screening 2. Renal angiography (gold standard): **"beads on a string"** (Fig. 20-1)	1. Avoid ACE and ARBs with bilateral renovascular disease due to increased risk of glomerular damage and precipitation of AKI secondary to hypoperfusion 2. **Percutaneous transluminal angioplasty**—curative
Retroperitoneal fibrosis	Increased scar tissue that blocks the ureters	1. HX of recurrent urinary tract infections 2. Back pain 3. Nausea, vomiting 4. Fever 5. Increased frequency and decreased urine output <u>Signs:</u> Lower extremity edema	CT abdomen/pelvis: bilateral renal hydronephrosis	1. Suprapubic or foley catheter • Drain the bladder

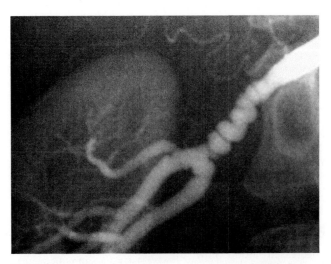

FIGURE 20-1. Fibromuscular dysplasia on arteriography showing classic "string of beads" appearance, which is due to alternating stenosis and dilation of the distal two thirds of the main renal artery. (From Upchurch GR Jr, Henke PK. *Clinical Scenarios in Vascular Surgery.* 2nd ed. Philadelphia: Wolters Kluwer; 2015.)

CHAPTER 21
Neurology

Refer to Family Medicine 👨‍⚕️ **for in-depth coverage of the following topics:**

Seizure Disorders, p 108
Syncope, p 107
Headaches and Migraines, p 120
Strokes: Transient Ischemic Attack, Cerebrovascular Accidents (CVA), p 111

Essential Tremor, Parkinson Disease, p 117
Bell Palsy, p 118
Delirium and Dementia, p 119

Recommended Supplemental Topics:
Loss of Coordination (Ataxia) ✳, p 408

Alzheimer Disease 👨‍⚕️, p 117

INTRACRANIAL TUMORS

- 50% are malignant and associated with high mortality
- Glial tumors (30% of all primary tumors)—80% are malignant
- Meningiomas (35%), schwannomas (10%), CNS lymphomas (2%)
- Brain metastases are 3× more common than all primary brain tumors
- RF: exposure to ionizing radiation (meningiomas, gliomas, schwannomas), immunosuppression (primary CNS lymphoma)

General	Focal

• Headache—worse in morning and improves throughout the day
  • Often holocephalic, but can be ipsilateral to side of the tumor
  • Can present as 'migraine' with unilateral throbbing pain associated with visual scotoma
• +/– Nausea or vomiting
• Cognitive difficulties
• Personality changes—apathy, withdrawal from social circumstances, mimicking depression
• Gait disorder
	• Subacute, progressive
	• Hemiparesis
	• Aphasia
	• Visual field defect—noticed by patient and revealed after it leads to injury (automobile accident in blind visual field)
	• Language difficulties—mistaken for confusion
	• Seizures (common)

- Cranial MRI (preferred) with gadolinium contrast
  - CT if unable to undergo MRI
  - PET—useful in determining the metabolic activity of the lesions seen on MRI
- Labs are rarely useful, although mets may have elevated tumor markers reflecting presence of brain mets (B-hCG) from testicular cancer
  - Also, rarely indicated or helpful—cerebral angiography, EEG, LP
- Treatment

- Symptomatic treatment
  - Edema (neurologic disability, high intracranial pressure)—steroids (dexamethasone 12 to 16 mg/d in divided doses PO or IV) with taper
  - Seizures—antiepileptic drug therapy (levetiracetam, topiramate, lamotrigine, valproic acid, lacosamide)
  - VTE—prophylactic anticoagulants during hospitalization and nonambulatory patients
- Definitive treatment—based on tumor type
  - Surgery, radiotherapy, chemotherapy

Intrinsic "Malignant" Tumors

Disease	Etiology, Prevalence, Risk Factors	Clinical Symptoms and Signs	Diagnostics	Therapy, Prognosis, and Health Maintenance
Astrocytoma (grade I-III)	Occur in children and young adults Most common in childhood: pilocytic (grade I), occurs in cerebellum	Grade II+ present with seizures	MRI—nonenhancing lesions with increased T2/FLAIR signal	1. Maximal surgical resection 2. Radiation therapy is helpful for grade II+ 3. Chemotherapy (temozolomide) 4. Median survival: 5 y
Glioblastoma (grade IV)	Most common malignant primary brain tumor Age: 60-70 y/o	1. Headache 2. Seizures 3. Focal neurologic deficits	MRI—ring-enhancing masses with central necrosis and surrounding edema • Highly infiltrative: increased T2/FLAIR signal	1. Maximal surgical resection + partial field external-beam RT + chemotherapy 2. 6-12 mo of adjuvant chemotherapy 3. Median survival: 14.6 mo, high recurrence rate Poor prognostic RF: Old age, histologic features of glioblastoma, poor Karnofsky performance status, unresectable tumor
Medulloblastoma	Most common malignant brain tumor of childhood (20%)	1. Headache 2. Ataxia 3. Brainstem involvement (signs)	MRI—dense enhancing tumors in posterior fossa + hydrocephalus	Maximal surgical resection + craniospinal irradiation + chemotherapy

Extrinsic "Benign" Tumors

Disease	Etiology, Prevalence, Risk Factors	Clinical Symptoms and Signs	Diagnostics	Therapy, Prognosis, and Health Maintenance
Meningiomas	Most common primary brain tumor (35%) Incidence increases with age, more common in women and patients with neurofibromatosis type II or history of cranial irradiation	1. Headaches 2. Seizures 3. Focal neurologic deficits	1. MRI: partially calcified, densely enhancing extraaxial tumor arising from the dura	1. If asymptomatic, no intervention necessary • Serial MRI studies 2. Complete resection = cure 3. External-beam RT or stereotactic radiosurgery (SRS)—tumors that cannot be resected
Acoustic neuroma (*vestibular schwannoma*)	Intracranial benign tumor affecting 8th cranial nerve Bilateral acoustic neuromas, associated with **neurofibromatosis type II**	1. **Unilateral, progressive** sensorineural hearing loss (may also be acute) 2. *Unsteadiness* 3. *Vertigo* (continuous, late): vestibular deficit compensated centrally as it develops 4. **Tinnitus** 5. Impaired speech discrimination 6. Headache Physical exam: Decreased corneal reflex sensitivity, diplopia, facial weakness	1. Head impulse test: deficient response when head rotated toward affected side 2. MRI: densely enhancing lesions, enlarging the internal auditory canal, and extending into the cerebellopontine angle 3. Lumbar puncture: elevated protein	1. Asymptomatic • Serial MRIs 2. Surgery or SRS for larger lesions Complication: Loss of corneal reflex from trigeminal involvement
Craniopharyngiomas	Rare Suprasellar, partially calcified, solid, or mixed Arises from remnants of Rathke's pouch Bimodal distribution: children and adults 55-65 y/o	1. Headaches 2. Visual impairment 3. Impaired growth (children) 4. Hypopituitarism (adults)		1. Surgery +/– RT
Pituitary Tumors	9% of brain tumors			

Functioning	Nonfunctioning

• Microadenomas (<1 cm in diameter)
• Secrete hormones producing specific endocrine syndromes
  • ACTH–Cushing disease
  • GH–Acromegaly
• Prolactin–galactorrhea, amenorrhea, infertility
	• Macroadenomas (>1 cm)
	• Produce symptoms by mass effect
	  • Headaches
	  • Visual impairment (bitemporal hemianopsia)
	  • Hypopituitarism

MULTIPLE SCLEROSIS

- Selective demyelination of CNS—multifocal zones of demyelination (plaques) scattered throughout white matter (angles of lateral ventricles)

- Demyelination—involves **white matter** of the brain and spinal cord; tends to spare the gray matter/axons and the PNS

- **Internuclear ophthalmoplegia**—lesion in the medial longitudinal fasciculus results in ipsilateral medial rectus palsy on attempted lateral gaze (adduction defect) and horizontal nystagmus of abducting eye (contralateral to side of lesion)

- Relapses of MS produce symptoms for >24 hours, once per year, decrease in frequency over time

- Prognosis: variable, normal life spans

  - Most never develop debilitating disease, one-third progress to severe disability

  - RF for severe: frequent attacks early in course, onset at old age, progressive course, early cerebellar or pyramidal involvement (Fig. 21-1A-B)

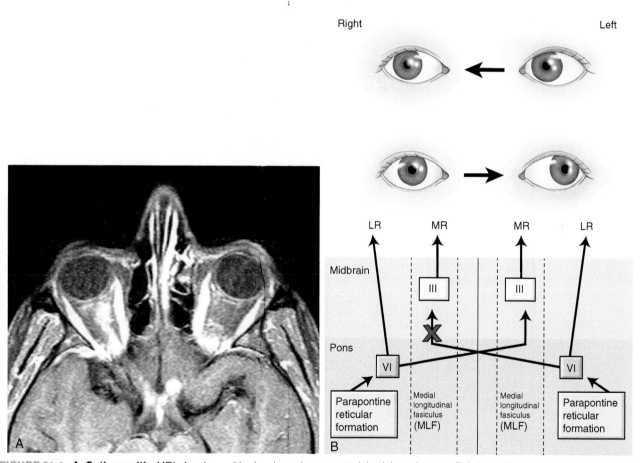

FIGURE 21-1. A, Optic neuritis. MRI of optic neuritis showing enhancement of the right optic nerve. **B, Internuclear ophthalmoplegia.** Adduction defect of the patient's right eye is shown in this example. (**A**, From Gerstenblith AT, Rabinowitz MP. *The Wills Eye Manual: Office and Emergency Room Diagnosis and Treatment of Eye Disease.* Philadelphia: Wolters Kluwer Health; 2013. **B**, Chern KC, Saidel MA. *Ophthalmology Review Manual*, 2nd Edition. Philadelphia: Lippincott Williams & Wilkins, 2012.)

Internal Medicine

Disease	Etiology, Prevalence, Risk Factors	Clinical Symptoms and Signs	Therapy, Prognosis, and Health Maintenance
Multiple sclerosis	Women (2×) > men Etiology: Unknown Most present in 20-30 y/o with localizing deficit such as optic neuritis, **one-sided** weakness, or numbness	1. Transient sensory deficits (most common), *decreased sensation* or paresthesias in upper or lower limbs 2. **Fatigue**—most common complaint 3. Motor symptoms: **weakness** or **spasticity** (insidious or acute) • Pyramidal tract involvement (UMN) • **Spasticity (legs)** can impair ability to walk and maintain balance • Leads to weakness → paraparesis, hemiparesis, quadriparesis 4. Visual disturbances • **Optic neuritis** (*monocular* visual loss, pain with movement of eyes, central scotoma, decreased pupillary reaction to light) • **Internuclear ophthalmoplegia** (strongly suggests MS): adduction defect, horizontal nystagmus of abducting eye 5. Cerebellar involvement: ataxia, intention tremor, dysarthria 6. *Loss* of bladder control—UMN injury 7. Autonomic involvement: impotence or constipation 8. Cerebral involvement: memory loss, personality change, emotional lability (**anxiety** and **depression** common) 9. Neuropathic pain: hyperesthesia, **trigeminal neuralgia**	DX: 1. Clinical definite • 2 episodes of SX • Evidence of 2 white matter lesions (imaging or clinical) 2. Lab-supported • 2 episodes of SX • Evidence of 1 white matter lesion on MRI • Abnormal CSF (*oligoclonal bands*) 3. Probable • 2 episodes of SX +1 white matter lesion OR + CSF: oligoclonal bands
Clinically silent	"Stable" or "benign"	Clinical DX 1. **MRI**—test of choice, most sensitive, diagnostic • Demyelinating lesions, number does not correlate to severity or speed of progression (Fig. 21-2) 2. **LP/CSF Analysis**: *oligoclonal bands* of IgG (90%) 3. Evoked potentials: slow sensory impulses	Acute attacks: 1. **High dose IV steroids**, shorten attack, but does not alter outcome or course, resolves in 6 wk with or without Disease-modifying: 1. **Recombinant interferon B-1α/1β** and glatiramer acetate • Can cause flu-like symptoms, but reduce relapse rates • Cyclophosphamide for rapidly progressive, but toxic Symptomatic therapy: • **Baclofen** or dantrolene for spasticity • Carbamazepine or **gabapentin** for neuropathic pain • Treat depression
Relapsing and remitting (R&R)	**Most common:** Exacerbations with remissions		
Secondary progressive	R&R disease with gradual worsening of SX that is progressive in later years		
Primary progressive	Steady progressive disease that appears later in life (>40), less visual and more axonal involvement		

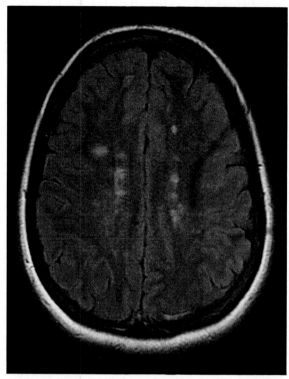

FIGURE 21-2. Multiple hyperintense white matter lesions, both ovoid and perpendicular to the lateral ventricles on axial FLAIR MRI. (From Sanelli P, Schaefer P, Loevner L. *Neuroimaging: The Essentials*. Philadelphia: Wolters Kluwer Health; 2016.)

MENINGITIS AND ENCEPHALITIS

- Kernig's sign—inability to fully extend the knees when patient supine with hip flexed 90°; caused by irritation of meninges (50%)

- Brudzinski sign—flexion of legs and thighs that is brought on by passive flexion of the neck (50%)

Disease	Etiology, Prevalence, Risk Factors	Clinical Symptoms and Signs	Diagnostics	Therapy, Prognosis, and Health Maintenance
Bacterial meningitis Acute—hours to days Chronic—within weeks to months, commonly caused by mycobacteria, fungi, Lyme disease, or parasites	Inflammation of the meningeal membranes that envelop the brain and spinal cord Infectious agents colonize the nasopharynx and respiratory tract MCC: ***Streptococcus pneumoniae Haemophilus influenzae, Neisseria meningitidis***	1. Triad: ***Fever, nuchal rigidity, change in mental status*** 2. ***Headache*** (more severe with lying down) 3. Nausea and vomiting 4. **Stiff, painful neck** 5. Malaise 6. Photophobia 7. AMS (**confusion, lethargy,** coma) Signs: 1. **Nuchal rigidity** (stiff neck with resistance to flexion) 2. **Rash** (maculopapular rash with petechiae for N. meningitidis) or vesicular lesions (varicella/HSV) 3. Increased ICP and its manifestations (papilledema, seizures) 4. Cranial nerve palsies 5. Kernig sign (+) Brudzinski sign (+)	1. **Lumbar puncture**– unless evidence of space-occupying lesion • Neutrophil predominant • Cell count >1000 • Low glucose level • Elevated protein 2. **CT scan of head**– recommended before performing LP if focal neurologic signs or evidence of space-occupying lesion with high ICP 3. **Blood cultures** prior to antibiotics	• Empiric therapy after LP • IV antibiotics immediately if CSF cloudy or bacteria suspected • Steroids if cerebral edema present Vaccinate adults >65 for *S. pneumo* Vaccinate asplenic patients Vaccinate immunocompromised for meningococcus Prophylaxis: • Rifampin or ceftriaxone for close contacts of meningococcal

(continued)

(continued)

Disease	Etiology, Prevalence, Risk Factors	Clinical Symptoms and Signs	Diagnostics	Therapy, Prognosis, and Health Maintenance
Aseptic (viral) meningitis	Caused by a variety of nonbacterial pathogens, frequently **viruses** (enterovirus 70 or 71, coxsackievirus A7 or A9 and HSV) MC in summer and fall temperatures	1. Acute onset of • **Subacute fever**, chills, **headache**, photophobia, pain on eye movement • Nausea, vomiting 2. Diarrhea, myalgias, rash, pleurodynia, myocarditis, herpangina Signs: 1. Meningismus without local neurologic signs 2. **Drowsiness** or irritability	1. Lumbar puncture: pleocytosis • Lymphocyte predom • Cell count <1000 • Normal glucose level • Elevated protein	• Supportive therapy • Analgesics and fever reduction • Better prognosis than acute bacterial meningitis
Encephalitis	Diffuse inflammation of the brain parenchyma and seen simultaneously with meningitis Usually **viral** in origin (HSV-1, arbovirus, *Enterovirus*) Nonviral infectious causes: Toxoplasmosis, cerebral aspergillosis RF: **AIDS** (*Toxo* if T-cell <200), immunosuppression, travel to underdeveloped countries, mosquito exposure, exposure to wild animals (bats)	1. Prodromal: headache, malaise, myalgias • Within hours-days, **acutely** ill • Headache, fever, photophobia, nuchal rigidity • Altered sensorium: **confusion**, delirium, disorientation, behavior abnormalities • **Focal neurologic findings:** hemiparesis, aphasia, CN lesions, and seizures	1. CXR, urine, and blood cultures, UTox, chemistry–r/o nonviral causes 2. **LP**: lymphocytosis, *normal* glucose (viral) • CSF cultures: usually negative • **CSF PCR**–most specific and sensitive for HSV-1, CMV, EBV, and VZV 3. **MRI brain:** Study of choice to r/o focal neuro causes (abscess): increased areas of T2 signal in frontotemporal localization (HSV) 4. EEG: diagnoses HSV-1, shows unilateral or bilateral temporal lobe changes 5. Brain biopsy: indicated in acutely ill patient with focal, enhancing lesion on MRI without clear diagnosis	1. Supportive care 2. Antivirals • HSV: acyclovir 2-3 wk • CMV: ganciclovir or foscarnet 3. Manage seizures and cerebral edema 4. 10% mortality

Age or RF	Likely Etiology	Empiric Therapy
Infants <3 mo	Group B Streptococci *E. coli*, *Klebsiella*, *Listeria*	Cefotaxime + vancomycin + **ampicillin**
3 M- 50 y	*N. meningitidis*, *S. pneumo*, *H. flu*	Ceftriaxone or cefotaxime + vancomycin
>50 y	*S. pneumo*, *N. meningitidis*, *Listeria*	Ceftriaxone or cefotaxime + vancomycin + **ampicillin**
Impaired cellular immunity (eg, HIV)	*S. pneumo*, *N. meningitidis*, *Listeria*, aerobic gram-negative bacilli (Pseudomonas)	*Ceftazidime* + vancomycin + **ampicillin**

Bacterial Meningitis	Aseptic Meningitis
• Neonates: Group B Streptococci *E. coli*, Listeria • Children >3M: N. meningitidis, *Strep pneumo*, H. flu • Adults: **S. pneumo**, *N. meningitidis*, H. flu • Elderly (>50): S. pneumo, N. meningitidis, L. monocytogenes • Immunocompromised: L. monocytogenes, gram-neg bacilli, S. pneumo	Caused by a variety of nonbacterial pathogens, frequently **viruses** (enterovirus and HSV) • Difficult to distinguish from acute bacterial meningitis • Better prognosis than acute bacterial meningitis
Complications: Seizures, coma, brain abscess, subdural empyema, DIC, respiratory arrest Permanent sequelae: deafness, brain damage, hydrocephalus	

Lumbar Puncture CSF Findings

- Order cell count, chemistry, gram stain, culture (include AFB) and cryptococcal antigen or India ink

	Normal	Bacterial	Aseptic (Viral)
WBC count	<5	>1000-5000/μL (250/cm³)	<1000
WBC differential	All lymphocytes or monocytes, no PMNs	Mostly PMNs (90%-100% **neutrophils**)	Mostly **lymphocytes** and monocytes
Glucose	50-75	**Low (35)**	Normal to high
Protein	<60	**High (150-250)**	NL to high
Gram stain		(+) in 75%-80%	

COMA

Depressed level of consciousness to extent that patient is completely unresponsive to any stimuli.

- Causes: structural brain lesions (bilateral), global brain dysfunction (metabolic or systemic disorders), psychiatric causes (conversion disorders, malingering)

- Initial steps
  - Vitals, ABCs
  - Assume underlying trauma (stabilize cervical spine) and assess for signs of underlying trauma
  - Assess level of consciousness using Glasgow Coma Scale, repeat serially

Glasgow Coma Scale (Fig. 21-3)		
Eye opening (E)—4	Does not open eyes	1
	Opens to painful stimulus	2
	Opens to voice (command)	3
	Opens spontaneously	4
Verbal response (V)—5	No sounds	1
	Incomprehensible sounds	2
	Inappropriate words	3
	Appropriate, but confused	4
	Appropriate and oriented	5
Motor response (M)—6	No movement	1
	Decerebrate posture	2
	Decorticate posture	3
	Withdrawals from pain	4
	Localizes pain stimulus	5
	Obeys commands	6

- Brainstem reflexes
  - Pupillary light reflex—should be round, symmetrical and reactive to light
    - If responsive, midbrain intact
    - Anisocoria (asymmetric pupils)—may be sign of uncal herniation
    - Pinpoint pupils—narcotics (morphine), ICH
    - Bilateral fixed, dilated pupils—severe anoxia
    - Unilateral fixed, dilated pupil—CN 3 compression
  - Eye movements—if cervical spine uninjured, perform oculocephalic test ("dolls eyes")
    - When head turned to one side, the eyes should move conjugately to opposite direction if brainstem intact
  - If breathing on own, brainstem is functioning
- Labs—CBC, electrolytes, calcium, BUN, creatinine, glucose, plasma osmolarity, ABG, EKG
- Toxicologic analysis of blood and urine

- CT or MRI of brain
- LP—if meningitis or SAH suspected

Treatment

- Correct reversible causes, treat underlying cause
  - Supplemental O_2
  - Naloxone for narcotic overdose
  - Dextrose for hypoglycemia, thiamine before glucose load
  - Correct electrolyte abnormalities
- Treat herniation—lower ICP

Criteria for Brain Death versus Persistent Vegetative State

- **Irreversible** absence of brain/brainstem function—unresponsive, apnea **despite adequate oxygenation and ventilation**, no brainstem reflexes (pupils, calorics, gag, cornea, doll's eyes)

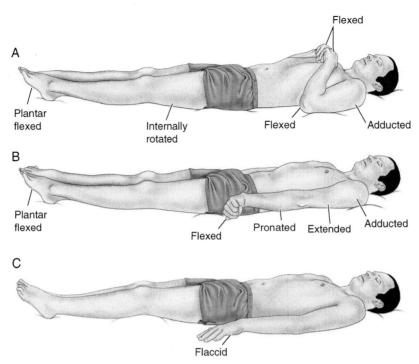

FIGURE 21-3. Glasgow coma scale. Abnormal posture response to stimuli: **A**, decorticate posturing; **B**, decerebrate posturing; **C**, flaccidity when patient makes no motor response to stimuli. (From Timby BK, Smith NE. *Introductory Medical-Surgical Nursing*. Philadelphia: Wolters Kluwer Health; 2018.)

- No drug intoxication or metabolic condition that can reversibly inhibit brain function
- Core body temperature >32°C (89.6°F), cannot be established in presence of hypothermia
- Clinical evidence or imaging study that provides causative explanation
- Exams must be repeated or EEG performed showing isoelectric activity
- Persistent vegetative state—completely unresponsive, but eyes are open and appear awake, may have random head or limb movements

MYASTHENIA GRAVIS

- Edrophonium chloride: acetylcholinesterase inhibitor with rapid onset (30 to 45 seconds) and short duration (5 to 10 minutes) → prolongs presence of acetylcholine in NMJ and results in immediate increase in muscle strength in affected muscles
  - Muscarinic effects of acetylcholine: increased salivation, GI cramping, bradycardia, bronchospasm, arrhythmia, syncope

- Pyridostigmine: acetylcholinesterase inhibitor with rapid onset (15 to 30 minutes) and peak action at 2 hours, effects lasting 3 to 4 hours
  - Adverse effects (muscarinic): abdominal cramping, diarrhea, increased salivation, bronchial secretions, nausea, sweating, bradycardia
  - Nicotinic effects: fasciculations, muscle cramping
  - Cholinergic crisis*: excess anticholinesterase medication = weakness (dose-limiting)
- Muscles involved: extraocular muscles, eyelids (ptosis), facial muscles (facial weakness, difficulty chewing, slurred speech)
- Limb muscles: proximal, symmetric
- Myasthenic crisis (15%)—diaphragm and intercostal fatigue results in respiratory failure, requiring mechanical vent
  - Low threshold for intubation—FVC of 15 mL/kg (1L) is indicated for intubation
- Meds that exacerbate: antibiotics (aminoglycosides, tetracyclines), BB, and antiarrhythmics (quinidine, procainamide, lidocaine)

Disease	Etiology, Prevalence, Risk Factors	Clinical Symptoms and Signs	Diagnostics	Therapy, Prognosis, and Health Maintenance
Myasthenia gravis	**Autoimmune disorder**—autoantibodies against nicotinic acetylcholine receptors of NMJ, leading to *reduced* **post-synaptic** response to *acetylcholine* → significant muscle fatigue Muscles that are stimulated frequently (EOM) prone to fatigue Peak incidence F: age 20-30 y/o M: age 50-70 y/o	1. **Skeletal muscle weakness**—preserved sensation and reflexes • Worse with continued use, better with rest, worse at end of day • Fluctuating (hallmark) • As disease progresses, symptom free periods are lost 2. **Ptosis and/or diplopia** (most common)—initial symptom 3. **Blurred vision** 4. Bulbar symptoms (15%): dysarthria, dysphagia, fatigable chewing • Quality of speech sounds nasal or low intensity (hypophonic) 5. Progresses slowly with periodic exacerbations Signs: 1. Myasthenic "sneer"—mid lip rises, but corners of mouth fail to move 2. Neck extensor and flexor muscles (dropped head syndrome)	1. The ice pack test: has sensitivity of 80% in patients with ptosis 2. Edrophonium (Tensilon) test • AChE meds cause improvement in SX, but high false (−/+) • Sensitivity 80%-90% • Use in patients with obvious ptosis who will benefit from drug administration 3. **Acetylcholine receptor antibody test** (most specific)—FIRST STEP • 10% antibody neg 4. **Repetitive nerve stimulation (RNS)**: progressive decline in CMAP amplitude with first 4-5 stimuli (decremental response) 5. Electromyography (EMG) • Less available, but most sensitive diagnostic test for MG • Abnormal if "jitter" detected 6. CT of thorax: r/o thymoma	1. AChE inhibitors: **pyridostigmine (Mestinon)** • Decreased AChE increases concentration of acetylcholine at synapses by decreasing breakdown 2. Thymectomy—symptomatic relief 3. Steroids, azathioprine, cyclosporine, and mycophenolate mofetil *Myasthenic crisis, bridging, adjuvant, or for refractory cases* 4. Plasmapheresis—removes antibodies 5. IVIG therapy for acute exacerbations 6. Monitoring 7. Monitor serial forced vital capacities
Ocular myasthenia gravis (OMG)	Symptoms isolated to levator palpebrae superioris, orbicularis oculi, and oculomotor muscles 50% of patients More likely to be seronegative for ACh-R antibodies than GMG	1. **Ptosis**—Weakness limited to eyelids and extraocular eye muscles • Variable throughout day • Can switch from one eye to other • Start bilaterally and improve in one eye, or start unilateral and become bilateral 2. Binocular **diplopia**—present when both eyes open • May be horizontal or vertical 3. Oculomotor paresis Signs: 1. May mimic internuclear ophthalmoplegia (INO) or a vertical gaze paresis 2. Pupils always spared 3. Ptosis may increase with sustained upward gaze or by holding up the opposite eyelid with examiner's finger (curtain sign)	1. **The ice pack test:** has sensitivity of 80% in patients with ptosis 2. Edrophonium (**Tensilon) test** • AChE inhibitors cause improvement in SX, but high false (−/+) • Sensitivity 80-90% • Use in patients with obvious ptosis who will benefit from drug administration 3. *Acetylcholine receptor antibody test* (most specific, first) • 50% antibody neg • MuSK antibodies are not present	1. Symptomatic and immunomodulatory therapy • Lubricating drops • Eye patch, opaque contact lens • **Mestinon** (pyridostigmine): AChE inhibitor • Prednisone 2. Thymectomy • For all patients with thymoma and MG 3. Corrective treatment of ptosis and strabismus • Consider strabismus surgery for patients 3 y after onset of OMG if deficits stable for at least 1 y 2/3 develop extremity weakness and bulbar muscle weakness, 1/3 maintain pure OMG Most (78%) who develop GMG do so in 1 y and all within 3 y

Internal Medicine

(continued)

(continued)

Disease	Etiology, Prevalence, Risk Factors	Clinical Symptoms and Signs	Diagnostics	Therapy, Prognosis, and Health Maintenance
Generalized myasthenia gravis (GMG)	98%-100% of patients with MG and **thymoma** are seropositive for antibodies MuSK-Ab (+): onset any age, female, oculobulbar form (not purely ocular), restricted myopathic form with prominent respiratory and/or proximal weakness, no thymoma, less responsiveness to AChE inhibitors, good response to PLEX and immunosuppression	Weakness commonly affects ocular muscles, but involves bulbar, limb, and respiratory muscles	1. *Acetylcholine receptor antibody test* (most specific, first) • 50% antibody neg • Present in 85% with generalized disease 2. MuSK antibodies • Present in 38%-50% of people who are AChR antibody negative	1. Plasmapheresis and IVIG for short-term management (no role in OMG)
Myasthenic crisis	Precipitators: surgery (thymectomy), infection, pregnancy, childbirth, medication, tapering of immunosuppression	Increasing respiratory muscle and/or bulbar muscle weakness from disorder that is severe enough to necessitate intubation, or in some cases, to delay extubation following surgery 1. SOB–described as "suffocation" or "drowning" worse when supine 2. Severe dysphagia with weak cough or difficulty clearing secretions 3. Hypophonia, pausing during speech to take a breath Signs: 1. Accessory muscle use 2. Poor respiratory effort, increased respiratory rate with shallow breaths 3. Paradoxical abdominal breathing	1. Low baseline vital capacity (VC) <30 mL/kg of ideal body weight: take a deep breath in and exhale maximally 2. Maximal inspiratory pressure (MIP)–inhale against closed valve	1. Admit to ICU and monitor respiratory rate 2. Intubation, if necessary and mechanical ventilation 3. Stop anticholinesterase inhibitors 4. Begin plasma exchange or IVIG 5. Begin Immunomodulating therapy with HD steroids, azathioprine, cyclosporine, or mycophenolate mofetil Complications: Aspiration (due to palatal weakness)

GIANT CELL (TEMPORAL) ARTERITIS

Vasculitis of unknown cause, may involve aorta or carotids, but typically temporal arteries.

Disease	Etiology, Prevalence, Risk Factors	Clinical Symptoms and Signs	Diagnostics	Therapy, Prognosis, and Health Maintenance
Giant cell arteritis	**Age >50** F (2×) >M **Increased risk of aortic aneurysm and dissection**	1. Constitutional symptoms: **malaise**, fatigue, weight loss, low grade **fever** 2. **New headaches**–severe 3. Visual impairment (25%-50%) • Optic neuritis → blindness (50%) 4. **Jaw pain** with chewing: intermittent claudication 5. **Tenderness** over temporal artery, absent pulse 6. **Palpable** nodules 7. 40% have **polymyalgia rheumatica**	1. Very **elevated ESR** 2. Biopsy temporal artery (90% sensitive)	1. High dose steroids to prevent blindness, start immediately, do not wait for biopsy results—treat 4 wk, then taper and maintain 2-3 y 2. Follow ESR levels 3. If untreated, most self-limiting

GUILLAIN-BARRE SYNDROME

Disease	Etiology, Prevalence, Risk Factors	Clinical Symptoms and Signs	Diagnostics	Therapy, Prognosis, and Health Maintenance
Guillain-Barré syndrome (*ascending polyneuropathy with areflexia*)	**Autoimmune** reaction against peripheral nerves Inflammatory demyelinating polyneuropathy affecting motor nerves Circulating antibodies against the <u>postsynaptic</u> nicotinic acetylcholine receptors at the NMJ of skeletal muscle cells Bimodal: 20-30 (F), 60-70 (M)	<u>HX:</u> Previous **viral infection** (or *C. jejuni*, CMV, hepatitis, HIV), surgery, or vaccination 1. *Abrupt onset* (12 h-28 d) and resolution 2. Rapidly **progressive bilateral and flaccid weakness** • Becomes more severe with repeated use of or during course of day • Loss of sensation in "stocking-glove" distribution of all 4 extremities • Usually symmetric • Progresses from distal to central muscles • Mild or severe 3. **Sphincter control** and **micturition** *spared* • Autonomic features: arrhythmias, tachycardia, postural hypotension 4. Absence of fever or other systemic symptoms <u>Signs:</u> Decreased or absent DTRs in weak limbs	See *Brighton Criteria* 1. Lumbar puncture • **Increased protein** • NL glucose, pressure • **WBC <50 cells/uL** 2. Electrodiagnostics: **decreased** motor nerve conduction velocity	1. Admit and monitor for respiratory failure • Start therapy ASAP 2. *High dose IVIg* • Initially use due to safety profile and ease of administration • Daily infusions for 5 d, total dose 2 g/kg body weight 3. **Plasmapheresis** for severe respiratory compromise or weakness • 40-50 mL/kg 4-5 × over 1 wk DO NOT GIVE STEROIDS → harmful 85% of patients achieve full recovery within several months to 1 y

HUNTINGTON DISEASE

Disease	Etiology, Prevalence, Risk Factors	Clinical Symptoms and Signs	Diagnostics	Therapy, Prognosis, and Health Maintenance
Huntington disease	Involuntary writhing of muscle groups Autosomal dominant disorder	1. Progressive **dementia** • Early age of onset • Subtle changes in cognitive functioning 2. **Choreiform** movements: restlessness • Expansive, dance-like movements in multiple limbs		Associated: depression

CEREBRAL ANEURYSM

Disease	Etiology, Prevalence, Risk Factors	Clinical Symptoms and Signs	Diagnostics	Therapy, Prognosis, and Health Maintenance
Cerebral (intracranial) aneurysm	• Develops from normal hemodynamic stress or HTN • Develops at junction of communicating branch with main cerebral artery (Ant Comm + Ant Cerebral) **AV malformation** 1. **Ruptured berry (saccular) aneurysm** (MC, 80%)–most located in anterior circulation 2. Fusiform (large) 3. Mycotic (bacterial endocarditis) Associated: polycystic kidney disease, Marfan syndrome	May manifest as compression as cranial nerves (CN III, IV, VI) Causes of rupture–strenuous activity (exercise, coitus, physical work)	1. **Noncontrast CT** head–if normal, do LP • Contrast CT or MRI for aneurysms >5 mm or AV malformations 2. Lumbar puncture 3. **Cerebral angiography** (gold standard)	1. Open surgical clipping 2. **Endovascular coiling** (preferred) Complication: Subarachnoid hemorrhage Of patients with aneurysms that rupture, 33% die before reaching the hospital, 20% die in the hospital, 30% recover without disability

CONCUSSION

Rapid onset of short-lived impairment of neurologic function resolving spontaneously.

Disease	Etiology, Prevalence, Risk Factors	Clinical Symptoms and Signs	Diagnostics	Therapy, Prognosis, and Health Maintenance
Concussion	Falls (28%), MVC (20%), struck by heavy object, assault	Minor head injury: GCS >13 Asymptomatic ~2 h, normal mental status No evidence of skull fracture Normal physical exam (+/−) LOC, seizure activity Vomiting, irritability, lethargy, headache, confusion, gait problems	Scalp hematoma, palpable crepitus Fundoscopic exam Neurologic exam SCAT2: MMSE + physical Imaging usually normal and NOT required CT if <48 h MRI if >48 h Especially image if: severe headache/worsening, prolonged recovery, focal deficits, seizures, slurred speech, unsteady gait, weakness, persistent vomiting, behavior changes, evidence of skull fracture	• Observe in ER × 4 h • Rest until asymptomatic • Light aerobic exercise • Sport-specific training, noncontact training drills, full contact after medical clearance, return to play 24 h for each stage

PERIPHERAL NEUROPATHIES

Related to duration and severity of hyperglycemia, but may be presenting symptom in diabetes → vascular insufficiency or nerve infarction.

Disease	Etiology, Prevalence, Risk Factors	Clinical Symptoms and Signs	Diagnostics	Therapy, Prognosis, and Health Maintenance
Peripheral neuropathy (polyneuropathy)	Refers to generalized relatively homogenous process affecting many peripheral nerves, with the distal nerves affected most prominently Causes: **Diabetes mellitus**, alcohol abuse, HIV	1. Symmetric distal sensory loss, burning or weakness 2. Paresthesias (numbness, tingling), burning or pain in feet, gait abnormality 3. Autonomic disturbances—most commonly in hands and feet (cold, sweating) 4. Weakness of lower legs and hand resulting in **'stocking and glove' distribution** of sensory loss Signs: 1. Decreased DTRs 2. Decreased vibration and two-point discrimination 3. Semmel-Weinstein (monofilament gauge)	1. **EMG and/or nerve conduction study** (initial) if no clear etiology or when symptoms rapidly progressive 2. Labs: blood glucose, serum B$_{12}$ with MMA (+/− homocysteine) and serum protein electrophoresis 3. Muscle or nerve biopsy 4. Skin biopsy 5. Autonomic testing 6. Quantitative sensory testing	If diabetic → tight diabetes control *Painful diabetic polyneuropathy* 1. Anticonvulsants: **Gabapentin** (first line) 2. Antidepressants: Amitriptyline (TCA) 3. α-lipoic acid

Disease	Etiology, Prevalence, Risk Factors	Clinical Symptoms and Signs	Diagnostics	Therapy, Prognosis, and Health Maintenance
Carpal tunnel syndrome (mononeuropathy)	Numbness and tingling and/or pain in median nerve distribution F>M (3:1) RF: Obesity, female, comorbidity (diabetes melitus, **pregnancy (3rd trimester)**, RA, hypothyroid), genetics, aromatase inhibitor use 65% bilateral Severe cases: Clumsiness "difficulty holding objects, turning keys or doorknobs, buttoning clothing, or opening jar lids"	1. **Pain** • Involvement of first 3 digits and radial half of 4th digit • Worse at night and awaken patient from sleep • Better by shaking or wringing hands or placing them under warm water 2. **Paresthesias** • May radiate proximally into forearm or above elbow to shoulder • Provoked by flexion or extension of wrist or raising arms (driving, reading, typing, holding phone) 3. **Weakness** (less commonly) Signs: 1. Weakness of thumb adduction and opposition 2. Thenar atrophy	Clinical DX: 1. **Phalen maneuver**: flex the wrist with elbow in full extension (backs of hands against one another to provide hyperflexion) • Positive if pain and/or paresthesia in median innervated fingers within one minute of wrist flexion 2. *Tinel Test*–percussion over proximal portion of carpal tunnel • Positive if pain and/or paresthesia • Less sensitive than Phalen sign (50%) 3. Nerve conduction study (NCS) with EMG • Excludes polyneuropathy, plexopathy, and radiculopathy • Delayed distal latencies and slowed conduction velocity	1. Mild (nonsurgical) • **Nocturnal wrist splinting** in neutral position × 1 mo • **Steroid injections** of methylprednisolone 40 mg, no more than 1/wrist q 6 mo • Oral steroids of 20 mg prednisone daily 10-14 d • PT/OT or yoga 2. Moderate–severe • Electrodiagnostic studies (first) • Surgical decompression *Note*: Should resolve postpartum in pregnancy

COMPLEX REGIONAL PAIN SYNDROME

- Usually begins after an operation, injury (fracture), or following a vascular event such as stroke or MI
- No identifiable neurologic lesion for pain, not well understood

Disease	Etiology, Prevalence, Risk Factors	Clinical Symptoms and Signs	Diagnostics	Therapy, Prognosis, and Health Maintenance
Complex regional pain syndrome: (reflex sympathetic dystrophy)	Characterized by regional pain in affected limb, restricted mobility, edema, color changes of skin, spotting bone thinning Follows soft tissue injury	1. Hallmark: **severe burning** or **throbbing pain** with associated allodynia in affected region/extremity 2. Cyanosis, abnormal sensitivity to temperature, abnormal skin temp, atrophy	Clinical DX: 1. Bone scintigraphy, plain x-rays, MRI 2. Regional nerve block–diagnostic	1. Early mobilization following injury 2. TCAs, gabapentin, pregabalin (Lyrica), lamotrigine for pain relief 3. NSAIDs in some patients 4. Calcitonin adjunctive 5. Bisphosphonates, IVIG, regional nerve blocks, dorsal column stimulation

Internal Medicine

CHAPTER **22**

Critical Care

ACUTE HYPOGLYCEMIA

Disease	Etiology, Prevalence, Risk Factors	Clinical Symptoms and Signs	Diagnostics	Therapy, Prognosis, and Health Maintenance
Fasting hypoglycemia	Consider insulinomas in healthy patients with fasting hypoglycemia Etiology: Hypopituitarism, Addison disease, myxedema, acute alcoholism, liver failure, ESRD MC: Adenoma of islets of Langerhans (90% benign), rare	1. Confusion 2. Blurred vision 3. Diplopia 4. Anxiety 5. Seizures	1. Serum glucose <45 mg/dL • Symptoms begin at plasma glucose levels <60 mg/dL • Impairment of brain function at 50 mg/dL 2. Serum insulin, proinsulin, and C-peptide: inappropriately high 3. Sulfonylurea screening (−) 4. Other labs: serum ketones, antibodies to insulin 5. Plasma BOH <2.7 mmol/L	1. Home glucose monitor • Measure time of symptoms and prior consumption of carbs 2. If high clinical suspicion despite outpatient trial • 72 h supervised inpatient fast 3. Surgical resection of insulin-secreting tumors
Medication-induced hypoglycemia	Common offenders: FQ, quinine, ACE inhibitors, salicylates, beta-blockers			1. Glucose administration to replenish glycogen stores until gluconeogenesis resumes

Disease	Etiology, Prevalence, Risk Factors	Clinical Symptoms and Signs	Diagnostics	Therapy, Prognosis, and Health Maintenance
Factitious hypoglycemia	Self-induced hypoglycemia	1. Patient has access to insulin or sulfonylureas taken by another family member 2. Hypoglycemia	1. Immunoreactive insulin: elevated 2. Low plasma C peptide 3. Insulin: C-peptide ratio > 1	
Postprandial hypoglycemia	Causes: s/p gastric surgery (gastrectomy, vagotomy, pyloroplasty, Nissen fundoplication, etc)	SX occur after eating high carb meal 1. Lightheadedness 2. Sweating 3. Confusion 4. Loss of consciousness 5. Anxiety Signs: 1. Palpitations 2. Diaphoresis		1. Dietary modification • Smaller meals of less rapidly digested carbs • Reduced intake of refined sugars • Increased dietary fiber intake 2. Octreotide 50 µg SQ 2-3 times/day, 30 min prior to meals
Insulin-induced hypoglycemia				1. Patient should carry glucose tablets or juice at all times 2. Ingestion of 15 g of carbs in most cases • Check glucose in 15 min and treat again if still low 3. IM 1 mg glucagon emergency kit • Inject SQ/IM into buttock, arm, or thigh • Turn patient on side to prevent aspiration of vomit 4. For severe hypoglycemia • 50 mL D5W rapid IV infusion or 1 mg IM glucagon

MYOCARDIAL INFARCTION

Suspect AMI in patients with CAD with acute onset hypotension and bradycardia.

- Acute infarction in left anterior descending artery (anterior distribution): ST elevations in leads V1-V2
  - Presents with acute, severe crushing or pressure-like chest pain associated with radiation to jaw or neck, as well as nausea and sweating

Cardiac Arrest

- V-tach or V-fib causes 75% of episodes of cardiac arrest

- β-blockers, O_2, morphine, NTG, and aspirin greet the patient at the door
- RCA distribution (right ventricular wall and inferior left ventricular wall, AV node): bradycardia due to AV nodal ischemia or infarction: ST elevation in leads II, III, and aVF

- Exception: "Pre-load dependent"—do not give NTG or morphine, treat with IV fluids first

Cardiac Arrest	Sudden Cardiac Death	Pulseless Electrical Activity (PEA)
Sudden loss of cardiac output • Potentially reversible if circulation and O_2 delivery promptly restored	Unexpected death within 1 h of symptom onset secondary to a cardiac cause	Occurs when electrical activity is on the monitor but there are no pulses (even with Doppler) • Treat possible causes: 5Hs and 5Ts

5 Hs: **H**ypoxia, **h**ypovolemia, **h**yperkalemia/hypokalemia, **H**$^+$ (acidosis), **h**ypothermia
5 Ts: **T**amponade, **t**ension pneumothorax, **t**oxins, **t**hromboembolism (PE), **t**hrombosis (MI)

ACUTE ABDOMEN

Refers to sudden, severe abdominal pain of unclear etiology less than 24 h duration.

- Also consider, acute peptic ulcer, DKA, acute diverticulitis, ectopic pregnancy with tubal rupture, ovarian torsion, acute pyelonephritis, adrenal crisis, AAA, sickle cell anemia, and kidney stones
- Work-up: KUB and/or CT scan
  - In unstable patient, IVF + FAST-ultrasound (if + free fluid, surgery)

SHOCK

Underperfusion of tissues.

- Presentation:
  - Tachycardia, hypotension
  - Malfunction of organ systems: lactic acidosis, renal (anuria/oliguria), CNS dysfunction (AMS)
- Initial steps: stabilize patient hemodynamically, determine cause

- Fluid bolus (500-1000 L NS or lactated Ringer's solution)
- CBC, CMP, Creatinine, PT/PTT, continuous pulse oximetry
- EKG, CXR
- Vasopressors (dopamine or norepinephrine) if hypotensive despite IVF
- Treatment
  - ABC assessment

Type of Shock	Cardiac Output	SVR	PCWP
Cardiogenic	Decreased	**Increased**	**Increased**
Hypovolemic	Decreased	**Increased**	Decreased
Neurogenic	Decreased	Decreased	Decreased
Septic	**Increased**	Decreased	Decreased

Type of Shock	General Characteristics & Causes	Clinical Features	Diagnosis	Treatment
Cardiogenic	Heart unable to generate CO to maintain tissue perfusion MCC: **Post-acute MI** Cardiac tamponade, tension pneumothorax, arrhythmias, PE, CM, myocarditis, valvular defects	SBP <90 Urine output <20 mL/h Altered sensorium, pale cool skin, hypotension, tachycardia JVD Pulmonary congestion	EKG: ST elevation (most common) Echo Hemodynamic monitoring	ABCs Identify underlying cause Vasopressors: Dopamine (initial) +/– dobutamine NTG or nitroprusside IVF–harmful if LV pressures elevated (may need diuretics)
Hypovolemic	Decreased circulatory blood volume → decreased preload and cardiac output Hemorrhage (trauma, GI bleed, retroperitoneal) Nonhemorrhagic–vomiting, diarrhea, dehydration, burns, third space loss	Vital signs and clinical picture	Central venous line or **pulmonary artery catheter**: decreased CVP/PCWP, decreased cardiac output, and increased SVR	AB: intubation, mech vent Circulation: direct pressure if acute bleed IV Hydration: class II (optional), class III/IV (required)
Neurogenic	Failure of sympathetic NS to maintain vascular tone SCI, head injury, spinal anesthesia, drug blockade	Vasodilation with decreased SVR (warm, flush skin) UOP: NL to LOW Bradycardia, hypotension		Judicious use of IV fluids Vasoconstrictors to restore venous tone Supine or Trendelenburg position Maintain temp
Septic	Hypotension induced by sepsis, persistent despite adequate IVF → Multi organ system failure Pneumonia, pyelo, meningitis, abscess, cholangitis, cellulitis, peritonitis	Severe decrease in SVR due to peripheral vasodilation (flush, warm skin) Signs of SIRS Signs of shock: hypotension, oliguria, lactic acidosis Fever or hypothermia	Decreased EF–reduced contractility Clinical DX: (+) blood cultures × 2 Source of infection	IV Antibiotics (broad spectrum) at max doses IVF: Increase mean BP Pressors: Maintain BP

CHAPTER 23

Infectious Diseases

Refer to Family Medicine 👪 **for in-depth coverage of the following topics:**

Chlamydia and Gonoccocal Infections, see Urology/Renal, p 182

Cholera, see GI, p 44

Tuberculosis, see Pulmonology, p 28

Salmonellosis, see GI, p 43

Tuberculosis, see Pulmonology, p 28

Parasitic Infections, see GI, p 59

Shigellosis, see GI, p 43

Refer to Pediatrics 👨‍👦 **for in-depth coverage of the following topics:**

Pertussis, see Pulmonology, p 315

HUMAN IMMUNODEFICIENCY VIRUS (HIV) INFECTION

- Targets of the virus are dendritic cells in the mucosa of the genital tract, which the virus uses to transport into lymph nodes and infect lymphocytes
- Infects cells expressing the T4 (CD4) antigen
- Chemokine coreceptors (CCR-5, CXCR-4 or both) are required for virus entry
- B-lymphocytes are also affected and can lead to hyper-gammaglobulinemia and can depress B-cell responses to new antigen challenges (such as vaccination)
- Macrophages act as a reservoir and can disseminate HIV to organ systems such as the CNS
- Virus is produced by newly infected lymphocytes (CD4, helper-inducer) and transported to tissues within days
  - **Primary HIV infection**, also known as acute retroviral syndrome or "seroconversion syndrome"
- **Immune response**: antibodies against HIV appear and cytotoxic T cells for HIV-infected cells proliferate, achieving partial control of the infection (plateau)

- The higher the plateau, the faster the development of AIDS
- Hallmark of HIV-induced immunodeficiency: *progressive reduction in CD4 T-cell count*
- Long-term nonprogressors or "elite controllers": survive many years (>10) with low viremia and normal CD4 counts
- Most opportunistic infections are caused by reactivation of latent pathogens (herpes virus, fungi, or bacteria) when CD4 cell counts drop below 200
- HIV has not been shown to be transmitted via respiratory droplets, mosquitoes, nonsexual contact, saliva, sweat, stool, or tears
- Women with HIV are at higher risk for recurrent candidal vaginitis, PID, and cervical dysplasia
- Low incidence of: listeriosis, aspergillosis
- High incidence of lymphoma, Kaposi Sarcoma
- HIV infected patients are at higher risk for CAD due to ART therapy with stravudine and several protease inhibitors

Disease	Etiology, Prevalence, Risk Factors	Clinical Symptoms and Signs	Diagnostics	Therapy, Prognosis, and Health Maintenance

HIV Infection (testing, presentation, opportunistic infections, treatment)	Infected: women younger than men 76% men: 65% of which were exposed through MSM contact, 14% IVDU, 12% heterosexual contact, 8% MSM and IVDU
	Transmission:
	Blood-blood, 1/300 needlestick, 30% for child of untreated infected mother, 0.01%-1% of vaginal or anal intercourse
	RF:
	Sexual contact with infected person, IV exposure to infected blood by transfusion or needle sharing, perinatal exposure
		Asymptomatic
		• Mean: 10 y
		"Primary HIV Infection"
		• Fever, night sweats, weight loss
		• Skin lesions
		• Pharyngitis
		• Swollen lymph nodes
		• Lasts days-weeks
		Signs:
		1. Hairy leukoplakia
		2. Disseminated Kaposi sarcoma
		3. Cutaneous bacillary angiomatosis
		4. Generalized lymphadenopathy
			1. **HIV ELISA** (enzyme-linked immunosorbent assay): screening
			  • Detectable in 95% within 6 wk after infection
			2. **Western blot** (confirmatory)
			  • 99.9% specific when combined with ELISA
			  • False positives with flu vaccine or connective tissue disease
			3. **HIV rapid antibody test** (screening): -Available within 10-20 min
			  • Must be confirmed with ELISA and WB
			4. CBC: anemia, neutropenia, thrombocytopenia
			5. **Absolute CD4** lymphocyte **count**: predicts HIV progression
			  • Monitor every 3-6 mo
			6. CD4 lymphocyte percentage: more reliable than count
			7. Viral load: correlates with disease progression and response to ART
			8. CXR–r/o PCP pneumonia, can present without respiratory symptoms
			9. Blood cultures if fever >38.5°C
			10. Serum cryptococcal Ag and myco-cultures of blood
			11. Sinus CT scan or XR
				1. Start treatment regardless of CD4 and perform resistance testing prior to ART initiation
				2. Primary goal is complete suppression of viral replication (low viral load)
				3. Combination therapy with at least 3 medications from at least 2 classes
				Prognosis:
				Age at time of infection (very young or older, rapid progression)

AIDS (with laboratory evidence of HIV)		1. Coccidioidomycosis 2. HIV encephalopathy 3. Histoplasmosis 4. Isosporiasis with diarrhea >1 mo 5. Kaposi sarcoma at any age 6. Lymphoma of the brain at any age 7. Other non-Hodgkin lymphoma of B cell 8. MAC, disseminated 9. Extrapulmonary TB 10. Salmonella septicemia, recurrent 11. HIV wasting syndrome 12. Pulmonary TB 13. Recurrent PNA 14. Invasive cervical cancer	1. HIV serology (+) 2. CD4 count <200 cells/uL or CD4 <14%	

Complications of Advanced Disease

Disease	Etiology, Prevalence, Risk Factors	Clinical Symptoms and Signs	Diagnostics	Therapy, Prognosis, and Health Maintenance
Kaposi sarcoma		Lesions anywhere: eyelids, conjunctiva, pinnae, palate, toe webs Signs: Purplish, nonblanching papules or nodules	(Fig. 23-1)	Resolves with effective ART

Disease	Etiology, Prevalence, Risk Factors	Clinical Symptoms and Signs	Diagnostics	Therapy, Prognosis, and Health Maintenance

Wasting syndrome	Decreased caloric intake, increased metabolic rate	1. Weight loss: disproportionate loss of muscle mass
		2. Anorexia, nausea, vomiting
		3. Diarrhea
				1. ART therapy
				2. Fever control
				3. Treat underlying opportunistic infections
				4. Food supplements, including TPN
				  • Megestrol acetate
				  • Dronabinol
				5. Growth hormone SQ × 12 wk
				6. Anabolic steroids IM q 2-4 wk

Primary non-Hodgkin lymphoma	Second most common space occupying lesion in HIV infected patients B-cell origin, 70% are extranodal	Diffuse large cell tumors	1. Lumbar puncture—(+) PCR assay of CSF for EBV 2. Brain biopsy	1. Radiation therapy 2. Combination EPOCH chemotherapy with Rituximab 3. G-CSF (granulocyte colony stimulating factor) to maintain WBC count

HIV-associated dementia		1. Difficulty with cognitive tasks (memory, attention)
		  • Waxes and wanes
		2. Diminished motor function
		  • Deterioration in handwriting
		3. Emotional or behavioral problems
			1. DX of exclusion
			2. CT/MRI
			3. Lumbar puncture
			4. Neuropsychiatric testing
			5. Hypoglycemia, hyponatremia, hypoxia	

Progressive multifocal leukoencephalopathy (PML)	Infection of the white matter of the brain seen in patients with very advanced HIV	1. Aphasia 2. Hemiparesis 3. Cortical blindness	1. MRI: nonenhancing white matter lesions without mass effect	
HIV myelopathy		1. Leg weakness 2. Incontinence Signs: 1. Spastic paraparesis 2. Sensory ataxia	DX of exclusion 1. MRI: vacuolation of white matter, r/o epidural lymphoma 2. Lumbar puncture: r/o CMV polyradiculopathy	
Peripheral neuropathy	Causes: HIV, ART therapy with stavudine and didanosine	1. Numbness, tingling, and pain in lower extremities	1. r/o alcoholism, thyroid disease, vitamin B_{12} deficiency, syphilis	1. Gabapentin 300 mg bedtime and increase to 300-900 mg PO TID

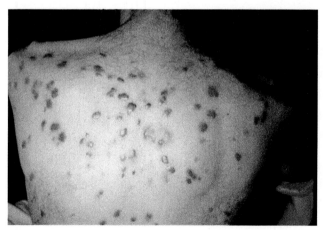

FIGURE 23-1. AIDS-related Kaposi sarcoma. (From Hinkle JL, Cheever KH. *Brunner & Suddarth's Textbook of Medical-Surgical Nursing.* 13th ed. Philadelphia: Wolters Kluwer Health; 2014.)

Health Maintenance for HIV

- Annual anal swabs (Papanicolaou smear) for cytologic examination of HPV
- Screen for cervical dysplasia in HIV-infected women—annually and if negative, every 3 years; continue beyond age 65 (unlike general population)
  - Perform when HIV diagnosed, annually thereafter, and after three negative exams, perform every 3 years
- Screen for HIV in adults aged 15 to 65
- *Annual* PPD testing
- Screen all men for syphilis with RPR or VDRL every *6 months*
- Vaccines—all should be given, including measles vaccination (even though live) and zoster vaccine if CD4 >200 and undetectable viral load
- Practice safe sex, avoid substance abuse, avoid consuming raw meat, eggs or shellfish, wash hands thoroughly after cleaning cat litter
- All patients taking protease inhibitors or NRTIs should have fasting serum cholesterol, LDL cholesterol, and TG levels annually

Prevention and Prophylaxis

- Pre-exposure ART Prophylaxis (PrEP)
  - Daily Truvada (emtricitabine/tenofovir) can reduce the risk of sexual transmission of HIV among uninfected individuals at high risk for infection
- Postexposure Prophylaxis
  - Healthcare workers with needle-stick injuries (risk 1:300), greater with deep punctures, large inoculum, and source patients with high VL
  - Tenofovir 300 gm with emtricitabine 200 mg daily with raltegravir 400 mg BID × 4 weeks
  - Provide ASAP no more than 72 hours after exposure
  - Follow up testing at 6 weeks, 3 months, and 6 months
- Prevention of Perinatal Transmission
  - HIV pregnant women should start ART therapy with at least three medications
  - Zidovudine, Lamivudine with either Ritonavir boosted Lopinavir or Ritonavir boosted Atazanavir
  - C-section delivery should be planned if viral load >1000 close to delivery
  - Zidovudine should be given to infant after birth for 6 weeks
  - Breastfeeding should be avoided

Prophylaxis for Common Opportunistic Infections In HIV (+) Patients

Infection/Organism	Treatment Indicated	Treatment
Pneumocystis pneumonia	If CD4 <200, <14%	1. Bactrim 2. Dapsone 3. Atovaquone 4. Aerosolized pentamidine
Toxoplasmosis	(+) IgG toxoplasma serology and If CD4 <100	1. Bactrim DS daily—D/C once CD4 >200 for 3 mo
Mycobacterium avium complex	If CD4 <75	1. Clarithromycin 2. **Azithromycin** (preferred)
CMV	If CD4 <50	1. Bactrim
Mycobacterium tuberculosis	If (+) PPD, without evidence of active disease (normal CXR)	1. Isoniazid + pyridoxine for 9-12 mo

CANDIDIASIS

Disease	Etiology, Prevalence, Risk Factors	Clinical Symptoms and Signs	Diagnostics	Therapy, Prognosis, and Health Maintenance
Candidiasis	***Candida albicans*** (MCC) RF: Antibiotics, diabetes, steroids, immunocompromised Oval, budding yeasts known for formation of hyphae and long pseudohyphae	1. Vagina **"yeast infection"**: thick, white, **"cottage cheese"** discharge, painless, itchy 2. Oropharynx/mouth **"thrush"**: thick, white plaques that adhere to oral mucosa, painless 3. Cutaneous: erythematous, eroded patches with satellite lesions (mostly diabetics) 4. GI tract (esophagus): odynophagia, asymptomatic 5. Disseminated/ invasive disease may occur in IC hosts: sepsis/shock, meningitis, abscesses Signs: 1. Vulva—erythematous, swollen, excoriation 2. White, clumpy discharge	CD4 <u><200</u> if AIDS Clinical DX: 1. KOH prep 2. Invasive—blood or tissue culture	1. Remove catheters or lines 2. Clotrimazole 5× daily, nystatin 3-5× daily, ketoconazole or fluconazole for esophagitis 3. Vagina: miconazole or clotrimazole cream 4. Skin: oral nystatin powder, keep skin dry 5. Systemic: ampho-B, **fluconazole**, flucytosine • Fluconazole 150 mg PO × 1 d
Esophagitis (esophageal candidiasis)	Immunosuppressed patients with AIDS, solid organ transplants, leukemia, and lymphoma MC pathogens: ***Candida albicans***, herpes simplex, CMV	1. 1 or more: Odynophagia, dysphagia • **Oral thrush** (75%) • Retrosternal or epigastric pain • Nausea, vomiting Signs: Normal oral mucosa	1. Endoscopy with biopsy and brushings	• Empiric • *Candida*: fluconazole 14-21 d • CMV: Ganciclovir 3-6 wk • AIDS—HAART • Herpetic: symptomatic TX unless immunocompromised, then acyclovir × 2-3 wk
Oral candidiasis (thrush)	RF: HIV, dentures, DM, exposure to broad spectrum antibiotics or inhaled steroids	1. **Sore** and painful, dry **mouth** 2. Burning mouth or tongue 3. Dysphagia 4. Unpleasant taste Signs: 1. Thick, whitish patches on oral mucosa • Easily rubbed off 2. Diffuse erythema	Clinical DX: KOH prep (wet mount): pseudohyphae or hyphae (Fig. 23-2)	1. Topical antifungal • **Clotrimazole troches** 10 mg 4-5 × daily • Nystatin 2. PO fluconazole 50-100 mg PO daily × 3-7 d

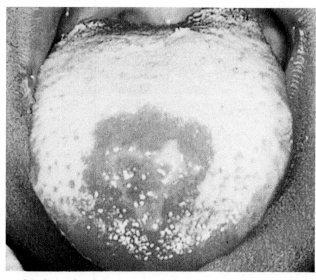

FIGURE 23-2. Thrush, seen as cream-colored pseudomembranous patches on the tongue, mouth, or pharynx. (From Weber J, Kelley JH. *Health Assessment in Nursing*. 2nd ed. Philadelphia: Lippincott Williams & Wilkins; 2003.)

FUNGAL: CRYPTOCOCCUS, HISTOPLASMOSIS, PNEUMOCYSTIS

Disease	Etiology, Prevalence, Risk Factors	Clinical Symptoms and Signs	Diagnostics	Therapy, Prognosis, and Health Maintenance
Cryptococcosis (Pneumonia)	MCC: ***Cryptococcus neoformans serotype A (AIDS),*** *Cryptococcus gattii* (70%-80%) Encapsulated budding *yeast* found in soil contaminated with dried **pigeon** dung, cockroaches, or bird droppings Transmission: 1. Inhalation 2. Common in immunocompromised and **solid organ transplant hosts** 3. most common areas for infection: lungs and CNS 4. CD4 <100 if AIDS	1. HX: Pulmonary disease if COPD, steroid use, posttransplant 2. **Fever** (low grade) • More common in HIV 3. Productive **cough** 4. **Dyspnea** 5. **Headache** 6. Weight loss 7. Pleuritic chest pain 8. Malaise Signs: 1. Pleural effusions 2. Lymphadenopathy Complications: Meningitis, meningoencephalitis	1. **CXR**: solitary or multiple nodules, granulomas, patchy pneumonitis 2. ***India ink prep*** (confirms) of CSF−variable pleocytosis (mostly lymphocytes), increased opening pressure, increased protein, decreased glucose 3. Culture of BAL Culture: Budding, encapsulated fungus CSF/serum: Cryptococcal antigen, india ink stain or serology with latex agglutination assay or cryptococcal antigen assay (CRAG) CT or MRI	1. Observation only if: • CSF normal • CSF culture, cryptococcal Ag, India ink, and serology (−) • Urine culture (−) • Lesion small, stable, or shrinking • No predisposing conditions for dissemination 2. **Oral fluconazole** 6-12 mo, itraconazole 1 y, or ampho-B 3. Severe = **Amphotericin-B** × 6-10 wk 4. +/− flucytosine
Histoplasmosis Fungal infection most commonly associated with being exposed to spelunkers and bat droppings causing an infection of the lung leading to granuloma formation	**Histoplasma capsulatum** (dimorphic fungus with septate hyphae) Exposure to bird/bat droppings, caves, chicken coops **Ohio and Mississippi river valleys** RF for disseminated disease: AIDS CD4 <150, use of steroids, hematologic malignancy, solid organ transplant	90% asymptomatic 1. Flu-like symptoms 3-14 d after exposure Acute: <1 mo Subacute: 1-3 mo Chronic: >3 mo • Fever, HA, **malaise**, myalgia, abdominal pain, chills 2. **Severe SOB**, *worsening cough*, hemoptysis, chest pain 3. Joint pain and skin lesions (5%-6%) 4. **Weight loss** 5. Diarrhea, abdominal pain 6. Cardiac: SOB, peripheral edema, angina, fever 7. CNS: HA, visual and gait disturbance, confusion, seizures, AMS, stiff neck, pain Signs: 1. **Erythema nodosum,** erythema multiforme, arthritis 2. HSM 3. Hilar and mediastinal nodes (5%-10%) 4. Rales/wheezes, hypoxemia 5. Pericarditis: rubs 6. Abdominal mass, intestinal ulcers 7. CN deficits, meningismus, muscle weakness, ataxia, AMS	1. **Urine and serum Ag testing** (60% sens, combined 80%) • Cross reactivity with blastomyces and coccidioides = false (+) 2. **BAL Ag testing** (96.8% sensitive) 3. CBC: pancytopenia (70%-90%) 4. AST/ALT: elevated, LDH: elevated (AIDS) 5. Sputum cultures (15% in acute, 60%-85% in chronic) 6. **Blood cultures** (50%-70% in progressive) 7. Antibodies • Anti-H (active) • Anti-M (chronic) 8. Complement fixing Ab (75%-90% positive at 6 wk) Imaging: 1. CXR: residual **hilar** and mediastinal **nodes** (coin lesions 1-4 cm in diameter), **cavitations** in upper lobes (90%) 2. CT−look for adrenal involvement (80%) 3. Echo: TEE or TTE if valvular involvement suspected Lumbar puncture	1. Acute asymptomatic: no treatment 2. Acute symptomatic: **PO itraconazole** 200 mg BID × 3 mo 3. Amphotericin B for severe or immunocompromised host

Disease	Etiology, Prevalence, Risk Factors	Clinical Symptoms and Signs	Diagnostics	Therapy, Prognosis, and Health Maintenance
Pneumocystis pneumonia	*Pneumocystis jiroveci–* caused by fungus found in lungs of mammals **Most common opportunistic infection** in HIV/AIDS (Fig. 23-3)	1. **Fever, SOB**, nonproductive **cough** 2. Exam findings disproportionate to imaging, showing diffuse interstitial infiltrates 3. Fatigue, weakness, weight loss	1. CXR (definitive): diffuse or **perihilar infiltrates, reticular interstitial** pneumonia or airspace disease that mimics pulmonary edema • 5%-10% normal CXR • Absent pleural effusions 2. **Sputum Wright-Giemsa stain or DFA (direct fluorescence Ab)** • Definitive in 50%-80% 3. **BAL** • Definitive in 95% 4. **CD4 <200** if AIDS 5. ABG: hypoxia, hypocapnia, reduced DLCO 6. LDH: increased, but nonspecific 7. Serum β-glucan • More sensitive and specific 8. WBC: low	1. **Bactrim**, add steroids if PaO_2 <70 mm Hg or A-a gradient >35 mm Hg if given in 72 h 2. Dapsone—if sulfa allergy All patients with CD4 <200 should undergo prophylaxis (Bactrim)

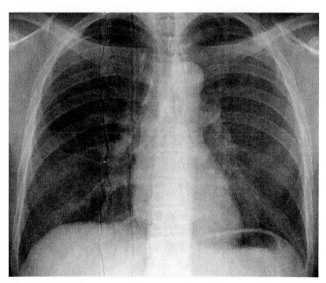

FIGURE 23-3. Pneumocystis pneumonia on chest x-ray showing perihilar ground-glass opacities. (From Webb WR, Higgins CB. *Thoracic Imaging: Pulmonary and Cardiovascular Radiology.* 3rd ed. Philadelphia: Wolters Kluwer; 2017.)

Internal Medicine

BACTERIAL: BOTULISM, DIPHTHERIA

Disease	Etiology, Prevalence, Risk Factors	Clinical Symptoms and Signs	Diagnostics	Therapy, Prognosis, and Health Maintenance
Botulism	*Clostridium botulinum* Results from ingestion of preformed toxins produced by spores of Clostridium botulinum Source: Improperly stored food (**home canned goods**)– inactivated by cooking food at high temps (212°F × 10 mins), wound contamination Incubation: 12 h-3 dd	1. **GI SX**: Abdominal cramps, nausea, vomiting, diarrhea (common) 2. Hallmark is **symmetric, descending flaccid paralysis** starting with dry mouth 3. **Double vision, ptosis**, and/or dysarthria, paralysis of limb musculature (late) 4. Respiratory distress → death	1. ***C. botulinum* toxin**– serum, stool, gastric bioassay (definitive) • Identifying in food alone is not reliable indicator	1. Admit patient and observe respiratory status; gastric lavage only in first few hours 2. If high suspicion–administer **antitoxin** (toxoid) 3. Contaminated wounds → wound cleansing and penicillin
Diphtheria	***Corynebacterium diphtheria*** Transmission: respiratory secretions Produces EXOTOXIN causing myocarditis and neuropathy	1. Nasal infection/discharge 2. Laryngeal infection 3. Pharyngeal infection: **tenacious gray membrane** covering tonsils and pharynx, mild sore throat, fever, malaise 4. Myocarditis, neuropathy involving cranial nerves	Clinical DX: Culture to confirm	1. **Horse serum antitoxin** from CDC 2. If airway obstruction → remove via laryngoscopy 3. PCN or erythromycin 4. Diphtheria toxoid as vaccine (DTaP) or Td

TETANUS

Disease	Etiology, Prevalence, Risk Factors	Clinical Symptoms and Signs	Diagnostics	Therapy, Prognosis, and Health Maintenance
Tetanus	Neurotoxins produced by spores of ***Clostridium tetani***, a gram positive anaerobic bacillus • *C. tetani* proliferates producing an exotoxin in contaminated wounds Incubation period: 2 d-2 wk, onset of symptoms gradual (1-7 d) RF: Incomplete or no tetanus immunization	• Hypertonicity and contraction of the masseter muscles resulting in **trismus** or "**lockjaw**" • Progresses to *severe*, generalized muscle contractions • **Risus sardonicus**: grin due to contraction of facial muscles • **Opisthotonos**–arched back due to contraction of back muscles • Sympathetic hyperactivity	Clinical DX: • Obtain wound cultures, but unreliable	1. Admit patient to ICU, provide respiratory support, give diazepam for tetany 2. Neutralize unbound toxin with passive immunization–give **single IM dose** of tetanus immune globulin (**TIG**)

Tetanus Sources

- Wounds contaminated in dirt, feces, or saliva
- Wounds with necrotic tissue
- Deep puncture wounds

Guide to Tetanus Immunization

History of Immunizations	Clean, Minor Wounds		Other Wounds	
	Give Td	Give TIG	Give Td	Give TIG
>3 known Td doses	No	No	No	No
<3 doses Td, unknown status, or >10 y since last boost	Yes	No	Yes	Yes

TOXOPLASMOSIS

Disease	Etiology, Prevalence, Risk Factors	Clinical Symptoms and Signs	Diagnostics	Therapy, Prognosis, and Health Maintenance
Toxoplasmosis (Fig. 23-4)	Organism: *Toxoplasma gondii* (obligate intracellular parasite) Active infection in immunocompromised hosts are due to the release of encysted parasites that undergo rapid transformation into tachyzoites within the CNS and are not contained by the immune system Definitive host: **Cat (feces)** → infects birds, rodents, grazing animals (lamb, pork), humans Transmission: Oral (ingestion of **contaminated soil, food, water**), by blood or organs, transplacental (⅓) • Lamb, beef, pork • Cat litter box Most common space-occupying lesion in HIV-infected patients	1. **Cervical lymph-adenopathy** (most common) • Single or multiple • Nontender, discrete, firm 2. **Headache**, malaise, fatigue, fever (20%-40%) 3. Myalgia, sore throat, abdominal pain, maculopapular rash, ***meningoencephalitis***, confusion 4. ***Encephalitis***–may be rapidly fatal if untreated • **Altered mental status**, fever, **seizures**, **headaches**, **focal neurologic findings** including motor deficits, CN palsies, movement disorders, dysmetria, visual-field loss, and aphasia Complications: Pneumonia, myocarditis, encephalopathy, pericarditis, polymyositis	Clinical diagnosis in AIDS pt–based on history of exposure (serology) and radiology 1. Serum IgG and **IgM** (acute) antibodies to toxoplasma • IgG titer detected 2-3 wk after infection, peaking at 6-8 wk • Serum IgG levels precede encephalopathy 2. Double-dose *contrast CT head*: multiple peripheral **ring-enhancing lesions** (<2 cm), usually in basal ganglia 3. MRI w/contrast: more sensitive • BG and corticomedullary junction most commonly involved 4. Brain biopsy–r/o primary CNS lymphoma 5. Labs **CD4 <100** if AIDS WBC: lymphocytosis ESR: high AST/ALT: high CSF: elevated intracranial pressure, mononuclear pleocytosis, increased protein and gamma globulin level	1. Recheck serum IgM titer in 3 wk 2. Presumptive encephalopathy treatment • **Pyrimethamine AND sulfadiazine** OR clindamycin, spiramycin 1. **Bactrim DS** daily is used as *prophylaxis* • Seropositive patients with **CD4 <100/uL** 2. Alternative: Dapsone-pyrimethamine • May discontinue prophylaxis if responsive to ART therapy and CD4 >200/uL x 3 months 50% improve by day 3, and 90% improve by day 7

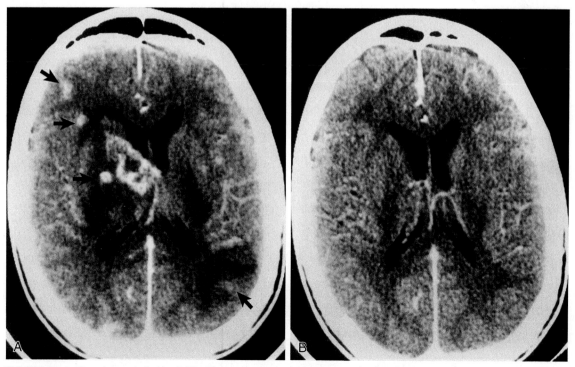

FIGURE 23-4. Toxoplasmosis **A,** Head CT with contrast shows a large right basal ganglion-enhancing mass (*arrow* in right hemisphere) and several other enhancing lesions (*arrows* in left hemisphere). Multiple small lesions favor the diagnosis of toxoplasmosis over lymphoma. **B,** The same patient after 2 weeks of antibiotics showing resolution of the lesions. (From Brant WE, Helms CA. *Fundamentals of Diagnostic Radiology.* 3rd ed Philadelphia: Lippincott Williams & Wilkins; 2007.)

LYME DISEASE AND ROCKY MOUNTAIN SPOTTED FEVER

- **Lyme**—most common vector borne illness in US

- RMSF—organisms enter host cells via tick bites, multiply in vascular endothelium and spread to different layers → damage to endothelium results in increased permeability, activation of complement, microhemorrhages, and microinfarcts

Lyme Disease	RMSF
Northeastern seaboard (Maine–Maryland), Midwest, West Coast Incubation: 3-32 d Transmission: vector-borne (**ticks**), white-footed mice, white-tailed **deer** Caused by spirochete **Borrelia burgdorferi**	Southeast, Midwest, and western US Spring and summer months Transmission: vector-borne (**dog ticks**), various mammals Intracellular bacteria **Rickettsia rickettsii**

Stage 1—early, localized (2-4 wk after bite)
• **Erythema chronicum migrans** (hallmark): large, <u>painless</u>, well-demarcated target shaped lesion on <u>**trunk**</u>, thigh, groin, axilla (Fig. 23-5)
Stage 2—early, disseminated (days to weeks)
• Intermittent **flu-like symptoms**: headaches, stiff neck, fever/chills, fatigue, malaise, myalgias
• After several weeks
  • Meningitis, encephalitis, cranial neuritis, peripheral radiculoneuropathy, **Bell palsy**
• Within weeks to months
  • Cardiac: **AV block**, pericarditis, **carditis**
Stage 3—late, persistent infection (months-years)
• **Arthritis** (60%), large joints (knee)
• Chronic CNS disease—subacute, mild encephalitis, transverse myelitis, or axonal polyneuropathy
• Acrodermatitis chronica atrophicans (rare): reddish-purple plaques and nodules on extensor surfaces of legs
	1. Onset of SX **within 1 wk** after bite
	2. Sudden onset **FEVER**, CHILLS
	  • Headache
	  • *Photophobia*
	  • *Nausea, vomiting*
	  • Malaise, myalgias
	3. **Papular rash** appears 4-5 d after fever
	  • **Begins peripherally** (wrists, forearms, ankles) and **spreads centrally** to rest of limbs, trunk, and face
	  • Becomes maculopapular → **nonblanching petechial rash** (Fig. 23-6)
	4. May lead to interstitial pneumonitis, **respiratory failure, and/or CNS involvement**

<u>Clinical DX:</u>
• Serologic studies: most important to confirm (IgM/IgG)
  • **ELISA** in first month
  • **Western blot** to confirm (+) or equivocal results
	<u>Clinical DX:</u>
	Labs: elevated **LFTs, thrombocytopenia**
	Acute and convalescent serology, **immunofluorescent staining** of skin biopsy (confirmatory)

<u>Early disease, localized:</u>
• 10 d of antibiotics
• If beyond skin, treat 20-30 d
  • **PO doxycycline × 21 d**–contraindicated in pregnant women and children <12
  • Amoxicillin and cefuroxime alternatives
  • *Erythromycin* for pregnant or PCN allergy
Treat complications: facial nerve palsy, arthritis, cardiac disease with antibiotic therapy (30-60 d)
For meningitis/encephalitis–treat with IV antibiotics × 4 wk
	1. **Doxycycline 100 mg PO BID × 7 d**, IV if vomiting
	2. If pregnant, treat with chloramphenicol (first line)
	  • Doxycycline associated with fetal bone and teeth malformations and hepatotoxicity to mother
	  • Doxycycline is first line for third trimester
	3. CNS manifestations or pregnant—give chloramphenicol

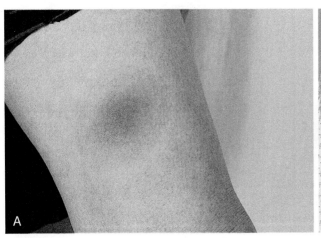
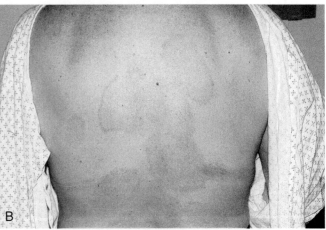

FIGURE 23-5. Dermatologic features of Lyme disease. **A**, Lyme disease. **B**, Erythema migrans. (From Goodheart HP. *Goodheart's Photoguide of Common Skin Disorders*, 2nd ed. Philadelphia, PA: Lippincott Williams & Wilkins; 2003.)

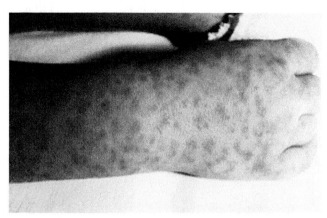

FIGURE 23-6. The pathognomonic lesion of Rocky Mountain spotted fever, described as a spotted rash with raised or palpable purpura. (From Kline-Tilford AM, Haut C. *Lippincott Certification Review: Pediatric Acute Care Nurse Practitioner*. Philadelphia: Wolters Kluwer Health; 2016.)

Lyme Serology

- IgM antibodies peak 3 to 6 weeks after onset of symptoms (acute)
- IgG antibodies slowly increase and remain elevated in patients with disseminated disease (acute or chronic)
  - Cross reacts with Treponema pallidum, but Lyme disease patients will <u>not</u> have positive VDRL

SYPHILIS

Treponema pallidum
spirochetes
Transmission: direct sexual contact with lesions
<u>Incubation:</u>
3 wk (Fig. 23--7)
	<u>Primary:</u>
	1. Chancre—indurated, **painless**, crater-like lesion with clean base appearing on genitalia *3-4 wk after* exposure; heals in 14 wk even without therapy, *highly infectious*
	2. **Inguinal lymphadenopathy**
	Secondary (*contagious*)
	1. Flu-like illness: headache, fever, sore throat, malaise
	2. Develops 4-8 wk after chancre has healed, **maculo-papular rash** beginning at sides of trunk
	3. *Aseptic meningitis*, alopecia, hepatitis
	4. 1/3 develop latent syphilis
	<u>Latent:</u>
	1. Presence of (+) serologic test results in *absence* of clinical *signs/symptoms*
	2. 2/3 remain asymptomatic and 1/3 develop tertiary
	3. Called "early latent" if serology (+) for <1 y, patient may relapse back to secondary
	4. Called "late latent" if serology (+) for >1 y, patients are contagious
	<u>Tertiary:</u>
	1. Occurs years after development of primary infection
	2. Major manifestations: **neurosyphilis**, cardiovascular syphilis, **gummas** (subcutaneous granulomas)
	3. Neurosyphilis: dementia, personality changes, **tabes dorsalis** (posterior column degeneration, loss of coordination of movement)
	4. Rare nowadays due to treatment with penicillin
		1. **Dark-field microscopy** (gold standard)
		2. Serologic tests (MC)
		 • <u>Nontreponemal tests:</u>
		RPR, VDRL
		  • Ideal for *screening*, 70% specific, if (+) use
		  • False positives with infection, age, HIV, rickettsia, pregnancy, lupus, and antiphospholipid syndrome
		  • Venereal disease research laboratory (VDRL)
		  • Rapid plasma reagin (RPR)
		 • <u>Treponemal tests:</u>
		FTA-ABS, MHA-TP (confirms)
		  • More specific, just to confirm (+) nontreponemal testing
		  • FTA-ABS = fluorescent treponemal antibody absorption test
		  • Positive in secondary syphilis
		3. Test all patients for **HIV**
		4. If FTA-ABS (+) → CSF-FTA-ABS should be checked

Treatment

- Antibiotics (early syphilis): **penicillin G benzathine** (one dose IM)
  - PCN allergy: doxycycline and tetracycline × 2 weeks
- Latent or tertiary syphilis—penicillin × 3 doses IM (1 week apart)
- Neurosyphilis: IV penicillin × 10 to 14 days, or PCN allergy: desensitization followed by penicillin
- Repeat nontreponemal tests q 3 months to ensure adequate response
  - Titers should decrease ×4 within 6 months

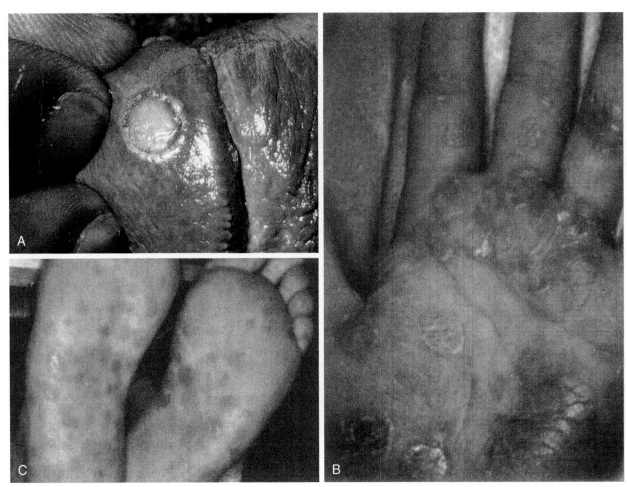

FIGURE 23-7. **Treponema pallidum. A,** Primary chancre of syphilis - a sharply bordered ulcer on the glans of the penis. **B,** Secondary syphilis - scaly papular lesions cover the trunk and extremities, including the palms and soles. (**A** and **B,** From Goldsmith LA, Papier A. *VisualDx: Essential Dermatology in Pigmented Skin.* Philadelphia: Wolters Kluwer Health; 2012. **C,** From Engleberg NC, Dermody T, DiRita V. *Schaechter's Mechanisms of Microbial Disease.* Philadelphia: Wolters Kluwer Health; 2013.)

CYTOMEGALOVIRUS

Disease	Etiology, Prevalence, Risk Factors	Clinical Symptoms and Signs	Diagnostics	Therapy, Prognosis, and Health Maintenance
Cytomegalovirus	**Human herpesvirus type 5**, double stranded DNA virus HIV or posttransplant CD4 <50 Asymptomatic → latent → reactivates <u>RF:</u> Daycare centers, blood transfusions, multiple sex partners, CMV mismatched organs or BMT <u>Transmission:</u> Person-person, placenta, blood transfusion, organ transplant, breast milk, sexual	1. Most asymptomatic 2. Flu-like symptoms: fever, malaise, myalgias, arthralgias (appears like mono) • Develops 9-60 d after primary infection <u>Signs:</u> 1. Fine crackles 2. Lymphadenopathy 3. +/− Pharyngitis 4. HSM <u>Complications:</u> Esophageal ulcers (CD4 <100), encephalitis (AMS), peripheral polyradiculopathy, retinitis (CD4 <50)	1. Antigen testing: CMV pp65 in WBCs 2. Qualitative PCR in blood and tissue 3. Labs • CBC: lymphocytosis or leukopenia, • LFTs: elevated 4. Culture: difficult, antigens in blood, urine, CSF via PCR 5. **BAL**—positive for CMV 6. Tissue biopsy: "owls' eyes" **intracytoplasmic inclusions** 7. CXR—consistent w/ pneumonia	1. Healthy without symptoms—no treatment 2. Immunocompromised: CMV immunoglobulin and IV **ganciclovir** • AE: fever, rash, diarrhea, heme effects (neutropenia, anemia, thrombocytopenia) <u>Prophylaxis:</u> Bactrim if CD4 <50

EPSTEIN-BARR INFECTION (MONONUCLEOSIS)

Disease	Etiology, Prevalence, Risk Factors	Clinical Symptoms and Signs	Diagnostics	Therapy, Prognosis, and Health Maintenance
Epstein-Barr virus	EBV, rarely by CMV (milder) Adolescents, college students or military recruit <u>Transmission:</u> Saliva (kissing, sharing food) 90% of adults infected previously and are carriers, lifelong immunity with 1 infection <u>Incubation:</u> 2-5 wk	1. Fever, LAD, pharyngitis • Fever (104°F) resolves in 2 wk • Sore throat • Malaise, myalgias, weakness <u>Signs:</u> 1. **Lymphadenopathy** (>90%), posterior cervical, tonsillar, enlarged, painful, tender 2. Pharyngeal erythema and/or exudate 3. **Splenomegaly** (50%) 4. Maculopapular rash (15%) 5. Hepatomegaly (10%) 6. Palatal petechiae and eyelid (periorbital edema)	1. Serology • **Monospot**: heterophile antibody (+) within 4 wk and undetectable by 6 mo • **WBC count with diff** • LFTs: **transaminitis** 2. EBV-specific antibody: indirect immunofluorescence or ELISA 3. Peripheral blood smear: lymphocytic leukocytosis with large, atypical lymphocytes 4. Throat culture	1. Supportive: rest, fluids, *avoid* strenuous activity, analgesics 2. Short course of steroids 3. Avoid sports 3-4 wk for splenic rupture <u>Complications:</u> Hepatitis, meningoencephalitis, Guillain Barré, Splenic rupture, thrombocytopenia, URTI <u>Health maintenance:</u> 1. Do not give amoxicillin or ampicillin—can cause maculopapular rash

HERPES SIMPLEX INFECTION

Disease	Etiology, Prevalence, Risk Factors	Clinical Symptoms and Signs	Diagnostics	Therapy, Prognosis, and Health Maintenance
Oral herpes simplex	Transmission: contact with active ulcerations or shedding of virus from mucous membranes Triggers: sunlight, stress, viral infections			Healing occurs over several days to 2 wk, usually without scarring
Herpes simplex virus, or herpes labialis, HSV-1	<u>Transmission:</u> Kissing Acquired in childhood >90% of people infected worldwide Lesions of oropharynx Resides in the trigeminal ganglion	<u>Asymptomatic</u> 1. Fevers, malaise 2. Vesiculopustular oral lesions in groups on patches of erythematous skin 3. Herpes labialis (cold sores): most common on lips, **painful**, heal in 2-6 wk 4. *Bell palsy* <u>Signs:</u> **Herpetic whitlow** may be seen in healthcare workers: infection of fingers from inoculation of abraded skin; vesicular and pustular with local erythema, pain and drainage	Clinical DX with lesions: "dewdrop on a rose petal" (vesicle on erythematous base) 1. **Tzanck smear**–swab base of ulcer and stain with Wright's sol'n: shows **multinucleated giant cells** (does not differentiate between VZV and HSV) • Quick, but nonspecific and insensitive 2. **Culture of HSV** (gold standard)–swab base of ulcer, available 2-3 d • Highly sensitive and specific 3. Direct fluorescent assay and ELISA (80% sensitive, results in minutes to hours) 4. PCR: more sensitive than culture	1. **PO acyclovir**, famciclovir, and valacyclovir 2. Recurrent—usually unsuccessful <u>Complications:</u> Herpes encephalitis (fever, personality changes, obtundation, seizures, 15% mortality), **HSV-keratitis** (tearing, pain, erythema, conjunctival swelling)

(continued)

Internal Medicine

(continued)

Disease	Etiology, Prevalence, Risk Factors	Clinical Symptoms and Signs	Diagnostics	Therapy, Prognosis, and Health Maintenance
Genital herpes, HSV-2	Lesions of genitalia Transmission: Sex Incidence from 10%-80% Resides in the sacral ganglion HSV 1 (30%), **HSV 2** (95%) Prior HSV-1 infection confers partial immunity to HSV-2 infection: less pain, fewer lesions, rapid resolution, shorter duration of shedding	1. Primary: severe, prolonged symptoms, lasting up to 3 wk • Recurrent: mild, shorter in duration, resolves in 10 d 2. Fever, headache, malaise 3. **Painful** vesicles (pustules, or ulcers) on genitals • Itching, dysuria • Multiple, bilateral 4. Tender inguinal LAD 5. Vaginal and/or urethral discharge Signs: 1. Tender vesicles progressing to tender, superficial, small ulcers on erythematous base	1. HSV-1 and HSV-2 Antibody negative 2. PCR: not routine 3. Culture if active lesion present	1. PO **acyclovir**, famciclovir, and valacyclovir 2. Sitz baths, perineal care, topical Xylocaine jellies or creams 3. Healing takes 14-21 d If recurrent—TX usually unsuccessful Complications: Aseptic meningitis, keratitis, blepharitis, keratoconjunctivitis

Herpes Simplex Infection

- After inoculation, HSV replicates in dermis and epidermis, then moves via sensory nerves to dorsal root ganglia → resides as latent infection in DRG where it can be reactivated at any time, reaching the skin through peripheral nerves
- May be asymptomatic and produce unrecognized symptoms—virus still sheds and still contagious
- Recurrences with stress, fever, infection, sun exposure

INFLUENZA

- The most extensive and **severe** outbreaks are caused by **influenza A** because of the propensity of H and N antigens to undergo periodic antigenic variation
- Designation is based on antigenic characteristics of the nucleoprotein (BP) and matrix (M) protein antigens
  - Further subdivided on basis of surface hemagglutinin (H) and neuraminidase (N) antigens
- Hemagglutinin is the site the virus binds to sialic acid cell receptors, whereas neuraminidase degrades the receptor and plays a role in the release of the virus from infected cells after replication has taken place
- Individual strains are designated according to site of origin, isolate number, year of isolation, and subtype
- Major variation—antigenic shifts (only seen with influenza A), associated with pandemics
- Minor variations—antigenic drifts

Disease	Etiology, Prevalence, Risk Factors	Clinical Symptoms and Signs	Diagnostics	Therapy, Prognosis, and Health Maintenance
Influenza	Orthomyxovirus Transmission: Respiratory droplets Winter months	1. Rapid onset of fever, chills, malaise, myalgia (legs or lumbosacral area) • **Fever** 100.4° to 105.8° 2. **Headache:** generalized or frontal 3. Nonproductive **cough:** may last more than 1 wk 4. Ocular signs/SX: pain with motion of eyes, photophobia, burning of eyes 5. Sore throat 6. +/− nausea Signs: 1. Cervical LAD 2. Rhonchi, wheezes, and scattered rales	1. Reverse transcriptase polymerase chain reaction (PT-PCR) = most sensitive and specific • Can differentiate subtypes and detect avian flu	Supportive care: • Tylenol or NSAIDs for headache, myalgias, fever • No cough suppressants • **Neuraminidase inhibitor:** zanamivir or oseltamivir for flu type A and B • Reduces symptoms by 1-1.5 d if started within 2 d of onset • Effective up to 5 d after onset • Adamantane agents: amantadine and rimantadine for flu type A Complications: Secondary bacterial pneumonia

Treatment

	Zanamivir (Relenza)	Oseltamivir (Tamiflu)
Indications	Prophylaxis in adults and pediatric patients >5 y/o Uncomplicated acute illness by influenza A and B in adults and pediatric patients >7 y/o who have been symptomatic for no more than 2 d	Prophylaxis: children >1 y of age and adults Treatment: >2 wk old and adults symptomatic for no more than 2 d
Adverse effects	Headache	Vomiting Nausea, abdominal pain, diarrhea
Contraindications	Hypersensitivity to milk or zanamivir	Hypersensitivity to oseltamivir Renal adjustment
Dosing	Prophylaxis: 2 inhalations (10 mg) 1/d × 10 d, begin within 36 h of onset Treatment: 2 inhalations daily × 5 d, separated by 2 h, begin within 48 h of onset	Prophylaxis: 75 mg PO daily × 10 d, start within 48 h of contact with infected individual Treatment: 75 mg PO BID × 5 d, start within 48 h of onset

RABIES

Disease	Etiology, Prevalence, Risk Factors	Clinical Symptoms and Signs	Diagnostics	Therapy, Prognosis, and Health Maintenance
Rabies	Incubation: 30-90 d Devastating, deadly viral encephalitis Contracted from a bite or scratch by infected animal; infection from corneal transplant as well More prominent in developing countries where rabies vaccination is not widespread	1. Once symptoms present, can be fatal • Pain at site of bite • **Prodromal symptoms** of sore throat, fatigue, headache, nausea, vomiting • **Encephalitis**: confusion, combativeness, hyperactivity, fever, seizures • **Hydrophobia**: inability to drink, laryngeal spasm with drinking, hyper-salivation (foaming at mouth), usually progresses to coma and death • **Ascending paralysis**	1. Virus or viral antigen from infected tissue or saliva 2. 4 × increase in serum antibody titers 3. Histology: **Negri bodies** 4. PCR detection of viral RNA	1. Clean wound thoroughly 2. Wild animal bites—send animal for immunofluorescence of brain tissue 3. If healthy animal—capture, place in observation × 10 d 4. Known rabies: • **Passive immunization**: human rabies IG 40 units/kg into the wound and gluteal region • **Active immunization**: human diploid cell rabies (HDCV) vaccine in 3 IM doses into deltoid or thigh over 28 d (days 3, 7, 14, 28)

VARICELLA ZOSTER

- Zostavax (live attenuated virus)
  - Approved for **adults 50 to 59** years old who are non-immunocompromised, nonpregnant, including those who have had a previous episode of zoster
  - Patients who are about to begin biologic therapy (should not be started while ON biologic therapy)
  - Contraindications: long-term steroid treatment, chemotherapy, radiation

- Varicella-zoster immune globulin (VZIG)
  - Recommended to prevent or modify clinical illness in persons with exposure to varicella or herpes zoster who are susceptible or immunocompromised
  - Reserved for patients at risk for severe disease and complications: neonates, immunocompromised, pregnant
  - Administer ASAP after presumed exposure or as late as 96 hours

Disease	Etiology, Prevalence, Risk Factors	Clinical Symptoms and Signs	Diagnostics	Therapy, Prognosis, and Health Maintenance

Varicella (herpes zoster)	Age >50 y/o
	Caused by reactivation of the varicella-zoster virus, which is dormant in the dorsal root ganglia and reactivated during stress, infection, or illness
	Occurs only in patients who have had chickenpox
	Contagious when open vesicles present and immunocompromised
		1. **Severe pain and rash** in dermatomal distribution (*pain before rash*)
		  • **Thorax (most common)** and trigeminal distribution, other CN and arms/legs
		2. On days 3-4, vesicles become more pustular
		3. Crust over by days 7-10 (no longer infectious)
		Signs:
		1. Grouped vesicles on erythematous base
		Complications:
		Postherpetic neuralgia, excruciating pain persisting after lesions have cleared and does not respond to analgesics, uveitis, meningoencephalitis, deafness
			1. Tzanck smear
			  • 60% sensitive
			2. **Culture of vesicular fluid** (confirmatory)
			Varivax—indicated for individuals >1 y/o
			Zostavax—indicated for prevention of zoster in patients who have no contraindications
				1. Keep lesions dry/clean
				2. **Analgesics** for pain (ASA or Tylenol), local triamcinolone in lidocaine
				3. **Antivirals**: Acyclovir, famciclovir, valacyclovir to reduce incidence of PHN, reduce pain and decrease length of illness
				4. Steroids to decrease incidence of PHN
				5. **Live vaccine (VariZIG)** to reduce severity and duration
				  • Administer within 10 d
				  • High-risk groups: immunocompromised children/adults, newborns of mothers with varicella shortly before or after delivery, premature infants, infants <1 y/o, adults without evidence of immunity, pregnant women

CHAPTER 24

Hematology

Recommended Supplemental Topics:

Splenomegaly, see Polycythemia Vera ✳, p 193
Hereditary Hemochromatosis, p 285

BLOOD CELL MORPHOLOGY AND LIFE CYCLE

	Function	Lasts	Smear
Neutrophils (polys, segs, grans)	Phagocytosis	Maturation: 7-14 d Duration in blood: 6 h	2-4 lobed nucleus
Lymphocytes	Chronic bacterial infection Acute viral infection	Most in lymph nodes, spleen, lymphatic vessels	Large round nucleus No granules NK cells—large granular lymphocytes

	Function	Lasts	Smear
Monocytes	Phagocytosis similar to neutrophils for bacteria Remove necrotic debris Produce interferon	Formed, mature in bone marrow Circulate 24-36 h → tissues (macrophages)	Bluish-grey cytoplasm with large cytoplasm to nuclear ratio **Kidney shaped nucleus**
Eosinophils	Allergic response No response for viral/bacterial infections Parasitic infections Main effector cells in asthma		Vibrant orange to beef red cytoplasmic granules **Bilobed nucleus**
Basophils	Allergic response No response for viral/bacterial infections Parasitic infections Cytoplasm contains heparin, histamine, and serotonin		Large cytoplasmic granules obscure the nucleus
Thrombocytes	Hemostasis	Circulate 8-10 d ⅓ sequestered in spleen	
Erythrocytes	Transport O_2	Circulate 120 d destroyed by liver/spleen	Small, non-nucleated cell with central pallor Flexible, donut shaped or inner tube

IRON DEFICIENCY ANEMIA

- **Transferrin**: major transporter for iron through the blood (HL = 8 days), made in the liver; increased in states of iron deficiency
  - A complete lack of transferrin is incompatible with life
- **TIBC** (total iron binding capacity) for Transferrin: measured directly using milligrams of iron per deciliter of plasma
- **Transferrin saturation**: circulating transferrin is approximately one-third saturated with iron
  - Reduced: IDA, anemia of chronic disease, etc
  - Increased: hemochromatosis, aplastic anemia, ineffective erythropoiesis, liver disease

- **Ferritin**: cellular storage protein for iron
- Serum ferritin <10 to 15 ng/mL is 99% specific for diagnosis of IDA
- Buchanan's Rules
  - Hgb: $11 + (0.1 \times age)$
  - MCV: 70 + age
- RBC life span: 120 days
- Hematocrit: the ratio of the volume of red cells to the total volume of a blood sample

Disease	Etiology, Prevalence, Risk Factors	Clinical Symptoms and Signs	Diagnostics	Therapy, Prognosis, and Health Maintenance

Iron deficiency anemia
A significant deficit in the mass of circulating red blood cells (oxygen carrying capacity of blood is low)
	Reduced cell mass or Hgb concentration (>2 SD below mean)
	Microcytic (MCV <80), hypochromic anemia with low H/H
		1. Fatigue with exercise
		2. Palpitations
		3. Shortness of breath
		4. Weakness
		5. Headaches, tinnitus
		<u>Signs:</u>
		1. Tachycardia
		2. Tachypnea on exertion
		3. Pallor
		4. Glossitis, angular cheilitis, pica, koilonychia
		5. Jaundice and splenomegaly
			1. CBC
			  • Reticulocyte count: **low**
			  • RDW: high
			2. Iron Studies
			  • Decreased serum iron, ferritin, and transferrin saturation
			  • **Increased TIBC**
			  • Ferritin **<15 ng/mL** (diagnostic)
			3. Check hemoglobin and Hematocrit
			  • Check at 12 and 18 mo, 12 y (females)
			  • Hgb/Hct <2× standard deviation of normal
			  • Hgb <13.5 g/dL or → Hct <39% (men)
			  • Hgb <12 g/dL or Hct <37% (women)
			4. Peripheral smear: poikilocytes **(pencil or cigar shaped cells)**
			5. Bone marrow biopsy
				1. Oral iron TID:
				  • 6 wk to correct anemia
				  • 6 mo to replete iron stores
				  • See treatment below
				  • Recheck blood counts every 3 mo × 1 y
				2. Vitamin C—helps to absorb iron

Anemia of Chronic Disease

Disease	Etiology, Prevalence, Risk Factors	Clinical Symptoms and Signs	Diagnostics	Therapy, Prognosis, and Health Maintenance

Anemia of chronic disease	Causes:
	Inflammation, cancer, RA, TB
	Inadequate iron delivery to marrow
			1. Low EPO
			2. Iron studies
			  • Decreased serum iron and TIBC, transferrin saturation
			  • NL to 3× increase serum ferritin
			3. Peripheral smear: normocytic, normochromic (cancer, CKD) to microcytic hypochromic (TB, RA)
			4. ESR: increased
				1. 50-150 U/kg IV EPO 3× weekly
				2. Treat underlying disease (CKD)

Iron Supplementation

1. **Ferrous sulfate** 3 mg/kg once or twice daily (20% elemental iron)
   • Give between meals with juice (not milk)
2. Ferrous fumarate (33% elemental iron) 100-200 mg/day in 2-3 doses
3. Ferrous gluconate (12% elemental iron) 3-6 mg/kg/day in 3 doses

Side Effects
1. Liquid preparations—gray staining of teeth or gums
   • Brush teeth or rinse with water after administration
2. GI upset

SICKLE CELL ANEMIA/CRISIS

• Hand-foot syndrome is caused by painful infarcts of the digits and dactylitis
• Stroke is especially common in children

Disease	Etiology, Prevalence, Risk Factors	Clinical Symptoms and Signs	Diagnostics	Therapy, Prognosis, and Health Maintenance

Sickle cell anemia	Mutation in the β-globin gene that changes the sixth amino acid from glutamic acid to valine	1. Acute pain
		  • Few hours to 2 wk
		  • RF: infection, fever, excess exercise, anxiety, abrupt change in temperature, hypoxia, hypertonic dyes
		Signs:
		1. Tenderness
		2. Fever, tachycardia
		3. Anxiety
		Complications:
		Pulmonary hypertension, ESRD, hand-foot syndrome, priapism → permanent impotence
			1. Hemolytic anemia
			  • Hct: 15%-30%
			  • Reticulocytosis
			  • Granulocytosis
			  • Peripheral smear: Elongated and crescent-shaped RBCs, target cells, nucleated RBC
			2. Hemoglobin electrophoresis, mass spectroscopy, sickling tests (confirms)
				Crisis:
				1. Vigorous hydration
				2. Aggressive pain medication (morphine)
				3. Nasal O_2
				Severe symptoms:
				1. **Hydroxyurea** (mainstay), for patients 3+ crises per year or repeated ACS
				  • Increases production of Hgb F (cannot sickle)
				2. BMT
				Health maintenance:
				1. Regular slit lamp exams: retinopathy
				2. Antibiotics for splenectomy patients undergoing dental or invasive procedures
				3. Vigorous oral rehydration during or in anticipation of periods of extreme exercise, exposure to heat/cold, emotional stress, or infection
				4. Pneumococcal and HiB vaccines early in life

Disease	Etiology, Prevalence, Risk Factors	Clinical Symptoms and Signs	Diagnostics	Therapy, Prognosis, and Health Maintenance
Acute chest syndrome	In situ sickling within the lung, producing pain and temporary pulmonary dysfunction	1. Chest pain 2. Fever 3. Cough Signs: Tachypnea	1. Arterial O_2 desaturation	1. Monitor hydration for pulmonary edema 2. O_2 therapy 3. Transfuse to Hct >30 Complications: Pulmonary hypertension, cor pulmonale

Variants of Sickle Cell

Condition	Clinical Abnormalities	Hemoglobin Level (g/L)	MCV	Hgb Electrophoresis
Sickle Cell Trait	None; rare painless hematuria; isosthenuria	NL	NL	HbS/A: 40/60
Sickle cell anemia (HbS/HbS) Most common and most severe	Vasoocclusive crises with infarction of spleen, brain, marrow, kidney, lung; aseptic necrosis of bone; gallstones; priapism; ankle ulcers	70-100	80-100	HbS/A: 100/0 **HbF: 2%-25%**
S/β thalassemia	Vasculoocclusive crises; aseptic necrosis of bone	70-100	60-80	HbS/A: 100/0 HbF: 1%-10%
S/β+ thalassemia	Rare crises and aseptic necrosis	100-140	70-80	HbS/A: 60/40
Hemoglobin SC	Rare crises, **aseptic necrosis**, painless hematuria; **retinopathy**	100-140	80-100	HbS/A: 50/0 HbC: 50%

- Hgb S—less soluble with deoxygenation and precipitates/polymerizes with other
- Hgb C—does not polymerize as readily as Hgb S

THALASSEMIA

Disease	Etiology, Prevalence, Risk Factors	Clinical Symptoms and Signs	Diagnostics	Therapy, Prognosis, and Health Maintenance

β-thalassemia	Only 2 β-globin genes on chromosome 11, but 4 α-globin genes on chromosome 16
	Disrupts ratio between α and β chains, changing stability of Hb → hemolysis
		1. Asymptomatic
		2. Mild anemia
		Signs:
		1. Hepatosplenomegaly
		2. Jaundice
			1. **Hgb electrophoresis**
			2. CBC: *microcytic* hypochromic anemia
			3. Iron studies
			  • NL to increased: serum iron, ferritin, and transferrin saturation
			  • Normal TIBC
			4. Peripheral smear: target cells, basophilic stippling, elliptocytes
				Acutely symptomatic:
				1. Transfusion
				Asymptomatic:
				1. PO iron repletion (200 mg per day) and B_{12}
				  • Only if concomitant iron deficiency anemia
				2. Allogeneic bone marrow transplant
				3. Folic acid 5 mg daily, iron, B_{12}
				4. Deferoxamine (iron chelator)
				5. Splenectomy for splenomegaly
				Poor prognostic factors:
				Chronic infection, liver or heart failure, die in 20-30 s

β-Thalassemia Treatment

Symptomatic, cardiovascular instability, continued/excessive blood loss—transfuse.

Asymptomatic —oral iron replacement (200 mg elemental iron/d) taken on an empty stomach to increase absorption to 25% absorption.

- Sustained treatment for 6 to 12 months after correction to achieve stores of at least 0.5 to 1 g/day
- Adverse effects: abdominal pain, nausea, vomiting, constipation → take delayed release

- Reticulocyte count increases within 4 to 7 days → peaks at 1 to 1.5 weeks

Unable to tolerate PO, acute therapy, chronic therapy—recombinant EPO therapy increases demand for iron.

- Sodium ferric gluconate (ferrlecit) 125 mg per injection
- Body weight (kg) × 2.3 × (15-patient's hemoglobin) + 500 or 1000 mg (for storage)
- Adverse effects: arthralgias, skin rash, low grade fever

β-thalassemias	Genotype	Disease
Thalassemia major	Homozygous (B0|B0, B0|B+, or B+|B+)	Severe, requires transfusion regularly
β-thalassemia trait	B|B0, or B|B+	Asymptomatic with mild microcytic anemia or microcytosis without anemia No transfusion needed
Alpha thalassemias		
Thalassemia major	(deletion of all 4 genes)	Almost total hemolysis of RBCs
Hydrops fetalis	-/- (deletion of all 4 genes)	Fatal in utero
HbH disease: Hgb precipitates → hemolysis → splenomegaly	--/-α (deletion of 3 genes)	Moderately severe microcytic anemia Smear with striking hypochromia, target cells, basophilic stippling
Alpha-thalassemia trait: deletion of 2 α genes	--/aa (asian) or -a/-a (black) deletion of 2 genes	Mild anemia
Thalassemia silent carrier	-a/aa	Asymptomatic, normal red cells

B = normal β chain gene
B0 = one completely deleted or inactive β chain gene
B+ = partially deleted or inactive β chain gene

VITAMIN B$_{12}$ AND FOLIC ACID DEFICIENCY ANEMIA

Disease	Etiology, Prevalence, Risk Factors	Clinical Symptoms and Signs	Diagnostics	Therapy, Prognosis, and Health Maintenance
Megaloblastic anemia	• MCV >100 • Inhibition of DNA synthesis during RBC production		1. CBC 2. Iron Studies • NL to increased: serum iron, ferritin, and transferrin saturation • NL to decreased: TIBC 3. Peripheral smear: macrocytic, megaloblastic	
Vitamin B$_{12}$ (cobalamin) deficiency	Autoimmune destruction of gastric parietal cells → atrophic gastritis → lack of intrinsic factor production (required for absorption in small intestines) Cofactor for 2 enzymatic reactions required for DNA synthesis, brain/nervous system function, formation of RBC Causes/RF: Chronic alcoholism, vegetarian, celiac and Crohn diseases, **gastric bypass surgery**, Parasites MCC: Pernicious anemia (lack of IF)	1. Anemia: weakness, fatigue, bruising/gum bleeding, **sore tongue** (unique) 2. Neuropsychiatric manifestations: peripheral neuropathy, balance probs, depression, dementia → can be irreversible if untreated 3. *Glossitis*: beefy red tongue Signs: 1. Loss of vibratory and fine touch	1. B$_{12}$ level: decreased, can be false (+) with folate deficiency 2. Homocysteine: *increased* 3. **Methylmalonic acid (MMA)**: increased 4. Hypersegmented neutrophils	1. Lifelong IM B$_{12}$: 1-3 ug/d (animal products, fortified cereal) for pernicious anemia • IV **Cyanocobalamin 1 mg** IM daily × 7 d, then weekly × 4 wk, then monthly for life 2. PO B$_{12}$ 1-2 mg PO daily for vegans and bariatric surgery Years to deplete stores
Folic acid deficiency	Cofactor for DNA synthesis Alcoholics and malnourished have smaller stores Decreased intake, increased requirement (pregnant), sickle cell anemia, thalassemia Sprue, Crohn, drugs	1. Less neuro-SX 2. Neural tube defects (spina bifida)	1. Homocysteine: *increased* 2. Serum folic acid: low 3. **RBC folic acid (more reliable show of stores): <150** (diagnostic) 4. Macro-ovalocytes and hypersegmented PMNs (pathognomonic)	1. **PO folic acid** 1-5 mg/d (first line) 2. Avoid ETOH and folic acid antagonists (Bactrim, phenytoin, sulfasalazine) Green leafy vegetables, yeast, legumes, fruits, animal proteins Prophylactic folic acid—pregnant/lactating women, contemplating pregnancy, sickle cell patients

HEMOLYTIC ANEMIAS: GLUCOSE-6-PHOSPHATE DEHYDROGENASE DEFICIENCY

- **Schistocytes**: intravascular hemolysis, RBCs fragmented by shear mechanism
- **Spherocytes**: extravascular hemolysis, RBC phagocytosis by macrophages

Internal Medicine

Disease	Etiology, Prevalence, Risk Factors	Clinical Symptoms and Signs	Diagnostics	Therapy, Prognosis, and Health Maintenance

Hemolytic anemias		1. Symptoms of acute/chronic anemia
		2. Dark urine
		3. Back pain
		Signs:
		Jaundice
			1. CBC
			  • Reticulocyte count: **high** (hallmark)
			2. Iron studies
			  • Increased: serum iron, ferritin, and transferrin saturation
			  • Decreased TIBC
			3. Check hemoglobin and hematocrit
			  • Check at 12 and 18 mo, 12 y (females)
			  • Hb/Hct <2× standard deviation of normal
			  • Hb < 13.5 g/dL or → Hct <39% (men)
			  • Hb <12 g/dL or Hct <37% (women)
			4. **Total (indirect) bilirubin increased, Haptoglobin decreased**
			5. Peripheral smear: microcytic, normochromic anemia, spherocytes
			6. Bone marrow biopsy	

Glucose-6 phosphate dehydrogenase deficiency	Oxidant sensitive hemolytic disease (depletion of reduced glutathione = oxidation of Hgb = precipitation of Hgb → Heinz bodies) + Bite cells → RBC destruction Most commonly seen in tropical geographic areas prevalent for malaria (Africa, China, and Mediterranean regions)	HX: Hemolysis only with **infection, metabolic acidosis,** and certain **medications** 1. Chronic hemolytic anemia 2. Jaundice 3. SX of hemolysis	1. Peripheral smear: Bite cells, Heinz bodies	1. Avoid potentially harmful drugs, monitor infection 2. Acute—blood transfusion

Hereditary spherocytosis
Congenital hemolytic jaundice, familial hemolytic anemia
	Inherited dysfunction or deficiency in one of the erythrocyte membrane proteins (spectrin, ankyrin, band 3 protein, or protein 4.2) → spherocytic erythrocytes are sequestered and destroyed in the spleen
	Autosomal dominant
		1. Mild **jaundice**
		2. Mild-moderate **anemia**
		3. Malaise, abdominal discomfort in LUQ
		Signs:
		Splenomegaly
			1. CBC: anemia
			  • MCV: decreased
			  • **Reticulocyte count**, LDH, indirect bilirubin, stool urobilinogen: **elevated**
			  • Wright stained smear: spherocytes
			2. Hgb: 4-6 g/dL (low)
			3. EDW: elevated
			4. Peripheral smear: spherocytes
			5. Osmotic fragility: increased
			6. Coombs test: negative
				1. **Splenectomy**
				  • Indicated even when anemia compensated and asymptomatic
				  • Delay operation until children are age 6
				2. Cholecystectomy if gallstones present
				Complications:
				Hypoplastic crises: follow acute viral illness → profound anemia, headache, nausea, abdominal pain, pancytopenia, hypoactive marrow, **pigmented gallstones** (85%)

ACUTE AND CHRONIC LEUKEMIA

Disease	Etiology, Prevalence, Risk Factors	Clinical Symptoms and Signs	Diagnostics	Therapy, Prognosis, and Health Maintenance
Acute myeloid leukemia (AML)	Neoplasm of myelogenous progenitor cells Mostly **adults** (80% of adult leukemias) **40-60** y/o RF: Exposure to radiation, myeloproliferative syndromes, Down syndrome, chemotherapy (alkylating agents)	1. **Anemia** (symptoms) 2. **Neutropenia–** Increased risk of bacterial infection 3. **Thrombocytopenia–** Abnormal mucosal or cutaneous bleeding 4. Splenomegaly, hepatomegaly, lymphadenopathy 5. Bone and joint pain 6. CNS involvement (meningitis, seizures) 7. Skin nodules (AML)	1. **Auer rods** (peroxidase + inclusions in cytoplasm) → leads to DIC 2. Bone marrow biopsy: increased myeloblasts, stain with myeloperoxidase	1. Transretinoic acid (vitamin A) If recurrent or refractory: **Bone marrow transplant** (best chance of remission or cure) Response to therapy not as favorable
Chronic myelogenous leukemia (CML)	Most common >40 Neoplastic, clonal proliferation of myeloid stem cells (+) for **Philadelphia** chromosome **t(9,22)** → mutation of BRC-ABL gene → unregulated cell production	Prolonged indolent course, before it transforms to acute leukemia (blast crisis) Most present in chronic phase–asymptomatic, discovered incidentally 1. Constitutional symptoms present 2. Recurrent infections, easy bruising and bleeding, anemia 3. Splenomegaly, hepatomegaly, lymphadenopathy	Marked leukocytosis: 50-200 k Small numbers of blasts and promyelocytes Eosinophilia Peripheral smear: leukemic cells (myelocytes, metamyelocytes, bands, segmented form) **Decreased leukocyte alkaline phosphatase activity** Thrombocytosis BMB: leukemic cells	**Imatinib**–oral tyrosine kinase inhibitor (TKI) targets the t(9,22) gene (Philadelphia chromosome) People with PC have shorter survival times and respond poorly to treatment Complications: Blast crisis
Acute lymphoblastic leukemia (ALL)	Neoplasm of early lymphocytic precursors MC in young children (<15) **MC childhood cancer** ALL: most common leukemia in childhood <15 (80%) Peak: 2-5 y RF: Initial WBC and age at diagnosis, rate of response, cytogenetics	1. **Anemia** (symptoms) 2. **Neutropenia–** Increased risk of bacterial infection 3. **Thrombocytopenia–** Abnormal mucosal or cutaneous bleeding 4. Splenomegaly, hepatomegaly, lymphadenopathy 5. Bone and joint pain 6. CNS involvement (meningitis, seizures) 7. Testicular involvement (ALL) 8. Anterior mediastinal mass (T-cell ALL)	1. Immuno • Fluorescence assay: **TdT (+)** 2. Histology: **lymphoblasts** 3. Bone marrow biopsy: required for DX -**Myeloblasts** Labs: 1. WBC: 1 k-100 k, large number of blasts in peripheral blood • **Hyperleukocytosis** 2. Anemia 3. Thrombocytopenia 4. Granulocytopenia 5. Electrolytes: hyperuricemia, hyperkalemia, hyperphosphatemia	Most responsive to **chemotherapy** 75% achieve complete remission, only 30%-40% of adults Relapses occur, but respond well With aggressive therapy, survival rates can be up to 15 y or longer, 50% cured Poor prognostic factors: Age <2 or >9, WBC >10^5/mm3, and CNS involvement (B-cell type, high LDG, or rapid proliferation)
Benign leukemoid reaction	Increased WBC count as a response to stress or infection	1. Usually no splenomegaly 2. Increased leukocyte alkaline phosphatase 3. History of precipitating infection		

Disease	Etiology, Prevalence, Risk Factors	Clinical Symptoms and Signs	Diagnostics	Therapy, Prognosis, and Health Maintenance
Chronic lympho-cytic leukemia (CLL)	Mostly adults (>65) Unknown cause Monoclonal proliferation of lymphocytes that are morphologically mature, but functionally defective Least aggressive type of leukemia	1. **Generalized painless lymphadenopathy** 2. Splenomegaly 3. Frequent respiratory or skin infections 4. Constitutional SX in advanced disease: fatigue, weight loss, pallor, skin rash, easy bruising, bone tenderness, abdominal pain	1. Discovered on routine CBC with lymphocytosis: 50-200 k 2. Anemia, thrombocytopenia, neutropenia 3. **Peripheral blood smear** (diagnostic) • Absolute lymphocytosis– most WBC are small and mature • **Smudge cells**–"fragile" leukemic cells that are broken when placed on slide 4. Flow cytometry–clonal population of B-cells 5. Bone marrow biopsy: infiltrating leukemic cells 6. CXR: normal	Survive longer than CML patients 1. Chemotherapy–little effect on survival, but given for symptomatic relief and reduction in infections

LYMPHOMA

Disease	Etiology, Prevalence, Risk Factors	Clinical Symptoms and Signs	Diagnostics	Therapy, Prognosis, and Health Maintenance
Hodgkin lymphoma Malignant proliferation of lymphoid cells from lymph nodes, thymus, spleen	Most common type: Nodular sclerosis Bimodal: Age 15-30, >50 y/o Associated with Epstein-Barr virus Typically have a HX of autoimmune disorders RF: Same sex siblings, identical siblings	1. MC: **painless lymphadenopathy** • Supraclavicular, **cervical**, axillary, **mediastinal** lymph nodes • Spreads from one node to another 2. **B symptoms**: • fever, night sweats • unintentional weight loss • itching • cough Signs: 1. **Mediastinal mass** (50%) 2. Abdominal mass	1. Lymph Node Biopsy (required): **Reed-Sternberg cells** • Neoplastic, large cell with 2+ nuclei ("owl's eyes") • Usually B-cell phenotype • Nonspecific • Presence of **inflammatory cell infiltrates**: distinguishes Hodgkin from NHL 2. CXR and CT chest/abdomen to detect LN involvement 3. Bone marrow biopsy 4. Labs: leukocytosis, eosinophilia 5. ESR sometimes corresponds with disease activity 6. Lymph node histology differentiates subtypes	1. **Radiation** therapy alone • Stage I, II, IIIA 2. **Chemotherapy with ABVD** • Adriamycin, bleomycin, vinblastine, decarbazine • Stages IIIB, IV 70% cure rates
Non-Hodgkin lymphoma (B-cell)	Most common type: diffuse **large B-cell (85%)** Starts in lymph nodes and spreads to blood and bone marrow, sometimes GI tract Group of solid tumors occurring with the *malignant* transformation and growth of B or T-cell lymphocytes or their precursors in the lymphatic system Unknown etiology RF: HIV/AIDS, immunosuppression, history of EBV, h/o H. pylori gastritis, autoimmune disease (Hashimoto thyroiditis, Sjögren syndrome, MALT)	1. **Nontender** Lymphadenopathy– supraclavicular, cervical, axillary • Painless, firm, mobile • Rapid enlargement 2. B-symptoms: less than Hodgkin lymphoma 3. HSM, abdominal pain or fullness 4. Recurrent infection, anemia or thrombocytopenia 5. SVC obstruction, respiratory involvement, bone pain, skin lesions "Virchow's node lymphadenopathy"	1. **Lymph node biopsy**: "Starry sky pattern" (*>1 cm, present >4 wk, not attributed to infection) 2. CXR: reveals hilar or mediastinal LAD CT scan 3. Bone marrow biopsy 4. Labs • Serum LDH and B₂ microglobulin– indirect indicators • Alk-Phos elevated LFTs or bilirubin elevated • CBC • Serum electrolytes, renal function tests	1. **Rituximab** (monoclonal antibody against CD-20 antigen) is used in combination PLUS 2. **CHOP therapy** • **C**yclophosphamide • **H**ydroxydaunomycin (doxorubicin) • **O**ncovin (vincristine) • **P**rednisone Prognosis 1. Indolent forms, not curable, 5-y 75% survival rate → observation, chemotherapy, radiation therapy 2. Intermediate and high grade NHLs → curable with aggressive therapy, survival less than 2 y if complete remission not achieved • CHOP and radiation therapy • Very high dose chemo + bone marrow transplant (last resort)

MULTIPLE MYELOMA

Second most common hematologic cancer.

Disease	Etiology, Prevalence, Risk Factors	Clinical Symptoms and Signs	Diagnostics	Therapy, Prognosis, and Health Maintenance
Multiple myeloma	Malignant plasma cell proliferation and secretion of monoclonal paraproteins (M-protein) 60-70 s, African American men Paraprotein levels are increased (IgG or IgA may cause hyperviscosity); light chain components may lead to renal failure	1. **Bone pain** (MC initial symptom) +/− pathologic fractures • Lumbar region 2. Constipation, nausea 3. Confusion, somnolence 4. Fatigue 5. **Infection** 6. Bleeding 7. Paresthesias (neuropathy) Signs: 1. Bone tenderness 2. Soft tissue plasmacytoma masses 3. Pallor 4. Ecchymoses, petechiae 5. Epistaxis 6. Lower extremity weakness or dysesthesias with incontinence, saddle anesthesia	1. Hypercalcemia 2. **Anemia: ROULEAUX** formation common (stacked RBCs) 3. Thrombocytopenia 4. Serum globulin protein: elevated 5. Protein electrophoresis: **monoclonal spike** (*confirms*) 6. CBC, PT/PTT, BUN/Cr, metabolic 7. Urinary protein excretion: **Bence Jones protein** (diagnosis) 8. XR: **lytic lesions** in skull and long bones, generalized osteoporosis	1. Melphalan and Prednisone 2. Irradiation and HD chemotherapy → hematopoietic stem cell transplant 3. Adjunct: bisphosphonates Complications: Renal impairment, amyloidosis, hypercalcemia, spinal cord compression

CLOTTING FACTOR DISORDERS

- vWF is a glycoprotein that, as opposed to most other coagulation factors, is synthesized, stored, and then secreted by the vascular endothelial cells. It is a cofactor for platelet adhesion and the carrier protein for factor VIII.

- Protective effect of hemophilia and for carriers of hemophilia for coronary heart disease (CHD) for which studies have shown up to an 80% reduction in coronary disease related mortality

Disease	Etiology, Prevalence, Risk Factors	Clinical Symptoms and Signs	Diagnostics	Therapy, Prognosis, and Health Maintenance
Disseminated intravascular coagulation (DIC)	Generalized activation of coagulation cascade → widespread **fibrin formation** (antithrombin + protein C) → **consumption of platelets and clotting factors** → microthrombosis → increased fibrinolysis Causes: infection, mechanical tissue injury, malignancy, pregnancy **Consumptive coagulopathy**—consumption of clotting factors 5 and 8, protein C, and low platelets Hereditary and acquired factors tip balance in favor of clotting → thrombophilic v. hypercoagulable state	1. Generalized **hemorrhage (bleeding)** • Petechiae and ecchymoses → GI bleed, GU bleed, surgical wound, mucocutaneous or venipuncture site bleed 2. Mental status changes 3. Focal ischemia or gangrene 4. Oliguria 5. Renal cortical necrosis 6. ARDS	1. **Thrombocytopenia** 2. FDP/**D-dimer**: increased (specific) 3. **Fibrinogen**: decreased (consumed) 4. PT/PTT: **prolonged** 5. Protein C: decreased	1. **Supportive care** and Manage underlying disease • IVF, RBCs, inotropic agents 2. Replete platelets or clotting factors *if going into surgery* • Fibrinogen repletion with cryoprecipitate • Platelet concentrates to replace platelets • **FFP** to replace coagulation factors • *Vitamin K and Folate* 3. Anticoagulation—only if DIC shifted toward hypercoagulability • Heparin Complications: Thrombosis, organ failure, purpura fulminans, **sepsis**, bacteremia

Disease	Etiology, Prevalence, Risk Factors	Clinical Symptoms and Signs	Diagnostics	Therapy, Prognosis, and Health Maintenance
Von Willebrand factor (vWF) deficiency or disease	Platelet dysfunction, impairment in synthesis or function; clots take longer to form or do not form properly, bleeding takes longer to stop **Autosomal dominant** (type 1 most common) F = M 2% of population (+) family history, surgical bleeding Most common congenital bleeding disorder	1. Recurrent epistaxis 2. Gingival bleeding 3. Unusual bruising 4. GI bleeding 5. Menorrhagia *Hemarthrosis is not typical unless severe	1. PTT–**prolonged (corrects with mixing)** • PT: normal 2. (+) **PFA-100**: prolonged 3. vWF antigen (ELISA): low to NL, low activity 4. Ristocetin cofactor assay–ability to induce plt aggregation 5. vWF multimer assay–differentiates different types	1. **DDAVP**–releases vWF and factor 8 from storage; 0.3 µg/kg IV q 12 h during bleed, 300 µg puff prophylaxis (watch for hyponatremia) 2. vWF concentrate (Humate P) 3. Avoid antiplatelet meds: aspirin, NSAID, heparin VWF protects factor 8 from proteolytic degradation, prolonging its half life in circulation
Hemophilia A (factor 8) hemophilia B (factor 9, Christmas disease)	**X-linked recessive** bleeding disorders Mostly **males** Male homozygote = always express Female heterozygote = carrier Generally presents in infancy or early childhood (3-10 y/o)	Neonates: 1. ICH, prolonged hemorrhage from circumcision (30%) or heel puncture Infancy: 1. SQ nodular hematoma Toddler (1-3 y): 1. **Hemarthrosis: Painful swelling around joint** (ankle, wrists) 2. Oral mucosa bleeding 3. ICH: Any child that sustains severe head bump or has persistent headache, lethargy, vomiting, seizures Complications: Retroperitoneal bleeding (back, thigh, groin, abdominal pain)	1. **Prolonged PTT** (corrects with mixing study) 2. Quantitative assay for individual factors 3. Normal: PT, thrombin time, INR 4. **CT scan** URGENTLY if signs of ICH	1. **Give factor concentrates** • Recombinate and BeneFIX, prophy 2-3× weekly 2. Antifibrinolytics–Amicar to stop/slow clot breakdown Hemophilia A 3. **DDAVP SQ or intranasal**: potentiates vWF and factor 8 release 4. Gene therapy for factor 8

HYPERCOAGULABLE STATE

Includes factor V Leiden, protein C/S deficiency, anti-thrombin III deficiency.

Disease	Etiology, Prevalence, Risk Factors	Clinical Symptoms and Signs	Diagnostics	Therapy, Prognosis, and Health Maintenance
Factor V Leiden	Point mutation (Arg506Gln)–factor 5 resistant to proteolysis by protein C This leads to overabundant conversion of prothrombin to thrombin Autosomal dominant	1. **Deep vein thrombosis** (7-20× increased risk) 2. Pulmonary embolism Complications: Pre-eclampsia, placental abruption, IUGR, stillbirth	1. DNA test 2. APC-resistance assay	1. Anticoagulation–prevent propagation of clot, dissolution of local clot, prevent recurrent VTE

IDIOPATHIC THROMBOCYTOPENIC PURPURA

Disease	Etiology, Prevalence, Risk Factors	Clinical Symptoms and Signs	Diagnostics	Therapy, Prognosis, and Health Maintenance

Idiopathic throm-bocytopenic purpura, immune thrombocytope-nic purpura (ITP)	Acquired **autoimmune** d/o, circulating antiplatelet IgG autoan-tibody (*produced in spleen*) directed against a membrane protein which is the fibrinogen receptor (glycoprotein IIb/IIIa) → clears com-plexes via macro-phages, *destroyed in spleen* → reduces life span of platelet
	Reduction in the number of circulating platelets, abundant megakaryo-cytes in the bone mar-row, and a shortened platelet life span
	Most common indication for splenectomy
		Acute—children <8
		HX:
		1-3 wk after viral URI
		1. **Bleeding gums,** vaginal bleeding, GI bleeding, hematuria, **epistaxis, easy bruising**
		2. **Petechiae, ecchymoses**
		3. NO splenomegaly (2%)
		4. CNS bleeding (3%)
		Chronic—any age, F
		1. Insidious onset, long HX of easy bruising and **menorrhagia**
		2. Petechiae over pres-sure areas
		3. Cyclic remissions and exacerbations
			No single diagnostic test, diagnosis of exclusion
			1. Bleeding time: **prolonged**
			2. **Thrombocytopenia** (new onset, severe, <30 k)
			3. CBC: iron deficiency anemia
			4. Assess bone marrow if: >60, other cytopenias, failure to respond to steroids, planning to undergo splenectomy
			  • Increased large megakaryocytes without platelet budding
			5. Capillary **fragility** (Rumpel-Leede test): **increased**
			6. PT/PTT: normal
				Mild-Mod: observation; avoid contact sports, elective surgery, and unnecessary meds
				1. First line: <20 k:
				Child: **IVIG**
				Adults: high dose **steroids** (prednisone 1 mg/kg/d)
				  • Should respond in 1 wk, taper to 20 mg/d, then slowly by 5 mg
				2. Second line: Rituximab (anti-CD20): clears active B-cells making antibodies
				3. **Splenectomy**—for persistently low platelet counts despite steroid therapy, long term
				  • Requires PCV vaccine
				  • Most effective therapy
				Better prognosis:
				Young age, short duration of disease

THROMBOTIC THROMBOCYTOPENIC PURPURA

Disease	Etiology, Prevalence, Risk Factors	Clinical Symptoms and Signs	Diagnostics	Therapy, Prognosis, and Health Maintenance
Microangiopathic hemolytic ane-mias (MAHA)	**Platelet aggregation** in the microvascular circulation via vWF Results from fragmentation of RBCs through occluded arterioles and capillaries			

Thrombotic thrombocyto-penic purpura, "platelet thrombi" **(TTP)**	MC:
	Adults, F, 30-50 y/o, African/Hispanic
	RF:
	1. *Pregnancy*, infection, inflammation, medication, HIV/AIDS
	2. Inappropriate platelet plug → thrombi → impede flow & cause isch-emia → multi organ failure and death
	3. Lack of ADAMTS13-acquired due to inhibitory antibody blocking enzyme activity
	Cause:
	Unknown
		Classic PENTAD
		1. **Thrombocytopenia**
		2. Fever
		3. **Anemia**
		4. Renal insufficiency
		  • AKI
		5. Mental status/neu-rologic changes: headache, sei-zures, hemiparesis, disorientation
		Signs:
		1. Nonpalpable pete-chial **purpura**
		2. Seizure, stroke, focal neurologic deficit, coma
			1. Microangiopathic hemolytic anemia (MAHA) = high LDH, indirect bili, and **ret-ics, low haptoglobin**
			2. Peripheral smear: **Helmet cells** and megakaryocytes, **schistocytes**
			  1. Thrombocytopenia <20 k
			3. **PT/PTT:** normal (*dis-tinguishes from DIC*)
			4. **ADAMTS13 test:** <10% normal (decreased)
			5. Direct Coombs test: negative
				1. **Plasma exchange and FFP**—Daily 40 mL/kg
				  • If not readily available, use FFP
				2. Refractory—IVIG, Vincristine, Cyclophosphamide, Splenectomy, Rituximab
				3. **Avoid platelet trans-fusion** unless ICH or life-threatening bleeding
				4. **Avoid aspirin**—worsens thrombocytopenia
				Severe:
				1. RBC transfusion, anticon-vulsants, antihypertensives, hemodialysis
				Prognosis:
				1. High mortality rate (>90%)

- ADAMTS-13 is made by hepatic stellate cells, glomerular podocytes, and vascular endothelial cells. Its function is to cleave von Willebrand factor that has been unfolded by shear stress within the microvasculature of arterioles and capillaries. Without this cleavage function, unfolded von Willebrand factor monomers can form large multimers that lead to formation of intravascular microthrombi

HEREDITARY HEMOCHROMATOSIS

Disease	Etiology, Prevalence, Risk Factors	Clinical Symptoms and Signs	Diagnostics	Therapy, Prognosis, and Health Maintenance
Hereditary **hemo-chromatosis** (iron overload) Also known as "bronze diabetes"(cirrhosis, diabetes, skin pigmentation)	Autosomal recessive, mutation in the *HFE* gene (MC) resulting in increased intestinal absorption of iron, iron overload and eventual tissue damage Men, 40-50 s, increased iron consumption RF: ETOH consumption Accumulation of iron → organ damage (**liver** → pancreas, heart, pituitary gland)	1. Unexplained fatigue 2. Arthralgias, weight loss 3. Abdominal pain 4. Reduced libido Signs: 1. Hepatomegaly, **cirrhosis** (95%) 2. Diabetes, hypogonadism (impotence, amenorrhea, osteoporosis) 3. Arthropathy: 2nd-3rd MCP and PIP joints 4. **Metallic or slate-gray hue** (bronzing) of skin • Volar forearms, face, neck, dorsum of hands, lower legs, genital regions • Cutaneous atrophy, flattening of nails, loss of body hair Complications: Atrial fibrillation, sinus sick syndrome	1. Screening • Serum iron/TIBC >45% • Ferritin: >200 ug/L 2. LFTs: elevated 3. Liver biopsy to assess iron concentration and hepatic iron index 4. XR: joint space narrowing, squared off bone ends, hook like osteophytes 5. Diagnosis of iron overload: • Ferritin >200-300 ng/mL in men, >150-200 ng/mL in women • Transferrin saturation >45%	1. **Phlebotomy** (mainstay) • Monitor Hgb and ferritin Prophylaxis: 1. Screen first degree relatives of C282Y homozygotes Health Maintenance: 1. **Recommended 1-2 units blood/weekly or every other week may be given to avoid iron overload** 2. Annual exam • Skin, heart, liver, joints, endocrine organs (hypothyroid, diabetes, hypogonadism) • Labs: iron, ferritin, transferrin saturation with LFTs and echocardiogram done when progression evident 3. Avoid vigorous exercise within 24 hours of phlebotomy and maintain hydration 4. Avoid excessive ETOH (increase absorption), vitamin C supplements, uncooked seafood5. Screen for HCC Prognosis Most deaths associated with complications decompensated cirrhosis (MC), hepatocellular carcinoma (HCC), diabetes, or cardiomyopathy

PRACTICE QUESTIONS

1. A 26-year-old patient with known history of type one diabetes mellitus presents with lethargy, nausea, vomiting, and abdominal pain. On examination, the patient has decreased skin turgor and a fruity odor to her breath. What is the best initial intervention for this condition?

   A. Infusion of isotonic saline

   B. Low dose IV insulin

   C. Potassium supplementation

   D. Oral glucose load

2. A 9-year-old patient presents with new onset sharp, pleuritic chest pain that improves with leaning forward. A pericardial friction rub is heard on examination. The patient's mother reports the patient had a sore throat and low-grade fever with painful oral ulcers and small "blisters and bumps" on the palms 2 weeks ago. What is the most likely etiology of this patient's diagnosis?

   A. Epstein Barr virus

   B. *Cytomegalovirus*

   C. Group A streptococcus

   D. Coxsackie virus

3. A patient presents with 4 days of fever, fatigue, headache, sore throat, and nonproductive cough. The patient tests positive for influenza A. What is the preferred treatment?

A. Oseltamivir (Tamiflu)

B. Supportive measures

C. Zanamivir (Relenza)

D. Peramivir (Rapivab)

4. A 56-year-old patient presents with complaints of morning stiffness, joint pain, and joint swelling of the metacarpophalangeal and proximal interphalangeal joints of the hands. What x-ray findings would one expect to see on work up of a patient with these findings?

A. Joint space widening and soft tissue swelling

B. Marginal osteophytes and subchondral sclerosis

C. Joint space narrowing, periarticular osteopenia, and bony erosions

D. Interosseous tophi, overhanging edges of bone at the joint, and small punched out erosions

5. A 42-year-old female patient with a history of migraines and depression presents with a 6-month history of chronic fatigue that is pronounced upon waking and in the afternoons, and widespread musculoskeletal pain. On examination, the patient reports tenderness in multiple soft tissue anatomic locations. A work up is done and is unrevealing. What is the first-line treatment for this patient's newly diagnosed fibromyalgia?

A. Amitriptyline

B. Sertraline

C. Gabapentin

D. Oxycodone

6. A 73-year-old patient presents with new onset dyspnea on exertion and exertional angina and dizziness. On physical examination, a crescendo-decrescendo systolic ejection murmur is heard over the right upper sternal border over the right second intercostal space with radiation to the carotid arteries. There is reduced intensity of the second heart sound. What is the most likely diagnosis?

A. Aortic stenosis

B. Aortic regurgitation

C. Pulmonary stenosis

D. Mitral regurgitation

7. A patient with a history of portal hypertension and cirrhosis is found to have esophageal varices on endoscopy. Which medication should be started for prophylaxis of variceal hemorrhage?

A. Propranolol

B. Lisinopril

C. Metoprolol

D. Misoprostol

8. A 21-year-old female with type one diabetes mellitus presents with a 3-day history of nausea, dysuria, and urinary frequency. On examination, there is suprapubic tenderness and costovertebral angle tenderness on the left, and urinalysis shows pyuria and bacteriuria. The patient is admitted to the hospital for management. What is an appropriate treatment for this patient pending culture results?

A. PO ciprofloxacin for 3 to 5 days

B. IV ceftriaxone for 7 to 14 days

C. PO amoxicillin for 7 to 14 days

D. IV ciprofloxacin for 3 to 5 days

9. A 28-year-old patient presents with new onset palpitations and presyncope. On examination, auscultation of the heart sounds reveals a harsh systolic crescendo-decrescendo murmur at the LLSB with increased intensity upon standing. Echocardiogram shows a stiff, hypertrophied left ventricle with systolic anterior motion of the mitral valve. What is the most likely diagnosis?

A. Hypertrophic cardiomyopathy

B. Restrictive cardiomyopathy

C. Dilated cardiomyopathy

D. Systolic congestive heart failure

10. A patient with recurrent, severe unilateral orbital headaches associated with restlessness and pacing has recently been diagnosed with cluster headaches. What is the first-line treatment that can be given to this patient for acute management of this condition?

A. Topiramate

B. Ergotamine

C. Oxygen

D. Verapamil

11. A 32-year-old pregnant patient in her first trimester has recently been diagnosed with Graves' disease. Assuming the patient has no drug allergies, what is the most appropriate treatment?

A. Radioactive iodine

B. PTU

C. Methimazole

D. Thyroidectomy

12. A patient presents with a week-long history of periorbital edema and generalized fatigue. The patient is found to have hypoalbuminemia, hyperlipidemia, and a spot urine sample of greater than 300 mg of protein per mmol creatinine. What is the most likely diagnosis?

A. Nephritic syndrome

B. Chronic kidney disease

C. Nephrotic syndrome

D. Urinary tract infection

13. A 59-year-old male with past medical history of HTN, coronary artery disease, and stable angina presents with gradual onset of substernal chest pain and discomfort, described as a "pressure" on the chest. The pain radiates to the shoulder and did not resolve with home sublingual nitroglycerin or rest. Troponins are positive. What is the most likely diagnosis?

    A. Stable angina

    B. Acute coronary syndrome (unstable angina or STEMI)

    C. GERD

    D. Pulmonary embolism

14. A 26-year-old male patient presents with a 1-week history of nonbloody urethral discharge and a painless genital ulcer. On examination, the patient is found to have mild bilateral inguinal lymphadenopathy. What is the most likely diagnosis of this lesion?

    A. Chancroid from infection with *Haemophilus ducreyi*

    B. A lesion from infection with herpes simplex virus

    C. Chancre from infection with *Treponema pallidum*

    D. A lesion from infection with human papilloma virus

15. A patient has been recently diagnosed with mild to moderate COPD. What is the best initial treatment for daily symptom management?

    A. SABA and anticholinergics

    B. LABA

    C. Smoking cessation and regular office visits only

    D. Oxygen

16. A 47-year-old Caucasian male with history of alcoholism presents with acute onset coffee ground hematemesis and epigastric pain after at least 7 separate bouts of vomiting this morning. On endoscopy, a single longitudinal mucosal tear at the esophagogastric junction is found. What is the most likely diagnosis?

    A. Barrett's esophagus

    B. Mallory-Weiss syndrome

    C. Esophageal varices

    D. Esophageal rupture

17. A 56-year-old female patient presents with a history of nausea, constipation, abdominal pain, fatigue, and bone pain. The patient also admits to some feelings of depression recently. On work up, the patient is noted to have renal calculi, and elevated serum calcium and parathyroid hormone levels. What is the most likely diagnosis?

    A. Hypoparathyroidism

    B. Secondary hyperparathyroidism

    C. Primary hyperparathyroidism

    D. Chronic renal failure

18. A patient presents with sudden onset right sided facial weakness that began this morning. She also reports decreased taste in the anterior two-thirds of the tongue. On examination, her right eyebrow and the right corner of her mouth are drooping, and she is unable to close her right eye completely. Her ear examination is unremarkable. On history, she does admit to having a cold a few weeks ago. What is the most likely diagnosis?

    A. Acute stroke

    B. Herpes zoster

    C. Bell's palsy

    D. Lyme disease

19. A patient was recently diagnosed with chronic myeloid leukemia. What genetic chromosomal abnormality is associated with this diagnosis?

    A. Trisomy 13

    B. Philadelphia chromosome

    C. Monosomy X

    D. Mutation of the *CEBPA* gene

20. A patient with a known seizure disorder presents with convulsive status epilepticus. After initial assessment, an IV line is placed. What is the recommended first-line pharmacologic treatment for this condition?

    A. Fosphenytoin (Cerebyx)

    B. Valproic Acid (Depakote)

    C. Levetiracetam (Keppra)

    D. Lorazepam (Ativan)

21. A 35-year-old male patient with a history of GERD for the last 2 years has failed treatment with lifestyle changes, H2 blockers, and most recently a PPI twice daily for the last 4 months. Evaluation of patient compliance with treatment and proper dosing times reveals no errors in treatment administration. What is the best next step for management and work up of this patient's refractory GERD?

    A. Esophageal impedance pH testing

    B. Esophagogastroduodenoscopy

    C. Nissen fundoplication

    D. Screening for psychological comorbidity

22. An 80-year-old female patient presents with a 3-day history of fever, fatigue, headache, jaw pain with chewing, and impaired vision of the right eye. On examination, the patient reports tenderness over the right temporal artery. What is the most likely diagnosis?

    A. Takayasu arteritis (TKA)

    B. Polyarteritis nodosa (PAN)

    C. Wegener's granulomatosis

    D. Giant cell arteritis

23. A patient is admitted to the hospital and diagnosed with new onset atrial fibrillation. It is unknown how long the patient has had this condition and she is not sure when her symptoms first started. How long should the patient be placed on anticoagulation prior to cardioversion?

A. 1 week

B. 48 hours

C. 24 hours

D. 3 weeks

24. A patient presents with purulent foul-smelling sputum, cough, and dyspnea that has been persistent over the last few months. Chest radiograph on initial work up reveals "tram track" lines representative of dilated and thickened airways. All other findings are nonspecific. What is the most likely diagnosis?

A. Bronchiectasis

B. Atypical pneumonia

C. Upper respiratory infection

D. Emphysema

ANSWERS

1. Clinical Intervention: Diabetic Ketoacidosis. Answer A: Infusion of isotonic saline is the first recommended step of treatment in patients with DKA to expand extracellular volume and correct volume depletion. B, Low dose IV insulin should be given only after administration of IVF and correction of hypokalemia as insulin will worsen hypokalemia by driving potassium into the cells. C, Correction of potassium deficit is the second step in treatment of DKA and should be done before insulin is given to avoid worsened hypokalemia. D, This is not recommended in treatment of DKA, although dextrose may be added to IVF once blood glucose reaches less than or equal to 200 mg/dL

2. Scientific Concepts: Pericarditis. Answer D: Coxsackie virus is a common cause of post-infectious pericarditis and causes hand foot and mouth disease. Although many other infectious agents may cause pericarditis including (A) Epstein Barr virus, (B) *Cytomegalovirus*, and (C) group A streptococcus, this is the most common and likely cause and is supported by the patient's history of infection.

3. Clinical Therapeutics: Influenza. Answer B: Supportive measures are indicated as (A) Tamiflu, (C) Relenza, and (D) Rapivab are only indicated for treatment of influenza in individuals with symptoms for less than 2 days or 48 hours

4. Scientific Concepts: Rheumatoid Arthritis. Answer C: Joint space narrowing, periarticular osteopenia, and bony erosions are classic findings of rheumatoid arthritis. A, Joint space widening and soft tissue swelling are not seen in rheumatoid arthritis. B, Marginal osteophytes and subchondral sclerosis are characteristic findings of osteoarthritis. D. Interosseous tophi, overhanging edges of bone at the joint, and small punched out erosions are characteristic findings of gout.

5. Clinical Therapeutics: Fibromyalgia. Answer A: Tricyclic antidepressants are indicated as first-line treatment of fibromyalgia, particularly amitriptyline. Duloxetine is used in management of fibromyalgia when patients fail to respond to first-line treatment

or present with severe disease. C, Gabapentin is used in management of fibromyalgia although it is not first line, and (B) sertraline and (D) oxycodone are not indicated for this condition.

6. Diagnosis: Aortic Stenosis. Answer A: These findings are common of aortic stenosis, which restricts outflow of blood through the aortic valve during systole, leading to the above symptoms due to reduced blood flow and a systolic ejection murmur. B, Aortic regurgitation produces a blowing diastolic decrescendo murmur that is best heard at the left upper sternal border. C, Pulmonary stenosis produces similar symptoms and a systolic ejection murmur as well, but the murmur is best heard over the left upper sternal border and is often associated with a jugular venous "A" wave, radiation to the back, splitting of the second heart sound, and a pulmonary ejection click. D, Mitral regurgitation produces a holosystolic murmur that is best heard over the apex and radiates to the axilla.

7. Clinical Therapeutics: Esophageal Varices. Answer A: A nonselective beta blocker such as propranolol is recommended for prophylaxis of variceal hemorrhage in patients with portal HTN and known esophageal varices. B, Lisinopril is an ACE inhibitor. C, Metoprolol is a selective β blocker and is therefore not recommended. D, Misoprostol is a synthetic prostaglandin E1 analogue used to treat stomach ulcers, postpartum bleeding due to poor contraction of the uterus and to induce labor or cause an abortion.

8. Clinical Therapeutics: Pyelonephritis. Answer B: While awaiting cultures, it is recommended to begin empiric IV antibiotics for complicated pyelonephritis, and to continue antibiotics such as ceftriaxone for 7-14 days. A, D, Ciprofloxacin (a fluoroquinolone) is commonly recommended as outpatient therapy. C, Amoxicillin is not a recommended treatment for complicated pyelonephritis.

9. Diagnosis: Hypertrophic Cardiomyopathy. Answer A: These findings are consistent with hypertrophic cardiomyopathy. B, In restrictive cardiomyopathy, you would see normal ventricular wall thickness. C, In dilated cardiomyopathy, you would see left ventricular wall dilation and systolic dysfunction. D, In systolic congestive heart failure, you would see dilated cardiomyopathy and systolic dysfunction.

10. Clinical Therapeutics: Cluster Headache. Answer C: Oxygen is the first-line treatment of choice for acute attacks. A, Topiramate and (D) Verapamil are both used for prevention of cluster headaches. B, Ergotamine can be used for acute relief.

11. Clinical Therapeutics: Graves' Disease. Answer B: PTU is recommended in pregnancy when hyperthyroidism is diagnosed in the first trimester as it has less incidence of teratogenic effects. A, Radioactive iodine is absolutely contraindicated in pregnancy. C, Methimazole has a higher incidence of teratogenic effects and is not recommended over PTU in the first trimester. D, Thyroidectomy is rarely necessary, and usually only done if the patient develops agranulocytosis from treatment or has an allergy to the treatment medication. It is only indicated for pregnancy if the patient's treatment with PTU is unsuccessful.

12. Diagnosis: Nephrotic Syndrome. Answer C. Nephrotic syndrome is defined by hypoalbuminemia and a urinary protein excretion of greater than 50 mg/kg per day, or a spot urine sample of greater than 300 mg of protein per mmol creatinine. Hyperlipidemia and periorbital edema are also common findings. A, Nephritic syndrome is defined by hematuria, varying levels of proteinuria although usually less than 3.5 g/24 hours, and edema in the late stages. The findings above support nephrotic pathology. B, Chronic kidney disease is defined by decreased GFR for at least 3 months, although proteinuria and edema occur in advanced disease. D, A urinary tract infection would not cause these findings.

13. Diagnosis: Acute Coronary Syndrome. Answer B: These findings are common in ACS (STEMI or unstable angina) and elevated troponins confirms the diagnosis. A, Stable angina occurs with increased oxygen demand and would improve with sublingual nitroglycerin. Troponins would be negative. C, GERD is ruled out with positive troponins although some minor chest pain can occur with this. D, Pulmonary embolism can cause chest pain, but is often associated with dyspnea, making this less likely. Troponins also confirm a cardiac source.

14. Diagnosis: Syphilis. Answer C: Chancres are typically painless lesions such as this one that occur at the site of inoculation and are commonly associated with bilateral inguinal lymphadenopathy. Urethral discharge is another common symptom with primary syphilis infection. A, Chancroids are classically painful, unlike this lesion, and only half of the time are associated with inguinal lymphadenopathy. This diagnosis is less likely than syphilis. B, HSV infection produces multiple painful genital pustules and ulcers and is often accompanied

by constitutional symptoms. D, HPV infection produces genital warts.

15. Clinical Therapeutics: COPD. Answer A: It is recommended to start treatment of mild COPD with short acting β agonists and short acting anticholinergics as needed for symptom relief. B, LABA and (D) oxygen are used for more severe disease. C, Smoking cessation is key as well, only observation with office visits would not be appropriate.

16. Diagnosis: Mallory-Weiss Tear. Answer B: Mallory-Weiss syndrome involves longitudinal tears of the esophagogastric junction mucosa, usually secondary to forceful vomiting. It often presents with hematemesis and epigastric pain. A, Barrett's esophagus is a condition in which the stratified squamous epithelium of the esophagus is replaced by metastatic columnar epithelium which predisposes the patient to cancer development. This is often asymptomatic. C, Esophageal varices are asymptomatic unless they have ruptured, in which case symptoms such as these would be present. D, Esophageal rupture involves a full thickness tear of the esophageal wall.

17. Diagnosis: Hyperparathyroidism. Answer C: Primary hyperparathyroidism is characterized classically by the symptom pattern of "painful bones, renal stones, abdominal groans, and psychiatric overtones." With primary hyperparathyroidism, PTH and calcium levels will be elevated, unlike in (B) secondary hyperparathyroidism where PTH will be low, such as with (D) chronic renal failure. A, Hypoparathyroidism will show low PTH levels.

18. Diagnosis: Bell's Palsy. Answer C: Bell's palsy is the most likely diagnosis in this patient as the clinical picture, including recent URI, loss of all facial movement including the forehead, and loss of some taste sensation are all known to be associated with this condition. A, A stroke can cause similar weakness involving the face, but more often does not involve the forehead and is usually associated with other signs, such as aphasia, contralateral hemiparesis or hemisensory loss, apraxia, hemiataxia, or homonymous hemianopsia depending on the location. B, Herpes zoster can cause similar symptoms but vesicles must be noted in the external meatus to make this diagnosis. D, Lyme disease commonly causes facial nerve palsies as well, but often presents with redness and edema of the face prior to symptom onset, and the clinical picture is not suggestive of this infection.

19. Scientific Concepts: Leukemia. Answer B: The Philadelphia chromosome confirms the diagnosis of CML. A, Trisomy 13, (C) monosomy X, and (D) mutation of the *CEBPA* gene are not associated with leukemia.

20. Clinical Therapeutics: Status Epilepticus. Answer D: First-line treatment for convulsive status epilepticus is a benzodiazepine, usually lorazepam. A, Fosphenytoin,

(B) valproate, and (C) levetiracetam can all be loaded intravenously to prevent recurrence, but are only used after benzodiazepines have been given.

21. Clinical Intervention: GERD. Answer A: Esophageal impedance pH testing is recommended after treatment-failure with a PPI twice daily for 2 months. B, Esophagogastroduodenoscopy and (C) Nissen fundoplication have a role in management for some patients but are not recommended until this work up is done first for patients with refractory GERD. D, It is not clear yet if screening for psychological comorbidity provides any value to management of patients with this condition.

22. Diagnosis: Giant Cell Arteritis. Answer D: These findings are classic for temporal or giant cell arteritis, including presentation in a female over 50 years old, making this the most likely diagnosis. A, TKA shares similar symptoms with giant cell or temporal arteritis, making it hard to distinguish the two. However, TKA commonly presents in younger patients under 40; whereas, temporal arteritis always presents in those over 50, making TKA less likely in this patient. B, PAN also presents with constitutional symptoms, although multiple organ systems including the skin and kidneys are often involved. Tenderness over the temporal artery, and the constellation of jaw pain, headache, and impaired vision are not seen, making this less likely. C. Similarly to PAN, Wegener's granulomatosis involves constitutional symptoms and a wide variety of symptoms and signs involving multiple organ systems. However, these specific findings and temporal artery tenderness would not be seen in this condition.

23. Health Maintenance: Atrial Fibrillation. Answer D. In patients with AF for more than 48 hours or unknown duration of AF, 3 weeks of anticoagulation is required prior to cardioversion.

24. Diagnosis: Bronchiectasis. Answer A: These symptoms are common of bronchiectasis. The radiographic findings of "tram track" lines are pathognomonic. B, Atypical pneumonia would show reticulonodular infiltrates or patchy areas of consolidation on CXR, not "tram track" lines. C, URI typically only last a few weeks, not a few months. D, Emphysema typically presents with these symptoms, although these radiographic findings would not be present. Instead, signs of COPD such as diaphragmatic flattening and hyperinflation would be present.

CHAPTER 25

Dermatology

 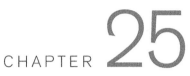
DERMATITIS

Disease	Etiology, Prevalence, Risk Factors	Clinical Symptoms and Signs	Diagnostics	Therapy, Prognosis, and Health Maintenance
Irritant diaper dermatitis (Fig. 25-1A)	Caused by overhydration of the skin, maceration, prolonged contact with urine/feces, retained diaper soaps, >3 diarrheal stools/d MC: Infants 9-12 mo Associated: history of eczema	1. Erythematous scaly diaper area 2. Genitocrural folds are **spared** in irritant dermatitis Signs: 1. Papulovesicular or bullous lesions, fissures, and erosions 2. Patchy or confluent 3. Genitocrural folds are spared	1. KOH preparation or culture	1. **Zinc oxide ointment** 2. Leave diaper area open to air or cover it with topical emollient • Petrolatum, Aquaphor®
Candidal diaper dermatitis (Fig. 25-1B)	Infection occurs after 48-72 h of active eruption MCC: *Candida albicans* Immunocompromised patients are more susceptible	1. Isolated to perineal area (92%) 2. Genitocrural folds are **involved** in primary candidal dermatitis Signs: 1. **Satellite lesions** (Miliaria rubra): tiny red papules and papulovesicles 2. Confluent diaper area with tomato-red plaques, papules, and pustules	1. KOH prep or culture (not necessary)	1. Hydrocortisone 1% BID AND 2. Antifungal: **nystatin cream**, powder, or ointment; clotrimazole 1% cream, miconazole 2% ointment after every diaper change • **Avoid** higher strength topical steroids, including clotrimazole/betamethasone and nystatin/triamcinolone 3. Leave diaper area open to air or cover it with topical emollient • Petrolatum, Aquaphor®

(continued)

(continued)

Disease	Etiology, Prevalence, Risk Factors	Clinical Symptoms and Signs	Diagnostics	Therapy, Prognosis, and Health Maintenance
Perioral dermatitis (Fig. 25-1C)	<u>MC:</u> Young women with history of prior topical steroid use in area	1. Papulopustules on erythematous base → confluent plaques and scales 2. Vermillion border spared 3. Satellite lesions common	Culture to r/o staphylococcal infection	1. Avoid topical steroids (aggravate!) 2. Topical flagyl or erythromycin 3. PO minocycline, doxycycline, tetracycline

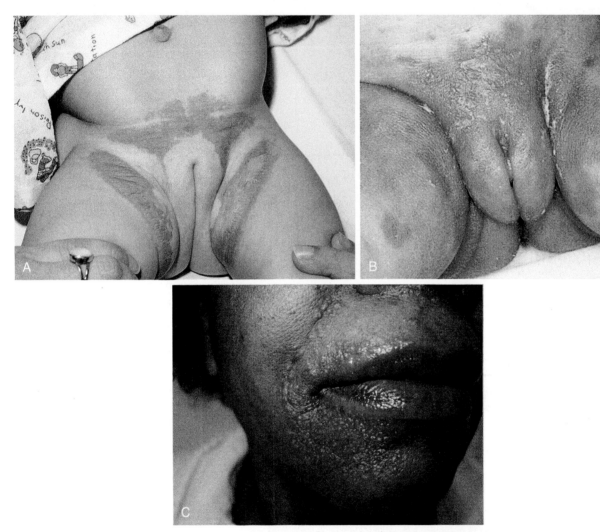

FIGURE 25-1. A, Irritant diaper dermatitis. Note the spared intertriginous areas without satellite lesions. **B**, Candidal diaper dermatitis. A bright red rash involving the intertriginous folds with satellite lesions along the edges. **C**, Perioral dermatitis due to steroid use. (**A**, Dr. Barankin Dermatology Collection. **B**, Fletcher M. *Physical Diagnosis in Neonatology*. Philadelphia: Lippincott-Raven Publishers; 1998. **C**, Image provided by Stedman's.)

DRUG ERUPTIONS

Disease	Etiology, Prevalence, Risk Factors	Clinical Symptoms and Signs	Diagnostics	Therapy, Prognosis, and Health Maintenance
Staphylococcal scalded skin syndrome	Diffuse erythema, superficial blistering, intraepidermal separation and sheetlike desquamation Only superficial layers involved ***Staphylococcus aureus*** producing exfoliative toxins	1. Initial infection in oral cavity or nasopharynx → spreads erythrodermalike rash 2. Diffuse sheetlike, superficial desquamation <u>Signs:</u> 1. Skin is warm, tender to touch	1. Shave biopsy *diagnostic*: superficial epidermal sloughing and intraepidermal separation	

BURNS (FIG. 25-2A-E)

- Parkland or Baxter formula, consists of 3 to 4 mL/kg/% burn of lactated Ringer, of which half is given during the first 8 hours after burn and the remaining half is given over the subsequent 16 hours

- Goals for urine output should be 30 mL/h in adults and 1 to 1.5 mL/kg/h in pediatric patients

Disease	Etiology, Prevalence, Risk Factors	Clinical Symptoms and Signs	Diagnostics	Therapy, Prognosis, and Health Maintenance
First degree (superficial)	MCC: Overexposure to sunlight and brief scalding Involves only epidermis	Painful but do not blister • Resolves in 48-72 h • Erythema and minor microscopic changes		Heals uneventfully • Damaged skin peels off in small scales in 5-10 d, no residual scarring
Second degree (partial thickness)	Involves all of epidermis and some of corium or dermis	Dermal involvement Extremely painful with weeping and blisters		
Superficial		Blister formation • Increase in size		Most heal with expectant management with minimal scarring in 10-14 d Complications: Severe pain
Deep		Reddish appearance or layer of whitish, nonviable dermis firmly adherent to remaining viable tissue		Excise and graft • Heal over 4-8 wk Complications: Conversion to full thickness burn by infection
Third degree (full thickness)	Prolonged exposure to heat, involvement of fat and underlying tissue	Leathery, painless, and nonblanching: 1. White, dry, waxy appearance (appears as unburned skin) 2. Fat—may be brown, dark-red, or black	**Lack of sensation in burned skin**, lack of capillary refill, leathery texture	Require skin grafting and escharotomy No potential for reepithelialization
Fourth degree		Affect underlying soft tissue		

- The "rule of nines" is a crude but quick and effective method of estimating burn size. In adults, the anterior and posterior trunk each account for 18%, each lower extremity is 18%, each upper extremity is 9%, and the head is 9%. In children under 3 years old, the head accounts for a larger relative surface area and should be taken into account when estimating burn size
- Follow American Burn Association criteria for transfer of a patient to a regional burn center
  - Partial thickness burns >10% BSA
  - Burns involving the face, hands, feet, genitalia, perineum, major joints
- Third-degree burns in any age
- Electrical burns, including lightning injury
- Chemical burns
- Inhalation injury
- Burn injury in patients with preexisting medical disorders
- Patients with burns and trauma in which burn is greatest risk
- Burned children without qualified personnel for care of children in hospital
- Patients who require social, emotional, or rehabilitative intervention

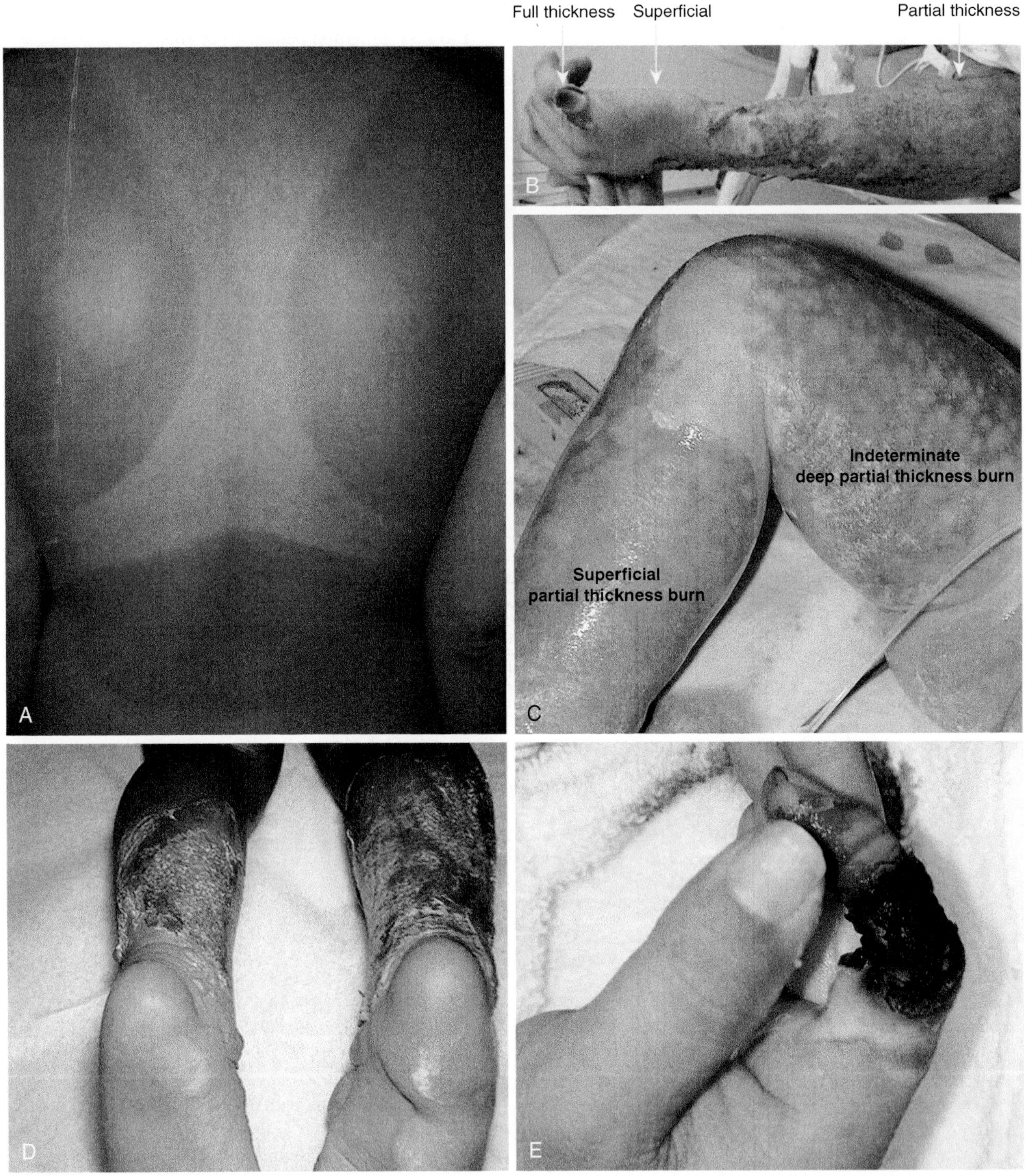

FIGURE 25-2. **A**, Superficial (first degree) burn. **B**, Partial thickness (second degree) burn. **C**, Deep burn. **D**, Full-thickness (third-degree) burn. **E**, Fourth-degree burn. (**A**, From Hinkle JL, Cheever KH. *Brunner & Suddarth's Textbook of Medical-Surgical Nursing*. Philadelphia: Wolters Kluwer Health; 2018. **B**, From Silbert-Flagg J, Pillitteri A. *Maternal and Child Health Nursing*. Philadelphia: Wolters Kluwer Health; 2018. **C**, From Werner R. *Massage Therapist's Guide to Pathology*. Philadelphia: Wolters Kluwer Health; 2013. **D**, From Werner R. *Massage Therapist's Guide to Pathology*. Philadelphia: Wolters Kluwer Health; 2013. **E**, From Doughty DB, McNichol LL. *Wound, Ostomy and Continence Nurses Society® Core Curriculum: Wound Management*. Philadelphia: Wolters Kluwer Health; 2016.)

CHAPTER 26

Head, Ears, Eyes, Nose, and Throat

Refer to Family Medicine for in-depth coverage of the following topics:

Otitis Media and Externa, p 81
Tympanic Membrane Perforation, p 79
Orbital Cellulitis, see Urgent Care, p 192
Bacterial, Viral, and Seasonal Allergic Conjunctivitis, p 84

Epistaxis, p 98
Acute Pharyngotonsillitis, p 99
Peritonsillar Abscess, p 100

Recommended Supplemental Topics:

Congenital Oral Malformations, p 301

HEAD

Mastoiditis (Fig. 26-1)

Disease	Etiology, Prevalence, Risk Factors	Clinical Symptoms and Signs	Diagnostics	Therapy, Prognosis, and Health Maintenance
Mastoiditis	MC pathogens: *S. pneumoniae, S. aureus*	<u>HX of antibiotic use without improvement:</u> 1. Spiking **fever**, malaise, hearing loss +/− headache 2. **Postauricular pain, erythema**, fluctuant painful mass, edema of the pinna 3. LAD 4. Posteriorly and downward displaced auricle	1. CT scan: loss of trabecular bone 2. MRI–r/o sigmoid sinus thrombosis, intracranial abscess	1. IV antibiotics, myringotomy + oral antibiotics 2. **Mastoidectomy** if ineffective • Debride necrotic bone 3. Myringotomy–adjunct to mastoidectomy 4. Tympanomastoidectomy if cholesteatoma present <u>Complications:</u> 1. Bony erosion 2. Temporal lobe abscess 3. Septic thrombosis of lateral sinus

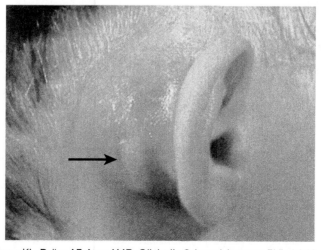

FIGURE 26-1. Mastoiditis. (From Moore KL, Dalley AF, Agur AMR. *Clinically Oriented Anatomy.* Philadelphia: Wolters Kluwer Health; 2014.)

EARS

Hearing Impairment/Hearing Loss

- Conductive—caused by impaired sound transmission to inner ear
- Sensorineural—damage or impairment of inner ear (cochlea) or neural pathways
- Most common causes—cerumen impaction, eustachian tube dysfunction (secondary to URI), increased age (presbycusis)

- Dilatory dysfunction is best differentiated by accompanying symptoms of hearing loss and abnormalities of the tympanic membrane such as retraction or middle ear effusion
- Patulous dysfunction should be suspected when the primary complaint is autophony (hearing one's own voice and breathing sounds), yet there is no complaint of hearing loss and the tympanic membrane appears normal

Disease	Etiology, Prevalence, Risk Factors	Clinical Symptoms and Signs	Diagnostics	Therapy, Prognosis, and Health Maintenance
Cerumen impaction	10% of children Buildup of secretions and sloughed epithelial cells and air from external auditory canal	1. Hearing loss 2. Ear pain or discomfort 3. Dizziness 4. Tinnitus 5. Chronic cough Complications: otitis externa, dizziness, syncope, tinnitus, tympanic membrane perforation, cardiac arrest	1. Direct visualization by otoscope	1. Irrigation alone • Contraindicated in patients with previous ear surgery or those with anatomic abnormalities 2. Ceruminolytics before Irrigation • **Saline** (first line): leave in for 15-30 min • Cerumenolytics improves irrigation success • Water-based preps more effective (triethanolamine) 3. Manual removal requires a cooperative patient and clinical skill • Quicker, allows direct visualization with handheld otoscope 4. Refer to ENT Avoid ear candling
Eustachian tube dysfunction The eustachian tube regulates middle ear pressure and allows for drainage of the middle ear. It must periodically open to prevent the development of negative pressure and effusion in the middle ear space	If opening does not occur, negative pressure leads to transudation of cellular fluid into the middle ear, as well as influx of fluids and pathogens from the nasopharynx and adenoids More prone to dysfunction if tube: shorter, higher compliance, and more horizontal than adults RF: 1. Down syndrome 2. Cleft palate	1. Ear pain 2. Sensation of ear fullness or pressure 3. Hearing loss 4. Tinnitus Signs: 1. Dull bluish gray or yellow TM = effusion 2. Red coloration and engorged vessels 3. Normal otoscopic exam does not rule out Associated: Vertigo	Clinical DX: 1. Nasal endoscopy (confirms) 2. Tympanometry (gold standard, confirms) 3. CT or MRI if unilateral symptoms for 3+ mo	1. Treat underlying condition, if known 2. Differentiate between dilatory dysfunction and patulous dysfunction (see above) Health maintenance: 1. Repeat tympanogram every 3 mo if persistent 2. Repeat tympanogram in 3-12 mo in adults, depending on severity 3. Referral to an allergist for children with persistent allergic symptoms who have not outgrown their eustachian tube dysfunction by age six Complications: AOM, hearing loss, tympanic membrane perforation, cholesteatomas

Treatment of Eustachian Tube Dysfunction

Dilatory Dysfunction	Patulous Dysfunction
Pharmacologic management 1. Decongestants (pseudoephedrine, phenylephrine) for congestive symptoms (ear fullness, pressure) 2. Oral methylprednisolone 3. Topical nasal steroids **Surgery** 1. Tympanostomy tubes—neutralize negative pressure in middle ear 2. Eustachian tuboplasty—reduces thickness of the mucosa and submucosa of the posterior medial wall of tubal orifice 3. Balloon dilation/tuboplasty	**Pharmacologic management** 1. Adequate hydration, nasal saline drops 2. Oral Potassium iodine TID—thickens mucosa 3. Decongestants and nasal steroids ineffective **Surgery** 1. Tympanostomy tubes 2. Intraluminal catheter placement 3. Cartilage grafting 4. Complete occlusion of eustachian tube

Pediatrics

Disease	Etiology, Prevalence, Risk Factors	Clinical Symptoms and Signs	Diagnostics	Therapy, Prognosis, and Health Maintenance
Conductive hearing loss	1. Blockage or obstruction due to cerumen impaction or exudate from otitis externa 2. Otitis media with effusion 3. Otosclerosis (bony growth of middle ear) 4. Ear trauma or injury		1. Weber test: lateralization to affected ear 2. Rinne test: bone > air conduction on affected side 3. Audiological testing unless obvious treatable cause	1. Ear curette or loop to remove cerumen or use detergent drops, suction, and irrigation
Sensorineural hearing loss	**Presbycusis**—most common cause		1. Weber test: lateralization to better hearing or unaffected side 2. Rinne test: air conduction > bone conduction 3. Audiological testing unless obvious treatable cause	

Cerumenolytics

Water-Based	Non–Water-Based Non–Oil-Based	Oil-Based
• Softens cerumen before irrigation	• Softens cerumen before irrigation or alternative to irrigation	• Softens cerumen before irrigation

1. **10% Triethanolamine**
  • Fill ear 15-30 min before irrigation
  • Can be irritative, not for prolonged use
2. Water or saline
  • If attempted irrigation without softening and ineffective → instill water and wait 15 mins before repeating
3. 3% Hydrogen peroxide
  • Fill affected ear 15-30 min prior to irrigation
  • If not completely removed, bubbling may interfere with visualization
4. Home: 2.5% acetic acid
  • Fill ear with 2-3 cc BID up to 14 d
  • More effective in children
	1. Carbamide peroxide (Debrox)
	  • Put 5-10 drops into affected ear twice daily × 7 d
		1. Olive oil, almond oil, or mineral oil
		  • 3 drops into affected ear at bedtime × 3-4 d

Tympanostomy tubes for children 6 months to 12 years:

- Indications—Offer bilateral tympanostomy tube insertion in children with
  - Bilateral OME for at least *3 months* AND documented hearing impairment
  - Recurrent AOM with effusion (**3 episodes in 6 months or 4 episodes in 1 year**)
  - Chronic symptomatic OME associated with balance problems, poor school performance, behavioral problems, or ear discomfort thought to be due to OME

- Recommendations
  - Obtain hearing test if OME persists >3 months or if tympanostomy tube insertion is being considered
  - Do not perform for children with
    - Single episode of effusion <3 months duration
    - Recurrent AOM without effusion
  - No need for prophylactic water precautions (use of earplugs or water sport restriction) for children with tympanostomy tubes

Types of Hearing Devices

- Assistive listening devices. A large variety of devices are available at much lower cost than hearing aids. Some of these are free. Telephone companies provide free amplifiers and ringers if patients present a physician or audiologist release. Hotels provide telephone amplifiers in 10% of rooms. Examples include devices that flash lights when the telephone rings, vibration devices when the doorbell sounds, flashing smoke alarms, television amplifiers

- Behind the ear (BTE). Cheapest, easiest to adjust, less feedback than other devices. Fairly visible. Most powerful. Fewest number of problems with wax or infections

- In the ear (ITE). Low visibility; harder to put in and adjust

- In the canal (ITC). Very low visibility. Clearer than assistive listening devices and BTE. Lower power. Patients with tremor or poor eyesight are not good candidates

- Completely in the canal (CIC). Cannot be seen. Requires tight fit. Hard to adjust and remove. Clearer than assistive listening devices and BTE. Patients with tremor or poor eyesight are not good candidates

- Cochlear implants—An exciting recent development is an ability to provide hearing to some bilaterally deafened individuals through implantation of a device that directly stimulates the hearing nerve (spiral ganglion). Although this device is not generally considered as a hearing aid, it performs the same purpose for individuals with severe hearing impairment involving both ears. Cochlear implants do not completely substitute for a normally hearing ear, and at very best, may allow someone who was previously totally deaf to understand conversation on a telephone

- Must be 12 months or older
- Bilateral severe-to-profound hearing loss
- No appreciable benefit with hearing aids
- Must be able to tolerate wearing hearing aids
- Enroll in aural/oral education program
- No medical or anatomic contraindications

EYES

Conjunctivitis

Inflammation of the bulbar and/or palpebral conjunctiva.

Disease	Etiology, Prevalence, Risk Factors	Clinical Symptoms and Signs	Diagnostics	Therapy, Prognosis, and Health Maintenance
Neonatal or hyperacute conjunctivitis	*C. trachomatis* and **N. gonorrhoeae** Suspect in newborns who may be exposed during vaginal delivery	Same as above 1. Preauricular lymphadenopathy (severe) Signs: 1. Copious purulence 2. Severe injection 3. Chemosis 4. Severe eyelid edema Complications: Blindness (8%)	1. ***Bacterial culture*** on Thayer-Martin agar, chocolate agar, and Gram stain 2. Giemsa stain: helpful to screen for intracellular inclusion bodies of chlamydia	Chlamydia: 1. **PO erythromycin** for neonate • 50 mg/kg/d in 4 divided doses × 2 wk 2. Treat mother and at-risk contacts with doxycycline 100 mg BID × 7 d Gonorrhea: 1. **IV aqueous penicillin G** for neonate • 100 U/kg/d in 4 divided doses × 1 wk 2. Mother and at-risk contacts get single-dose IM ceftriaxone (Rocephin) and doxycycline as above 3. Prophylaxis against ophthalmia neonatorum: 1% silver nitrate solution, 1% tetracycline or 0.5% erythromycin ointment

Strabismus (Fig. 26-2A-D)

- Cover-uncover test
  - Child fixates on a point (small toy, penlight)
  - Cover one eye for 1 to 2 seconds
  - Rapidly uncover the eye
- Observe for movement of previously covered eye from a deviated position back to fixation on object
  - Abnormal or (+) test suggests latent strabismus (phoria)
  - Cover other eye and repeat

Disease	Etiology, Prevalence, Risk Factors	Clinical Symptoms and Signs	Diagnostics	Therapy, Prognosis, and Health Maintenance
Strabismus	Intermittent alternating convergent strabismus frequently noted in first 6 mo	Can result in vision loss in one eye (*amblyopia*)	Screening–corneal light reflex (reflected light should appear symmetrically in both corneas)	REFER–infants >6 mo with intermittent alternating convergent strabismus
Esotropia	Esotropia is inward turning of the eyes ("crossed eyes")		Cover-uncover test: eye moves outward to pick up fixation	
Exotropia	Exotropia is the term used to describe outward turning of the eyes ("wall-eyed")		Cover-uncover test: eye moves inward to pick up fixation	
Hypotropia	Abnormal eye higher than the normal eye			
Hypertropia	Abnormal eye higher than the normal eye			

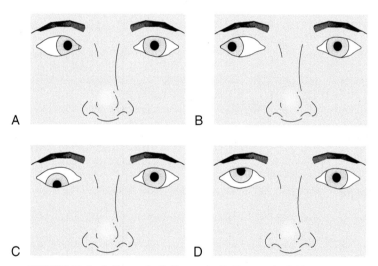

FIGURE 26-2. **A**, Esotropia. **B**, Exotropia. **C**, Hypotropia. **D**, Hypertropia.

THROAT AND MOUTH

Oral Candidiasis

Disease	Etiology, Prevalence, Risk Factors	Clinical Symptoms and Signs	Diagnostics	Therapy, Prognosis, and Health Maintenance
Oral candidiasis (thrush)	<u>RF</u>: HIV, dentures, DM, exposure to broad-spectrum antibiotics, or inhaled steroids	1. **Sore** and painful, dry **mouth** 2. Burning mouth or tongue 3. Dysphagia 4. Unpleasant taste <u>Signs</u>: 1. Thick, whitish patches on oral mucosa • Easily rubbed off 2. Diffuse erythema	<u>Clinical DX</u>: 1. KOH prep (wet mount): pseudohyphae or hyphae	1. Topical antifungal • **Clotrimazole troches** 10 mg 4-5 × daily • Nystatin 2. PO fluconazole 50-100 mg PO daily × 3-7 d

Acute Epiglottitis

- Dysphagia: subjective sensation of difficulty or abnormality of swallowing

- Odynophagia: pain with swallowing

Disease	Etiology, Prevalence, Risk Factors	Clinical Symptoms and Signs	Diagnostics	Therapy, Prognosis, and Health Maintenance
Acute epiglottitis (*supraglottitis*) 1. Ds: **d**ysphagia, **d**rooling, **d**istress (Figs. 26-3 and 26-4)	Pathogen: ***H. influenzae* type B** (MCC, now rare due to vaccination, though still occurs in immunized children), *S. pneumoniae*, GAS, MRSA IC: *Pseudomonas aeruginosa*, candida Noninfectious causes: thermal injury, FB, caustic ingestion Median age: 6-12 y/o RF: Incomplete/lack of immunization for Hib, immune deficiency Inflammation of the epiglottis and adjacent supraglottitis structures Results from bacteremia or direct invasion of epithelial layer (posterior nasopharynx)	Rapid, abrupt onset in children: 1. Difficulty breathing (80%) 2. Muffled speech (79%) • "Hot potato" voice 3. **Sudden onset high fever (38.8°–40°C)** 4. **Severe sore throat** (mostly adults) 5. **Dysphagia**, odynophagia 6. Absent cough (30% with cough) or hoarseness 7. Anxiety, restless, irritable Signs: 1. Respiratory **distress (stridor)** 2. Copious oral secretions **(drooling)** 3. **Difficulty swallowing** 4. **Pharyngitis** 5. Lean forward to prevent full obstruction of airway • **Tripod position** or "sniffing" posture 6. Neck hyperextended, chin thrust forward 7. Inspiratory retractions 8. Appear toxic	1. **Direct or fiberoptic laryngoscopy** (gold standard) • Erythematous, edematous epiglottis 2. Lateral x-ray • **Thumb sign** (77%-88% of adults) • Loss of vallecular air space • Thickened aryepiglottic folds • Distended hypopharynx • Used to confirm if direct examination unsafe or unsuccessful • Labs–not routinely performed if clinical diagnosis is clear 3. CBC, blood cultures 4. Throat/epiglottis cultures	MEDICAL EMERGENCY 1. **Stabilize airway** (mainstay, precedes diagnostic evaluation) • BVM • Supplemental O$_2$ • Endotracheal tube • Emergent tracheostomy 2. Antibiotics × **7-10 d** • **3rd generation cephalosporin** (ceftriaxone or cefotaxime) AND **Antistaph agent** (vancomycin or clindamycin) Prevention: 1. Hib vaccine 2. Pneumococcal vaccine–to prevent secondary infection Complications: Airway obstruction, epiglottic abscess, secondary infection, necrotizing epiglottitis, death

Tonsillectomy Indications:

- Tonsillar hypertrophy with sleep disordered breathing
- Recurrent throat infections for

- >= 7 episodes of recurrent throat infection in last year
- >= 5 episodes per year in last 2 years
- >= 3 episodes per year in last 3 years

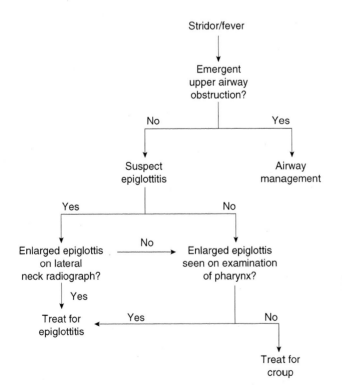

FIGURE 26-3. Approach to the child with suspected epiglottitis. (From Fleisher GR, Ludwig S. *Textbook of Pediatric Emergency Medicine.* Philadelphia: Wolters Kluwer Health; 2011.)

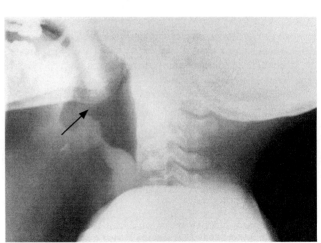

FIGURE 26-4. Epiglottitis thumb sign *(arrow).* (From Kline-Tilford AM, Haut C. *Lippincott Certification Review: Pediatric Acute Care Nurse Practitioner.* Philadelphia: Wolters Kluwer Health; 2016.)

Congenital Oral Malformations (Fig, 26-5)

Disease	Etiology, Prevalence, Risk Factors	Clinical Symptoms and Signs	Diagnostics	Therapy, Prognosis, and Health Maintenance
Tongue-tied (ankyloglossia) (Fig. 26-5A-C)	A short lingual frenulum can hinder both protrusion and elevation of the tongue	1. Puckering of midline tongue tip with movement 2. Feeding difficulties, speech problems, dental problems		1. Referral to ENT if tongue cannot protrude past teeth or alveolar ridge or move between the gums and cheek 2. Frenulectomy if having difficulty breastfeeding
Submucous *cleft palate*	Separation of the levator palatini muscles but intact mucosa 40% risk of developing persistent MEE, also at risk for velopharyngeal incompetence (hypernasal speech)	1. Nasal regurgitation of food during feeding 2. Abnormal speech (most do not have) Signs: 1. A translucent zone in the middle of the soft palate (zona pellucida): **central thinning of soft palate** 2. **Palpation of hard palate**: absence of posterior bony protrusion 3. **Bifid uvula**		Refer to ENT for surgical repair • **Furlow double-opposing Z-plasty**
High-arched palate	Chronic mouth breathers, premature infants who undergo prolonged oral intubation, Marfan syndrome, Ehlers-Danlos syndrome, Treacher Collins syndrome	Signs: Visualization on examination		Orthodontic treatment Complications: OSA

Pediatrics

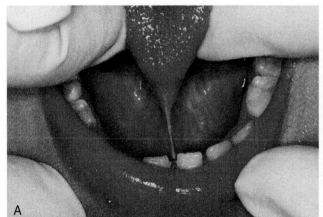
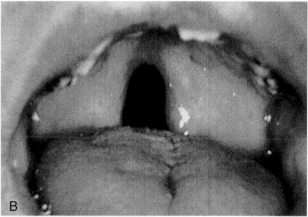
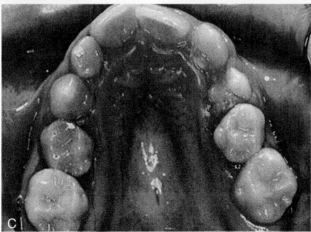

FIGURE 26-5. **A**, Tongue-tied (ankyloglossia). **B**, Cleft palate. **C**, High-arched palate (**A**, From Chung EK, Atkinson-McEvoy LR, Lai NL, Terry M. *Visual Diagnosis and Treatment in Pediatrics*. Philadelphia: Wolters Kluwer Health; 2015. **B**, From Wilkins EM. *Clinical Practice of the Dental Hygienist*. Philadelphia: Wolters Kluwer; 2017. **C**, Courtesy of Dr. Kasey Li.)

CHAPTER **27**

Pulmonology

Refer to Family Medicine 👪 for in-depth coverage of
the following topics:

Asthma, p 18

CROUP (LARYNGOTRACHEOBRONCHITIS)

- Laryngotracheitis (croup) refers to inflammation of the larynx and trachea
- Laryngotracheobronchitis (LTB) refers to inflammation beyond the bronchi resulting in lower airway signs, such as wheezing, crackles, tachypnea, and air trapping; used interchangeably with laryngotracheitis
- Bacterial tracheitis (bacterial croup) refers to bacterial infection of the trachea resulting in thick, purulent exudate and symptoms of upper airway obstruction

Croup Severity Score (Westley Croup Score)		Treatment

Mild (score <2)	• No stridor at rest (may be present with crying or upset)
	• Barking cough
	• Hoarse cry
	• Mild to no chest wall or subcostal retractions
		1. **Supportive care**
		  • Humidifier or Cool Mist
		  • Antipyretics
		  • Oral fluids
		AND
		1. **Single dose of PO dexamethasone** (0.15-0.6 mg/kg, max 10 mg)
		OR
		2. Nonpharmacologic management with anticipatory guidance about potentially worsening symptoms/signs and instructions on when to seek care or return for follow-up

Moderate (score 3-7)	• Stridor at rest
	• Mild retractions
	• Other symptoms/signs of respiratory distress
	• No agitation
		1. **Supportive care**
		  • Anxiety can worsen airway obstruction, humidified air or O_2
		  • Antipyretics
		  • PO intake
		  • Instruct parent to hold or comfort child as anxiety can worsen airway obstruction
		AND
		2. **Dexamethasone** (0.6 mg/kg, max 10 mg) by least invasive route tolerated: PO, IV, or IM
		AND
		3. Nebulized epinephrine in all patients with mod-severe
		  • **Racemic epinephrine** 0.05 mL/kg per dose (max 0.5 mL) of a 2.25% solution diluted to 3 mL total volume with normal saline, given over 15 min
		    • Can be repeated every 15-20 minutes
		    • Close cardiac monitoring if 3+ doses given in 2–3 h time frame
		OR
		  • L-epinephrine 0.5 mL/kg per dose (max 5 mL) of a 1:1000 solution over 15 min

Severe (score >8)	• Significant stridor at rest • Severe retractions (indrawing of sternum) • Anxious, agitated, or pale and fatigued child	

Respiratory failure (score >12)	• Fatigue and listlessness
	• Marked retractions
	• Decreased to absent breath sounds
	• Decreased level of consciousness
	• Tachycardia out of proportion to fever
	• Cyanosis or pallor
		1. Treatment as above
		2. Consider admission to PICU if
		  • Requires endotracheal intubation
		  • Persistent symptoms requiring frequent nebulized epinephrine
		  • Underlying comorbid conditions

When to Admit Croup

- Stridor at rest
- Rapid progression of symptoms (symptoms of upper airway obstruction <12 hours of illness)
- Inability to tolerate PO fluids
- Underlying airway abnormality (subglottic stenosis or hemangioma, previous intubation)
- Previous episodes of moderate to severe croup
- Comorbid respiratory illnesses (bronchopulmonary dysplasia)
- Parental concern not amenable to reassurance
- Prolonged symptoms (3 to 7 days) or atypical course

Disease	Etiology, Prevalence, Risk Factors	Clinical Symptoms and Signs	Diagnostics	Therapy, Prognosis, and Health Maintenance
Croup (**laryngotra-cheobronchitis**)	**6 mo–3 y**, fall or early winter, M > F MC pathogen: Parainfluenza virus type 1 Parainfluenza virus, type 2, milder than type 1 Parainfluenza, type 3; sporadic, severe Mucosal inflammation, increased secretions with edema (narrowed subglottic airway) 8%-15% presenting to ED with croup require hospitalization <u>RF:</u> FH (+) croup	1. URI prodrome: nasal discharge, congestion, coryza • Gradual onset • Progresses over 12-48 h 2. Low fever 3. **Seal-like barking cough** • Resolves in 3 d 4. **Hoarseness** Signs: 1. Inspiratory **stridor** 2. Subcostal retractions	1. AP x-ray of neck: Steeple sign (Fig. 27-1) Note: narrow subglottic airway 2. Utilize the Croup Severity Score when patient is seen outpatient or in the ED	See treatment above based on severity <u>If seen in ED:</u> 1. Patients should be observed for 3-4 h after initial treatment 2. If symptoms persist or worsen, consider admission 3. Follow-up with PCP in next 24 h after discharging home <u>Complications:</u> Hypoxemia, respiratory failure, pulmonary edema, pneumothorax, pneumomediastinum, secondary bacterial infections (tracheitis, bronchopneumonia, pneumonia)

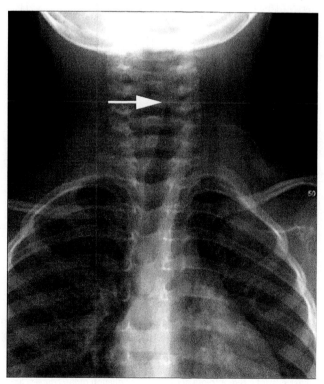

FIGURE 27-1. Steeple sign (*arrow*) on chest x-ray, seen in pediatric patients with croup. (From Sherman SC, Ross C, Nordquist E, Wang E, Cico S. *Atlas of Clinical Emergency Medicine.* Philadelphia: Wolters Kluwer Health; 2016.)

Pediatrics

BRONCHIOLITIS

Disease	Etiology, Prevalence, Risk Factors	Clinical Symptoms and Signs	Diagnostics	Therapy, Prognosis, and Health Maintenance
Acute bronchiolitis (Fig. 27-2)	Pathogen: **RSV** (MCC in children, late fall/winter), rhinovirus (spring, fall), parainfluenza virus type 3 (early spring, fall) Mostly during fall/winter <2 y (peak 2-6 mo) RF: Premature, low birth weight, age <12 wk, CHD, CLD, immunodeficient, severe neuromuscular disease A nonspecific inflammatory injury that affects the lower respiratory tract (2 mm or less in diameter)	Preceding 1-3 d URI (Nasal congestion +/− discharge, cough) 1. Fever <101°F 2. **Respiratory distress or SOB** • Insidious onset 3. **Dry cough** 4. Rhinorrhea 5. Irritability 6. **Feeding difficulty** • SX peak at 3-5 d Signs: 1. End-inspiratory crackles 2. **High-pitched inspiratory wheezing** 3. Prolonged expiratory phase 4. Tachycardia, **tachypnea** 5. Hyperresonant to percussion 6. Cyanosis/pallor 7. Hypoxemia (O_2 <95%) 8. Retractions, nasal flaring, grunting, sunken fontanelle, low UOP in children Associated: AOM, pharyngitis, conjunctivitis	Clinical DX: 1. CXR: not required—**Hyperinflation** and diffuse interstitial infiltrates, **peribronchial thickening** • Best for infants and young children with mod-severe disease 2. PCR—confirms diagnosis, if necessary 3. RAT for RSV or other viruses	1. Mostly self-limited 2. Moderate/severe: O_2 **(nasal cannula)**, IVF, PO, or NG feedings +/− bronchodilators 3. Monitor q 1-2 h Prophylaxis: 1. See below • **Palivizumab** (Synagis) 15 mg/kg IM once per month, max 5 doses with 35 d between Prognosis: 1. Longer length of admission with RSV compared to rhinovirus 2. Prolonged course in infants <6 mo or those with CLD 3. Worse prognosis if mechanical ventilation required 4. Mortality <0.1% Complications: Apnea, respiratory failure, dehydration, aspiration pneumonia, secondary bacterial infection

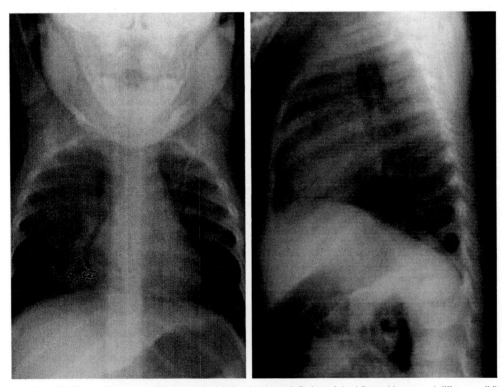

FIGURE 27-2. Acute bronchiolitis on chest x-ray of a 6-month-old showing hyperinflation of the bilateral lungs and diffuse perihilar infiltrates. (From Kline-Tilford AM, Haut C. *Lippincott Certification Review: Pediatric Acute Care Nurse Practitioner*. Philadelphia: Wolters Kluwer Health; 2016.)

Pediatrics

Management of Bronchiolitis

Nonsevere
Mild: O$_2$ >93%, no apnea, minimal accessory muscle use, treat at home
	1. **Supportive care**
	  • Maintenance of adequate hydration
	  • Nasal congestion relief
	  • Monitor for disease progression
	2. **Anticipatory guidance**
	  • Bronchiolitis starts as a URI and develops into a LRTI on days 2–3 (peak 3–5 d), then resolves over 2–3 wk
	  • Suction nose with syringe bulb after administration of nasal saline
	  • Monitor fluid intake and output
	  • Avoid OTC decongestants and cough medicines (not effective)
	  • Return to ER for: apnea, cyanosis, poor feeding, new fever, increased breathing rate, or increased WOB, decreased fluid intake (<75% normal, no wet diapers × 12 h), exhaustion
	  • Follow-up with PCP in 1–2 d
	3. **Antibiotics**
	  • For otherwise healthy infants/children, no pharmacologic intervention necessary (no proven benefit)
	  • Only indicated if coexisting bacterial infection exists
	  • No nebulized hypertonic saline indicated
	4. If not improving, consider a chest x-ray to rule out foreign body aspiration, heart failure, etc

Severe	Requires treatment in ER, ICU, or inpatient setting: 1. Supportive care and anticipatory guidance as above (mainstay) 2. ER management—trial of bronchodilator, nebulized hypertonic saline or steroids (not for first time bronchiolitis) 3. Inpatient management—contact precautions, IV fluids, monitor UOP, nasal suctioning, supplemental O$_2$, HFNC, and/or CPAP, +/– intubation • Not recommended: chest physiotherapy, inhaled bronchodilators, nebulized hypertonic saline, leukotriene inhibitors, or steroids—especially for first-time bronchiolitis
When to admit	1. Toxic appearance, poor feeding, lethargy, dehydration 2. Moderate to severe respiratory distress 3. Apnea 4. Hypoxemia +/– hypercapnia 5. Parents unable to care for their child at home
Prophylaxis	Primary prevention: 1. Hand hygiene, minimize passive smoke exposure, avoid ill contacts 2. Immunoprophylaxis with palivizumab (humanized monoclonal Ab against RSV F glycoprotein) • Side effects: hypersensitivity reaction (rare) 3. Annual flu vaccine for everyone >6 mo

Indications for Palivizumab

- Infants <1 year old with bronchopulmonary dysplasia (BPD)

- Preterm infants without BPD born at <28 weeks, 6 days of gestation, and younger than 12 months of age at start of RSV season

- Children with CHD: infants <12 months with (1) acyanotic heart disease and receiving medication for heart failure and require surgical correction (2) moderate to severe pulmonary hypertension

- Children with Down syndrome

- Case-by-case basis for: children with neuromuscular diseases (impairing ability to clear secretions), pulmonary malformations, tracheoesophageal fistula, tracheostomies, immunocompromised children (lung transplant or stem cell transplant)

- As of 2014, the AAP recommends against prophylaxis for infants born >29 weeks gestation with no additional RSV disease risk factors

- As of 2014, the AAP recommends only for children <12 months with cystic fibrosis and evidence of CLD and/or nutritional compromise or children <2 with cystic fibrosis and manifestations of severe lung disease

Disease	Etiology, Prevalence, Risk Factors	Clinical Symptoms and Signs	Diagnostics	Therapy, Prognosis, and Health Maintenance
Respiratory syncytial virus (RSV)	Paramyxoviridae family, single-stranded, RNA virus (type A = more severe) Highest incidence in infants 1-6 mo (peak 2-3 mo) Peak in Jan-Feb Transmission: inoculation of nasopharyngeal or ocular mucous membranes, fomites, direct contact (MC), aerosol droplets Incubation: 4-6 d (range: 2-8 d) MCC of LRTI in children <1 y/o RF: Infants <6 mo (born during first half of RSV season, attend daycare, older siblings), underlying CLD, born before 35 wk gestation, CHD, Down syndrome, immunocompromised, asthma, live at altitude >2500 m, adults with cardiopulmonary disease or COPD	Infants/children: 1. LRTI/bronchiolitis or pneumonia 2. Apnea (20%) 3. Wheezing (20%) 4. Hyponatremia–due to SIADH Adults: URI or tracheobronchitis 1. Wheezing (35%) 2. SOB 3. URI: cough, coryza, rhinorrhea, conjunctivitis General: 1. Rhinorrhea 2. Low-grade fever 3. Mild systemic symptoms 4. Cough 5. Wheezing 6. Dyspnea (severe) Signs: 1. Tachypnea (severe) 2. Wheezing, rales, rhonchi	Clinical DX: 1. CXR: Diffuse interstitial infiltrates to segmental or lobar consolidation 2. Sputum culture or throat swab (PCR) 3. BAL	1. **Supportive care**–Hydration, suctioning of secretions, humidified O_2 • Hand washing, contact precautions • Most recover gradually over 1-2 wk 2. Nebulized **ribavirin** • Nucleoside analog • Reserved for immunocompromised patients with severe illness • Recommended in adults with stem cell transplant • CI: pregnant women Prognosis: 1. Children with Down syndrome at an increased risk for severe RSV Health maintenance: 1. Avoid tobacco or smoke exposure 2. Restrict child care 3. Hand washing 4. Cough hygiene Complications: Sinusitis, AOM

PNEUMONIA (BACTERIAL, VIRAL)

Age Group	Most Common Pathogens and Treatment	Age Group	Most Common Pathogens and Treatment
Neonates (<28 d)	*E. coli*, GBS, **S. aureus**, *Listeria, C. trachomatis*	**2 wk–4 mo**	**C. trachomatis**, *S. pneumoniae*, CMV, *Mycoplasma hominis, Ureaplasma urealyticum*
	Treatment duration: 10-21 d: 1. Amp + Gent or Amp + cefotaxime 2. Blood culture, drain effusion		Treatment duration: 10 d: 1. *Erythromycin, azithromycin, or cefotaxime*
6 W–4 Y LOBAR	**S. pneumoniae**	>4 Y LOBAR	**S. pneumoniae**
	Treatment duration: 7-10 d: 1. *Amoxicillin, clindamycin* 2. Ceftriaxone or cefotaxime		Treatment duration: 7-10 d: 1. *Amoxicillin, clindamycin* 2. Ceftriaxone or cefotaxime AND 3. Macrolide (clarithromycin, azithromycin)
6 W–4 Y ATYPICAL	*B. pertussis*	>4 Y ATYPICAL	Mycoplasma or chlamydia, influenza
	1. Erythromycin × 14 d 2. Azithromycin × 5 d 3. Clarithromycin × 7 d		Treatment duration: 14-21 d: 1. *Clarithromycin, azithromycin, erythromycin, doxycycline* 2. Zanamivir or oseltamivir

- 50% of children <5 years of age with CAP require hospitalization
- Pneumonia is most prevalent during colder months, due to transmission being via droplets worse with indoor crowding
- RF: low economic status, environmental crowding, congenital heart disease, bronchopulmonary dysplasia, cystic fibrosis, asthma, sickle cell disease, neuromuscular disorders, GI disorders (GERD), cigarette smoke exposure
- Prevention: vaccination with Hib and pneumococcal conjugate vaccines

- Children with cystic fibrosis frequently infected with *S. aureus, P. aeruginosa*, and *H. influenzae*
- Children with sickle cell anemia are also at an increased risk of acute chest syndrome with pneumonia pathogens including *S. pneumoniae, S. aureus*, and *H. influenzae*
- No single sign or symptom is pathognomonic for pneumonia in children
- **Tachypnea**—most sensitive and specific sign of radiographically confirmed pneumonia in children (absence rules out pneumonia)

Tachypnea as Defined by the WHO

<2 mo	2-12 mo	12 mo–5 y	>5 ys
>60 breaths/min	>50 breaths/min	>40 breaths/min	>20 breaths/min

- **Walking pneumonia**: a term that describes pneumonia that does not interfere with normal activity

Disease	Etiology, Prevalence, Risk Factors	Clinical Symptoms and Signs	Diagnostics	Therapy, Prognosis, and Health Maintenance

Community acquired pneumonia in children	Typically follows a URI that permits invasion of LRT by other pathogens, triggering an immune response and inflammation
	MCC of bacterial pneumonia in children:
	S. pneumoniae
	Viruses (50%) of cases in young children <5
	MC viral cause in children <5: **RSV** (fomites)
	Transmission:
	Respiratory droplets
		Onset after 1-2 d of flu-like symptoms:
		1. **Cough** +/– sputum production
		2. Dyspnea (SOB)
		  • Apnea (newborns)
		3. **Fever**
		4. **Abdominal pain**, **vomiting**
		5. Anorexia
		Signs:
		1. **Tachypnea** and tachycardia
		2. **Increased work of breathing**
		3. **Retractions, nasal flaring**, grunting
		4. Dullness to percussion, egophony
		5. Bronchial breath sounds
		6. Inspiratory **crackles**, rhonchi, **wheezing**
		7. Increased fremitus, whispered pectoriloquy
		8. Head bobbing
		9. Nuchal rigidity
		10. Fever
		11. **Hypoxemia**
			Clinical DX:
			1. **CXR** (not required): bilateral hilar interstitial infiltrates
			  • Indications: severe disease, low suspicion, history of recurrent PNA, prolonged illness, resistant PNA, fever, and leukocytosis +/– cough
			  • Radiographic findings should not be used alone and lag behind clinical findings
			  • Confirms if compatible clinical findings
			2. WBC: elevated/NL
			  • <15k = nonbacterial
			  • >15k = bacterial
			3. ESR/CRP, serum procalcitonin
			  • Distinguish bacterial from viral causes
			4. Electrolytes–assesses degree of dehydration
			5. Blood cultures and sputum cultures
			  • If admitted
			6. PCR for *S. pneumoniae*, RSV, flu, adenovirus, *M. pneumoniae*, *Chlamydia* spp
				1. See treatment below
				Complications:
				Pleural effusion, empyema, pneumatoceles, necrotizing pneumonia, lung abscess

	Mild Pneumonia	Severe Pneumonia
Capillary refill	Normal	≥2 s
Heart rate	Normal	Tachycardic
Feeding	Normal (infants); No vomiting	Not feeding (infants) or Signs of dehydration (older children)
Mental status	Normal	Altered
O₂ saturation	≥92% in room air	<90% in room air at sea level
Skin color	Normal	Cyanotic
Temperature	<38.5°C (101.3°F)	≥38.5°C (101.3°F)
	Mild or absent respiratory distress: • Increased RR, but less than the age-specific RR that defines moderate-to-severe respiratory distress • Mild or absent retractions • No grunting, nasal flaring, or apnea • Mild SOB	Moderate to severe respiratory distress • RR >70 breaths/min for infants; RR >50 breaths/min for older children • Moderate/severe suprasternal, intercostal, or subcostal retractions (if <12 mo) • Severe difficulty breathing (if ≥12 mo) • Grunting, nasal flaring, or apnea may all be present • Significant SOB

RR, respiratory rate.

Modified from UpToDate: Barson MD. *Community-acquired pneumonia in children: Clinical features and diagnosis*. In: Post TW, ed. *UpToDate*. Waltham, MA: UpToDate Inc. http://www.uptodate.com. Accessed February 2018.

Pediatrics

Admission Indications	ICU Admission Indications
1. Age 3-6 mo or younger 2. Family cannot provide appropriate care or compliance issues, any age 3. Hypoxemia <90% at room air 4. Dehydration, inability to feed 5. Moderate-to-severe respiratory distress 6. Toxic or ill appearance 7. Complications 8. Failure of outpatient therapy: worse or no response after 2-3 d	<u>Two or more of the following:</u> 1. RR > 70 breaths/min (infants <12 mo) and >50 breaths (>12 mo) 2. Apnea, increased WOB (retractions, nasal flaring, grunting, SOB) 3. PaO_2/FiO_2 <250 (NL: 500) 4. Multilobular infiltrates 5. Altered mental status 6. Hypotension 7. Pleural effusion 8. Comorbidities (sickle cell, immunodeficient) 9. Metabolic acidosis 10. Pediatric Early Warning Score >6

Treatment of Community Acquired Pneumonia in Children

Outpatient	Inpatient

1. Supportive therapy
2. Antibiotics as below
  • Neonates: discussed separately
  • 1-6 mo: admit to hospital for empiric therapy
  • 6 mo–5 y: HD amoxicillin 90-100 mg/kg/d in 2-3 divided doses (alt: cefdinir, PCN allergy: clindamycin, macrolide)
	1. Antipyretics, analgesics, respiratory support (supplemental O_2), oral/IV fluids
	2. See *Antibiotic Therapy* below

Antibiotic Therapy for Uncomplicated Pneumonia in Children

Age	Suspected Pathogens	Inpatient Empiric Regimens	Outpatient Empiric Regimens

1-6 mo	Bacterial (nonchlamydia or *S. aureus*)	1. One of the following
		  • Ceftriaxone 50-100 mg/kg/day in 1-2 divided doses
		  • Cefotaxime 150 mg/kg/d in 3-4 divided doses
			1. Hospitalize

	Chlamydia trachomatis	1. Azithromycin 10 mg/kg on days 1-2 of therapy → oral therapy	1. Azithromycin

>6 mo
Up to 5 y (for outpatient)
	Uncomplicated bacterial (not *Mycoplasma* or *Chlamydophila pneumoniae*, or *S. aureus*)	1. One of the following
		  • Ampicillin 150-200 mg/kg/d in 4 divided doses
		  • Penicillin G 200-250 000 units/kg/d in 4-6 divided doses
		  • Cefotaxime 150 mg/kg/d in 3 divided doses
		  • Ceftriaxone 50-100 mg/kg/d in 1-2 divided doses
			1. One of the following:
			  • Amoxicillin 90 mg/kg/d in 2-3 divided doses
			  • Augmentin 90 mg/kg/d in 3 divided doses
			2. Non-type I hypersensitivity
			  • Cefdinir 14 mg/kg/d in 2 doses
			3. Type I hypersensitivity
			  • Levofloxacin 16-20 mg/kg/d in 2 doses
			  • Clindamycin 30-40 mg/kg/d in 3-4 doses
			  • Erythromycin 30-50 mg/kg/d in 4 doses
			  • Azithromycin 10 mg/kg on day 1 → 5 mg/kg/d × 4 d
			  • Clarithromycin 15 mg/kg/d in 2 doses

	Mycoplasma or *Chlamydophila pneumoniae*	1. One of the following
		  • Azithromycin 10 mg/kg once per day × 2 d → oral therapy 5 mg/kg/d
		  • Erythromycin 20 mg/kg/d in 4 divided doses
		  • Levofloxacin 16-20 mg/kg/d in 2 divided doses (6 mo–5 y/o), 8-10 mg/kg/d (5-16 y/o)	

Age	Suspected Pathogens	Inpatient Empiric Regimens	Outpatient Empiric Regimens

>5 y/o	Typical bacteria		1. One of the following:
			  • Amoxicillin 90 mg/kg/d in 2-3 doses
			2. Non-type-I hypersensitivity
			  • Cefdinir 14 mg/kg/d in 2 doses
			3. Type I hypersensitivity
			  • Levofloxacin 8-10 mg/kg/d (5-16 y/o), 750 mg/d (16+)
			  • Clindamycin 30-40 mg/kg/d in 3-4 doses
			  • Erythromycin 40-50 mg/kg/d in 4 doses
			  • Azithromycin 10 mg/kg on day 1 → 5 mg/kg/d × 4 d
			  • Clarithromycin 15 mg/kg/d in 2 doses

	Mycoplasma or *Chlamydophila pneumoniae*		1. One of the following:
			  • Erythromycin 40-50 mg/kg/d in 4 doses
			  • **Azithromycin** 10 mg/kg/d on day 1 → 5 mg/kg/d × 4 d
			  • **Clarithromycin** 15 mg/kg/d in 2 doses
			  • Doxycycline 4 mg/g/d in 2 doses
			    • For children 8+ y/o

Age 18+ y/o	Atypicals		1. One of the following
			  • Levofloxacin 8-10 mg/kg/d (5-16 y/o), 500 mg/d (16+ y/o)
			  • Moxifloxacin 400 mg/d

Aspiration pneumonia			1. One of the following:
			  • Augmentin 40-50 mg/kg/d in 2-3 doses
			  • Type-I hypersensitivity clindamycin 30-40 mg/kg/d in 3-4 doses

Inpatient Empiric Therapy for Various Pneumonias

Severe pneumonia	1. One of the following
	  • Ceftriaxone 100 mg/kg/d in 2 doses
	  • Cefotaxime 150 mg/kg/d in 4 doses
	AND
	2. One of the following
	  • Azithromycin 10 mg/kg/d × 2 days → oral therapy 5 mg/kg/d
	  • Erythromycin 20 mg/kg/d in 4 doses
	  • Doxycycline 4 mg/kg/d in 2 doses
	    • For children 8+

Severe, requiring ICU admission	1. **Vancomycin** 60 mg/kg/d in 4 doses
	AND
	2. One of the following
	  • Ceftriaxone 100 mg/kg/d in 2 doses
	  • Cefotaxime 150 mg/kg/d in 4 doses
	AND
	3. Azithromycin 10 mg/kg/d × 2 d → oral therapy 5 mg/kg/d
	4. If necessary, add nafcillin or antiviral therapy

Nosocomial (hospital acquired)	1. Gentamicin 7.5 mg/kg/d in 3 doses (<5), 6-7.5 mg/kg/d in 3 doses (>5)
	AND
	2. One of the following
	  • Zosyn 300 mg/kg/d in 4 doses
	  • Meropenem 60 mg/kg/d in 3 doses
	  • Ceftazidime 125-150 mg/kg/d in 3 doses
	  • Clindamycin 30-40 mg/kg/d in 3-4 doses

Aspiration pneumonia	1. Ampicillin-sulbactam 150-200 mg/kg/d in 4 doses AND 2. If MRSA suspected, clindamycin 30-40 mg/kg/d in 3-4 doses

Hospital acquired
Gram-negative pathogens
	1. One of the following
	  • Zosyn 300 mg/kg/d in 4 doses
	  • Meropenem 60 mg/kg/d in 3 doses

Pediatrics

Disease	Etiology, Prevalence, Risk Factors	Clinical Symptoms and Signs	Diagnostics	Therapy, Prognosis, and Health Maintenance
Pneumonia in neonates	RF: Prolonged rupture of fetal membranes (>18 h), maternal amnionitis, prematurity, fetal tachycardia, maternal intrapartum fever Pathogens: Group B streptococcus (MC bacteria), *L. monocytogenes, M. tuberculosis* MC virus: HSV	1. Difficulty feeding 2. Restlessness, fussiness 3. Fever 4. Respiratory distress 5. Lethargy 6. Apnea 7. Jaundice 8. Vomiting Signs: 1. Ill-appearance 2. Cyanosis 3. Fever (common, not required) 4. Tachypnea, tachycardia 5. Poor perfusion 6. Abdominal distention	1. CBC—leukocytosis 2. Blood and CSF cultures 3. PCR studies 4. Gram stain and culture of tracheal aspirates 5. CXR (confirms) • Bilateral alveolar densities with air bronchograms • Irregular patchy infiltrates	1. Supplemental O2, mechanical ventilation 2. Empiric Antibiotics • Started until culture results available • For <3 d old: ampicillin and gentamicin • For >3 d old: • Vancomycin and aminoglycoside • Ribavirin—for RSV pneumonia • IV acyclovir for HSV pneumonia
Atypical pneumonia	*Mycoplasma* and *Chlamydophila pneumoniae* Mostly in children >5 These pathogens attach to respiratory epithelial membranes through which they enter cells for replication	Gradual onset: 1. Prodrome: headache, malaise, low grade fever, chills 2. Hacking, nonproductive cough 3. Sore throat 4. Myalgias, arthralgias Extrapulmonary: Hemolysis, skin rash, joint involvement, GI distress, CNS involvement, heart disease Signs: 1. Rales, wheezes 2. Sinus tenderness 3. Erythema of posterior pharynx 4. Erythema or bullae of tympanic membrane 5. Cervical adenopathy	Clinical DX: 1. CXR • Peribronchial pneumonia pattern (thick bronchial shadow, streaks of interstitial infiltration, areas of atelectasis) 2. CBC—neutrophilia 3. ESR—elevated 4. Other tests: PCR, serology, Ag-EIA, Gram stain and culture, cold agglutinins	See treatment above Complications: Pleural effusions (20%)

Clinical and Radiographic Clues to Etiology of Pneumonia

Etiology	Clinical Features	Radiographic Features
Bacteria (MC: *Streptococcus pneumoniae*)	Children of all ages Abrupt onset Ill-appearance Chills Moderate-to-severe respiratory distress Focal auscultatory findings Localized chest pain WBC count >15 000/microL (if obtained) Elevated acute phase reactants (if obtained)	Alveolar infiltrates Segmental consolidation Lobar consolidation "Round" pneumonia Complications: Pleural effusion/empyema Lung abscess Necrotizing pneumonia Pneumatocele
Atypical bacterial (*Mycoplasma pneumoniae, Chlamydophila pneumoniae*)	Children of all ages (most common in children >5 y) Abrupt onset with constitutional findings (malaise, myalgia, headache, rash, conjunctivitis, photophobia, sore throat, headache) Gradually worsening nonproductive cough Wheezing Extrapulmonary manifestations or complications (eg, urticaria, Stevens-Johnson syndrome, hemolytic anemia, hepatitis, pancreatitis, myocarditis, pericarditis)	Interstitial infiltrates

Pediatrics

Etiology	Clinical Features	Radiographic Features
Viral	Usually children <5 y Gradual onset Preceding upper airway symptoms Nontoxic appearing Diffuse, bilateral auscultatory findings Wheezing May have associated rash (eg, measles, varicella)	Interstitial infiltrates
Afebrile pneumonia of infancy (MC: *Chlamydia trachomatis*)	Usually in infants 2 wk–4 mo Insidious onset Rhinorrhea, tachypnea Staccato cough pattern Diffuse inspiratory crackles +/– Conjunctivitis Peripheral eosinophilia (if CBC obtained)	Hyperinflation with interstitial process
Fungal	Appropriate geographic or environmental exposure	Mediastinal or hilar adenopathy
Mycobacterium tuberculosis	Children of any age Chronic cough Constitutional symptoms Exposure history	Mediastinal or hilar adenopathy

FOREIGN BODY (ASPIRATION) (FIG. 27-3)

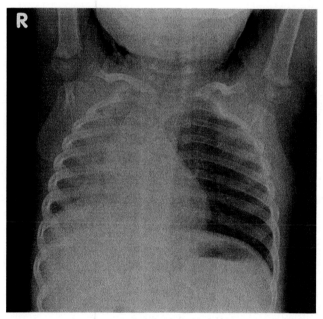

FIGURE 27-3. A 2-year-old child with respiratory distress after choking on a peanut. Chest x-ray shows hyperinflation of the left lung, tracheal deviation, and mediastinal shift, atelectasis of the right lung (air trapping) secondary to foreign body aspration. (From Fleisher GR, Ludwig S. *Textbook of Pediatric Emergency Medicine.* Philadelphia: Wolters Kluwer Health; 2011.)

Disease	Etiology, Prevalence, Risk Factors	Clinical Symptoms and Signs	Diagnostics	Therapy, Prognosis, and Health Maintenance
Foreign body aspiration	6 mo–4 y HX: playing with small toys Nasal: "seeds and beads" (nasal foreign body); MCC of halitosis	1. Acute (sudden onset) choking or coughing episode 2. Rhinorrhea 3. Bleeding 4. Halitosis, foul smell Signs: 1. Expiratory wheeze, **unilateral** 2. Asymmetrical decreased breath sounds, localized wheeze	1. AP expiratory XR: tracheal deviation and mediastinal shift AWAY from affected side, **hyperinflation, and air trapping** in affected lung	1. EMERGENT Rigid bronchoscopy

HYALINE MEMBRANE DISEASE

Disease	Etiology, Prevalence, Risk Factors	Clinical Symptoms and Signs	Diagnostics	Therapy, Prognosis, and Health Maintenance
Hyaline membrane disease (respiratory distress syndrome)	Deficiency of surfactant: decreased production and secretion Peak: **48-72 h after delivery** Most common cause of respiratory distress in PREMATURE INFANT	1. **SOB (dyspnea)** 2. Expiratory grunt Signs: 1. **Cyanosis** and poor response to oxygen 2. Poor breath sounds 3. Decreased pulses 4. Tachypnea 5. Nasal flaring 6. Retractions: suprasternal, subxiphoid, intercostal, subcostal	1. CXR (nonspecific): diffuse **reticular granularity, air bronchograms**, bell-shaped thorax, diffuse bilateral atelectasis (ground glass appearance) 2. ABG: low O_2, high CO_2	1. Mechanical ventilation, O_2 2. **Tracheal surfactant** admin 3. Supportive care, maternal steroids (prophy) 4. Complications pneumothorax, interstitial emphysema, pulmonary hemorrhage, BPD, subglottic stenosis
Sudden infant death syndrome (SIDS)	Leading cause of death 1 mo–1 y Peak: 2-4 mo, males RF: Low birth weight, premature, multiple births, siblings with SIDS, recent infection Maternal RF: smoking, drug use, poor prenatal care, low education level, single mom, multiparous, young (<20)	Unexplained or unexpected death of infant <1 y: 1. Sleeping on soft mattress 2. Over bundling 3. Bed sharing	Clinical DX	1. Back to sleep 2. Firm mattress, keep head uncovered 3. Sleep in room with caregiver until 6 mo 4. Good prenatal care and nutrition

CYSTIC FIBROSIS

Disease	Etiology, Prevalence, Risk Factors	Clinical Symptoms and Signs	Diagnostics	Therapy, Prognosis, and Health Maintenance
Cystic fibrosis	Defective gene on chromosome 7, which codes for CFTR Abnormal transport across epithelial cells of exocrine glands in respiratory tract and pancreas MC mutation: Delta F580 Autosomal **recessive** First 3 mo: *H. Flu* or *S. Pneumo* Young child (>3 mo): **Pseudomonas** 1:3000-1:4000, Caucasians Most common lethal genetic disorder	Infant: 1. Meconium ileus 2. Prolonged jaundice 3. **Recurrent respiratory infections** 4. Malabsorption, steatorrhea 5. **FTT** (50% present) Young child: 1. Persistent loose 2. Cough, sputum production, dyspnea 3. Coarse breath sounds, wheezing 4. **Steatorrhea, diarrhea, abdominal pain** Complications: rectal prolapse (intestinal obstruction), nasal polyps, sinusitis, **infection, terminal respiratory failure (cor pulmonale)**	1. Trypsinogen test–screening 2. **Sweat test** (definitive) • Abnormal if above 60, 2+ tests on separate days required 3. CXR: hyperinflation 4. Spirometry (FEV1): decreased	1. Enema +/– surgery 2. High calorie diet, fat vitamins, oral pancreatic enzymes 3. Daily exercise 4. Bronchodilator 5. Mucolytics 6. Antibiotic: tobramycin, dornase (pulmozyme), hypertonic saline 7. Prophy: **Palivizumab** (Synagis)

28

Infectious Disease

Refer to Internal Medicine 🩺 for in-depth coverage of the following topics:

Epstein-Barr Disease, see Mononucleosis, p 271
Herpes Simplex, p 271
Influenza, p 272

Refer to Family Medicine 👪 for in-depth coverage of the following topics:

Erythema Infectiosum, see Dermatology for Family Medicine, p 154
Mumps, see Mumps Parotitis on ENOT/Ophthalmology for Family Medicine, p 101

Roseola, Rubella, and Measles, see Dermatology for Family Medicine, p 154

Recommended Supplemental Resources:

Pertussis, see below, p 315
Trichuriasis (Whipworm), see below, p 314
Lyme Disease and Rocky Mountain Spotted Fever 🩺, p 268
Gingivostomatitis, see below, p 317
Onychomycosis, see below, p 317

ATYPICAL MYCOBACTERIAL DISEASE

Disease	Etiology, Prevalence, Risk Factors	Clinical Symptoms and Signs	Diagnostics	Therapy, Prognosis, and Health Maintenance
Atypical mycobacterial disease	*Mycobacterium avium* complex (MAC), *M. fortuitum* complex, *M. kansassi* No airborne contact, noncontagious MAC survives in vacuole and uses macrophage as launch pad for infection	Indolent or subacute course: 1. Most common SX: **fever** 2. Cough 3. SOB 4. Fatigue 5. Weight loss 6. Hemoptysis	Runyon criteria: 1. Nonchromogens (MAC): produce no pigment, rapid growers; produce visible growth on standard agar in 1 wk, which usually takes 2 2. Ziehl-Neelsen: AFB (+) 3. PPD: (+) or (−) 4. AFB smear and culture	In AIDS patients, affects bone marrow and blood stream, rather than lung → 1. *Clarithromycin, azithromycin* 2. Rifampin and **rifabutin** 3. Ethambutol

PINWORMS

- Two most common nematode infections worldwide

Pinworms (enterobiasis)	Transmission: Fecal-oral Humans are ONLY natural host RF: Close living quarters, crowding MC: Children 5–10 Occurs in both temperate and tropical climates MC helminthic infection in the US Pathogen: Enterobius vermicularis	1. MC: Perianal pruritus at night (pruritus ani) 2. Abdominal pain 3. Nausea, vomiting	1. Pinworm paddle test—place cellophane tape on anus and microscopically examine for ova • Performed at night or first thing in the morning, prior to bath • Eggs "bean shaped"	1. One of the following: • Albendazole 400 mg, repeat in 2 wk • 100 mg **mebendazole**, repeat in 2 wk • Pyrantel pamoate 11 mg/kg, max 1 g • AE: anorexia, nausea, vomiting, cramps, diarrhea, neurotoxic effects, increased LFTs • Okay for pregnant women, with significant symptoms only Health maintenance: 1. Treat entire family at once, wash bedding and clothes, clip fingernails, hand hygiene Prognosis: 1. Reinfection common Complications: Secondary bacterial infections
Trichuriasis (whipworm)	*Trichuris trichiura* MC in tropical climates RF: Poor hygiene Transmission: Via food or hands contaminated with soil	Most asymptomatic: 1. Loose stool +/– mucous or blood 2. Nocturnal stooling Signs: 1. Pica 2. Finger clubbing Associated: Secondary anemia, colitis, rectal prolapse	1. Stool examination for eggs • "Barrel shape" with smooth thick walls and hyaline plug at ends 2. Proctoscopy or colonoscopy: worms protruding from bowel 3. PCR	1. One of the following: • Mebendazole 100 mg PO × 3 d • Albendazole 400 mg PO × 3 d • Avoid both in first trimester of pregnancy Health maintenance: 1. Adequate disposal of feces, good sanitation, good hygiene, wash vegetables and fruits Prognosis: 1. Reinfection common

VARICELLA INFECTION

Disease	Etiology, Prevalence, Risk Factors	Clinical Symptoms and Signs	Diagnostics	Therapy, Prognosis, and Health Maintenance
Varicella (chickenpox)	Incubation: 14 d	1. Fever 2. Rash on face/scalp → trunk/extremities Signs 1. Papules and vesicles, crusts "dew drop on a rose petal"	1. Tzanck smear to confirm herpes simplex, varicella, and zoster infections	1. Valacyclovir (Valtrex)—decreases incidence of varicella pneumonia

HAND-FOOT-AND-MOUTH DISEASE

Disease	Etiology, Prevalence, Risk Factors	Clinical Symptoms and Signs	Diagnostics	Therapy, Prognosis, and Health Maintenance
Hand-foot-and-mouth disease **(herpangina)**	Coxsackie virus group A type 16	1. Low fever (38°C–39°C) for 24-48 h 2. *Sore mouth or throat* 3. Fatigue, **malaise** 4. URI +/– *abdominal pain* Signs: 1. Dehydration 2. Petechiae 3. Vesicular or papular lesions on mouth, palms and soles that become shallow ulcers in 3 d • Can also involve buttocks, genitalia	Clinical diagnosis	1. Adequate fluid intake (cold liquids) • Avoid spicy or acidic substances 2. Ibuprofen (Motrin) 3. Magic mouthwash Prognosis 1. Virus clears in 10 d

PERTUSSIS

Disease	Etiology, Prevalence, Risk Factors	Clinical Symptoms and Signs	Diagnostics	Therapy, Prognosis, and Health Maintenance
Pertussis (whooping cough), also known as "the cough of 100 d"	***Bordetella pertussis***: Gram-negative coccobacillus Highly contagious during catarrhal stage, transmitted via respiratory droplets Incubation period: 7-10 d More than 50% of cases occur in adolescents and adults—**serve as reservoir for infection of infants and children**	1. Catarrhal stage (1-2 wk) • Insidious onset of sneezing • Rhinorrhea • Loss of appetite • Malaise • **Hacking cough at night** (most infectious state) Signs: Gagging, cyanosis, increased work of breathing, sweating 1. Paroxysmal stage (2-8 wk) • Spasms of rapid **coughing fits** during expiration followed by • **Deep, high-pitched inspiratory** (whoop), last several minutes • Posttussive emesis or syncope 2. Convalescent stage: • Decrease in frequency and severity of paroxysms • Begins 4 wk after onset of cough and lasts for several weeks	1. Diagnostic testing • Most accurate during Catarrhal phase • Diagnosis is mostly clinical (cough 2+ wk required) • Microbiological testing required to confirm 2. **Culture and PCR assays** - if cough for 2-4 wk • Culture (gold standard) • Must use Dacron (polyester) or calcium alginate swab to obtain from posterior nasopharynx 3. Serology—alternative to culture, for cough after 4+ wk (best test) 4. WBC count: elevated, lymphocytosis	Antibiotics during catarrhal phase • Decreases severity and duration of cough • Indicated for cough <3 wk or 6 wk for pregnant women, health care workers, or child care workers 1. **Macrolides**—treat close contacts prophylactically • **Azithromycin or clarithromycin** • Erythromycin 2. Macrolide intolerant: • **Bactrim DS** BID × 14 d • Ampicillin Prophylaxis: • Single Tdap booster recommended for adults 19-64 y/o • Postexposure prophylaxis for close contacts, especially infants with chronic lung disease or immunocompromised Complications: Infection (pneumonia, otitis media), subconjunctival hemorrhage, abdominal wall hernia, rib fracture, urinary incontinence, lumbar strain Prognosis: 1. Morbidity and mortality highest in infants and young children

(continued)

Pediatrics

(continued)

Disease	Etiology, Prevalence, Risk Factors	Clinical Symptoms and Signs	Diagnostics	Therapy, Prognosis, and Health Maintenance
Pertussis in infants and children	<4 mo of age Often has a close contact with prolonged cough and no fever Known triggers for cough: exercise, cold temperatures, nasopharyngeal suctioning Pathogen: *B. pertussis* Close contacts: 1. Living in same household 2. Face-to-face exposure within 3 ft 3. Direct contact with respiratory, oral, or nasal secretions of affected patient 4. Sharing same confined space with patient for >1 h High risk individuals: 1. Infants <1 y (<4 mo, highest risk) 2. Pregnant women 3. Immunodeficient 4. Chronic lung diseases, cystic fibrosis 5. Contact with infants	1. Catarrhal stage (short or absent) • Insidious onset of sneezing • Absent fever • Watery coryza • **Mild cough** 2. *Paroxysmal stage (2-8 wk)* • Gagging • Gasping • Vomiting Signs: 1. Cyanosis 2. Bradycardia 3. Eye bulging	1. DX Testing: • Most accurate during Catarrhal phase • Diagnosis is mostly clinical (cough 2+ wk required) • Microbiological testing required to confirm 2. **Culture and PCR assays** - if cough for 2-4 wk • Culture (gold standard) • Must use Dacron (polyester) or calcium alginate swab to obtain from posterior nasopharynx 3. Serology–alternative to culture, for cough after 4+ wk (best test) 4. WBC count: elevated, lymphocytosis	1. Supportive care (mainstay) • Bronchodilators, steroids, antihistamines, or anti-tussive agents are ineffective 2. Antibiotics for (+) cultures or PCR within 3 wk of cough onset, or infants <6 mo • Treat infants <21 d regardless of labs • See therapy below Health maintenance: 1. No school until 5 d of therapy has been completed, or if untreated, 21 d after onset of cough Indications for hospitalization: 1. Respiratory distress 2. Evidence of pneumonia 3. Inability to feed 4. Cyanosis or apnea 5. Seizures 6. Age <4 mo • Standard and droplet precautions × 5 d after therapy initiated • Monitor fluid and nutritional status • IV fluids or NG feeds Prophylaxis: 1. Recommended for all close contacts and household contacts in individuals at high risk for severe or complicated pertussis, even if immunized • Best in first 21 d of onset of cough • DTap immunization Complications: Apnea, seizures, respiratory distress, pneumonia, pulmonary hypertension, shock, renal failure, death

Pertussis Therapy Based on Age

Infants <1 mo	Infants + Children >1 mo	Children >2 mo
1. Azithromycin (first line) 10 mg/kg/d, single dose × 5 d 2. Erythromycin • Both associated with an increased risk of hypertrophic pyloric stenosis	1. Azithromycin 10 mg/kg/d × 5 d, single dose 2. Clarithromycin 15 mg/kg/d × 7 d, divided in 2 doses	1. Macrolides 2. Macrolide alternative: Bactrim • TMP 8 mg/kg/d, SMX 40 mg/kg/d divided in 2, for 14 d • Not for children <2 mo: risk of kernicterus

GINGIVOSTOMATITIS

- After the initial infection, herpes virus travels to the terminal ganglion where it is latent unless reactivation occurs. This can be induced by sun exposure, trauma, stress, cold air, or immunosuppression

- Magic mouthwash: consists of diphenhydramine, magnesia-alumina (Maalox), kaolin pectin (Kaopectate), and/or viscous lidocaine

Disease	Etiology, Prevalence, Risk Factors	Clinical Symptoms and Signs	Diagnostics	Therapy, Prognosis, and Health Maintenance
Herpes simplex stomatitis	MC manifestation of primary HSV infection in childhood Ulcerative lesions on gingiva and mucous membranes of mouth with perioral vesicular lesions MCC: HSV-1 Mainly children 6 mo–5 y but can occur anytime Transmission: direct contact with infected oral secretions or lesions (symptomatic or asymptomatic individuals with primary or recurrent HSV) Shedding occurs × 1 wk Incubation: 2 d–3 wk (mean: 4 d)	1. Prodrome: 4 d • Fever (>100.4°F) • Anorexia • Irritability • Malaise • Sleeplessness • Headache 2. Painful lesions in oral cavity or perioral area Signs: 1. Red, edematous marginal gingivae that bleed easily 2. Clusters of small vesicles • Turn yellow after they rupture • Red halo • Coalesce to form large, painful ulcers • Involve buccal mucosa, tongue, gingiva, hard palate, pharynx Associated: Halitosis, refusal to drink, anorexia, fever, arthralgia, headache, submandibular or cervical LAD	**Clinical DX:** 1. Viral culture, serology, immunofluorescence, or PCR (confirms) 2. Tzanck smear • Limited use, only good for active lesions • Cannot distinguish between HSV1 or 2	1. Supportive care • Fluid intake • Oral rinses • Tylenol or ibuprofen • Magic mouthwash not routinely recommended 2. Topical therapy • Barrier cream (petroleum jelly) on lips 3. PO Acyclovir • Immunocompetent who present within 3-4 d of onset, unable to drink, or significant pain • 15 mg/kg/d × 5-7 d • AE: nausea/vomiting, diarrhea, headaches, renal failure 4. Antibiotics if underlying bacterial infection 5. Amoxicillin or clindamycin Prognosis: 1. Mild lesions heal in 1 wk (but may take 2-3 ws if severe) Complication: Dehydration (MC), herpetic whitlow or keratitis, secondary bacteremia, esophagitis, epiglottitis, pneumonitis, HSV encephalitis, eczema herpeticum, lip adhesions

- Indications for admission:
  - Unable to maintain adequate hydration
  - Immunocompromised
  - Eczema herpeticum
  - Encephalitis, epiglottitis pneumonitis

- Prevention
  - Avoid child care or school if oral secretions not controlled
  - Contact precautions if admitted

ONYCHOMYCOSIS

Disease	Etiology, Prevalence, Risk Factors	Clinical Symptoms and Signs	Diagnostics	Therapy, Prognosis, and Health Maintenance
Tinea unguium (onychomycosis)	MC: *T. rubrum* Infection of the finger or toenails Subset of onychomycosis RF: Associated tinea pedis, improperly fitting shoes, diabetes		Recommended nail scraping for KOH microscopy +/– culture	1. Topical antifungals (**terbinafine**) 2. Oral antifungals—if severe

CHAPTER 29

Cardiovascular

Refer to Family Medicine 👥 **for in-depth coverage of the following topics:**

Acute Rheumatic Fever, see Cardiology, p 208
Infective Endocarditis, see Cardiology for Family Medicine, p 5

Refer to Emergency Medicine ✴ **for in-depth coverage of the following topics:**

Syncope, p 372

Refer to Appendices for the following topics:

Heart Murmurs, including Atrial Septal Defect, Coarctation of the Aorta, Patent Ductus Arteriosus, Tetralogy of Fallot, Ventricular Septal Defect, Hypertrophic Cardiomyopathy, Functional and Innocent Murmurs, Mitral Regurgitation, Bicuspid Aortic Valve, Functional Murmur, Innocent Murmur, Physiologic Murmur, p 665 (Fig. 29-1)

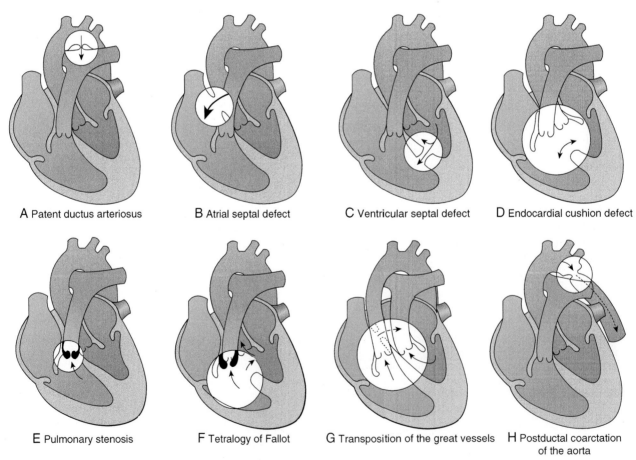

A Patent ductus arteriosus   B Atrial septal defect   C Ventricular septal defect   D Endocardial cushion defect

E Pulmonary stenosis   F Tetralogy of Fallot   G Transposition of the great vessels   H Postductal coarctation of the aorta

FIGURE 29-1. Congenital heart disorders. (From Porth C. *Essentials of Pathophysiology.* Philadelphia: Wolters Kluwer Health; 2015.)

Pediatrics

KAWASAKI DISEASE (FIG. 29-2A-E)

Disease	Etiology, Prevalence, Risk Factors	Clinical Symptoms and Signs	Diagnostics	Therapy, Prognosis, and Health Maintenance
Kawasaki disease	Primarily in children 6 mo–4 y Unknown etiology Vasculitis → aneurysms	1. **Fever >5 d** + any 2. 4 of the following: • Bilateral conjunctivitis • Red mucous membranes (red, cracked lips) • Swelling of hands/feet with red palms and soles • Transverse grooves on nails • Polymorphous rash • Cervical nodes >1.5 cm <u>Signs:</u> 1. Strawberry tongue 2. Red lips 3. Injected throat 4. Conjunctivitis 5. Peeling rash–fingers and toes	1. CBC: Anemia, WBC <15k, platelet >450k 2. Albumin <3 3. Increased AST 4. Urine >10 WBC/HPF 5. ASO titer and strep = negative 6. Echocardiogram	1. **Aspirin** for thrombosis prophylaxis 2. Immune globulin (IVIG) in first 10 d 3. Plasmapheresis 4. Corticosteroids <u>Complications</u> 1. **Coronary artery aneurysms** 2. **Polymorphous exanthema** 3. Arteritis

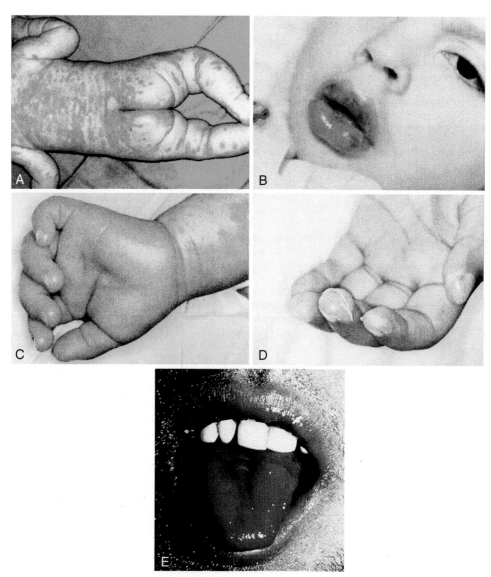

FIGURE 29-2. Manifestations of Kawasaki disease. **A**, Rash of Kawasaki disease in a 7-month-old child on the fourth day of illness; **B**, conjunctival injection, lip edema in a 2-year-old boy on the sixth day of illness; **C**, erythema and edematous hand of a 1.5-year-old girl on the sixth day of illness; **D**, periungual desquamation in a 3-year-old child on the 12th day of illness; **E**, strawberry tongue. (From Coombs C, Kirk AS. *Oski's Pediatric Certification and Recertification Board Review.* Philadelphia: Wolters Kluwer Health; 2011.)

CHAPTER **30**

Gastrointestinal

Refer to Family Medicine 🩺 for in-depth coverage of the following topics:

Gastroenteritis, p 42
Gastroesophageal Reflux Disease, p 60
Constipation, p 62
Hepatitis, p 63
Jaundice, p 52
Anal Fissure, p 35

Inguinal Hernia, see Urology and Renal for Family Medicine, p 173

Supplemental Recommend Reading:

Liver Function Tests, p 34 🩺
Volvulus, p 48 🩺
Foreign Body Ingestion, see Pulmonology for Pediatrics, p 21

GASTROENTERITIS AND DEHYDRATION

- **Norovirus:** MCC of gastroenteritis in patients >2 years old

Disease	Etiology, Prevalence, Risk Factors	Clinical Symptoms and Signs	Diagnostics	Therapy, Prognosis, and Health Maintenance
Rotavirus	3-15 mo of age Winter <u>Transmission:</u> Fecal, oral <u>Incubation:</u> 1-3 d **Most common cause of gastroenteritis in children <2 y/o**	1. **Vomiting** 2. Diarrhea (watery, non-bloody, nonmucous) lasting 4-8 d 3. Low-grade fever 4. Nasal symptoms + coryza precede GI symptoms <u>Signs:</u> 1. Metabolic acidosis form bicarbonate loss in stool 2. Ketosis from poor intake 3. Lactic academia from hypotension/perfusion	1. Hypo-or hypernatremia with dehydration 2. PCR of stool	1. Supportive care • Pedialyte 2. Reduced fat intake to decrease N/V 3. Antidiarrheal ineffective <u>Health Maintenance:</u> 1. Vaccinate: 2, 4, 6 mo
Dehydration or hypovolemia Loss of plasma free water compared to loss of electrolytes	<u>RF:</u> Higher incidence with gastroenteritis (vomiting, diarrhea), fever, burns, young children unable to communicate needs <u>Etiology:</u> Large number wet diapers, vomiting, bleeding, oliguria/anuria, diarrhea, sick contacts, diuretic therapy, diabetes insipidus, glycosuria, fever, burns Volume depletion is measured by change in weight from baseline	1. HX: increased thirst, decreased UOP 2. Lethargy 3. Irritable <u>Signs:</u> 1. Volume depletion - change from baseline weight (2 kg = 2 L) 2. Increased pulse or respirations 3. Low blood pressure 4. Decreased skin turgor 5. Delayed capillary refill See Dehydration Table below	1. Hypernatremia 2. HCO_3 <17 mEq/L indicates moderate to severe hypovolemia or metabolic acidosis 3. Urine sodium <25 mEq/L and Osmolality >450 mosmol/kg indicates hypovolemia 4. Severe: BMP, VBG, lactic acid, CBC, glucose, HCO_3	1. Maintenance fluids • See later

Pediatrics

Signs and Symptoms of Dehydration

Dehydration	Pulse	Systolic Pressure	Respirations	Buccal Mucosa	Anterior Fontanelle, Eyes	Skin Turgor	Urine Output	Systemic
Mild 3%-5%	Full, NL	NL	NL	Tacky, slightly dry	NL	NL	NL	Inc. thirst
Moderate 6%-9%	Rapid	NL-low	Deep, +/− tachy	Dry	Sunken	Reduced, cool	Markedly reduced	Listless, irritable
Severe >10%	Rapid and weak, or absent	LOW	Deep, tachy or dec-absent	Parched	Markedly sunken	**Cool, tenting, mottled**, cyanosis Increased capillary refill >3 s	Anuria	Grunting, **lethargy**, coma

Calculation of Repletion Fluids

- Replaces any current existing water and electrolyte deficits, replaces any ongoing abnormal losses; returns patient to normal volume and electrolyte status

Mild 3-5%	1. Oral rehydration therapy (ORT) • Mild: 50 mL/kg over 4 h • Moderate: 100 mL/kg over 4 h + maintenance fluids
Moderate 6%-9%	2. No bowel rest, resume feeding all ages 3. 10 mL/kg ORT for each stool
Severe >10%	1. **Rapid IV 20 mL/kg** isotonic saline only, repeat PRN • Reassess during and after saline bolus • Isotonic saline: 0.9% saline or NSS 2. Oral rehydration therapy (ORT) 3. Rate of elevation (hypernatremia): NOT to exceed 12 mEq/L over 24 h → can cause osmotic demyelination if inc. too quick

Calculation of Daily Maintenance Fluids

- Maintenance fluids replace expected ongoing losses of water and electrolytes from normal physiologic processes and maintains normal volume and electrolyte status

Weight (kg)	mL/kg	Plus Additional mL
3.5-10	100	0
11-20	50 (for every kg over 10)	1000
>20	20 (for every kg over 20)	1500

- Divide daily volume by 24 to calculate fluid rate
- Maximum 2400 mL daily
- Does not apply to newborn infants (0-28 days)
- Or use **Holliday-Segar (4-2-1) Method:** 4 mL/kg per hour first 10 kg, 2 mL/kg per hour next 10 kg, then 1 mL/kg

APPENDICITIS

- **McBurney point:** approximately one-third of the distance along a line from the anterior superior iliac spine to the umbilicus (most sensitive sign of acute appendicitis)
- Early appendicitis: appendicitis without evidence of perforation or gangrene

Pediatrics

Disease	Etiology, Prevalence, Risk Factors	Clinical Symptoms and Signs	Diagnostics	Therapy, Prognosis, and Health Maintenance
Neonates (0-30 d)	Rare Attributed to anatomic differences, soft diet, infrequent diarrheal illness, and recumbent positioning	1. **Abdominal distention <48 h** 2. **Vomiting** 3. **Decreased feeding** 4. Fever 5. Lethargy or irritability 6. Hematochezia Signs: 1. Abdominal tenderness 2. Abdominal wall cellulitis 3. Respiratory distress 4. Abdominal mass	Clinical DX: 1. WBC count: >18k • Nonspecific 2. ANC: elevated • Nonspecific 3. CRP: elevated • More sensitive for symptoms 24-48 h 4. Urinalysis • R/o UTI or nephrolithiasis 5. Urine B-hCG in postmenarchal females Imaging: 1. Ultrasound • For patients with atypical or equivocal clinical findings • NL appendix must be seen to r/o appendicitis 2. Contrast enhanced CT scan 3. MRI with or without contrast • Just as accurate as CT 4. Abdominal x-ray • Confirms bowel obstruction or perforation	1. **Laparoscopic appendectomy** • Complications: infection, paralytic ileus 2. Single prophylactic dose of **broad spectrum ABX** • 30-60 min prior to incision • **Cefoxitin** • **Ceftriaxone and Flagyl** • Cefotetan • Gentamicin + Clindamycin or Flagyl • Zosyn 3. **IV fluids** • Correct electrolyte abnormalities prior to surgery • 20 mL/kg bolus of isotonic crystalloid • 0.45% NS + 10-20 mEq/L KCl at 1-1.5 maintenance doses 4. **IV analgesics**: opioids or ketorolac (Toradol) Nonoperative treatment (NOT) • For abdominal pain <48 h, WBC <18k, normal CRP, minimal concern for rupture • 1-2 d of IV ABX • Zosyn • Ceftriaxone • Flagyl • Ciprofloxacin and Flagyl Prognosis: 1. Mortality: 28% Complications: Bowel perforation, bowel obstruction, **sepsis**
Young children <5 y	Uncommon Rule out intussusception, acute gastroenteritis	1. **Abdominal pain** 2. **Fever** 3. **Vomiting** 4. Anorexia 5. Abdominal distention 6. Diarrhea: low volume, frequent, +/– mucus Signs: 1. Fever 2. **Diffuse > localized abdominal tenderness** • Localized RLQ tenderness (50%) 3. Rebound or guarding 4. Grunting respirations 5. Irritability 6. Difficulty or refusal to ambulate		
School age (5-12 y)	More frequent in this age group compared to younger children Typical periumbilical pain migrating to RLQ may not occur	1. **Abdominal pain over RLQ** 2. **Difficulty walking** 3. **Nausea** 4. **Anorexia** 5. Vomiting 6. Fever 7. Diarrhea Signs: 1. RLQ tenderness 2. Guarding or rebound • Indicates perforation 3. Pain with percussion, hopping or coughing		
Adolescents and adults	Most common 15-30 y/o High incidence in childhood, especially <2 y/o Rule out: Mittelschmerz, ovarian cysts, ectopic pregnancy, pelvic inflammatory disease	1. **Fever** 2. Period of **anorexia** 3. **Periumbilical pain** shifting to RLQ • Onset before vomiting (sensitive) 4. **Nausea, vomiting** followed by low fever 5. Diarrhea (nonbloody and no mucous), infrequent Signs: 1. (+) Peritoneal signs **McBurney point** tenderness, rigidity—most sensitive 2. Rebound, guarding • Seen with perforation 3. Psoas sign—more specific 4. Obturator sign—more specific	1. **CBC: leukocytosis** 2. U/A: Pyuria 3. Fecal leukocytes 4. (+) guaiac stool sometimes present 5. **CRP: elevated** 6. Ultrasound: noncompressible, thick appendix or localized fluid	1. IV Hydration, correction of electrolyte abnormalities 2. Preoperative ABX • 60 min prior to incision • Single dose of IV • **Cefoxitin** 1-2 g • Unasyn 3 g • **Cefazolin 2-3 g + Flagyl 500 mg** • PCN allergy: **Clindamycin + FQ**, gentamicin or aztreonam 3. Laparoscopic appendectomy (gold standard) • Postoperative ABX are not necessary Perforated appendix: 1. Postop antibiotics (a) Zosyn • 3rd gen cephalosporin + Flagyl • FQ + Flagyl MC Complications: Infection (abscess or wound)

GASTROESOPHAGEAL REFLUX DISEASE

- Gastroesophageal reflux (GER) is a normal physiologic process that occurs in healthy individuals

- Gastroesophageal reflux disorder (GERD) occurs when reflux is associated with complications like esophagitis, poor weight gain or respiratory complications

Disease	Etiology, Prevalence, Risk Factors	Clinical Symptoms and Signs	Diagnostics	Therapy, Prognosis, and Health Maintenance

Gastroesophageal reflux (GER)	Weak LES
	Well nourished "happy spitter"
	Rule out torticollis or seizures
	MC around 4 mo of age
		1. Frequent **regurgitation**
		2. Good weight gain
		3. Feeds well
		4. Not usually irritable
		5. Nasal congestion or difficulty sleeping while supine
		Signs:
		1. Cyanosis
		2. Apnea
		3. Burping
		4. Reswallowing
		Sandifer syndrome:
		1. Arching of the back, torsion of the neck, chin lifting
		2. Screaming/fussy (2-6 h)
		3. Spitting up, choking
			<u>Clinical DX—no lab testing required:</u>
			1. Esophageal pH monitoring
			  • Rarely useful
			2. Upper GI series—r/o anatomic abnormalities
			3. Endoscopy
			  • For infants who do not respond to empiric clinical trials or suspected dietary protein intolerance
				1. **Lifestyle changes**
				  • Change to hypoallergenic formula
				  • Consider introducing a milk-free/soy-free diet and eliminate beef from mother's diet if breastfeeding
				  • Smaller, more frequent feedings
				  • Concentrate the formula
				  • Thicken feeds
				  • Keep infant upright (on shoulder) for 20-30 min after feeding
				  • 2-wk trial of acid suppression therapy
				  • Burp infants more frequently, after each ounce
				  • Avoid exposure to tobacco smoke
				2. **Acid suppression**
				  • Not useful in children <1 y/o with uncomplicated GER
				  • 2-wk trial for infants with: mild esophagitis on endoscopic biopsy, infants who have failed conservative measures with significant symptoms
				    • PPI preferred
				    • H2 receptor antagonist
				Prognosis
				1. **Resolves between 9 and 12 mo of age**, can continue up to 18-24 mo
				  • No intervention if gaining weight/thriving
				Complications: strictures, Barrett's esophagus

GERD in preschool age children	Prevalence: 1.8%-8.2%	1. Intermittent regurgitation
		  • Usually past the age of 2
		2. Decreased PO intake
		3. Poor weight gain
		4. Food aversion, especially solids
		5. Dysphagia
		6. Severe or progressive asthma unresponsive to therapies
		7. Recurrent pneumonia
		8. Chronic hoarseness or stridor
		Sandifer syndrome—also appears in this population, in developing or delayed children
			Clinical Diagnosis
			1. Empiric treatment with acid suppression → persistence of symptoms →
			2. Upper endoscopy with biopsy, especially if (+) dysphagia or odynophagia
			  • Rule out esophagitis
			3. pH monitoring or multichannel intraluminal impedance (MII) monitoring
			  • Only useful for particular situations
			4. Barium contrast radiography
			  • Used to exclude anatomic abnormalities
			5. Barium esophagram, for children with dysphagia to r/o motility disorders
				1. Lifestyle changes
				2. Acid suppression therapy × 2-4 wk
				  • PPI
				  • H2 receptor antagonists
				    • Short-term relief
				3. Prokinetic agents
				4. Refer to gastroenterology for alarm symptoms: dysphagia, weight loss, hematemesis, recurrent vomiting

Pediatrics

(continued)

(continued)

Disease	Etiology, Prevalence, Risk Factors	Clinical Symptoms and Signs	Diagnostics	Therapy, Prognosis, and Health Maintenance
Gastroesophageal reflux disorder (GERD) in school age children and adolescents (mimics adults)	Children with neurogenic impairment (cerebral palsy, muscular dystrophy), Down syndrome, obesity, or cystic fibrosis at increased risk	1. **Heartburn, dyspepsia**–retrosternal pain, burning shortly after eating, worse with lying down after meals, *mimics cardiac chest pain* 2. **Regurgitation** • Waterbrash (reflex salivary hypersecretion) 3. **Cough**–due to aspiration of refluxed material 4. **Hoarseness, sore throat**, feeling a lump in the throat • Early satiety, postprandial nausea, vomiting 5. Poor weight gain, esophagitis **Warning signs:** hematemesis, hematochezia, onset **after** 6 mo of age, pneumonia, FTT	1. Upper GI series (**barium contrast study**): identifies complications or r/o malignancy, but does not DX → FIRST LINE • Indications: patients with persistent symptoms, GERD with complications, alarm symptoms (dysphagia, odynophagia, weight loss, bleeding), suspicion of malignancy, new onset GERD in >50 y/o 2. **Endoscopy (EGD)** with biopsy: if refractory to TX, dysphagia, odynophagia, GI bleed, persistent nausea/vomiting, heartburn and chronic acid reflux, persistent dyspepsia >45, unexplained anemia, IBD → CONFIRMATORY 3. **24-h pH monitor** (gold standard) • Indications: persistent cases after lifestyle modifications or pharmacologic therapy are attempted and definitive diagnosis needed 4. Impedance-pH monitoring: determines the frequency of reflux episodes and relationship of reflux episodes and symptoms 5. Manometry (if motility d/o suspected)	1. **Phase I: Diet changes**– avoid spicy or fatty food, orange juice, coffee, ETOH, chocolate, large meals before bed; elevation of head of bed and avoid recumbency after meals • Stop smoking • Antacids - after meals and at bedtime 2. Phase II: add H2 blocker • Indications: mild to moderate GERD who have failed lifestyle modifications 3. Phase III: switch to PPI • Indications: severe disease, lifestyle modification or H2 blocker therapy failure, documented case of esophagitis 4. Phase IV: add promotility (metoclopramide or Reglan, bethanechol) 5. Phase V: H2 + promotility 6. PPI + promotility 7. Phase VI: **Nissen fundoplication** for intractable cases, aspiration, other complications Complications: 1. **Barrett esophagus** (*squamous epithelium replaced with columnar*) → esophageal adenocarcinoma, get EGD 2. Dental erosion, gingivitis 3. Laryngitis, pharyngitis 4. Recurrent pneumonia 5. Peptic stricture: dysphagia, dilation with EGD 6. Erosive esophagitis–long-term PPI therapy

PYLORIC STENOSIS, INTUSSUSCEPTION, HIRSHSPRUNG DISEASE, DUODENAL ATRESIA

Disease	Etiology, Prevalence, Risk Factors	Clinical Symptoms and Signs	Diagnostics	Therapy, Prognosis, and Health Maintenance
Pyloric stenosis	Forceful vomiting caused by hypertrophy and spasm of pylorus Most common cause of obstruction in neonate MC: **3-6 wk of life** Mostly males Common presentation 1. Hungry infant that wants **feeding after vomiting**, constipation	1. **Blood streaked, NON-bilious** projectile vomiting 2. **Weight loss** 3. Anorexia 4. Steady periumbilical pain → RLQ 5. Nausea, vomiting 6. Low fever Signs: 1. L-R peristaltic waves in LUQ after feeding 2. **Palpable olive shaped mass** superior to right of umbilicus in **midepigastrium** 3. **Dehydration**	1. **Ultrasound** (initial) thickened, enlarged pylorus, antral nipple sign, cervix sign 2. (+) peritoneal signs 3. **UGI:** "string sign" (long, narrow pyloric lumen); required for diagnosis 4. Venous pH: hypo-chloremic alkalosis 5. Laboratory findings: hypochloremia, hypokalemia, meta-bolic alkalosis	1. IVF 2. Surgical: **pyloromyotomy**
Intussusception	Males, most common abdominal emergency in early childhood MCC: **Intestinal obstruction** in first 2 y of life Etiology: 1. 75% idiopathic, most common location is ileocolic 2. Adhesions in adults	Infant: 1. **Paroxysmal abdominal pain, bilious vomiting**, diar-rhea progressing into bloody stool 2. **Inconsolable crying, draws legs toward abdomen** Child: 1. Follows VIRAL illness 2. Sudden onset, intermittent, severe, **colicky abdominal pain** 3. Pain → **vomiting**, becomes bilious with time 4. **Currant jelly stool:** blood + mucous Signs: 1. Palpable **sausage shaped mass** in RUQ	1. Abdominal **ultra-sound:** target/bull's eye/coiled spring sign 2. CT scan: target lesion representing layers of intussus-cepted segment	1. **Barium/air enema:** diagnostic + therapeu-tic 2. NPO, IVF, NG, ABX 3. Manual reduction or resection with primary anastomosis
Hirschsprung disease	MC: Short segment of distal colon (**tran-sition zone in rectosigmoid**) M > F FH or genetic mutations Associated: **Trisomy 21,** kidney or urinary tract anomalies Congenital absence of Meissner and Auerbach autonomic plexus → functional obstruction	Infant: 1. Failure to pass meconium in **first 24 h** (meconium ileus) 2. **Bilious** vomiting, distention Older child: 1. Chronic Constipation • Acute enterocolitis or chronic constipation 2. Foul-smelling stool that is ribbon-like Signs: 1. Distended abdomen with veins 2. Pencil-like stools	1. DRE: "Squirt sign" 2. KUB: transition zone 3. **Barium enema** w/ XR: cone-shaped transition zone, **nar-rowed distal colon with proximal dilation** 4. **Full-thickness rectal biopsy:** no ganglion cells (definitive) 5. Acute enterocolitis: bowel stasis and bacterial over-growth, sepsis-like (F, V/D, distention)→ toxic megacolon 6. Chronic consti-pation: pencil-like stools, no fecal incontinence, FTT, distention	1. Acute: NPO, IVF, NG, ABX, **surgery** (diverting colostomy or ileostomy) 2. Colonic lavage: mechanical irrigation with large bore rectal tube and large volume irrigant 3. Surgery: diverting colostomy 4. Chronic: stimulant lax-atives, osmotic laxative, enema, rectal irrigation, anal botox

Pediatrics

(continued)

(continued)

Disease	Etiology, Prevalence, Risk Factors	Clinical Symptoms and Signs	Diagnostics	Therapy, Prognosis, and Health Maintenance
Duodenal atresia	Congenital absence or complete closure of a portion of lumen of duodenum Associated: *Trisomy 21*	1. HX: **Polyhydramnios** during pregnancy 2. Bilious vomiting **first day** of life 3. Lethargy Signs: 1. Upper abdominal distention 2. Respiratory difficulty	1. XR: **double bubble sign**	1. IVF 2. NG tube 3. **Duodeno- duodenostomy**, not urgent

COLIC, CONSTIPATION, ENCOPRESIS

Disease	Etiology, Prevalence, Risk Factors	Clinical Symptoms and Signs	Diagnostics	Therapy, Prognosis, and Health Maintenance
Infantile colic	**2 wk to 3-4 mo** (peak: 6 wk) Prevalence: 8%-40% M = F Unknown etiology, thought to be related to: • Faulty feeding techniques: underfeeding, overfeeding, infrequent burping, swallowing air • Cow's milk protein intolerance • Lactose intolerance • GI immaturity • Intestinal hypermotility • Alterations in fecal microflora Persistent or excessive crying during infancy Benign, self-limiting condition that resolves with time	"Rule of Threes" (Wessel Criteria) 1. Child **cries for for 3+ h/d, 3+ d/wk** for **at least 3 wk** • Loud, high pitched • Screaming > crying • Unable to console 2. Occurs suddenly in the late evening • May occur while happy, fussy, feeding, or sleeping 3. Otherwise healthy and well fed 4. Aggravators: hungry, hurt, sick, too hot or cold, tired; allergy to formula or breastmilk Signs: 1. **Hypertonia** 2. Facial flushing, circumoral pallor 3. Tense and distended abdomen 4. Knees drawn up 5. Fists clenched 6. Stiffening and tightening of arms 7. Arching of back	Clinical DX	1. **Soothing techniques** • Rub infant's abdomen • Provide "white noise": vacuum cleaner, clothes drier, dishwasher • Rhythmic stimulation: gentle swinging, rocking, drives in the car, walks in stroller • Use a pacifier • Warm bath 2. **Change feeding habit** • Do not rush eating • Give ample opportunity to burp • Bottle fed in vertical position (curved bottle) 3. **If refractory:** • Trial of changing the feedings • Eliminate cow's milk Prognosis: 1. Resolves by age 3-4 mo in 60%-80%, respectively Health maintenance: 1. It is normal for infants to cry up to 2 h a day, especially in the first 3 mo of life 2. Simethicone, herbal teas, and probiotics not proven to help 3. Do not treat with: dicyclomine, phenobarbital
Constipation	95% **functional**, no path MCC: Painful BM with voluntary withholding of feces Triggers: Toilet training, changes in routine/diet, stress, illness, unavailable toilets, too busy Most nonorganic causes: toilet phobia, avoidance, excessive parental intervention, developmental, genetics, reduced stool volume/dryness	1. 2 or more of the following for 2 mo • <3 BMs per wk • More than one episode of encopresis per week 2. Impaction of the rectum with stool 3. Passage of stool so large it obstructs the toilet 4. Retentive posturing and fecal withholding 5. Pain with defecation - painless rectal bleeding		Infants (<1 y) 1. Glycerin suppository Children (1 y/o +) 1. Rapid disempaction: enemas, **mineral oil**, normal saline, milk and molasses Slower disimpaction: 1. HD mineral oil, PO Senna, PO Mg Citrate Adults: 1. Dietary fiber + fluids 2. Osmotic stool softener: milk of magnesia, lactulose, Miralax (PEG) 3. Stimulants: Senna (ExLax)

Pediatrics

Disease	Etiology, Prevalence, Risk Factors	Clinical Symptoms and Signs	Diagnostics	Therapy, Prognosis, and Health Maintenance
Encopresis	Males: 3-6× more common Age 5-6 y **Constipation** (90%), retention, colon dilation, overflow	1. Repeated voluntary/involuntary passage of feces in inappropriate places (soiling) 2. 1 event per mo, at least 3 mo 3. At least 4 y/o <u>Signs</u>: 1. Dark, foul smelling, liquid stool	1. T4/TSH 2. IgA TG antibodies 3. Calcium and lead 4. KUB	1. Evacuation behavior strategies • Sit on toilet after meals to stimulate gastrocolic reflex • Increased fluid intake ≤1 y/o: osmotic laxative, glycerin suppository, enema ≥1 y: osmotic laxative, lubricants, stimulants, enema

JAUNDICE

Disease	Etiology, Prevalence, Risk Factors	Clinical Symptoms and Signs	Diagnostics	Therapy, Prognosis, and Health Maintenance
Jaundice	<u>RF</u>: Birth weight <2500 g, breast feeding, gestational age <37 wk, sibling with previous phototherapy, cephalohematoma or bruising, east Asian	1. Yellow face, sclera <u>Signs</u>: 1. *Splenomegaly* with hereditary spherocytosis	1. **Bhutani nomogram** 2. **Hyperbilirubinemia** >35 wk gestation is **TB >95%** on nomogram • If extends below umbilicus, measure total bilirubin (TB) • At risk if TB > 25 mg/dL (kernicterus with encephalopathy)	
Acute			Chronic	
Poor feeding, lethargy High pitched cry Hyper or hypotonia Decerebrate posturing Seizures Sensorineural hearing loss Incomplete Moro reflex Setting sun sign Fever			Motor delay Choreoathetosis Asymmetric spasticity Paresis of upward gaze Dental enamel dysplasia MR, cognitive dysfunction Sensorineural hearing loss	
Overproduction: blood group desensitization (Rh isoimmunization, ABO incompatibility), hereditary spherocytosis, G6P deficiency			Decreased **rate of conjugation**: BREAST FEEDING, physiologic jaundice, prematurity, inborn errors of metabolism, Gilbert syndrome	
ABO incompatibility	First 24 h after birth	Coombs (+) Retic: high, H&H: low	Transfusion Phototherapy	
Rh isoimmunization		Coombs (+) Retic: ?, H&H: low	Transfusion Phototherapy	
Hereditary spherocytosis		Coombs (-) Retic: high, (+) osmotic fragility test Spherocytes on peripheral smear	Transfusion Phototherapy	
G6PD deficiency		Coombs (-) Test for G6PD	**Phototherapy**	
Physiologic jaundice	**After 24 h**, peaks at *3-5 d*	Bili increases by <5 mg/dL per day	**Phototherapy** if >15 or not descending	
Breast feeding jaundice	Peaks at *2-3 d* of life	Bili increases and persists 6-8 wk!	*Supplement breast milk*, feed every 2 h **Phototherapy** if >15	

Pediatrics

HERNIAS

Disease	Etiology, Prevalence, Risk Factors	Clinical Symptoms and Signs	Diagnostics	Therapy, Prognosis, and Health Maintenance
Inguinal hernia	**Processus vaginalis** remains open and peritoneal fluid or abdominal structure forced into it (**INDIRECT** inguinal hernia) Boys > Girls, any age Preterm male infants: 5% Males weighing <1000 g (ELBW): 30%	1. **Painless** inguinal swelling • Retracts when cold, active, frightened or agitated 2. +/− Vomiting, abdominal distention Signs: 1. Inguinal fullness with coughing or long periods of standing, or presence of firm, globular, tender swelling		1. Manual reduction of incarcerated hernias attempted AFTER infant sedated and placed in−Trendelenburg position with ice bag on affected side 2. Manual reduction contraindicated if incarceration present for 12+ h or if bloody stool present • **Refer to surgery if ever incarcerated** 3. Complications: more likely in boys <10 mo old
Umbilical hernia	MC: **Full-term, African American infants**	1. Increasing in size • Usually contain omentum, but small and large bowel may be present 2. Sharp pain on coughing or straining • Large hernias produce dragging or aching sensation		1. Most regress spontaneously if fascial defect has diameter of <1 cm 2. If **4 y or older**: SURGERY NOTE: reducing the hernia and strapping the skin over the abdominal wall does NOT accelerate healing

VITAMIN/MINERAL DEFICIENCIES

Disease	Etiology, Prevalence, Risk Factors	Clinical Symptoms and Signs	Diagnostics	Therapy, Prognosis, and Health Maintenance
(Niacin) **Vitamin B$_3$ deficiency**	Synthesized from tryptophan foods and cereals, vegetables, and dairy products Causes: Corn-based diets, alcoholism Occurs due to inborn error of metabolism Lowers LDL and VLDL, raises HDL	Early: 1. Anorexia 2. **Weakness** 3. Mouth soreness 4. Weight loss **Signs:** 1. **Glossitis**, stomatitis 2. Irritability 3. Advanced (pellagra): pigmented **dermatitis, diarrhea, dementia** • Dermatitis affects the sun exposed areas	1. **N-methylnicotinamide** measured in urine Dermatitis: symmetric, sun-exposed areas, dark, dry, scaly Dementia: insomnia, irritable, apathetic → confusion, memory loss, hallucinations, psychosis Diarrhea: severe, malabsorption	1. **Niacinamide** 10-150 mg/d−has no lipid lowering effects
Vitamin A deficiency	Leading cause of preventable blindness in children Causes: Inadequate dietary intake (rice diet) and malabsorption Sources: Fish, liver, egg yolk, butter, cream, dark green leafy vegetables, yellow fruits Iron deficiency can affect vitamin A absorption Increased susceptibility to infections	1. **Nyctalopia** (dim light or night blindness) 2. **Xerophthalmia** (dry eyes) **Signs:** 1. **Bitot spots** (white conjunctiva patches) 2. Kerophthalmia 3. Keratomalacia 4. Conjunctival and corneal xerosis 5. Pericorneal and corneal opacities 6. Complete blindness 7. Xeroderma, hyperkeratotic skin lesions	Clinical DX: 1. Measure serum retinol levels (<20 ug/dL = deficiency) • Fasting recommended	1. Infants 6-12 mo: 100k IU PO once 2. High-dose vitamin A (200k IU) PO, repeat dose every 4-6 mo Health maintenance: 1. Vegetarians do not need to supplement if they eat adequate variety of vegetables containing carotenoids

Disease	Etiology, Prevalence, Risk Factors	Clinical Symptoms and Signs	Diagnostics	Therapy, Prognosis, and Health Maintenance
Vitamin C deficiency (scurvy, ascorbic acid)	Weakened capillaries and impaired formation of connective tissue Causes: Inadequate intake, pregnancy and lactation (increase requirements) Sources: Citrus fruits (orange, lemon, tangerine), tomato, potato	HX: **anemia**, impaired wound healing: 1. Nonspecific malaise and weakness Signs: 1. *Perifollicular hemorrhages* and follicular **Hyperkeratotic papules** 2. Petechiae and purpura 3. Splinter hemorrhages on nails 4. Bleeding gums: swollen, friable 5. *Hemarthroses*, subperiosteal hemorrhages 6. Loose teeth Late: Edema, oliguria, neuropathy, intracerebral hemorrhage, death	1. Ascorbic acid: low (<0.1 mg/dL)	1. Ascorbic acid (vitamin C): 300-1000 mg PO daily 2. Supplement with citric fruits and vegetables

Vitamin D deficiency (rickets)	Due to **deficient intake or defective metabolism** (lack of sunlight) of vitamin D, results in low serum calcium
	Vitamin D deficiency or low intake of calcium and phosphorous
	Med HX: phenobarbital, phenytoin, aluminum antacids
		HX:
		1. Dental caries, diarrhea/fat malabsorption, poor growth, pneumonia, hypocalcemia symptoms, GI/renal disease
		2. **Inability to walk**: muscle weakness, delayed walking, waddling gait
		Signs:
		1. Observe gait
		2. Listen to lungs for atelectasis or PNEUMONIA
		3. Plot growth
		4. **Rachitic rosary**
		5. **Genu valgum/varum**
		6. **Craniotabes**
			1. Calcium: NL to low
			2. PTH: elevated
			3. PA x-ray: wrist shows thick growth plate, **fraying, cupping**, widening of distal metaphysis
			4. Other labs
			  • Serum phos/alk-phos
			  • 25-hydroxyvitamin D
			  • 1,25 dihydroxyvitamin D_3
			  • Creatinine, electrolytes
			  • U/A: glycosuria, aminoaciduria (Fanconi syndrome)
			  • -24-h urinary excretion of urine
				1. **High-dose vitamin-D** 2000-5000 IU/d for 4-6 wk
				Then daily vitamin D 400 IU/d (multivitamin)
				2. Dietary calcium/PO_4: milk, formula
				Breast-fed infants:
				should get at least 400 IU/d of vitamin D

Lactose intolerance	Lactose is digested by lactase (produced in small intestine) For most people, lactase production ceases after age of 12	1. Explosive watery diarrhea, borborygmi • With milk ingestion 2. Abdominal distention 3. Flatulence (gas) Signs: 1. Excoriated diaper area	1. Genetic testing 2. Lactose breath test with rise in hydrogen content, lactose load test (1 g/kg)	1. Restrict dietary lactose or supplement with lactase
Vitamin B_1 (thiamine) deficiency, beriberi	Associated with beriberi, characterized by high output cardiomyopathy and polyneuritis Occurs in infants 1-4 mo of age who have protein-energy malnutrition and are either (1) breastfed by mothers deficient in thiamine or (2) getting unsupplemented hyperalimentation fluid or boiled milk	1. Bilateral symmetric peripheral neuropathy beginning in legs 2. Wernicke-korsakoff syndrome: nystagmus, ophthalmoplegia, ataxia, memory loss, confabulation 3. Congestive heart failure: tachycardia, peripheral edema, cardiomegaly Infants 1. Hoarseness 2. Aphonic cry		Supplementation

(continued)

Pediatrics

(continued)

Disease	Etiology, Prevalence, Risk Factors	Clinical Symptoms and Signs	Diagnostics	Therapy, Prognosis, and Health Maintenance
Vitamin B_2 (riboflavin) deficiency	Inadequate dietary intake (milk, cheese, meat, enriched cereal) Rare	1. Angular stomatitis 2. Cheilosis Signs: 1. Pale 2. Atrophic glossitis 3. **Glossitis** (magenta tongue) 4. Seborrheic dermatitis: greasy material in nasolabial folds, alae nasi, and genitals 5. Vascularization of cornea		Supplementation with milk, meat, eggs, cereal, and green leafy vegetables
Vitamin B_6 (pyridoxine) deficiency	Causes: Malabsorption, medications (isoniazid, penicillamine) Sources: Liver, legumes, whole grain cereals, meats	1. Irritability 2. Confusion 3. Weight loss 4. Depression 5. Peripheral neuropathy (adolescents) 6. Seborrheic dermatosis 7. Glossitis 8. Cheilosis 9. Encephalopathy with seizures (younger children)	1. CBC: anemia, lymphopenia	Supplementation with bananas, nuts, many common vegetables (potatoes, green beans, cauliflower, carrots) Supplementation 1. Infants: 0.1-0.3 mg/d 2. Children and adolescents: 0.5-1.3 mg/d
Vitamin B_{12} (cobalamin deficiency)	Causes: Pernicious anemia, blind loop syndrome, fish tapeworm infestation, vegetarian diets Sources: Liver, beef, eggs, milk Uncommon, but can occur exclusively in **breastfed infants of mothers who are strictly vegetarian or vegan** or with vitamin B_{12} malabsorption due to gastric bypass, short bowel syndrome, or pernicious anemia	1. SX of anemia: fatigue, lightheadedness, syncope, pallor 2. Poor weight gain and linear growth 3. Weakness 4. Failure to thrive 5. Developmental delay 6. Afebrile seizures 7. Involuntary movements, nystagmus, tremors 8. Irritability Signs: 1. Neurologic: **ataxia**, paresthesias, decreased proprioceptive and vibratory sensations in lower limbs 2. Atrophic glossitis	1. CBC: macrocytic cells 2. Acylcarnitines, propionylcarnitine (C3) and/or methylmalonylcarnitine elevated	Supplementation with liver, milk, fish, meat
Vitamin K deficiency	Results in a bleeding diathesis seen in skin, GI tract, GU tract, gingiva, lungs, joints, or CNS	1. Epistaxis 2. Menorrhagia 3. Hematuria	1. PT and aPTT: prolonged	Supplementation
Iron deficiency	Most common nutritional deficiency in children	1. Weakness, lethargy 2. Dizziness 3. Fatigue 4. Syncope 5. Irritability 6. Poor feeding Signs: 1. Pale conjunctiva 2. Koilonychia (spooning of nails) 3. Pallor 4. Tachypnea	1. Microcytic hypochromic anemia	Supplementation

Pediatrics

Disease	Etiology, Prevalence, Risk Factors	Clinical Symptoms and Signs	Diagnostics	Therapy, Prognosis, and Health Maintenance
Vitamin E deficiency	Causes: Limited placental transfer of vitamin E, deficiency in diet Sources: Wheat germ, vegetable oils, egg yolk, leafy vegetables	Infants: 1. Hemolytic anemia	1. Plasma tocopherol: low 2. Hgb: low 3. Reticulocytosis, hyper-bilirubinemia, creatinuria	Supplementation with sunflower seeds, wheat germ oil, corn, and nuts
Folic acid deficiency	Malabsorption, inadequate intake by alcoholics, increased demand in pregnancy and chronic hemolytic anemias; also found in children with zinc and vitamin B_{12} deficiencies Sources: Green leafy vegetables, liver, yeast Phenobarbital increases the need for folate	1. Anemia 2. Fatigue 3. Weakness 4. Syncope Signs: Pale	1. CBC: macrocytic RBCs 2. Hgb: <12 g/dL	Supplementation: 1. Green leafy vegeta-bles, fruits, cereals, grains, nuts, meats
Zinc deficiency	Malabsorption, alcoholism, prolonged parenteral nutrition Sources: Beef, liver, eggs, oysters	1. **Hypogeusia** (decreased taste sensation) 2. Anorexia 3. Delayed sexual maturation 4. Night blindness 5. Hair loss Signs: 1. Alopecia 2. Growth retardation 3. Delayed sexual maturation 4. Hypogonadism	1. Hypospermia	Supplementation
Iodine deficiency	Sources: Iodized table salt, seafood, eggs, dairy products	1. Anterior neck swelling that rises with deglutition (colloid goiter) 2. Hearing impairment 3. Spastic diplegia 4. Strabismus 5. **Intellectual disability** Complications: Cretinism (infants), impaired brain development and fetal growth	1. TSH/T3/T4: euthyroid, some hypothyroid	Supplementation
Copper deficiency	Malabsorption, infants with persistent diarrhea fed on milk, copper-free TPN, excess intake of zinc salt dietary supplements Menkes syndrome: inherited form of copper deficiency caused by X-linked gene, male infants Sources: Organ meats, oysters, nuts, dried legumes, whole grain cereals	1. Intellectual disability 2. Kinky hair 3. Hypopigmentation 4. Vascular aneurysms	1. Hypocupremia 2. Decreased ceruloplasmin	Supplementation

Pediatrics

CHAPTER 31

Psychiatry and Behavioral Medicine

Refer to Psychiatry 🖼️ **for in-depth coverage of the following topics:**

Attention Deficit/Hyperactivity Disorder, see Conduct, Developmental, Impulse and Attention-related Disorders, p 572

Autism Spectrum Disorder, see Conduct, Developmental, Impulse and Attention-related Disorders, p 575

Feeding or Eating Disorders, see Feeding or Eating Disorders, p 588

Depressive Disorders, see Depressive and Mood Disorders, p 536

Anxiety Disorders, see Anxiety, Trauma, and Stress-related Disorders, p 544

Disruptive, Impulse Control, and Conduct Disorders, see Conduct, Developmental, Impulse and Attention-related Disorders, p 572

Suicide, see Depressive and Mood Disorders, p 543

Recommended Supplemental Topics:

Temper Tantrums, p 333

Breath-Holding Spells, p 333

All of the following topics are currently updated with criteria from the fifth edition of the American Psychiatric Association's *Diagnostic and Statistical Manual (DSM-5)*, which utilizes specific criteria with which to objectively assess symptoms, rather than purely discrete diagnostic categories. For example, personality dimensions are more prominent than they were in *DSM-IV*. Nonetheless, the diagnosis is still based on a solid history and examination.

CHILD ABUSE AND NEGLECT

- Physical abuse most often afflicted by a caregiver or family member

Disease	Etiology, Prevalence, Risk Factors	Clinical Symptoms and Signs	Diagnostics	Therapy, Prognosis, and Health Maintenance

Child abuse	History of abuse in caregiver's childhood, inappropriate effect of caregiver, increasing severity or number of injuries, stress or crisis in the family
	Children <3 y/o
	MC form of child abuse: **neglect**
	Shaken baby syndrome—lethargy, coma—seizure, vomiting, respiratory distress
		1. Implausible mechanism for injury
		2. Discrepant, evolving, or absent history
		3. Delay in seeking care
		4. Event/behavior in child that triggers loss of control by caregiver
		5. Social/physical isolation of the caregiver or child
		6. Unrealistic expectations of the caregiver for the child
		7. Behavioral changes in child
		Signs:
		1. Ocular trauma (40%)—**retinal hemorrhage** from shaking violently
		2. Bruises, bites, abrasions, alopecia, dental trauma, lacerations, scars, burns, fractures, head trauma, abdominal injuries
		  • In multiple stages of healing
		  • Patterns, **found in soft tissue areas**
		  • Toddlers: **bruises over bony prominences**
		  • Lacerations of the frenulum or tongue and bruising of the lips
		  • Burns in stocking or glove distribution, immersion burns (doughnut hole sparing)
			1. XR
			  • Metaphyseal corner or bucket handle **fractures in long bones**
			  • Spiral fracture in nonambulatory infants
			  • Rib fractures
			  • Spinous process fractures
			2. CT/MRI: subdural hemorrhage
			3. Labs: CBC, coagulation studies, LFTs
				1. Home visitor services to families at risk for prevention
				2. Anticipatory guidance
				  • How to handle stressful situations (colic, crying, toilet training), age appropriate discipline, and developmental issues

Disease	Etiology, Prevalence, Risk Factors	Clinical Symptoms and Signs	Diagnostics	Therapy, Prognosis, and Health Maintenance
Child (emotional) neglect	Rejection, ignoring, criticizing, isolation, or terrorizing of children <u>MC:</u> Verbal abuse (denigration)	1. Nutritional failure to thrive 2. Causes loss of self-esteem or confidence, sleep disturbance, somatic symptoms, hypervigilance, avoidance, or phobic behavior		
Child (physical) neglect and failure to thrive	Failure to provide necessary food, clothing, shelter, and safe environment to grow MC form of abuse	1. Infants in significant deceleration in growth 2. Depression 3. Short stature <u>Signs</u> 1. Absence of subcutaneous fat in cheeks, buttocks, extremities	1. Assess growth curve 2. Labs: CBC, U/A, CMP, TFT, LFTs	1. Evaluation of home and entire family

TEMPER TANTRUMS AND BREATH-HOLDING SPELLS

Disease	Etiology, Prevalence, Risk Factors	Clinical Symptoms and Signs	Diagnostics	Therapy, Prognosis, and Health Maintenance

Temper tantrums	12 mo–4 y	1. Child throws themselves down, kicks and screams, strikes out at people or objects in the room, holds their breath		1. Minimize need to say "no" by childproofing environment—less restrictions enforced
				2. Use distraction when frustration increases; redirect child and reward positive response
				3. Present options within child's capabilities
				4. Fight only battles that need to be won
				5. Do not abandon preschool child
				  • No threats
				  • Tell them to go to room
				  • Restrain small children
				6. Do not use negative terms, praise when they regain control
				7. Never let them hurt themselves or others
				8. Do not hold a grudge

Breath-holding spells	Occurs during expiration and is reflexive, not volitional 6 mo–6 y	1. Start in first year of life in response to anger or mild injury 2. Child is provoked or surprised, starts to cry and then falls silent 3. Color change—cyanotic or acyanotic 4. Loss of consciousness followed by seizure-like activity (stiffening and jerking, eyes rolled back)	1. **Iron studies** • TIBC, serum iron, serum ferritin, CBC 2. EKG—rule out any cardiac anomalies or arrhythmias	1. Help child control their responses to frustration 2. If LOC → place on side to protect against injury and aspiration 3. Iron supplementation, if signs of anemia or low iron

CHAPTER 32

Neurology and Developmental

Refer to [icon] for in-depth coverage of the following topics:

Seizure Disorders, p 108

Recommended Supplemental Topics:

Lennox-Gastaut Syndrome, p 336

Macrocephaly, p 341

IMMUNIZATION GUIDELINES

	Routine	Boosters	Contraindications	"Cautions"
Hepatitis B: 3 doses	Birth-1 mo 1-2 mo 6-18 mo		1. Severe allergic reaction after previous dose	1. Mod/severe illness +/− fever 2. Infant weighs <2000 g (4 lbs., 6.4 oz)
Rotavirus: 2-3 doses	2, 4, and 6 mo		1. Severe allergic reaction after previous dose 2. Severe combined immunodeficiency 3. History of **intussusception**	1. Mod/severe illness +/− fever 2. Immunocompetence 3. Chronic GI disease 4. Spina bifida or bladder dystrophy
DTaP: 5 doses	2, 4, and 6 mo 15-18 m/o, 4-6 y/o TdAP booster at 11-12 y		1. Severe allergic reaction after previous dose	1. If after last dose: • Fever >105 F within 48 h • Crying inconsolably 3+ h within 48 h • Seizure within 3 d (*not* febrile sz) • Encephalopathy within 7 d • Collapse/shock (hypotonic hyporesponsive) within 48 h
Pneumococcal (PCV13): 2-3 doses + booster (3-4)	2,4, and 6 mo	12-15 mo	1. Severe allergic reaction after previous dose	
HiB:3 doses	2, 4 and 6 mo	12-15 mo	1. Severe allergic reaction after previous dose 2. **Age <6 wk**	
Polio (IPV): 3 doses	2, 4, and 6-18 mo		1. Severe allergic reaction after previous dose	
MMR Varicella	12-15 m/o, 4-6 y /o		1. Severe allergic reaction after previous dose (egg anaphylaxis) 2. Known immunodeficiency 3. Pregnancy	1. Mod/severe illness +/− fever 2. Recent (within 11 m) Ab-containing blood product 3. History of thrombocytopenia or TTP 4. Needs Tb-Test 5. Receipt of specific antivirals 24 h before vaccination • Avoid use of acyclovir, famciclovir, or valaciclovir × 14 d after

	Routine	Boosters	Contraindications	"Cautions"
Hepatitis A: 2 doses	Both 12-23 mo Separate by 6-18 mo		1. Severe allergic reaction after previous dose	
Influenza:1-2 doses	6 mo, annual		1. Severe allergic reaction after previous dose (egg anaphylaxis)	1. Mod/severe illness +/– fever 2. Guillain-Barre within 6 wk after previous dose 3. Only hives with exposure to eggs (not contraindicated)
HPV: 3 doses (0, 2, 6 mo)	F: 11-12 y to 26 M: 11-12 y to 21		1. Severe allergic reaction after previous dose	1. Mod/severe illness +/– fever 2. Pregnancy
Tdap	11-12 y		1. Severe allergic reaction after previous dose	1. Mod/severe illness +/– fever 2. Guillain-Barre within 6 wk after previous dose 3. Arthus-type hypersensitivity reaction after previous dose 4. Progressive or unstable neuro disorder (uncontrolled seizures or progressive encephalopathy)
Meningococcal (MenACWY, conjugate) or polysaccharide (MPSV4)	11-12 y		1. Severe allergic reaction after previous dose	1. Mod/severe illness +/– fever

Pediatrics

ANTICIPATORY GUIDANCE

- The primary cause of death in children in the US is motor vehicle injuries

Infants and toddlers	1. Rear-facing car safety seat until 2 y of age or until they reach height/weight limits for convertible car safety seats (35 lb.) 2. Infants may ride in infant-only seats (handle and snap into a base that is secured in the car) until they reach the height/weight limit for that seat
2 y	1. Forward facing car safety seat with harness → 2. Belt-positioned booster
Age 8-12, height of 4 ft. 9 in	1. Vehicle's lap and shoulder belt fits properly (child can sit with back against vehicle seat, bend knees at edge of seat, have belt positioned in center of shoulder and across the chest, have lap belt touching thighs)
<13 y/o	Restrained in rear seats of vehicle

- Wear a helmet when riding a bicycle
- A gun in the home doubles the likelihood of a lethal suicide attempt
  - Adolescents with history of depression or violence are at higher risk
  - Lock them in a drawer/cabinet and store ammunition in a separate locked location

- Recreational swimming should always be supervised
- Scalding is the most common type of burn in children
- Most fire-related deaths result from smoke inhalation
- Sunburn is the most common thermal injury
  - Avoid sun between 10 AM and 4 PM
  - Use sunscreen with SPF of 15 or higher that protects against UVA and UVB rays
  - Wear hats, sunglasses, and long-sleeved swim shirts
  Children <3 are at high risk for choking because they have not fully coordinated chewing and swallowing and are able to put small objects into their mouths.

TEETHING

- Primary teeth eruption occurs symmetrically and bilaterally
- First teeth to erupt: central incisors at 6 to 10 months
- Primary dentition is typically fully erupted by 30 months
- Girls develop their teeth earlier than boys, black children earlier than white children
- Permanent tooth eruption occurs at 6 years of age.

Disease	Etiology, Prevalence, Risk Factors	Clinical Symptoms and Signs	Diagnostics	Therapy, Prognosis, and Health Maintenance
Teething	Infants with primary teeth eruption who is cranky, chewing on objects, excessive drooling	1. **Irritable** 2. **Drooling** 3. Increased temperature (NOT fever or temperature >38.5°C) 4. Diarrhea 5. Other systemic symptoms	Clinical DX	1. Palliative: chewing on chilled teething ring or other teething device, systemic analgesics Health maintenance: 1. Do not recommend OTC or prescription strength analgesics (lidocaine, benzocaine) as they may be harmful and risk > benefit

FEBRILE SEIZURE

Disease	Etiology, Prevalence, Risk Factors	Clinical Symptoms and Signs	Diagnostics	Therapy, Prognosis, and Health Maintenance
Simple febrile seizures	Children <5 y/o Increases the risk of developing epilepsy later in life Peak: 12-18 mo Seizure occurring with fever No CNS infection	1. Fever >38°C (100.4°F) 2. Must meet all 3: • Lasts <15 min • **Generalized tonic-clonic seizure** • *Once* in 24 h period	1. No blood studies, neuroimaging, or EEG for most 2. **LP in infants <12 mo** (strongly recommended) 3. LP in infants 12-18 mo (somewhat recommended) • If previous febrile seizure, do not r/o meningitis as cause	1. Antipyretics (**Tylenol, Motrin**) will NOT prevent subsequent seizures, although indicated 2. Anticonvulsant therapy NOT recommended—AE outweigh risk of recurrence 3. 30% recur before age 1 or if family history of febrile seizures
Complex febrile seizures	HHV-6 (86%), magnitude of temperature or rate of temperature may precipitate seizure RF: CP, MR, early onset febrile seizure <1 y, FH of epilepsy	1. Fever >38°C (100.4°F) 2. One or more: • Lasts >15 min • **Focal seizure** • *Recurs* within 24-h period 3. No serious signs of infection 4. DX of exclusion	1. CBC with blood culture 2. U/A with culture 3. LP: CSF with culture 4. EEG 5. MRI	1. If negative results, discharge without antibiotics 2. Follow-up in 24 h to review cultures and repeat physical 3. **Antipyretics (Tylenol)** will NOT prevent subsequent seizures, although indicated 4. Prophylaxis: **phenobarbital or valproic acid** • Do not use: diazepam, phenytoin, carbamazepine

SEIZURE DISORDERS

Disease	Etiology, Prevalence, Risk Factors	Clinical Symptoms and Signs	Diagnostics	Therapy, Prognosis, and Health Maintenance
Lennox-Gastaut syndrome	Generalized epilepsy caused by diffuse or multifocal brain dysfunction Age: 2-10 60% have preexisting encephalopathy and developmental delay, 20% have infantile spasms Associated: MR	1. Akinetic (atonic) 2. Myoclonic seizures ('drop attacks') 3. Developmental delay	1. EEG: 2.5 Hz or slower generalized spike and slow wave with bursts of diffuse fast rhythms during sleep indicating tonic-atonic seizures	1. Requires supervision and most live in group homes 2. If drop seizures are present, helmets must be prescribed 3. **Valproic acid** (initial) 4. Added: Lamotrigine, topiramate, levetiracetam, zonisamide 5. Vagus nerve stimulator

Pediatrics

MENINGITIS

Disease	Etiology, Prevalence, Risk Factors	Clinical Symptoms and Signs	Diagnostics	Therapy, Prognosis, and Health Maintenance
Bacterial meningitis Acute—hours to days Chronic—within weeks to months, commonly caused by mycobacteria, fungi, Lyme disease, or parasites	Inflammation of the meningeal membranes that envelop the brain and spinal cord Infectious agents colonize the nasopharynx and respiratory tract Neonatal: listeria monocytogenes MCC: ***Streptococcus pneumoniae H. influenza, N. meningitidis***	1. Triad: ***fever, nuchal rigidity, change in mental status*** 2. ***Headache*** (more severe with lying down) 3. Nausea and vomiting 4. **Stiff, painful neck** 5. Malaise 6. Photophobia 7. AMS (***confusion, lethargy***, coma) Signs: 1. **Nuchal rigidity** (stiff neck with resistance to flexion) 2. **Rash** (maculopapular rash with petechiae for *N. meningitidis*) or vesicular lesions (varicella/HSV) 3. Increased ICP and its manifestations (papilledema, seizures) 4. Cranial nerve palsies 5. Kernig sign (+) 6. Brudzinski sign (+)	1. **Lumbar puncture–** unless evidence of space-occupying lesion • Neutrophil predom • Cell count >1000 • Low glucose level • Elevated protein 2. **CT scan of head–** recommended before performing LP if focal neurologic signs or evidence of space-occupying lesion with high ICP 3. **Blood cultures** prior to antibiotics	Bacterial: • Empiric therapy after LP • IV antibiotics immediately if CSF cloudy or bacteria suspected • Steroids if cerebral edema present 1. Early onset (<7 d): ampicillin 2. Late onset (7 d-3 mo): ampicillin + cefotaxime 3. Late late (>3 mo): ***Cefotaxime (3rd gen) + vancomycin*** Health maintenance: 1. Vaccinate asplenic pts and immunocompromised for meningococcus 2. Prophylaxis: • Rifampin or ceftriaxone for close contacts of meningococcal
Aseptic (viral) meningitis	Caused by a variety of non-bacterial pathogens, frequently **viruses** (enterovirus 70 or 71, coxsackievirus A7 or A9 and HSV) MC in summer and fall temperatures	1. Acute onset of • **Subacute fever**, chills, **headache**, photophobia, pain on eye movement • Nausea, vomiting 2. Diarrhea, myalgias, rash, pleurodynia, myocarditis, herpangina Signs: 1. Meningismus without local neurologic signs 2. **Drowsiness** or irritability	1. Lumbar puncture: pleocytosis • Lymphocyte predom • Cell count <1000 • Normal glucose level • Elevated protein	Aseptic meningitis: • Supportive therapy • Analgesics and fever reduction • Better prognosis than acute bacterial meningitis

Age or RF	Likely Etiology	Empiric Therapy
Infants <3 mo	GBS, *E. coli*, *Klebsiella*, *Listeria*	Cefotaxime + vanc + **ampicillin**
3 mo-50 y	*N. meningitidis*, Strep pneumo, *H. influenza*	Ceftriaxone or cefotaxime + vanc
>50 y	*S. pneumoniae*, *N. meningitidis*, Listeria	Ceftriaxone or cefotaxime + Vanc + **ampicillin**
Impaired cellular immunity (eg, HIV)	*S. pneumoniae*, *N. meningitidis*, Listeria, aerobic Gram-negative bacilli (*Pseudomonas*)	*Ceftazidime* + vanc + **ampicillin**

Bacterial Meningitis	Aseptic Meningitis
• Neonates: GBS, *E. coli*, Listeria • Children >3 mo: *N. meningitidis*, Strep pneumoniae, *H. influenza* • Adults: **S. pneumoniae**, *N. meningitidis*, *H. influenza* • Elderly (>50): *S. pneumoniae*, *N. meningitidis*, *L. monocytogenes* • Immunocompromised: *L. monocytogenes*, Gram-neg bacilli, *S. pneumo*	Caused by a variety of nonbacterial pathogens, frequently **viruses** (enterovirus and HSV) • Difficult to distinguish from acute bacterial meningitis • Better prognosis than acute bacterial meningitis
Complications: Seizures, coma, brain abscess, subdural empyema, DIC, respiratory arrest Permanent sequelae: deafness, brain damage, hydrocephalus	

Pediatrics

Lumbar Puncture CSF Findings

	Normal	Bacterial	Aseptic (Viral)
WBC count	<5	>1000-5000/mcL (250/cm³)	<1000
WBC differential	All lymphocytes or monocytes, no PMNs	Mostly PMNs (90%-100% **neutrophils**)	Mostly **lymphocytes** and monocytes
Glucose	50-75	**Low (35)**	Normal to high
Protein	<60	**High (150-250)**	NL to high
Gram stain		(+) in 75%-80%	

- Order cell count, chemistry, Gram stain, culture (include AFB) and cryptococcal antigen or India ink

TURNER SYNDROME AND DOWN SYNDROME

Disease	Etiology, Prevalence, Risk Factors	Clinical Symptoms and Signs	Diagnostics	Therapy, Prognosis, and Health Maintenance
Turner syndrome (gonadal dysgenesis)	**45, XO karyotype**—no X or Y from father Complications: Coarctation of the aorta	1. Primary amenorrhea (no period) 2. Short stature 3. Infertility 4. Congenital cardiac malformations common Signs: 1. Short and stocky build 2. *Micrognathia* 3. Shield chest (broad, flat) 4. *Webbed neck* 5. Widely spaced nipples, scant pubic hair 6. High palate 7. Short 4th metacarpal 8. *Low posterior hairline* 9. *Hand/foot edema* 10. *Multiple pigmented nevi* 11. *Increased carrying angle* 12. Ptosis and strabismus 13. Cubitus valgus	Not GH deficient, but may improve final height with treatment: 1. Normal growth hormone levels 2. Karyotype, echocardiogram, renal ultrasound 3. Blood pressure, hearing screen, scoliosis screen 4. TSH—annually 5. Screen for learning disability	1. Growth hormone at 2-5 y 2. Estrogen replacement 12-13 y 3. TSH replacement 4. Repair CoA 5. Psych referral 6. Complications: pulmonary stenosis, **gonadal dysgenesis (90%)** 7. Renal anomalies: horseshoe **kidney, ectopic kidney (60%)** 8. Hypothyroid (10%-30%) 9. Glucose intolerance 10. Cardiac defects (20%): **CoA**, bicuspid aortic valve 11. **Hearing loss 50%**
Down syndrome	Trisomy 21 (three copies of 21) Due to nondisjunction in meiosis RF: Advanced maternal age during pregnancy	1. Mild to severe mental retardation 2. Congenital heart disease Signs: 1. Flat nasal bridge 2. Folded or dysplastic ears 3. Transverse palmar crease (**simian crease**) 4. Upward slanting palpebral fissure 5. Protruding, large wrinkled tongue 6. Wide gap between first and second toes 7. Umbilical hernia 8. Dysplasia of the mid phalanx 5th digit (**clinodactyly**)	1. Karyotype 2. Echocardiogram 3. Annual blood testing: TSH, LFT, CBC 4. Annual hearing test 5. Eye exam by 3-5 y 6. X-ray atlantoaxial junction 7. Special growth charts	1. Refer to ECI 2. Associated: **Mental retardation (100%), hearing loss (75%), eye disease (60%), serous otitis media (50%-70%)**, cardiac (AV canal, ASD/VSD), thyroid (15%), atresia (12%), atlantoaxial instability (12%), leukemia (1%)

NORMAL GROWTH AND DEVELOPMENT

Primitive Reflexes

Reflex	How to Elicit	Description	Disappears
Asymmetric tonic neck reflex (ATNR)	Lying supine, turn infant's head to side	Fencing posture with one arm outstretched Baby will extend limbs on that side; others flex	2-3 mo
Galant's Reflex	Support baby prone; stroke one side of back	Spine will curve toward stimulated side	
Rooting/sucking	Stimulus near or in mouth	Turning of head toward stimulus, sucking	
Palmar/plantar grasp	Object placed in palm/sole	Flexion of fingers/toes	3-4 mo
Moro	Sudden head extension	Symmetrical extension, then flexion (all limbs)	4-6 mo
Placing/stepping	Infant held vertically, dorsum of feet brought into contact with surface	Lifts one foot, placing it on surface, then other	
Positive supporting	Infant held vertically, feet on surface	Legs take body weight, push against (jumping)	

Postural Reflexes

Postural Reaction	Description	Importance	Appears
Head righting	Chin lift when prone	Head control	6 wk–3 mo
Anterior propping	Arm extension anterior when sitting	Tripod sitting	4-6 mo
Landau response	Extension of head, trunk, and legs when prone	Trunk Control	
Lateral propping	Arm extension laterally	Independent sitting	6-7 mo
Parachute	Arm extension when falling	Facial protection when falling	8-9 mo Remains for life
Posterior propping	Arm extension posteriorly	Pivot in sitting	8-10 mo

	Motor	Vision	Hearing	Social
Birth	Follows to midline, fisted hand	Distance between breast and face	Mature, **recognizes voices**	Smile, not social
Red flags: birth-2 mo	Poor suck, slow feeder Stiff, **floppy (hyper/hypotonic)**	No reaction to light	No response to loud noise (no startle reflex to clap)	
2 mo	**Raise head, chest off ground** Hands in mouth, bats objects, **grasps toys, sucks fingers**	**Watches face, tracks objects past midline**, begins hand-eye coord	**Coos** (vowels), **turning head to sounds**	Social smile "plays" with people
4-5 mo	**Rolls front to back, holds head**, no head lag, tripod position (5 mo) Brings hands to midline/mouth, reaches for objects with both hands		Belly laughs, turns to sounds	Enjoys looking around
Red flags: 2-5 mo	Head lag at 3 mo, not noticing hands or bringing stuff to mouth, constant fisted hands or flexed/stiff arms/legs	Not tracking objects	No coos by 3-4 mo	No social smile
6-7 mo	**Rolls over front to back, back to front** Sits unsupported, unilateral reaching, transfers objects, shakes toys, radial palmar grasp (7 mo)		Babbles (syllables)	Finds partially hidden objects, explores hands/feet and mouth, tries for things out of reach

(continued)

Pediatrics

(continued)

	Motor	Vision	Hearing	Social
Red flags: 6-7 mo	Not reaching for things, cannot roll over in either direction or sit with support by 9-10 mo, stiff/floppy Scissoring		No laughing or vowel sounds	No affection for caregiver
9-10 mo	**Crawls, sitting** (8 mo) **Pull to stand** (9 mo) **Cruising** (10 mo), **radial grasp** (Pincer grasp)		Mama/dada nonspecific, babbles multiple syllables, understands "no"	Stranger anxiety starts (9 mo) Plays gesture games, waves bye-bye
Red flags: 9-10 mo	No sitting without support, not bearing weight on legs Not transferring objects		Not responding to name, no babbling	
12 mo	Stands/walks alone with **wide gait, fine pincer grasp**		Using **mama/dada** correctly **1-step commands** with gesture	Imitates actions, stranger anxiety continues
Red flags: 12 mo	Not standing, pointing, or searching for hidden objects, not developing handedness		No single words or saying mama/dada specifically	Does not learn gesture games: patty cake
15 mo	Walks well, creeps up steps, imitates scribbles, tower of 2 blocks		4-6 words 1-step commands, no gesture	Drinks from cup
18 mo	Running, throwing objects without falling Tower of 3-4 blocks, scribbles spontaneously		10-25 words	Parallel play Spoon/fork use, imitates parent, turns pages in book, plays in company of others
Red flags: 15-18 mo	Does not walk or takes few steps		Has not said first words or learned any new ones	Not imitating others Does not notice or mind when caregiver leaves or returns or show affection
2 y	**Runs, kicks ball, walks up/down stairs** using rail Tower of 4-8 blocks, imitates stroke with pencil, **able to remove most clothing**		**2-word sentences** **2-step commands** 50 words, 50% understandable	More defiant behavior Enjoys company of others Increased independence **Toilet training begins**
3 y	Alternates feet going up steps, **rides tricycle** **Balances on one foot 1-2 s** Tower of 9-10 cubes, draws person with head and 1 body part		250 words, long sentences 75% understandable	**Puts on clothing, knows name/age/gender** Names playmate, concern for crying friend, imaginative play
Red flags: 2-3 y	Difficulty walking, frequent falls	No eye contact	Speech not understandable, few words Does not understand simple instruction	Does not want to interact or play with others/toys No pretend play, does not know what to do with common things
4 y	**Balances on 1 foot for 3-4 s, hop, skip** Draws person with 3-6 body parts, copies square		**100% understandable** 3-4 colors, asks questions Complex sentences	**Dresses completely and buttons** Pretend play Plays with kids, tells stories
Red flags: 4 y	Can not jump in place or throw ball well		Poor speech, cannot use pronouns properly Not following commands well	No interest in games or make-believe Little interaction with children or strangers Difficulty dressing, toileting

Pediatrics

	Motor	Vision	Hearing	Social
5-8 y	Organized sports begin			Home relationships most important, pay attention to friends, think about future Talk about feelings Fundamentals in K-2 Grade 3–abstract, progress reports, conferences
9-12 y	Development of strength/coordination, improved sports performance Increased attention span, academics more complex, increased independence, abstract reasoning			Complex friendships, prefer friends of same gender, move away of body, peer pressure
Red flags: school age	Poor/borderline grades, easily distracted, spending excessive time completing HW, difficulty spelling/word structure, poor handwriting, acting out/embarrassed, difficulty expression self			Difficulty entering/joining group, keeping friends, dealing with teasing/bullying, managing minor conflicts, handling failure or disappointment, responding to success, considering others feelings

MACROCEPHALY

- Differential: autism, hydrocephalus, neurofibromatosis, achondroplasia, intracranial hemorrhage, genetic syndrome (Fragile X), neoplasm, congenital infection, caput succedaneum, cephalohematoma, dolichocephaly, scaphocephaly, rickets, osteogenesis imperfecta
- Relies on the measurement of the occipitofrontal circumference (OFC) of the head

Disease	Etiology, Prevalence, Risk Factors	Clinical Symptoms and Signs	Diagnostics	Therapy, Prognosis, and Health Maintenance
Macrocephaly	OFC should be measured in all children between birth and 3 y/o and at neurologic or developmental visits Caused by increase in size of any cranial component (brain, CSF, blood, or bone) or increased ICP	1. An OFC greater than 2 standard deviations above the mean for given age, sex, and gestation (>97 percentile) Signs: 1. Bulging anterior fontanelle (MC) 2. Papilledema 3. Skin findings 4. Abnormal tone or DTRs, hypotonia, or spasticity	1. LP–rule out increased ICP 2. MRI/CT/XR/ultrasound 3. Metabolic evaluation 4. Genetic testing 5. Ophthalmologic testing	Treat underlying cause Referral if: 1. Syndromic features 2. Seizures or abnormal MRI 3. Hydrocephalus or mass lesions 4. Developmental problems

CHAPTER **33**

Orthopedics and Rheumatology

Recommended Topics (see Appendix G: Fractures, Dislocations, Tears):

Nursemaid's Elbow (Radial Head Subluxation), p 712
Slipped Capital Femoral Epiphysis (SCFE), p 726

Osgood-Schlatter Disease (Osteochondritis of Tibial Tubercle), p 721
Congenital Hip Dysplasia, see Developmental Dysplasia of the Hip (DDH), p 729
Avascular Necrosis (Osteochondroses), also see Legg-Calve-Perthes (LCP) Disease, p 726

OSTEOCHONDRITIS DISSECANS

Disease	Etiology, Prevalence, Risk Factors	Clinical Symptoms and Signs	Diagnostics	Therapy, Prognosis, and Health Maintenance
Osteochondritis dissecans	Wedge-shaped necrotic area of bone and cartilage develops adjacent to articular surface MC sites: Knee (medial femoral condyle), elbow (capitellum), talus (superior lateral dome)	1. Joint pain (first) 2. Local swelling or locking	1. Normal labs	1. Protect the involved area from mechanical damage 2. Stable/attached lesions–decrease activity and immobilize 3-6 mo 3. Unstable/dislodged lesions–surgery with arthroscopic drilling

NEOPLASIA OF THE MUSCULOSKELETAL SYSTEM

Disease	Etiology, Prevalence, Risk Factors	Clinical Symptoms and Signs	Diagnostics	Therapy, Prognosis, and Health Maintenance
Osteosarcoma	Malignant bone tumor Most common primary pediatric bone tumor MC in metaphyses of long bones	1. Pain and swelling in a LONG BONE • 50% in knee joint (distal femur or proximal tibia) • Persistent **bone pain that worsens at night or with activity** 2. May present with loss of function, mass, or limp	1. X-ray: lytic lesion with cortical destruction near metaphysis (**sunburst** appearance) 2. Biopsy (required)	No improvement with conservative therapy: 1. Chemotherapy • Radiation resistant 2. Limb sparing surgery (excision) or amputation 3. 20% have metastases at time of diagnosis: **lungs**, bone
Ewing sarcoma	Malignant bone tumor MC older children and adolescents MC sites: Long bones (femur, tibia, humerus) and axial skeleton (pelvis, ribs, spine)	1. Increasing **pain** and swelling at tumor site • No prior history of injury or trauma 2. Wakes child up at night 3. Fever Signs: 1. **Tenderness** 2. Swelling	1. X-ray: lytic mass with multi-laminated **periosteal "onion skin" reaction** (or moth-eaten appearance) 2. CBC: leukocytosis 3. Biopsy (required)	No improvement with conservative therapy: 1. Chemotherapy 2. Radiation therapy 3. Surgery 4. Metastasis in 25%: lungs, bone, marrow

Pediatrics

Disease	Etiology, Prevalence, Risk Factors	Clinical Symptoms and Signs	Diagnostics	Therapy, Prognosis, and Health Maintenance
Osteochondroma	Benign—most common benign tumor in children Bone mass capped with cartilage M > F	1. <u>Painless</u> mass • Pain caused by bursitis or tendinitis • Single or multiple	1. X-ray: stalk or broad-based projection from surface of bone	1. Excise if interfering with function 2. Good prognosis
Osteoid osteoma	Benign bone forming lesion of unclear etiology, children 5-20 y/o	1. Increasing pain, worse at night • **Relieved by NSAIDs or Aspirin** • Upper femur can cause referred pain to knee <u>Signs</u>: 1. Tenderness over lesion	1. X-ray: round lucency surrounded by sclerotic bone 2. CT scan (confirms)	1. Surgical excision or radiofrequency ablation 2. Good prognosis
Osteoblastoma	Benign, rare Presents in 20s M > F <u>MC location</u>: posterior column of spine Unknown etiology	1. Involves the spine 2. Dull aching chronic pain • No change at night 3. Nonresponsive to NSAIDs 4. Limp or neurologic symptoms secondary to cord compression	1. XR: variable findings 2. CT 3. MRI • Appears similar to osteoid osteoma, but larger (>2 cm diameter)	1. Curettage and bone grafting 2. En block excision for aggressive lesions 3. Radiation for spinal lesions that cannot be fully resected <u>Prognosis</u>: 1. Untreated, may cause progressive neurologic symptoms 2. Good prognosis if removed completely 3. 20% recurrence if expansion outside bone

JUVENILE RHEUMATOID ARTHRITIS (JRA)

- **Polyarthritis**: Five or more small or large joints
- **Pauciarticular**: Four or less medium to large joints
- **Enthesitis**: Inflammation of sites at which ligaments, tendons, or other fibrous structures insert to bone
- **Dactylitis**: Swelling within a digit that extends beyond borders of joints; "sausage digit"

- JRA is distinct from adult-onset arthritis and the term "rheumatoid" was removed to emphasize that childhood arthritis most often has no relationship to seropositive rheumatoid arthritis
- All definitions above and terms below are utilizing the International League of Associations for Rheumatology's (ILAR) guidelines revamped in the 1990s.

Disease	Etiology, Prevalence, Risk Factors	Clinical Symptoms and Signs	Diagnostics	Therapy, Prognosis, and Health Maintenance
Juvenile idiopathic arthritis (JIA), previously juvenile rheumatoid arthritis (JRA)	Most common arthritis in children <17 y/o Rheumatoid factor (+) in: infection, lupus, liver disease, malignancy – but most common cause is **VIRAL INFX** (+) ANA in liver disease, infection, malignancy and healthy	1. Arthritis lasting >6 wk to 3 mo in any **ONE joint (DIP)** 2. Onset age **16 y or less** 3. **Pain** 4. **Joint *swelling*** 5. +/– Gait disturbance (limp) 6. Difficulty with ADLs (writing, buttons) 7. Joint ***stiffness***, morning stiffness	1. DX of EXCLUSION 2. **RF (−)** in 95% with arthritis 3. ANA (+) in 95% of Lupus • 80% pauciarthritis 4. ESR (+) infection, malignancy, pregnancy, obesity 5. X-rays—least helpful for ruling out	<u>Goals</u>: 1. Control pain 2. Improve function 3. Prevent joint damage <u>Complications</u>: Uveitis, growth inhibition
Polyarticular JIA	**Diagnosis: Involvement of 4+ joints after 6 mo of illness** Divided according to presence or absence of rheumatoid factor Additional subgroups: age at onset, symmetric vs. asymmetric, presence/absence of ANA 30%-40% of JRA Complications: bony erosions and joint destruction, osteopenia, osteoporosis, TMJ, difficulty with ambulation; uveitis			

(continued)

(continued)

Pediatrics

Disease	Etiology, Prevalence, Risk Factors	Clinical Symptoms and Signs	Diagnostics	Therapy, Prognosis, and Health Maintenance
Polyarthritis-rheumatoid **factor positive (RF+)**	**Female**, 10%-14 y/o **Hispanic or black**	1. Rapid onset of **multiple** affected joints, including many **small** joints of **hands and feet** • Symmetric 2. Pain > stiffness or inflammation 3. Affects fingers, wrists, elbows, cervical spine, hips, knees, ankles 4. Severe morning **stiffness** 5. Fatigue, malaise Signs: 1. **Subcutaneous *nodules*** 2. *Multiple **swollen**, **painful*** joints	Clinical DX: 1. CBC: anemia, thrombocytosis 2. ESR: elevated 3. **ANA: (+)** 4. **Rheumatoid factor: (+)** 5. Joint films: erosions	1. NSAIDs (initial), may be used alone if low activity 2. DMARD (initial) in low disease with no response to NSAIDs in 2 mo 3. Methotrexate for severe disease Prognosis: 1. If RF (+), more likely to be female with more severe disease, may be HLA-DR4 (+) and/or anti-CCP Ab (+) = at risk for aggressive disease in absence of therapy 2. If ANA (+) or RF (−) at young age, screen more for anterior uveitis; higher risk Health maintenance: 1. Periodic slit-lamp examination for asymptomatic uveitis
Polyarthritis-rheumatoid **factor negative (RF−), sero-negative** polyarthritis	**Female** 2-5 y/o **White** Generalized: impaired development of normal bone mass, cortical > trabecular, failure accentuated at puberty, correlates with severity/activity of disease (prednisone) Localized: TMJ, overgrowth (leg-length discrepancy, premature closure of epiphyses (fingers)	1. Begins with 1-2 joints, indolent 2. Disease progresses rapidly after concurrent infection precipitates, then involves 5+ joints in first 6 mo • Difficulty with tasks, otherwise healthy 3. Symmetric involvement: wrist, knees, ankles 4. Morning **stiffness**, **swelling** in *multiple* **large** joints Signs: 1. Multiple **symmetric** swollen **large** joints, involvement of small joints of hands/feet 2. ***TMJ** and **c-spine*** involvement	Clinical DX: 1. CBC: normal or anemia, thrombocytosis 2. ESR: elevated or normal 3. **ANA: mostly (-)**, sometimes (+) 4. **RF: negative**, rarely (+) 5. Joint films: normal	

Juvenile *psoriatic* arthritis (psJIA) Children with arthritis + psoriasis OR Children with arthritis + (+) FH of psoriasis in 1st degree relative, plus dactylitis or pitting/onycholysis	**MC: White females** Bimodal distribution
	  • First peak in females (1-3 y/o), similar to early-onset oligoarticular
	  • Second peak during late childhood (9-11 y/o), resembles adult psoriatic arthritis
	Skin rash absent in 50% at onset, may lag 10 y behind onset of joint complaints
	7% of all JIA patients
	If younger, more likely to be female with (+) ANA
	MC joints affected: **Knee and ankle**, hip (30%)
	Highly suggestive: Isolated **DIP involvement** (though uncommon)
		1. May involve 1 joint or many (<5 in 80% of children)
		2. May present with
		  • *Single* swollen toe **(dactylitis)**
		    • Usually 2nd toe or index finger
		  • **Large** joint involvement **(knee)**
		  • *Asymmetric* oligoarticular picture with small/large joints
		3. +/− involvement of sacroiliac joints, spine, or peripheral entheses
		Young children:
		1. **Dactylitis** (common)
		2. Involvement of wrists and small joints of hands/feet
		Older children:
		1. **Enthesitis**
		  • Insertion of Achilles tendon, plantar fascia into calcaneus
		  • Hallmark of adult psoriatic arthritis
		2. **Spondylitis** or sacroiliitis (10%-30%)
		Other Signs:
		1. Chronic **painless Uveitis** (10%-15%)
		2. **Psoriatic rash** (40%-60%)
		  • Hairline, umbilicus, behind ears, intergluteal fold
		3. **Nail pitting** (50%-80%)
			Clinical DX:
			1. **Rheumatoid factor (−)**
			2. ESR/CRP: elevated
			3. Thrombocytosis
			4. ANA: low titer in 60%
			5. X-ray: bony changes, joint space narrowing
			6. MRI—rule out enthesitis or sacroiliitis
			7. (+) FH psoriasis excludes patients with rheumatoid factor (+) disease for diagnosis of polyarthritis
				1. **NSAIDs**
				  • First line, but not monotherapy >2 mo
				2. DMARDs:
				  • **Methotrexate**
				  • Leflunomide
				    • Initiate at DX
				    • For patients with multiple joint involvement
				3. TNF antagonists
				Prognosis:
				1. In absence of treatment, 60%-80% will develop arthritis in 5+ joints
				2. Sacroiliitis occurs in older patients (+) for HLA-B27 Ag
				3. Remission achieved in majority of patients

Disease	Etiology, Prevalence, Risk Factors	Clinical Symptoms and Signs	Diagnostics	Therapy, Prognosis, and Health Maintenance
Oligoarticular JIA or **pauciarticular**–onset JRA	Bimodal: 1-4 or 20-30 y/o **Female** White Typical presentation: toddler girl noticed to be limping without complaint "Pain in both knees and R-ankle" 50% of JRA cases (+) rheumatoid factor or FH of psoriasis or spondyloarthropathy excludes disease	1. Fussy or "walks funny" in the morning • May *refuse* to walk 2. Later plays normally and sometimes with a limp 3. Otherwise healthy (no constitutional SX) Signs: 1. Swollen and tender: **knees** > **ankles** > wrist, elbow • Warm, no erythema • 50% **monoarticular** 2. Associated: Chronic **uveitis, iridocyclitis** (20%), leg-length discrepancy Complications: TMJ arthritis (75%), uveitis (20%), leg-length discrepancy, short stature	No diagnostic tests: 1. ANA: (+) in 80% 2. Rheumatoid factor (−) 3. CBC, ESR, x-ray = normal DX criteria: • Arthritis in 4 or less joints in first 6 m after r/o other causes	1. **NSAIDs**: Naprosyn, ibuprofen • Relief within 2 wk 2. Intra-articular corticosteroid injections: methylprednisolone acetate, triamcinolone acetate • Used to prevent leg-length discrepancy • First line for moderate to high disease activity 3. DMARDs: methotrexate Prognosis: 1. 50% progress to polyarticular 2. 36% remiss 3. If ANA (+), increased risk of iridocyclitis or uveitis Poor prognostic factors: • Hip or spine arthritis • Ankle or wrist, marked elevation of ESR/CRP • Radiographic evidence of joint damage
Systemic JIA (Still disease) Difficult to diagnose: • Arthritis not always evident early on • Systemic symptoms not always typical • No diagnostic tests • Mimics infection or malignancy first with no response to antibiotics	Any age, white M: F (50:50) Can start as early as 1 y/o or less Refers to patients with rash and intermittent fever in addition to arthritis of any number of joints **Autoinflammatory**, unrelated to other forms of childhood arthritis 10%-15% of JRA Adult-onset Still disease: if begins age 16+ y	1. Intermittent daily **fever** (>38.5°C) for at least **2 wk** 2. Persistent **arthritis 6+ wk** (88%) • Most oligoarthritis or polyarthritis • Affects wrists, ankles, knees mostly • May start in hips and rapidly progress • Required for diagnosis 3. **Rash** (81%) 4. Lymphadenopathy (31%) 5. Arthralgias 6. No response to antibiotics Signs: 1. High–grade fever: 102°–106°F 2. Macular, salmon-pink rash • Round to oval macules of differing size • Found in axillae and around waist • Prominent with fever, fades when afebrile • Koebnerizes 3. *Multiple* swollen joints or no arthritis for months 4. Micrognathia 5. Cervical spine fusion Complications: Pericarditis (effusion), HSM, pleural effusion, Kawasaki disease, lymphadenoapthy, uveitis (rare)	DX of exclusion: 1. WBC >15 000– left shift, granulocytosis 2. Anemia (common, profound) 3. Thrombocytosis: >1 million 4. ESR/ferritin: very elevated 5. ANA, RF: negative 6. U/A: normal	1. **NSAIDs**, then refer to rheumatology 2. Adjunct **biologics** • IL-1 Receptor Antagonist: Daily Anakinra Injection • Anti-IL-6 Receptor Monoclonal Ab: tocilizumab • Anti-IL-1-beta Monoclonal Ab: canakinumab 3. Steroids if persistent 4. If refractory, DMARDs Health maintenance: 1. Limited steroid use 2. PT, OT, nutrition, psychosocial support Prognosis: 1. Better if response to adequate therapy 2. Poor prognosis with pulmonary complications MC complications: **Macrophage activation system (MAS)**, severe growth retardation, osteoporosis; others include ILD, pulmonary HTN, lipoid PNA, alveolar proteinosis
Enthesitis-related arthritis	Arthritis + enthesitis in children with 2+ of following: • Sacroiliac joint tenderness • Inflammatory spinal pain • HLA-B27 (+) • (+) FH anterior uveitis with pain, spondyloarthropathy, or IBD • Anterior uveitis with pain, redness, or photophobia			

Eye Exam Screening Recommendations from AAP for Patients with JIA

	ANA (+)	ANA (−)
Onset of JIA <6 y/o	1. Disease <4 y/o: every 3 mo 2. Disease 4-7 y/o: every 6 mo 3. Disease >7 y/o: every 12 mo	1. Disease <4 y/o: every 6 mo 2. Disease >4 y/o: every 12 mo
Onset of JIA >6 y/o	1. Disease <2 y/o: every 6 mo 2. Disease >2 y/o: every 12 mo	1. Every 12 mo
Enthesitis-related JIA RF (+) polyarticular JIA systemic JIA	Every 12 mo, regardless of ANA status, age of onset, or disease duration	

SCOLIOSIS

Disease	Etiology, Prevalence, Risk Factors	Clinical Symptoms and Signs	Diagnostics	Therapy, Prognosis, and Health Maintenance
Scoliosis	F, 8-10 y/o Lateral curvature of the spine associated with rotation of the involved vertebrae and classified by its anatomic location, in either the thoracic or lumbar spine, with rare involvement of the cervical spine 80% idiopathic 5%-7% congenital	1. No significant pain • If pain, r/o infection or tumor 2. Deformity of rib cage or asymmetry of waistline Signs: 1. Forward bending test 2. Scoliometer or inclinometer: good screening tool for angle of rotation	1. Calculate the **Cobb angle** using AP and lateral x-ray films of entire spine 2. *60-90 degrees*: respiratory complaints, or neuromuscular cause: **PFT**, especially if surgery being considered; at high risk for cardiopulmonary compromise and secondary restrictive lung disease	Treatment—based on Cobb angle and symptoms *<10 degrees*: observation only *<20 degrees*: no treatment, unless they show progression *20-40 degrees*: Bracing *40-60 degrees*: surgical *fusion*

CHAPTER 34

Endocrinology

Refer to Internal Medicine 🩺 for in-depth coverage of the following topics:

Refer to Appendices for the following topics:

Recommended Supplemental Topics:

SHORT STATURE (FIG. 34-1)

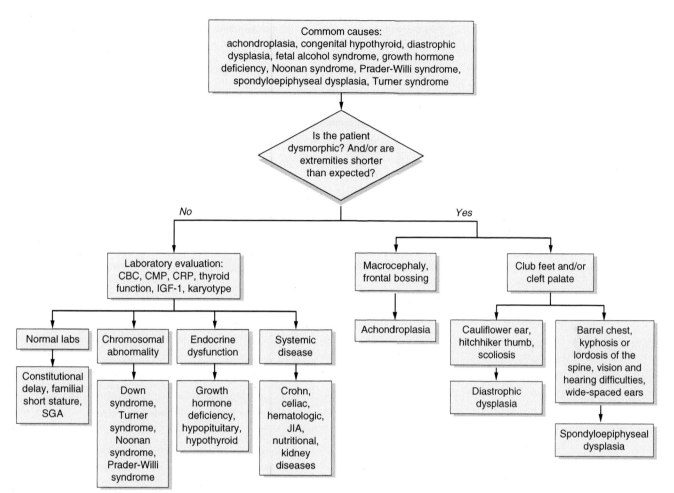

FIGURE 34-1. Workup for short stature. (From Michols NJ, Baldwin A. *5-Minute Clinical Consult 2018*. Philadelphia: Wolters Kluwer Health; 2017.)

- Infantile growth (first 1 to 2 years): linear growth, rapid, gradually decelerates
- Childhood growth: growth at constant velocity, slowing later in childhood
  - Age 2 to 4 years: 5.5 to 9 cm/year
  - Age 4 to 6 years: 5 to 8.5 cm/year
  - Age 6 to puberty: 4 to 6 cm/year (boys); 4.5 to 6.5 cm/year (girls)

- Children with height velocity above these cutoff points have a nonpathologic cause of short stature, but below these points are likely to have pathologic causes requiring further evaluation
- Adolescent growth: growth spurt of 8 to 14 cm/year due to synergistic effects of increasing gonadal steroids and growth hormone
  - Puberty starts at age 10 in girls (as early as 8)
  - Puberty starts at age 12 in boys (as early as 10)

Disease	Etiology, Prevalence, Risk Factors	Clinical Symptoms and Signs	Diagnostics	Therapy, Prognosis, and Health Maintenance
Short stature	<u>MCC</u> (beyond 1-2 y): Familial (genetic) short stature, constitutional short stature (constitutional delay of growth and puberty)	1. Height 2 standard deviations below the mean for individuals of same sex and chronological age • Ht < 2/3rd percentile 2. Do not require further evaluation unless: • Progressively declining height percentiles (growth failure) • Dysmorphic features • Evidence of underlying systemic disease <u>Signs</u>: 1. Height velocity • Serial measurements of height/length	1. Evaluate growth rate (**height velocity**) • More sensitive indicator 2. Check **bone age** if: • Normal growth rate • No other symptoms • Delayed: 2+ SD below mean 3. Check nutrition: albumin 4. CBC, electrolytes, BUN/Cr, calcium, phosphate, alk-phos, urinalysis, ESR/CRP, celiac serologies, thyroid testing, LH/FSH 5. Karyotype–females • CMA if dysmorphic	1. Growth hormone therapy for children with ISS (below) • Diagnosis of exclusion • Height predicted by the mid-parental height • Given SQ daily <u>Health maintenance</u>: 1. Serial growth measurements
Achondroplasia (Fig. 34-2A-F)	Autosomal dominant, mutation in *FGFR3* gene, 80% arise de novo Most common bone dysplasia in humans <u>Prevalence</u>: 0.005%	1. Disproportionate **short stature** 2. **Large head** 3. Delayed motor development 4. Brachydactyly: shortened fingers and toes <u>Signs</u>: 1. **Rhizomelic shortening**: Short limbs (upper arms) compared to trunk • Redundant skin folds in upper extremities • Difficulty with extension of UE and supination 2. **Trident hands** (broad, space between middle fingers) • Joint laxity 3. **Macrocephaly** 4. Flat nasal bridge (**saddle nose deformity**) 5. Frontal bossing and midface retrusion 6. Kyphoscoliosis 7. **Accentuated lumbar lordosis** after 1.5 y 8. Narrow chest	Clinical/radiographic DX: 1. AP x-ray • Large calvaria, narrowed foramen magnum • Short long bones with metaphyseal abnormalities • Progressive caudal narrowing • Round pelvis with flat, round iliac bones • Short, narrow chest • Proximal scooping of femoral metaphyses 2. Molecular testing (<u>confirmatory</u>)	1. Physical therapy for delayed motor development 2. Occupational therapy for ADLs 3. Limb lengthening surgery 4. Weight management: nutrition and physical activity 5. Referral to ENT for tonsillectomy and adenoidectomy 6. Leg bowing–PT and braces (rare) 7. Referral to neurosurgery for spinal stenosis or cervical compression <u>Health maintenance</u>: 1. Plot linear growth and head circumference 2. C-section for pregnant women with achondroplasia due to small pelvic size <u>Prognosis</u>: 1. Adult height: ~4 ft 2. When both parents have achondroplasia, the risk of their children having homozygous achondroplasia (lethal) is 25%, and 50% nonhomozygous achondroplasia 3. Stenosis of lumbar spine during 20-30s 4. Delayed motor development • Hold head at 4-7 mo • Sit alone 9-11 mo • Crawl 9-10 mo • Walk 16-22 mo <u>Complications</u>: Recurrent otitis media, OSA, obesity, genu varum, spinal stenosis, cervical medullary compression
Growth hormone deficiency	Decreased growth velocity Delayed skeletal maturation in *absence of other explanation* <u>MC</u>: **Idiopathic** GHD	<u>Infants</u>: 1. Normal birth weight or slightly reduced length 2. *Hypoglycemia* 3. Micropenis 4. Excess truncal adiposity	1. **IGF-1 and GH** stimulation testing 2. GH: low (not really helpful) 3. IGF-1: helpful in nourished child	1. SQ GH 0.15-0.3 mg/kg/d 2. Approved for: GHD, chronic renal failure, Turner syndrome, Prader-Willi, and Noonan, SGA

Pediatrics

Disease	Etiology, Prevalence, Risk Factors	Clinical Symptoms and Signs	Diagnostics	Therapy, Prognosis, and Health Maintenance

Turner syndrome (gonadal dysgenesis)	**45, XO karyotype**—no X or Y from dad (loss of X chromosome)
	Prevalence:
	0.04%-05%
	All or part of 1 of the X chromosomes is missing
	Lack of gonadal estrogen → failed breast development (Tanner 1-2)
		1. **Primary amenorrhea** (no period)
		2. **Short stature**
		  • Growth velocity <10th percentile
		3. **Infertility**
		4. Congenital cardiac malformations common
		Signs:
		1. **Short and stocky** build
		2. Micrognathia
		3. **Shield chest** (broad, flat)
		4. *Webbed neck*
		5. Widely spaced nipples
		6. High arched palate
		7. Short 4th metacarpal
		8. Low posterior hairline
		9. **Hand/feet lymphedema**
		10. Multiple pigmented nevi
		11. **Cubitus valgus**—increased carrying angle of arm
		12. **Madelung (bayonet)** deformity of forearm and wrist
		13. Genu valgum (knocked knees) or varum (bowlegged)
		14. Strabismus
		15. Scant pubic hair
		Associated:
		Recurrent otitis media nail dysplasia, learning difficulties, hearing loss, hypothyroidism, scoliosis (20%), kyphosis (50%), **primary hypogonadism** (common, AKA gonadal dysgenesis)
			Clinical DX:
			1. Diagnosed incidentally during prenatal testing and confirmed by **karyotype** (FISH)
			2. TSH, free or total T4
			  • Begin at 4 y/o, check for autoimmune thyroid disorders (15%)
			3. **FSH: increased** (20-40); measure **AMH**
			  • Measure at 10-11 y to estimate ovarian function and predict need for ERT
			  • **AMH: most sensitive**
			4. Renal ultrasound—look for renal abnormalities (30%-40%)
			5. Check tTG-IgA for Celiac disease
			6. Complications:
			Coarctation of the aorta (17%), **bicuspid aortic valve**, **aortic dissection**, hypoplastic left heart syndrome, Pulmonary stenosis, **Hypertension** (common), hypothyroidism, celiac disease, strabismus, amblyopia, ptosis, lymphedema, primary hypogonadism
				1. Cardiology eval
				  • EKG and echo, BP, **cardiac MRI** (most sensitive)
				2. Treat HTN >140/90
				  • β blockers or ACE inhibitors
				3. Support stockings, lymphatic drainage massage, PT, or vascular surgery for lymphedema
				4. Short stature—recombinant human GH
				  • Start if height <5th percentile
				5. Primary hypogonadism—ERT at 10-11 y/o if no breast development
				  • Use transdermal estradiol patch
				Health maintenance:
				1. Not GH deficient but may improve final height with treatment
				2. Repeat cardiac imaging every 5-10 y
				3. Monitor BP regularly
				4. Neuropsychological testing
				  • Prior to pre-K or kindergarten, again prior to middle and high school
				5. Serial audiological evaluations
				  • Every 1-5 y
				6. Surveillance of scoliosis and kyphosis
				7. Eye exam at age 12-18 mo or at diagnosis
				  • R/o strabismus, amblyopia, ptosis
				8. Monitor growth curves
				9. Annual physical and testing (thyroid, glucose tolerance, lipid panel, LFTs), hearing loss, CV disease
				Prognosis:
				1. Patients with Y chromosome mosaicism have increased risk for **gonadoblastoma**
				  • Requires prophylactic oophorectomy or salpingooophorectomy
				2. CHD and CVA account for 41% of deaths

(continued)

Pediatrics

(continued)

Disease	Etiology, Prevalence, Risk Factors	Clinical Symptoms and Signs	Diagnostics	Therapy, Prognosis, and Health Maintenance

Neonatal Down syndrome		Signs:
		1. Flat facial profile
		2. Slanted palpebral fissures
		3. Anomalous ears
		4. Hypotonia
		5. Poor Moro reflex
		6. Dysplasia of midphalanx of 5th digit
		7. Transverse palmar (Simian) crease
		8. Excessive skin at nape of neck
		9. Hyperflexible joints
		10. Dysplasia of pelvis
			1. Diagnosis made by **prenatal screening in utero**
			  • Combined test at 11-13 and 6/7ths wk gestation
			    • Detects 85%, 5% false positive rate
			  • Full integrated test
			    • Detects 85%, 1% false-positive rate
			    • Results in 2nd trimester
			  • If screen *positive*: Amniocentesis >15 wk or CVS through 14 wk for definitive or secondary screening test on cell free DNA
				Prognosis:
				1. Developmental impairment
				  • Sitting and walking occurs at twice normal age
				  • Language development at twice normal age
				Associated: polycythemia (65%), IDA

Down syndrome in children and adults	Trisomy 21 (three copies of 21) Most common chromosome abnormality among infants Comorbidities: autism (7%) Most have CHD (50%) • 37% CVASD • 31% VSD • 15% ASD • Most frequent form of intellectual disability	1. Mild to severe mental retardation 2. Congenital heart disease Signs: 1. Flat nasal bridge 2. Folded or dysplastic ears, low set, small 3. Transverse palmar crease (**Simian crease**), short 5th digit 4. Upward slanting palpebral fissure 5. Epicanthic folds 6. Open mouth; protruding, large wrinkled tongue 7. Wide gap between first and second toes (**sandal gap**) 8. Brachycephaly 9. Brushfield spots 10. Short neck, excessive skin at nape of neck 11. Narrow palate, abnormal teeth 12. Hyperflexible joints 13. Short broad hands Associated: Umbilical hernia	Clinical DX: 1. **Karyotype** (confirmatory) 2. CBC at birth • R/o myeloproliferative d/o and polycythemia, monitor for leukemia 3. Hgb—annually starting at age 1 for IDA 4. Neurologic abnormalities—get MRI to r/o spinal compression 5. Polysomnography—monitor for sleep apnea 6. Associated: ADHD, conduct disorder, ODD, aggressive behavior, Alzheimer disease, celiac disease, short stature, obesity, eye problems (refractive errors, strabismus, nystagmus), hearing impairment (38%-78%), otitis media, hypo or hyperthyroidism, type I diabetes, leukemia (1%-1.5%), OSA (30%-75%), palmoplantar hyperkeratosis (41%)	1. Pediatric cardiology evaluation incl. echo 2. Newborn hearing screen 3. Ophthalmologic evaluation before 6 mo, then annually 4. Thyroid function testing in newborn period: 6 mo, 12 mo, then annually 5. Monitor for celiac at 1 y Health maintenance: 1. Plot growth, monitor for growth disorders, weight gain, hypothyroidism, celiac 2. Monitor for otitis media 3. Monitor for hearing impairment Prognosis: 1. Nearly all males are infertile, women are fertile and may become pregnant 2. Shorter life expectancy: 50-60s
Noonan syndrome	Autosomal dominant	Signs: 1. Triangular face 2. Downward slanting eyes, ptosis 3. Low-set ears with thick helices 4. High nasal bridge 5. Pectus carinatum or excavatum 6. Webbed neck		

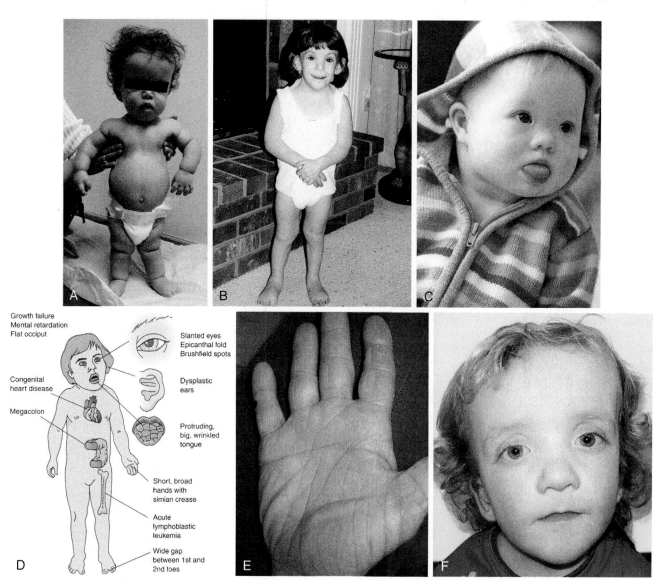

FIGURE 34-2. A, Achondroplasia. **B,** Characteristic facies of Turner syndrome. **C,** Characteristic facies of neonatal down syndrome. **D,** Characteristics in Down syndrome. **E,** Simian crease. **F,** Characteristic facies of Noonan syndrome. (**A,** From Coombs C, Kirk AS. *Oski's Pediatric Certification and Recertification Board Review.* Philadelphia: Wolters Kluwer Health; 2011. **B,** From Nettina SM. *The Lippincott Manual of Nursing Practice.* 7th ed. Philadelphia, PA: Lippincott Williams & Wilkins; 2000. **C,** From Beall M, Ross MH. *Lippincott's Obstetrics Case-Based Review.* Philadelphia: Wolters Kluwer Health; 2012. **D,** From Rubin R, Strayer DS, Rubin E. *Rubin's Pathology.* Philadelphia: Wolters Kluwer Health; 2012. **E,** Image provided by Stedman's. **F,** From Allen HD, Driscoll DJ, Shaddy RE, Feltes TF. *Moss & Adams' Heart Disease in Infants, Children, and Adolescents.* Philadelphia: Wolters Kluwer Health; 2013.)

Normal Variants of Growth

- Familial short stature—also known as genetic short stature is most often a normal variant; low to normal growth velocity throughout life
- Constitutional delay of growth and puberty (CDGP)—also known as constitutional short stature for prepubertal children results in childhood short stature but relatively normal adult height; normal size at birth with a decline in growth rate at 3 to 6 months of age, but tends to be more severe and prolonged; by 3 to 4 years of age they grow at a low to normal growth rate; growth remains below 3rd percentile; marked height discrepancy during early teenage years, but followed by catch-up growth during puberty
  - Hallmark: delayed skeletal age
  - Height data interpreted according to bone age, rather than chronological age
  - Often a FH of delayed growth and puberty in one or both parents "late bloomer"
- Idiopathic short stature—definition of short stature above, in absence of any endocrine, metabolic or other diagnosis; normal height velocity; Short Stature HOmeoboX (*SHOX*) gene mutations in 1% to 4%

Pathologic Causes of Growth Failure

- Systemic disorders with secondary effects on growth
  - Undernutrition—delayed pattern of growth that can be isolated by inadequate food supply or self-imposed restriction, or underlying disease interfering with food intake/absorption (hallmark: low weight for height)
  - Steroid therapy—can occur with or without features of Cushing syndrome; suppresses growth through endogenous GH secretion, nitrogen retention, and collagen formation
- Gastrointestinal disease (IBD), JIA, CKD, malignancy, cystic fibrosis, heart disease, HIV, inborn errors of metabolism, type 1 diabetes, vitamin D deficiency, hypothyroidism, GH deficiency, precocious puberty, Turner Syndrome, SHOX mutations, Prader Willi syndrome, Noonan syndrome, Russell-Silver syndrome, skeletal dysplasias
- BA = bone age; CA = chronological age

	CA > BA	CA = BA	CA < BA
Normal growth velocity (Fig. 34-3)	1. **Constitutional delay of growth** (normal variant) = 2. NON-pathologic (LATE BLOOMER) 3. Delay in skeletal maturity and onset of puberty 4. Growth continues beyond time the average child stops growing	1. **Familial genetic short stature** = NON-pathologic	
Abnormal growth velocity	1. Malnutrition, chronic disorder, endocrine – height level curves off, weight NL or increases (**pathologic**)	Malnutrition, chromosomal disorder	1. Precocious puberty

HYPERTHYROIDISM AND HYPOTHYROIDISM

- T4 is converted to T3 by deiodination outside of the thyroid
- T3 is more biologically active than T4
- Most of T4 (and T3) is reversibly bound to TBG and is inactive - highly bound to protein, especially albumin and can cause hypoalbuminemia if given in too high of quantity
- Factors that increase TBG (and total T4): pregnancy, liver disease, OCPs and ASA

Disease	Etiology, Prevalence, Risk Factors	Clinical Symptoms and Signs	Diagnostics	Therapy, Prognosis, and Health Maintenance
Hyperthyroidism in infants	F > M Children: MC cause is Graves (see below)	1. Jittery 2. Loose stool 3. Worsening school performance, poor concentration, hyperactivity 4. Fatigue 5. Emotionally labile 6. Nervous, personality disturbance 7. Insomnia 8. **Weight loss** 9. **Palpitations** 10. Heat intolerance, sweating Signs: 1. **Tachycardia**, tremor, proximal muscle weakness, warm skin	1. **Thyroid function tests (TFTs)** 2. TSH: low 3. Total T3: high 4. Free T4: high 5. **Autoantibody tests** • Antithyroid peroxidase Ab • TS-immunoglobulin	1. Symptomatic relief A. **Propranolol**– Relieves tachycardia, tremor, sweating, anxiety 2. **Anti-thyroid meds** • Methimazole • Potent, long acting • Propylthiouracil (PTU)
Hypothyroidism in infants	Severe cretinism (congenital hypothyroid), mental impairment AAP recommends screening between days **2-4 of birth** (newborn)	1. Round face, hirsute forehead, large anterior/posterior fontanelle, wide suture 2. Protruding tongue 3. Hoarse cry 4. Distended abdomen 5. Prolonged jaundice 6. **Lethargy** 7. Poor weight gain 8. **Constipation** Signs: 1. Dry skin 2. Hypoactivity, poor feeding, mottling 3. Hypothermia 4. Poor muscle tone 5. Macroglossia (large tongue) 6. Hypertelorism	1. Thyroid function tests 2. Serum TSH: **high** (most sensitive), if low → secondary 3. Free T4: **low** in clinically overt 4. Antibody Testing 5. CBC: **Normocytic anemia (MC)**	See Treatment of Hypothyroidism in Adults

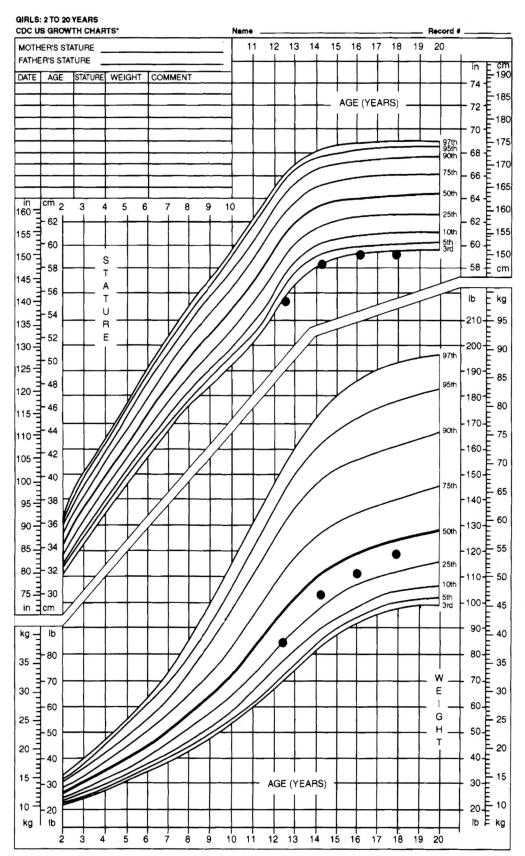

FIGURE 34-3. Growth chart of patient with familial genetic short stature. (From Sabella C, Cunningham RJ. *Cleveland Clinic Intensive Review of Pediatrics.* Philadelphia: Wolters Kluwer Health; 2014.)

CONGENITAL ADRENAL HYPERPLASIA

Disease	Etiology, Prevalence, Risk Factors	Clinical Symptoms and Signs	Diagnostics	Therapy, Prognosis, and Health Maintenance
Congenital adrenal hyperplasia (CAH) Deficiency in 1 of 5 enzymes to produce cortisol = cortisol deficiency	Autosomal recessive MC: **21-hydroxylase deficiency** No cortisol produced, which normally inhibits hypothalamus Overproduces ACTH without feedback suppression → hypertrophy	1. Females: Virilization with mild clitoromegaly to complete fusion of labioscrotal folds 2. Adrenal insufficiency—salt loss 3. Hyperpigmentation of skin on labial/scrotal folds and nipples History: 2nd week of life, lethargy, irritable, poor feeding, vomiting, poor weight gain	1. Bedside glucose level: low 2. Serum electrolytes: **hyponatremia, hyperkalemia** 3. Elevated urinary and plasma androgens (DHEA, androstenedione), ketosteroids 4. Decreased aldosterone • No effect on estrogen, LH, FSH 5. Definitive: serum hormone levels	1. **Steroid hormone replacement**: glucocorticoids, mineralocorticoids, reconstructive surgery • **Hydrocortisone urgently** Neonates: 25 mg IV/IO Toddlers: 50 mg IV/IO Adolescent: 100 mg IV/IO If hyperkalemic—IV calcium gluconate 100 mg/kg DO NOT GIVE insulin/glucose → hypoglycemia

CUSHING SYNDROME (HYPERCORTISOLISM)

Disease	Etiology, Prevalence, Risk Factors	Clinical Symptoms and Signs	Diagnostics	Therapy, Prognosis, and Health Maintenance
Cushing syndrome (hypercortisolism)	Excessive cortisol production Most common cause: **iatrogenic** due to prescribed prednisone (steroids), androgen excess absent (exogenous steroids suppress production by adrenals) Second most common cause: ACTH-secreting **adenoma** → bilateral adrenal hyperplasia (androgen excess common) Children: Poor growth rate, short stature, delayed skeletal maturation	1. Purple striae, buffalo hump, central **obesity** 2. "Moon" facies, lanugo hair, acne, easy bruising 3. **Proximal muscle weakness** and wasting, osteoporosis, AVN of femoral head 4. Headache 5. Depression, mania Signs: 1. Hypertension 2. **Diabetes** (decreased glucose tolerance) 3. **Menstrual irregularity, infertility** (hypogonadism) 4. Masculinization (androgen excess)	1. **HD dexamethasone suppression test** • Decrease by 50% unless ACTH or adrenal tumor 2. Midnight serum cortisol, late night salivary cortisol • Specific and sensitive 3. **24-h urinary free cortisol**: high, primary test 4. CT or MRI Sustained elevated cortisol: Hypercortisolism *Hypokalemia* *Hyperglycemia* *Glucosuria*	If iatrogenic → taper steroids: 1. **Oral glucocorticoids and mineralocorticoids** 2. If ACTH-secreting pituitary adenoma → transsphenoidal resection of tumor 3. Adrenal adenoma → pituitary radiation, medical adrenalectomy 4. Bilateral adrenalectomy Complications: Ectopic ACTH production (**2/3 SCC from lungs**)

OBESITY

Disease	Etiology, Prevalence, Risk Factors	Clinical Symptoms and Signs	Diagnostics	Therapy, Prognosis, and Health Maintenance
Obesity	12-19: BMI >95th percentile for age and gender (obese), 85%-95% (overweight) RF: Obesity, HTN, tobacco use, high lipid levels Comorbidities: Social marginalization, poor self-esteem, depression, poor QOL	1. Altered consciousness 2. Deep breathing 3. Fruity breath odor Complications: DVT, PE, asthma, OSA, proteinuria, gallstones, risk for cirrhosis and colon cancer, Blount disease, SCFE, flat feet, dyslipidemia, HTN, LVH, type 2 DM, PCOS, hypogonadism	1. 85-94th percentile: fasting lipid levels, no RF necessary 2. 94-95th + RF: fasting lipids, AST/ALT, serum glucose 3. >95th: fasting lipids, AST/ALT, serum glucose Weight goals (if obese) <12: maintenance 1 lb/mo >12: 2 lb/wk Only med for >12: Orlistat (lipase inhibitor)	1. Recommend ≥5 servings of fruits and vegetables per day 2. No more than 2 h of screen time per day • No television in room where teen sleeps 3. Minimize or eliminate sugar-sweetened beverages 4. Address eating behaviors (eg, avoid skipping breakfast) 5. Recommend ≥1 h of moderate intensity physical activity per day 6. Involve whole family in lifestyle changes and acknowledge cultural differences

DIABETES MELLITUS

- 1.7 times higher risk of CV disease
- Leading cause of blindness (30% with diabetic retinopathy)
- All endogenous glucose comes from **hepatic** output
  - Glycogenolysis: breakdown of glycogen (stored in the liver)
  - Gluconeogenesis: glucose made from carbohydrates and proteins (dietary sources)
- Glucose homeostasis (carbohydrate homeostasis)
  - Mouth—amylase in saliva
  - Upper GI tract—amylase released from pancreas
    - Brush border enzymes on intestinal wall
    - Monosaccharides taken to blood, liver, other organs
  - Pancreas
    - Alpha cells—respond to low blood sugar → glucagon release → stimulates liver to break down glycogen and release glucose into the blood
    - Beta cells—respond to high blood sugar → insulin release → stimulates muscle and fat cells to take glucose from blood
      - *Insulin*—stores glucose, impacts lipids, ketones, and proteins
      - *Amylin*—inhibits glucagon secretion by binding receptors in the brain, slows gastric emptying, promotes feelings of satiety
  - Releases glucose into the blood
  - Releases free fatty acids from stored fat
- Definitions
  - Insulin sensitivity—insulin's ability to lower circulating glucose
  - Insulin resistance—low insulin sensitivity to tyrosine kinase receptors
    - Increased with aging, sedentary lifestyle, and abdominovisceral obesity

- Incretin hormones
  - GLP-1: peptide hormone secreted in the gut, release stimulated by ingestion of food, stimulates insulin release, and suppresses glucagon release (inactivated by DPP-4)
- **Dawn phenomenon**: increased resistance to insulin in the early morning due to counter-regulatory hormones
  - Increase overnight basal insulin, exercise, metformin, TZD
- **Somogyi phenomenon**: rebound fasting hyperglycemia following undetected hypoglycemia overnight
  - Excessive hunger, weight gain, worsening hyperglycemia
  - Decrease overnight basal insulin or eat a snack at bedtime
- Effects of insulin
  - Liver—decreased gluconeogenesis and glycogenolysis
  - Muscle—increased glucose uptake
  - Endothelium—increased vasodilation
  - Adipose—decreased lipolysis
  - Brain—decreased appetite
  - Lipids—increased HDL, decreased triglycerides
  - Kidney—decreased gluconeogenesis, albuminuria, and glomerulosclerosis

Screening children

- BMI for age/sex >85th percentile
- Weight for height >85th percentile
- Weight >120%
- PLUS 2 risk factors
- Start at age 10 (onset of puberty), screen with A1C, fasting glucose, or 2 hours OGTT
- Use OGTT if patient is prediabetic
- If normal results → repeat at least every 3 years

CHAPTER **35**

Urology and Renal

Refer to Family Medicine [icon] **for in-depth coverage of the following topics:**

Glomerulonephritis, p 177
Cystitis, p 175

Refer to Internal Medicine [icon] **for in-depth coverage of the following topics:**

Testicular Torsion, Hydrocele, p 241

Recommended Supplemental Topics:

Nephrotic Syndrome, p 177 [icon]

CRYPTORCHIDISM

Disease	Etiology, Prevalence, Risk Factors	Clinical Symptoms and Signs	Diagnostics	Therapy, Prognosis, and Health Maintenance
Cryptorchidism	**Increases risk for testicular cancer** 1%-2% of males after 1 y of age Underlying hypogonadism, including hypogonadic hypogonadism	1. One or both testes absent from scrotum at birth 2. Distinguish from retractile testes – which requires treatment	1. **MRI** > Ultrasound 2. 1500 units IM hCG × 3 d should cause significant rise in testosterone if testes present	1. Therapy with hCG works in 25% 2. Surgery: orchiopexy • Reduces risk of infertility • Decreases risk of neoplasia

HYPOSPADIAS, PARAPHIMOSIS, PHIMOSIS

Disease	Etiology, Prevalence, Risk Factors	Clinical Symptoms and Signs	Diagnostics	Therapy, Prognosis, and Health Maintenance
Paraphimosis Due to chronic inflammation under redundant foreskin, leading to contracture of the preputial opening and formation of tight ring of skin when foreskin is retracted behind the glans	Foreskin, once retracted over the glans, cannot be replaced into normal position RF: Frequent catheterization without reducing foreskin, forcibly retracting constricted foreskin, vigorous sexual activity	1. Pain, edema, tenderness, erythema of glans and foreskin Signs: 1. Skin ring causes venous congestion leading to EDEMA and enlargement of the GLANS 2. Arterial occlusion and necrosis of the glans may also occur	None required	1. Manual reduction: firmly squeeze the glans for 5 min to reduce edema and size of glans 2. Surgery: may require incision under local anesthesia 3. Emergent urologic referral and circumcision 4. Antibiotics and circumcision should be completed after inflammation goes away
Phimosis	Foreskin that *cannot* be retracted Congenital: children, adolescents, physiologic Acquired: adults with poor hygiene and chronic balanitis	1. **EDEMA**, erythema, tenderness of prepuce 2. Presence of purulent discharge 3. Inability to retract foreskin over glans penis 4. Obstructed urinary stream, hematuria, pain of prepuce	None required	1. Asymptomatic → watch and wait 2. Symptomatic → refer for circumcision 3. Initial infection treated with broad spectrum antibiotics 4. Circumcision should be avoided in <2 y until reach age when general anesthesia can be administered

Disease	Etiology, Prevalence, Risk Factors	Clinical Symptoms and Signs	Diagnostics	Therapy, Prognosis, and Health Maintenance
Hypospadias	Associated with chordee: ventral curvature of penis Both genetic and environmental RF: Subfertility in father, maternal age, IUGR, fetal exposure to oral progestins or combined progestins and estrogens	1. Urethra is abnormally placed where the meatus is proximal and ventral to its normal or anterior location	1. Bilateral renal ultrasound to r/o ascending pathology 2. If severe, evaluate: gonadotropin, AMG, inhibin B, testosterone secretion at 1-3 mo or response to hCG	1. Do not circumcise 2. Refer to pediatric urologist

ENURESIS

- Differential: cystitis, diabetes insipidus, diabetes mellitus, seizure disorders, neurogenic bladder, anatomic abnormalities (urethral obstruction), constipation, psychological stress, and child maltreatment
- Nocturnal polyuria: production of urine >130% of expected bladder capacity for age
  - Calculated (mL) = 30 × (age in years +1)
- Relapse: more than one wet night per month after a period of dryness

Disease	Etiology, Prevalence, Risk Factors	Clinical Symptoms and Signs	Diagnostics	Therapy, Prognosis, and Health Maintenance
Enuresis	Urination into the clothing during the day and into the bed at night by a child to who is chronologically and developmentally older than 5 y/o RF: Boys, first-degree relative	1. Must occur at least twice per week for 3 mo	1. Primary: R/O UTI, constipation, polyuria from DM or renal failure 2. Daytime: U/A, culture +/− U/S of bladder, x-ray of spine 3. Secondary: U/A, culture	1. **Behavioral strategies** • Praise, star chart, nonblaming • No drinking excess fluid during evening meal and afterward • Void before bedtime • If no improvement after 3-6 mo, move to step 2 2. **Alarm devices** (conditioning therapy) • Most effective long-term therapy • First line if no response to behavioral strategies 3. **Desmopressin** (DDAVP)—response within 2 wk • Monitor fluid intake if on DDAVP due to hyponatremia • Children 5+ • Contraindicated: hyponatremia, hx of hyponatremia • AE: dilutional hyponatremia • 30% achieve total dryness, 40% have a decrease • Given 1 h before bedtime, 0.2 mg up to 0.4 mg 4. Third line: TCAs—Imipramine • Amitriptyline • Desipramine 5. If UTI, PO Bactrim, cefixime × 7 d
Primary enuresis	Primary nocturnal: bedwetting	1. One bedwetting incident weekly for a boy >6 y/o or girl >5 y/o 2. Child has never had a "dry" night	1. Voiding diary (mainstay) 2. Urinalysis • First morning void 3. Renal sonogram or voiding cystourethrogram • For children with daytime complaints, hx of UTI, or possible structural abnormality	See treatment above
Secondary enuresis	Secondary: previously dry, emotional upset/ family stress	1. Child previously dry for period >6 mo 2. Bed wetting		See treatment above

VESICOURETERAL REFLUX

Disease	Etiology, Prevalence, Risk Factors	Clinical Symptoms and Signs	Diagnostics	Therapy, Prognosis, and Health Maintenance
Vesicoureteral reflux (VUR)	Abnormal retrograde flow of urine from bladder into one or both ureters and kidneys because of mislocated and incompetent ureterovesical valves Cause: Recurrent UTI? High pressure sterile reflux impairs growth of the kidneys + recurrent UTIs = patchy interstitial scarring and tubular atrophy Loss of functioning nephrons → hypertrophy of remaining glomeruli MCC: **Weakness of the trigone** and its contiguous intravesical ureteral musculature Young children, girls > boys	1. Prolonged bed wetting or recurrent UTIs 2. Renal insufficiency 3. Hypertension 4. Mild to mod proteinuria 5. Unremarkable urine sediment	1. **VCUG** (voiding cystourethrogram) • Clubbed calyces and dilated tortuous ureters entering the bladder 2. RNC (radionuclide cystography) 3. Renal U/S 4. DMSA: first UTI in all children <5, febrile UTI any child, any boy with UTI	1. **Spontaneous resolution** common in younger children, less with puberty/severity—watch and wait 2. Aggressive control of BP with ACE or ARB to reduce proteinuria Health maintenance: • Long-term **antibiotic prophylaxis** recommended if recurrent UTI: • Neonates—amoxicillin • Child/adult: Bactrim, nitrofurantoin • ¼ therapeutic dose at PM, D/C once VUR resolved, corrected, or outgrows need • Follow-up renal U/S/VCUG/RNC every 1-1.5 y • Surgery as needed: breakthrough febrile UTI, severe reflux, persistent in females, poor med compliance, poor renal growth Complications: Pyelonephritis, hydroureteronephrosis

URINARY TRACT INFECTION, CYSTITIS, AND PYELONEPHRITIS (FIG. 35-1)

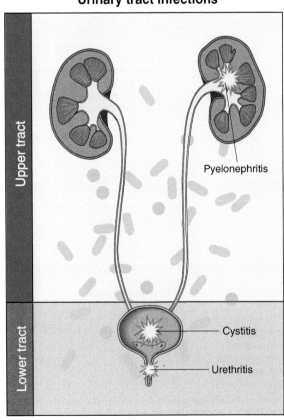

Urinary tract infections

FIGURE 35-1. The lower urinary tract consists of the bladder and urethra, while the upper tract consists of the ureters and the kidneys. (LifeART image copyright (c) [2018]. Lippincott Williams & Wilkins. All rights reserved.)

- Urinary tract infection: denotes symptomatic disease
- Boys tend to get UTIs more in the first months of life compared to girls because of initially lower voiding pressures and residual volumes
- Cystitis: inflammation of the urinary bladder, usually caused by an infection
- Pyelonephritis: symptomatic infection of the kidneys (renal parenchyma) without inflammatory mass or abscess
- Pyuria: (+) leukocyte esterase on dipstick; >5 WBC/hpf on standard microscopy; or >10 WBC on enhanced urinalysis
- Bacteriuria: (+) nitrites on dipstick, though negative dipstick nitrite does not rule out; any bacteria on standard microscopic urinalysis, any bacteria on Gram-stained smear

Disease	Etiology, Prevalence, Risk Factors	Clinical Symptoms and Signs	Diagnostics	Therapy, Prognosis, and Health Maintenance

UTI in neonates (term infants <30 d old)	Presents in 2-3rd week after birth
	MC pathogen (term): *E. coli*
	MC pathogens (preterm): coagulase-negative *Staph* and *Klebsiella*
	M (75% of cases) >>> fF
	RF:
	Preterm, low birth weight (<1000 g), uncircumcised males (10×), kidney and urinary tract anomalies (pelviectasis, mild hydronephrosis)
		1. Fever (20%-40%)
		2. Failure to thrive
		3. Jaundice
		4. Vomiting
		5. Loose stools
		6. Poor feeding
		7. Other: Lethargy, irritability
		Signs:
		1. Tachypnea
		2. Cyanosis
		3. Ill appearing
		4. Jaundice (may be initial sign)
		Associated:
		Bacteremia, congenital anomalies of the kidney and urinary tract (CAKUT), conjugated hyperbilirubinemia
			1. CBC with diff
			2. Urinalysis
			  • Not sensitive or specific enough alone to make diagnosis
			  • 10-50k CFU/mL
			  • (+) leukocyte esterase
			3. (+) Urine culture (diagnostic)
			4. Blood cultures—obtain in every infant with suspected UTI, r/o urosepsis
			5. Renal ultrasound
			  • Recommended in all neonates with UTI to r/o structural anomalies
			  • Obtain after antibiotics initiated
			  • NL U/S does not rule out VUR or renal scarring
			6. VCUG
			  • Recommended in all neonates with UTI to r/o VUR
				Treatment as below
				Health maintenance:
				1. Routine surveillance cultures for asymptomatic children not indicated
				2. Antibiotic prophylaxis for children without VUR and frequent UTIs (3 febrile UTIs in 6 mo, or 4 total in 1 y)
				  • Bactrim 2 mg TMP/kg single daily nose × 6 mo
				  • OR
				  • Nitrofurantoin 1-2 mg/kg daily × 6 mo
				3. Cranberry juice or probiotics *not* routinely recommended for prevention of recurrent UTI
				Prognosis:
				1. 8%-30% experience reinfection (mostly in females)
				2. Renal scarring associated with recurrent pyelonephritis
				Complications: urosepsis (4%-7%)

UTI in neonates (preterm infants <30 d old)	As above	1. Feeding intolerance 2. Lethargy 3. Abdominal distention Signs: 1. Apnea 2. Bradycardia 3. Hypoxia 4. Tachypnea	As above	Treatment as below

UTI in infants and children >1 mo old	MC pathogen: *E. Coli* (80%)
	Other Gram-negative pathogens: *Klebsiella, Proteus, Enterobacter, Citrobacter*
	Gram positives: *Staph saprophyticus, Enterococcus, Staph aureus* (rare)
	RF: hx of UTI/VUR, **lack of circumcision,** chronic urinary symptoms (incontinence, lack of proper stream, frequency, urgency, withholding maneuvers), chronic constipation, VUR, antenatally dx renal anomaly, non-black race
		Infants:
		1. Fever (MC) > 39 C or >24 h
		  • No apparent source
		2. Less common: irritability, poor feeding, failure to thrive
		3. Not diagnostic: Foul smelling urine, vomiting, diarrhea
		>1 mom old:
		1. Fever
		2. Urinary symptoms
		  • Urgency, dysuria, frequency, incontinence
		3. Abdominal pain
		Signs:
		1. Fever >39 C or fever >24 h
		2. Suprapubic tenderness
		3. Ill appearing
		Associated: hyperbilirubinemia
			1. Urinalysis
			  • Via catheterization or suprapubic aspiration, if not toilet trained (otherwise, clean catch)
			  • Dipstick
			(+) nitrite and/or (+) leukocyte esterase
			  • Urine culture (standard):
			    • Clean catch: >100k CFU/mL
			    • Catheter: >50k CFU/mL
			  • May be diagnosed in absence of pyuria (>5 WBC/hpf) if culture shows growth of *Enterococcus, Klebsiella,* or *Pseudomonas*
			2. RBUS
			  • Indications: Image children 2 mo–2 y with first UTI, recurrent febrile UTIs, family hx of urologic disease, poor growth or HTN, and when not improving at 48 h
			3. VCUG (gold standard to dx VUR)
			  • Indications: Image children 2 mo–2 y with first UTI, recurrent febrile UTIs, hydronephrosis or scarring on RBUS, high grade VUR or obstructive uropathy
				1. Antibiotics given within 72 h to prevent renal damage
				  • 3rd gen cephalosporins: cefpodoxime, **cefixime,** cefdinir, ceftibuten, cefotaxime, ceftriaxone
				  • Aminoglycosides: gentamicin, amikacin
				    • Assess hydration status and renal function
				2. Add *Enterococcus* coverage, if suspected
				  • Amoxicillin or ampicillin
				Indications for admission:
				1. Age <2 mo
				2. Clinical urosepsis (toxic, hypotension, poor capillary refill)
				3. Immunocompromised
				4. Vomiting, inability to tolerate PO meds
				5. Chance of inadequate follow-up
				6. Failure to respond
				Inpatient therapy:
				1. Ampicillin and gentamicin
				Health maintenance:
				1. No prophylaxis recommended for first febrile UTI in children 2 mo–2 y
				Prognosis:
				1. 25%-30% with first UTI have VUR
				Complications:
				Renal abscess, death (uncommon)

(continued)

(continued)

Disease	Etiology, Prevalence, Risk Factors	Clinical Symptoms and Signs	Diagnostics	Therapy, Prognosis, and Health Maintenance
Cystitis in children and adolescents	<u>MC pathogen:</u> ***E. coli*** Other pathogens: *Enterococcus, P. mirabilis, P. aeruginosa, Enterobacter, Adenovirus, Schistosoma haematobium* <u>RF:</u> Female, uncircumcised males (mostly in infants), sexual intercourse (especially in females), unprotected insertive anal intercourse in males, abnormalities of the urinary system (bladder stones, neurogenic bladder), indwelling catheter, sickle cell disease, diabetes, immunodeficiency	>2 y: urgency, dysuria, frequency, abdominal pain Pain in bladder, groin, lower abdomen during urination Cloudy or dark urine, excessive urination at night, foul smelling, blood in urine	1. R/o if unexplained fever in less than 2 y/o 2. U/A with microscopy: pyuria (WBC >5) • Suprapubic aspiration (+) >1K • Cath: (+) if >10K • Voided: (+) if >100K 3. Urine culture 4. (+) leuk-esterase and nitrites 5. Catheter: > 10-50K 6. Clean catch: >100K	1. Hygiene, close follow-up 2. PO Bactrim, **cefexime**, **augmentin**, amoxicillin × 10-14 d–3rd gen ceph (*first line*) 3. If toxic/dehydrated: IM or IV after U/A and culture obtained (refer to ER) <u>Older:</u> Nitrofurantoin
Uncomplicated acute cystitis	Usually adults and children >2 with lower urinary tract symptoms <u>MCC:</u> ***E. coli* (80%)**, *Proteus, Klebsiella, S. saprophyticus* Hemorrhagic cystitis: caused by adenovirus	1. **Dysuria, urgency, frequency** 2. Hematuria 3. New onset incontinence (in toilet trained children) 4. Abdominal or suprapubic pain 5. Absence of fever, chills, or flank pain <u>Signs:</u> 1. Change in urine color/odor 2. **Suprapubic pain** 3. Fever (**absent**)	1. Urine dipstick: nitrite, leukocyte esterase 2. Urinalysis: pyuria, bacteriuria +/− hematuria +/− nitrites 3. CBC: leukocytosis 4. **Urine culture** (*standard*): only obtain if **symptomatic** • >100k CFU/mL (women) • >1000 CFU/mL men or cath patients • → takes 24 h to obtain results 5. Blood cultures: obtain in febrile Pts; consider in complicated UTI	See Treatment Below <u>Complications:</u> Hemorrhagic cystitis 1. Microscopic hematuria 2. Bladder hemorrhage with clot formation 3. Dysuria, frequency → hematuria 12-24 h after 4. Preceding URI
Complicated acute cystitis: Infection in patient with structural or functional abnormality that would reduce the efficacy of antibiotic therapy	Adults and children >2 **MCC:** ***E. coli* (30%)**, enterococci, PsA, *Staphylococcus epidermidis* Catheter-associated pathogens: *P. aeruginosa, Candida albicans* Complicated defined as children, men, nosocomial or nursing home acquired, kidney allograft, pregnancy, immunosuppression <u>RF:</u> DM, sickle cell disease, BPH, recurrent UTI, indwelling catheter, neurogenic bladder, polycystic kidney disease	Same as uncomplicated UTI	1. Urine culture (clean-catch midstream or straight cath): only get if **symptomatic** • >10^5 CFU/mL	See Treatment Below

Disease	Etiology, Prevalence, Risk Factors	Clinical Symptoms and Signs	Diagnostics	Therapy, Prognosis, and Health Maintenance
Recurrent UTI	Relapse: Recurrence of UTI within 2 wk of treatment caused by same organism Refinection: Recurrent UTI caused by different bacteria; more common than relapse	1. 2 uncomplicated UTI in 6 mo OR 3+ uncomplicated UTIs in previous year	1. Urine culture (clean-catch midstream or straight cath)	1. Empiric treatment 2. Refer to PCP for repeat culture in 1-2 wk 3. Prophylaxis × 6 mo Once daily low-dose Bactrim, nitrofurantoin, cephalexin or ciprofloxacin + Postcoital dose + Contraception, topical estrogen (postmenopausal women 3× weekly), postcoital voiding, liberal fluid intake, cranberry tablets
Pyelonephritis in children	RF: sexual intercourse, a new sexual partner, a UTI in the previous 12 mo, a maternal history of UTI, diabetes, and incontinence **E. coli** (most common)	Older children: 1. Presents with fever 2. Chills 3. Flank pain 4. Cystitis: **dysuria, urgency, frequency** 5. Fever + chills 6. Nausea, vomiting, diarrhea Signs: 1. **Flank** or back pain, 2. CVA tenderness	1. U/A: **pyuria, bacteriuria, WBC casts** +/− hematuria +/− nitrites 2. CBC: leukocytosis, left shift 3. Urine culture (clean-catch midstream or straight cath): only get if symptomatic • >10^5 CFU/mL (women) • >10^3 CFU/mL men or cath patients 4. Blood cultures: obtain in febrile Pts; consider in complicated UTI 5. Abdominal CT: r/o abscess in patients with pyelo who fail to defervesce after 72 h 6. Urologic w/u (renal U/S, abd CT, VCUG): recurrent UTI in men	1. First line: **fluoroquinolones** • Ciprofloxacin PO 500 mg BID +/− initial IV 400 mg load

Treatment of Urinary Tract Infections in Children

Neonates	Infants >1 mo and Children	Children 2+ and Adolescents: Uncomplicated	Children 2+ and Adolescents: Complicated
Same as for sepsis, as difficult to discern DX based on presentation Duration: 10-14 d 1. Term babies • Ampicillin 50 mg/kg/dose every 8 h AND • Gentamicin 4 mg/kg/dose every 12 h • For birthweight >2 kg 2. Preterm babies (7 d and younger) • Ampicillin 150 mg/kg/dose every 12 h 3. If admitted, vancomycin substituted for ampicillin	Duration: 7-14 d Outpatient: 1. **Cefixime** 16 mg/kg on day 1, then 8 mg/kg daily 2. Cefdinir 14 mg/kg daily 3. Ceftibuten 9 mg/kg/day Inpatient: 1. Ampicillin 100 mg/kg/d in 4 doses 2. Gentamicin 7.5 mg/kg/d in 3 doses 3. Cefotaxime 150 mg/kg/d in 3-4 doses 4. Ceftriaxone 50-75 mg/kg/d	Initiate for pending cultures: • Febrile, immunocompromised, ill-appearing, or indwelling catheter, GU abnormalities, or previous UTI • Afebrile, immunocompetent, well-appearing, without urinary catheter, GU abnormalities, or previous UTI, IF they have (+) bacteriuria (+/− pyuria) on dipstick or microscopic analysis • Positive urine culture in patients meeting criteria in previous list (afebrile) Based on coverage: 1. E. coli–2nd (cefuroxime, cefprozil) or 3rd-generation cephalosporin (cefdinir, cefixime, cefpodoxime, ceftibuten) 2. S. saprophyticus–**Bactrim DS PO × 3 d** • OR **nitrofurantoin (Macrobid) 100 mg × 5 d** • OR **fluoroquinolones** 3. Enterococcus–Amoxicillin; PCN allergy: nitrofurantoin	IV therapy duration: • 5 d if: first episode of uncomplicated, afebrile cystitis in girls 2+ or boys 2-13 y/o • 7-14 d: (a) 5 d if: recurrent, febrile, or complicated cystitis in children 2+ y/o Based on coverage: 1. E. coli–2nd (cefuroxime, cefprozil) or 3rd-generation cephalosporin (cefdinir, cefixime, cefpodoxime, ceftibuten) 2. S. saprophyticus–**Bactrim** 3. OR **nitrofurantoin (Macrobid)** 4. OR **fluoroquinolones** 5. Enterococcus–amoxicillin; PCN allergy: nitrofurantoin

Pediatrics

Treatment of Pyelonephritis in Adults

Outpatient	Inpatient	Pregnant	Men
1. **FQ** × 7 d **OR** 3. **Bactrim DO** × 14 d	1. **IV 1-g ceftriaxone** OR 2. Amp/sulbactam OR 3. Aminoglycoside × 14 d (change to PO if clinically improved and afebrile 24-48 h)	1. IV B-lactam (**ampicillin**) +/– 2. Aminoglycoside (**gentamicin**) × 14 d → Increased risk of PTB, low birth weight, and perinatal mortality, if untreated	1. FQ or Bactrim × 7-14 d

CHAPTER **36**

Hematology

Refer to Internal Medicine 🩺 for in-depth coverage of the following topics:

Anemia, see Iron Deficiency Anemia, Thalassemia, Vitamin B$_{12}$ and Folic Acid Deficiency Anemia, Sickle Cell Anemia, and Hemolytic Anemias, p 275
Bleeding Disorders, see ITP and TTP; DIC, vWF Disease, p 262
Lymphomas, p 281

Neutropenia, see also Multiple Myeloma in Internal Medicine, p 282
Hemophilia, see Hemophilia A and B, p 283

Recommended Supplemental Material:

Hereditary Spherocytosis, see Hemolytic Anemias in Hematology for Internal Medicine, p 279
Blood Cell Morphology and Life Cycle, p 274 🩺

BLEEDING DISORDERS

- **Microangiopathic hemolytic anemia (MAHA)—platelet aggregation** in the microvascular circulation via vWF

  - Results from fragmentation of RBCs through occluded arterioles and capillaries

Disease	Etiology, Prevalence, Risk Factors	Clinical Symptoms and Signs	Diagnostics	Therapy, Prognosis, and Health Maintenance
Hemolytic-uremic syndrome (HUS)	<u>MC:</u> Children Common cause of acute renal failure <u>MCC:</u> Shiga toxin producing *E. coli* (serotype 0157:H7) <u>Sources:</u> Contaminated food or water Toxin-mediated microvascular injury promotes platelet aggregation → thrombus formation	<u>HX:</u> Infectious diarrhea (bloody, without fever), infectious colitis → 2-4 d after diarrhea, abdominal cramps 1. **Thrombocytopenia** 2. **A**nemia 3. **R**enal insufficiency 4. Hyperglycemia (new onset diabetes): microthrombi in pancreas = B cell death = decreased insulin	1. Stool culture: fecal leukocytes and *E. coli* 0157:H7 2. Electrolyte and renal function panels - check for nephropathy 3. U/A: check for RBCs, RBC casts, protein	1. **Supportive care**: hydration, pain control, RBC or platelet transfusion 2. AKI–hemodialysis may be required 3. Do not use antimotility agents or antibiotics 55%-70% develop renal failure 5%-15% mortality

ACUTE LEUKEMIA

- **Terminal deoxynucleotidyl transferase (TdT)**, also known as DNA nucleotidylexotransferase or terminal transferase is a specialized DNA polymerase expressed in immature, pre-B, pre-T, lymphoid cells, and ALL/lymphoma cells

Disease	Etiology, Prevalence, Risk Factors	Clinical Symptoms and Signs	Diagnostics	Therapy, Prognosis, and Health Maintenance
ALL (acute lymphoblastic leukemia)	Neoplasm of early lymphocytic precursors MC in young children (<15) **MC childhood cancer** ALL: most common leukemia in childhood <15 (80%) Peak: 2-5 y RF: Initial WBC and age at diagnosis, rate of response, cytogenetics	1. **Anemia** (symptoms) 2. **Neutropenia** - Increased risk of bacterial infection 3. **Thrombocytopenia**—Abnormal mucosal or cutaneous bleeding 4. Splenomegaly, hepatomegaly, lymphadenopathy 5. Bone and joint pain 6. CNS involvement (meningitis, seizures) 7. Testicular involvement (ALL) 8. Anterior mediastinal mass (T-cell ALL)	1. Immunofluorescence assay: **TdT (+)** 2. Histology: **lymphoblasts** 3. Bone marrow biopsy: required for DX • **Myeloblasts** Labs: 1. WBC: 1k–100k, large number of blasts in peripheral blood • **Hyperleukocytosis** 2. Anemia 3. Thrombocytopenia 4. Granulocytopenia 5. Electrolytes: hyperuricemia, hyperkalemia, hyperphosphatemia	Most responsive to **chemotherapy** 75% achieve complete remission, only 30%-40% of adults Relapses occur, but respond well With aggressive therapy, survival rates can be up to 15 y or longer, 50% cured Poor prognostic factors: age <2 or >9, WBC >10⁵/mm³, and CNS involvement (B-cell type, high LDG, or rapid proliferation)
Benign leukemoid reaction	Increased WBC count as a response to stress or infection	1. Usually no splenomegaly 2. Increased leukocyte alkaline phosphatase 3. History of precipitating infection		

LYMPHOMA

Disease	Etiology, Prevalence, Risk Factors	Clinical Symptoms and Signs	Diagnostics	Therapy, Prognosis, and Health Maintenance
Indolent or low-grade				
Small lymphocytic lymphoma	Closely related to CLL More common in elderly **Indolent course**			Eventually results in widespread involvement with dissemination to liver, spleen, and bone marrow
Follicular, small, cleaved-cell lymphoma	**Most common form on NHL** • Mean age onset 55 y • May transform into diffuse, large cell; associated with translocation t(14,18) • Indolent course	Presents with **painless, peripheral lymphadenopathy**		Most present with localized disease Cured with radiotherapy but only 15% have localized disease Median survival: 10 y
Intermediate				
Diffuse, large B-cell lymphoma	Predominantly B-cell origin Middle-aged and elderly Locally invasive	Presents as **large, extranodal mass**		85% cure rate with CHOP therapy
High grade				
Lymphoblastic lymphoma (T-cell)	More common in children May progress to T-ALL	50% have B-symptoms		Aggressive with rapid dissemination, but may respond to combo chemotherapy
Burkitt lymphoma	African and American versions African—linked to **EBV** Translocation t(8,14)	African—involves facial bone and jaw American— 1. **Rapidly expanding abdominal mass** 2. GI SX 3. Marrow or CNS disease	1. **Starry sky appearance**	Grave prognosis unless treated aggressively with chemotherapy Treatment cures 50%-60%

Pediatrics

NEUTROPENIA

- Differential: *ALL, AML, Aplastic Anemia, Bacterial Sepsis, CML, CMV, Folic Acid Deficiency, Wegener Granulomatosis, Hodgkin Lymphoma, Infectious Mononucleosis, Multiple Myeloma, NHL, Viral Hepatitis*

Disease	Etiology, Prevalence, Risk Factors	Clinical Symptoms and Signs	Diagnostics	Therapy, Prognosis, and Health Maintenance
Aplastic anemia	? autoimmune 50% idiopathic Radiation, infection, toxins, drugs <u>Inherited</u>: Fanconi anemia	1. Weakness, fatigue 2. Palpitations 3. DOE 4. Tinnitus 5. Bleeding and bruising 6. Infections	1. CBC: Normocytic **A**nemia, **N**eutropenia, **T**hrombocytopenia 2. Peripheral smear: Peripheral pancytopenia with marrow **hypocellularity** (<25%) 3. Bone marrow biopsy–r/o MDS	1. Transfusion dependent with **growth factors** (temp) 2. **Immunosuppression**: ATG (stops T-cell response), Cyclosporin × 1 y, steroids 3. Cure is **allogeneic stem cell transplant**

- Reticuloendothelial system (extravascular hemolysis in spleen)
- Within circulation (intravascular hemolysis)
- Symptoms: acute/chronic anemia, jaundice, dark urine, back pain
  - Increased retic count, LDH and indirect bilirubin

- Decreased Haptoglobin - Hgb converted to indirect bilirubin in spleen (extravascular) or bound by haptoglobin in plasma (intravascular)
  - Hgb-haptoglobin complex cleared quickly by liver → decreased haptoglobin levels = intravascular hemolysis

BRAIN TUMORS AND LEAD POISONING

Disease	Etiology, Prevalence, Risk Factors	Clinical Symptoms and Signs	Diagnostics	Therapy, Prognosis, and Health Maintenance
Brain tumors	Age <15 60% infratentorial Pilocytic astrocytoma— most common overall; benign, cystic, slow growing, 6.5-9 y, surgical resection **Medulloblastoma**— most common, malignant, XRT/chemo, resection	**Infant:** Large head, bulging fontanelle, anorexia/FTT, loss of milestones, irritable/shrill cry, resistance to being held <u>**Child:**</u> Morning headaches, vomiting (no nausea), drowsiness, decreased academics, personality change <u>**Others:**</u> Vision change/papilledema, altered speech and handwriting, CN deficit, head tilt, altered gait and ataxia, diabetes insipidus	Neurological exam Head CT or MRI head/spine Biopsy	Surgery—mainstay
Lead poisoning	<u>RF:</u> Inner city low income, recent immigrants, exposure, adult workers employed in lead exposure jobs, Ayurvedic meds	<u>Asymptomatic:</u> 1. Pica 2. Anorexia 3. Colicky abdominal pain <u>Signs:</u> 1. Lead lines in gingiva 2. Failure to thrive, mental delay, CNS symptoms	1. Lead: if (+), get venous CBC 2. AAP recommends checking at **9-12 m** and **24 m** 3. Questionnaire: annual 3-6 y 1. CBC: **basophilic stippling**, hypochromic anemia 2. XR: lead lines on x-rays of knee/wrist (metaphysis)	<u>Blood levels:</u> 1. 10-15: low IQ, impaired development, hearing and growth → survey, follow-up 2. 25-55: more severe, renal, hematopoietic damage → IM/IV **EDTA** (edetate calcium disodium versenate) 3. 45-69: IM EDTA + PO DMSA 4. >70: IV EDTA + IM DMSA

Pediatrics

PRACTICE QUESTIONS

1. A 14-year-old woman with a history of contact lens use presents to the clinic with left eye pain and photophobia. She admits that she has been sleeping in her contacts. On physical exam, you note pupils are equal and reactive to light, conjunctival injection in the left eye, and no discharge bilaterally. Which should be performed next?

    A. Visual acuity

    B. Fluorescein exam with slit lamp

    C. CT of the face

    D. Patch the left eye

2. What intervention is indicated for a reducible umbilical hernia in a 15-month-old female?

    A. Surgical repair

    B. Taping the hernia down

    C. Watchful waiting

    D. Abdominal binders

3. A 9-month-old male with Down Syndrome presents for his well child check with concerns that he is not meeting any developmental milestones. During the visit, it is noted that he has dry skin, thin hair, and puffy eyes. What is the most likely diagnosis?

    A. Diabetes

    B. Anemia

    C. Hypothyroidism

    D. Hyperparathyroidism

4. During a clinic visit with a 14-year-old patient, her mother reports that the patient recently broke up with her boyfriend and since then she no longer wants to participate in her dance class, she is constantly tired and sleeping, and she will not come out of her room. You note that she has lost 15 pounds since her last clinic visit 3 months ago. Which of the following is the treatment of choice?

    A. Fluoxetine

    B. Amitriptyline

    C. Selegiline

    D. Paroxetine

5. An 11-year-old boy with asthma currently on budesonide once daily has been using his albuterol inhaler 2 times a day while playing sports with some limitation and 3 times per week before going to bed. What is the best medication to add at this time?

    A. Omalizumab

    B. Fluticasone propionate

    C. Formoterol

    D. Prednisone

6. While completing the newborn exam on a 2-day old female infant with an uncomplicated gestational history, but a prolonged vaginal delivery, you note she has a boggy edematous swelling extending over the occipital and left temporal bones. What is the most likely diagnosis?

    A. Cephalohematoma

    B. Subcutaneous fat necrosis

    C. Caput succedaneum

    D. Subarachnoid hemorrhage

7. A 7-year-old boy presents for his wellness exam and a harsh crescendo-decrescendo systolic murmur is heard at the left lower sternal border. What else do you expect to find on physical exam?

    A. The murmur increases with a handgrip

    B. The murmur decreases with a Valsalva maneuver

    C. The murmur increases after raising the leg while supine

    D. The murmur decreases with going from standing to squatting

8. What is the most common source for posterior epistaxis?

    A. Kiesselbach Plexus

    B. Sphenopalatine artery

    C. Greater Palatine Artery

    D. Superior labial artery

9. A child is brought in for their newborn evaluation. Patients are concerned about a diffuse accumulation of yellowish, greasy scale on his scalp and eyebrows that did not go away after repeatedly cleaning the area. At what age will this condition most likely resolve?

    A. 1 week

    B. 3 weeks

    C. 3 months

    D. 9 months

10. A female infant has paroxysm episodes of high pitching crying that can last for hours and most commonly occurs at night. During the crying episodes, she becomes flushed, draws her legs up to her abdomen, and stiffens her arms. What is the best way to reduce these episodes?

    A. Start Keppra

    B. Feed the infant in an upright position

    C. Start Prilosec

    D. Reduce frequency of burping during feeding

11. A 5-year-old boy presents to your clinic with a new onset erythematous malar rash. For the past 3 days he has had a low-grade fever (100.4°F), headache, congestion, and runny nose. What is the most likely etiology of his condition?

    A. Parvovirus B19

    B. Rhinovirus

    C. Coxsackievirus

    D. Parainfluenza

12. A 6-year-old girl presents for her well child check. During the visit, the mother reports that she has recently started to wet the bed at night 1-2 times per week when she was previously dry throughout the night. There have been no recent changes to the household and she will be starting Kindergarten this fall. Physical exam is consistent with a normally developing 6-year-old girl with no abnormalities or delays. What is the recommended initial treatment?

   A. Motivation therapy
   B. Nitrofurantoin
   C. Starting pull-ups
   D. Desmopressin

13. A 15-year-old boy presents with nonerythematous vesicles in different healing stages under his armpits. Some of the vesicles are filled with a clear yellow fluid, while others have already ruptured leaving a thin yellowish-brown crust. What is the treatment of choice for his condition?

   A. 1% hydrocortisone cream
   B. Amoxicillin
   C. Cephalexin
   D. Levofloxacin

14. A 4-year-old girl presents to the ED with her mother with fever and a sore throat. Upon entering the room you note that she is sitting on the exam table with a tripod posture, excessively drooling, with inspiratory stridor. What intervention should come first?

   A. Chest x-ray
   B. Draw blood cultures
   C. Begin bag-valve-mask ventilation
   D. Start IV prednisone and empiric antibiotics.

15. For a health infant, at what age you expect the Moro reflex to disappear?

   A. 1 to 2 months old
   B. 2 to 3 months old
   C. 5 to 6 months old
   D. 9 to 10 months old

16. An 8-year-old boy is complaining of fever (T_{max} 102 F), a sore throat, and a couple episodes of diarrhea for the past three days. Physical exam is notable for cervical lymphadenopathy, bilateral bulbar injection without discharge, cracked red lips, and indurated edema on his palms. What is the most appropriate treatment for him?

   A. Oseltamivir (Tamiflu)
   B. Supportive care
   C. IVIG with ASA
   D. HD amoxicillin

17. During a newborn exam you note the mother has epilepsy and was treated with valproic acid until the second trimester. What is the most likely complication?

   A. Cleft palate
   B. Short palpebral fissures
   C. Excessive skin on the nape of the neck
   D. Leukocoria

18. An inconsolable infant is brought into the ED with intermittent bilious vomiting episodes and drawing his legs up toward his abdomen for the past couple hours. A sausage-shaped abdominal mass is palpable. What test should be done next?

   A. Abdominal ultrasound
   B. KUB
   C. Rectal exam
   D. Fecal occult blood test

19. Which of the following do you expect to find in a patient with hereditary spherocytosis?

   A. Elevated indirect bilirubin
   B. Decreased mean corpuscular hemoglobin concentration
   C. Decreased lactate dehydrogenase
   D. Elevated haptoglobin

20. A 16-year-old boy presents to the ED with a 2-day history of fever, headache, and anorexia with new onset of a redness and swelling of his left cheek. What is the most likely complication of the diagnosis?

   A. Sjögren syndrome
   B. Orchitis
   C. Pancreatitis
   D. ST segment elevation

21. A 7-year-old girl with a recent acute otitis media infection on Amoxicillin presents with protrusion of the left auricle, ear pain and erythema, and postauricular tenderness. What is the treatment of choice given the most likely diagnosis?

   A. Ampicillin + cefotaxime
   B. Vancomycin + cefepime
   C. Doxycycline
   D. Piperacillin tazobactam

22. Which of the following best describes the murmur of an atrial septal defect?

   A. A midsystolic murmur heard best in the right upper sternal border with radiation to the carotids
   B. A midsystolic ejection click with a wide, fixed split S2 that is best heard at the left upper sternal border
   C. A crescendo-decrescendo machinery like murmur that is best heard at the left upper sternal border
   D. A vibratory systolic murmur that is best heard at the left lower sternal border while the patient is supine

23. An 8-year-old male patient is evaluated for hyperactivity and is diagnosed with attention deficit hyperactivity disorder. When starting methylphenidate, which of the following should you recommend?

   A. Limiting TV before bed
   B. Taking the medication before meals
   C. Obtaining liver function test before initiation
   D. Monitoring EKG every 6 months

24. A 14-year-old girl presents to the clinic for two potential syncopal episodes. Her mother reports that on two different occasions she was talking to her mother at the house when she suddenly fell to the floor, her head deviated to the right, and she had jerking movements of her bilateral upper and lower extremities. She also reports urinary incontinence and tongue biting with the event. You obtain an EEG, which is abnormal indicating increased risk for seizures. What is the best initial treatment for this patient?

   A. Valproic acid (Depakote)
   B. Levetiracetam (Keppra)
   C. Tetrabenazine
   D. Ethosuximide (Zarontin)

25. A 4-year-old boy presents with pain immediately below his right knee for the last 3 days and a limp. He has had multiple complaints about this pain in the past year. It is not relieved with Tylenol or Motrin. On examination, there is swelling noted in the area. His mother states that this pain worsens at night or when he is playing soccer. An x-ray is obtained of the femur, tibia, and fibula. What is most likely to be seen on x-ray given the most likely diagnosis?

   A. A lytic mass with multi-laminated periosteal "onion skin" reaction
   B. A "sunburst" appearance
   C. A stalk or broad-based projection
   D. A round lucency surrounded by sclerotic bone

ANSWERS

1. Diagnostic Studies: Corneal Abrasion. Answer A: Visual acuity should be performed next before performing the fluorescein exam to confirm corneal abrasion. B, Fluorescein exam with slit lamp is used to confirm corneal abrasion but should be performed after a visual acuity exam and funduscopic exam. C, CT of the face will not provide any help to diagnose a corneal abrasion. D, Corneal abrasions caused by contact lens should not be patched due to infection risk.

2. Clinical Intervention: Umbilical Hernia. Answer C: Watchful waiting is indicated in this situation. The child is less than 5 years old and is reducible at this time. No intervention is indicated. A, Surgical repair is indicated if the hernia becomes incarcerated, strangulated, the hernia ceases to decrease in size with age, or the hernia does not spontaneously close by 5 years old. B, Taping the hernia down is an old folklore and can lead to skin irritation and infection. D, Abdominal binders are not recommended to treat umbilical hernias.

3. Diagnosis: Hypothyroidism. Answer C: Hypothyroidism and other thyroid disorders are common in children with Down syndrome. Hypothyroidism can present with pallor, dry skin, hair thinning, cold intolerance, weight gain, and pale puffy eyes. A, Children with Down syndrome do have an increased risk of type 1 diabetes, but diabetes typically presents with a child in diabetic ketoacidosis or hyperosmolar hyperglycemic state. B, Anemias are common in children with DS but the symptoms described above do not match with an anemic state. D, Hyperparathyroidism typically presents with complaints of bone pain, kidney stones, abdominal symptoms, and psychiatric/mood abnormalities.

4. Clinical Intervention: Major Depressive Disorder. Answer A: Fluoxetine is the first-line treatment when treating unipolar depression in pediatric patients. B, Amitriptyline and other tricyclic antidepressants are not indicated to treat unipolar depression in the pediatric population. C, Selegiline and other MAOIs are not indicated to treat unipolar depression in pediatric patients. D, Paroxetine is an SSRI that does not have a proven efficacy to treat unipolar depression in pediatric patients

5. Clinical Therapeutics: Asthma. Answer C: Formoterol is a long-acting beta agonist (LABA) that is indicated as an add-on medication to ICS for step 3-6 on the stepwise asthma management protocol. In the scenario above, the patient is classified as moderate persistent asthma because he is using the rescue inhaler 2 times a day and still having activity limitation, and greater than 1 time a night but not nightly. He is already on an ICS, so a long-acting β agonist (LABA) is indicated to add on to his current medication regimen. A, Omalizumab is used to treat severe asthma that are inadequately controlled with inhaled corticosteroids (ICS) and other treatments. The scenario describes a patient with moderate persistent asthma. B, Fluticasone propionate is an inhaled corticosteroid (ICS) that is used in different dosages for all types of asthma. The scenario above indicates that the patient is already on an ICS, and it is not indicated to add another ICS. D, Prednisone is indicated to give to patients who are not well controlled on high-dose ICS + LABA who is classified as a step 6 on the stepwise approach. The patient in the scenario is classified as a moderate persistent asthmatic, and it is therefore not indicated to treat with systemic steroids at this time.

6. Diagnosis: Caput Succedaneum. Answer C: Caput succedaneum a boggy edematous swelling extending over the presenting part due to prolonged engagement of the infant's head on the cervix or vaginal wall during a prolonged spontaneous vaginal delivery. It usually resolves within a few days and requires no treatment. A, Cephalohematoma is a subperiosteal hematoma present after delivery that does not cross suture lines and rarely expands after delivery. It is most commonly caused by forceps or vacuum-assisted deliveries. Most will resolve spontaneously within a few weeks without treatment needed. B, Subcutaneous fat necrosis is characterized as multiple erythematous, blue, or flesh-colored nodules

or plaques found most commonly on the cheeks, back, forearms, buttocks, or thighs that develop within the first weeks of life due to ischemia of the adipose tissue following a traumatic delivery. No treatment is usually required and the nodules/plaques will resolve in 6 to 8 weeks. D, A subarachnoid hemorrhage is the second most common type of intracranial hemorrhage in neonates and is due to the rupture of veins in the subarachnoid space during vaginal deliveries assisted with vacuum or forceps. Infants present between 24 to 48 hours after birth with apnea, respiratory distress, or seizures. It is best diagnosed with a CT scan followed by conservative treatment.

7. Scientific Concepts: HCM. Answer D: HCM decreases with going from standing to squatting due to increasing preload to the heart. Squatting squeezes blood up into the heart, increasing blood return to the heart. A, Hypertrophic Cardiomyopathy (HCM) decreases with hand grip due to increase in afterload. Handgrip causes the contraction of muscles in the arms, which compresses those arteries and increases resistance. In effect, increasing afterload means it is more difficult for blood to be ejected from the left ventricles due to this increased resistance the blood faces. B, HCM increases with valsalva maneuver due to decrease in preload. Valsalva increases intrathoracic pressure and decreases blood return to the heart. C, HCM decreases after raising the leg while supine because preload is increased. More blood is returning to the heart this way.

8. Scientific Concepts: Posterior Epistaxis. Answer B: Sphenopalatine artery is the most likely source for a posterior nosebleed. A, Kiesselbach's Plexus is the most likely source for an anterior nosebleed. C, The Greater Palatine Artery mainly supplies the hard palate. D, The superior labial artery supplies Kiesselbach's plexus.

9. Health Maintenance Seborrheic Dermatitis. Answer C: Seborrheic dermatitis, also known as cradle cap in infants, is a self-limiting accumulation of yellowish greasy plaques that most commonly develops on an infant's scalp, external ear, eyebrows, eyelids, cheeks, and nasolabial folds. Parents can apply vegetable oil or baby oil to the scalp before bath time to loosen the scales and then gently remove the scales with a soft brush during bath time. It most commonly resolves (A, B) several weeks to (D) months after birth.

10. Health maintenance: Colic. Answer B: Changes in feeding technique are the first line intervention for colic in attempts to soothe the infant. These interventions address potential etiologies, such as swallowed air or overstimulation. Bottle feeding the baby in a vertical position in combination with frequent burping may reduce swallowed air. A, Keppra is indicated to treat seizures, not for the treatment of colic. C, Prilosec is indicated to treat GERD, not to treat colic. D, For the treatment of colic, increasing the frequency of burping is a recommended technique to treat colic.

11. Scientific Concepts: Fifth Disease. Answer A: Erythema infectiosum, or Fifth disease, is caused by parvovirus B19 and presents with prodromal nonspecific flu-like symptoms for 2 to 5 days before an erythematous rash with circumoral pallor appears classically on the face (slapped cheek). A lacelike rash can also appear on the trunk and extremities several days after it appears on the face. B, The Rhinovirus causes the common cold with symptoms that include fever, nasal congestion, nasal discharge, and cough. A rash is usually not present. C, Hand, foot, and mouth is caused by the coxsackievirus A16. Symptoms include fever below 101 with mouth or throat pain due to vesicles surrounded by a halo of erythema on the tongue or buccal mucosa. Macular, maculopapular, or vesicular clear lesions with an erythematous halo may also be present on the palms or soles. D, Laryngotracheitis is caused by the parainfluenza virus and is most common in children 3 months to 3 years old. Common signs and symptoms include nasal discharge, congestion, fever, hoarseness, and a barking cough with stridor.

12. Clinical Therapeutics: Nocturnal Enuresis. Answer A: The initial treatment for nocturnal enuresis includes reassurance, limiting fluids in the afternoon/evening, and motivation therapy with sticky charts, prizes for getting up to go to the bathroom at night. B, Nitrofurantoin is used to treat urinary tract infections. The scenario above does not give an indication that an infection is the cause of the nocturnal enuresis because his physical exam was normal. C, Using pull ups or diapers in a previously potty trained child with nocturnal enuresis is discouraged because it can interfere with their motivation to get up to use the restroom at night when they have the sensation to go. D, Desmopressin is recommended to treat nocturnal enuresis when motivational therapy, decrease in afternoon/evening fluid intake, and alarm system have failed. Desmopressin can also be initiated when the patient's social life is affected by the enuresis like for sleepovers.

13. Clinical Therapeutics: Bullous Impetigo. Answer C: Treatment of bullous impetigo should cover *Staphylococcus aureus* and streptococcal sources. Cephalexin covers for both possible etiologies. A, 1% hydrocortisone cream is used to treat skin conditions like atopic dermatitis and psoriasis. It is not effective against impetigo. B, Amoxicillin is less effective in treating bullous impetigo than cephalosporins. D, Fluoroquinolones should not be used to treat impetigo due to MRSA resistance.

14. Clinical Intervention: Epiglottitis. Answer C: Bag-Valve-Mask ventilation is the first step that should be performed for a child with Epiglottis with airway obstruction with plans for endotracheal intubation. A, Chest x-ray is an alternative way to diagnose epiglottitis and direct visualization is not performed but should be done after the airway is secured. B, Blood

cultures should be drawn before initiation of antibiotic treatment but first secure an airway. D, Glucocorticoids have not been proven to benefit in the treatment of patients with epiglottis. Antibiotics should be initiated after the airway is secured.

15. Scientific Concept: Moro reflex. Answer C: At 5 to 6 moths the Moro reflex disappears. A, At 1 to 2 months, the Galant reflex disappears. B, At 2 to 3 months, the asymmetric tonic neck reflex disappears. D, At 9 to 10 months, the Plantar grasp disappears.

16. Clinical Therapeutics: Kawasaki Disease. Answer C: IVIG with aspirin is the treatment of choice for Kawasaki disease to decrease the risk of coronary artery aneurysms. A, Oseltamivir is the medication of choice to start for patients diagnosed with flu within the first 48 hours of symptom onset. Flu is not characterized with cracked red lips, conjunctivitis, or indurated edema on the palms or soles. B, Supportive care is not the best treatment for Kawasaki disease because of the possible complication of the patient to develop coronary artery aneurysm. Supportive care can be an adjuvant therapy to IVIG + ASA therapy. D, High-dose amoxicillin is the treatment of choice for acute otitis media, not for the treatment of Kawasaki disease.

17. H&P: Cleft Palate. Answer A: Cleft palate is a complication seen in newborns whose mother's were on anti-convulsant medications like valproic acid (Depakote). B, Short palpebral fissures is a feature of fetal alcohol syndrome. C, Excessive skin on the nape of the neck is a feature of Down syndrome. D, Leukocoria is a diagnostic feature of retinoblastoma.

18. Diagnostic Studies: Intussusception. Answer A: Abdominal ultrasound is the initial test of choice for a patient suspected to have intussusception because it has a high sensitive and specificity. B, KUB is normally performed routinely for patients presenting with abdominal symptoms but it is not the preferred initial study for patients with intussusception because radiographs are less sensitive and specific than ultrasound. C, Rectal exam is not indicated for this patient and will not provide a lot of information for a patient with intussusception. D, Fecal occult blood test is used to test for microscopic blood in the stool/rectum. This will not be very much help to diagnose intussusception. It is better utilized as a screening tool for colorectal cancer.

19. Diagnosis: Hereditary Spherocytosis. Answer A: Indirect bilirubin is elevated in hereditary spherocytosis because of the hemolysis of the red blood cells. B, Mean corpuscular hemoglobin concentration is increased in hereditary spherocytosis, and it is the most helpful red cell index. C, Lactate dehydrogenase is increased in hereditary spherocytosis and other hemolytic processes. D, Haptoglobin is decreased in hereditary spherocytosis and other hemolytic processes.

20. Scientific Concept: Mumps. Answer B: Orchitis is one of the most common complications of a mump infection. A, Sjögren syndrome is not a complication of a mumps infection. C, Pancreatitis a possible complication of a mumps infection, however is it not as common as Orchitis. D, ST segment elevation is not a possibly complication of a mumps infection. ST segment depression is a less common myocardial complication of a mumps infection.

21. Clinical Therapeutics: Mastoiditis. Answer B: Vancomycin + cefepime is used to treat mastoiditis in a patient who has been treated for acute otitis media within the last 6 months. A, Ampicillin + cefotaxime is used to treat meningitis in patients less than 1 month old, not for the treatment of mastoiditis. C, Doxycycline is not used to treat mastoiditis. D, Piperacillin-tazobactam (Zosyn) is not used to treat mastoiditis.

22. H&P: Atrial Septal Defect. Answer B: Atrial septal defect is a midsystolic ejection click with a wide, fixed split S2 that is best heard at the left upper sternal border. A, Aortic stenosis is a midsystolic murmur heard best in the right upper sternal border with radiation to the carotids. C, Patent ductus arteriosus is a crescendo-decrescendo machinery-like murmur that is best heard at the left upper sternal border. D, An Innocent or Still's murmur is a vibratory systolic murmur that is best heard at the left lower sternal border while the patient is supine.

23. Health Maintenance: ADHD. Answer A: A routine bedtime and good sleep hygiene is important to establish while on stimulants for ADHD because of the risk of insomnia. Good sleep hygiene includes going to bed and waking up at the same time every day, avoiding caffeine in the afternoon, avoiding TV or electronics at least 1 to 2 hours before bedtime, and sleeping in a dark and quiet room. B, Stimulants can cause anorexia and therefore should be taken after meals to avoid decreased appetite and skipping meals. C, A complete blood count (CBC) is recommended before starting and periodically while on the medication long term, not liver function tests. D, EKG is recommended before starting a stimulant medication, but is not a continuous monitoring parameter while on methylphenidate.

24. Clinical Therapeutics: Generalized Epilepsy. Answer B: Levetiracetam is a first-line treatment for both generalized and focal epilepsy and does not require frequent blood monitoring. It is relatively safe in terms of its side effect profile, which are mainly behavioral, in comparison to other seizure medications. A, Valproic acid is not a first line medication and should not be the first therapy used in girls of child bearing age, though it is a broad-spectrum anticonvulsant and covers a variety of seizure types. It is often used to treat headaches and is also a mood stabilizer. The side effects of Valproic acid include weight gain (increased appetite), decreased platelet count, liver damage, tremor, hair loss, and ataxia. It has many interactions with other medications

Pediatrics

and frequent blood monitoring is required every 6 to 12 months. C, Tetrabenazine is used to treat dystonias not epilepsy. D, Ethosuximide is used to treat absence epilepsy only. In patients with focal EEG changes, this medication can worsen their seizures. The EEG results were not clearly given to us, but given the history, we can assume that the patient might have complex partial seizures, making ethosuximide a terrible choice for this patient.

25. Diagnosis: Osteosarcoma. Answer B: The description fits Osteosarcoma, which is a malignant bone tumor and the most common primary pediatric bone tumor. It is most common in the metaphysis of long bones. It requires chemotherapy and possibly limb sparing surgery or amputation. 20% of children have metastases at the time of diagnosis, often to the lungs or other bones. A, This x-ray finding is typical of Ewing sarcoma, which is a malignant bone tumor seen in older children and adolescents. It presents with increasing pain and swelling at the tumor site, which is often the long bones (femur, tibia, humerus) and there is no prior history of trauma or injury. It often wakes the child up at night and the child also presents with fever. C, This x-ray finding is consistent with Osteochondromas, which is a benign tumor in children. It is mostly seen in males. It presents as single or multiple painless mass(es) and can have associated surrounding bursitis or tendinitis. D, This x-ray finding is most consistent with Osteoid Osteoma, which is a benign bone-forming lesion of unclear etiology seen in children ages 5-20. It presents as increasing pain, worse at night, relieved by NSAIDs or aspirin. There will be tenderness over the lesion.

CHAPTER 37

Cardiovascular

Refer to Internal Medicine 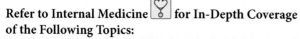 for In-Depth Coverage of the Following Topics:

Refer to Family Medicine for In-Depth Coverage of the Following Topics:

Refer to Appendices for the Following Topics:

Recommended Supplemental Material:

HYPOTENSION (CARDIOGENIC SHOCK, ORTHOSTATIC HYPOTENSION)

Shock: Underperfusion of tissues

- Presentation
  - Tachycardia, hypotension
  - Malfunction of organ systems: lactic acidosis, renal dysfunction (anuria/oliguria), CNS dysfunction (AMS)

- Initial steps: stabilize patient hemodynamically, determine cause
  - Fluid bolus (500-1000 L NS or lactated Ringer)
  - CBC, CMP, creatinine, PT/PTT, continuous pulse oximetry
  - EKG, CXR
  - Vasopressors (dopamine or norepinephrine) if hypotensive despite IVF
- Treatment
  - ABC assessment

Type of Shock	Cardiac Output	SVR	PCWP
Cardiogenic	Decreased	**Increased**	**Increased**
Hypovolemic	Decreased	**Increased**	Decreased
Neurogenic	Decreased	Decreased	Decreased
Septic	**Increased**	Decreased	Decreased

Disease	Etiology, Prevalence, Risk Factors	Clinical Symptoms and Signs	Diagnostics	Therapy, Prognosis, and Health Maintenance
Cardiogenic shock	Heart unable to generate CO to maintain tissue perfusion MCC: **post-acute MI** Cardiac tamponade, tension pneumothorax, arrhythmias, PE, CM, myocarditis, valvular defects	1. Altered sensorium Signs: 1. SBP <90 2. Urine output <20 mL/h 3. Pale cool skin 4. Hypotension 5. Tachycardia 6. JVD 7. Pulmonary congestion	1. EKG: ST elevation (most common) 2. Echo 3. Hemodynamic monitoring	1. ABCs 2. Identify underlying cause • Vasopressors: dopamine (initial) +/− dobutamine • NTG or nitroprusside • IVF−harmful if LV pressures elevated (may need diuretics)

SYNCOPE

Loss of consciousness/postural tone secondary to acute decrease in cerebral blood flow; rapid recovery of consciousness without resuscitation.

- Almost 20% of patients who present with "syncope" have a primary diagnosis of mood, anxiety, or substance abuse disorder, the most common being panic disorder
- Differential
  - Seizure disorder
  - Cardiac—sudden, no prodromal symptoms (face hits floor)
    - Arrhythmias (sick sinus syndrome, v-tach, AV block, rapid SVT)
    - Obstruction of blood flow (aortic stenosis, HCM, mitral valve prolapse)
    - Massive MI
  - **Vasovagal syncope** ("neurocardiogenic, simple faints, vasodepressor"): paradoxical withdrawal of sympathetic stimulation and enhanced parasympathetic stimulation
    - Most common cause (50%)
    - Emotional stress, pain, fear, extreme fatigue, claustrophobic situations
    - Premonitory SX: pallor, sweating, lightheadedness, nausea, dimming of vision, roaring in ears
    - First episode usually >40
    - **Tilt-table study** to reproduce symptoms
    - Treatment: supine posture, elevate legs, β-blockers
  - Orthostatic hypotension: ganglionic blocking agents, diabetes, old age, prolonged by bed rest; defect in vasomotor reflexes

- Posture is main cause, sudden standing or prolonged standing
- (+) Tilt-table test
- Premonitory symptoms: lightheaded, nausea, etc
- Treat with increased sodium and fluids, fludrocortisone
- Severe cerebrovascular disease—rare
  - TIA involving vertebrobasilar circulation
- Noncardiogenic causes: hypoglycemia, hyperventilation, hypersensitivity (wearing tight collar or turning head), mechanical reduction of venous return (Valsalva or postmicturition), medicines (BB, NTG, antiarrhythmics)
- Evaluation—r/o life-threatening causes (MI, hemorrhage, arrhythmias)
  - History: events before, during, and after; check medicines, witness reports
  - Physical: orthostatics, postictal mental status, murmurs, carotid pulses, apply pressure to carotid sinus (reflex bradycardia and hypotension)
  - **EKG**—for all patients
  - CBC, CMP
  - A 24-hour ambulatory EKG (Holter)
  - Tilt-table testing
  - CT or EEG—if seizure suspected
  - Echo—if evidence of structural heart disease or abnormal EKG
  - Electrophysiologic studies
  - Serum prolactin—although it may not differentiate between syncope or seizures, measurement after an event may rule out nonepileptic psychogenic events if performed within 10 to 20 minutes after an event; will be elevated after syncope or seizures

Disease	Etiology, Prevalence, Risk Factors	Clinical Symptoms and Signs	Diagnostics	Therapy, Prognosis, and Health Maintenance
Subclavian steal syndrome	Stenosis of the subclavian artery proximal to the takeoff of the vertebral artery	1. Vertigo 2. *Syncope* 3. Left arm exertion, angina, or ulcerated/gangrenous findings	1. **Unequal blood pressures in upper extremities**: ~45 mm Hg decrease in systolic pressure in arm supplied by stenotic vessel	1. Vascular consult 2. Elective hospitalization 3. Bypass grafting from common carotid to subclavian artery distal to lesion or transposition of subclavian beyond the lesion to the side of the nearby common carotid

AORTIC ANEURYSM OR DISSECTION (FIG. 37-1)

- An *aneurysm* is defined as a pathologic dilation of a segment of a blood vessel. A *true aneurysm* involves all 3 layers of the vessel wall and is distinguished from a *pseudoaneurysm*, in which the intimal and medial layers are disrupted and the dilated segment of the aorta is lined by adventitia only and, at times, by perivascular clot

- Aneurysms of the descending thoracic aorta are usually contiguous with infradiaphragmatic aneurysms and are referred to as *thoracoabdominal aortic aneurysms*

- Chronic cocaine or amphetamine use accelerates atherosclerosis, increasing the risk for dissection

- Most common complication of Marfan syndrome: aortic root disease and type A dissection (ascending)

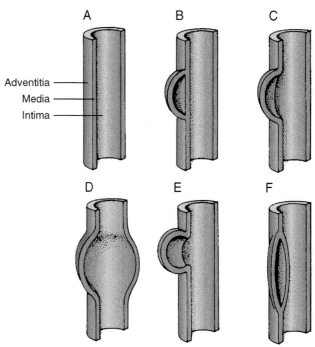

FIGURE 37-1. Types of aortic aneurysms. **A**, Normal artery. **B**, False aneurysm–actually a pulsating hematoma. The clot and connective tissue are outside the arterial wall. **C**, True aneurysm. One, two, or all three layers may be involved. **D**, Fusiform aneurysm–symmetric, spindle-shaped expansion of entire circumference of involved vessel. **E**, Saccular aneurysm–a bulbous protrusion of one side of the arterial wall. **F**, Dissecting aneurysm–this usually is a hematoma that splits the layers of the arterial wall. (Reprinted with permission from Morton PG, Fontaine DK, eds. *Critical Care Nursing: A Holistic Approach.* 11th ed. Philadelphia: Wolers Kluwer; 2018.)

Disease	Etiology, Prevalence, Risk Factors	Clinical Symptoms and Signs	Diagnostics	Therapy, Prognosis, and Health Maintenance

Aortic dissection Ascending: type A Descending: type B	Weakening of the aortic wall that may lead to the development of aneurysmal dilatation Bimodal:
	• Young patient with connective tissue disorders
	• Age 50+ with chronic hypertension
		Presentation predicts the intimal disruption:
		1. Abrupt, severe **chest pain**, radiates to the area between the scapulae
		  • Feeling of impending doom
		  • Anterior chest pain: type A
		  • Abdominal pain: type B
		  • 64% describe as sharp, 50% describe as tearing or ripping
		2. Syncope (10%), type A
		3. Dysphagia, hoarseness, Horner syndrome
		Signs:
		1. **Hypertension**
		2. Aortic insufficiency
		3. Pulse deficit in radial or femoral arteries
			1. EKG–r/o ACS
			2. Biomarkers–D dimer
			3. CXR: widened mediastinum, abnormal aortic contour
			4. **CT with and without (preferred)**
			  • Anatomy, location, extension, signs of rupture, end organ damage
			5. TEE–as sensitive and specific as CT
			6. CT angiography–DX CAD, PE, and aortic dissection
			  • Requires special contrast, increased radiation
			7. MRI (gold standard)
				1. Negative inotropic agent to lower BP without increasing the shear force on intimal flap
				  • **β-Blockers**: propranolol, labetalol, esmolol
				  • Goal: 100-120 systolic
				2. **Definitive: segmental resection of the dissection with interposition of a synthetic graft**
				Complications:
				Stroke, cardiac tamponade, paraplegia, back, flank, abdominal pain, death

(continued)

Emergency Medicine

(continued)

Disease	Etiology, Prevalence, Risk Factors	Clinical Symptoms and Signs	Diagnostics	Therapy, Prognosis, and Health Maintenance

Thoracic aortic aneurysm	Ascending aneurysms: medial degeneration
	Descending aneurysms: atherosclerosis
		Asymptomatic:
		1. Chest pain, SOB, cough
		2. Hoarseness, dysphagia
			1. CXR: widened mediastinal shadow, displacement of trachea or left main stem bronchus
			2. Echo (TEE)
			3. Contrast CT, MRI, invasive aortography
				1. If asymptomatic, follow with contrast CT or MRI every 6-12 mo
				2. β-Blockers for Marfan syndrome
				3. Prosthetic graft if symptomatic ascending AA, >5.5 cm
				  • With Marfan syndrome or bicuspid aortic valve, repair 4-5 cm
				  • Descending: >6 cm
				  • Increasing 1 cm/y
				Prognosis: worse if associated Marfan syndrome or dissection

Abdominal aortic aneurysm (AAA)	Aortic aneurysms result from conditions that cause degradation or abnormal production of the structural components of the aortic wall: elastin and collagen
	MC pathology:
	Atherosclerosis
	Older males, >50 y
	RF:
	Smoking, high cholesterol, aging, hypertension, male sex
		Asymptomatic:
		If ruptured → acute pain and hypotension
		Signs:
		1. Palpable, pulsatile, expansile, and nontender mass → becomes painful with expansion (chest, back, lower scrotum)
			1. **CXR**: calcified outline of aneurysm
			2. **Abdominal ultrasound**: serial documentation of size
			3. CT with contrast, MRI– determine location and size
				1. Medical emergency
				2. Endovascular placement of aortic stent graft or open surgical repair with prosthetic graft
				  • Expanding rapidly
				  • Asymptomatic >5.5 cm
				3. Serial noninvasive follow-up for <5 cm
				Prognosis:
				1. Related to size (>5 cm) and severity of coexisting CAD and CVD
				Screening:
				1. Screen in men aged 65-75 who have ever smoked
				2. Siblings of individuals with thoracic aortic or peripheral arterial aneurysms

ARTERIAL EMBOLISM OR THROMBOSIS

- Emboli that arise from a ventricular aneurysm or from a dilated cardiomyopathy can be very large and can lodge at the aortic bifurcation (saddle embolus), thus rendering both legs ischemic

- A palpable femoral pulse and absent popliteal and distal pulses may either be due to distal common femoral embolus (the pulse being palpable above the level of occlusion) or embolus to the superficial femoral or popliteal arteries

Thrombolysis	Embolectomy
1. Absolute CI: **Recent stroke, intracranial malignancy, brain metastases, or intracranial surgical intervention** 2. Relative CI: renal disease, allergy to contrast, cardiac thrombus, diabetic retinopathy, coagulopathy, recent arterial puncture, or surgery	Absolute contraindications to thrombolysis: 1. Established cerebrovascular events (including transient ischemic attack, stroke) within last *2 mo* 2. Active bleeding diathesis 3. Recent (*<10 d*) gastrointestinal bleeding 4. Neurosurgery (intracranial or spinal) within last *3 mo* 5. Intracranial trauma within last *3 mo* 6. Intracranial malignancy or metastasis

ACUTE LIMB ISCHEMIA (ACUTE ARTERIAL OCCLUSION)

- Patients found to have an ischemic but viable extremity on clinical examination should undergo urgent arteriography to plan surgical or percutaneous revascularization.

Catheter-directed thrombolytic therapy (mechanical and/ or pharmacologic) is a safe and effective alternative to surgery for appropriately selected patients

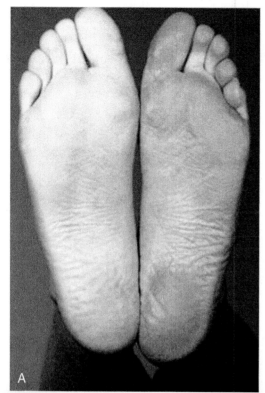

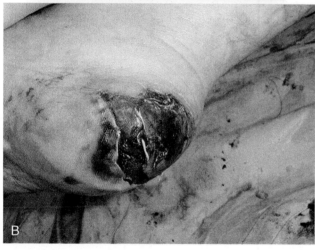

FIGURE 37-2. A, Acute limb ischemia. **B**, Blue toe syndrome. (**A**, Reprinted with permission from Topol EJ, Califf RM, Prystowsky EN, Thomas JD, Thompson PD, eds. *The Topol Solution*. 3rd ed. Philadelphia: Lippincott Williams & Wilkins; 2007. **B**, Reprinted with permission from Upchurch GR, Henke PK, eds. *Clinical Scenarios in Vascular Surgery*. 2nd ed. Philadelphia: Wolters Kluwer; 2015.)

Disease	Etiology, Prevalence, Risk Factors	Clinical Symptoms and Signs	Diagnostics	Therapy, Prognosis, and Health Maintenance

Acute limb ischemia (ALI) *or* acute arterial occlusion *or* threatened limb *or* critical limb ischemia (Fig. 37-2A)	Sudden loss of limb perfusion up to 2 wk after initiating event
	1%-2% of patients with **PAD age 50+**
	MCC:
	Embolism, native vessel thrombosis, reconstruction thrombosis, trauma, and complications of peripheral aneurysm
	MC location: femoral bifurcation
	RF:
	Diabetes (4×), smoking (3×), hypercholesterolemia (2×)
		1. **Pain**–foot/calf
		  • Abrupt, severe
		  • Gradually increasing in severity
		  • Progresses proximally
		2. **Paresthesias**: loss of *sensory* or *motor* function
		  • **Numbness**, tingling
		Signs:
		1. Pulselessness
		2. Pallor (severe)
		3. Paralysis
		4. Poikilothermia or perishing cold
			1. Ankle-brachial index
			  • 0.5-0.9 = claudication
			  • <0.5 = rest pain, necrosis
			2. **Contrast *angiography*** (gold standard) if prior vascular procedure or history of lower extremity claudication
			3. Baseline laboratory tests and Cr
				1. ***Thrombolysis*** less effective if it is of >2 wk duration
				  • Anticoagulation with ***IV heparin bolus*** → continuous heparin infusion ASAP
				  • Start IVF and Foley
				  • Gradual clot dissolution
				2. ***Embolectomy*** or thrombectomy
				3. Amputation if nonviable limb
				Complications:
				Stroke

(continued)

(continued)

Disease	Etiology, Prevalence, Risk Factors	Clinical Symptoms and Signs	Diagnostics	Therapy, Prognosis, and Health Maintenance
Blue toe syndrome (Fig. 37-2B)	Embolic occlusion of foot (digital) arteries with atheroembolic material from proximal source: *aorta* Small vessel occlusion	1. Sudden-onset, cool, painful, cyanotic toe, or forefoot Signs: 1. **Normal pedal pulses** and warm foot 2. Scattered petechiae or cyanosis of soles		Same as acute limb ischemia
Arterial embolism	MC source: Heart (90%) Associated: **Atrial fibrillation**, subacute endocarditis and acute bacterial endocarditis, rheumatic heart disease	1. No history of prior vascular disease	1. EKG: diagnose atrial fibrillation 2. TEE: look for cardiac source—presence of mobile plaque 3. CT scan: look for descending thoracic and abdominal sources	1. Embolectomy
Arterial thrombosis	RF for atherosclerosis, hypercoagulable status		1. Duplex imaging	1. Thrombectomy
Phlebitis	Inflammation at entry site due to needle or catheter insertion MCC of fever after postoperative day 3 Most common in lower extremity veins	1. Induration 2. Edema 3. Tenderness 4. Visible signs minimal: redness		Remove catheters at earliest signs Prevention: Aseptic technique during insertion, frequent change of tubing (48-72 h), rotation of insertion sites (every 4 d) Use silastic catheters (least reactive), and hypertonic solutions in veins with substantial flow
Suppurative phlebitis	MC bug: **Staphylococci** Presence of infected thrombus around indwelling catheter	Local signs of inflammation + pus from venipuncture site High fever	1. (+) Blood cultures	Excise affected vein Extend incision proximally to first open collateral Leave wound open

CLAUDICATION

- Differential: atherosclerosis obliterans, arteritis (Takayasu, giant cell), embolic disease (acute arterial occlusion), degenerative joint disease, spinal stenosis, myopathy, thromboangiitis obliterans, popliteal entrapment, venous claudication or varicosities, Baker cyst, deconditioning, aortic dissection, aortic coarctation, retroperitoneal fibrosis

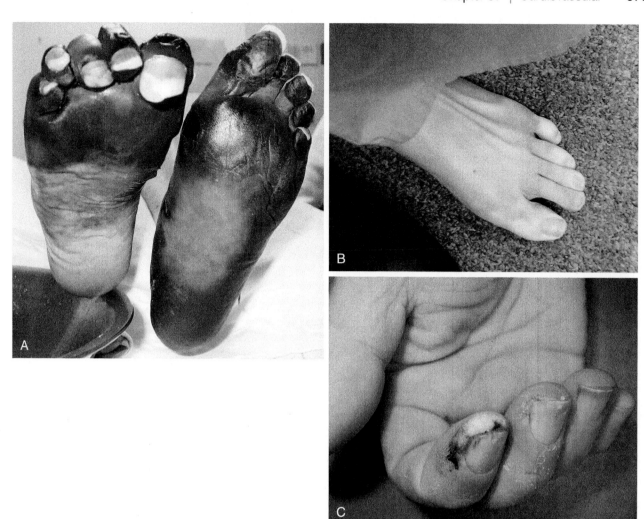

FIGURE 37-3. **A**, Thromboangiitis obliterans, Buerger disease. **B**, Raynaud phenomenon. **C**, Acrocyanosis. (**A**, Reprinted with permission from *Stedman's Medical Dictionary for the Health Professions and Nursing*. 6th ed. Philadelphia: Wolters Kluwer Health/Lippincott Williams & Wilkins; 2008. **B**, Reprinted with permission from Zierler RE, Dawson DL, eds. *Strandness's Duplex Scanning in Vascular Disorders*. 5th ed. Philadelphia: Wolters Kluwer; 2016. **C**, Image provided by Stedman's.)

Emergency Medicine

Disease	Etiology, Prevalence, Risk Factors	Clinical Symptoms and Signs	Diagnostics	Therapy, Prognosis, and Health Maintenance

Intermittent claudication	Means "limping" Occurs distal to the level of stenosis or occlusion For example, calf pain with walking 10%-35% of people with PAD	1. Reproducible pain in single or multiple muscle groups
		  • **Aggravated by** sustained **exercise**
		  • **Relieved with rest**
		  • Aching, dull pain
		  • Leg pain that occurs after certain walking distance causing patient to stop walking, resolving within 10 min
		2. Cramping
		3. Numbness, weakness, giving way
		Physical:
		1. **Hair loss** on bilateral lower extremities
		2. Thinning of skin
		3. Diminished pulses
			1. Treadmill testing using **ABIs** at rest and after exercise protocol (confirms)
			  • <0.9 (diagnostic)
				Stop smoking (first line):
				1. Graduated exercise—walk to point of claudication, rest, then continue walking
				2. Foot care
				3. Control HLD, HTN, weight, DM
				4. Avoid extremes of temperature
				5. **ASA + ticlopidine** or clopidogrel (symptomatic relief)
				6. Cilostazol (PDE inhibitor)
				Surgery:
				1. *Angioplasty*
				2. Bypass grafting

(continued)

(continued)

Disease	Etiology, Prevalence, Risk Factors	Clinical Symptoms and Signs	Diagnostics	Therapy, Prognosis, and Health Maintenance
Thromboangiitis obliterans, Buerger disease Difficult to differentiate from PVD, but lesions on toes and patient younger than 40 (Fig. 37-3A)	Nonatherosclerotic, segmental, inflammatory disease affecting small- to medium-sized arteries and veins of extremities **Typically, younger heavy smokers** MC arteries affected: plantar, digital vessels of foot and lower leg → fingers/hands in advanced stages	1. Digit ischemia (MC) 2. Intermittent claudication uncommon, but rest pain in toes frequent	1. MRA or invasive angiography	1. Stop smoking (mainstay) Prognosis: 1. Pain progresses to tissue loss and amputation, unless patient stops smoking 2. Prognosis better than PVD if smoking ceases
Takayasu arteritis	A granulomatous vasculitis of the aorta and its major branches Rare Females > males, early adulthood	1. Nonspecific constitutional symptoms • Malaise, fever, weight loss Signs: 1. Diminished pulses 2. Unequal blood pressure in both arms 3. Bruits over carotids and subclavian arteries 4. Limb claudication 5. Hypertension	1. ESR/ CRP–elevated 2. MRI–establishes diagnosis • Thickening of vessel walls 3. CT angiography–shows stenosis, occlusions, and dilations	1. Corticosteroids • Prednisone 1 mg/ kg × 1 mo → taper to 10 mg daily over several months 2. Adjunct: methotrexate or mycophenolate mofetil Prognosis: 1. Chronic relapsing and remitting course
Raynaud phenomenon (RP) (Fig. 37-3B)	Exaggerated response to **cold temperature or emotional stress** Provoking factors: • Cold temperature, emotional stress, sudden startling • Primary RP: idiopathic, Raynaud disease • Onset 15-30 y • Young women, family history (+) • Symmetric, involves fingers of both hands • No digital pitting, ulceration, or gangrene Secondary RP: • Rheumatic disease (scleroderma, SLE, Sjögren syndrome, polymyositis) • Unilateral, involves 1-2 fingers • Nailfold capillary abnormalities	1. Sharply demarcated color changes of skin of digits • Mostly affects the hands, but can occur in toes • Begins in single finger and spreads to other digits symmetrically in both hands 2. Sensation of pins and needles, numbness, and/or clumsiness of hand, finger aching Signs: 1. ***Pallor and cyanosis*** required, **erythema** 2. Reversible with rewarming or reduction of stress 3. Pain or ulceration of skin from ischemia 4. Livedo reticularis: violaceous mottling or reticular pattern of the skin of arms and legs	Clinical DX: 1. Nailfold capillaroscopy– distinguishes primary from secondary RP	1. Preventative • Wear gloves or mittens when outside • Keep body warm (mainstay) • Wear warm shirts, coats, and hats • Stop smoking • Lubricate with lotion frequently • Avoid sympathomimetics (decongestants, diet pills, amphetamines) For severe symptoms or tissue injury/ischemia: 1. Calcium channel blockers (first line) • More effective for primary than secondary RP • Nifedipine 30-180 mg/d • Amlodipine 5-20 mg/d 2. ACE inhibitors 3. Sympatholytic agents • Prazosin 4. Topical nitrates 5. PDE inhibitors • Sildenafil, tadalafil 6. SSRIs, bosentan, statins, prostaglandin E1, misoprostol or: 1. Sympathectomy (surgery)–for attacks that are frequent and severe, interfere with work/life Prognosis: 1. Primary RP–benign 2. Secondary RP–depends on severity

Disease	Etiology, Prevalence, Risk Factors	Clinical Symptoms and Signs	Diagnostics	Therapy, Prognosis, and Health Maintenance
Acrocyanosis (Fig. 37-3C)	Functional PVD Cyanosis of hands is permanent and diffuse	1. Symmetrical painless and persistent blue discoloration of hands or feet • Worse with cold Signs: 1. Absence of pallor 2. Hyperhidrosis	Seen in patients with scleroderma	1. Avoid cold exposure and Trauma

PALPITATIONS AND EDEMA

Disease	Etiology, Prevalence, Risk Factors	Clinical Symptoms and Signs	Diagnostics	Therapy, Prognosis, and Health Maintenance
Palpitations	Unpleasant awareness of forceful, rapid, or irregular beating of the heart Mostly benign, but can be lethal arrhythmias Rule out: panic, stress, anxiety, arrhythmia, presyncope, syncope, hyperthyroidism, hypovolemia, atrial fibrillation, other valvular defect, drug use	1. Described as • Stop and start • Fluttering • Pounding in the neck Signs: 1. "Cannon" A waves in the JVP, visible neck pulsations 2. Signs of hyperthyroid: tremulousness, brisk DTRs, hand tremor 3. Signs of drug use: dilated pupils, skin, or nasal septal perforations 4. Auscultate for midsystolic clicks, holosystolic murmurs, and changes with Valsalva, displaced PMI, etc	1. 12-Lead EKG and ambulatory EKG (Holter monitor) → inpatient continuous monitoring	1. Abstain from caffeine and tobacco 2. Reassurance if normal workup 3. If abnormal, treat underlying condition Refer for: 1. Electrophysiologic studies 2. Advice regarding treatment of arrhythmias When to admit: 1. Palpitations with near syncope or syncope, especially if >75 years old and abnormal EKG, Hct < 30%, SOB, RR >24/min, of Hx of CHF 2. High suspicion for arrhythmias
Edema	Lower extremity: either increased venous or lymphatic pressures, decreased intravascular oncotic pressure, increased capillary leak or infection/local injury MCC: Chronic venous insufficiency Common complication of DVT	1. MC symptom: sensation of "heavy legs" 2. Itching 3. Pain Signs: 1. Hyperpigmentation, stasis dermatitis 2. Lipodermatosclerosis (thick, brawny skin), atrophie blanche (small depigmented macules) 3. Measure size of calves 10 cm below tibial tuberosity 4. Check for tenderness and pitting 5. Ulcer located over medial malleolus (hallmark finding)	1. If low suspicion–D dimer indicated 2. Use Wells' criteria to rule out DVT or go to step 3 3. Color duplex ultrasound, as well as ABI 4. Urine dipstick to rule out nephrotic syndrome 5. SCr to check kidney function	1. Treat underlying cause 2. If chronic venous insufficiency without volume overload, avoid diuretics • May enhance sodium retention through increased secretion of renin and angiotensin → AKI and oliguria 3. Supportive care • Leg elevation above heart × 30 min TID and during sleep • Compression stockings • Ambulatory exercise

• Other causes of lower extremity edema: cellulitis, musculoskeleton-related disorders (Baker cyst rupture, diabetic myonecrosis, gastrocnemius rupture, or tear), lipoedema, heart failure, lymphedema, cirrhosis, nephrotic syndrome, medication side effects (CCB, minoxidil, pioglitazone), left common iliac vein compression, prolonged airline flights (>10 hours)

• Note: The left calf is normally slightly larger than the right because of the left common iliac vein coursing under the aorta (Fig. 37-4).

Emergency Medicine

DYSPNEA (FIG. 37-4)

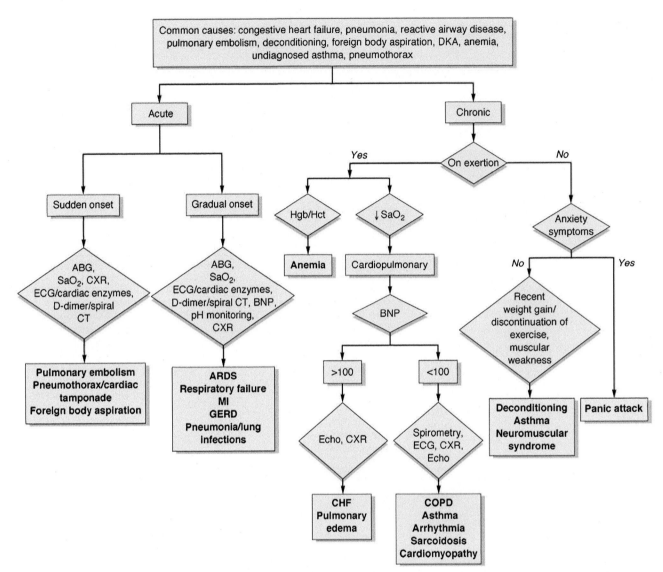

FIGURE 37-4. Dyspnea workup. (From Domino FJ. *The 5-Minute Clinical Consult 2019*. 27th ed. Philadelphia: Wolters Kluwer; 2019.)

ORTHOPNEA

Orthopnea—inability to breathe (SOB) in the horizontal (lying down) position that improves with sitting upright.

- Differential: COPD, acute asthma, gross obesity, heart failure

CHAPTER **38**

Orthopedics and Rheumatology

SPINAL CORD LEVELS—SENSORY EXAMINATION

- C6 (thumb), C7 (middle finger), C8 (pinky)
- T4 (nipple line), T10 (umbilicus)
- L3 (upper thigh), L4 (anterior knee, medial malleolus), L5 (dorsal aspect of foot, lateral malleolus), S1 (heel)

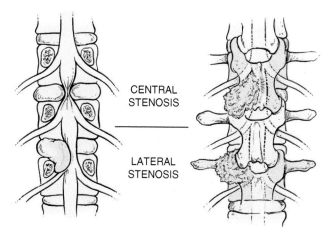

CENTRAL STENOSIS

LATERAL STENOSIS

FIGURE 38-1. Spinal stenosis. Lateral stenosis results from an overgrowth of the superior articular process and affects the spinal nerve root at the disk level, whereas central stenosis develops at the disk level because of a bulging disk with facet joint overgrowth from the inferior articular process. (Reprinted with permission from Anderson MK. *Foundations of Athletic Training: Prevention, Assessment, and Management.* 6th ed. Philadelphia: Wolters Kluwer; 2017.)

Disk	Root	Reflex	Muscle	Sensation
C4-C5	C5	Bicep reflex	Deltoid/bicep	Lateral arm
C5-C6	C6	Brachioradialis	Wrist extension/bicep	Thumb, index finger
C6-C7	C7	Triceps reflex	Wrist flex, triceps, finger extensors	Middle finger
C7-T1	C8	–	Grip strength	Ring/ulnar
T1-T2	T1	–	Finger abductors	Medial arm

- **Radicular** (root) **pain** differs from referred pain in that it is much greater in intensity; has distal radiation, circumscribed to the surrounding root; and has certain factors that excite it. It is caused by stretching, irritation, or compression of a spinal root within or central to the intervertebral foramen. The pain is often sharp, intense, and usually superimposed on the dull ache of referred pain; it nearly always radiates from a paracentral position near the spine to some part of the lower limb

    - Coughing, sneezing, and straining characteristically evoke this sharp radiating pain, although each of these actions may also jar or move the spine and enhance local pain

- The most common pattern is **sciatica**—pain that originates in the buttock and is projected along the posterior or posterolateral thigh.

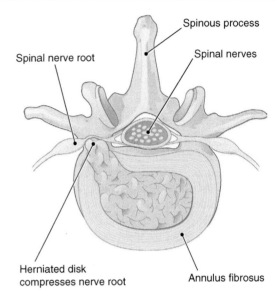

FIGURE 38-2. Herniated disk. The spinal nerve root experiences the pressure of the protruding central disk into the spinal canal. (Reprinted with permission from Cohen BJ. *Medical Terminology: An Illustrated Guide.* 6th ed. Philadelphia: Wolters Kluwer Health/Lippincott Williams & Wilkins; 2011.)

Disease	Etiology, Prevalence, Risk Factors	Clinical Symptoms and Signs	Diagnostics	Therapy, Prognosis, and Health Maintenance
Cauda equina lesion	Lesions below spinal cord termination at the L1 vertebral level (L4-L5)	1. Flaccid, areflexic asymmetric paraparesis • Bilateral lower extremity weakness 2. **Bowel and bladder incontinence** 3. Sensory loss below L1 (**saddle anesthesia**) • Numbness and/or paralysis 4. Leg pain (common) • Projected to perineum or thighs	1. XR 2. MRI (preferred)	1. Emergent surgery
Herniated disk (lumbar disk) (Figs. 38-1 and 38-2)	Most common: **L5-S1**, L4-L5, L3-L4, L2-L3, L1-L2 Major cause of severe and chronic or recurrent low-back and leg pain Mostly 30-40 y/o Sudden movement causes the weakened and frayed nucleus pulposus to prolapse and protrude through the annulus where they impinge on one or more nerve roots and cause sciatica or radicular pain	1. Pain referral (**sciatica**) • Midgluteal sciatica, posterior thigh, posterolateral leg, lateral foot, heel, or toes • Mild aching discomfort to severe knifelike stabbing, **radiating down the leg**, superimposed on intense ache 2. **Stiff or unnatural posture** 3. Some combination: • *Weakness* • Plantar flexor and hamstring weakness • *Reflex change* • Absent or diminished ankle jerk • *Paresthesias* Signs: • Pain with straight leg raise and tenderness over lumbosacral joint and sciatic notch • Discomfort walking on heels • Drop foot (L5) and weakness with plantar flexion (S1)	1. **Straight leg raise** with healthy leg (Lasègue maneuver): flexion at hip, extension at knee • Produces sciatic pain on contralateral side 2. **MRI of lumbar spine:** herniated nucleus pulposus • Not needed unless persistent pain for weeks 3. CT with myelography	1. Most comfortable lying supine with legs flexed at knees and hips, shoulders raised on pillows 2. Analgesics—**NSAIDs or opioids** for a few days • Repeated epidural injections of steroids with unconfirmed efficacy 3. Surgical decompression—emergent if: • Bilateral sensorimotor loss • Sphincteric paralysis

Disease	Etiology, Prevalence, Risk Factors	Clinical Symptoms and Signs	Diagnostics	Therapy, Prognosis, and Health Maintenance

Osteomyelitis	Inflammation of the bone
	MCC:
	S Staphylococcus aureus
	Streptococcus pyogenes (10%), other gram-negative organisms
	Puncture wounds:
	Pseudomonas aeruginosa
	Cause may be hematogenous, exogenous, surgical, true contiguous spread
	May be a complication from otitis externa or sinusitis, sickle cell anemia, diabetic ulcers, stasis ulcers, and arterial leg ulcers
		1. Acute: Worsening **pain**, swelling, tenderness, decreased ROM
		 • Chronic: recurrent acute flare-ups of tender, warm, swollen areas with constitutional symptoms (malaise, anorexia, fever, weight loss, night sweats)
		  • Duration: acute or chronic
		  • Site: spine, hip, other
		  • Extent: size of defect
		  • Specify type of patient: infant, child, adult, or immunocompromised
		2. **Fever**
		3. Drainage–rare
		Signs:
		Point tenderness over vertebral bodies or spinous processes
			Laboratory tests:
			1. CBC, CRP/ESR– elevated if chronic
			2. X-ray: **periosteal new bone** (involucrum)–signs lag behind symptoms and changes take 7-10 d
			3. 2× Blood culture or open **bone biopsy** (most accurate)
			4. Ultrasound for acute cases
			5. **MRI** shows changes before x-ray or bone scan; good for patients with diabetes with symptoms related to foot
				1. Acute
				 • 1-wk IV fluoroquinolone
				 • 2-wk PO FQ
				 • Adjunct: hyperbaric oxygen, negative pressure wound therapy (vacuum-assisted closure)
				2. Chronic
				 • Minimum 4 wk-24 mo IV and PO antibiotics
				 • PO rifampin and Bactrim
				3. Immobilization and surgical debridement may be required
				 • Indefinite oral antibiotics if known or presumed infected hardware
				4. Surgery
				 • Remove sequestra, sinus tract, infected bone, scar tissue
				5. Most common tumor associated with chronic osteomyelitis: **squamous cell carcinoma**

SEPTIC (INFECTIOUS) ARTHRITIS

Disease	Etiology, Prevalence, Risk Factors	Clinical Symptoms and Signs	Diagnostics	Therapy, Prognosis, and Health Maintenance
Septic arthritis	45% older than 65, also common in **immunosuppressed and elderly** 56% males Direct inoculation or contiguous spread from periarticular tissue, via **bloodstream** (MC): Intra-articular injections MCC: S. aureus	1. **Acute onset joint pain** (75%) • Pain superimposed on chronic pain • Previous Hx of joint disease of trauma • Recent catheterization or IVDU • Extra-articular symptoms 2. **Fever** (40%-60%), low grade <102°F, chills 3. **Impaired range of motion** Signs: • MC involved joint: **knee** (50%), hip, shoulder, ankle, wrists • **Swelling** (90%), **erythema, warmth, tenderness** • Effusion with marked limited ROM	1. **Synovial fluid for analysis** (r/o infection or crystals) • Typically, yellow green • Most septic joints have **WBC >50 000, >75% PMNs** • Low synovial glucose • If (+) crystals, gram stain (–) treat for crystal arthritis • If (–) crystals, treat patient for presumed infection even if (–) gram stain 2. Send fluid for culture regardless of result 3. **2 sets of blood cultures**–r/o bacteremia (40% +) 4. ESR/CRP: elevated 5. XR: periarticular soft tissue swelling → imaging not helpful	1. Drainage 2. Antibiotics • Native joint: **IV ceftriaxone (Rocephin) × 2 wk or** • **Dicloxacillin** 3. Immobilization of joint to control pain: no movement × 3 d, physical therapy 4. Arthrotomy and arthrocentesis often required 5. Poor prognosis: age >60, infection of hip or shoulder, underlying RA, (+) synovial fluid cultures after 7 d of therapy, delay of 7 d in starting therapy Complications: Dysfunctional joints, osteomyelitis, sepsis

(continued)

Emergency Medicine

(continued)

Disease	Etiology, Prevalence, Risk Factors	Clinical Symptoms and Signs	Diagnostics	Therapy, Prognosis, and Health Maintenance
Gonococcal	MC pathogen among young, sexually active: **Neisseria gonorrhoeae** (75%)	1. **Polyarticular, fever**, multiple skin **lesions** (dermatitis) developing after gonococcal infection from cervix, urethra, or pharynx • Hands (most), knee, wrist, ankle, elbow • Lesions: papular, pustular, vesicular, necrotic • May recur over several months 2. *Monoarticular*, tenosynovitis, lesions 3. *Septic bursitis*—olecranon or prepatellar bursae, swelling, pain		1. Add chlamydia TX: 2 g azithromycin or 7 d doxycycline twice weekly
Nongonococcal	**S. aureus** in adults and children >2, *Viridans streptococci, Streptococcus pneumoniae*, GBS GU infections with *Chlamydia trachomatis*	1. Monoarticular (85%-90%) • If >1 joint, most likely *S. aureus*		1. IV linezolid + rifampin × 4 wk, especially for prosthetic joint infections where CoNS is suspected

CHAPTER **39**

Pulmonology

Refer to Family Medicine 👥 for In-Depth Coverage of the Following Topics:

Refer to Pediatrics 👤 for In-Depth Coverage of the Following Topics:

Recommended Supplemental Topics:

SHORTNESS OF BREATH (DYSPNEA) (FIG. 37-4)

- **Dyspnea** (per American Thoracic Society): "a term used to characterize a subjective experience of breathing discomfort that is comprised of qualitatively distinct sensations that vary in intensity. The experience derives from interactions among multiple physiological, psychological, social, and environmental factors, and may induce secondary physiological and behavioral responses"

- The peripheral chemoreceptors, located in the carotid bodies and aortic arch, sense changes in the partial pressure of oxygen in arterial blood and are also stimulated by acidosis and hypercapnia. The central chemoreceptors, located in the medulla, respond to changes in pH and arterial tension of carbon dioxide ($Paco_2$).

- Clues to the need for an urgent evaluation include heart rate >120 beats/min, respiratory rate >30 breaths/min, pulse oxygen saturation (Spo_2) <90%, use of accessory respiratory muscles, difficulty speaking in full sentences, stridor, asymmetric breath sounds or percussion, diffuse crackles, diaphoresis, and cyanosis

Cardiovascular Causes	Respiratory Causes
1. Acute myocardial infarction 2. Heart failure 3. Cardiac tamponade	1. Bronchospasm 2. Pulmonary embolism 3. Pneumothorax 4. Pulmonary infection 5. Upper airway obstruction

History and Physical Examination in the Emergent Setting

History	Physical
1. PMH: new or recurrent, preexisting conditions, medication list 2. Events leading up to episode (recent symptoms), triggers (medication noncompliance or diet noncompliance, exposure to cold or allergen, onset after eating a particular food, new-onset cough, recent surgery or immobilization, trauma) 3. Prior intubation 4. Time course (sudden or insidious) 5. Severity 6. Associated: chest pain, trauma, fever, hemoptysis, sputum, cough 7. Tobacco or drug use 8. Psychiatric conditions	**Danger signs:** 1. Depressed mental status 2. Inability to maintain respiratory effort 3. Cyanosis 4. Tachypnea 5. Tripod position 6. Diaphoresis 7. Use of accessory muscles 8. Stridor or wheezing **Severe respiratory distress:** 1. Retractions 2. Fragmented speech 3. Inability to lie supine 4. Profound diaphoresis 5. Agitation or other AMS **Other:** 1. Peripheral edema 2. Heart murmur 3. Pulsus paradoxus 4. Crackles, augmented breath sounds

Workup in the Emergent Setting for Acute Dyspnea

1. EKG and CXR

2. Ancillary testing: cardiac biomarkers, ultrasound, BNP, D dimer, ABG/VBG, CO_2 monitoring, chest CT or VQ scan, peak flow and PFTs

3. EKG and pulse oximetry monitoring

4. Airway management

5. Establish most likely cause of dyspnea and initiate further treatment

Management

1. Oxygen provided

2. Establish IV access and obtain blood for measurements

Differential Diagnosis for Dyspnea

Head, Eyes, Ears, Nose, and Throat	Neurologic
Angioedema Anaphylaxis Pharyngeal infections Deep neck infections Foreign body Neck trauma	Stroke Neuromuscular disease
Chest wall	**Toxic/metabolic**
Rib fractures Flail chest	Organophosphate poisoning Salicylate poisoning CO poisoning Toxic ingestion Diabetic ketoacidosis Sepsis Anemia Acute chest syndrome
Pulmonary	
COPD exacerbation Asthma exacerbation Pulmonary embolism Pneumothorax Pulmonary infection **Acute respiratory distress syndrome** (ARDS) Pulmonary confusion or other lung injury Hemorrhage	**Miscellaneous**
	Hyperventilation Anxiety Pneumomediastinum Lung tumor Pleural effusion Intra-abdominal process Ascites Pregnancy[a] Massive obesity[a]
Cardiac	
ACS ADHF Flash pulmonary edema High-output failure Cardiomyopathy Arrhythmia Valvular dysfunction Cardiac tamponade	

[a]Although these conditions do not cause acute dyspnea directly, they can exacerbate symptoms or contribute to other underlying causes.
From *Differential diagnosis of acute dyspnea. UpToDate.* 2018. https://www.uptodate.com/contents/image?imageKey=EM%2F52926&topicKey=EM%2F292&source=outline_link&search=dyspnea&selectedTitle=2~150.

WHEEZING

- Differential: status asthmaticus, bronchiolitis, lower airway foreign body, allergic reaction
  - If inspiratory: croup or upper airway foreign body
  - Wheezing without fever—atypical pneumonia, atelectasis, bronchiolitis, asthma, anaphylaxis, pulmonary edema, chronic pulmonary disease exacerbation, heart failure, foreign body, mediastinal mass
- Diffuse expiratory wheezes are a sign of lower airway intrathoracic obstruction typically caused by asthma or bronchiolitis. They are musical in tone with higher pitched wheezes indicative of more severe obstruction
- Unilateral wheezes may be appreciated if there is a foreign body in the lower airway
- Inspiratory wheezes indicate an upper airway extrathoracic obstruction or a severe fixed intrathoracic obstruction, and are most commonly due to laryngeal edema or a foreign body
- In severe cases, wheezes can be appreciated without a stethoscope. However, if asthma is so severe that air movement is poor, wheezes may not be heard

- Evaluation
  - Pulse oximetry
  - CBC with differential—rule out infection or anemia
  - Blood glucose, electrolytes, and blood gas—in suspected diabetic ketoacidosis
  - Blood, urine, CSF cultures—if child with fever and altered mental status
  - ABG—for severe respiratory distress
  - XR—neck, chest, abdominal based on history
  - EKG—rule out cardiac causes
  - Ultrasound—rule out pulmonary causes
  - CT—r/o intra- or extrathoracic structural abnormalities, masses, vascular processes
- Stabilization and treatment—depends on history, physical examination, and evaluation

HEMOPTYSIS

- **Massive hemoptysis**: bleeding that is potentially life threatening, defined as a range from 100 mL to more than 600 mL of blood over 24 hours (generally >500 mL over 24 hours)

- Bleeding from a bronchial artery is the cause of massive hemoptysis in 90% of cases, as 1 to 2 of them typically provide blood supply to each lung. They most commonly arise from the aorta and are under high systemic pressure, but carry only a portion of the cardiac output
- Most common causes: bronchitis, bronchogenic carcinoma, and bronchiectasis in developed countries

Disease	Etiology, Prevalence, Risk Factors	Clinical Symptoms and Signs	Diagnostics	Therapy, Prognosis, and Health Maintenance
Hemoptysis	The expectoration of blood	History: 1. How much blood coughed up in 24-48 h? 2. Is blood mixed with white or purulent phlegm? 3. What is the frequency of hemoptysis? 4. Is this a new or recurrent symptom? 5. Is the patient dyspneic? 6. Are there other symptoms to suggest infection (eg, fever, chills or night sweats)? 7. Are there any symptoms to suggest systemic disease (rash, hematuria, joint pain, or swelling)? Signs: 1. Sputum color or purulent secretions 2. Tachypnea, tachycardia, accessory muscle use, cyanosis, diaphoresis 3. Focal wheeze or diffuse crackles? 4. Heart murmur 5. Palpable purpura, telangiectasia 6. Peripheral edema, joint effusions, or periarticular warmth	1. Hgb/Hct–assess magnitude and chronicity of bleed 2. CBC white/differential–r/o infection 3. Urinalysis and renal function–r/o Goodpasture syndrome or Wegener granulomatosis 4. LFTs and coag–r/o thrombocytopenia or other coagulopathy 5. Sputum culture or serologic testing for ANA, ANCA, or other Ab 6. *CXR* (most important for all persons) 7. BNP or pro-BNP–if cardiac causes suspected 8. Consider D dimer	1. Cause and location guide treatment • Mild to moderate with good gas exchange: no hospitalization required 2. Supportive care • Adequate ventilation • Airway support • Control hemoptysis • Monitor pulse oximetry

PLEURITIC CHEST PAIN

- **Pleuritic chest pain** (pleurisy): pain with forceful breathing movement (taking a deep breath, talking, coughing, or sneezing)
- Most common potentially life-threatening cause: pulmonary embolism (5%-20% of patients who present to the ED with pleuritic pain)
- Differential: pericarditis, pneumonia, myocardial infarction, pneumothorax, etc

- Treatment
  - Control the pleuritic chest pain with **NSAIDs** (first line)—typically indomethacin (Indocin)
  - Treat underlying cause

Emergency Medicine

ACUTE BRONCHITIS

- DDx: Upper respiratory tract infection

Disease	Etiology, Prevalence, Risk Factors	Clinical Symptoms and Signs	Diagnostics	Therapy, Prognosis, and Health Maintenance

Upper respiratory tract infection (common cold)	Viral
	Incubation period: 1-3 d
		1. Nasal congestion, discharge (rhinorrhea), sneezing
		2. Sore throat
		3. Cough
		4. Low-grade fever
		5. Headache
		6. Malaise
			Clinical DX	<u>Symptoms are self-limited:</u>
				1. Mild—no treatment
				2. Moderate to severe: symptomatic therapy
				  • Analgesics for headache, ear pain, muscle/joint pains, malaise, sneezing
				  • Antihistamines and decongestants, intranasal or inhaled cromolyn sodium, or intranasal ipratropium bromide
				  • Cough: dextromethorphan
				  • Nasal saline sprays
				  • Expectorants: guaifenesin
				<u>Complications:</u>
				Sinusitis, lower respiratory tract disease, asthma exacerbations, acute otitis media

PERTUSSIS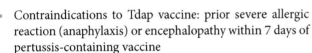

- Contraindications to Tdap vaccine: prior severe allergic reaction (anaphylaxis) or encephalopathy within 7 days of pertussis-containing vaccine

INFLUENZA

- The most extensive and *severe* outbreaks are caused by **influenza A** because of the propensity of H and N antigens to undergo periodic antigenic variation

  - Designation is based on antigenic characteristics of the nucleoprotein (BP) and matrix (M) protein antigens

- Further subdivided on the basis of surface hemagglutinin (H) and neuraminidase (N) antigens
- Hemagglutinin is the site where the virus binds to sialic acid cell receptors, whereas neuraminidase degrades the receptor and plays a role in the release of the virus from infected cells after replication has taken place
- Individual strains are designated according to the site of origin, isolate number, year of isolation, and subtype
- Major variation—antigenic shifts (only seen with influenza A), associated with pandemics
- Minor variations—antigenic drifts

Disease	Etiology, Prevalence, Risk Factors	Clinical Symptoms and Signs	Diagnostics	Therapy, Prognosis, and Health Maintenance

Influenza	Orthomyxovirus
	<u>Transmission:</u>
	Respiratory droplets
	Winter months
		1. Rapid onset of fever, chills, malaise, myalgia (legs or lumbosacral area)
		  • **Fever** 100.4-105.8°F
		2. **Headache**: generalized or frontal
		3. Nonproductive **cough**: may last more than 1 wk
		4. Ocular signs/SX: pain with motion of eyes, photophobia, burning of eyes
		5. Sore throat
		6. +/− Nausea
		<u>Signs:</u>
		1. Cervical LAD
		2. Rhonchi, wheezes, and scattered rales
			1. Reverse transcriptase polymerase chain reaction (RT-PCR) is the most sensitive and specific
			  • Can differentiate subtypes and detect avian flu
				1. Supportive care
				  • Tylenol or NSAIDs for headache, myalgias, fever
				  • No cough suppressants
				2. **Neuraminidase inhibitor**: zanamivir or oseltamivir for flu types A and B
				  • Reduces symptoms by 1-1.5 d if started within 2 d of onset
				  • Effective up to 5 d after onset
				3. Adamantane agents: amantadine and rimantadine for flu type A
				<u>Complications:</u>
				Secondary bacterial pneumonia

	Zanamivir (Relenza)	Oseltamivir (Tamiflu)
Indications	Prophylaxis in adults and pediatric patients >5 y old Uncomplicated acute illness by influenza A and B in adults and pediatric patients >7 y old who have been symptomatic for no more than 2 d	Prophylaxis: children >1 y of age and adults Treatment: >2 wk old and adults symptomatic for no more than 2 d
Adverse effects	Headache	Vomiting Nausea, abdominal pain, diarrhea
Contraindications	Hypersensitivity to milk or zanamivir	Hypersensitivity to oseltamivir Renal adjustment
Dosing	Prophylaxis: 2 inhalations (10 mg) once daily × 10 d, begin within 36 h of onset Treatment: 2 inhalations daily × 5 d, separated by 2 h, begin within 48 h of onset	Prophylaxis: 75 mg PO daily × 10 d, start within 48 h of contact with infected individual Treatment: 75 mg PO BID × 5 d, start within 48 h of onset

PLEURAL EFFUSION

A pleural effusion is present when there is an excess of fluid in the pleural space. It accumulates when pleural fluid formation exceeds pleural fluid absorption. Normally, fluid enters the pleural space from the capillaries in the parietal pleura and is removed via the lymphatics in the parietal pleura. The lymphatics have the capacity to absorb 20 times more fluid than is formed normally. Accordingly, a pleural effusion may develop when there is excess pleural fluid formation (from the interstitial spaces of the lung, the parietal pleura, or the peritoneal cavity) or when there is decreased fluid removal by the lymphatics.

- Diagnostics: chest U/S has replaced lateral decubitus CXR in the evaluation of suspected pleural effusions, and guides thoracentesis
- Differentiate between transudative and exudative: the primary reason for making this differentiation is that additional diagnostic procedures are indicated with exudative effusions to define the cause of the local disease
  - Indications for thoracentesis
    - Lack of resolution of pleural effusion in the setting of CHF (without symptoms of fever, chest pain, or *dyspnea*)
    - Regression of symptoms in the first days of diuretic therapy
    - Unilateral effusion
    - Presence of fever or chest pain

- Indications for thoracostomy
  - Gram (+) stain of pleural fluid, (+) pleural fluid culture, pus
  - → Remove when <100 mL fluid drains in 24 hours
- Remove no more than 1.5 L per procedure
- **Video-assisted thoracoscopic surgery** may be required to lyse extensive intrapleural adhesions
- If 1+ exudative criteria are met and the patient is clinically thought to have a condition producing a transudative effusion, measure the difference between protein levels in pleural fluid versus serum
- If a patient has an exudative pleural effusion, the following tests on the pleural fluid should be obtained: description of the appearance of the fluid, glucose level, differential cell count, microbiologic studies, and cytology
- **Light criteria**—helps you differentiate between a transudative and exudative pleural effusion; not enough to formulate a diagnosis by itself
  - **Pleural fluid [protein]: serum [protein] ratio >0.5 (less protein in the blood)**
  - **Pleural fluid [LDH]: serum [LDH] >0.6 (less LDH in the blood)**
  - Pleural fluid [LDH] > 2/3 ULN serum [LDH]
  - Exudate if any 1 of the above criteria is met, otherwise usually transudate

Transudative (Imbalance of Pressure in Vessels)	Exudative (Injury and Inflammation)
• Increase in <u>hydrostatic pressure</u> of pleural membrane microvessel • Decrease in serum <u>colloid osmotic pressure</u> (nephrotic syndrome) eg, **hepatic hydrothorax** (5%-10% patients with cirrhosis and portal HTN): transdiaphragmatic movement of abdominal ascitic fluid from peritoneal compartment to pleural space via diaphragmatic openings • Ascites, jaundice, LFT abnormalities • Confirm with radionuclide scan • TX: paracentesis to drain ascites, **sodium restriction, diuresis** Refractory hepatic hydrothorax (10%) • TX: transjugular intrahepatic portosystemic shunt (TIPS)–decreases portal venous pressure and rate of ascites formation	• Increased <u>permeability</u> of microvessels in pleural membranes, can be due to pleural inflammation in neoplasia • Fibrin deposits limit outflow rate via lymphatics • <u>Increased protein</u> and other biomarkers • Clinical features of parapneumonic effusion: protracted respiratory SX (7-10 d to wk) despite antibiotics Complicated examination findings: large effusions (>40%-50% of hemithorax), loculated or multiloculated fluids on chest CT with thick or enhancing visceral pleura, pH < 7.3, LDH > 1000 unit/L, glucose <40 mg/dL • Stage 1 (capillary leak): 2-5 d after onset → TX: tube thoracostomy • Stage 2 (fibrinopurulent or bacterial invasion stage): 3-14 d after onset • Stage 3 (organizational, empyema stage): 10-21 d *Thoracic empyema*: overt pus in pleural space; end result of complicated examination findings

Transudative (Imbalance of Pressure in Vessels)	Exudative (Injury and Inflammation)
• Mnemonic: transudate is transparent (no proteins) • Low pleural fluid concentrations of plasma protein (albumin), LDH, cholesterol • Bilateral inspiratory crackles • MCC: **left ventricular heart failure** and cirrhosis • Examples: **cirrhosis**, hepatic hydrothorax, **pulmonary embolism, nephrotic syndrome**, hypothyroidism, peritoneal dialysis	Mnemonic: exudate exudes proteins • MCC: **parapneumonic effusion** (40%-50% of bacterial pneumonias) • Examples: **pneumonia, empyema, malignancy, pulmonary embolism**, connective tissue disease, pancreatitis, tuberculous pleurisy, esophageal rupture, drug reaction • Uncomplicated parapneumonic effusion: exudative, free-flowing effusion developing with infectious pneumonia → treat pneumonia, requires **thoracentesis** • Complicated parapneumonic effusion: requires pleural space drainage for resolution → intrapleural adhesions, loculated fluids, trapped lung

Serum albumin ascites gradient (SAAG) is used for finding out the cause of ascites.

- **SAAG = albumin in serum—albumin in ascitic fluid**

- If SAAG > 1.1, it is portal hypertension

- If SAAG < 1.1, it could be cancer, nephrotic syndrome, tuberculosis, etc

Pleural Effusion and Foreign Body Aspiration
(Fig. 39-1)

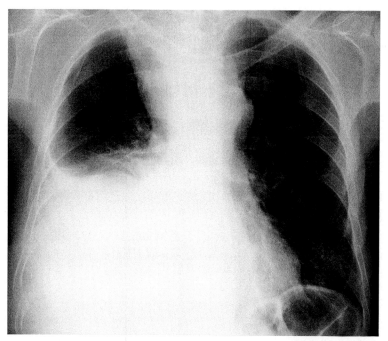

FIGURE 39-1. Right-sided pleural effusion and a right superior mediastinal mass on chest x-ray in a patient with non-Hodgkin lymphoma. (Reprinted with permission from Webb WR, Higgins CB. *Thoracic Imaging: Pulmonary and Cardiovascular Radiology*. 3rd ed. Philadelphia: Wolters Kluwer; 2017.)

Disease	Etiology, Prevalence, Risk Factors	Clinical Symptoms and Signs	Diagnostics	Therapy, Prognosis, and Health Maintenance
Pleural effusion	Common after upper abdominal operations Highest risk: patients with free peritoneal fluid and postoperative atelectasis May suggest subdiaphragmatic inflammation (subphrenic abscess, acute pancreatitis) Abnormal collection of fluid in pleural space resulting from excess fluid production, decreased absorption, or both	1. Dyspnea (MC) 2. **Cough**—mild, nonproductive 3. Chest pain—mild to severe, sharp and stabbing, worse with deep inspiration, localized or referred to ipsilateral shoulder 4. Other SX: increasing lower extremity edema, orthopnea, PND <u>No physical examination findings if ≤300 mL, otherwise:</u> 1. Dullness to percussion 2. Decreased tactile fremitus 3. Egophony changes in superior aspect 4. Decreased breath sounds 5. Asymmetrical chest expansion 6. Mediastinal shift away from the effusion if >1000 mL 7. Pleural friction rub		If not compromising airway function, leave alone If suspicious for infection, sample by needle aspiration If respiratory compromise, drain with thoracostomy tube <u>Indications for urgent drainage:</u> 1. Frank purulent fluid 2. Pleural fluid pH <7 3. Loculated effusions 4. Bacteria on gram stain or culture

(continued)

(continued)

Disease	Etiology, Prevalence, Risk Factors	Clinical Symptoms and Signs	Diagnostics	Therapy, Prognosis, and Health Maintenance
Pulmonary aspiration	Aspiration of oropharyngeal and gastric contents High risk: pregnant, intestinal obstruction, a person who has had a trauma, thoracic or abdominal surgery, tracheostomy Basal segments affected most	1. Tachypnea 2. Rales 3. Hypoxia within hours 4. Less common: cyanosis, wheezing, apnea, hypovolemia		1. Preoperative fasting, proper positioning of patient, careful intubation 2. H2 or PPI before anesthesia if high risk Prognosis: 1. Death rate is 50%

PULMONARY EMBOLISM/DEEP VEIN THROMBOSIS, ACUTE RESPIRATORY DISTRESS/FAILURE, PNEUMOTHORAX

- Consider pulmonary embolism (PE) and deep vein thrombosis (DVT) as a continuum of one clinical entity (venous thromboembolism—VTE)—diagnosing either is an indication for treatment

- Modified Wells' Criteria—decision rule for suspected acute PE

Wells' Criteria for Risk of Pulmonary Embolism				
DVT			**PE**	
Variable	Score		Variable	Score
Active cancer	1.0		Clinical evidence of DVT	3.0
Paralysis/immobilization	1.0		Other DX less likely than PE	3.0
Bedridden for >3 d or major surgery within 4 wk	1.0		Heart rate >100	1.5
Entire leg swollen	1.0		Immobile >3 d or major surgery within 4 wk	1.5
Tenderness along deep vein	1.0		Previous DVT/PE	1.5
Calf swelling >3 cm	1.0		Hemoptysis	1.0
Pitting edema (unilateral)	1.0		Malignancy	1.0
Collateral superficial veins	1.0			
Alternative DX more likely than DVT	−2			
Score and Probability–DVT			**Score and Probability–PE**	
High: 3 or greater (75% risk of DVT)			High: 6 or greater (70% risk of PE)	
Moderate: 1 or 2 (20% risk of DVT)			Moderate: 2-6 (20%-30% risk of PE)	
Low: 0 (3% risk of DVT)			Low:<2 (2%-3% risk of PE)	

From Goldhaber SZ, Bounameaux H. Pulmonary embolism and deep vein thrombosis. *Lancet*. 2012;379:1835.

The Presence or Absence of Hemodynamic Stability

The first step in working up a patient for probable pulmonary embolism is to determine if he or she is hemodynamically stable.

Unstable "Massive" (hemodynamic effect, not size) **"High risk"**	Stable "Submassive" or **"Intermediate risk"** Presence of right ventricular strain	Stable **"Low risk"** Absence of right ventricular strain
• Results in hypotension • SBP <90 mm Hg or • A drop of ≥40 mm Hg from baseline × 15 min or • Hypotension requiring vasopressors or inotropic support unexplained by sepsis, arrhythmia, LVD from AMI or hypovolemia • More likely to die of obstructive shock (severe right ventricular failure) • Death within first 2 h • Elevated risk 72 h after initial presentation	• Mild or borderline hypotension that stabilizes with fluid therapy • Present with right ventricular dysfunction • Do not meet criteria for unstable PE	• Mildly symptomatic or asymptomatic patients • Do not meet criteria for unstable PE

Risk for Bleeding and Empiric Anticoagulation

Unacceptably "High Risk" of Bleeding	"Intermediate Risk" for Bleeding	"Low Risk" of Bleeding
• Absolute contraindications to anticoagulant therapy (recent surgery, hemorrhagic stroke, active bleeding) or patients with high risk of bleeding (aortic dissection, intracranial or spinal cord tumors)[a]	• 1+ risk factor for bleeding	• No risk factors for bleeding (age >65, previous history of bleeding, cancer, liver or renal failure, thrombocytopenia, previous CVA, diabetes, anemia, antiplatelet therapy, poor anticoagulant control, recent surgery in last 10 d (for IV therapy), frequent falls, alcohol abuse)
• Do not administer empirical anticoagulation, if high bleeding risk or contraindicated • Consider IVC filter or embolectomy if PE confirmed	• Risk of bleeding 3%-13% • Therapy individualized based on clinical assessment and patient preferences	• Bleeding risk <2% • Empirical anticoagulation if clinical suspicion for PE • High (Wells' >6) • Moderate (Wells' 2-6), diagnostic studies expected to yield result >4 h • Low (Wells' <2), diagnostic studies expected to give result >24 h[b] • Do not administer thrombolytics
1. If hemodynamically unstable—immediate anticoagulation, unless contraindicated (see bleeding risks above) • IV **unfractionated heparin** (in anticipation of IVC filter versus embolectomy) • UFH 1 bolus + continuous infusion × 5-10 d (a**PTT 1.5-2.5 × ULN**) or • Oral warfarin (INR 2-3) + heparin day 1 • **Thrombolytics** for massive PE and hypotensive, RHF • IVC placement, if high risk of recurrent DVT and anticoagulation contraindicated 2. Do not use factor Xa inhibitors or DTI	• Therapy individualized based on clinical assessment and patient preferences	1. **Low-molecular-weight heparin**—if no renal insufficiency • Lovenox (enoxaparin) • Fragmin (dalteparin) • Innohep (tinzaparin)

[a]Presence of minor hemoptysis, epistaxis, or menstruation is not contraindication but should be monitored.
[b]Regardless of risk, if hemodynamically stable.

Indefinite and long-term anticoagulation: administered beyond 3 months if the patient has persistent risk factors or unprovoked VTE.

• Do not administer for patients with provoked VTE episode with major transient risk factors (surgery, cessation of hormonal therapy) or in patients with high bleeding risk

• Must follow-up at least annually

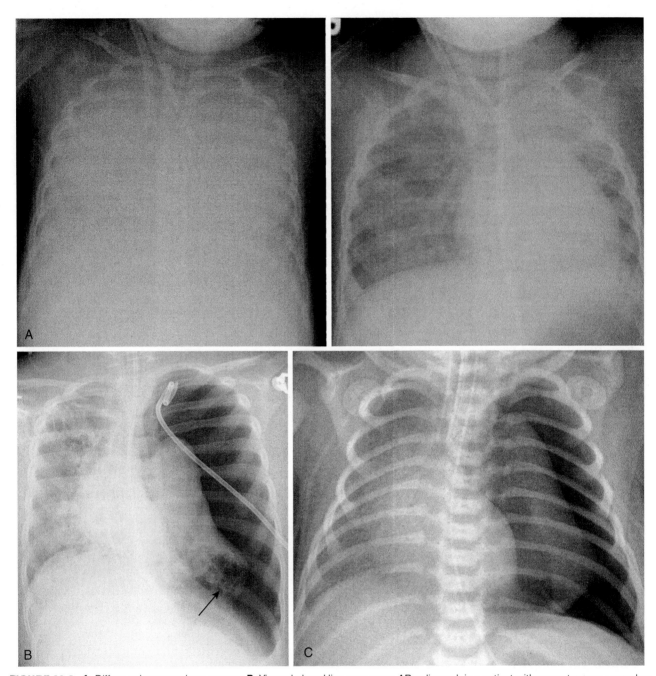

FIGURE 39-2. A, Diffuse pulmonary edema on x-ray. **B,** Visceral-pleural line seen on an AP radiograph in a patient with a spontaneous secondary pneumothorax. In this image, you can see a large left pneumothorax with a right mediastinal shift *(arrow)*. **C,** Tension pneumothorax on chest x-ray showing collapse of the left lung and mediastinal shift to the right. (**A,** Reprinted with permission from Gravlee GP, Davis RF, Hammon J, Kussman B, eds. *Cardiopulmonary Bypass and Mechanical Support: Principles and Practice.* 4th ed. Wolters Kluwer; 2016. **B,** Reprinted with permission from Collins J, Stern EJ. *Chest Radiology: The Essentials.* 2nd ed. Philadelphia: Lippincott Williams & Wilkins/Wolters Kluwer Business; 2008. **C,** Reprinted with permission from Kline-Tilford AM, Haut C. *Lippincott Certification Review: Pediatric Acute Care Nurse Practitioner.* Philadelphia: Wolters Kluwer; 2016.)

Emergency Medicine

Disease	Etiology, Prevalence, Risk Factors	Clinical Symptoms and Signs	Diagnostics	Therapy, Prognosis, and Health Maintenance

Pulmonary embolism	Thrombus in another region of the body embolizes to pulmonary vascular tree via RV and pulmonary artery → blood distal obstructed → increased PVR → increased pulmonary artery pressure → increased RV pressure → cor pulmonale (severe)
	
	MC site:
	1. Most lodge distal to bifurcation of main pulmonary artery in main lobar, segmental, or subsegmental branches of pulmonary artery
	2. Saddle: bifurcation of main pulmonary artery (3%-6%)
	
	Incidence:
	Males > females
	
	RF:
	Age >60 y, malignancy, prior history, hypercoagulable states (factor 5 Leiden, protein C/S deficiency, antithrombin III deficiency), prolonged **immobilization or bed rest**, **long-distance travel**, cardiac disease (CHF), **obesity**, nephrotic syndrome, major surgery (pelvic) or major trauma in prior 4 wk, pregnancy, estrogen use (OCP)
	
	Virchow's triad: hypercoagulable state, venous stasis, endothelial injury
		Mostly asymptomatic:
		1. **Dyspnea (MC)**
		  • At rest or with exertion
		  • Rapid onset
		2. **Pleuritic chest pain**
		  • Worse with inspiration
		3. Cough
		4. Calf or thigh pain +/− swelling
		5. Wheezing
		6. Hemoptysis
		7. Syncope (large PE)
		
		Signs:
		1. **Tachypnea**
		2. Calf or thigh: swelling, erythema, edema, tenderness, palpable cords
		3. Tachycardia >100 bpm
		4. Rales
		5. Decreased breath sounds
		6. Accentuated pulmonic component of S2
		7. JVD
		8. Fever (3%)
		
		Signs of RVHF:
		1. **Hypotension and JVD**
		2. R-sided S3
		3. Parasternal lift
		4. Cyanosis
			Screening:
			1. CXR−normal, +/− atelectasis or pleural effusion
			2. D dimer−if low clinical suspicion, do first (sensitive)
			3. EKG: commonly shows tachycardia and non-specific ST and T-wave changes
			  • <10% show S1Q3T3
			1. **(+) CT pulmonary angiogram** with contrast (gold standard), invasive
			  • Presence of a filling defect in any branch of pulmonary artery
			2. V/Q scan: normal CXR required prior, treat if high probability
			  • Test of choice in pregnancy, contrast allergy, and patients with renal insufficiency
			3. Doppler U/S of lower extremity−helpful when (+), useless when negative, perform if renal insufficiency
			4. Increased A-a gradient: PAo2-Pao2 due to VQ mismatch
			5. ABG−respiratory alkalosis, low Pao2 and Paco2, pH high
				Treatment options:
				1. Supplemental O_2, target ≥90%
				2. If hemodynamically **unstable**
				  • IVF
				  • Vasopressors: norepinephrine
				3. Anticoagulation (as above)
				
				Prognosis:
				1. Recurrence common → chronic pulmonary HTN and cor pulmonale
				2. 10% mortality when diagnosed, 30% if undiagnosed
				3. Poor prognostic factors
				  • Hyponatremia
				  • Elevated lactate
				  • Leukocytosis
				  • Age ≥65
				
				Complications:
				1. In patients with PE who survive initial event: recurrent PE or pulmonary HTN (in two-thirds)
				2. 50% with DVT have concurrent PE at presentation

Alteplase (tPA)	Indications: massive pulmonary embolism, STEMI, acute ischemic CVA (within 3 h) Contraindications to tPA: head trauma, hemorrhagic stroke Antidote: aminocaproic acid			

Emergency Medicine

(continued)

(continued)

Disease	Etiology, Prevalence, Risk Factors	Clinical Symptoms and Signs	Diagnostics	Therapy, Prognosis, and Health Maintenance
ARDS	An acute hypoxemic respiratory failure following a systemic or pulmonary insult without evidence of heart failure Effects of increased pulmonary fluid same as cardiogenic pulmonary edema, but the cause is different RF: 1. **Sepsis (MC)** due to pneumonia, urosepsis, wounds 2. Aspiration 3. Severe trauma, fractures, acute pancreatitis, multiple or massive transfusions 4. Drug OD/toxins 5. Intracranial HTN 6. Cardiopulmonary bypass	1. Rapid-onset dyspnea, 12-48 h after initial event Signs: 1. Labored breathing, tachypnea, tachycardia, retractions, crackles 2. Progressive **hypoxemia**—unresponsive to O_2 (**Pao2:Fio2<300 mm Hg**) 3. Difficulty ventilating due to high peak airway pressures (stiff, noncompliant lungs)	1. CXR–**diffuse bilateral pulmonary infiltrates** with air bronchograms 2. ABG: respiratory alkalosis (Paco2<40) initially → respiratory acidosis due to *tachypnea* If septic–respiratory acidosis +/– compensation 3. Pulmonary artery catheter: **PCWP low** (<18 mm Hg), if high (>18 mm Hg) suspect cardiogenic pulmonary edema 4. Bronchoscope with bronchoalveolar lavage–if acutely ill; culture fluid and analyze (cell diff, cytology, gram stain, silver stain)	1. $O_2 > 90\%$, tracheal intubation 2. **Mech vent with PEEP** (usually required)–opens collapsed alveoli and decreases shunting • Lowest levels of PEEP and O_2 should be used for Pao2>55 mm Hg 3. Volume overload–diuretics versus vasopressors (PCWP 12-15 goal) 4. Treat underlying cause 5. Nutrition–tube fees > parenteral feeds Prognosis: 1. Mortality rate: 30%-40% 2. If complicated by epsis, rate is 90%
Acute respiratory failure	Respiratory dysfunction resulting in abnormalities of oxygenation or ventilation severe enough to threaten function of vital organs	SX of hypoxemia or hypercapnia: 1. Dyspnea 2. Headache 3. Anxiety, delirium Signs: 1. Cyanosis, peripheral and conjunctival hyperemia 2. Restlessness 3. Confusion 4. Tachypnea, bradycardia, or tachycardia 5. Hypertension 6. Tremor, asterixis 7. Papilledema	1. ABG criteria • $PO_2 <60$ mm Hg • $PCO_2 >50$ mm Hg	1. Treat underlying cause 2. Respiratory support • Adequate oxygenation of organs • Do not withhold O_2 therapy for fear of causing progressive respiratory acidosis • Ventilator support • NPPV, BiPAP preferred • Tracheal intubation 3. Supportive care • Parenteral nutrition • Hypnotics and opioids • Neuromuscular blockade • Skin care, avoid ulcers • Sucralfate to prevent stress ulcers or gastritis • SQ heparin, DVT prophylaxis
Pulmonary edema	ARDS–An increase in alveolar capillary permeability versus cardiogenic pulmonary edema–congestive hydrostatic forces	1. Cough 2. SOB Signs: 1. Volume overload 2. JVD 3. Peripheral edema 4. Hepatomegaly Associated: CHF	(Fig. 39-2A)	

Disease	Etiology, Prevalence, Risk Factors	Clinical Symptoms and Signs	Diagnostics	Therapy, Prognosis, and Health Maintenance
Pneumothorax (PTX)	Air in the pleural space: 1. Spontaneous Primary (simple)—without underlying disease (healthy), spontaneous rupture of sub-pleural blebs, **MC in tall, lean men**, 50% recurrence in 2 y • Secondary (complicated)—underlying lung disease (MC: COPD), asthma, ILD, neoplasm, CF, TB, life threatening 2. Traumatic—iatrogenic	1. **Ipsilateral chest pain**, sudden onset 2. **Dyspnea** 3. Cough 1. Decreased/absent tactile fremitus 2. Mediastinal shift *toward* affected side 3. **Decreased breath sounds** over affected side 4. **Hyperresonance**	1. CXR–confirms DX, **visceral-pleural line (Fig. 39-2B and C)**	Primary: 1. Small and asymptomatic: observe 10 d +/– small chest tube 2. Large +/– symptoms: O_2 with chest tube 3. Secondary–chest tube drainage Repeat CXR daily until resolved
Tension pneumothorax	Air in pleural space; tissue surrounding opening acts as valve: air may enter, but not leave Accumulation of air under (+) pressure → collapse of ipsilateral lung, shifts mediastinum away from affected side Causes: Mechanical ventilation, CPR, trauma	1. **Hypotension**–cardiac filling impaired due to compression 2. **Distended neck veins** 3. Shift of trachea away from affected side 4. Decreased breath sounds 5. Hyperresonance	1. XR–not necessary, as this is a medical emergency Collapse of ipsilateral lung with mediastinal shift to contralateral lung	1. Chest decompression with **large-bore needle** (2nd or 3rd ICS MCL) 2. Followed by **chest tube placement**

Emergency Medicine

Indications for Tracheal Intubation

- Hypoxemia despite supplemental oxygen, upper airway obstruction, impaired airway protection, inability to clear secretions, respiratory acidosis, progressive general fatigue, tachypnea, use of accessory muscles, or change in mental status, and apnea

Indications for Mechanical Ventilation

- (1) Apnea, (2) acute hypercapnia not easily reversed by appropriate therapy, (3) severe hypoxemia, (4) progressive fatigue despite adequate therapy
- Complications: atelectasis, barotrauma, volutrauma, acute respiratory alkalosis, hypotension, ventilatory-associated pneumonia

CHAPTER 40

Gastrointestinal System and Nutrition

Refer to Family Medicine 👥 **for In-Depth Coverage of the Following Topics:**

Liver Function Tests, p 34

Heartburn, refer to Gastroesophageal Reflux Disease, p 60

Jaundice, p 52

GI Bleed/Melena/Bleeding Per Rectum, refer to GI Bleed, p 47

Constipation/Change in Bowel Habits, refer to Constipation, p 62

Esophagitis, p 61

Mallory-Weiss Tear, p 60

Peptic Ulcer Disease, p 41

Acute Cholecystitis, p 50

Cholangitis, p 51

Acute Hepatitis, p 63

Acute Pancreatitis, p 44

Acute Appendicitis, p 47

Ischemic Bowel Disease, see Emergency Medicine, p 400

Inflammatory Bowel Disease, refer to Ulcerative Colitis/Crohn Disease, p 45

Obstruction (Small Bowel, Large Bowel, Volvulus), p 48

Anal Fissure/Fistula, p 35

Hemorrhoids (Thrombosed), p 38

Hernia (Incarcerated/Strangulated), p 172

Gastritis, p 42

Gastroenteritis

Diarrhea/Constipation, p 42

Cirrhosis, p 56

Giardiasis and Other Parasitic Infections, p 59

Refer to Psychiatry 🧠 **for In-Depth Coverage of the Following Topics:**

Anorexia, p 588

Refer to Internal Medicine 🩺 **for In-Depth Coverage of the Following Topics:**

Diverticular Disease, p 216

Supplementary Recommended Reading:

Hepatitis B, see Family Medicine, p 64 👥

Colorectal Cancer, p 40 👥

Reye Syndrome, as below, p 404

Foreign Body, see Pulmonology, p 311 👪

ABDOMINAL PAIN

- Rule out immediate life-threatening conditions: abdominal aortic aneurysm, mesenteric ischemia, perforated bowel, peptic ulcer, appendicitis, esophageal perforation, acute bowel obstruction, ectopic pregnancy, volvulus, placental abruption, myocardial infarction, splenic rupture
- Others: acute cholecystitis, pancreatitis, diverticulitis, incarcerated hernia, gastroenteritis, foodborne disease, complications of bariatric surgery, inflammatory bowel disease, hepatitis, spontaneous bacterial peritonitis, irritable bowel syndrome, UTI or pyelonephritis, adnexal torsion, preeclampsia, ruptured ovarian cyst, pelvic inflammatory disease, endometriosis, Fitz-Hugh Curtis Syndrome, Tubo-ovarian abscess, testicular torsion, malignancy
- Extra-abdominal: DKA, alcoholic ketoacidosis, pneumonia, pulmonary embolus, herpes zoster

- History and physical examination are crucial for determining cause and workup
- Should perform pelvic and testicular examinations when appropriate for lower abdominal pain
- High-risk features:
  - Age >65, immunocompromised, alcoholism, cardiovascular disease, major comorbidities (cancer, diverticulosis, gallstones, IBD, pancreatitis, renal failure), prior surgery or recent GI instrumentation, early pregnancy
  - Pain characteristics: sudden onset, maximal at onset, pain with subsequent vomiting, constant pain of <2 days duration
  - Examination findings: tense or rigid abdomen, involuntary guarding, signs of shock
- Testing may include: pregnancy test, blood glucose, CBC, pancreatic enzymes, urinalysis, CXR or abdominal XR, abdominal ultrasound, CT scan, angiography, type and cross

- Treat patients judiciously with appropriate analgesics
  - For example, morphine 0.05 to 0.10 mg/kg IV every 15 minutes until pain is well controlled
  - For example, fentanyl 0.1 to 0.3 µg/kg IV in 5-minute intervals until well controlled
  - Goal is to reduce pain to manageable levels, making patient more cooperative and improving accuracy of examination, not to alleviate all pain and make them somnolent

ANOREXIA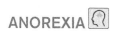

NAUSEA/VOMITING

- Acute nausea and vomiting (hours to a few days) typically presents to ER

- Rule out life-threatening causes: bowel obstruction, mesenteric ischemia, acute pancreatitis, and myocardial infarction
- Workup may include pregnancy test, electrolytes, EKG, abdominal ultrasound, abdominal CT, chemistry, CBC, Hgb, endoscopy
- Treat complications: fluid depletion, hypokalemia, metabolic alkalosis
- Target therapy by cause

Selection of Antiemetics by Clinical Situation		
Situation	**Associated Neurotransmitters**	**Recommended Antiemetic**
Migraine headache	Dopamine (probably a primary mediator)	For headache and nausea: metoclopramide or prochlorperazine
		For nausea: oral antiemetics, metoclopramide, prochlorperazine, serotonin antagonists
Vestibular nausea	Histamine, acetylcholine	Antihistamine and anticholinergics (equally effective)
Pregnancy-induced nausea	Unknown	For nausea: ginger, vitamin B$_6$
		For hyperemesis gravidarum: promethazine (first-line agent); serotonin antagonists and corticosteroids (second-line agents)
Gastroenteritis	Dopamine, serotonin	First-line agents: dopamine antagonists
		Second-line agents: serotonin antagonists
		Use in children is controversial
Postoperative nausea and vomiting	Dopamine, serotonin	Prevention: serotonin antagonists, droperidol, dexamethasone
		Treatment: dopamine antagonists, serotonin antagonists, dexamethasone

Adapted from Flake ZA, Scalley RD, Bailey AG. Practical selection of antiemetics. *Am Fam Physician.* 2004;69:1169.

- Serotonin antagonists: prochlorperazine (Compazine)
- Dopamine antagonists: metoclopramide (Reglan)
- 1st generation antihistamine: promethazine (Phenergan)

ISCHEMIC BOWEL DISEASE AND TOXIC MEGACOLON

Acute abdomen—refers to sudden, severe abdominal pain of unclear etiology of less than 24 hour duration.

- DDX: acute peptic ulcer, DKA, acute diverticulitis, ectopic pregnancy with tubal rupture, ovarian torsion, acute pyelonephritis, adrenal crisis, AAA, sickle cell anemia pain crisis, and kidney stones
- Workup: KUB and/or CT scan
  - In unstable patient, IVF + FAST ultrasound (if + free fluid, surgery)

Emergency Medicine

Disease	Etiology, Prevalence, Risk Factors	Clinical Symptoms and Signs	Diagnostics	Therapy, Prognosis, and Health Maintenance
Acute peritonitis	Inflammation or irritation of the peritoneum that causes rebound tenderness	Signs: 1. Rebound tenderness 2. Rigidity (specific)		
Ischemic bowel disease	Can be acute or chronic AMI: arterial embolus/thrombus, venous thrombosis >50 y Other CV or collagen vascular disease	AMI: Sudden-onset severe abdominal pain CMI: Abdominal angina, pain occurs 10-30 min after eating, relieved by squatting or lying down Intestinal infarction more common in small bowel than large CMI: Normal physical examination AMI: Pain out of proportion to examination findings → involuntary guarding, rebound, heme-(+) stool	1. Plain film radiography and CT—r/o other causes 2. Duplex ultrasound of mesenteric arteries 3. Confirmed by *CT angiography*	AMI: emergency, high mortality 1. **Abdominal laparotomy** • Immediate surgery indicated for AMI with clinical signs/symptoms of advanced ischemia (peritonitis, sepsis, pneumatosis intestinalis)
Acute mesenteric ischemia (interstitial ischemia)	SMA supplies small bowel and **ascending** and **proximal two-thirds of transverse colon** IMA supplies: distal one-third of transverse colon, descending and sigmoid Consider with a patient with **A-fib** (cardioembolus) "**Watershed area**"—splenic flexure most vulnerable to ischemia during systemic hypoperfusion	1. *Diffuse* abdominal pain, severe and out of proportion to examination • Visceral in nature, poorly localized • Worse after eating (postprandial) 2. Bowel distention 3. Bloody diarrhea 4. Nausea, vomiting Signs: 1. Rebound tenderness 2. Bowel sounds absent	1. CBC—neutrophilic leukocytosis +/− left shift 2. Serum amylase: high 3. *CT angiography* (gold standard)—diagnostic and therapeutic, distinguishes between arterial embolic and thrombotic causes KUB—**air-fluid levels**, widespread edema	1. Mesenteric angiogram: vasodilator therapy, thrombectomy, and embolectomy 2. Emergent laparotomy • Remove bowel with infarction, anastomosis of healthy tissue Highest mortality from arterial thrombosis: 70%-100%
Toxic megacolon	Extreme dilation and immobility of the colon, true emergency Presents as a complication of UC, Crohn disease, pseudomembranous colitis, infections (amebiasis, *Shigella*, *Campylobacter*, *Clostridium difficile*)	1. **Fever** 2. Prostration 3. Severe cramps 4. Abdominal distention Signs: 1. Rigid abdomen, *diffuse*, rebound abdominal tenderness	1. Abdominal x-ray: **colonic dilation**	1. **Decompression** of colon, in some cases colostomy or complete colonic resection 2. Monitor fluid and electrolytes

Ranson Criteria

- Prognosis and mortality rates of pancreatitis

Admission Criteria (GA LAW)	Initial 48 h (C HOBBS)	Mortality
Glucose > 200 mg/dL	**C**alcium < 8 mg/dL decrease in **h**ematocrit >10%	<3 criteria (1%)
Age > 55	Pa**o**$_2$ < 60 mm Hg	3-4 criteria (15%)
LDH > 350	**B**UN increased >8 mg/dL	**5-6 criteria (40%)**
AST > 250	**B**ase deficit >4 mg/dL	**>7 criteria (100%)**
WBC > 16 000	Fluid **s**equestration >6 L	

ANORECTAL ABSCESS

- Dentate line: divides the squamous epithelium distally and the columnar epithelium proximally

- Obstruction of anal glands by debris leads to stasis, bacterial overgrowth and abscess formation extending into intersphincteric groove between internal and external sphincters

- Most common locations: perianal, ischiorectal, intersphincteric, supralevator

Disease	Etiology, Prevalence, Risk Factors	Clinical Symptoms and Signs	Diagnostics	Therapy, Prognosis, and Health Maintenance
Anorectal (perianal) abscess Anaerobes: *Bacteroides fragilis,* *Peptostreptococcus,* *Prevotella,* *Fusobacterium,* *Porphyromonas,* *Clostridium* Aerobes: *Staphylococcus aureus,* *Streptococcus,* *Escherischia coli*	Originates from an infection arising in the cryptoglandular epithelium lining the anal canal Most common: **Perianal (60%)**, ischiorectal, intersphincteric, supralevator 30% have previous history Mostly 30-40 y old, males	Correlates with anatomic location: 1. **Severe perirectal pain** that is indolent, dull • Constant, not associated with bowel movement • Increased pressure with sitting or defecation 2. **Itching** 3. **Fever, malaise**, chills, severe pain, and fullness 4. Constipation due to pain with defecation Signs: 1. Tender, fluctuant mass around anus 2. Drainage—bloody, purulent, mucoid 3. Small, red, indurated subcutaneous mass	1. DRE—fluctuant, indurated mass 2. CT scan 3. MRI (gold standard)	1. **Incision and drainage** • If acutely tender, fluctuant • Collect pus and send for culture • Manual pressure for hemostasis, pack with iodoform gauze • Remove gauze after 24 h 2. Antibiotics for: SIRS, sepsis, extensive cellulitis, diabetes, immunosuppression, heart valve abnormalities 3. Sitz baths TID and after bowel movements 4. Postoperative analgesics and stool softeners Complications: Fistula **(30%-60%) formation**, bacteremia, sepsis, fecal incontinence, malignancy

HERNIA (INCARCERATED/STRANGULATED)

- A **reducible hernia** is one in which the contents of the sac return to the abdomen spontaneously or with manual pressure when the patient is recumbent

- An **irreducible (incarcerated) hernia** is one whose contents cannot be returned to the abdomen, usually because they are trapped by a narrow neck. The term "incarceration" does not imply obstruction, inflammation, or ischemia of the herniated organs, although incarceration is necessary for obstruction or strangulation to occur

- Compromise to the blood supply of the contents of the sac (eg, omentum or intestine) results in a **strangulated hernia**, in which gangrene of the contents of the sac has occurred

Disease	Etiology, Prevalence, Risk Factors	Clinical Symptoms and Signs	Diagnostics	Therapy, Prognosis, and Health Maintenance
Indirect inguinal hernia	Obliteration of the **processus vaginalis** (peritoneal extension accompanying the testis in its descent into the scrotum) fails to occur • Hernial sac passes through internal inguinal ring, a defect in the transversalis fascia halfway between the ASIS and pubic tubercle • Sac located antero-medially in spermatic cord • Descends into scrotum	1. Asymptomatic 2. Lump or swelling in groin with sudden pain and bulge that occurred while lifting or straining 3. "Dragging" sensation, radiation of pain into scrotum 4. With enlargement → discomfort, aching pain, must lie down to reduce	1. Mass that may or may not be reducible 2. Examine patient both supine and standing, with cough and strain 3. Ask patient to cough/strain while finger directed laterally and upward into inguinal canal → protrudes against tip of finger 4. Tissue must be felt protruding the inguinal canal during coughing in order for diagnosis • Posterior wall of inguinal canal is firm and resistant	1. All symptomatic groin hernias should be repaired if patient can tolerate **surgery** • Especially painful or tender hernias • Repair may be deferred if hernia reduces with gentle manipulation and no evidence of strangulation (gangrenous tissue) 2. Nonsurgical management: Truss • Use if patient refuses operative repair or when absolute contra-indications to operation • Fit to provide adequate external compression over defect • Take off at night at put on in the morning before arising • Does not preclude later repair of hernia 3. Sedentary workers return to work in few days, no heavy manual labor for 4-6 wk 4. Recurrence rate after hernia repair: 4%
Direct inguinal hernia	A weakness or defect in the transversalis fascia • Funicular type more likely to become incarcerated since it has distinct borders	Same as above	1. Appears as symmetric, circular swelling at external ring with standing and straining 2. Ask patient to cough/strain while finger directed laterally and upward into inguinal canal → protrudes against side of finger • Bulges forward through Hesselbach triangle 3. Disappears when lying supine • Posterior wall of inguinal canal is relaxed or absent	
Hiatal hernia Congenital or acquired Acquired may be non-traumatic (common) or traumatic Nontraumatic: 1. Sliding hiatal hernia 2. Paraesophageal hiatal hernia	A portion of the stomach herniates through the diaphragmatic esophageal hiatus RF: Pregnancy, obesity, ascites, muscle weakening	Most asymptomatic, discovered incidentally: 1. **GERD symptoms**—reflux or worsening reflux 2. Pain radiates to chest, not back Signs: 1. No palpable mass Complications: • Intermittent bleeding from esophagitis, erosions, discrete ulcers, or IDA • Incarcerated hernia (rare) • Barrett esophagus • Tumor	1. **Upper GI series (barium swallow):** outpouching of barium at lower end of esophagus, wide hiatus, free reflux of barium • Distinguishes sliding from paraesophageal 2. **Upper GI endoscopy (EGD):** diagnoses hiatal hernia and complications, good for biopsy of suspicious areas	1. Lifestyle modification 2. **PPI therapy** 3. Surgical treatment—remove hernial sac and close wide hiatus—only necessary if refractory to PPI • Nissen fundoplication, Belsey fundoplication, hill repair
Femoral hernia	Acquired protrusion of a peritoneal sac through the femoral ring • Passes beneath the iliopubic tract and inguinal ligament into upper thigh Predisposing factor: small empty space between lacunar ligament medially and femoral vein laterally	1. Bulge near groin or thigh		**Highest incidence of strangulation and incarceration** >>> inguinal hernias

| Umbilical hernias | Due to gradual yielding of the cicatricial tissue closing the ring
Females > males
RF:
Multiple pregnancies with prolonged labor, ascites, obesity, large intra-abdominal tumors | 1. Increasing in size
• Usually contain omentum, but small and large bowel may be present
2. Sharp pain on coughing or straining
• Large hernias produce dragging or aching sensation | | 1. Requires emergency repair because neck is usually narrow compared to the size of herniated mass → incarceration and strangulation common
• Mesh = lowest recurrence rate, use for all but smallest
• Control significant ascites preoperatively: medically or TIPS
• Correct fluid and electrolyte imbalances
2. RF for high complication and recurrence—large size, old age, debility of patient, obesity, intra-abdominal disease |

HEPATITIS B VACCINATION

- The hepatitis B vaccine consists of recombinant hepatitis B surface antigen (HBsAg) produced in yeast. A series of 3 injections may achieve HBsAg antibody (anti-HBs) levels greater than 10 million International Units/mL in approximately 95% of vaccinated individuals. Vaccination with a single dose must be **repeated every 5 to 10 years**

- **All newborns** must be vaccinated against hepatitis B. For infants born to mothers with active hepatitis B, a passive-active approach (hepatitis B immunoglobulin [HBIG] and vaccination) is recommended

- **Health care workers** should be vaccinated against HBV. Individuals who have had a **needle stick accident from a patient with active hepatitis B infection** must receive *active-passive* immunization (HBIG and the first dose of the vaccine at the same time). These individuals must be monitored with blood tests

- Current guidelines recommend that **all previously unvaccinated adults aged 19 through 59 years with diabetes mellitus (types 1 and 2) be vaccinated against** **hepatitis B** as soon as possible after a diagnosis of diabetes is made. Clinicians may use their discretion in determining whether to vaccinate elderly diabetic patients (age ≥60 years)

- The New York State Department of Health recommends vaccination with the hepatitis B vaccine series in **patients infected with human immunodeficiency virus (HIV)** who are negative for anti-HBs, unless they have chronic infection

- It is recommended that testing for anti-HBs be done 4 to 12 weeks following vaccination

- Revaccinate nonresponders, (HBsAb levels <10 International Units/L) with another series of 3-dose hepatitis B vaccine

- Consider delaying revaccination for several months after initiation of antiretroviral therapy in patients with CD4 counts below 200 cells/mm^3 or those with symptomatic HIV disease. The delay in these individuals is an attempt to maximize the antibody response to the vaccine. Do not defer vaccination in pregnant patients or patients who are unlikely to achieve an increased CD4 count

Emergency Medicine

REYE SYNDROME

Disease	Etiology, Prevalence, Risk Factors	Clinical Symptoms and Signs	Diagnostics	Therapy, Prognosis, and Health Maintenance

Reye syndrome	<u>Rapidly progressive encephalopathy with</u>:
	1. Liver dysfunction-begins several days after viral illness (varicella or influenza A or B)
	2. Most cases occur in winter or spring
		1. Vomiting
		2. Confusion
		3. Rapidly evolves to seizures and coma
		<u>Signs</u>:
		1. Hepatomegaly (common)
		2. +/− Icterus
			1. Elevated LFTs
			2. Increased PT
			3. Hyperammonemia
			4. Hypoglycemia
			5. Metabolic acidosis
			6. **CT head**/ultrasound: steatosis of liver and other visceral organs
			7. Consider LP if concern for **elevated ICP**
			  • Macrocephaly, bulging anterior fontanelle
			  • Irritability
			  • Lethargy, lack of interest in surroundings, poor feeding
			  • Nausea and vomiting
			  • Older children: vision changes, headaches, poor coordination, abnormal gait, papilledema
				1. External ventricular drain−to measure ICP
				  • If >20 mm Hg, confirms intracranial HTN
				2. LP with elevated opening pressure of >27 cmH$_2$O can establish a diagnosis of pseudotumor cerebri
				3. Stabilize airway, breathing, and circulation
				4. Consider endotracheal intubation for patients with refractory hypoxia, hypoventilation, GCS of <8 or <12 with rapid decline, loss of airway protective reflexes, acute herniation requiring controlled hyperventilation
				  • Paco$_2$ should be maintained 35-40 mm Hg
				5. Treat hypovolemia with isotonic fluids (normal saline)
				6. Treat with antipyretics (avoid fever)
				7. Neurosurgical consult
				8. Manage underlying condition
				  • Brain herniation
				    • Mannitol or hypertonic saline
				  • Vasogenic edema
				    • Dexamethasone
				<u>Health maintenance</u>:
				1. Caution use of salicylates in children, especially aspirin in febrile children

CHAPTER **41**

Neurology

 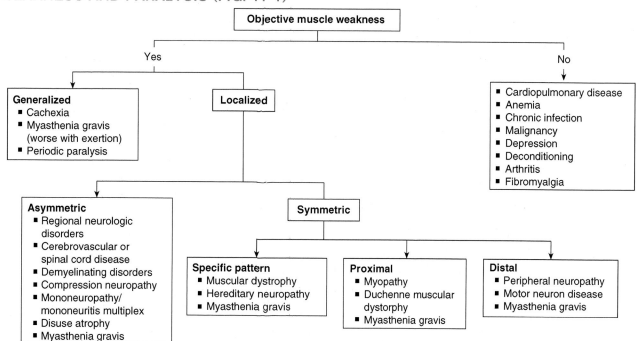
Emergency Medicine

WEAKNESS AND PARALYSIS (FIG. 41-1)

FIGURE 41-1. Approach to the adult patient complaining of weakness. (From Castillo M. *Neuroradiology Companion: Methods, Guidelines, and Imaging Fundamentals.* 4th ed. Philadelphia: Lippincott Williams & Wilkins; 2012.)

- **Asthenia** (not true weakness)—Many patients who complain of weakness are not objectively weak when muscle strength is formally tested. A careful history and physical examination will permit the distinction between asthenia, motor impairment due to pain or joint dysfunction, and true weakness

- True muscle weakness is documented by formal muscle testing. The strength of each muscle can be assessed by determining how much force is required by the examiner to overcome maximal contraction by the patient

- Asymmetric weakness most likely reflects disease of the central or peripheral nervous system; furthermore, lesions of the motor cortex, spinal cord, spinal nerve root, and peripheral nerve each have distinct distribution patterns. Symmetric patterns of weakness can be divided into distal, proximal, or specific distributions

- Distal weakness is characterized by decreased grip strength, weakness of wrist flexion or extension, decreased plantar flexion strength, and foot drop. These patients have difficulty walking on their heels or toes. Foot drop can be detected by opposing the patient's attempt to dorsiflex the ankle. Distal symmetric weakness is characteristic of early motor neuron disease or peripheral neuropathy

- Proximal weakness involves the axial muscle groups, deltoids, and hip flexors. Affected patients may have difficulty flexing or extending the neck against resistance. One way to detect the presence of neck flexor weakness is to observe the patient sitting up from the supine position. In this setting, the head will lag behind as the patient sits up. Sitting up may be difficult or even impossible in patients with more severe proximal muscle weakness or, at times, may be the only objective evidence of weakness. Deltoid muscle strength can be assessed by pressing down on the patient's fully abducted arms with the elbows flexed. The examiner should not be able to overcome the patient's resistance if strength is normal

Disease	Etiology, Prevalence, Risk Factors	Clinical Symptoms and Signs	Diagnostics	Therapy, Prognosis, and Health Maintenance
Upper motor neuron lesion	Degeneration of frontal motor neurons located in the motor strip (Brodmann area 4) and their axons traversing the corona radiata, internal capsule, cerebral peduncles, pontine base, medullary pyramids, and the lateral corticospinal tracts of the spinal cord	1. **Weakness** with slowness, incoordination, stiffness • Poor dexterity 2. **Hyperreflexia** • Ankle clonus 3. **Spasticity** • Spastic gait with poor balance and leg flexor spasms		
Lower motor neuron lesion	Degeneration of lower motor neurons in the brainstem and spinal cord producing muscle denervation	1. **Weakness** • Hand: difficulty manipulating small objects (buttons, zippers, coins) and writing • Proximal arm: difficulty bathing, dressing, grooming, eating • Foot/ankle: tripping, slapping gait, falling • Proximal leg: cannot arise from chair, climb stairs, or get up off floor • Upper face: incomplete eye closure 2. **Atrophy** (amyotrophic) 3. **Fasciculations** 4. **Muscle cramps**		

Emergency Medicine

Disease	Etiology, Prevalence, Risk Factors	Clinical Symptoms and Signs	Diagnostics	Therapy, Prognosis, and Health Maintenance
Amyotrophic lateral sclerosis (Lou Gehrig disease)	Amyotrophy with the pathologic finding of lateral sclerosis 65-70 y old: Males > females peak: 70-80 y old, but can occur in 20s Sporadic Only 10% familial	1. Asymmetric limb weakness (80%) - • Upper extremity onset: **hand weakness**, but may begin in **shoulder girdle** • Lower extremity: weakness of foot dorsiflexion (**foot drop**) 2. *Bulbar symptoms*: dysarthria, dysphagia • Coughing, choking • Increased masseter tone and difficulty opening mouth (trismus) • Laryngospasm 3. **Autonomic symptoms**: constipation, urgency without incontinence, excessive sweating • Early satiety, bloating 4. Parkinsonism and supranuclear gaze palsy • Facial masking, tremor, bradykinesia, postural instability 5. Sensory (20%-30%): tingling 6. Respiratory: muscle weakness, generalized weakness 7. Weight loss	**Clinical** <u>DX</u>: 1. Upper and lower MN signs and symptoms 2. Progressive spread 3. EMG: fibrillations, positive sharp waves 4. Electrodiagnostics: decreased motor conduction velocity 5. MRI (preferred) to r/o other causes 6. Unilateral arm onset (MC) → contralateral arm → ipsilateral leg → contralateral leg → bulbar muscles 7. Unilateral leg → contralateral leg → ipsilateral arm → contralateral arm → bulbar muscles	1. **Riluzole** 50 mg BID 2. AE: asthenia, dizziness, GI upset, elevated LFTs 3. MCC death: progressive respiratory failure <u>Complications</u>: Aspiration <u>Median survival</u>: 3-5 y
Organophosphate and carbamate poisoning Bind to acetylcholinesterase (AChE) and render this enzyme nonfunctional; responsible for hydrolysis of acetylcholine to choline and acetic acid, and inhibition → overabundance of acetylcholine at the neuronal synapses and the neuromuscular junction	Insecticides, neuromuscular blockades (neostigmine, pyridostigmine), treatment of glaucoma, myasthenia gravis, Alzheimer (pyridostigmine, tacrine, donepezil) Agent undergoes conformational change (aging) → enzyme becomes irreversible (resistant to antidote oxime) Risk highest in elderly	<u>Signs/SX within 3 h of ingestion</u>: 1. **D**iarrhea 2. **U**rination 3. **M**iosis (constriction) 4. **B**ronchorrhea, bronchospasm, bradycardia 5. **E**mesis (vomiting) 6. **L**acrimation 7. **S**alivation, sweating *Nicotinic effects*: fasciculations, muscle weakness, paralysis • Central respiratory depression, lethargy, seizures, coma *Intermediate neurologic syndrome* (10%-40%): 24-96 h after exposure • Neck flexion weakness, decreased DTRs, CN abnormalities, proximal muscle weakness, respiratory insufficiency Neuropathy (OPIDN) • Transient, painful "stocking glove" paresthesias → symmetrical polyneuropathy with flaccid weakness of lower extremities → upper extremities	<u>Clinical Diagnosis</u>: 1. EKG: heart block, QTc prolongation 2. Red blood cell (RBC) AChE levels—measures degree of toxicity	1. 2-5 mg *Atropine* 2. Pralidoxime (2-PAM) 3. Moderate-severe: • 100% O_2, endotracheal intubation • IVF: isotonic crystalloid (NS or LR) • Activated charcoal within 1 h of ingestion: 1 g/kg • Do not do gastric lavage

Emergency Medicine

(continued)

(continued)

Disease	Etiology, Prevalence, Risk Factors	Clinical Symptoms and Signs	Diagnostics	Therapy, Prognosis, and Health Maintenance
Temporal (giant cell) arteritis	Inflammatory condition affecting small- and medium-sized intra- and extra-cranial vessels Age 50+ y, history of polymyalgia rheumatica	1. **New headache** 2. Throat pain 3. Jaw, tongue, or upper extremity claudication 4. **Fever** 5. Transient ischemic attack symptoms (especially **transient visual loss**) 6. **Scalp tenderness** 7. Proximal **muscle weakness** of the shoulder and pelvic girdle 8. Malaise Signs: 1. Temporal artery tenderness (tender scalp)—may be enlarged or pulseless 2. Afferent pupillary defect if optic nerve circulation affected	1. **ESR/CRP–elevated** 2. CBC–normochromic normocytic anemia, thrombocytosis 3. **Biopsy** of temporal artery (after initiating steroids, confirms) • Still +1 wk after steroid therapy 4. Check IOP to rule out glaucoma DX criteria: (must meet 3 of 5): 1. Age >50 2. New-onset headache 3. ESR >50 mm/h 4. Abnormal arterial biopsy	1. High-dose IV steroids to prevent visual impairment and stroke 2. Low-dose aspirin 3. Consult ophthalmologist and rheumatologist Complications: 1. Can affect contralateral eye if not treated 2. Profound visual loss

- The "split-hand syndrome" describes a frequent pattern of weakness and atrophy in ALS that predominantly involves the median- and ulnar-innervated lateral (thenar) hand intrinsic muscles with relative sparing of the medial (hypothenar) muscles

- Like organophosphorus agents, carbamates are rapidly absorbed via all routes of exposure. Unlike organophosphates, these agents are **transient** cholinesterase inhibitors, which spontaneously hydrolyze from the cholinesterase enzymatic site within 48 hours. Carbamate toxicity tends to be of shorter duration than that caused by equivalent doses of organophosphates, although the mortality rates associated with exposure to these chemical classes are similar

Loss of Coordination or Ataxia

- Ataxia: disturbance in the smooth, accurate coordination of movements; most commonly manifested as unsteady gait

- Truncal ataxia: inability to sit unsupported by arms

- Alcohol intoxication is the most common cause of acute walking difficulty

- Dystonia is a disorder characterized by sustained muscle contractions resulting in repetitive twisting movements and abnormal posture

Disease	Etiology, Prevalence, Risk Factors	Clinical Symptoms and Signs	Diagnostics	Therapy, Prognosis, and Health Maintenance

Cerebellar ataxia	Causes: stroke, trauma, tumor, multiple-system atrophy, fragile X (older men)	Hx: difficulty maintaining balance when turning:
		1. Wide base of support
		2. Lateral instability of the trunk
		3. Erratic foot placement
		4. Decompensation of balance when attempting to walk on a narrow base
		Signs:
		1. Unable to tandem heel-to-toe
		2. Truncal sway in narrow based or tandem stance
			1. Laboratory tests
			  • UTox–most useful for acute ataxia
			  • Blood glucose
			  • CMP, urine and serum amino acids, CBC, serum lactate, pyruvate, and ammonia; urine organic acids
			2. Lumbar puncture
			3. CT head <<< MRI–especially if trauma or stroke suspected
			4. EEG
				Treat underlying cause

Sensory ataxia	Causes: Vitamin B$_{12}$ deficiency	1. Stance destabilized with eye closure 2. Look at feet when walking and do poorly in dark		Treat underlying cause

Emergency Medicine

Disease	Etiology, Prevalence, Risk Factors	Clinical Symptoms and Signs	Diagnostics	Therapy, Prognosis, and Health Maintenance
Spinocerebellar ataxia (SCA)	Only 60%-75% of patients with SCA have mutations in known loci MC autosomal dominant ataxias: SCA1 (3%-16%), SCA2 (6%-18%), SCA3 (21%-23%), SCA6 (15%-17%) Due to CAG repeats in disease-causing alleles	1. Dysarthria 2. Bulbar symptoms 3. Cerebellar ataxia Signs: 1. Hyperreflexia 2. Increased tone 3. Extensor plantar responses 4. UMN findings: wasting and generalized fasciculations 5. Slow saccadic eye movements (SCA2 only) 6. Nystagmus (may be horizontal or vertical) Associated: hypotonia or rigidity, developmental delay, infantile spasms, autonomic dysfunction, dysphagia, retinitis pigmentosa, dystonia, cognitive impairment, insomnia	MRI: cerebellar atrophy	1. No effective treatment Prognosis: 1. Most patients require a wheelchair by 10-15 y after onset
Friedreich ataxia	The only autosomal **recessive** ataxia Associated: diabetes (20%), vitamin E deficiency Mixed sensory and cerebellar ataxia Onset: Age <25	1. Staggering gait, frequent falling, titubation • Difficulty standing and running • Clumsy hands • Patient stands with feet wide apart, constantly shifting position to maintain balance 2. **Dysarthria** (presenting symptom) Signs: 1. Scoliosis (rarely), pes cavus, pes equinovarus 2. Truncal titubation (nodding movement of head) 3. Nystagmus, loss of fast saccadic eye movement 4. Hammertoes: retraction of the toes at the MTP joints and flexion at the ITP joints 5. (+) Romberg sign 6. Speech: dysarthria 7. Dysmetria 8. Absence of DTRs 9. Weakness: distal > proximal 10. Loss of vibratory and proprioceptive sensation Complications: **Cardiomyopathy** (50%)	1. Nerve conduction studies: NL 2. EKG and echo: heart block and ventricular hypertrophy 3. MRI of spinal cord: cerebellar **atrophy;** small spinal cord	1. Oral 5-hydroxytryptophan 2. Treat underlying heart failure, arrhythmias, and diabetes, surgery for scoliosis Prognosis: 1. Median age of death: 35 y 2. Better prognosis if female

INTRACEREBRAL HEMORRHAGE (ICH)

Disease	Etiology, Prevalence, Risk Factors	Clinical Symptoms and Signs	Diagnostics	Therapy, Prognosis, and Health Maintenance
Hemorrhagic Stroke (15%)				

Intracerebral hemorrhage (ICH): bleeding into the brain parenchyma, also known as parenchymal hemorrhage
 	
Note: in the acute phase, the mass effect of a cerebral hematoma is far greater than in a large cerebral infarction with a greater risk of herniation and death
 	
In chronic phase, prognosis is much better for those with hemorrhage than those with ischemia
	Causes:
	HTN (sudden increase) is most common cause
	• Ischemic stroke convert to → hemorrhagic stroke
	Patient develops edema around lesion or expansion of hematoma → herniation of brain tissue
	Locations:
	Putamen (40%), thalamus, lobar white matter, caudate, pons, cerebellum
	RF:
	Smoking, advanced age, anticoagulant use
		1. **Abrupt** onset of a focal neurologic deficit worse steadily over 30-90 min
		   • Pinpoint pupils–pons
		   • Poorly reactive pupils–thalamus
		   • Dilated pupils–putamen
		   • Decreased level of consciousness
		2. **Headache, nausea, vomiting**
		   • Severity of headache correlates with size of lesion
		3. Confusion, aphasia, hypersomnolence
		Signs:
		1. Increased ICP
		2. Respiratory failure
		3. **Hypertensive**
		4. Hyperconvergence, absent vertical gaze, horizontal gaze paresis
		5. Sensorimotor: hemiparesis, hemisensory or hemimotor loss, quadriplegia, ataxia
		6. Stupor, coma
			1. Noncontrast **CT scan of head** (90% of ICH): hyperintense area with mass effect and (later) hyperintense surrounding edema
			2. CT angiography
			   • Coagulation panel and platelets
			   • Ophthalmologic examination is mandatory to rule out papilledema
				1. Admit, supportive care, control BP
				   • **IV labetalol,** esmolol, or nicardipine (Cardene)
				     • Target: SBP <180
				     • MAP <130
				   • Reverse anticoagulants: FFP + vitamin K, protamine
				   • **Mannitol** (osmotic agent) and diuretics to reduce ICP
				   • Steroids harmful, not recommended
				   • Rapid surgical evacuation of cerebellar hematomas only
				2. Emergent neurosurgery consult
				   • High mortality rate (50% at 30 d)
				3. Surgery if >3 cm
				4. Steroids contraindicated
				Complications:
				Increased ICP, seizures, rebleeding, vasospasm, hydrocephalus, SIADH

Subarachnoid hemorrhage (SAH): bleeding into the CSF; outside brain parenchyma	RF:
	Smoking, hypertension, cocaine, and alcohol use, first-degree relative with SAH, female, African-American, connective tissue disorders
	"Thunderclap headache"
	Locations: saccular aneurysms at bifurcations of arteries of the Circle of Willis
		1. **Sudden-onset severe headache** (excruciating)
		   • Absence of focal neurologic deficit
		   • *"Worst headache of my life"*
		   • Sudden, transient loss of consciousness
		2. Nausea, **vomiting** (common)
		3. **Neck pain, nuchal rigidity**
		4. Photophobia, visual changes
		5. *Decreased level of consciousness* (53%)
		6. Seizure (20%)
		Signs:
		1. **Hypertensive**
		2. Retinal hemorrhage (30%)
			1. Fundoscopic examination: retinal hemorrhage
			2. **Non-contrast CT** (first line): negative in 10%
			   • if negative, follow with CSF
			     • Most are negative<2 h, most sensitive >12 h
			3. *Lumbar puncture*
			   • CI: elevated ICP, thrombocytopenia, suspected epidural abscess
			   • Xanthochromia, elevated RBCs
			
			1. **Blood in CSF** (hallmark)
			2. **Xanthochromia** (yellow CSF) is the gold standard for diagnosis, resulting from RBC lysis by 6 h
			3. CT angiography
			4. Once diagnosed → cerebral angiogram (definitive)
				1. Supportive care, admit
				   • Bed rest in quiet, dark room
				   • Stool softeners to avoid straining
				   • Analgesia for headache (Tylenol)
				   • IV fluids for hydration
				   • Lower BP gradually using CCB (nifedipine) for vasospasm
				2. Craniotomy and clipping–definitive
				   • Coiling: alternative
				3. **Treat BP aggressively,** if severe and unresponsive
				   • PO nimodipine 60 mg should be given × 21 d after to prevent vasospasm
				4. High mortality (40%-50% at 30 d)
				5. Most rebleeding occurs within first 3 d after rupture
				Complications:
				Rerupture (30%), vasospasm (50%), hydrocephalus, SIADH, hypertension

ALTERED LEVEL OF CONSCIOUSNESS OR COMA

- **Locked-in syndrome:** patients are fully awake, yet quadriplegic and can communicate only by means of vertical eye movements and blinking

HEAD TRAUMA/CONCUSSION/ CONTUSION

- **Concussion:** rapid onset of short-lived impairment of neurologic function resolving spontaneously
- Brain Injury occurs from rotational acceleration-deceleration of the head, which results in shearing forces causing mechanical disruption of nerve fibers, the end result of which is a diffuse axonal injury

- **Moderate TBI:** initial Glasgow Coma Scale (GCS) scores between 9 and 12
- **Severe TBI:** GCS scores less than or equal to 8
- **Contusion:** typically, a bruise of the scalp with no other clinical symptoms (substantial if >1 cm in diameter or more than 1 site affected)
- **Acceleration:** a moving object strikes a stationary head; least injurious
- **Deceleration:** moving head strikes a stationary surface; most severe brainstem injuries
- **Rotational acceleration-deceleration:** rotation of the brain, such as shaking an infant vigorously; causes large subdural hematomas

Disease	Etiology, Prevalence, Risk Factors	Clinical Symptoms and Signs	Diagnostics	Therapy, Prognosis, and Health Maintenance
Mild traumatic brain injury (TBI) or concussion in adults	Etiology: Falls (28%), MVC (20%), struck by heavy object or person, assault	1. Asymptomatic for up to 2 h 2. No evidence of skull fracture 3. +/–**Brief LOC** 4. +/– seizure activity 5. **Vomiting** 6. Irritability 7. Lethargy 8. Headache 9. Confusion or **disorientation** 10. Gait problems Signs: 1. Normal mental status and neurologic examination 2. Scalp hematoma, palpable crepitus 3. Funduscopic examination 4. GCS score of 13-15, measured 30 min after injury	Imaging usually normal and not required 1. **CT if <48 h** 2. MRI if > 48 h Image if: Severe headache/ worsening, prolonged recovery, focal deficits, seizures, slurred speech, unsteady gait, weakness, persistent vomiting, behavior changes, evidence of skull fracture	1. Observe in ER for at least 4 h 2. Treatment as below 3. Admit criteria: • GCS <15 • Seizures • Abnormal CT • Bleeding diathesis or from oral anticoagulation • Other neurologic deficit • Recurrent vomiting Health maintenance: 1. Light aerobic exercise 2. Sport-specific training, noncontact training drills, full contact after medical clearance, return to play 3. Return to work after period of 24 h with physical and cognitive rest Prognosis: 1. Postconcussion syndrome symptoms occur within 7-10 d for most of people

Emergency Medicine

Disease	Etiology, Prevalence, Risk Factors	Clinical Symptoms and Signs	Diagnostics	Therapy, Prognosis, and Health Maintenance
Minor head trauma in children and adolescents	Note: Concussion is a type of minor head trauma +/− brief loss of consciousness[a]	<u>≤2 y old</u>: 1. Frequently asymptomatic 2. History of blunt trauma to the scalp, skull, or brain 3. Scalp hematoma 4. Altered mental status (5%) 5. Vomiting 6. Irritability <u>≥2 y old</u>: 1. GCS of 14-15 2. Scalp hematoma 3. Altered mental status (13%) 4. Vomiting (13%) 5. Headache (46%) <u>Signs</u>: 1. Awake and alert to voice or light touch 2. Normal neurologic examination without focal deficits 3. No physical evidence of skull fracture (no palpable skull defect or signs of basilar skull fracture) 4. Signs of basilar skull fracture: hemotympanum, Battle sign, CSF otorrhea or rhinorrhea, periocular or posterior auricular hematomas 5. Bulging fontanelle 6. Altered mental status (lethargy, irritability)	Most do not need neuroimaging and clinical judgment should be exercised 1. **Noncontrast CT head** for GCS 13+ with altered mental status	<u>Treatment as below</u>: <u>Prognosis</u>: 1. Skull fractures or clinically important TBI may occur despite only minor head trauma <u>Complications</u>: 1. Seizures (<0.6%) 2. Skull fractures (10%)

Disease	Etiology, Prevalence, Risk Factors	Clinical Symptoms and Signs	Diagnostics	Therapy, Prognosis, and Health Maintenance
Concussion (minor TBI) in children and adolescents	1. Trauma-induced brain dysfunction without structural injury on neuroimaging that may or may not involve loss of consciousness 2. Most are young males 3. Mostly due to **falls** (MC), MVC, pedestrian and bicycle accidents, projectiles, assaults, sports-related trauma, abuse 4. Caused by direct blow to head, face, neck, or elsewhere on body with an impulsive force transmitted to the head 5. Rapid-onset short-lived neurologic impairment, that resolves spontaneously 6. Cannot be explained by other phenomena (eg, drugs) Concussion is a synonym used for a mild TBI, but is used to describe the symptoms and signs associated after a TBI occurs	1. **Headache** 2. **Nausea** or vomiting 3. Unsteadiness with walking or standing 4. **Fatigue** 5. **Dizziness** 6. Feeling mentally slow or foggy, difficulty with concentration 7. Sleep disturbance (drowsiness, insomnia, sleeping more or less) 8. Emotional lability, irritability, sadness, nervousness 9. Anterograde amnesia: cannot remember events after 10. Retrograde amnesia: cannot remember events before Signs: 1. **Confusion** and disorientation (walking in wrong direction, not aware of date/time/place) 2. **Amnesia** or memory changes (asking same questions) 3. Blank stare or "stunned" appearance 4. Inattentive (cannot follow directions or focus on a task) 5. Slow or incoherent speech 6. Gait abnormalities and imbalance (stumbling, or falling) 7. Emotional lability (inappropriate laughing or crying) 8. +/− Preceding **loss of consciousness**	Clinical DX: 1. Neuroimaging: CT preferred to MRI • Though neither will reveal a concussive brain injury and should not be performed unless concern or intracranial injury	In ER: 1. Observe and evaluate for other traumas and life-threatening injuries • Zofran for nausea • Avoid promethazine or metoclopramide in children due to side effects of drowsiness, orthostatic hypotension, and acute dystonic reaction • Encourage sleep hygiene, and if necessary, trial melatonin 2. Cervical spine—immobilize if patient has paresthesias, numbness, or paralysis 3. No participation in sports until cleared for play by athletic trainer, PCP, or concussion specialist (neurologist, neurosurgeon, sports medicine specialist) • Minimum of **1-2 d of rest** from physical activity, neurocognitive rest, and competition; gradual advance to increased level of activity and minimum of 5 d before full return to competition Health maintenance: 1. It is not necessary to awaken most children—no evidence to address this question • Unless the patient had a concerning mechanism of injury or prolonged symptoms and did not undergo neuroimaging: awaken every 4+ h to assess neurological status • Follow-up within 24 h by phone • Avoid activities that make symptoms worse (reading, video games, screen time) • Return to school if they can tolerate 30-45 min of concentration Worse prognosis if: 1. Persistent or worsening vomiting or headache 2. Change in mental status or behavior 3. Unsteady gait or clumsiness, incoordination 4. Seizure 5. Inability to arouse the child from sleep Complications: 1. Chronic traumatic encephalopathy 2. Second-impact syndrome

Emergency Medicine

(continued)

(continued)

Disease	Etiology, Prevalence, Risk Factors	Clinical Symptoms and Signs	Diagnostics	Therapy, Prognosis, and Health Maintenance

Acute severe TBI	As above	As above	As above
			1. Blood work: CBC, electrolytes, glucose, coagulation parameters, blood alcohol level, urine toxicology
			  • Correct coagulopathy if INR elevated
			2. CT head without contrast ASAP
			  • In all patients with GCS <14
			  • Follow-up scanning for deterioration in clinical status
				Prehospital:
				1. Prevent hypotension and hypoxia
				2. Early endotracheal intubation for GCS 8 or less
				3. IV fluid resuscitation using isotonic crystalloids
				4. Assume spinal fracture until proven otherwise
				ER–ATLS protocol:
				1. O_2, monitor vitals
				2. Neurologic examination
				3. Examine for other trauma
				4. Reverse any signs of coagulopathy
				5. If possible herniation suspected, elevate the head + osmotic therapy (mannitol) with CT

aGCS: Glasgow Coma Scale (see chapter 21).

• In the past, concussions were graded numerically (1, mild; 2, moderate; or 3, severe), based on the presence and duration of loss of consciousness. This was changed by the Concussion in Sport Group and American Academy of Neurology (AAN) because the brief loss of consciousness associated with concussion does not predict the clinical long-term prognosis. In addition, the absence of loss of consciousness in a person who has sustained a concussion should not be used to justify a more rapid return to play

EPIDURAL OR SUBDURAL HEMATOMA (FIG. 41-2A-B)

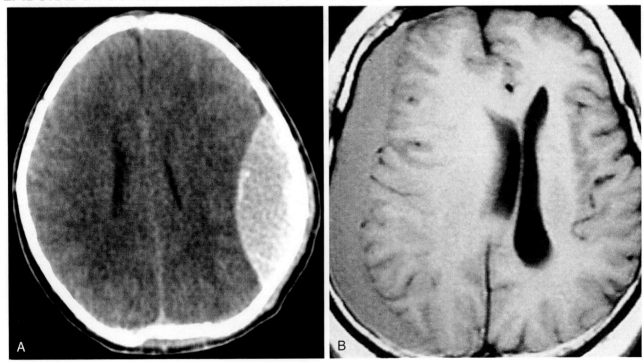

FIGURE 41-2. A, Epidural hematoma on axial CT scan. **B,** Large acute subdural hematoma on T1-weighted MRI. Note the crescent-shaped extra-axial hematoma covering the right cerebral convexity. The midline shift compresses the right lateral ventricle, and subsequently there is enlargement of the contralateral ventricle, likely causing obstructive CSF outflow. (From Linn-Watson T. *Radiographic Pathology*. Philadelphia: Wolters Kluwer Health; 2015.)

Disease	Etiology, Prevalence, Risk Factors	Clinical Symptoms and Signs	Diagnostics	Therapy, Prognosis, and Health Maintenance
Epidural hematoma	Classic: "talk and die" Collection of blood between dura and bones of the skull MCC: Trauma MC affects temporoparietal region, 2/2 laceration of **middle meningeal artery**	Progressive symptoms: 1. History of trauma with overlying skull fracture 2. **Brief loss of consciousness** 3. Return to alertness (**lucid interval**) 4. **Headache, vomiting**, lethargy, hemiparesis → coma (20%) Signs: Associated hematoma	1. Noncontrast CT: **lens-shaped** (lenticular, biconvex) extra-axial collection of blood that does not cross suture lines (differentiates it from subdural)	1. Urgent neurosurgery consult 2. If evidence of herniation (pupil dilation or contralateral hemiparesis) → burr hole ipsilateral to the trauma 3. Decrease ICP Complications: Herniation
Acute Subdural hematoma	MCC: Trauma Other RF: Alcoholism, seizures, coagulopathies Collection of blood between the dura and arachnoid mater; source is bridging veins	Nonspecific, nonlocalizing symptoms, or absent, stable, or rapidly progressive; 1. Headache 2. Confusion 3. Depressed level of consciousness 4. +/− Seizures Signs: 1. Hemiparesis–contralateral to the lesion (60%) 2. Ipsilateral pupillary dilation (75%)	1. CT head with contrast–hyperdense **crescent-shaped** (biconcave) extra-axial collection of blood, rarely crosses the falx or tentorium • Subacute lesions (2-3 wk): isodense • Chronic lesions: 4-6 wk: hypodense	1. Immediate hospitalization 2. Emergent neurosurgery consult 3. Unstable patients with rapidly worsening neurologic deficits → treat for increased ICP

SPINAL CORD INJURY

- **Anterior cord syndrome**: loss of pain and temperature below the level with preserved joint position/vibration sense

- **Central cord syndrome**: loss of pain and temperature sensation at the level of the lesion, where the spinothalamic fibers cross the cord, with other modalities preserved (dissociated sensory loss)

- **Complete cord transection**: rostral zone of spared sensory levels (reduced sensation caudally, no sensation in levels below injury); urinary retention and bladder distention

- **Brown-Sequard syndrome** (hemisection of the cord): loss of joint position sense and vibration sense on same side as lesion and pain and temperature on opposite side a few levels below the lesion

  - Lesion of half-ipsilateral cervical cord lesion
  - Contralateral sensory findings: pain and temperature loss

Disease	Etiology, Prevalence, Risk Factors	Clinical Symptoms and Signs	Diagnostics	Therapy, Prognosis, and Health Maintenance
Cauda equina	Midline herniation below spinal cord termination at the L1 vertebral level (typically the L4-L5 level or the L5-S1 level) Loss of motor and sensory function occurs	1. Flaccid, areflexic asymmetric paraparesis • Bilateral lower extremity weakness 2. **Bowel and bladder incontinence**–severely impaired 3. Sensory loss below L1 (**saddle anesthesia**) • Numbness and/or paralysis 4. Leg pain (common) • Projected to perineum or posterior thighs, or lateral leg (sciatica) • Worse with coughing, sneezing, or straining • Lying flat relieves pain Signs: 1. Straight leg raise limited on side of lesion 2. Dorsiflexion of foot at limit of straight leg raise worsens pain 3. Tenderness to palpation of central back or buttock 4. +/− Sensory loss and muscle weakness 5. +/− Knee or ankle reflexes absent	1. Plain x-rays (lateral, AP, +/− oblique views) of thoracic, lumbar, or other parts of the spine • Narrowing of the intervertebral space 2. Helical CT with coronal and sagittal reconstructions • Higher sensitivity 3. MRI–indications have not been defined	1. Bed rest, application of heat or ice, NSAIDs and muscle relaxants 2. **Emergent surgery** (definitive) Indications: • Acute disabling neurologic deficit (bladder dysfunction) • Intractable severe pain

BELL'S PALSY

DYSTONIA

• Defined as a movement disorder characterized by sustained or intermittent muscle contractions causing abnormal, often repetitive, movements, postures, or both

• Typically patterned, twisting, or tremulous

Disease	Etiology, Prevalence, Risk Factors	Clinical Symptoms and Signs	Diagnostics	Therapy, Prognosis, and Health Maintenance
Cervical dystonia (spasmodic torticollis)	Most common isolated focal dystonia; affects muscles of neck and shoulders	1. Torticollis: horizontal turning of head • Laterocollis: lateral tilt of neck • Anterocollis: flexion of head • Retrocollis: extension of head 2. Pain (50%)		1. **BoNT-A** (first line) • Improves posture, pain, and disability 2. BoNT-B
Blepharospasm	Focal dystonia involving the orbicularis oculi muscles	1. Increased blinking 2. Spasms of involuntary eye closure 3. Bilateral, synchronous, symmetric 4. Increased spasms under bright light or stress (driving in car in traffic)		1. **BoNT-A** (first line) • Improves posture, pain, and disability

Treatments for Dystonia

Oral medications	1. Levodopa 2. Anticholinergics (trihexyphenidyl): for focal and generalized dystonia • AE: dry mouth (dental caries), blurred vision, constipation, urinary hesitancy/retention, tachycardia, pupil dilation, increased IOP, dizziness, confusion, memory impairment, nausea, vomiting, anxiety • CI: narrow-angle glaucoma, confusion, dementia 3. Tetrabenazine • AE: sedation, parkinsonism, depression, akathisia, nervousness, insomnia
Botulinum toxin injection (BoNT)	1. Potent neurotoxin produced by *Clostridium botulinum* that causes regional muscle weakness through action as zinc endopeptidase-cleaving protein involved in vesicular fusion → release of acetylcholine at NMJ → localized muscle weakness 2. Benefits 50%-85% of patients with cervical dystonia (spasmodic torticollis) and blepharospasm; treatment of choice for spasmodic dysphonia (laryngeal dystonia), limb dystonia, and oromandibular dystonia 3. AE: neck weakness, dysphagia, dry mouth/sore throat, voice changes or hoarseness 4. Most patients continue to respond to long-term treatment with BoNT
Deep brain stimulation	1. For patients with severe dystonia who have failed treatment with pharmacologic agents or botulinum toxin injections

TRIGEMINAL NEURALGIA

Disease	Etiology, Prevalence, Risk Factors	Clinical Symptoms and Signs	Diagnostics	Therapy, Prognosis, and Health Maintenance
Trigeminal neuralgia (tic douloureux)	Unilateral facial pain in sensory distribution of CN V (maxillary or mandibular)	1. Severe, **lancinating**, unilateral facial pain in distribution of one or more branches of trigeminal nerve (V2, V3) 2. Worse with chewing, talking, smiling • Drinking cold or hot fluids • Touching, shaving, brushing teeth, blowing nose, cold air 3. Localized pain	1. Paroxysmal attacks of pain last from a fraction of a second to 2 min, affecting 1 or more divisions of trigeminal nerve 2. Pain has at least 1 of the following: (a) intense, sharp, superficial, or stabbing (b) trigger areas or factors 3. Attacks stereotyped in individual patient 4. No clinically evident neurologic deficit 5. Not attributable to another disorder	1. Carbamazepine 100 mg BID

CHAPTER 42

Head, Ears, Eyes, Nose, and Throat

EARS

Ear Pain, Vertigo

Disease	Etiology, Prevalence, Risk Factors	Clinical Symptoms and Signs	Diagnostics	Therapy, Prognosis, and Health Maintenance
Vertigo	Sensation of movement (spinning, tumbling, or falling) in the absence of actual movement or an overresponse to movement Central etiology: Multiple sclerosis, brain tumor, head injury, medications	1. Duration and presence of hearing loss or nystagmus 2. Peripheral vertigo–sudden onset, intermittent, nausea/vomiting, tinnitus, hearing loss, nystagmus (horizontal with rotary component) 3. Central vertigo–gradual onset, continuous, nausea or vomiting, vertical nystagmus, **no auditory symptoms**; motor, sensory, or cerebellar deficits	1. **Dix-Hallpike maneuver**–non-fatigable nystagmus = central cause 2. Audiometry, caloric stimulation, ENG, MRI, evoked potentials	Peripheral: 1. Vestibular suppressants help with acute symptoms • Diazepam (Valium) • Meclizine • Less helpful for chronic dizziness 2. Epley maneuver Central–treat the source: 1. Deep head-hanging maneuver

Disease	Etiology, Prevalence, Risk Factors	Clinical Symptoms and Signs	Diagnostics	Therapy, Prognosis, and Health Maintenance
Acute prolonged vertigo (vestibular neuritis)	Due to sudden asymmetry of inputs from 2 labyrinths or in central connections, stimulating continuous rotation of the head Central (cerebellar, brainstem infarct, hemorrhage) can be life threatening Peripheral—affects vestibular nerve or labyrinth	1. Sudden, unilateral vertigo • **Persists even when head remains still** 2. Nausea, vomiting 3. Oscillopsia—motion of the visual scene 4. Imbalance 5. Central symptoms: diplopia, weakness, numbness, dysarthria	1. Head impulse test	Spontaneously resolves: 1. Steroids within 3 d of symptom onset 2. Antivirals non-beneficial unless herpes zoster oticus (Ramsay Hunt syndrome) suspected 3. Vestibular suppressant medications for acute symptoms 4. Resume normal activity ASAP and directed vestibular rehabilitation
Benign paroxysmal positional vertigo (BPPV)	Common cause of recurrent vertigo Caused by free floating otoconia (calcium carbonate crystals) dislodged from utricular macula and moved to semicircular (posterior) canal	1. Brief episodes (**<1 min**), last 15-20 s • Provoked by changes in head position relative to gravity (lying down, rolling over in bed, rising from supine position, extending head to look upward) 2. Posterior canal BPPV: **upward, torsional nystagmus** 3. Horizontal canal BPPV: horizontal nystagmus when lying ear down 4. Superior (anterior) BPPV: rare	1. **(+) Dix-Hallpike maneuver** produces delayed fatigable nystagmus 2. Posterior canal BPPV: **Epley maneuver**	1. Dix-Hallpike maneuver (quickly turn patient's head 90° while supine) 2. Avoid using meclizine or similar medicines
Meniere disease (endolymphatic hydrops)	Excessive endolymph fluid in cochlea overstimulates hairs causing vertigo and sudden hearing loss with aural fullness Unknown etiology	1. **Sudden**, *recurrent* **vertigo** (lasting *minutes to hours*) 2. **Tinnitus** 3. One-sided aural pain, pressure, and/or fullness (unilateral) 4. **Hearing loss (low frequency)** 5. Nausea, vomiting Signs: 1. Nystagmus on impaired side	1. Audiometry at the time of attack 2. Caloric testing	1. **Low-sodium, high-water diet** 2. **Diuretics** (acetazolamide) 3. Intratympanic gentamicin 4. Referral to ENT Health maintenance: 1. Avoid alcohol, caffeine, and tobacco
Acoustic neuroma (vestibular schwannoma)	Intracranial benign tumor affecting eighth cranial nerve Bilateral acoustic neuromas, associated with **neurofibromatosis type II**	1. **Unilateral, progressive** sensorineural *hearing loss* (may also be acute) 2. *Unsteadiness* 3. *Vertigo* (continuous, late): vestibular deficit compensated centrally as it develops 4. **Tinnitus** 5. Impaired speech discrimination 6. Headache 7. Diplopia Signs: 1. Decreased corneal reflex sensitivity 2. Facial weakness	1. Head impulse test: deficient response when head rotated toward affected side 2. **MRI**: densely enhancing lesions, enlarging the internal auditory canal and extending into the cerebellopontine angle 3. Lumbar puncture: elevated protein	1. Asymptomatic • Serial MRIs 2. Surgery or SRS for larger lesions Complication: Loss of corneal reflex from trigeminal involvement
Labyrinthitis (otitis externa)	Unknown etiology Likely viral, head injury, stress, or allergy related	1. Acute severe vertigo, lasting several *days to a week* • Improves over a few weeks, but hearing loss may or may not resolve • Imbalance 2. Hearing loss 3. Nausea or vomiting Signs: 1. Severe nystagmus		1. Antibiotics for fever or signs of infection 2. Vestibular suppressants for acute symptoms • Diazepam • Meclizine 3. Symptoms regress after 3-6 wk

(continued)

Emergency Medicine

(continued)

Disease	Etiology, Prevalence, Risk Factors	Clinical Symptoms and Signs	Diagnostics	Therapy, Prognosis, and Health Maintenance
Tinnitus		1. Ringing in the ears	1. Comprehensive audiologic examination for unilateral persistent tinnitus or associated hearing impairment 2. Imaging for unilateral tinnitus, pulsatile tinnitus, asymmetric hearing loss, or focal neuro deficits	1. Hearing aids for tinnitus with hearing loss 2. CBT or sound therapy for persistent, bothersome tinnitus

Drugs that cause vertigo (MALES-TIP)

- Methanol, alcohol, lithium, ethylene glycol, sedative hypnotics/solvents

- Thiamine depletion/carbamazepine (Tegretol), isopropanol, PCP/phenytoin (Dilantin)

Barotrauma

| Barotrauma | Inability to equalize barometric changes on the middle ear when encountering quick changes in pressure, such as flying, diving, or altitude change
Etiology:
Congenital narrowing or acquired mucosal edema | 1. Ear pain
2. Hearing loss | Clinical DX | 1. Swallow or yawn to autoinflate the Eustachian tube
2. Systemic or PO decongestants
3. Myringotomy
Health maintenance:
1. If left unequalized, can cause TMP or AOM |

Trauma/Hematoma (External Ear)

Disease	Etiology, Prevalence, Risk Factors	Clinical Symptoms and Signs	Diagnostics	Therapy, Prognosis, and Health Maintenance
Trauma/hematoma (external ear)	Develops between cartilage and perichondrium	1. Purplish swelling of upper part of ear 2. Obscured cartilage folds	Clinical DX	1. Referral to ENT 2. Aspiration of area with applied pressure dressing 3. Recurrent—requires I&D

EYES

Vision Loss: Blurred Vision and Decreased Visual Acuity

- Transient loss
  - Differential: TIA, emboli (amaurosis fugax), or giant cell (temporal) arteritis

- Sudden loss
  - Differential: central retinal vein or branch vein occlusion, optic neuropathy, papillitis, or retrobulbar neuritis
- Gradual loss
  - Differential: macular degeneration, tumors, cataracts, glaucoma

Senile (age-related) cataract	Leading cause of blindness in the world
	Opacity of lens to the eye, which causes partial or total blindness
	<u>MCC:</u>
	Age-related nuclear sclerosis
	<u>Other RF besides age:</u>
	Smoking (2×), ETOH, sunlight exposure, low education, malnutrition, physical inactivity, metabolic syndrome, diabetes, steroid use, statin use
		1. Painless, progressive loss of vision
		2. Bilateral, asymmetrical field of vision
		3. Difficulty driving at night, reading road signs, or reading fine print
		<u>Signs:</u>
		1. Funduscopic examination: darkening of red reflex, obscured ocular fundus
				1. Nonurgent referral to ophthalmologist
				2. Conservative: change in glasses prescription
				3. Surgery
				  • Indications: if symptoms interfere with the ability to perform ADLs; no criteria based on level of visual acuity
				  • No advantage to removing sooner
				  • Extracapsular cataract extraction versus phacoemulsification

Amaurosis fugax	Etiology: **atherosclerosis** (emboli to the ophthalmic artery), carotid stenosis	"Fleeting blindness" or "curtain coming down" vertically into the field of vision 1. Painless, transient 2. *Unilateral* (monocular) vision loss 3. Seconds of a *graying out* of vision in one eye	Retinoscopy: refractile arterial lesions (**Hollenhorst plaques,** cholesterol crystals)	Annual risk of stroke is 1%-2%

Blowout Fracture

Disease	Etiology, Prevalence, Risk Factors	Clinical Symptoms and Signs	Diagnostics	Therapy, Prognosis, and Health Maintenance
Blowout fracture	Fracture of the floor of the orbit resulting in increased IOP Blunt force trauma against the eye	1. Intraocular muscles and fat pads caught in fracture <u>Signs:</u> 1. Enophthalmos 2. Upward gaze diplopia (inferior rectus entrapment) 3. Infraorbital rim, upper lip, cheek anesthesia 4. Step off of infraorbital rim <u>Complications:</u> Retinal detachment, lens dislocation, ruptured globe, hyphema	1. Orbital CT	1. Tetanus vaccination 2. Pain control 3. Prophylactic antibiotics 4. Avoid blowing nose and Valsalva 5. Consult ophthalmology and maxillofacial surgeon

THROAT

Dental Abscess

Disease	Etiology, Prevalence, Risk Factors	Clinical Symptoms and Signs	Diagnostics	Therapy, Prognosis, and Health Maintenance

Dental abscess: periodontal	Chronic gingival disease	1. Swelling of cheek, mouth, or neck
		2. Adjacent tooth tender to percussion
		3. More localized
			Clinical DX	1. Rinse abscessed area with warm saltwater × 10 min every 2 h
				2. Apply ice to face, NSAIDs, opioids
				3. Incision and drainage
				4. Antibiotics
				  • Penicillin VK 500 PO qid
				  • Erythromycin 500 mg PO qi
				  • Clindamycin 300 mg PO TID

Periapical	Dental caries	1. Increased pain when supine 2. Bad "taste" in mouth or tooth "feels longer" than other teeth Gumboil: abscess under gum	Clinical DX	<u>Complications:</u> Facial cellulitis

Emergency Medicine

Acute Epiglottitis

Disease	Etiology, Prevalence, Risk Factors	Clinical Symptoms and Signs	Diagnostics	Therapy, Prognosis, and Health Maintenance
Acute epiglottitis–adults	Adults: bacterial (MC: Hib), viral, fungi, noninfectious causes	Slow progression: 1. **Sore throat** (MC) or odynophagia (90%-100%) 2. Fever >37.5°C 3. Muffled voice 4. Hoarseness Signs: 1. Drooling 2. Stridor, respiratory compromise Associated (adults): HTN, DM, substance abuse, immune deficiency	Refer to Pediatrics, p 10	Refer to Pediatrics, p 10

FOREIGN BODY (EAR, EYE, NOSE)

Disease	Etiology, Prevalence, Risk Factors	Clinical Symptoms and Signs	Diagnostics	Therapy, Prognosis, and Health Maintenance
Foreign body (FB)–ear	Children FB of metallic origin, plant, or organic matter	1. Conductive hearing loss 2. Otalgia or discharge if secondarily infected 3. Bleeding if object is sharp	None	1. Solids–loop, hook, or alligator forceps may be used • Irrigate if rounded object (bead) 2. Do not put water in ear if the FB is organic matter (can swell) 3. If insect is the FB, lidocaine or mineral oil can be used to immobilize before removal 4. Irrigation (sterile room temperature water or normal saline) if TM intact 5. After removal, otic topical antibiotics with steroid

FB–eye (corneal)	Trauma to cornea by FB on surface of, or embedded into, cornea
	FB sets off inflammatory reaction → if not removed → infection, necrosis, or both
		1. Pain
		2. Erythema
		3. Photophobia, excessive tearing
		4. Foreign body sensation
		5. Blurred vision
		6. Hx recent trauma
		Signs:
		1. Eyelid closed
		2. Ring infiltrate surrounding site of FB if embedded >24 h
			1. Check visual fields and acuity
			2. Slit lamp examination
			3. Fluorescein staining
			  • FB appears dark with area of green surrounding it under black light
				1. Tetanus immunization
				2. Topical anesthetic
				3. Use moistened cotton-tipped applicator, sterile 22 G needle or Alger brush to remove
				4. Antibiotic ophthalmic drops
				  • Trimethoprim/polymyxin (Polytrim), sulfacetamide sodium (Sulamyd), tobramycin (Tobrex)
				5. Apply eye patch with firm pressure
				6. Reassess in 24 h
				7. Refer to ophthalmology

FB–nose	Bead or seed in nose	1. Foul smelling discharge from affected nostril 2. Rhinorrhea 3. Bleeding 4. Halitosis 5. Nasal obstruction		1. Older child can attempt to blow nose to dislodge 2. Remove FB with topical anesthetic, nasal decongestion, restraints, good lighting 3. If wedged-in, refer to ENT 4. If battery operated, must be removed within 4 h • Battery is true emergency

HORNER SYNDROME (FIG. 42-1)

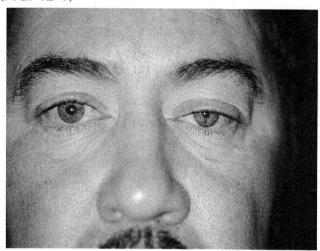

FIGURE 42-1. Horner syndrome. Ptosis with miosis on the left side. The amount of ptosis is more than is often seen in Horner syndrome, and there may be some aponeurotic dehiscence as well. (Reprinted with permission from Penne RB, ed. *Oculoplastics*. 2nd ed. Philadelphia: Lippincott Williams & Wilkins/Wolters Kluwer Business; 2012.)

Disease	Etiology, Prevalence, Risk Factors	Clinical Symptoms and Signs	Diagnostics	Therapy, Prognosis, and Health Maintenance
Horner syndrome	Associated with posterior, inferior cerebellar artery occlusion Results from the destruction of the ipsilateral superior cervical ganglion below the level of entry to the skull Causes (adults): CVA, tumors, internal carotid artery dissection, herpes zoster, trauma Causes (children): Neuroblastoma, lymphoma, metastasis	1. Ipsilateral facial **anhidrosis** (loss of sweating) 2. Ipsilateral **ptosis** 3. Ipsilateral **miosis** (constricted pupil) 4. Associated with apical lung cancers or neuroblastomas (children)	1. CXR 2. CT head and cervical neck 3. CT angiogram or MRA of the head and neck—rule out carotid dissection	Treat underlying cause

CHAPTER 43
Urology and Renal

Emergency Medicine

HEMATURIA (FIGS. 43-1 TO 43-4)

- **Gross hematuria**: blood in the urine visible to the naked eye

- **Microscopic hematuria**: blood in the urine detectable only on microscopic examination of the urine sediment.

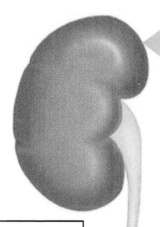

RENAL
Benign renal mass (angiomyolipoma,
    oncocytoma, abscess)
Malignant renal mass (renal cell
    carcinoma, transitional cell carcinoma)
Glomerular bleeding (IgA nephropathy,
    thin basement membrane disease, hereditary
    nephritis - Alport's syndrome)
Structural disease (polycystic kidney
    disease, medullary sponge kidney)
Pyelonephritis
Hydronephrosis/ distension
Hypercalciuria/ hyperuricosuria
Malignant hypertension
Renal vein thrombus/ renal artery embolism
Arteriovenous malformation
Papillary necrosis (sickle cell disease)

URETER
Malignancy
Stone
Stricture
Fibroepithelial polyp
Postsurgical conditions
    (ureteroiliac fistula)

**MIMICS OF
HEMATURIA**

Menstruation
Drugs (pyridium,
    phenytoin, rifampin,
    nitrofurantoin)
Pigmenturia
Beeturia

**Renal and/or upper or
lower collecting system:**

Infection (bacterial, fungal,
    viral)
Malignancy
Urolithiasis
Tuberculosis
Schistosomiasis
Trauma
Recent instrumentation
    including lithotripsy
Exercise-induced hematuria
Bleeding diathesis/
    anticoagulation*

Upper collecting system
Lower collecting system

BLADDER
Malignancy (transitional
    cell carcinoma, squamous
    cell carcinoma)
Radiation
Cystitis

PROSTATE/URETHRA
Benign prostatic hyperplasia
Prostate cancer
Prostatic procedures (biopsy,
    transurethral resection of
    the prostate)
Traumatic catheterization
Urethritis
Urethral diverticulum

Emergency Medicine

FIGURE 43-1. Etiology of hematuria. (From: Kurtz M. *Causes of hematuria. UpToDate.* 2018. https://www.uptodate.com/contents/
image?imageKey=NEPH%2F63501&topicKey=NEPH%2F7208&source=outline_link&search=hematuria&selectedTitle=1~150.)

Disease	Etiology, Prevalence, Risk Factors	Clinical Symptoms and Signs	Diagnostics	Therapy, Prognosis, and Health Maintenance
Hematuria	<u>MCC:</u> Inflammation or infection of the prostate or bladder, stones, and in older patients, kidney or urinary tract malignancy or BPH Common and frequently benign in young patients	1. Unilateral flank pain 2. Red or brown urine <u>Signs:</u> 1. Hypertension 2. Edema and weight gain (with glomerular disease due to fluid retention or impaired water excretion)	1. Urinalysis with culture—rule out infection • Follow-up in 6 wk 2. **Urine dipstick** (gold standard for detection of microscopic hematuria): urine sediment (counting of RBC per mL of uncentrifuged urine) • Hematuria: 3+ RBCs per high-power field (HPF) • Confirm with microscopic examination of urine • Repeat U/A if: menstruating woman, recent vigorous exercise (after 4-6 wk), or acute trauma (after 6 wk) 3. Non-contrast helical CT scan or ultrasound—if unilateral flank pain 4. Renal biopsy • Indicated for glomerular hematuria (presence of dysmorphic RBC and/or red cell casts) in the presence of proteinuria and/or elevated serum Cr	Treat underlying cause <u>Health maintenance:</u> 1. Repeat urine culture in 6 wk to determine if hematuria has resolved

Quick Guide: Evaluation of Hematuria

Gross Hematuria		Microscopic Hematuria		
With visible clots	Without visible clots	Nonpregnant No risk factors for malignancy (kidney or bladder) or Hx of urologic disorder (BPH, nephrolithiasis)	Nonpregnant With risk factors for malignancy (kidney or bladder) or Hx of urologic disorder (BPH, nephrolithiasis)	Pregnant
1. CT urography (CTU) 2. Urgent urology evaluation for cystoscopy	1. If AKI or glomerular bleeding: refer to nephrology 2. Nonpregnant without AKI or glomerular bleeding: CTU and urology referral for cystoscopy 3. Pregnant: renal and bladder ultrasound to r/o ureteral obstruction or urolithiasis	1. No imaging or cystoscopy 2. Nephrology evaluation if persistent, unexplained microscopic hematuria for several years	1. CTU 2. Urology referral for cystoscopy	1. Renal and bladder ultrasound

• **Risk factors for malignancy:** age >35, smoking history, occupational exposure to chemicals or dyes (printers, painters, chemical plant workers), history of gross hematuria, history of chronic cystitis or irritative voiding symptoms, history of pelvic irradiation, history of exposure to cyclophosphamide, history of chronic indwelling catheter, history of analgesic abuse

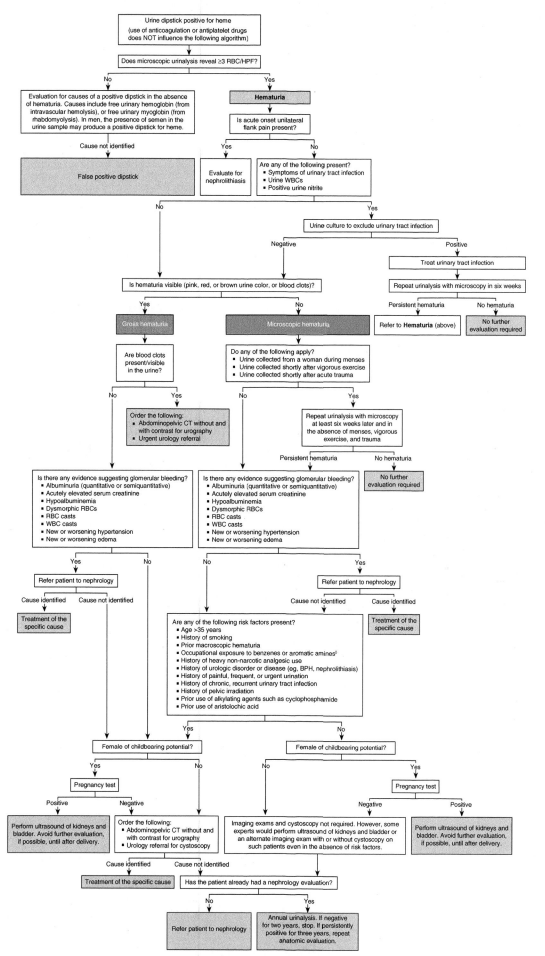

FIGURE 43-2. Evaluation of gross hematuria in adults. (From *Evaluation of the adult with asymptomatic hematuria. UpToDate.* 2018. https://www.uptodate.com/contents/image?imageKey=NEPH%2F107857&topicKey=NEPH%2F7208&source=outline_link&search=hematuria&selectedTitle=1~150.)

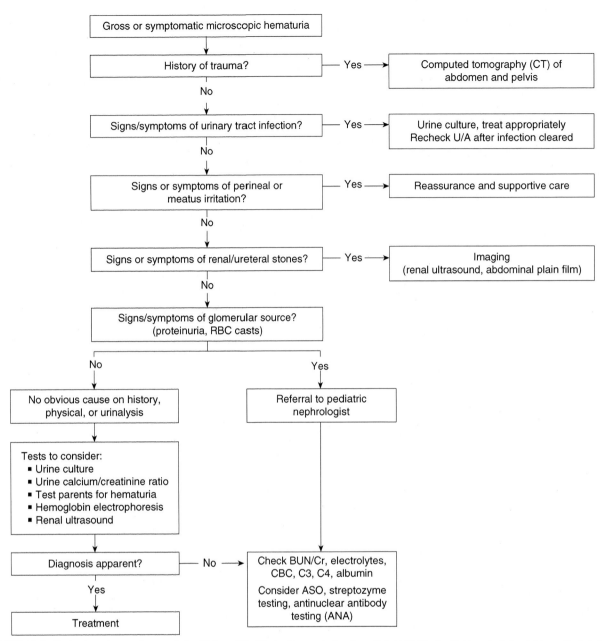

FIGURE 43-3. Evaluation of gross hematuria in children. (Modified with permission from Patel HP, Bissler JJ. Hematuria in children. *Pediatr Clin North Am.* 2001;48:1519.)

Emergency Medicine

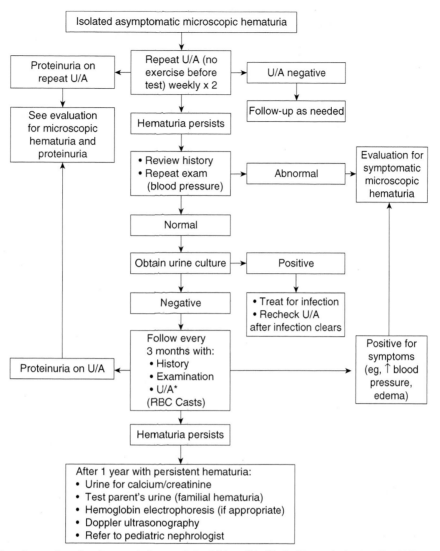

FIGURE 43-4. Evaluation of asymptomatic microscopic hematuria in children. (Modified with permission fromPatel HP, Bissler JJ. Hematuria in children. *Pediatr Clin North Am.* 2001;48:1519.)

INCONTINENCE

- Evaluation: three incontinence questions, assess other medical problems, review voiding diary, postvoid residual urine volume (if overflow incontinence)

  - Check serum creatinine (elevated with urinary retention)
  - Urinalysis

- Identify transient or reversible causes of incontinence: DIAPPERS (**Delirium, Infection, Atrophic, Pharmaceuticals, Psych, Excessive, Reduced, Stool**)

  - Delirium, infection (UTI), atrophic vaginitis, pharmaceuticals, psych disorder (depression), excessive urine output (hyperglycemia), reduced mobility (functional), stool impaction

- Three questions: ask if, when, and how often they experience urine leakage

- **Red flags:** hematuria, obstructive symptoms (straining to void, sensation of incomplete bladder emptying), recurrent UTI → urology referral

- Pelvic organ prolapse (with cystocele, urethral polyps, or rectocele) may not lead to incontinence, but accompanies atrophic vaginitis

- Indications for referral to urology: marked prostate enlargement, persistent hematuria, or proteinuria, postvoid residual volume >200 mL, previous pelvic surgery or radiation, pelvic pain, pelvic organ prolapsed past introitus, recurrent UTI, new-onset neurologic symptoms or muscle weakness

Disease	Etiology, Prevalence, Risk Factors	Clinical Symptoms and Signs	Diagnostics	Therapy, Prognosis, and Health Maintenance
Urge incontinence (overactive bladder): detrusor overactivity (uninhibited bladder contractions) caused by irritation within the bladder or loss of inhibitory neurologic control of bladder contractions	Females 75+ y old (31%) **Males 75+ y old** (42%) Causes: Cystitis, prostatitis, atrophic vaginitis, bladder diverticulum, pelvic radiation therapy Loss of neurologic control from stroke, dementia, spinal cord injury, Parkinson disease	1. Loss of urine preceded by a sudden and severe desire to pass urine • Loss of urine on way to toilet • Loss ranges from minimal to flooding 2. Contractions with change in body position (supine to upright) or with sensory stimulation (running water, hand washing, cold weather) 3. **Frequency** and **nocturia** common 4. **Urgency** w/o urinary loss (OAB)	1. Voiding diary: variable 2. Cough stress test: may show delayed leakage after cough 3. PVR: <50 mL 4. Check serum creatinine: elevated	
Stress incontinence: Sphincter weakness (urethral sphincter and/or pelvic floor weakness)	Primarily **females >30 y** Causes: may occur after prostatectomy or after childbirth in obese women	1. Loss of small amount of urine during physical inactivity or intraabdominal pressure (**cough, sneeze, jump, lift, exercise**) • Can occur with minimal activity, such as walking or rising from a chair	1. Voiding diary: small volume leakage (5-10 cc) with activity 2. **Cough stress test** (+): leakage with coughing (most reliable) 3. PVR: <50 mL	
Overflow incontinence (urinary retention): overdistention of bladder caused by impaired detrusor contractility or bladder outlet obstruction	Primarily men with prostate problems 5% of patients with chronic incontinence Causes: Anticholinergic medicines, BPH, pelvic organ prolapse, DM, multiple sclerosis, spinal cord injuries	1. **Dribbling** 2. Inability to empty bladder 3. Hesitancy 4. Urine loss without recognizable urge or sensation of fullness or pressure in lower abdomen	1. Voiding diary: varies 2. Cough stress test: no leakage 3. **Postvoid residual urine measurement: >200-300 mL**	
Functional incontinence: caused by environmental or physical barriers to toileting	Non-GU factors: cognitive or physical impairment resulting in patient's inability to void independently	History of severe dementia, physical frailty, or inability to ambulate, mental health disorder (depression)	1. Voiding diary: pattern in circumstances of incontinence 2. Cough stress test: no leakage 3. PVR: varies	
Detrusor (bladder) sphincter dyssynergia	Consequence of neurologic pathology: SCI or multiple sclerosis Urethral sphincter muscle dyssynergically contracts during voiding causing the flow to be interrupted and bladder pressure to arise Obstructive cause	1. Daytime and nighttime wetting 2. Urinary retention 3. History of UTI/bladder infections 4. Associated: constipation and encopresis	1. Postvoid residual urine volume (PVR) >150 mL	1. Botulinum A toxin injections 2. Surgical incision of bladder neck • Can result in incontinence

PRIAPISM

Disease	Etiology, Prevalence, Risk Factors	Clinical Symptoms and Signs	Diagnostics	Therapy, Prognosis, and Health Maintenance
Priapism	Urologic emergency Persistent, painful, pathologic erection Etiology: • Intracavernosal injection of prostaglandin E, etc • Oral agents for hypertension (hydralazine, prazosin, CCB) • Neuroleptic medications (chlorpromazine, **trazodone**, thioridazine) In children: • Hematologic disorders, such as **sickle cell**: sickling of RBC in sinusoids of corpus cavernosum causes decreased venous outflow • 27% of males have at least one episode by age 20 Bimodal peak: 1. Age 5-13 y 2. Age 21-29 y	1. Typically painful persistent erection 2. Difficulty with urinating Signs: 1. Painful, swollen, edematous, tender penis	1. Doppler ultrasound: distinguishes the type of priapism (whether ischemic/low flow or arterial/high flow) 2. Aspirate blood from the cavernosal arteries (confirmatory) for ABG If low flow: • Darker • PO_2 <30 mm Hg • PCO_2 >60 mm Hg • pH <7.25	1. IV fluids and opioid analgesics, supplemental O_2, NPO status (for possible sedation) 2. Corporal aspiration of blood with irrigation (plain saline or phenylephrine) 3. Urologic consult and surgery, if above fails to work If due to sick cell crisis: 1. IV venous hydration, consider RBC exchange transfusion Complications: 1. Impotence results in 35% of untreated prolonged erections • If duration >4 h, risk for permanent damage increases

CHAPTER

44

Endocrinology

Emergency Medicine

Refer to Internal Medicine 🩺 for In-Depth Coverage of the Following Topics:

Refer to Appendices for In-Depth Coverage of the Following Topics:

Supplemental Material:

PALPITATIONS

- DDx: hyperthyroidism, pheochromocytoma

HEAT AND COLD INTOLERANCE

- Heat intolerance DDx: hyperthyroidism
- Cold intolerance DDx: myxedema (hypothyroidism)

TREMORS

- DDx: hyperthyroidism, thyrotoxicosis

HYPERPARATHYROIDISM AND HYPERTHYROIDISM

- **Increased parathyroid hormone (PTH)** stimulates the osteoclasts to increase bone resorption, **elevating calcium levels**

- Works in the kidney to increase calcium reabsorption
- Increases renal excretion of phosphorous
- Hematocrit unaffected by parathyroid hormone
- Causes a proximal renal tubular acidosis (a **hyperchloremic metabolic acidosis**), increasing bicarbonate loss
- **High calcium levels**

- **Suppresses PTH** secretion (be aware that a normal PTH level is "abnormal" in the setting of high calcium levels)
- Can cause **nephrogenic diabetes insipidus** because the renal tubule becomes unresponsive to the action of ADH
- Asymptomatic patients with primary hyperparathyroidism have defects in their ability to concentrate urine

DIABETIC KETOACIDOSIS AND NONKETOTIC HYPERGLYCEMIA

Disease	Etiology, Prevalence, Risk Factors	Clinical Symptoms and Signs	Diagnostics	Therapy, Prognosis, and Health Maintenance
Diabetic ketoacidosis	Most common acute life-threatening complication of diabetes MC: Type 1 diabetes, but may occur with type 2 Precipitating factor: Omission/inadequate insulin, **infection** (most common), new-onset T1 DM, pancreatitis, AMI, CVA, drugs Acidosis drives K$^+$ out of cells → hyperkalemia	1. Fatigue and weakness • *Hours to days* 2. **Abdominal pain** 3. Vomiting (25%) 4. Polyuria, polydipsia Signs: 1. Rapid deep respirations (**Kussmaul respirations**) 2. Tachycardia, hypotension 3. Decreased turgor 4. **Fruity** or acetone breath 5. If severe—altered mental status → Stupor/coma	Diagnostic studies: 1. ABG • Arterial pH: <7.3 2. Glucose >250 3. Serum HCO$_3^-$ <15 4. Serum ketones or ketonuria: (+) Check 1. Serum K$^+$ 2. Anion gap—assess severity of acidosis and follow progress of therapy >12 (typically >20 mEq/L) 3. **β-Hydroxybutyrate** (primary ketone body) 4. Serum osmolality: >250	1. Restore circulation: **IV saline** 2. Treat insulin deficiency: IV insulin infusion until urinary ketones resolve → **SQ insulin** 3. Treat electrolyte disturbances • Na—initially low, increases with IVF/IVI • K/PO$_4$—initially high, decreases with IVF/IVI • Mg—low 4. Search for underlying causes of metabolic decompensation
Hyperosmolar hyperglycemic state (nonketotic hyperglycemia)	Precipitating factors: infection, AMI, CVA, trauma, decreased access to water, medication effects or interactions RF: >65 y, nursing home, change in diabetes medicines, infection, dementia Sufficient insulin activity to prevent lipolysis and ketogenesis Results from gradual diuresis → severe dehydration and electrolyte depletion	1. Polyuria, polydipsia, or polyphagia 2. Generalized weakness 3. Nausea, vomiting • No abdominal pain • Develops over *days-weeks* 4. **Mental status changes** (most common), stupor/coma Signs: 1. Severe dehydration • Dry mucus membranes, poor skin turgor, delayed capillary refill 2. Tachycardia 3. Orthostatic hypotension	Diagnostic studies 1. ABG • Arterial pH: **>7.3** (no acidosis) 2. Glucose: **>600** 3. Serum HCO$_3^-$: >15 4. Serum ketones or ketonuria: small 5. Glucosuria Check: 1. Serum osmolality: **>320-380** 2. Anion gap: variable <10 3. Sodium: hyponatremia (125-130) 4. K$^+$: low/NL 5. BUN: elevated	1. Restore circulation: IV saline • **1-1.5 L 0.9% saline** infused over first hour • 500 mL/h • 250-500 mL/h • 150-300 mL/h 2. Treat insulin circulation: • **IV regular insulin** infusion 0.1 units/kg per hour → SQ insulin 3. Treat electrolyte disturbances • Recheck hourly 4. Search for underlying causes of metabolic decompensation

Potassium Repletion for Insulin Administration

Potassium Range	Insulin Administration	Potassium Administration
K <3.3 mEq/L	No insulin	40 mEq KCl IV or ⅔ KCl + ⅓ KPO_3
K 3.3-5.0 mEq/L	No insulin	20-30 mEq KCl in each L of IVF
K >5.0 mEq/L	If levels remain elevated, or EKG changes noted → Regular insulin bolus 8-12 units with standard treatment of hyperkalemia	Hold, recheck in 1 h

CHAPTER 45

Dermatology

Refer to Family Medicine 👪 for In-Depth Coverage of the Following Topics:

Refer to Pediatrics 🧍 for In-Depth Coverage of the Following Topics:

Refer to Surgery ✎ for In-Depth Coverage of the Following Topics:

Recommended Supplemental Topics 👪 :

Emergency Medicine

ITCHING (PRURITUS) (FIG. 45-1)

Algorithm for the evaluation of pruritus

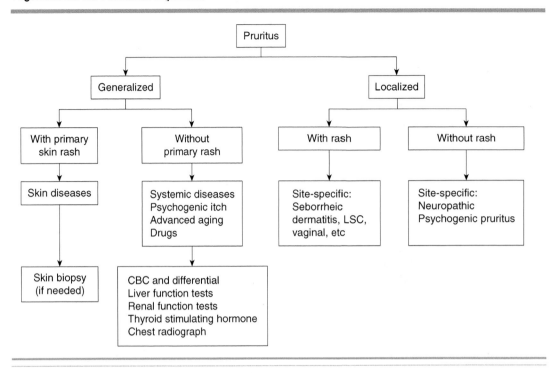

CBC: complete blood count; LSC: lichen simplex chronicus.

FIGURE 45-1. Evaluation of pruritus (itching). (From Yosipovitch G, Dawn AG, Greaves MW, Pathophysiology and clinical aspects of pruritus. In: Wolff K, Goldsmith LA, Katz SI, et al, eds. *Fitzpatrick's Dermatology in General Medicine.* 7th ed. New York: McGraw Hill; 2008.)

- Primary cutaneous diseases: scabies, eczema, insect bites, pediculosis, contact dermatitis, drug reactions, urticaria, psoriasis, and lichen planus
- Consider drugs such as calcium channel blockers
- Persistent itching not explained by skin disease should prompt workup for systemic causes
  - Most common cause associated with systemic disease: uremia in conjunction with hemodialysis

DERMATITIS (ECZEMA, CONTACT)

Disease	Etiology, Prevalence, Risk Factors	Clinical Symptoms and Signs	Diagnostics	Therapy, Prognosis, and Health Maintenance
Irritant diaper dermatitis	Caused by overhydration of the skin, maceration, prolonged contact with urine/feces, retained diaper soaps, >3 diarrheal stools/d MC: Infants 9-12 mo Associated: History of eczema	1. Erythematous scaly diaper area 2. Genitocrural folds are **spared** in irritant dermatitis Signs: 1. Papulovesicular or bullous lesions, fissures, and erosions 2. Patchy or confluent 3. Genitocrural folds are spared	1. KOH preparation or culture	1. **Zinc oxide ointment** 2. Leave diaper area open to air or cover it with topical emollient • Petrolatum, Aquaphor

Disease	Etiology, Prevalence, Risk Factors	Clinical Symptoms and Signs	Diagnostics	Therapy, Prognosis, and Health Maintenance

Candidal diaper dermatitis	Infection occurs after 48-72 h of active eruption
	MCC: *Candida albicans*
	Immunocompromised patients are more susceptible
		1. Isolated to perineal area (92%)
		2. Genitocrural folds are *involved* in primary candidal dermatitis
		Signs:
		1. **Satellite lesions** (miliaria rubra): tiny red papules and papulovesicles
		2. Confluent diaper area with tomato-red plaques, papules, and pustules
			1. KOH prep or culture (not necessary)	1. Hydrocortisone 1% BID
				2. AND
				3. Antifungal: **nystatin cream**, powder, or ointment; clotrimazole 1% cream, miconazole 2% ointment after every diaper change
				  • *Avoid* higher strength topical steroids, including clotrimazole/betamethasone and nystatin/triamcinolone
				4. Leave diaper area open to air or cover it with topical emollient
				  • Petrolatum, Aquaphor

Perioral dermatitis	MC: Young females with history of prior topical steroid use in area	1. Papulopustules on erythematous base → confluent plaques and scales 2. Vermillion border spared 3. Satellite lesions common	1. Culture to r/o staphylococcal infection	1. Avoid topical steroids (aggravate!) 2. Topical Flagyl or erythromycin 3. PO minocycline, doxycycline, tetracycline
Contact	**Irritant**: nonimmune modulated skin irritation caused by skin injury, direct cytotoxic effects, or cutaneous inflammation from contact with irritant **Allergic**: *type IV, T-cell-mediated, delayed hypersensitivity* reaction from foreign substance Most common: Poison ivy, nickel, fragrances	1. Not painful, but **red** and itchy 2. Onset after contact with irritant or allergen 3. Distribution patterns from irritant or allergen Signs: 1. **Scaly** occurring on thin areas of skin (flexural surfaces, eyelids, face, anogenital region) 2. Acute = erythema, vesicles, and bullae 3. Chronic = lichenification with cracks and fissures	1. Determine if problem resolves with removal of substance	1. Localized = mid- or high-potency topical steroids (triamcinolone 0.1%/Kenalog or clobetasol 0.05%) 2. If >20% of BSA, systemic steroids recommended with resolution in 12-24 h • 5-7 d of prednisone 0.5-1 mg/kg per day

Atopic **(eczema)**	More susceptible to skin infections, *Staphylococcus aureus* (most common)
	Associated **allergic triad**: asthma, allergic rhinitis, atopic dermatitis
		Onset before age 2 y, 10% diagnosed after age 5 y
		Acute phase:
		Vesicular, weeping, crusting eruption
		Subacute:
		Dry, scaly, red papules, and plaques
		Chronic:
		Excoriations and lichenification of skin, xerosis, hyperpigmentation
		Flexural lichenification in adults: anterior and lateral neck, eyelids, forehead, face, wrists, dorsa of feet, hands
		Facial and extensor involvement in children and infants
			Clinical DX:
			Complications:
			Secondary bacterial infections—pustules and crusts
				1. Moisturizers or **emollients** (mainstay): Cetaphil or Eucerin
				  • Ointments: Aquaphor, petroleum jelly
				2. Bathing—removes scale, crust, irritants, allergens
				  • Limit use of nonsoap cleansers (hypoallergenic, no fragrance)
				3. **Topical steroids** (first line)—flare ups
				4. Topical calcineurin inhibitors—second line moderate to severe (pimecrolimus 1% or tacrolimus 0.03%)
				5. Antibiotics to reduce flare-ups
				6. UV phototherapy for severe or refractory

Emergency Medicine

NECROTIZING FASCIITIS

Disease	Etiology, Prevalence, Risk Factors	Clinical Symptoms and Signs	Diagnostics	Therapy, Prognosis, and Health Maintenance
Necrotizing fasciitis	Affects young, healthy patients RF: Increased age, immunocompromised, chronic illness, alcoholism, and IV drug use Arises at sites of recent tattoos Pathogens: **Group A β-hemolytic strep** Pathophysiology not fully understood, but bacteria produce enzymes that degrade fascia and allow rapid proliferation of bacteria → local thrombosis, progressive ischemia, liquefaction necrosis, superficial gangrene	1. Early (stage 1): painful at first, then swelling, **erythema**, warmth, tenderness, resembles cellulitis • Constitutional SX: high fever, toxicity 2. Stage 2: **induration worsens, bullae develop** 3. Stage 3: skin color becomes purple, frank cutaneous gangrene • No longer tender, nonpainful	1. XR: subcutaneous air caused by gas-forming organisms within the fascia	1. **Urgent irrigation and debridement** 2. Antibiotics • PCN G 3. Adjunctive therapies: hyperbaric O_2

BURNS

- Patients who require social, emotional, or rehabilitative intervention
- The **zone of coagulation** is the most severely burned portion and is typically in the center of the wound; likely needs excision and grafting
- Peripheral to that is a **zone of stasis**, with variable degrees of vasoconstriction and resultant ischemia, much like a second-degree burn
- The last area of a burn is called the **zone of hyperemia**, which will heal with minimal or no scarring and is most like a superficial or first-degree burn
- Appropriate resuscitation and wound care may help prevent conversion to a deeper wound, but infection or suboptimal perfusion may result in an increase in burn depth
- Burn wounds evolve over the 48 to 72 hours after injury
- One of the most effective ways to determine burn depth is full-thickness biopsy, but this has several limitations; the procedure is painful and potentially scarring and accurate interpretation of the histopathology requires a specialized pathologist and may have slow turnaround times
- Prognosis is directly related to the extent of injury, both size and depth

SHINGLES (HERPES ZOSTER)

Disease	Etiology, Prevalence, Risk Factors	Clinical Symptoms and Signs	Diagnostics	Therapy, Prognosis, and Health Maintenance
Shingles (herpes zoster)	Age >50 y Caused by reactivation of the varicella-zoster virus, which is dormant in the dorsal root ganglia and reactivated during stress, infection, or illness Occurs only in patients who have had chickenpox Contagious when open vesicles present and immunocompromised	1. **Severe pain and rash** in dermatomal distribution (*pain before rash*) • **Thorax (most common)** and trigeminal distribution, other CN and arms/legs 2. On days 3-4, vesicles become more pustular 3. Crust over by days 7-10 (no longer infectious) Signs: 1. Grouped vesicles on erythematous base Complications: **Postherpetic neuralgia**, excruciating pain persisting after lesions have cleared and does not respond to analgesics, uveitis, meningoencephalitis, deafness	1. Tzanck smear • 60% sensitive 2. **Culture of vesicular fluid** (confirmatory) 3. Varivax–indicated for individuals >1 y old 4. Zostavax–indicated for prevention of zoster in patients who have no contraindications	1. Keep lesions dry/clean 2. **Analgesics** for pain (ASA or Tylenol), local triamcinolone in lidocaine 3. **Antivirals**: acyclovir, famciclovir, valacyclovir to reduce incidence of PHN, reduce pain, and decrease length of illness 4. Steroids to decrease incidence of PHN 5. **Live vaccine (VariZIG)** to reduce severity and duration • Administer within 10 d • High-risk groups: immunocompromised children/adults, newborns of mothers with varicella shortly before or after delivery, premature infants, infants <1 y old, adults without evidence of immunity, pregnant women

Emergency Medicine

Disease	Etiology, Prevalence, Risk Factors	Clinical Symptoms and Signs	Diagnostics	Therapy, Prognosis, and Health Maintenance
Ramsay-Hunt syndrome (herpes zoster oticus)	Polycranial neuropathy (CN V, IX, and X) Reactivation of latent VZV residing within facial nerve and geniculate ganglion with spread involving CN VIII HSV type 2 infection?	1. Itching → face and ear pain pain (out of proportion to examination) 2. Ipsilateral facial paralysis 3. Decreased salivation and loss of taste sensation over posterolateral tongue, hearing (tinnitus, hyperacusis), vertigo, and lacrimation Signs: 1. Vesicles in auditory canal and auricle and face	1. Clinical DX 2. Tzanck smear—usually not helpful 3. MRI with contrast: enhancement of geniculate ganglion and facial nerve	1. PO antivirals and steroids 2. Lubricating drops to protect involved eye from corneal abrasions and ulcerations 3. Referral to ophthalmology Prognosis: 10% with full paralysis recover fully 66% with partial paralysis recover fully
Trigeminal neuralgia (tic douloureux)	Unilateral facial pain in sensory distribution of CN V (maxillary or mandibular)	1. Severe, **lancinating**, unilateral facial pain in distribution of one or more branches of trigeminal nerve (V2, V3) 2. Worse with chewing, talking, smiling • Drinking cold or hot fluids • Touching, shaving, brushing teeth, blowing nose, cold air 3. Localized pain	1. Paroxysmal attacks of pain last from a fraction of a second to 2 min, affecting 1 or more divisions of trigeminal nerve 2. Pain has at least 1 of the following features: (a) intense, sharp, superficial, or stabbing (1b) trigger areas or factors 3. Attacks stereotyped in individual patient 4. No clinically evident neurologic deficit 5. Not attributable to another disorder	1. Carbamazepine

- Zostavax (live attenuated virus)
  - Approved for **adults aged 50 to 59** who are nonimmunocompromised, nonpregnant, including those who have had a previous episode of zoster
  - Patients who are about to begin biologic therapy (should not be started while ON biologic therapy)
  - Contraindications: long-term steroid treatment, chemotherapy, radiation
- Varicella-zoster immune globulin (VZIG)
  - Recommended to prevent or modify clinical illness in persons with exposure to varicella or herpes zoster who are susceptible or immunocompromised

- Reserved for patients at risk for severe disease and complications: neonates, immunocompromised, pregnant
- Administer ASAP after presumed exposure or as late as 96 hours

Urticaria
Pilonidal Disease
Pressure Ulcers
Drug Eruptions, Stevens Johnson Syndrome, Toxic Epidermal Necrolysis
Erythema Multiforme, Bullous Pemphigoid

PEMPHIGUS VULGARIS

Disease	Etiology, Prevalence, Risk Factors	Clinical Symptoms and Signs	Diagnostics	Therapy, Prognosis, and Health Maintenance
Pemphigus (vulgaris)	An autoimmune disease that causes formation of blisters, or bullae Caused by autoantibodies to adhesion molecules in the skin and mucous membranes Occurs in middle=aged adults More common in patients of Jewish or Mediterranean ancestry May be drug induced: Penicillamine, Captopril, others More fragile than bullous pemphigoid	1. Flaccid bullae in the oropharynx • Skin lesions develop 6-12 mo later on the scalp, chest, axillae, and groin • Spontaneously rupture 2. Pain or burning 3. Absence of itching 4. Weakness, malaise Signs: 1. Nikolsky sign: applying pressure to skin causes superficial skin to separate from deeper layers 2. Round vesicles that contain clear fluid and easily rupture; discrete and scattered diffusely; erosions and crusts occur	1. Immunofluorescence or serum ELISA of blister contents shows IgG **(confirmatory)** 2. Biopsy shows acantholysis	1. IV therapy and feeds • Prednisone 2. Immunosuppressive agents 3. Azathioprine +/− methotrexate Complications: 1. Secondary infection 2. Fluid and electrolyte imbalance and disturbances in nutritional intake due to painful oral ulcers Prognosis: 1. Chronic course in most, one-third experience remission 2. Infection is the most common cause of death, due to *S. aureus* septicemia

KAPOSI SARCOMA

Disease	Etiology, Prevalence, Risk Factors	Clinical Symptoms and Signs	Diagnostics	Therapy, Prognosis, and Health Maintenance
Kaposi sarcoma	Caused by human herpesvirus 8 (HHV-8) Associated with AIDS RF: Homosexual men with HIV infection Complicates: Immunosuppressive therapy and stopping therapy may improve it	1. Lesions anywhere: eyelids, conjunctiva, pinnae, palate, toe, webs 2. May involve the GI tract 3. May involve the lungs • SOB, cough, hemoptysis, or chest pain Signs: 1. Purplish or red, nonblanching papules or nodules 2. Marked edema	1. FOBT—screen for GI lesions 2. CXR—may screen for lung lesions 3. Bronchoscopy, may be indicated if suspicious for lung lesions	1. Reduction of immunosuppressive medications in setting of iatrogenic immunosuppression 2. In patients with AIDS—treat with ART 3. Cryotherapy or intralesional vinblastine 4. Radiation therapy 5. Laser surgery 6. ART therapy + chemotherapy

CHAPTER **46**

Psychiatry

Emergency Medicine

SPOUSE OR PARTNER NEGLECT/VIOLENCE

Disease	Etiology, Prevalence, Risk Factors	Clinical Symptoms and Signs	Diagnostics	Therapy, Prognosis, and Health Maintenance
Intimate partner violence (IPV)	Abusive behavior (physical, sexual, emotional) by a person in an intimate relationship with the victim Females > males to be victims Goal of abuser: Gain control over victim RF: Young (<35 y old), pregnant; being single, divorced, or separated; ETOH or drug abuse in victim or partner, smoking, low economic status	1. Explanation of injuries that do not fit with examination findings 2. Frequent visits to ED 3. Somatic complaints: headache, abdominal pain, fatigue Signs: 1. Vague during history 2. Minimal eye contact 3. Abuser in room answers all questions or declines to leave room 4. Injuries to central area of body, forearms 5. Bruises in various stages of healing	Screening tools: 1. HITS (Hurt, Insult, Threaten, Screamed at tool) 2. WAST (Women Abuse Screening Tool) 3. PVS (Partner Violence Screen) 4. AAS (Abuse Assessment Screen) 5. WEB (Women's Experience with Battering) scale	1. Most important: speak with patient alone 2. Document all history and findings carefully 3. US Preventative Services Task Force recommends screening women of childbearing age for IPV including domestic violence and refer women who screen (+) to intervention services • Interventions: leave abusive situation ensuring a safe place to go, counseling to assess risk of danger, create plan for safety

CHAPTER **47**

Hematology

Refer to Internal Medicine 🩺 **for In-Depth Coverage of the Following Topics:**

Easy Bruising and Bleeding, see ITP, TTP, and HUS, p 284

Sickle Cell Anemia/Crisis, see Sickle Cell Anemia, p 276

Clotting Factor Disorders, p 282

Hypercoagulable States, p 283

Thrombocytopenia, see ITP and TTP, p 284

Acute Leukemia, p 280

Anemia, see Iron Deficiency Anemia, Beta Thalassemia, Vitamin B$_{12}$, and Folic Acid Deficiency Anemia, and Hemolytic Anemias, p 275

Lymphomas, p 281

Refer to Family Medicine 👥 **for In-Depth Coverage of the Following Topics:**

Polycythemia, p 193

Recommended Supplemental Material:

Aplastic Anemia, see Pediatrics, 👪 p 364 🔍

Neutropenia, see Pediatrics, 👪 p 364 👥

Blood Cell Morphology and Life Cycle, see Internal Medicine, p 274 🩺

EASY BRUISING AND BLEEDING

Disease	Etiology, Prevalence, Risk Factors	Clinical Symptoms and Signs	Diagnostics	Therapy, Prognosis, and Health Maintenance
Heparin-induced thrombocytopenia (HIT)	In 3% of patients trigger immune response between platelet *factor 4* and heparin → forms antibodies that cross-react with platelets (*antibody-induced process*) Most common thrombocytopenia in postoperative period: Occurs **4-7 d after** initiation of heparin prophylaxis or therapy	Occurs **4-7 d after** initiation of heparin prophylaxis or therapy 1. Thrombocytopenia + **50% drop in platelets from baseline** (not below 30 000) • Bleeding is *not* common 2. **Venous or arterial thrombosis**—activated platelets render patient hypercoagulable	1. PT/PTT: normal 2. Check ELISA for PF4-heparin–associated IgG 3. Doppler LE to r/o DVT 4. CBC: thrombocytopenia	1. ***Discontinue heparin*** and heparin-coated products • Avoid platelet transfusion (this will provide a substrate) 2. ***Anticoagulate***: Use lepirudin or argatroban • Lepirudin: avoid in renal failure • IV argatroban: avoid in hepatic failure 3. Long-term anticoagulation on warfarin 4. Higher incidence with UFH than enoxaparin sodium (Lovenox) 5. 50% reduction in total platelet volume 6. Surgical patients (orthopedic/cardiac) at increased risk

FATIGUE

Difficulty or inability to initiate activity and is a perception of generalized weakness.

- Other definitions: easy fatigability (or reduced capacity to maintain activity)
- Associated with: concentration and memory difficulties, emotional fatigue/stability

Major Causes of Chronic Fatigue	
Psychologic	**Infectious**
Depression	Endocarditis
Anxiety	Tuberculosis
Somatization disorder	Mononucleosis
Malnutrition or drug addiction	Hepatitis
Pharmacologic	Parasitic disease
Hypnotics	HIV infection
Antihypertensives	Cytomegalovirus
Antidepressants	**Cardiopulmonary**
Drug abuse and withdrawal	Chronic heart failure
Endocrine-metabolic	Chronic obstructive pulmonary disease
Hypothyroidism	**Connective tissue disease**
Diabetes mellitus	Rheumatoid arthritis
Apathetic hyperthyroidism	**Disturbed sleep**
Pituitary insufficiency	Sleep apnea
Hypercalcemia	Esophageal reflux
Adrenal insufficiency	Allergic rhinitis
Chronic renal failure	Psychologic causes
Hepatic failure	**Idiopathic (diagnosis by exclusion)**
Neoplastic-hematologic	Idiopathic chronic fatigue
Occult malignancy	Chronic fatigue syndrome
Severe anemia	Fibromyalgia

Adapted from Gorroll AH, May LA, Mulley AG Jr, eds. *Primary Care Medicine: Office Evaluation and Management of the Adult Patient. 3rd ed.* Philadelphia: JB Lippincott; 1995.

ACQUIRED HEMOLYTIC ANEMIA

- A group of disorders characterized by hemolysis of red blood cells (RBCs) *not* due to congenital or inherited disorders of hemoglobin synthesis or of the RBC membrane
- AIHA is also divided into "warm" and "cold" categories, based on the temperature at which the autoantibodies exert their effect
- Intravascular hemolysis of RBCs releases hemoglobin into the bloodstream that then binds to haptoglobin and other serum proteins. The hemoglobin-haptoglobin complex travels to the liver for processing, thus decreasing the amount of free haptoglobin in the serum—an important laboratory finding of intravascular hemolysis
- The **direct Coombs test** (direct antigen test) is performed by combining the patient's anticoagulated, washed RBCs with anti-immunoglobulin G and anti-C3d (complement) antibodies to detect the presence of immunoglobulin G (IgG) and/or complement on the RBC surface
  - A **positive** direct antigen test consists of the detection of either immunoglobulin G or complement on the RBC surface; it does not require the detection of both
  - Differential: AIHA, hemolytic transfusion reaction, hemolytic disease of the newborn, sickle cell disease, β-thalassemia, multiple myeloma, Hodgkin lymphoma
- The **indirect Coombs test** looks for the presence of auto-antibodies in the patient's serum, testing against a panel of RBCs bearing specific surface antigens

Emergency Medicine

Disease	Etiology, Prevalence, Risk Factors	Clinical Symptoms and Signs	Diagnostics	Therapy, Prognosis, and Health Maintenance
Warm Ab autoimmune hemolytic anemia (AIHA) 70%-80% of AIHA cases 2:1 (females > males)	Extravascular; antibody-coated RBCs consumed by splenic macrophages MC: Females, 40s-50s Primary: 50% Idiopathic Secondary: 50% (Lymphoproliferative, autoimmune disease, postinfection)	1. Mild **jaundice** or dark urine 2. **Anemia**: weakness, fatigue, dizziness, SOB, dyspnea on exertion, palpitations, chest pain 3. **Splenomegaly** (33%-50%) Signs: 1. Palpable spleen 2. Tachycardia 3. New or accentuated heart murmur 4. Pallor	1. CBC: anemia, reticulocytosis • Elevated: bilirubin, LDH, K$^+$ 2. Peripheral smear: schistocytes, **spherocytes** 3. Haptoglobin: low 4. (+) **Direct Coombs test** (confirms)	Severe symptomatic: 1. Transfuse allogeneic RBCs Otherwise: 1. Plasma exchange (PLEX)—interim • Adjunct IVIG 2. HD *corticosteroids* • Continue until rise in Hct or decrease in reticulocyte count (3 wk) • PO 1-2 mg/kg per day × 3-4 wk 3. Splenectomy • After failure of steroids or anti-CD20 antibody • 60% Benefit • Removes major site of hemolysis and autoantibody production • AE: postsplenectomy infection (sepsis) • Patients should get regular pneumococcal and meningococcal vaccinations • Daily penicillin prophylaxis
Cold-Ab autoimmune hemolytic anemia (AIHA) **cold agglutinin disease**	Intravascular and extravascular; hepatic macrophages (Kupffer cells) destroy RBCs IgM autoantibody against I antigen Primary: Females, 70s Secondary disease: **Lymphoproliferative disorders** (CLL, lymphoma) (50%)	1. Severe symptoms uncommon • Attacks precipitated by cold exposure (seen in winter) Signs: 1. Raynaud phenomenon 2. Vascular occlusion → acrocyanosis → tissue necrosis/gangrene 3. Livedo reticularis	1. Peripheral smear: spherocytes, anisocytosis, poikilocytosis, polychromasia, agglutination 2. (+) Direct Coombs	1. Keep extremities (nose and ears) warm in cold weather 2. Not steroid responsive 3. Splenectomy never indicated 4. PLEX + immunosuppression: chlorambucil, cyclophosphamide, interferon alpha, Rituximab Prophylaxis: 1. Daily folate supplement

POLYCYTHEMIA

- Primary polycythemia (polycythemia vera): bone marrow disorder characterized by autonomous overproduction of erythroid cells

Disease	Etiology, Prevalence, Risk Factors	Clinical Symptoms and Signs	Diagnostics	Therapy, Prognosis, and Health Maintenance
Secondary polycythemia (secondary erythrocytosis or erythrocythemia)	Typically, due to increased erythropoietin (EPO) production in response to chronic hypoxia or from an EPO-secreting tumor MCC: **Obstructive sleep apnea, COPD, and obesity hypoventilation syndrome**; also, heavy cigarette smoking, testosterone replacement therapy, EPO-secreting tumors (HCC, RCC, adrenal adenoma)	1. Impaired alertness 2. Dizziness 3. Headaches 4. Compromised exercise intolerance 5. Confusion Signs: 1. Lethargic 2. Skin erythema (palms and soles) and redness of mucosa 3. Acrocyanosis 4. Obtunded 5. Signs of stroke, DVT, or heart attack 6. Less likely if signs of hepatosplenomegaly Associated: CVA, MI, DVT, thrombosis	1. Check JAK2 V617F mutation and EPO levels–r/o primary polycythemia • Will be positive for mutation and low EPO level in primary 2. RBC count and plasma volume • Hct >52% in men and 47% in women • Note that increased Hgb and Hct can also be seen in severe dehydration 3. Red blood cell mass • Elevated if >35 mg/kg in men and 31 mg/kg in women • Will show a decreased plasma volume with normal RBC mass 4. Renal CT to rule out tumor	1. If hematocrit >60%-65%, treat with **phlebotomy** until symptoms resolve 2. Treat underlying cause • Recommend weight loss in patients with obesity and hypoventilation • Recommend smoking cessation in patients with carboxyhemoglobin • Recommend O$_2$ supplementation in patients with COPD

PRACTICE QUESTIONS

1. A 48-year-old woman presents with chest pain and a headache. Vitals reveal a blood pressure of 205/165, pulse of 88, and a respiratory rate of 16. Which of the following would you expect on physical examination?

   A. Carotid bruit

   B. Papilledema

   C. Systolic murmur

   D. Water hammer pulse

2. A 17-year-old male presents with new-onset headache, nuchal rigidity, fever of 39°C, and disorientation. Which finding supports the diagnosis?

   A. Blood cultures positive for *Listeria monocytogenes*

   B. Opening pressure of 200 mm H$_2$O

   C. CSF glucose to serum glucose ratio of 0.3

   D. Generalized 3 Hz spike wave on EEG

3. A 67-year-old woman presents to the ED after falling on an outstretched hand with volar displacement of the distal fragment. What is the best clinical intervention?

   A. Sugar tong splint

   B. Immediate surgery

   C. Ulnar gutter splint

   D. Thumb spica splint

4. A 25-year-old woman with no past medical or surgical history presents with sudden onset of nausea, vomiting, fever, and right upper quadrant pain. Ultrasound is positive for Murphy sign. Which of the following is the treatment of choice?

   A. IV fluids and morphine drip

   B. Endoscopic retrograde cholangiopancreatography (ERCP)

   C. Cholescintigraphy

   D. Surgical removal

5. A 28-year-old G1 woman presents to the ED at 10 weeks' gestation after a brief episode of vaginal bleeding. She denies abdominal pain, fever, or dysuria. On examination, there is a small amount of blood in the vaginal vault and the cervical os is closed. Bimanual examination reveals a uterus sized for date, but softer than normal, no adnexal tenderness or cervical motion tenderness. What is the most likely diagnosis?

   A. Inevitable abortion

   B. Cervicitis

   C. Bacterial vaginosis

   D. Threatened abortion

6. A 65-year-old man presents to the ED with bright red blood per rectum for the past 3 days. On examination the patient is ill appearing, pale, generally weak, and on rectal examination has frank rectal bleeding. CBC reveals hemoglobin of 6 and a serum iron of 50. Which of the following is the most appropriate treatment at this time?

   A. PO iron supplementation
   B. Packed red blood cell transfusion
   C. IV iron transfusion
   D. PO B$_{12}$ supplementation

7. A 50-year-old man with no previous medical history presents to the ED with severe left sided flank pain with radiating pain around to his groin. He also notes a pinkish tint to his urine. He has experienced some nausea secondary to his pain. What is the diagnostic study of choice to confirm his most likely diagnosis?

   A. CT abdomen pelvis without contrast
   B. KUB
   C. MRI pelvis
   D. Urinalysis

8. A 42-year-old woman presents to the ED with a 1-week history of progressively worsening cough, shortness of breath, fatigue, and intermittent fevers. On examination the patient is ill appearing, diaphoretic, and has coarse breath sounds in the right upper lung field. Vital signs include temperature 101°F, pulse 102, BP 125/80, respiratory rate 24, and pulse ox of 94% in room air. Chest x-ray reveals a right upper lobe consolidation. The patient has no significant previous medical history or recent admissions. What is the recommended outpatient treatment?

   A. Penicillin
   B. Vancomycin
   C. Cefepime
   D. Azithromycin

9. A 45-year-old man patient that was recently discharged from the hospital with pneumonia presents to the ED complaining of dehydration and profuse foul-smelling diarrhea for the last 2 days. What else do you expect to find to support the diagnosis?

   A. Colonic dilation >7 cm on x-ray
   B. Accordion sign on x-ray
   C. Positive PCR
   D. Flat mucosa with loss of villi on biopsy

10. A 58-year-old man with a past medical history of hypertension and diabetes complains of severe headache and blurred vision. Blurred disk margin, diminished cup, optic nerve elevation, and vascular congestion are noted on funduscopic examination. What is the most likely diagnosis?

    A. Optic neuritis
    B. Papilledema
    C. Acute angle-closure glaucoma
    D. Ocular migraine

11. A 9-year-old boy presents to the ED with mother with concern for an intensely itchy scalp. Upon examination, there are many nits fixed to hair shafts that fluoresce a pale blue with use of a Wood's lamp. What is the most likely diagnosis?

    A. Scabies
    B. Lice
    C. Arthropod assault
    D. Ants

12. A 29-year-old IV drug user presents with chest pain and petechiae on his fingers and toes. On physical examination, a new-onset murmur at left second intercostal space is appreciated. What is the most common etiology for his condition?

    A. *S. aureus*
    B. *S. pyogenes*
    C. *S. pneumoniae*
    D. *S. epidermidis*

13. A 30-year-old homosexual man presents with dysuria, urinary frequency and urgency, malodorous urine for the last 48 hours after having unprotected anal sex with his male partner, with whom he is monogamous. He denies sexual activity with others. This morning he noticed scant white discharge from his penis noticed once this morning after urination. He has no known drug allergies or prior medical history. His vital signs are unremarkable. Examination of the abdomen, genitalia, and prostate are unremarkable. You order standard STI testing and a urinalysis. Urinalysis is remarkable for nitrite (+) and pyuria, bacteriuria, negative for leukocyte-esterase. NAAT, RPR, and HIV testing is negative.

    A. Penicillin
    B. Nitrofurantoin (Macrobid)
    C. Clindamycin
    D. Cephalexin

14. A 42-year-old male patient is newly diagnosed with type II diabetes mellitus with a HbA1c of 9.2%. You provide him with patient education regarding appropriate screenings and suggest that he see an ophthalmologist for a dilated funduscopic examination at what intervals to evaluate for diabetic retinopathy?

    A. Now and then annually if retinopathy is present
    B. Within 5 years of diagnosis and then annually if retinopathy is present
    C. Now and then biannually if retinopathy is present
    D. Within 5 years of diagnosis and then biannually if retinopathy is present

15. A 65-year-old man with a past medical history of diabetes mellitus type II and hypertension is brought to the emergency room complaining of sudden-onset chest pain that radiates to this back and left arm for the past hour. Vitals reveal a HR of 115, BP of 190/90 in his left arm and 160/70 in his right arm, RR of 22, and temperature of 99.1°F. Physical examination reveals a high-pitched decrescendo diastolic murmur best heard along the left mid-sternal border. What is the most likely diagnosis?

    A. Acute myocardial infarction

    B. Aortic dissection

    C. Right subclavian arterial embolus

    D. Coarctation of the aorta

16. Which of the following is caused when there is inadequate fixation of the testis to the tunica vaginalis?

    A. Epididymitis

    B. Prostate cancer

    C. Prostatitis

    D. Testicular torsion

17. A 58-year-old man with a 25 pack-year smoking history is being seen for an annual physical. He has a family history of colon cancer in his father who was diagnosed at 72 years. He reports quitting smoking when he was 30 years old. Which of the following health screenings are recommended?

    A. Colonoscopy now and every 5 years if normal

    B. Annual low-dose CT screenings for lung cancer

    C. A one-time ultrasound to screen for AAA at 65-years-old

    D. Annual PSA screenings

18. A 30-year-old woman complains of 1-year history of depressed mood, decreased appetite, apathy, and withdrawn behavior. You decide to start her on an SSRI. What is the most common side effect she might experience?

    A. Sexual dysfunction

    B. Nausea

    C. Diarrhea

    D. Insomnia

19. A patient presenting with hyponatremia and hypoosmolality consistent with syndrome of inappropriate anti-diuretic hormone secretion will present with which of the following examination findings?

    A. Metabolic acidosis

    B. Elevated serum uric acid concentration

    C. Reduction in total body water

    D. Low plasma sodium concentrations

20. A 30-year-old woman presents to the emergency department 4 weeks postpartum with gradually worsening right wrist pain that is exacerbated when she tries to grip and open objects around the house. She denies history of trauma, numbness, or tingling. Physical examination reveals right radial styloid swelling and tenderness that is exacerbated with ulnar deviation of a fist clenched over the abducted thumb. What is the most likely diagnosis?

    A. de Quervain tendinopathy

    B. Radial nerve entrapment

    C. Carpal tunnel syndrome

    D. Game Keeper's thumb

21. A 68-year-old woman presents with sudden unilateral lower extremity pain and heart palpitations. EKG is significant for an irregularly irregular rhythm at a rate of 180 bpm. What other characteristics would you expect to see in this limb?

    A. Ischemic ulcer

    B. Loss of hair

    C. Pale limb

    D. Atrophic skin

22. A 35-year-old overweight woman presents to the ED complaining of painful menstrual cycles with heavy bleeding. She reports that her periods have gotten worse over the past few years. She also reports pain with intercourse. Which of the following may the patient have?

    A. Endometriosis

    B. Uterine fibroids

    C. Pelvic inflammatory disease

23. An otherwise healthy 24-year-old man presents to the ED with shortness of breath, chest discomfort, and mild chest pain that began while mowing the lawn. EKG shows a narrow QRS tachycardia, regular rhythm, with a heart rate of 170. Vitals are as follows: BP, 130/80, RR, 18, pO_2, 99% on room air. What is the most appropriate management at this time?

    A. Adenosine

    B. Amiodarone

    C. Epinephrine

    D. Vasovagal maneuver

24. A 16-year-old male presents to the ED after hearing a popping sound during his soccer game. He reports that he was running for the ball when he planted his left foot and pivoted to the left to avoid a defender. His knee immediately began to swell and felt as if it was going to give out. Which of the following tests would support the diagnosis of his condition?

    A. Knee x-ray

    B. Lachman test

    C. Posterior drawer test

    D. CT scan

25. A 35-year-old man presents to his PCP with complaints of reoccurring pain in his big toe so much so that he cannot wear a shoe. Fluid is aspirated from the joint and reveals needle-shaped urate crystals. What is the best maintenance therapy?

    A. Prednisone

    B. Colchicine

    C. Allopurinol

    D. Ibuprofen

ANSWERS

1. History and Physical: Malignant Hypertension. Answer B: Malignant hypertension is characterized by a blood pressure $\geq$ 180/120 and signs of end organ damage such as papilledema, encephalopathy, or nephropathy. A, Carotid bruits are a result of turbulent flow in the carotid artery due to stenosis. A soft bruit is usually audible at 50% stenosis and increases in volume as the degree of stenosis increases. C, Systolic murmurs are usually caused by regurgitation of the AV valves or by a ventricular septal defect. D, Water hammer pulse is typically a sign of aortic regurgitation.

2. Diagnostic studies: Acute Bacterial Meningitis. Answer C: Acute bacterial meningitis presents with new-onset headache, nuchal rigidity, high fever, and altered mental status. It is differentiated from viral meningitis with a lumbar puncture with elevated white blood cell counts between 1000 and 5000/μL, protein greater than 200 mg/dL, glucose less than 40 mg/dL with a CSF glucose to serum glucose ratio less than or equal to 0.4. A, *Listeria monocytogenes* is not a common cause of acute meningitis in adolescents and young adults. It is more common in infants and older adults. B, Opening pressure is considered normal up to 200 mm H_2O. In acute bacterial meningitis, the opening pressure is elevated approximately greater than or equal to 350 mm H_2O. D, Generalized 3-Hz spike wave on EEG is seen with absence epilepsy.

3. Clinical intervention: Smith fracture. Answer A: Sugar tong splint is indicated for Smith fractures, as well as Colles fractures. B, Surgery is indicated for vascular injuries, which are rare for Smith fractures. C, Ulnar gutter splinting is indicated for fractures involving fourth and fifth metacarpals or phalanges. D, Thumb spica splinting is indicated for scaphoid, lunate, or ulnar collateral ligament injuries.

4. Clinical Therapeutics: Acute Cholecystitis. Answer D: Cholecystectomy is the treatment of choice for low-risk patients diagnosed with acute cholecystitis. A, IV fluids and morphine drip can be used to help control the symptoms but does not correct acute cholecystitis. B, ERCP is the treatment of choice for choledocholithiasis. C, Cholescintigraphy or a HIDA scan is used to diagnose cholecystitis if the ultrasound is uncertain.

5. Diagnosis: Threatened Abortion. Answer D: Threatened abortion is identifiable by closed cervical os, vaginal bleeding before the 20th week of gestation without loss of POC, and a uterus that is softer than normal and size for date. A, Inevitable abortion would have open cervical os, possibly with passing products of conception (POC). B, Cervicitis and (C) bacterial vaginosis often present with vaginal discharge and irritation.

6. Clinical Therapeutics: Iron Deficiency Anemia. Answer B: Given Hgb <7, replete packed RBCs is the first line of treatment at this time while determining and treating the source of bleeding. A, Oral iron supplementation may be necessary if the hemoglobin does not return to normal after transfusion. C, IV iron transfusion not indicated in this setting. D, B_{12} supplementation not indicated in this setting.

7. Diagnostic Studies: Nephrolithiasis. Answer A: The presentation is typical of nephrolithiasis and CT A/P without contrast is the test of choice. B, KUB may identify radiopaque stones, but can often miss small stones or those that are radiolucent. C, MRI of the pelvis may be performed if symptoms do not subside but is not the initial study of choice. D, Urinalysis may be performed in addition to a CT scan, but the CT scan is used to confirm the presence of stones.

8. Clinical Therapeutics: Community Acquired Pneumonia. Answer D: The recommended empirical treatment of community-acquired pneumonia is azithromycin, or other macrolides, including clarithromycin. An alternative is doxycycline. A, Penicillin, (B) vancomycin, and (C) cefepime are not indicated for outpatient treatment of CAP.

9. H&P: *Clostridium difficile*. Answer C: Laboratory testing with PCR is the recommended diagnostic study for a patient suspected to have *C. difficile*. The scenario above is characteristic of a patient at risk of developing *C. difficile* due to recent hospitalization and concurrent antibiotic use. A, Colonic dilation >7 cm on abdominal x-ray is characteristic of toxic megacolon. Toxic megacolon is a serious complication of untreated *C. difficile* infection. B, Accordion sign on x-ray is characteristic of pseudomembranous colitis and indicates that further testing is needed to investigate for *C. difficile* etiology. D, Flat mucosa with loss of villi on biopsy is characteristic of celiac disease.

10. Diagnosis: Papilledema. Answer B: Based on the patient's history, the patient is likely presenting with a hypertensive emergency and papilledema due to increased intracranial pressure. A, Optic neuritis refers to inflammation of the optic nerve, which can occur because of demyelinating or infectious disease processes. The optic nerve head is occasionally swollen and usually pale. C, Acute angle-closure glaucoma patients may complain of seeing halos of light, severe headache, severe eye pain, and nausea and vomiting. On physical examination, the patient may present with corneal cloudiness, mid-dilated pupil that poorly responds to light, and ciliary flush. On funduscopic examination, cupping of the optic disk may be present if narrow-angle glaucoma is present. D, Ocular migraine or retinal migraine is a rare condition that leads to repeated attacks of monocular scotomata or blindness lasting less than 1 hour that is typically followed by a headache. There are no distinct funduscopic findings for this condition.

11. Diagnosis: Lice. Answer B: This presentation is typical of lice and is often common in school-aged children. A, Scabies typically presents with burrow tracks, often in webbed spaces or creases. C, Arthropods often leave 3 small bite marks near one another, often unwitnessed. D, This is not a typical presentation of any bite.

12. Scientific Concepts, Bacterial endocarditis. Answer A: Skin flora such as *S. aureus* is the most common organism involved in IVDU with infective endocarditis. B, *S. pyogenes* is the main organism responsible for GAS infections such as strep throat, rheumatic fever, impetigo, erysipelas, and cellulitis. C, *S. pneumoniae* is the most common cause of lobar pneumonia. D, *S. epidermidis* is a common organisms involved in prosthetic valve endocarditis.

13. Clinical Therapeutics: Uncomplicated UTI. Answer B: First-line treatments for uncomplicated UTI include nitrofurantoin, Bactrim, and fosfomycin. Urethritis is less likely as the patient has negative NAAT and urethritis does not typically present with urinary frequency. Prostatitis is less likely given being afebrile, having a negative prostate and abdominal examination, and lack of obstructive symptoms.

14. Health Maintenance: Diabetic retinopathy. Answer A: The American Diabetic Association recommends a comprehensive ophthalmologic examination for type II diabetics shortly after diagnosis and then annually if retinopathy is present and biannual if no signs of retinopathy are present. B, The American Diabetic Association recommends a comprehensive ophthalmologic examination for type I diabetic patients 10 years of age or older within 5 years of diagnosis and then annually if retinopathy is present and biannually if no signs of retinopathy are present.

15. Diagnosis: Aortic Dissection. Answer B: This is the classic presentation for aortic dissection with an aortic insufficiency murmur. A, AMI would does not manifest with unequal blood pressures of the upper extremities. C, This patient would present with a cold, painful, pulseless upper extremity and may be preceded by upper extremity claudication with exertion. D, Coarctation of the aorta is typically a congenital condition resulting in discrepancies between blood pressures of upper and lower extremities or lack of palpable pulses in the lower extremities. Infants usually present with poor feeding, tachypnea, and lethargy.

16. Scientific Concepts: Testicular Torsion. Answer D: Testicular torsion occurs due to faulty fixation of the testis and tunica vaginalis.

17. Health Maintenance: Abdominal Aortic Aneurysm. Answer C: The USPSTF recommends a one-time screening for abdominal aortic aneurysms with ultrasonography for men aged 65 to 75 years who have ever smoked. Follow-up ultrasonography may be required to monitor aneurysms <5.5 cm. A, The American College of Gastroenterology recommends a colonoscopy screening every 10 years starting at age 50 for adults with no family history of colon cancer or with a first-degree relative diagnosed at ≥60 years. In adults with a first-degree relative who was diagnosed with colorectal cancer at <60 years, or with two first-degree relatives with colorectal cancer, the ACG recommends colonoscopy every 5 years beginning at age 40 years or 10 years younger than the diagnosis of the youngest affected relative, whichever is earlier. B, The US Preventative Services Task Force (USPSTF) recommends annual low-dose CT lung cancer screenings in adults aged 55 to 80 years who have a 30 pack-year history of smoking and have been currently smoking for the past 15 years. Screenings can be discontinued after the patient has not smoked for 15 years. D, The USPSTF no longer recommends annual PSA screenings, and the American Cancer Society recommends screenings based on a patient's risk and after outweighing the risks and benefits with their health care provider.

18. Clinical Therapeutics: Major Depressive Disorder. Answer A: Fluoxetine, an SSRI, is the first-line medication for the treatment of major depressive disorder. B, Trazadone is indicated for psychotic disorders. C, Lisinopril is an ACE inhibitor used for blood pressure control and renal protection. D, Zyprexa is indicated for psychotic disorders.

19. H&P: SIADH. Answer D: SIADH presents with low plasma sodium concentrations secondary to the increase in total body water due to the uninhibited release of antidiuretic hormone. A, SIADH does not present with acid-base disturbances. B, SIADH presents with **reduced** serum uric acid levels. C, SIADH presents with an **increase** in total body water.

20. H&P: De Quervain Tenosynovitis. Answer A: De Quervain tendinopathy is atraumatic radial wrist pain characterized by radial styloid tenderness and enlargement that is exacerbated by actively or passively flexing the thumb. A (+) Finkelstein test, which is characterized by pain reproduced with ulnar deviation of a fist clenched over an abducted thumb, is typical. It most commonly affects postpartum women aged 30 to 50 years. B, Radial nerve entrapment involves the superficial radial sensory nerve that causes a burning sensation of pain and paresthesias over the dorsal aspect of the hand, wrist, middle finger, index finger, and thumb. C, Carpal tunnel syndrome is characterized by median nerve pain and numbness/tingling involving the index, middle, ring, and radial aspect of the little fingers. Symptoms are worse at night and tend to wake patients up from sleep. D, Game Keeper's thumb is also known as ulnar collateral ligament injury that is exacerbated with thumb extension and abduction. Swelling is present along the ulnar aspect of the thumb MCP joint.

Emergency Medicine

21. History and Physical: Acute arterial occlusion. Answer C: This patient most likely has an acute arterial occlusion secondary to atrial fibrillation. Patients typically present with a cold, painful, pale pulseless extremity with a mottled appearance. A, Ischemic ulcers are usually secondary to arterial insufficiency and are mostly located on the lateral ankles or toes. They result from peripheral artery disease, a chronic process, not an acute one. B, Hair loss can be seen in venous stasis ulcers, which is also a chronic process. D, Atrophic skin is most commonly due to chronic venous insufficiency but may also be due to chronic steroid use or autoimmune processes like systemic lupus erythematosus or vasculitis.

22. Diagnosis: Endometriosis. Answer A: Endometriosis presents with pelvic pain, dysmenorrhea, and dyspareunia. B, Uterine fibroids may cause pain when they grow to be very large, but do not typically cause dyspareunia. C, Patient with pelvic inflammatory disease may experience pelvic pain, but is typically more acutely ill, including fever.

23. Clinical Therapeutics: Supraventricular tachycardia. Answer D: Patient is currently hemodynamically stable, so carotid sinus massage and vasovagal maneuver is indicated before administration of pharmaceuticals. PSVT may occur in healthy patients following exercise and is usually benign. A, Adenosine is indicated when carotid sinus massage or vasovagal maneuver has failed. B, Amiodarone is indicated in the rate control of atrial fibrillation. C, Epinephrine is an α- and β-adrenergic agonist indicated for asystole or pulseless ventricular tachycardia/ventricular fibrillation.

24. Diagnostic Studies: ACL tear. Answer B: Noncontact ACL tears occur with deceleration and rotational injury while running, cutting, or jumping. Contact ACL tears involve hyperextension and/or valgus forces from a direct blow to the knee. Lachman test is one of the most valuable clinical evaluation that can be used to diagnose anterior cruciate ligament (ACL) tears. A, Knee x-ray can identify fractures of the knee but will not be useful to diagnose anterior cruciate ligament tears. An MRI would be necessary to visualize an ACL tear. C, Posterior drawer test is used to assess for a posterior cruciate ligament tear. D, CT scan is not indicated to diagnose suspected anterior cruciate ligament tears. MRI is the test of choice for a definitive diagnosis.

25. Health Maintenance: Gout. Answer C: Allopurinol is a urate-lowering therapy that is indicated for reoccurring gout flares as a maintenance medication. It is not indicated for acute flares. A, Prednisone is used for acute gout flares along with use of NSAIDs like naproxen or indomethacin. B, Colchicine is used for acute gout flares when patients have failed steroid and NSAID treatment. D, NSAIDs like naproxen or indomethacin are indicated for acute gout flares.

CHAPTER 48

Prenatal Care

Recommended Supplemental Topics:

Mastodynia/Breast Tenderness, see Breast Disorders, p 499

Candidiasis, see Infections, Vaginitis, p 484

Gonorrhea, see Infections, Cervicitis, p 487

Urinary Tract Infection, see Urology for Family Medicine, p 175

Cholasma, see Dermatology for Family Medicine, p 162

KEY PREGNANCY DEFINITIONS

- **Nulligravida**: woman who currently is not pregnant or has ever been pregnant

- **Gravida**: woman who is currently pregnant or who has been in the past, irrespective of the outcome; first (primigravida), successive multiples (multigravida)

- **Parity**: number of births, both before and after 20 weeks of gestation (includes full term, preterm, abortions, and living children)

  - Term: born between 37 0/7 and 40 0/7 weeks of gestation
  - Post term infant: born after 42 weeks of gestation

- **Nullipara**: woman who has never completed a pregnancy beyond 20 weeks (may not have been pregnant or may have had a spontaneous or elective/ectopic abortion/pregnancy)

- **Primipara**: woman who has been delivered only once of a fetus or fetuses born alive or dead with a gestation of 20+ weeks

- **Multipara**: completed 2+ pregnancies reaching 20+ weeks

- **Macrosomia** (large for gestational age): fetal weight at or beyond 90th percentile at any gestational age

- Low-birth weight infant: any live birth in which the infant's weight is less than or equal to 2500 g

- **Fetal growth restriction**: at or below 10th percentile for any gestational age

PRENATAL DIAGNOSIS AND CARE

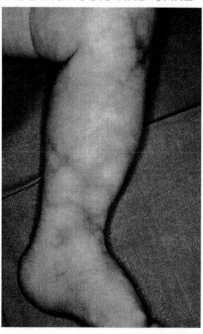

FIGURE 48-1. Cutis marmorata. (From Requena L, Requena L, Kutzner H. *Cutaneous Soft Tissue Tumors*. Philadelphia: Wolters Kluwer Health; 2015.)

Disease	Etiology, Prevalence, Risk Factors	Clinical Symptoms and Signs	Diagnostics	Therapy, Prognosis, and Health Maintenance
Intrauterine pregnancy		Note: none of these are diagnostic 1. Amenorrhea 2. Nausea, vomiting 3. Breast tenderness, tingling 4. Urinary frequency, urgency 5. "*Quickening*" (first movement at week 18) 6. Weight gain Signs: 1. Breast changes: enlargement, vascular engorgement, colostrum 2. Vagina—cyanosis 3. Cervix—portio, softening (7th wk), cervicouterine junction (8th wk), enlargement and softening of corpus (>8 wk) 4. Abdominal enlargement: 16 wk 5. Palpable uterine fundus above pubic symphysis: 12-15 wk • Umbilicus by 20-22 wk 6. FHT heard at 10-12 wk of gestation	1. Urine pregnancy test 2. Serum β-hCG, should double every 48 h, peak at 50-75 d, fall in 2-3 trimesters • **Progesterone**: remains stable during first trimester (best indicator of viable pregnancy) >25 ng/mL	1. Prenatal vitamins and/or folic acid 2. 0.4-0.8 mg of folic acid, unless prior child with NTD (4 mg, 1 mo prior to conception)
Hyperemesis gravidarum (HEG)	Unexplained intractable nausea, retching or vomiting beginning in first trimester Peaks during weeks 8-12 MC: Young mothers and patients w/HX of motion sickness, migraines, N/V associated w/OCPs	1. Severe intractable nausea and vomiting during pregnancy 2. Weight loss >5% 3. Starts during 3-5 wk Signs: 1. Dehydration 2. **Ptyalism**: excessive salivation Complications: Wernicke encephalopathy, ATN, central pontine myelinolysis, Mallory-Weiss tear, pneumomediastinum, splenic avulsion	1. **Hypokalemia** 2. **Alkalosis** 3. U/A: ketonuria 4. TFTs: elevated T3 5. LFTs, bilirubin, amylase, lipase: elevated	1. **Supportive** • Hydration • Vitamin supplementation • Acupuncture, hypnotherapy, avoid triggers, herbal teas, vitamin B_6, ginger 2. >50% resolve by 16 wk, 80% by 20 wk
Cutis marmorata (Fig. 48-1)	Persistent coarse cutis marmorata, telangiectasia, and sometimes atrophy and ulceration Incidence: Sporadic Etiology: Obscure Variant: **Cutis marmorata telangiectasia congenita** (persists despite rewarming)	1. Net-like, reticulated, pink patches seen in premature newborns • **Better with rewarming of the skin** • **Worse with cooling** Signs 1. Atrophic, dusky, stellate patches with overlying telangiectasias 2. Associated anomalies: limb asymmetry, hemangiomas, vascular birthmarks, pigmented nevi, aplasia cutis congenita (ACC)	Clinical DX	1. Rewarming of the skin 2. 50% improve over the first 2 y
Vulvovaginal **Candidiasis** (VVC, candida vaginalis) **yeast infection**	Second MCC (20%-25%) Path: **C. albicans**, *C. glabrata, C. tropicalis* 75% F RF: High-dose OCP, diaphragm use, DM, recent ABX, pregnant, immune suppression, *tight fitting clothing*	1. Vulvar or vaginal *itching* and *burning*, external *dysuria* 2. Dyspareunia 3. Odorless thick **"cottage cheese"** curd-like discharge Signs: 1. Erythema of vulva and vagina 2. Excoriations from scratching	1. Wet mount (saline or 10% KOH): **Budding yeast (snowman)** 2. Gram stain: pseudohyphae or tangles **(spaghetti and meatballs)** 3. Vaginal culture (+) for yeast 4. Microscopy only (+) in 50% 5. pH: <4.7 (acidic)	1. **Fluconazole** 150 mg PO once—repeat in 1 wk • Treat uncircumcised partners • Short-course topical Azole (1-3 d) for 80%-90% of patients 2. Recurrent – weekly topical/PO • 5% recurrence rate 3. Resistant – boric acid 600 mg gel capsules TID × 7 days

Disease	Etiology, Prevalence, Risk Factors	Clinical Symptoms and Signs	Diagnostics	Therapy, Prognosis, and Health Maintenance
Murmur of pregnancy	Most common reason for cardiologic assessment during pregnancy Correlate with increased blood volume across the aortic and pulmonic valves	1. Most occur at 10-12 wk of gestation 2. Chest pain, palpitations 3. SOB 4. Fatigue Signs: 1. MC: **soft mid-systolic ejection murmur** heard with greatest intensity at the left sternal border 2. Increased second heart sound split with inspiration 3. Distended neck veins 4. S3 gallop and third heart sound normal after midpregnancy	1. EKG and echo– unhelpful to assist in diagnosis and do not substantially alter management	1. Most resolve spontaneously by 1 wk after delivery 2. *Note*: Diastolic murmurs should not be considered normal in pregnancy

Antiemetics in Pregnancy

Nausea or vomiting interfering with daily routine	1. **Vitamin B$_6$ 10-30 mg TID–QID PO** 2. Continued symptoms after 48 h: add doxylamine 12.5 mg TID–QID PO 3. Continued symptoms after 48 h: substitute doxylamine with other antihistamine: 4. Promethazine 12.5-25 mg every 4 h PO or PR 5. Dimenhydrinate 50-100 mg every 4-6 h PO or PR 6. Consider alternative therapies at any point in this sequence: acupuncture or acustimulation, ginger tablets 250 mg QID
Persistent symptoms, with or without dehydration	1. **Prochlorperazine** 25 mg every 12 h PR OR 2. **Metoclopramide** 5-10 mg every 8 h PO or IV OR 3. Trimethobenzamide 200 mg every 6-8 h PR
Dehydration or weight loss	1. **Thiamine 100 mg IV daily for 3 d; continue thiamine in MVI daily** 2. **Ondansetron** 8 mg every 8-12 h IV or PO OR 3. Methylprednisolone up to 16 mg TID for 3 days; taper over 2 wk to lowest effective dose; total duration of therapy 6 wk
Unable to maintain weight	1. Institute **total enteral or parenteral nutrition**

- **Naegele rule** (expected delivery date): add 7 days to first day of LMP and count back 3 months
- **Gestational age:** calculated using clinically performed uterine size and LMP
  - 6-week gestation: small orange
  - 8-week gestation: large orange
  - 12-week gestation: grapefruit
  - First trimester crown-rump length: most accurate tool for calculating gestational age
- **Prenatal visits**
  - Prenatal visits at 4-week intervals until 28 weeks, then every 2 weeks until 36 weeks, weekly thereafter

- Initial screening labs: CBC, blood type with Rh status, Ab screen, hepatitis B, syphilis, and immunity to rubella, +/– HIV testing
  - If not hypertensive, routine U/A beyond first visit is not necessary (only screen for asymptomatic bacteriuria)
- At return visits (surveillance): well-being of mother and fetus; determine fetal heart rate, growth, amniotic fluid volume, and activity
  - Assess maternal blood pressure and weight
  - Assess symptoms: headache, altered vision, RUQ abdominal pain, nausea, vomiting, bleeding, vaginal fluid leakage, and dysuria
  - Measure fundal height (symphysis to fundus)
- Fundal height: 20 to 34 weeks within 3 cm
- Fetal heart tones: 10 weeks (110 to 160)
- Gestational diabetes (GDM): screen with labs at 24 to 28 weeks
  - Screening for gestational diabetes is performed using a 50-g glucose load (Glucola) and a 1-hour post-Glucola blood glucose determination.
  - Abnormal values (greater than or equal to 140 mg/dL or 7.8 mmol/L) should be followed up with a 3-hour glucose tolerance test
- Group B streptococcal infection (GBS): 35 to 37 weeks with intrapartum antimicrobial prophylaxis for (+) cultures
  - A single standard culture of the distal vagina and anorectum
  - Patients whose cultures are positive receive intrapartum penicillin prophylaxis during labor
  - Patients who have had a previous infant with invasive group B streptococcal disease or who have group B streptococcal bacteriuria during this pregnancy should receive intrapartum prophylaxis regardless, so rectovaginal cultures are not needed
- Fetal aneuploidy testing: 11 to 14 weeks and/or at 15 to 20 weeks, serum screening at 15 to 20 weeks
- Hep-B/HIV repeat testing before 36 weeks for women at risk

OB/GYN

- D (Rh) negative: repeat at 28 to 29 weeks with administration of anti-D immune globulin
- Hematocrit or Hgb and syphilis (if suspected) should be repeated at 28 to 32 weeks
- Repeat HIV testing during the third trimester if suspected, before 36 weeks
- Pregnant women may fly safely up to 36 weeks of gestation
- The mean duration of pregnancy calculated from the first day of the last normal menstrual period is very close to 280 days or 40 weeks
- **Biophysical profile:** prenatal ultrasound evaluation of fetal well-being involving Manning score
  - Performed when a nonstress test (NST) is nonreactive
- **Fundal height:** height of the fundus in centimeters measured between 20 to 34 weeks correlates with gestational age in weeks
  - Monitors fetal growth and amniotic fluid volume
  - Bladder must be emptied before measurement
  - Distance along abdominal wall from top of symphysis pubis to top of fundus
- **Fetal heart tones:** measured using Doppler ultrasound, detected by 10 weeks
  - Normal fetal heart rate: 110 to 160

FETAL ANEUPLOIDY SCREENING

- If a woman first seeks OB care after the 14th week of pregnancy, only the second trimester tests can be offered (triple or quad)
  - Nuchal translucency—ultrasound measurement of space under the skin behind the neck, performed only during first trimester. Component of the combined, integrated, and sequential tests

- Chorionic villus sampling (CVS) is removal of a small piece of placental tissue in order to obtain fetal cells in order to obtain the fetal karyotype. This identifies the number of chromosomes the fetus has inherited and usually only performed after an abnormal Down syndrome screening test. Performed in the first trimester because amniocentesis cannot be performed this early in pregnancy
- Combined test—gives a woman the earliest results compared to any other test but does not perform as well. On average, combined test detects about 85% of all Down syndrome fetuses at a 5% false-positive rate
- Sequential test—if woman desires early risk assessment but is willing to wait for test results if needed (ie, not too concerned); reports results in the first trimester only if the risk of having Down syndrome is very high. If risk is not high, results are not reported until second trimester test is completed
- Integrated test—if she can wait until second trimester, the best screening test is the Integrated test, which gives the highest DS detection rate (95%). Even without nuchal translucency, it provides the same detection rate with a slightly higher false-positive rate
- Offered when NT and CVS not available.
  - Fetal aneuploidy testing: 11 to 14 weeks and/or at 15 to 20 weeks, serum screening at 15 to 20 weeks
  - Nuchal translucency at 11 to 13 weeks combined with serum markers at 10 to 13 weeks
  - Quadruple test at 15 to 19 weeks (but may be offered 14 to 21 weeks) for women who first attend after 13 weeks 6 days, optimal for NTD screening using AFP
  - The use of maternal fetal age alone to assess fetal DS risk is insufficient

Disease	Etiology, Prevalence, Risk Factors	Clinical Symptoms and Signs	Diagnostics	Therapy, Prognosis, and Health Maintenance

Edwards syndrome (trisomy 18)	Incidence: 1:8000
	RF: advanced maternal age
	MC due to maternal nondisjunction
	Can screen for in first and second trimester
		1. Severe cognitive impairment
		Postnatal signs:
		  1. Clenched fists and overlapping digits
		  2. Hypoplastic nails
		  3. Rocker bottom feet
		  4. VSD and tetralogy of Fallot
		  5. Omphalocele
		  6. Congenital diaphragmatic hernia
		  7. Neural tube defects
		  8. Choroid plexus cysts
		  9. Small for gestational age at birth
		  10. Short sternum
		  11. Prominent occiput
		  12. Low set, structurally abnormal ears
		  13. Micrognathia
		  14. Cystic and horseshoe kidneys
		  15. Failure to thrive
		  16. Seizures
		  17. Hypertonia
		  18. Severe developmental delays
			1. First trimester screening with follow-up testing if increased risk
			  • Noninvasive prenatal diagnosis with fetal circulating DNA in maternal serum
			  • Karyotype (definitive) at birth or prenatally by amniocentesis or CVS
			2. U/S:
			  • Intrauterine growth restriction
			  • Polyhydramnios
				Prognosis:
				Less than 10% survive past 1 y

NORMAL LABOR AND DELIVERY

Stages, Duration, Mechanism of Delivery, Monitoring

- **Labor** is a sequence of uterine contractions that results in effacement and dilatation of the cervix and voluntary bearing-down efforts, leading to the expulsion per vagina of the products of conception
- **Delivery** is the mode of expulsion of the fetus and placenta
- **Lightening**: settling of the fetal head into the brim of the pelvis 2 or more weeks before the onset of labor → decreased heartburn and SOB, increased pelvic discomfort, and urinary frequency
- **Braxton Hicks contractions**: *painless* uterine contractions that begin at 28 weeks of gestation and increase in regularity with advancing gestation; disappear with walking or exercise
- Several days to weeks prior to true labor: cervix softens, effaces, and dilates
- With effacement, **bloody show** occurs (blood-tinged mucus) with release of mucus plug

	True Labor	False Labor (Braxton Hicks)
Contractions		
Rhythm	Regular	Irregular
Intervals	Gradually shorten	Unchanged (every 10-20 min)
Intensity	Gradually increases	Unchanged
Discomfort		
Location	Back and abdomen	Lower abdomen
Sedation	No effect	Usually relieved
Cervical dilation	**Yes** (usually 1-3 cm)	**No**
FHT	130-140 (lowers FHT)	Normal (110-160)

Mechanisms of Labor (Fig. 48-2)

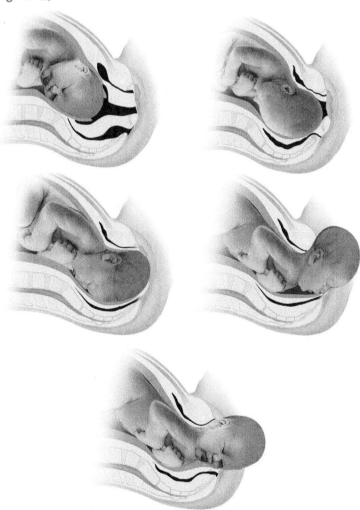

FIGURE 48-2. Mechanisms of labor.

- The mechanism of labor in the vertex position consists of **engagement** of the presenting part, **flexion**, **descent**, **internal rotation**, **extension**, **external rotation**, and **expulsion**

- *Engagement*: the head enters the superior strait in the **occiput transverse** position in 70% of women with a gynecoid pelvis

- *Flexion*: Good flexion is noted in most cases. Flexion aids engagement and descent (Extension occurs in brow and face presentations.)

- *Descent*: Depends on pelvic architecture and cephalopelvic relationships. Descent is usually slowly progressive

- *Internal rotation*: Takes place during descent. With the descent of the head into the midpelvis, rotation occurs so that the sagittal suture occupies the anteroposterior diameter of the pelvis

- *Extension*: Follows distention of the perineum by the vertex. Head concomitantly stems beneath the symphysis. Extension is complete with the delivery of the head.

  - **Crowning** occurs when the largest diameter of the fetal head is encircled by the vulvar ring

- *External rotation (restitution)*: After delivery, head normally rotates to the position it originally occupied at engagement. Next, the shoulders rotate **anteroposteriorly** for delivery. Then, the head swings back to its position at birth

  - Delivery of the **anterior** shoulder is aided by gentle **downward traction** on the externally rotated head
  - The **posterior** shoulder is then delivered by gentle upward traction on the head
  - Delayed cord clamping can result in neonatal hyperbilirubinemia as additional blood is transferred to the newborn infant

- Expulsion

Effacement, Dilation, and Station

Effacement

- The cervix will gradually soften, shorten, and become thinner. You might hear phrases like "ripens" or "cervical thinning," which refer to effacement (Fig. 48-3)

Dilation

- Opening of the cervix (Fig. 48-4)

Station

- The relationship of the bony portion of the fetal head to the level of the maternal ischial spines (Fig. 48-5)

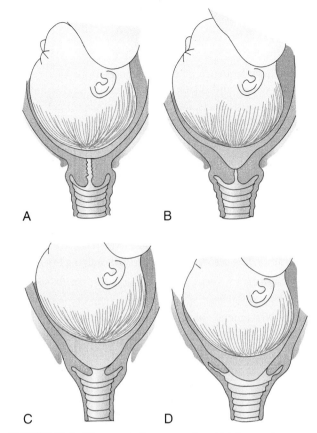

FIGURE 48-3. Effacement—the process by which the cervix prepares for delivery, characterized by softening, shortening, and thinning, also known as cervical ripening. **A**, 0% effacement. **B**, 30% effacement. **C**, 100% effacement. **D**, 100% effacement + dilation. (From Weber JR, Kelley JH. *Health Assessment in Nursing.* Philadelphia: Wolters Kluwer Health; 2014.)

Fetal Position (Fig. 48-6)

- Fetal **position** is the orientation of the fetus in the womb, identified by the location of the presenting part of the fetus relative to the pelvis of the mother

- **LOA (vertex position)**: occiput against the buttocks, facing anteriorly, toward the left (most common position and lie)

  - ROA: occiput faces anteriorly and toward right
  - LOP: posteriorly, toward left
  - ROP: posteriorly, toward right
  - LOT: occiput faces left
  - ROT: occiput faces right

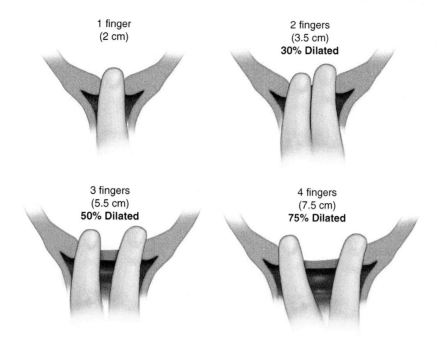

FIGURE 48-4. Cervical dilation by vaginal examination.

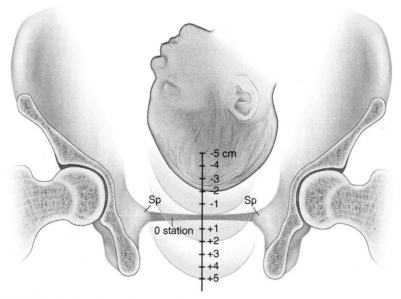

FIGURE 48-5. Station–descent of the fetal head by vaginal examination. (From *Assessing descent of the fetal head by vaginal examination. UpToDate.* 2018. https://www.uptodate.com/contents/image?imageKey=OBGYN%2F67068&topicKey=OBGYN%2F4445&source=outline_link&search=effacement&selectedTitle=1~22.)

OB/GYN

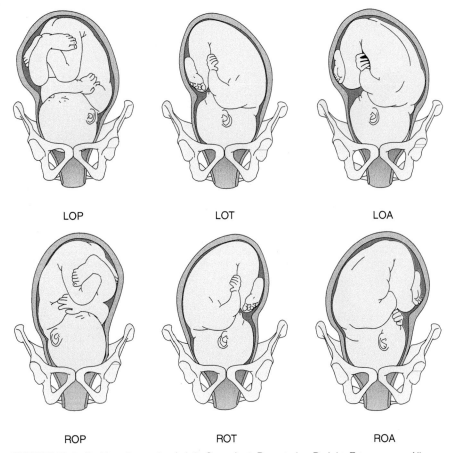

LOP   LOT   LOA

ROP   ROT   ROA

FIGURE 48-6. Position. A, anterior; L, left; O, occiput; P, posterior; R, right; T, transverse. All are vertex presentations. (From Pillitteri A. *Maternal and Child Health Nursing*. Philadelphia: Wolters Kluwer Health; 2014.)

Four Stages of Labor

First Stage	

Interval between the onset of labor and full cervical dilation
 	
Evaluated by the *rate of change* of cervical effacement, dilatation, and descent of fetal head
	1. **Latent phase**—may send women home
	  • Begins when mother feels regular contractions
	  • Ends with 3-5 cm dilation
	    • **Nulliparous:** longer interval (epidural); 6-18 h
	      • Affected by sedation, epidural analgesia, unfavorable cervical condition, false Labor
	    • **Multiparous:** shorter interval; 2-10 h
	2. **Active phase**
	  • Begins with *cervical dilation* of 3-5 cm (monitor every 2 h)
	    • at 9 cm—very active/fast → monitor and augment with oxytocin
	  • Ends with complete dilation (10 cm)
	    • **Protraction:** not changing at rate we expect women to
	      • Nulliparous women—Less than 2 cm/h dilation or <1 cm/h descent
	      • Multiparous: less than 1.5 cm/h dilation or <2 cm/h descent
	        • **Arrest of dilation:** no cervical change over 2 h
	        • **Arrest of descent:** no fetal descent over 1 h
	        • Factors: sedation, epidural, fetal malposition, cephalopelvic disproportion (CPD)
	    • CPD: baby does not fit in the pelvis because they are too large
	    • Oxytocin is used in arrest disorders, except with CPD
	3. Management: follow cervical change
	  • **Oxytocin,** unless large baby (C-section)
	  • Monitor fetal well-being, uterine contractions, and maternal VS (every 2-4 h)
	    • Contractions measured in Montevideo units (MVUs)
	    • **Required: 200 MVUs to deliver infant**
	    • Add them up in 10-min measured interval
	    • Limit oral intake: only clear liquids and ice chips
	    • +/− IV fluids and pain control
	  • Continuous monitoring of fetus recommended if HTN, IUGR, diabetes, multiple gestation
	  • Uterine contractions—use external tocodynamometer or IPC in amniotic cavity for abnormal progression of labor or oxytocin requirement for augmentation
	    • Palpation: every 30 min (frequency, duration, intensity)
	    • Tocodynamometer
	    • Internal pressure catheter (IPC)

Second Stage	Time from *complete dilation* (effacement 100%, dilation 10 cm) **to fetal delivery**
Interval between full cervical dilation and delivery of the infant Measured by descent, flexion, and rotation of presenting part	1. Median duration: 30 min-3 h (nulliparous), 5-30 min (multiparous); HIGHLY VARIABLE 　• Allow 2 h for nulliparous and 1 h for multiparous 　• Epidural = 1 additional hour 　• Fetal heart tracing may be nonexistent 2. Begin pushing: coached or uncoached, supine, legs hyperflexed (**dorsal lithotomy**)
Third Stage	**Time from delivery of the infant to delivery of the placenta**
Period between delivery of the infant and delivery of the placenta	1. Placental separation: uterus becomes globular and firm, sudden gush of blood, uterus rises in abdomen, umbilical cord lengthens 　• Must NOT exert excess traction on umbilical cord—do not want to cause uterine inversion 　　• Uterine inversion—uterus does not let go of placenta and inverts 　　　• Rare, but when you do not resuscitate, mother dies (4 U lost) 　　　• Do not remove, SEDATE patient, push with force to replace placenta with uterus still attached → retained placenta occurs 　　• **Retained placenta**: placenta does not deliver >30 min after the delivery, still bleeding 　　　• RF: Previous uterine surgery 　　• Absence of decidua allows placenta to become densely anchored to myometrium, resulting in **placenta accreta** (placenta that grows through uterus) 　　• RF: Prior history of C-section, history of retained placenta, preterm delivery, age 35+ (AMA), parity (>5), labor induction (extended) 2. Management—place sterile gloved hand into uterine cavity and manually remove placenta from uterus within 30 min, DO NOT SEDATE
Fourth Stage *Hour immediately following the delivery*	1. Postpartum hemorrhage MOST LIKELY TO OCCUR 2. Check maternal BP and pulse immediately after the delivery and every 15 min during this time

- Artificial rupture of the membranes increases the risk of chorioamnionitis and the need for antibiotics (especially if labor is prolonged), as well as the risk of cord prolapse if the presenting part is not engaged

- Amniotomy may provide information on the volume of amniotic fluid and the presence of meconium

  - Indicated when internal fetal or uterine monitoring is required and when enhancement of uterine contractility in active phase is indicated

- Rupture of the membranes may cause an increase in uterine contractility

- Once the head is delivered, the airway is cleared of blood and amniotic fluid using a bulb suction device. The oral cavity is cleared initially, followed by clearing of the nares

- After the airway is cleared, an index finger is used to check whether the umbilical cord encircles the neck. If so, the cord can usually be slipped over the infant's head. If the cord is too tight, it can be cut between two clamps

- **Signs of placental separation** are as follows: (1) a fresh show of blood appears from the vagina, (2) the umbilical cord lengthens outside the vagina, (3) the fundus of the uterus rises up, and (4) the uterus becomes firm and globular

Induction and Augmentation of Labor

- **Induction** of labor is the process of initiating labor by artificial means

  - The **Bishop Method** of pelvic scoring should be used for elective induction of labor
  - Common *indications* for induction
    - Maternal: preeclampsia, DM, heart disease
    - Fetal: prolonged pregnancy, Rh incompatibility, chorioamnionitis, PROM, placental insufficiency, suspected IUGR, fetal abnormality
- *Contraindications*: **contracted pelvis**, placenta previa, uterine scar from previous C-section, myomectomy, hysterectomy, unification surgery; transverse lie

- **Augmentation** is the artificial stimulation of labor that has begun spontaneously

The Bishop Method of Pelvic Scoring			
	Points		
Examination	**1**	**2**	**3**
Cervical dilation (cm)	1-2	3-4	5-6
Cervical effacement (%)	40-50	60-70	80
Station of presenting part	−1, −2	0	+1, 2
Consistency of cervix	Medium	Soft	–
Position of cervix	Middle	Anterior	–

Cervical Ripening

- Ripening before induction of labor facilitates the onset and progression of labor and increases the chance of vaginal delivery, particularly in primigravid patients

- Two forms of prostaglandins are commonly used for cervical ripening before induction at term: misoprostol (PGE1, Cytotec) and **dinoprostone** (PGE2, **Cervidil**, FDA approved)

- **Contraindications**: Cervidil should *not* be used in patients with a *history of asthma, glaucoma, or myocardial infarction*

OB/GYN

- For cervical ripening and induction at term, misoprostol is given vaginally at a dose of 25 μg every 4 to 6 hours. With Cervidil, usually 12 hours should be allowed for cervical ripening, after which oxytocin induction should be started
- PGE1 and PGE2 have similar side effect and risk profiles, including *fetal heart rate deceleration,* fetal *distress,* emergency caesarean section, *uterine hypertonicity,* nausea, vomiting, fever, and peripartum infection
- Balloon catheter: passed into endocervix above internal os, inflated with sterile saline, and withdrawn gently to the level of internal os (induces over 8 to 12 hours), balloon falls out after dilation of 2 to 3 cm → amniotomy possible

Oxytocin

- IV administration of a very dilute solution of oxytocin is the **most effective** medical means of inducing labor
- In most cases, it is sufficient to add 1 mL of oxytocin (10 units of oxytocin to 1 L of 5% dextrose in water [1 mU/min]) → increase at 2-milliunit increments at 15-minute intervals
- When contractions of 50 to 60 mm Hg (per the internal monitor pressure) or lasting 40 to 60 seconds (per the external monitor) occur at 2.5- to 4-minute intervals, the oxytocin dose should be increased no further
- Oxytocin infusion is discontinued whenever *hyperstimulation* or **fetal distress** is identified but can be restarted when reassuring fetal heart rate and uterine activity patterns are restored

Amniotomy (Artificial Rupture of Membranes)

- Early and variable decelerations of the fetal heart rate are noted to be relatively common
- Induce labor in cases with high Bishop scores using an amnihook
- Release of amniotic fluid shortens the muscle bundles of the myometrium; the strength and duration of the contractions are thereby increased, and a more rapid contraction sequence follows
- Because amniotomy has not been proven effective in augmenting labor uniformly, it is recommended that the **active phase of labor be entered before performing**

MATERNAL PHYSIOLOGY DURING PREGNANCY

- **Physiologic Changes**
  - Increased
    - Blood volume increases, plateauing at week 30; hypervolemia of pregnancy compensates for maternal blood loss at delivery, which averages 500 to 600 mL for vaginal and 1000 mL for caesarean delivery
    - Utilization of iron (can promote iron-deficiency anemia)
    - Leukocytosis during last trimester
    - Thrombocytosis, clotting factors (fibrinogen, factor 8, plasminogen)
    - Plasma volume increases by 50%, **increased red cell mass** by 30%
    - Estrogen production by placenta → RAAS → increased aldosterone → renal Na+ reabsorption and water retention
    - Prolactin levels >200 ng/mL
    - Cardiac output (40%), stroke volume (25%-30%), maternal HR, venous pressure in lower extremities (compression of IVC by gravid uterus), renal blood flow
    - Tidal volume, inspiratory capacity, minute ventilation (50%) (Fig. 48-7)
    - Progesterone → reduced GI motility
    - GFR, aldosterone, renin activity
    - Production of gastrin = acidic gastric secretions
    - Hyperpigmentation (linea nigra, melasma), spider angiomas, palmar erythema, cutis marmorata
    - Hemorrhoids
    - Thickening of the hair during pregnancy is caused by an increased number of follicles in anagen (growth) phase
  - Decrease
    - Systemic arterial pressure (nadir at 24 to 28 weeks)
    - Peripheral vascular resistance
    - Blood viscosity
    - Expiratory reserve and residual volume
    - Esophageal peristalsis, emptying of gallbladder (bile stasis → gallstone formation)
- **Respiratory alkalosis** and compensated metabolic acidosis
- **Chadwick sign**: During pregnancy, the vaginal mucosa usually appears dark bluish red and congested
  - Increased cervical softening as pregnancy advances
- **Hegar sign**: At 6 to 8 weeks of menstrual age, the firm cervix contrasts with the now softer fundus and the compressible interposed softened isthmus
- Increased pigmentation and visual changes in abdominal striae
- During first pregnancy, a woman may first perceive fetal movements between 16 and 18 weeks of gestation
  - At about 20 weeks, depending on maternal habitus, an examiner can begin to detect fetal movements
- Syncytiotrophoblast produces hCG in amounts that increase exponentially during the first trimester following implantation
  - This can be detected in maternal serum or urine by 8 to 9 days after ovulation
  - The doubling time of serum hCG concentration is **1.4 to 2.0 days**
  - Serum hCG levels increase from the day of implantation and reach peak levels at 60 to 70 days, then begins to decline
  - A plateau is reached at approximately 16 weeks

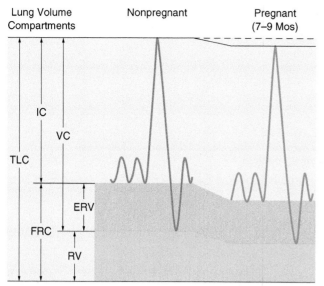

TLC = Total Lung Capacity   IC = Inspiratory Capacity
FRC = Functional Residual Capacity   VC = Vital Capacity
ERV = Expiratory Reserve Volume   RV = Residual Volume

FIGURE 48-7. Respiratory changes in pregnancy. Tidal volume (*TV*) increases by approximately 35%-50%. Inspiratory reserve (IRV) decreases. Expiratory reserve and residual volume decrease by 20%. Inspiratory lung capacity increases by 5%-10%. Total lung capacity and functional residual capacity decrease by 5% and 20%, respectively. Vital capacity is the only lung capacity that remains the same. (From Barash PG, Cullen BF, Stoelting RK, Cahalan M, Stock MC. *Clinical Anesthesia*. Philadelphia: Wolters Kluwer Health; 2010.)

- Transvaginal sonography is used to establish gestational age and confirm pregnancy location
  - A small anechoic fluid collection within the endometrial cavity may be seen by 4 to 5 weeks of gestation
  - **Intradecidual sign:** An anechoic center surrounded by a single echogenic rim
  - **Double decidual sign**: Two concentric echogenic rings surrounding the gestational sac
  - Visualization of the yolk sac—a brightly echogenic ring with an anechoic center—confirms with certainty an intrauterine location of the pregnancy and can normally be seen by the middle of the fifth week
  - Up to 12 weeks of gestation, the crown-rump length is predictive of gestational age within 4 days
- Pica and ptyalism (profuse salivation): may be triggered by iron deficiency
- **Quickening** (18 to 20 weeks): maternal perception of fetal movement

CHANGES AND MONITORING DURING PREGNANCY

6-12 gestational weeks	• Uterine size and growth are determined by pelvic examination • **Fetal heart tones audible at 10-12 wk** • Urinalysis; culture of a clean, voided, midstream, urine sample; random blood glucose; complete blood count (CBC) with red cell indices; serologic test for syphilis, rubella antibody titer; varicella immunity; blood group; Rh type; antibody screening for anti-Rho(D), hepatitis B surface antigen (HBsAg), and the HIV should be performed • Cervical cultures are usually obtained for *Chlamydia trachomatis* and possibly *Neisseria gonorrhoeae*, along with a Papanicolaou smear of the cervix • All black women should have sickle cell screening • Fetal aneuploidy screening is available in the first and second trimesters and should be offered to all women, ideally before 20 wk of gestation • For pregnancies at high risk for aneuploidy, noninvasive testing with cell-free fetal DNA from maternal plasma can be performed. It screens only for trisomy 13, 18, and 21 • If indicated and requested by the patient, chorionic villus sampling can be performed during this period (11-13 wk).
12 gestational weeks	• Uterus palpable above the symphysis pubis • Fetus begins to make spontaneous movements
14 gestational weeks	• **Gender can be determined** by inspection of external genitalia
16 gestational weeks	• Eye movements begin • The "quad screen" and amniocentesis are performed as indicated and requested by the patient during this time
20 gestational weeks	• Midpoint of pregnancy
24 gestational weeks	• Lungs are almost fully developed • The patient should be instructed about the symptoms and signs of preterm labor and rupture of membranes • U/S examination is performed as indicated

(continued)

(continued)

28 gestational weeks	• **Glucose tolerance test must be done by 28 wk** • Neonate born at this age has 90% chance of survival • If initial antibody screen for anti-Rho(D) is negative, repeat antibody testing for Rh-negative patients is performed, but the result is not required before Rho(D) immune globulin is administered • A CBC is done to evaluate for anemia of pregnancy • Screening for syphilis and HIV is also performed at this time • Fetal position and presentation are determined • The patient is asked about symptoms or signs of preterm labor or rupture of membranes at each visit. Maternal perception of fetal movement should be assessed at each visit. Antepartum fetal testing in the form of nonstress tests and biophysical profiles can be performed as medically indicated
36 gestational weeks	• Repeat syphilis and HIV testing (depending on state laws) and cervical cultures for *N. gonorrhoeae* and *C. trachomatis* should be performed in at-risk patients • The indicators of onset of labor, admission to the hospital, management of labor and delivery, and options for analgesia and anesthesia should be discussed with the patient
35-37 gestational weeks	• Prenatal culture-based screening for group B streptococcal colonization in pregnancy
41 gestational weeks	• Cervical examination to determine the probability of successful induction of labor • Induction is undertaken if the cervix is favorable (generally, cervix 2 cm or more dilated, 50% or more effaced, vertex at −1 station, soft cervix, and midposition)

Weight Gain in Pregnancy

BMI	Total Weight Gain Range (lb)	Weight Gain in 2nd and 3rd Trimesters (lb/wk)
Underweight (<18.5)	28-40	1
Normal (18.5-24.9)	25-35	1
Overweight (25-29.9)	15-25	0.6
Obese (>30)	11-20	0.5

Uterine Size

- 8 weeks: palpable at the pubic symphysis
- 16 weeks: palpable midway between the pubic symphysis and umbilicus
- 20 weeks: Palpable at the umbilicus

Fetal Position

- In late pregnancy, vaginal examination often provides valuable information that includes confirmation of the presenting part and its station, clinical estimation of pelvic capacity and its general configuration, amniotic fluid volume adequacy, and cervical consistency, effacement, and dilatation

Multiple Gestation

- Complications
  - First trimester bleeding can indicate threatened or spontaneous abortion
  - In second or third trimester, demise of 1 fetus can trigger DIC
- Anemia develops because of greater demand for iron by fetuses
  - Hypochromic normocytic anemia 2 to 3 times more common in multiple gestation
- Fetal malpresentation more common in multiple gestation; both twins present in cephalic presentation in 50% of cases
- Prolapse of the cord occurs 5 times more often in multiple than singleton pregnancy

Disease	Etiology, Prevalence, Risk Factors	Clinical Symptoms and Signs	Diagnostics	Therapy, Prognosis, and Health Maintenance
Multiple gestation	• Routine U/S screening, then again at 18-20 wk	1. Earlier and more severe pressure in pelvis, nausea, backache, varicosities, constipation, hemorrhoids, abdominal distention, and difficulty breathing 2. History of assisted reproduction Signs: 1. Uterus larger than expected (>4 cm for dates) 2. Excessive maternal weight gain, not explained by edema or obesity 3. Polyhydramnios (10× more common) 4. Palpation of 1 or more fetuses in fundus after delivery of 1 infant	1. **MSAFP:** elevated 2. **Ultrasound:** • Outline or ballottement of more than 1 fetus • Multiplicity of small parts 3. Fetal heart tones • Recording of different fetal rates simultaneously, varying by 8 beats/minute 4. Hemoglobin/Hct and RBC reduced compared to blood volume (anemia) 5. Tidal volume increased	1. Increased iron and calcium supplementation, vitamin and folic acid, high-protein diet, and more weight gain 2. Tocolytics to suppress PTL and extend gestation 48 h, so effects of steroids realized • Start with $MgSO_4$ 3. Admit at first sign of suspected labor or PTL, whether leakage or bleeding, >4 contractions/h at 34 wk 4. Vaginal delivery, unless complicated, then immediate C-section Complications: Morbid course of pregnancy (5×), maternal anemia (2-3×), UTI (2×), preeclampsia-eclampsia (3×), hemorrhage, uterine atony Higher rates of gestational DM and hypoglycemia Operative intervention more likely due to malpresentation, prolapsed cord, and fetal distress

APGAR SCORING

- Scores between 0 and 2 in each of 5 different categories are assigned at 1 and 5 minutes of life
- The score reflects the cardiorespiratory and neurologic status at those time points. If the score is <7 at 5 minutes, scores should be assigned every 5 minutes until the baby has a score of 7 or greater or has reached 20 minutes of life
- The Apgar score is <u>not</u> what determines the need for resuscitation
- Although scores are based on the same elements used to evaluate the newborn's status, the assessment of the need for intervention with PPV (positive pressure ventilation) should ideally already have been made by the time the 1-minute Apgar score is assigned
- It is important to know that factors such as prematurity, maternal medications, and congenital disease can adversely affect scores

Signs	0	1	2
Appearance (color)	Blue/pale	Body pink, extremities blue	Completely pink
Pulse	Absent	Slow (<100)	>100
Grimace (reflex)	No response	Grimace	Cry or cough
Activity (muscle tone)	Limp	Some flexion	Active motion
Respiratory effort	Absent	Slow, irregular	Good, crying

OB/GYN

CHAPTER 49

Menstruation

Refer to Family Medicine 👪 for In-Depth Coverage of the Following Topics:

Osteoporosis and Osteopenia, p 74

Recommended Supplemental Topics:

Gonadal Dysgenesis (including **Turner Syndrome**), see Endocrinology, p 338 👥

NORMAL PHYSIOLOGY

The Menstrual Cycle (Fig. 49-1)

- **Menstruation**: cyclic vaginal bleeding that occurs with shedding of uterine mucosa
- The "typical" menstrual cycle is defined as **28 ± 7 days** with menstrual flow lasting 4 ± 2 days and an average blood loss of 20 to 60 mL
- By convention, the first day of vaginal bleeding is considered day 1 of the menstrual cycle
- Mean cycle length: 35 days (age 15), 30 days (age 25), and 28 days (age 35)
  - Decrease due to shortening of follicular phase, with luteal phase remaining constant
- When viewed from a perspective of ovarian function, the menstrual cycle can be defined as a preovulatory follicular phase and postovulatory luteal phase. Corresponding phases in the endometrium are termed the proliferative and secretory phases
- For most women, **the luteal phase of the menstrual cycle is stable, lasting 13 to 14 days.** Thus, variations in normal cycle length generally result from variations in the duration of the follicular phase

Ovarian Function and Cycle

- Ovaries have two interrelated functions: (1) the generation of mature oocytes and (2) the production of steroid and peptide hormones that create an environment in which fertilization and subsequent implantation in the endometrium can occur
- No new ova formed after birth (most germ cells during fetal development) → ova undergo first meiotic division and **arrest in prophase** until adulthood → just before ovulation, first meiotic division is complete
  - Secondary oocyte: receives most of cytoplasm → begins second meiotic division and **stops at metaphase** → completed only when sperm penetrates → second polar body cast off and ovum proceeds
  - First polar body: fragmented; disappears
- **Mittelschmerz**: "ovulation pain" or "midcycle pain" that appears suddenly and subsides within hours; occurs midcycle and pelvic exam shows no abnormalities
- **Follicular phase**: primordial follicles → antrum formation → dominant follicle (day 6)
  - The follicle most responsive to FSH is likely to first produce estradiol
  - Graafian follicle (mature ovarian follicle) layers
    - Antrum (follicular fluid): high estrogen content that comes from granulosa cells
    - Granulosa cells
    - Theca interna: source of circulating estrogen
    - Theca externa
- **Ovulation**: on the 14th day of the cycle, the **distended follicle ruptures and ovum is extruded into abdominal cavity**; picked up by fimbriated ends of uterine tubes
  - Unless fertilization occurs, the ovum degenerates and passes through the uterus out of the vagina

- Corpus hemorrhagicum: follicle that ruptures fills with blood; bleeding into abdominal cavity can cause peritoneal irritation (**mittelschmerz**)
- Granulosa and theca cells rapidly proliferate, clotted blood replaced by yellow, lipid-rich luteal cells, forming the **corpus luteum**
- **Luteal phase:** luteal cells produce estrogen and progesterone
  - If pregnancy occurs, corpus luteum persists and no more menstrual cycles until after delivery
  - If no pregnancy, corpus luteum degenerates 4 days before next menses (day 24) and is replaced by fibrous tissue (**corpus albicans**)

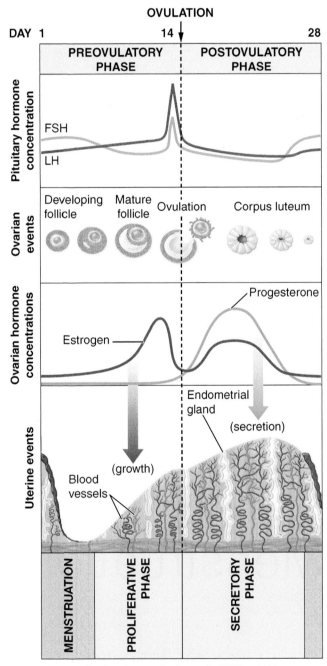

FIGURE 49-1. The female reproductive cycle. FSH and LH are secreted by the anterior pituitary controlling the follicle and corpus luteum, which in turn secrete ovarian hormones. These hormones (estrogen and progesterone) control uterine endometrial changes. (From Cohen BJ, Hull K. *Memmler's The Human Body in Health and Disease.* Philadelphia: Wolters Kluwer Health; 2015.)

- **Proliferative phase** (preovulatory or follicular phase): Under the influence of estrogen secreted from the developing follicles, the endometrium regenerates from the deep layer and increases rapidly in thickness during the period from the fifth to 16th days of the menstrual cycle

- **Secretory phase** (luteal phase, **14 days**): After ovulation, the endometrium becomes more highly vascularized and slightly edematous under the influence of estrogen and progesterone from the corpus luteum. The glands become coiled and tortuous, and they begin to secrete clear fluid. Late in the luteal phase, the endometrium, like the anterior pituitary, produces prolactin

Vascular Supply of the Endometrium

- Two arteries: (1) long, coiled spiral arteries (supply superficial ⅔ of endometrium, stratum functionale, shed during menstruation), (2) short, straight basilar arteries (supply deep layer, stratum basale, not shed)

- After the **corpus luteum regresses**, hormonal support for the endometrium is withdrawn, causing vascular spasms in the spiral artery, ultimately leading to endometrial ischemia and thinning of the endometrium

Cyclic Changes in the Uterine Cervix, Vagina, Breasts

- Mucosa does not undergo cyclic desquamation

- Estrogen makes mucus much thinner and more alkaline to support survival and transport of sperm

- Progesterone makes mucus thick, tenacious, cellular

- **Mucus is thinnest at the time of ovulation** and elasticity (spinnbarkeit) increases

- After ovulation and during pregnancy, mucus becomes thick and fails to form fernlike pattern

- Vaginal epithelium becomes cornified (peripheral smear) and thick mucus secreted (due to progesterone)

- Breast swelling, tenderness, and pain during 10 days preceding menstruation

- Increased body temperature during luteal phase and ovulation (thermogenic effect of progesterone)

- Ovulation occurs 9 hours after peak of LH surge at midcycle

ABNORMAL UTERINE BLEEDING DEFINITIONS

- **Me*nor*rhagia (hypermenorrhea)**: irregularly *prolonged* or *heavy* menstrual period that maintains a **normal** menstrual cycle (21 to 35 days)

  - Differential: coagulopathy (ITP, hemophilia, vWD), endometriosis, leiomyoma, neoplasm

- **Metrorragia (intermenstrual bleeding)**: abnormal vaginal bleeding in between normal cycles that recurs at irregular intervals

  - Commonly seen with contraceptive medications, called "breakthrough bleeding" or underlying disorders such as leiomyomas, endometriosis, or GU neoplasms

- **Menometrorrhagia**: heavy or prolonged uterine bleeding AND occurs at irregular intervals (more frequently than normal)

- **Polymenorrhea**: regular menstruation cycles occurring at irregularly shortened intermenstruation intervals (<21 days); shortened *luteal* phase

- **Hypomenorrhea (cryptomenorrhea)**: unusually light menstrual flow, sometimes just spotting

- **Oligomenorrhea**: menstrual cycles that occur >35 days apart (decreased amount of bleeding and possibly anovulation) or <9 cycles per year

- **Amenorrhea**: no menstrual period for more than 6 months

- **Contact (postcoital) bleeding**: can be considered a sign of cervical cancer until proven otherwise

- **Postmenopausal bleeding**: bleeding that occurs after 12 months of amenorrhea in a middle-aged woman

- For many years, **dilatation and curettage (D&C)** has been regarded as the gold standard for the diagnosis of abnormal uterine bleeding

DYSFUNCTIONAL UTERINE BLEEDING

- Exclusion of all possible pathologic causes of abnormal bleeding establishes the diagnosis of dysfunctional uterine bleeding

OB/GYN

Disease	Etiology, Prevalence, Risk Factors	Clinical Symptoms and Signs	Diagnostics	Therapy, Prognosis, and Health Maintenance
Dysfunctional uterine bleeding	AUB in the **absence of an anatomic lesion,** caused by a problem with the hypothalamic-pituitary-ovarian axis Occurs shortly after menarche and during perimenopause because of **increased anovulatory cycles** Other causes: PCOS, obesity, adrenal hyperplasia Very young (20%) or perimeno-pausal woman (40%)	1. Abnormal uterine bleeding (AUB) Signs: 1. Unremarkable physical exam	1. Urinary β-hCG levels–r/o pregnancy 2. Labs: CBC, iron studies, PT, PTT, TSH, progesterone, Prolactin, FSH, LFTs 3. **Progestin** trial–if bleeding stops, anovulatory cycles confirmed 4. Ovulation journal 5. Pap smear 6. **Pelvic U/S,** endo-metrial biopsy, HSG, hysteroscopy	Adolescents: 1. Pelvic U/S, serum hCG 2. OCPs, 3-4× normal dose 3. IV high-dose estrogen for acute hemorrhage • Then medroxyprogesterone × 7-10 d Premenopausal: 1. Hysteroscopy and EMB **D&C:** • Indications: bleeding not controlled with OCPs, symptomatically anemic, lifestyle restricted by persistence of irregular bleeding • If persistent → Mirena IUD or endo-metrial ablation • If failure → consider hysterectomy Postmenopausal: 1. D/C use of exogenous hormones 2. EMB 3. Endocervical curettage 4. D&C if diagnosis not established 5. Hysterectomy

Management of Dysfunctional Uterine Bleeding

	Mild	Moderate	Severe
Hgb Value (g/dL)	**>12**	**9-12**	**<9**

Acute treatment	1. Monitor menstrual calendar
	2. Iron supplementation
	3. NSAID with menses may help reduce flow
	4. Consider OCPs if patient is sexually active and desires contraception
		1. OCP BID until bleeding stops
		2. Continue active pill daily × 21 d, followed by 1 wk of placebo pills
			1. Admit to hospital if
			  • Hgb <7 g/dL or
			  • hemodynamically unstable
			  • Transfusion based on the degree of hemodynamic instability and ability to control bleeding
			2. Conjugated estrogens
			  • 25 mg IV every 4 h for up to 48 h
			  • Provide scheduled IV antiemetic
			    When bleeding stops, step down to 50 µg OCP PO QID (or TID), then taper as below
			  • If bleeding does not stop, gynecology consulta-tion for further evaluation and possible dilation and curettage
			OR
			1. One 30-35 µg OCP PO QID until bleeding stops, then decrease to TID × 2 d (and up to 7 d), then daily (skipping placebo pills) until Hct >30%
			  • Antiemetic 2 h prior to OCPs as needed for nausea

Long-term management	1. Monitor menstrual calendar and Hgb
	2. Follow-up in 2-3 mo
		1. Iron supplementation
		2. Monitor Hgb closely for improvement
		3. May need to revert to BID OCP dosing if bleeding persists
		4. If bleeding controlled, cycle with OCPs (28-d pack) or other combined hormonal contracep-tive agent for minimum 3-6 mo
			1. Iron supplementation
			2. Serial hematocrits
			  • If Hct >30%, cycle with OCPs (28-d pack) or other combined hormonal contraceptive agent for minimum 3-6 mo
			  • Consider placement of levonorgestrel intrauterine (IUD) system once anemia improved as alternative to short-acting method

From Richards MJ, Kaplan DW, Sass AE. Adolescence. In: Hay WH, Levin MJ, Deterding, RR, Abzug MJ, eds. *Current Diagnosis & Treatment: Pediatrics.* 23rd ed. New York: McGraw-Hill; 2014 [chapter 4]. https://accessmedicine.mhmedical.com/content.aspx?bookid=1795&sectionid=125736260.

OB/GYN

AMENORRHEA

- Although there are unique cases of primary amenorrhea, all causes of secondary amenorrhea can also cause primary disease
- 15% of girls with primary amenorrhea will have an anatomic abnormality on ultrasound

- Presence or absence of breast development is a marker of estrogen activity and function of the ovary (except in case of complete androgen insensitivity syndrome)
- Presence or absence of uterus (by ultrasound or MRI) is useful for evaluation
- FSH (follicle stimulating hormone) level crucial for evaluation

Evaluation of Primary Amenorrhea

	Gonadal Dysgenesis	Mullerian Agenesis	Androgen Insensitivity Syndrome	Hematometra	Hematocolpos	Congenital GnRH Deficiency
Serum FSH	Elevated	Normal	Normal	Normal	Normal	Low to NL
Ultrasound findings	–	Absent uterus	Absent uterus	Blood in uterus	Blood in vagina	–
Testosterone level	–	NL range for women	Range for men	–	–	–
Next steps	Karyotype AMH	Karyotype	Karyotype			

Sexual Maturity Rating of Secondary Sexual Characteristics

Boys–Development of external genitalia

Stage 1: Prepubertal

Stage 2: Enlargement of testes and scrotum; scrotal skin reddens and changes in texture

Stage 3: Enlargement of penis (length at first); further growth of testes

Stage 4: Increased size of penis with growth in breadth and development of glans; testes and scrotum larger, scrotal skin darker

Stage 5: Adult genitalia

Girls–Breast development (Fig. 49-2)

Stage 1: Prepubertal

Stage 2: Breast bud stage with elevation of breast and papilla; enlargement of areola

Stage 3: Further enlargement of breast and areola; no separation of their contour

Stage 4: Areola and papilla form a secondary mound above level of breast

Stage 5: Mature stage: projection of papilla only, related to recession of areola

Boys and girls–Pubic hair

Stage 1: Prepubertal (the pubic area may have vellus hair, similar to that of forearms)

Stage 2: Sparse growth of long, slightly pigmented hair, straight or curled, at base of penis and along labia

Stage 3: Darker, coarser, and more curled hair, spreading sparsely over junction of pubes

Stage 4: Hair adult in type, but covering smaller area than adult; no spread to medial surface of thighs

Stage 5: Adult in type and quantity, with horizontal upper border

From *Sexual Maturity Rating of Secondary Sexual Characteristics*. *UpToDate*. 2018. https://www.uptodate.com/contents/image?imageKey=ENDO%2F55329&topicKey=PEDS%2F5849&source=outline_link&search=tanner%20staging&selectedTitle=1~88.

OB/GYN

Tanner staging of breast development in girls

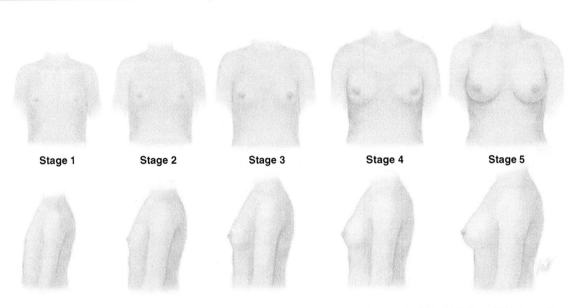

Stage 1	Stage 2	Stage 3	Stage 4	Stage 5

FIGURE 49-2. Tanner staging–breast development. (From *Tanner Staging of Breast Development in Girls. UpToDate.* 2018. https://www.upto-date.com/contents/image/print?imageKey=ENDO%2F67072&topicKey=ENDO%2F7403&rank=1~43&source=see_link&search=primary%20amenorrhea&utdPopup=true.)

Primary and Secondary Amenorrhea

Disease	Etiology, Prevalence, Risk Factors	Clinical Symptoms and Signs	Diagnostics	Therapy, Prognosis, and Health Maintenance
Primary amenorrhea	Absence of menarche by age 15 y	1. Presence of normal growth and secondary sex characteristics		
Müllerian agenesis (Mayer-Rokitansky-Kuster-Hauser syndrome) Cause of 15% of primary amenorrhea	Congenital absence of the vagina, cervix, uterus, and fallopian tubes (**ovaries present**) **46 XX**, female karyotype "Short or absent vagina"	1. Primary amenorrhea Signs: 1. Small vaginal opening with "blind pouch" 2. Normal secondary sex characteristics 3. **Renal anomalies**	1. TSH: Normal 2. Pelvic U/S: normal ovaries, absence of uterus and cervix 3. Karyotype 4. **Renal U/S**: check for renal anomalies (25%-35%)	1. **McIndoe procedure–** skin graft to create artificial vagina
Androgen insensitivity syndrome (AIS)	No uterus; testes present Receptor defect **46 XY, female** phenotype Testes cause MIF secretion lead to no Müllerian structures; resistant to testosterone due to a defect in the androgen receptor → fail to develop male sexual characteristics X-linked recessive disorder	1. Primary amenorrhea 2. Normal breast development Signs: 1. Little to no axillary or pubic hair 2. Tall 3. Blind vaginal pouch	1. TSH: High 2. Testosterone: **high** (adult male range >200 ng/dL) 3. Pelvic U/S: normal ovaries, absence of uterus and cervix 4. Karyotype	1. **Gonadectomy** required–to prevent gonadal neoplasia • Surgery delayed until puberty in patients with complete AIS as tumors develop after puberty/growth spurt Prognosis: 1. Increased risk of malignancy – remove after puberty 2. Testes should be excised after puberty because of increased risk of testicular cancer after age 25 y

OB/GYN

Disease	Etiology, Prevalence, Risk Factors	Clinical Symptoms and Signs	Diagnostics	Therapy, Prognosis, and Health Maintenance
Imperforate hymen	Lower genital tract malformation At birth, due to vaginal secretions stimulated by maternal estradiol, causing a bulging introitus	1. Primary amenorrhea 2. Cyclical abdominal or pelvic pain during adolescence 3. Back pain, pain with defecation, or difficulty urinating Signs: 1. Perirectal mass (**hematocolpos**): bluish mass pushing labia open 2. "Difficulty inserting speculum" 3. Normal secondary sex characteristics	1. β-hCG–r/o pregnancy first	1. If diagnosis not made in infancy and hymen remains imperforate, mucus will be reabsorbed and child will be asymptomatic until menarche 2. Surgical correction preferred during infancy, postpuberty, or premenarchal
Secondary amenorrhea	Absence of menses for 3 mo (girls) or women who previously had regular menstrual cycles or 6 mo in girls or women who had irregular menses MCC: 1. Pregnancy 2. PCOS (40%) 3. Functional hypothalamic amenorrhea (35%) 4. Hyperprolactinemia (13%)		1. β-hCG–r/o pregnancy first 2. TSH level 3. FSH: normal 4. Serum estradiol (E2) 5. Prolactin level 6. Serum DHEAS to r/o hyperandrogenism	1. Correct underlying pathology, if possible 2. Help women achieve fertility, if desired 3. Prevent complications of disease processes

Chronic anovulation with estrogen *present* (**MCC: PCOS**), **polycystic ovarian syndrome**	Higher GnRH = higher androstenedione and testosterone and estrogen = higher LH
	Higher estrogen decreases FSH release no **LH surge**
	Insulin resistance–direct insulin stimulation of theca cells
	Chronic anovulation
	Pubertal women
	RF:
	First-degree relatives
	Ovaries contain multiple follicular cysts that are inactive
		1. **Menstrual irregularities** (amenorrhea → menorrhagia)
		2. **Infertility**: ovulation induction yields increased risk for multifetal pregnancy
		3. **Hirsutism**: due to peripheral androgen excess
		4. **Metabolic syndrome**: DM or insulin resistance, hypertension, central obesity
		Signs:
		1. Hirsutism (coarse facial hair)
		2. Male alopecia
			DX of exclusion:
			1. R/o pregnancy
			2. Thyroid function
			  • TSH: NL or increased
			  • **Free T3: high**
			  • FSH: **low** (or NL with low E2)
			3. Gonadotropins
			  • LH: high (in response to increased estrogens)
			  • FSH <<< LH
			  • Prolactin: NL to high
			  • Androstenedione and DHEA: high
			4. Progestin admin: bleeds (withdrawals)
			5. **ACTH (17-HPG)**: definitive
			6. Dexamethasone suppression test or 24-h urinary cortisol to r/o Cushing's
			7. Pelvic U/S: if high risk
				1. **OCPs**
				2. Clomid (clomiphene citrate)–induces ovulation
				3. Metformin
				4. Spironolactone
				Complications:
				1. Endometrial hyperplasia and cancer (due to unopposed estrogen)
				Rotterdam criteria:
				requires 2 of 3
				1. **H**yperandrogenism (Clinical or biochemical)
				2. **O**ligo/amenorrhea
				3. **P**CO (12+) on U/S

OB/GYN

(continued)

(continued)

Disease	Etiology, Prevalence, Risk Factors	Clinical Symptoms and Signs	Diagnostics	Therapy, Prognosis, and Health Maintenance
Hypogonadotropic hypogonadism (chronic anovulation with estrogen *absent*) "Functional hypothalamic-pituitary amenorrhea"	Inherited hypothalamic abnormalities: lack of normal pulsatile secretion of GnRH leads to decreased stimulation of pituitary gland to produce FSH and LH, leading to anovulation and amenorrhea The result of ovarian failure or follicular resistance to gonadotropin stimulation Etiology: 1. Disorders of anterior pituitary: pituitary adenomas 2. Drugs: marijuana, tranquilizers 3. Psychogenic: chronic anxiety, anorexia nervosa 4. Functional abnormalities: weight loss, obesity, excessive exercise 5. Chronic debilitating disease	HX: excessive **exercise, stress, anorexia** nervosa, or significant weight loss: 1. Anovulation, **amenorrhea** 2. Cycles previously regular since menarche 3. Normal SSC and external genitalia 4. +/– **Dyspareunia** due to vaginal dryness (estrogen deficiency)	1. R/o pregnancy 2. β-hCG: normal 3. Prolactin: normal 4. TSH: normal 5. FSH and LH: LOW • FSH >>> LH 6. HbA1C–r/o diabetes 7. Progestin withdrawal test: no bleeding 8. tTG-IgA antibodies– screen for Celiac disease 9. MRI with contrast–r/o pituitary adenoma	1. Treat underlying issue • Bromocriptine, if prolactinoma • Weight gain • Reduction in exercise • Resolution of illness or emotional stress 2. Estrogen replacement therapy (ERT): for women who want to continue to exercise and not seeking fertility; prevents osteoporosis and heart disease 3. Exogenous gonadotropins • For women who wish to become pregnant
Asherman syndrome (intrauterine adhesions)	**Intrauterine scarring (synechiae)**, normal cycles with cyclic premenstrual symptoms → defect located at uterus	HX: uterine instrumentation (**dilation and curettage**) following vaginal delivery or pregnancy termination, including h/o endometritis: 1. Secondary amenorrhea 2. Infertility	1. *Progestin challenge*: no withdrawal bleeding 2. Administer estrogen and progestin • Failure to bleed upon cessation of this therapy suggests endometrial scarring 3. **Hysterosalpingogram** (confirmatory): shows webbed pattern	1. Excision of synechiae (scars) using D&C (curettage) 2. Long-term high-dose estrogen (Premarin) or IUD administration to stimulate regrowth of endometrial tissue
Sheehan syndrome: postpartum hypopituitarism (necrosis) due to ischemic necrosis	Due to blood loss and hypovolemic shock during and after childbirth (severe postpartum hemorrhage leading to pituitary apoplexy)	1. Amenorrhea, breast atrophy 2. Loss of pubic and axillary hair 3. Hypothyroidism 4. ACTH insufficiency 5. Failure to lactate	1. R/o pregnancy 2. T4: decreased • TSH: decreased 3. Estrogen: decreased • LH surge: absent • FSH: low to normal 4. Cortisol: low 5. Prolactin: low 6. Progestin admin: withdrawal bleeding	
Prolactinoma	Most common pituitary tumor causing amenorrhea	1. Amenorrhea (anovulation) 2. **Galactorrhea** 3. **Visual field defects:** bitemporal hemianopsia 4. Normal secondary sex characteristics	1. Prolactin: high (hyperprolactinemia) 2. TRH: increased TSH: increased T4: decreased (hypothyroidism)	

DYSMENORRHEA

Refers to pain associated with menses, which can either be primary or secondary.

• Reserved for women whose pain prevents normal activity and requires medication, whether an over-the-counter or a prescription drug

OB/GYN

Disease	Etiology, Prevalence, Risk Factors	Clinical Symptoms and Signs	Diagnostics	Therapy, Prognosis, and Health Maintenance
Dysmenorrhea				
Primary dysmenorrhea (no organic cause)	Painful uterine muscle activity due to an excess of prostaglandins (F2a) Incidence: teens-early 20s, declines with age No associated pelvic pathology RF: menarche before age 12, nulliparity, smoking, family history, obesity	1. **Pain with menstruation** • Described as: lower abdominal, intermittent, "labor-like" • Days **1-3** 2. Nausea, vomiting, diarrhea (smooth muscle contraction) 3. Headache Signs: 1. Normal pelvic exam 2. Patient appears ill, in fetal position		1. **NSAIDs (first line):** mefenamic acid (Ponstel), **600 mg ibuprofen** (Motrin) **q 4-6 h**, naproxen (Anaprox) 2. OCPs (POPs)–progestin causes endometrial atrophy ═ less prostaglandins • Given for 6-12 mo 3. Support: heat application, exercise, psychotherapy
Secondary dysmenorrhea (pathologic cause)	Painful menstruation caused by clinically identifiable cause Causes: Endometriosis, adenomyosis, polyps, fibroids, IUD, **infection**, tumors, adhesions, cervical stenosis/lesions, non-Gyn, psych Common women age **(20-40 s)**	1. **Pain with menstruation** • Begins **mid cycle** and increases in severity until end **Differential:** 1. Heavy flow with pain: adenomyosis, myomas, polyps 2. Pelvic fullness: myomas, tumors 3. Uterine enlargement: Adenomyosis, myomas, tumor 4. Restricted uterus: adhesions, inflammation 5. Discharge: GC/CT 6. Posterior cul-de-sac: endometriosis	1. GC/CT testing	Treat underlying condition: 1. Surgery 2. Antibiotics 3. Cervical dilation 4. NSAIDs 5. OCPs

MENOPAUSE

- **Menopause (natural):** 12 months of amenorrhea with no obvious pathologic cause
  - Oocytes responsive to gonadotropins disappear from the ovary
  - The few remaining oocytes do not respond to gonadotropins
- **Induced (artificial) menopause:** Permanent cessation of menstruation after bilateral oophorectomy or ablation of ovarian function (chemotherapy, radiation)
  - Used as treatment for endometriosis, estrogen-sensitive neoplasms of the breast and endometrium (rarely)
- **Perimenopause/menopause transition:** menstrual cycle and hormonal changes that occur a few years before and 12 months after the final menstrual period resulting from natural menopause
- **Premature menopause (spontaneous premature ovarian failure):** menopause reached at or before age 40
- The early rise of FSH in menopause is related to **inhibin** (polypeptide synthesized and secreted by granulosa cells), which causes negative feedback on FSH release by pituitary → as oocyte number decreases, inhibin levels decrease resulting in elevated FSH

- Note: during the menopausal transition, high FSH stimulates follicles to secrete estradiol (2 to 3 times higher than normal)

Changes in Hormone Metabolism

- In postmenopausal women, there is a reduction in circulating androstenedione to approximately 50% of the concentration found in young women, reflecting the absence of follicular activity
- The level of testosterone found in postmenopausal women is only minimally lower than that found in premenopausal women before oophorectomy and is distinctly higher than the level observed in young women who have had ovaries removed
- Levels of the adrenal androgens dehydroepiandrosterone (DHEA) and dehydroepiandrosterone sulfate (DHEAS) are reduced by 60% and 80%, respectively, with age
- A decrease of *estradiol* occurs up to 1 year after the last menstrual period
  - Although both estrone and testosterone are converted in peripheral tissues to estradiol, its conversion from estrone that accounts for most estradiol in older women (adrenal gland is major source)
  - Last hormonal change associated with loss of ovarian function

OB/GYN

- In young women, the major source of *progesterone* is the ovarian corpus luteum after ovulation. During the follicular phase of the cycle, progesterone levels are low. With ovulation, the levels rise greatly, reflecting the secretory activity of the corpus luteum. Because postmenopausal ovaries do not contain functional follicles, ovulation does not occur and progesterone levels remain low
  - Dexamethasone suppresses level, ACTH increases level, hCG has no effect
- Gonadotropins: with menopause, both LH and FSH levels rise substantially, with FSH usually higher than LH

Disease	Etiology, Prevalence, Risk Factors	Clinical Symptoms and Signs	Diagnostics	Therapy, Prognosis, and Health Maintenance
Menopause	**Average age: 51.3** Range: 44-56 RF (early menopause): genetics, **smoking**, cancer therapies Consider in differential: pregnancy and hypothyroidism, premature ovarian failure (if <35) Most common SX: hot flash or flush	Early menopause: 1. **Menstrual irregularity** (more frequent) 2. Vasomotor symptoms: hot flashes, night sweats, 3. Sleep disturbances 4. Irritability, mood disturbances 5. Vaginal dryness → dyspareunia Vulvovaginal atrophy/**GSM** (intermediate): 1. Vaginal atrophy, loss of urogenital integrity, loss of skin elasticity Late menopause: 1. Osteoporosis 2. CVD 3. Macular degeneration 4. Periodontal disease 5. Decreased hearing, balance, skin integrity 6. Alzheimer disease, memory and cognition,	DX: **1 y of no periods** (amenorrhea) after age 40 with no pathologic cause: 1. **FSH: elevated** (21-100 mU/mL) • Elevated during early follicular phase, decrease during follicular maturation 2. **Estradiol <20 pg/mL, low** • Establishes diagnosis of menopause • Determines ovarian status of patient 3. Progesterone levels: same as younger women • No clinical use in postmenopausal women 4. AMH, inhibin B: low 5. LH: elevated, but not necessary to measure	1. Estrogens • Used to treat hot flashes • Woman with **intact uterus** should **not** use estrogen alone because of the increased risk of endometrial cancer 2. Progestins • Hot flashes • Increased risk of breast cancer 3. SSRI and SNRIs • Caution use with tamoxifen 4. Black cohosh 5. HRT—severe menopausal symptoms (hot flashes, night sweats, vaginal dryness) • "Smallest dose for shortest possible time and annual reviews of the decision to take hormones" • HRT should not be used to prevent cardiovascular disease due to slight increased risk of breast cancer, MI, CVD, DVT • Hormone therapy effect on lipid profile: HDL and *TG levels increase*, LDL levels decrease
Spontaneous premature ovarian failure (**premature menopause**)	Spontaneous cessation of menses before age 40 Prevalence: 1%-5% Causes: Unknown, iatrogenic (chemotherapy, surgery of ovaries, pelvic irradiation) Ovaries fail secondary to depletion of ova	1. Cessation of menstruation (**amenorrhea**) before age 40 2. Development of climacteric symptoms	1. Increased gonadotropin levels 2. Estrogen deficiency 3. Karyotype - r/o sex chromosome translocations, short arm deletions, or occult Y chromosome fragment (16% have Fragile X)	

PREMENSTRUAL SYNDROME

- "The cyclic occurrence of symptoms that are of sufficient severity to interfere with some aspects of life and that appear with consistent and predictable relationship to the menses."
- Although the symptoms themselves are not unique, the restriction of the symptoms to the **luteal phase** of the menstrual cycle is pathognomonic of PMS
- Serotonin (5-hydroxytryptamine [5-HT]), a neurotransmitter, is important in the pathogenesis of PMS/PMDD

- GABA levels are decreased in women with PMS/PMDD during the late luteal phase compared with normal women
- One of the most common symptoms of PMS is **mastodynia**, or mastalgia (pain, and usually swelling, of the breasts caused by edema and engorgement of the vascular and ductal systems)
- The most common associated psychiatric illness is **depression**, which generally responds to antidepressant drugs and psychotherapy

OB/GYN

Disease	Etiology, Prevalence, Risk Factors	Clinical Symptoms and Signs	Diagnostics	Therapy, Prognosis, and Health Maintenance
Premenstrual syndrome (PMS)	RF: FH of PMS, vitamin B$_6$, calcium, or magnesium deficiency Up to 75% of women experience some recurrent PMS symptoms Highest incidence: 20-30s	1. Headache 2. Breast tenderness 3. Pelvic pain 4. Bloating 5. Premenstrual tension 6. More severe: irritability, dysphoria, mood lability 7. Other: abdominal discomfort, clumsiness, lack of energy, sleep changes, mood swings 8. Behavior: social withdrawal, altered daily activities, marked change in appetite, increased crying, changes in sexual desire	ACOG criteria: 1. At least 1 affective and 1 somatic symptom during the **5 d preceding menses** in each of the 3 prior cycles with: • Symptoms relieved within 4 d of onset • Without recurrence until cycle day 13 • Reproducible during any 2 cycles	1. Must keep a daily calendar See Treatment below

Criteria for PMS

Affective/Behavioral	Somatic/Physical
1. **Depression** 2. Anxiety 3. **Angry outbursts** 4. **Irritability** 5. **Confusion** 6. Changes in libido 7. **Social withdrawal** 8. Food cravings 9. Poor concentration 10. Loss of motor skills	1. **Breast tenderness (mastodynia)** 2. **Abdominal bloating** 3. Diarrhea/constipation 4. **Swelling of extremities** 5. **Headache** • Can be migraine like with scotomas and vomiting 6. Fatigue

Treatment for PMS

Step 1 (mild symptoms)	1. Education, supportive therapy • Limit caffeine, alcohol, tobacco, and chocolate intake • Eat small, frequent meals high in complex carbohydrates • Decrease sodium intake to alleviate edema • Supplements (Ca^{2+}, Mg, vitamins A, E, B$_6$) • Calcium carbonate (1000–1200 mg/d) for bloating, food cravings, and pain • Magnesium (200-360 mg/d) for water retention • NSAIDs • Bromocriptine for mastalgia • Spironolactone for cyclic edema 2. Stress management: CBT, aerobic exercise
Step 2 (moderate symptoms)	1. First line: **SSRIs** (fluoxetine, sertraline, citalopram, paroxetine) • Give 14 d prior to the onset of menstruation and continue through the end of cycle 2. Anxiolytics: alprazolam and buspirone

Step 3 (severe symptoms)	1. Hormonal ovulation suppression 2. OCPs: **drospirenone** (Yaz, approved PMDD) or continuous levonorgestrel (Implanon) 3. GnRH agonist: leuprolide/leuprorelin (Lupron) 4. Danazol for mastalgia 5. Definitive surgical treatment: bilateral oophorectomy

PREMENSTRUAL DYSPHORIC DISORDER

• Severe PMS with functional impairment
• PMS and PMDD are highly associated with unipolar depressive disorder and anxiety disorders, such as obsessive-compulsive disorder, panic disorder, and generalized anxiety disorder

OB/GYN

Disease	Etiology, Prevalence, Risk Factors	Clinical Symptoms and Signs	Diagnostics	Therapy, Prognosis, and Health Maintenance
Premenstrual dysphoric disorder (PMDD)	Type of **depression** in which symptoms such as depressed mood, marked anxiety, affective lability, and anhedonia regularly occur during the **luteal** phase of the menstrual cycle RF: previous anxiety, depression, or other MH problems	1. In most menstrual cycles during past year, **5+ of symptoms** were present most of the cycle and during the **last week of luteal phase** • Begin to remit within a few days after the onset of menstruation • Absent in the week postmenses	A. At least 1 of the following was 1, 2, 3, or 4 (affective/ behavioral criteria as below) B. Disturbance markedly interferes with work or school or social activities/relationships C. Disturbance not merely an exacerbation of the symptoms of another disorder (depression, panic, dysthymia) D. Criteria A, B, C must be confirmed by prospective daily ratings during at least 2 consecutive symptomatic cycles	1. First line: **SSRI** 2. Second line: OCP, Xanax, GnRH agonists

Criteria for PMDD

Affective/Behavioral	Somatic/Physical
1. Depression 2. Anxiety, **tension, feeling of being "on edge"** 3. **Affective lability (suddenly sad)** 4. **Persistent/marked anger**, irritability, angry outbursts 5. Poor concentration 6. **Lethargy, fatigability, or marked lack of energy** 7. Marked **change in appetite, overeating**, or food cravings 8. Hypersomnia or insomnia 9. Feeling overwhelmed NOT: Changes in libido, social withdrawal, loss of motor skills	1. Breast tenderness 2. Abdominal bloating 3. Headache 4. **Joint pain** NOT: Diarrhea/constipation Swelling of extremities Fatigue

CHAPTER 50

Complications of Pregnancy

Recommended Supplemental Topics:

Erythroblastosis Fetalis (Fetal Hydrops), p 481

Intrauterine Growth Restriction, p 483

ABORTION

- **Abortion**: A pregnancy that ends spontaneously before the fetus has reached a viable gestational age (**before 20 weeks of gestation or <500 g**)

Disease	Etiology, Prevalence, Risk Factors	Clinical Symptoms and Signs	Diagnostics	Therapy, Prognosis, and Health Maintenance

Spontaneous abortion (SAB), also known as a miscarriage	Occurs in the absence of intervention
	Incidence:
	15%-25%
	Most:
	First 12 wk (80%)
	Fetal RF:
	Chromosomal abnormalities (MC: **trisomy**, monosomy X), congenital anomalies
	Maternal RF:
	1. **AMA**
	2. Previous SAB
	3. *Smoking*
	4. Maternal infection
	5. Anatomic anomalies (large **uterine fibroids**), Asherman syndrome
	6. Maternal disease
	7. Gravidity
	8. Fever
	9. Prolonged ovulation to implantation interval
	10. Prolonged time to achieving pregnancy
	11. BMI <18.5 or >25
	12. Celiac disease
		1. Vaginal bleeding
		2. Pain
		Type of abortion is defined by:
		1. Whether all products of conception (POC) have passed
		2. Whether cervix is dilated or not
			1. Quantitative β-hCG
			2. CBC
			3. Blood type
			4. Antibody screen
			5. U/S to assess fetal viability and placentation
				1. Expectant management (<13 wk): allow complete abortion to occur
				2. >13 wk: medical abortion
				  • Mifepristone (antiprogestin)
				  • Misoprostol (prostaglandin)
				    • 96% safe and effective
				3. D&C (first trimester)
				4. Dilation and evacuation (2nd)
				5. Surgery required if ineffective or excessive blood loss

Complete abortion	Known pregnancy with passage of **ALL products of conception before 20-wk gestation** Passage of all products of conception, no symptoms of pregnancy, test (−) Consider ECTOPIC	1. Can still present with small amount of vaginal bleeding Signs: 1. SSE: cervical os **closed** 2. BME: uterus **firm**, well contracted, **small for dates**, no CMT or adnexal tenderness	1. U/S: empty uterus	1. Does not require evacuation of uterus, still needs monitoring 2. Curettage is nearly 100% successful in completing early pregnancy losses Health maintenance: 1. Vaginal rest (no tampons, douches, or intercourse) to decrease the risk of infection
Missed abortion	Retention of **nonviable** pregnancy for a prolonged period (2+ menstrual cycles) Patient presents with smaller gestational size by examination than by dates and no fetal heart tones	1. Missed menses (**persistent amenorrhea**), (+) pregnancy test or inappropriately rising hCG levels 2. No bleeding 3. Loss of earlier symptoms of pregnancy (nausea, breast tenderness) Signs: 1. No cramping, 2-3 wk lag 2. SSE: cervical os **closed** 3. BME: uterus small for dates, no CMT or adnexal tenderness	1. UCG, hCG 2. CBC 3. Type and screen 4. Check fibrinogen weekly for coagulation 5. U/S: **fetal demise, no cardiac activity, macerated**	1. Resuscitation, observation 2. Serial exams (fever, tenderness) 3. Medical, surgical, or expectant management

OB/GYN

(continued)

(continued)

Disease	Etiology, Prevalence, Risk Factors	Clinical Symptoms and Signs	Diagnostics	Therapy, Prognosis, and Health Maintenance
Threatened abortion	Consider ectopic pregnancy in differential diagnosis Vaginal bleeding (first trimester) **before 20th wk** without loss of fluid or tissue (ie, a normal pregnancy with bleeding)	1. **Bleeding** 2. Followed by **cramping** abdominal pain (hours or days later) 3. Pain: may present as anterior and rhythmic cramps; persistent low backache with pelvic pressure, or dull midline suprapubic discomfort Signs: 1. SSE: cervical os **closed** 2. BME: uterus sized for date, **softer** than normal, no CMT or adnexal tenderness	1. (+) UPT 2. CBC 3. Type and screen	1. No intervention if no abnormality on imaging Prognosis: 1. 50% proceed to spontaneous 2. Increased risk of PTB and LBW
Inevitable abortion	Presents during **first 20 wk** of pregnancy with bleeding and crampy abdominal pain with associated dilated cervix or gush of fluid *without* passage of POC	1. **Heavy bleeding** • No passage of POC = no tissue 2. **Painful cramps** and contractions (reach peak as time passes) Signs: 1. SSE: cervical os **dilated** 2. BME: uterus hard, tender, gestational tissue felt through internal os, no adnexal tenderness	1. UCG, hCG 2. CBC 3. Type and screen 4. Transvaginal U/S—early pregnancy 5. U/S: IUP, slow cardiac activity, abnormal yolk sac, abnormal gestational sac	1. Resuscitation, observation 2. Serial exams 3. Send home to run natural course or may elect for surgical or medical management
Incomplete abortion	Involves passage of products of conception—"looks like pieces of skin or liver" Products of conception (POC) can be at the open os with partial expulsion Intermittent pain and continued bleeding	1. **Heavy bleeding** • Passage of POC = tissue 2. **Painful cramping**, cervical dilation Signs: 1. SSE: cervical os **dilated**, POCs seen 2. BME: uterus soft, tender, not well contracted, small for date	1. UCG, hCG 2. CBC 3. Type and screen 4. U/S: retained POCs, clot	1. Surgery but can be expectant management • Surgery not necessary for all women and is invasive 2. Persistent, heavy bleeding with significant pain requires D&C • If infection, uterine evacuation
Recurrent abortion	First: usually genetic Second: autoimmune (antiphospholipid lupus anticoagulant) or anatomic (Asherman) Etiology: **Septate uterus**, factor V Leiden, unexplained	1. More than 2 consecutive losses or >3 spontaneous losses before 20 wk 2. 2-3+ successive spontaneous abortions in the first or early second trimester (<15 wk)	1. **Anticardiolipin** and β-2 glycoprotein antibody status, PTT, Russell viper venom time 2. Check **antiphospholipid antibodies**—associated with recurrent pregnancy loss 3. Karyotyping—recommended for both parents when recurrent early abortion occurs (parent may carry a chromosomal translocation)	1. **17-hydroxyprogesterone** treatment—indicated if history of prior preterm birth 2. Lupus anticoagulant and anticardiolipin antibody syndromes: treat with low-dose **aspirin** + unfractionated **heparin** Recurrence: 1st pregnancy: 0%-30% 2nd pregnancy: 30% 3rd pregnancy: 33%

OB/GYN

Disease	Etiology, Prevalence, Risk Factors	Clinical Symptoms and Signs	Diagnostics	Therapy, Prognosis, and Health Maintenance
Induced abortion	Medical or surgical termination of an intact pregnancy before the time of viability Mifepristone and methotrexate: increase uterine contractility by reversing the progesterone-induced inhibition of contractions Misoprostol: stimulates the myometrium directly	1. Medical abortion—first trimester (up to 49 d gestation) and second trimester 2. Surgical abortion: recommended at >49 d gestation		1. First trimester • **Suction curettage** using vacuum aspiration 2. Second trimester • **Mifepristone** (RU 486) = antiprogestin PLUS • Methotrexate = antimetabolite • **Misoprostol** = prostaglandin OR • Suction or extraction forceps 3. Last line: D&E (dilation and evacuation) <u>Complications:</u> Uterine perforation, cervical laceration, hemorrhage, incomplete removal, infection
Septic abortion	Infected abortion, whether complete or incomplete More common with illegal abortions under unsterile conditions by persons who have little or no knowledge of medicine or anatomy	1. Bleeding, **Sanguinopurulent drainage (strawberry milkshake)** +/− passage of POCs 2. **Fever, chills** 3. **Abdominal pain** 4. Amenorrhea <u>Signs:</u> 1. Tachycardia, tachypnea, fever 2. SSE: cervical os **dilated** 3. BME: uterus soft and boggy, **cervix soft and dilated**	1. UCG, hCG 2. CBC 3. Type and screen 4. Blood and endometrial cultures 5. U/S: retained POCs, clot, foreign body	1. **Broad spectrum antibiotics** 2. Fluid resuscitation 3. **Uterine evacuation,** assess for perforation 4. Pain: NSAIDs, narcotics, sedation 5. Lacerations: iatrogenic 6. Immediate laparotomy if failure to respond, suspicion of pelvic abscess, or clostridial necrotizing myonecrosis Perforations: iatrogenic Bleeding: retained POCs, hematometra Fever: retained POCs (endometritis), pyometra, sepsis Rhogam (anti-D antibody): 300 mg IM × 1 (if RH negative) **Methergine** (methylergonovine): decreases postabortal bleeding **Doxycycline**: reduce postabortal infection Contraception

PLACENTAL ABRUPTION AND PLACENTA PREVIA

• Do not forget: if preterm between 24 to 34 weeks of gestation, give antenatal steroids FIRST! This reduces the risk of respiratory distress syndrome, intraventricular hemorrhage, and neonatal death

Disease	Etiology, Prevalence, Risk Factors	Clinical Symptoms and Signs	Diagnostics	Therapy, Prognosis, and Health Maintenance

Placenta previa	Placenta implants over the internal cervical os
	Most common abnormality of placental implantation
	RF:
	Advanced maternal age
	Multi*parity*, multiple gestation
	Prior previa
	C-section, D&C
	Smoking
		1. **Painless** vaginal bleeding
		  • Light spotting to profuse hemorrhage
		  • Latter half of pregnancy, occasional contractions
		Signs:
		1. Uterus: rarely tender
		2. Breech/transverse lie common, lie often abnormal or head high and tachycardic
		Consequences:
		PPH, required C-section, placenta accreta, increta, or percreta, abruption, and growth restriction
			1. If DX in first or second trimester, repeat U/S
			2. U/S: TAUS or **TVUS: placenta low**
			3. CBC, coags
			Type and screen
			4. Fetal HR monitoring
			DO NOT PERFORM DIGITAL—can cause severe hemorrhage
				1. Hospitalization for extended evaluation (initial)
				2. If 37+ wk with continued bleeding, delivery is indicated
				3. <36 wk expectant management
				Asymptomatic/mild (preterm <37 wk): close observation, steroids
				Mature fetus +/− contractions/labor: base on fetal testing, document lung maturity, schedule *36-38 wk*
				Delivery regardless of gestational age: severe fetal status, life threatening hemorrhage, bleeding *after 34 wk*

Placental abruption (abruptio placentae)	Premature separation of the placenta from its implantation site before delivery
	Vascular RF: preeclampsia, chronic **HTN**, smoking, cocaine, thrombophilia
	Maternal-fetal RF: prior abruption, **AMA, multiparity**, multifetal gestation, **prior uterine surgery,** polyhydramnios, fibroid, PPROM
		1. Painful vaginal bleeding
		  • Common, severe, constant with exacerbations
		  • Bleeding: absent or dark
		2. **Uterine tenderness**
		3. Frequent contractions
		Signs:
		1. **Uterine tenderness**
		  • Tender, "**woody**"
		2. *Fetal distress*
		3. Shock: tachycardia, hypotension
		4. Cervix: dilation from labor
			Clinical DX:
			1. U/S: exclude previa
			2. CBC, coags, fibrinogen, type and screen, BUN/Cr
			3. Tocodynamometry
			  • Fetal HR monitoring
			4. Monitor urine output/blood
			Profound coagulopathy and acute hypovolemia from blood loss
				1. **Immediate delivery** due to high risk of fetal death
				2. Preterm/no distress (34-37): induce labor
				3. Term/no distress: vaginal delivery
				4. Fetal distress: emergent CS regardless of age
				5. Fetal demise: vaginal delivery, induction;
				D&E if 2nd trimester
				Complications:
				Life-threatening PPH and increased need for emergent hysterectomy

Invasive placenta	Abnormally adherent placenta that has invaded the uterus—does not separate after delivery and bleeding can be torrential RF: **Prior uterine scar** (invasive placenta or C-section, placenta previa), AMA, multiparity	Suspect in patients with 1 or more prior cesarean deliveries and an anterior placenta previa	U/S: intraplacental lacunae, bridging vessels into the bladder, loss of the retroplacental clear space	1. Emergent **hysterectomy** 2. Transfusion

Further classified depending on the depth of invasion.

1. **Placenta accreta**—limited to endometrium (*accreta adheres* to myometrium)

2. Placenta increta—extends into myometrium (*increta invades* the myometrium)

3. Placenta percreta—invades beyond the uterine serosa (possibly bladder), *percreta penetrates*

ECTOPIC PREGNANCY, GESTATIONAL TROPHOBLASTIC DISEASE (MOLAR PREGNANCY, CHORIOCARCINOMA)

Disease	Etiology, Prevalence, Risk Factors	Clinical Symptoms and Signs	Diagnostics	Therapy, Prognosis, and Health Maintenance
Ectopic pregnancy	MC site: **Ampulla** RF: An **ECTOPIC** **A**MA n **E**xposure to DES in utero **Ci**garette smoking **T**ubal ligation **O**vulation induction **P**rior PID/ectopic **I**nfertility **C**ontraceptive IUD Classic: reproductive age women with AUB and/or pain + RF	**Abdominal pain** **Vaginal bleeding**—varies in amount/pattern, pain varies Associated symptoms: nausea, breast swelling, tenderness Ominous findings: vertigo/ syncope, shoulder pain worse with inspiration Prior to rupture: diagnosis based on lab and imaging After rupture: lab, imaging, + physical exam findings (50%-90% abdominal tenderness, CMT and adnexal tenderness, 1/3 pelvic mass, FEVER, bleeding or open cervix **Signs:** 1. Abdomen: generalized, unilateral tenderness 2. BME: cervical *os closed*, **adnexal tenderness, CMT** (50%), uterus **smaller than dates**	**(+) UPT** as early as 14 d after conception **Serum β-hCG** as early as 5 d, **repeat every 48 h** × 3 (inappropriately rising levels, less than 50% in 48 h = ectopic)* ***Serum rises until 60-90 d following last menses, then plateaus at 100k IU/L In normal pregnancy, it should rise 66% every 48 h, but if not, consider abnormal pregnancy Gestational sac on TVUS: 4-5 wk after LMP Yolk sac: 5-6 wk after LMP Fetal pole with cardiac activity: 5. 5-6 wk **β-hCG discriminatory zone**: lower limit of hCG to visualize pregnancy on U/S = **2000** Below this#, an early IUP may not be visualized on U/S, difficult to establish a diagnosis of ectopic, missed AB or IUP Serum progesterone: <5 ng/ mL = nonviable pregnancy (>20 = normal)	**Methotrexate IM 50 mg:** adverse effects include nausea/vomiting, dizziness, GI discomfort, stomatitis Check baseline kidney and liver function Must be motivated and willing to follow-up at days 4 and 7, then weekly until negative for hCG levels Gestational sac <3.5 mm No embryonic cardiac motion Initial hCG levels (best predictor of success): <5000 (92% success) Contraindications: Breastfeeding, immunodeficient, liver disease, blood dyscrasias, pulmonary disease, PUD, renal disease Exploratory laparotomy or laparoscopy if ruptured ectopic (eg, unstable VS/ exam, anemia)
Ruptured ectopic		1. Lightheaded, weak 2. Shoulder pain 3. Urge to defecate 4. Sudden acute or chronic pain 5. Collapse (**syncope**) Signs: 1. Pallor 2. Abdominal distention, rebound, rigidity, shifting dullness 3. Shock: tachycardia, hypotension 4. Tachypnea		
Gestational trophoblastic disease	RF: Asian race, 2+ miscarriages		FIGO criteria: • Plateau of 4 hCGs over 3+ wk • Rise of 3 weekly consecutive hCGs over 2+ wk (by at least 10%) • Persistently elevated hCG >6 mo after D&C • Histologic diagnosis of choriocarcinoma	

(continued)

OB/GYN

(continued)

Disease	Etiology, Prevalence, Risk Factors	Clinical Symptoms and Signs	Diagnostics	Therapy, Prognosis, and Health Maintenance
Molar pregnancy Partial mole: May contain fetus/ fetal parts, placenta/cord; triploid karyotype 69XXY, 69XXX, 69XYY resulting from fertilization of egg by dispermy; marked villi swelling; lower hCG levels, affect older patients, longer gestations, diagnosed as missed or incomplete abortions Complete moles: do not contain fetal or placental parts; diploid, resulting from fertilization of empty egg by single sperm (46XX, 90%) or by two sperm (X & Y = 46XY, 6%-10%); trophoblastic proliferation with Hydropic degeneration, larger uteri, pre-eclampsia, post-molar GTD	Presence of villi Excessively edematous immature placentas, including: complete Hydatidiform mole, partial Hydatidiform mole, and malignant INVASIVE mole (malignant, metastases) RF: History of previous mole, women at both age extremes, vitamin A and carotene deficiency, long term use of OCPs, previous unsuccessful pregnancies Presents during 11-25 wk gestation (avg 16 wk)	HX: 1-2 mo of amenorrhea: 1. 50% asymptomatic, 50% vaginal bleeding 2. **Vaginal bleeding:** Spotting to profuse hemorrhage as gestation advances 3. **Nausea, vomiting** significant Signs: 1. **Large uterus for dates (25%-50%)** Complications: Anemia, preeclampsia *(hypertension)*, hyperemesis, hyperthyroidism *(tachycardia)*	1. CBC, SCr, AST, type and screen, PT/PTT 2. **β-hCG levels:** +1 million IU/mL 3. **Sonogram (TVUS):** "snowstorm" • Hydropic chorionic villi 4. Elevated free-T4 and decreased TSH Moderate iron deficiency anemia No FHM NOTE: a single β-hCG value is not diagnostic for a molar pregnancy but will determine whether a TVUS will be helpful in confirming gestation (based on levels) Discriminatory zone (>1500): IUP easily identified	1. Chest x-ray: lungs (MC site of metastasis) 2. **Suction dilatation and curettage** (preferred) with preoperative cervical dilation (osmotic agent) OR • hysterectomy with ovarian preservation 3. **Repeat β-hCG 48 h after evacuation** • Repeat quantitative β-hCG every 1-2 wk until levels become undetectable (median: 7-9 wk), then monthly for 6 mo • Contraception: Depo Recurrent risk for molar pregnancy: 1%-2%
Nonmolar	No villi Includes: choriocarcinoma, placental site trophoblastic tumor, and epithelioid trophoblastic tumor			
Choriocarcinoma: most common type of trophoblastic neoplasm following a term pregnancy or miscarriage, only 1/3 of cases follow molar gestation	Placental tumors, aggressive invasion into myometrium and propensity to metastasize Cells follow early cytotrophoblast and syncytiotrophoblast	1. Irregular bleeding (spotting)—most common finding • Continuous or intermittent, sudden or massive hemorrhage • *After* any pregnancy	1. **Serum *β-hCG* levels (+) in reproductive age woman with h/o recent pregnancy required for diagnosis** 2. Hemogram 3. TVUS 4. CXR **DO NOT BIOPSY**	1. **Chemotherapy:** methotrexate or actinomycin D Most common metastases are: **lungs** and **vagina** Do not repeat evacuation—risk for perforation, bleeding, infection, or intrauterine adhesion!

OB/GYN

INCOMPETENT CERVIX

Disease	Etiology, Prevalence, Risk Factors	Clinical Symptoms and Signs	Diagnostics	Therapy, Prognosis, and Health Maintenance
Incompetent cervix (cervical insufficiency)	Inability of the uterine cervix to retain a pregnancy in the second trimester, in the absence of uterine contractions RF: Previous cervical trauma (**laceration**, D&C, **conization**, cold knife, laser, LEEP) from **history of CIN**, congenital Müllerian anomalies, or collagen d/o (Ehlers-Danlos), prior abortion	HX: previous midtrimester pregnancy loss: 1. **Painless cervical dilation** in the second trimester • **Absence of contractions**, infection, placental abruption, or uterine anomaly 2. Pelvic pressure, cramping, back pain, increased vaginal discharge 3. PPROM 4. Can be followed by prolapse and ballooning of membranes into the vagina and expulsion of the fetus	1. Sonogram: decreased cervical length <30 mm 2. Fetal fibronectin (fFN) testing (+) 3. Evaluate for infectious process: CBC, amniocentesis 4. Evaluate for placental abruption	1. **Cerclage placement**: reinforces a weak cervix by a purse-string suture • History of cervical insufficiency with cerclage placement • History of spontaneous PTB and **short cervical length <25 mm prior to 24 wk** • Painless dilation on exam Contraindications to Cerclage: bleeding, uterine contractions, ruptured membrane

PREGNANCY-INDUCED HYPERTENSION AND PREECLAMPSIA/ECLAMPSIA, GESTATIONAL DIABETES

Disease	Etiology, Prevalence, Risk Factors	Clinical Symptoms and Signs	Diagnostics	Therapy, Prognosis, and Health Maintenance
Mild gestational hypertension	Considered mild until the following thresholds are exceeded	1. Blood pressure • Systolic ≤160 mm Hg • Diastolic ≤110 mm Hg 2. Must make at least 2 readings at least 4 h apart		1. Treatment does not alter course of pre-eclampsia or diminish perinatal morbidity/mortality and should be avoided
Chronic (pre-existing) hypertension	HTN that was pre-existing, preceding pregnancy	1. HTN present <20 wk gestation or predating conception 2. Persistent >12 weeks postpartum	Work-up is the same as primary or secondary HTN depending on etiology	1. Uncomplicated Mild (140-150/90-100 mm Hg) • No treatment 2. Persistent (>150, 95-99 mm Hg) or organ damage • **Methyldopa** or Labetalol
Gestational (pregnancy induced) hypertension HTN diagnosed >20 wk gestation **in absence of proteinuria**	MCC: HTN during preg. RF: **Extremes of age, nulliparity,** chronic HTN, underlying vascular disease, multifetal gestation, obesity, **African American (3.5×)** RF for progression: 1. Gest age <34 wk 2. Mean SBP: >135 3. High serum uric acid	1. BP >140/90 2. No proteinuria or evidence of end-organ damage 3. Normotensive by 12 wk postpartum→ diagnosis changes to transient HTN of pregnancy (otherwise, considered Chronic HTN = 15% of cases)	Goal: Distinguish from pre-eclampsia 1. 24 h urine – r/o proteinuria 2. Eval. for severe signs: HA, visual changes, RUQ/epigastric pain, vag. Bleeding, dec. fetal movement 3. CBC w/diff, LFTs, SCr 4. Biophysical profile	BP <160/110 1. Expect. management 2. Bed rest: slows freq. but does not prevent progression 3. No HTN TX, but goal is 130-150/80-100 mm Hg 4. No seizure prophy. BP >160/110: anti-HTN drugs below + seiz. proph Health Maintenance 1. No weight lifting 2. Week/Bi-week visits, measure BP/urine prot. 3. Serial US q 3-4 wk

OB/GYN

(continued)

(continued)

Disease	Etiology, Prevalence, Risk Factors	Clinical Symptoms and Signs	Diagnostics	Therapy, Prognosis, and Health Maintenance
Preeclampsia Pregnancy-specific hypertensive disease with multisystem involvement Photopsia: flashes of light Scotomata: dark areas or gaps in visual field Pearl: Women who smoke cigarettes have lower risk than non-smokers	Typically occurs after 20 wk gestation in previous normo-tensive women Prevalence: 4.6% of pregnancies worldwide RF: **history of pre-eclampsia, pre-existing HTN** or DM, multifetal gestation, CKD, auto-immune (lupus, anti-phospho-lipid), **AMA** (40+), **nulliparity**	1. **New onset HTN:** BP >140/90 2. **+/- Proteinuria:** ≥ 300 mg/24-h or 1+ on urine dipstick **PLUS 1+ Severe Signs:** (a) severe HA, photopsia +/- scotomata, AMS (b) Pulm. edema (10%) (c) Severe, persistent RUQ pain or LFT >2xULN (d) PLT <100k (e) Renal insufficiency Exam Findings 1. Hyperreflexia Complications: acute pan-creatitis, stroke, seizures, placental abruption, cere-bral hemorrhage, hepatic rupture, renal failure, IGUR, oligohydramnios, CVD for mother	1. AST: 2× baseline (impaired liver function) 2. SCr: >1.1 or 2× baseline (renal insufficiency) 3. PLT <100K **(thrombocytopenia)**	1. Conservative mgmt. if no severe features and 24 to <34 wk gest. • Steroids and deliver if severe features develop • Continuous mat-fetal monitoring • Fluid management • If BP >150/100: IV **Labtetalol** or **Hydralazine** • All get **Mag-Sulfate** 2. Delivery for >37 wk NOT an indication for C-section 3. Urgent delivery if: Persistent/severe HA, visual abnormalities, upper/epigastric pain, AMS, or dyspnea Health Maintenance 1. Monitor BP 72 h PPM, then after 7-10 days 2. Low dose aspirin for some groups
Pre-eclampsia with severe features	New onset proteinuria, signifi-cant end organ dysfunction, or both AFTER 20+ wk gesta-tion in woman with pre-exist-ing (chronic) HTN	1. BP >160/110 2. Proteinuria: 2 g or 2+ on dipstick 3. Evidence of end organ damage	Magnesium Toxicity: 1. Loss of DTRs (7-10 mEq)/abs. patellar reflex 2. Bradypnea (10-13 mEq), <12/min 3 Cardiac conduction altered 4. Cardiac arrest (>25 mEq) -> Calc. gluconate	1. Only treat HTN if BP >160/110, otherwise deliver 2. Seizure prophylaxis: **Magnesium sulfate** +24 h postpartum • Check Mag q 6 h • CI: myasthenia gravis • AE: sweat, flush, warmth 3. DELIVERY
HELLP syndrome **H**: hemolysis (increased LDH, schistiocytes) **EL**: elevated LFTs **LP**: low platelets	Most severe form of pre-eclampsia • 15-20% have no preceding HTN or proteinuria • Incidence: 0.1-0.2% world-wide· Onset during 28-36 wk RF: previous pre-eclampsia or HELLP (nulliparity NOT a RF)	1. +/- **Proteinuria** 2. +/- **HTN** 3. MC: **RUQ/epigastric pain** 4. **Nausea/vomiting** 5. Headache 6. Visual changes 7. Jaundice/ascites Complications: hepatic hematoma or infarction or rupture, DIC (21%), placental abruption	1. CBC w/ platelet count • Increased LDH not required for diag-nosis, non-specific 2. Peripheral smear 3. AST (2xULN), bilirubin 4. Hepatic imaging (CT or MRI) if indicated	1. **Stabilize** mom, assess fetal condition, det. Freq. of delivery 2. **Treat severe HTN**: Same as pre-eclampsia 3. Seizure prophylaxis 4. **Delivery** (curative, only effective TX): fetal demise, NRFHT, Mat complications, >34 wk or <23 wk gestation 5. Maternal steroids NOT indicated
Superimposed severe preeclampsia	20% of women with chronic HTN not on meds and 35% women on meds DX after 20+ wk gest.	Preexisting CHRONIC HTN with BP above baseline, new onset proteinuria, new onset end-organ damage	BP monitoring: q 30 min 24-h urine Fetal surveillance Labs: AST, SCr, CBC	If severe → DELIVERY IV Apresoline (hydralazine) and Labetalol

Disease	Etiology, Prevalence, Risk Factors	Clinical Symptoms and Signs	Diagnostics	Therapy, Prognosis, and Health Maintenance
Eclampsia RF: nonwhite, **nulliparous**, low socioeconomic status	Onset of new convulsions or coma in a woman with preeclampsia, in absence of other neurologic causes Occurs preterm in 50% of pregnancies	1. NEW onset: coma or GTC seizures (antepartum intrapartum or postpartum) - most occur in first 48 h Preceding Signs: 1. HTN (75%) 2. HA - front/occip (66%) 3. Vision changes (27%) 4. RUQ pain (25%) 5. Asymptomatic (25%) Signs: 1. Ankle clonus	1. Neuroimaging: findings similar to posterior reversible leukoencephalopathy syndrome (PRES) 2. EEG – low utility Complications: cerebral hemorrhages	1. Seizure precautions 2. Treat severe HTN as above: consider Nifedipine for CVA prophy. 3. Seizure prophy. with Mag. sulfate 4. PROMPT Delivery Prognosis: 1. 10% will have repeated seizures 2. 90% of PP-seizures occur w/in 1 w
Gestational diabetes mellitus (GDM) *Non-stress test with amniotic fluid index **Data from National Diabetes Data Group	RF: history of prior GDM or impaired glucose tolerance, nonwhite, FH diabetes in first-degree relative, age >25 y/o, glycosuria at first prenatal visit, medical condition associated with DM (PCOS), multiple gestation, prior unexplained perinatal loss, pre-preg. BMI >30: Most common associated anomaly: cardiac Prevalence: 6-7% in US	Term is based on gestational age at diagnosis: diagnosis at 24-28 wk is gestational **Overt**: diagnosis occurs at first prenatal visit (early in pregnancy) = A1C 6.5% Complications: MC: **LGA/Macrosomia**, pre-eclampsia, shoulder dystocia, polyhydramnios, still birth	Screening at 24-48 wk gestation: 1. 1-h 50 g OGTT (+, if >140) if positive, then… 2. 3-h 100 g OGTT (+ if 2 elevated: 105,190, 165, 145)** If positive screening: 3. 24-h urine 4. Evaluation by ophthalmology 5. Fetal u/s and ECHO 6. EKG	1. Nutritional counseling and diet: 30 kcal/kg/d • If BMI > 30, 30-33% caloric restriction • Induce at 41 weeks 2. Insulin recommended, goal FBG <95 mg/dL • Avoid maternal hyperglycemia • Induce labor at 39 weeks 3. Twice weekly NST* starting at 32 weeks Health Maintenance: 1. 2 h 75 g OGTT at 6 & 12 weeks post-partum 2. Post-partum: half dose insulin regimen, assess at 6 and 12 wk (2-h GTT), then every 3 y

Diabetes in Pregnancy

Class	Age at Onset	Duration (Years)	Vascular Disease	
A (gestational)				
B	20+	<10	None	
C	10-19	10-19	None	
D	<10	>20	Benign retinopathy	30% have progression despite sugar control
F (5%)	Any	Any	Nephropathy (>500 mg protein)	50% develop preeclampsia (>300)
R	Any	Any	Proliferative retinopathy	
H	Any	Any	Heart/CAD	

RH-INCOMPATIBILITY AND ERYTHROBLASTOSIS FETALIS (FETAL HYDROPS)

• If enough fetal cells cross into the maternal blood, a maternal antibody response may be provoked. If these maternal antibodies cross the placenta, they then can enter the fetal circulation and destroy the fetal erythrocytes, causing hemolytic anemia

• Rh antigens are lipoproteins that are confined to the red cell membrane

• The major antigen in this group, Rh (D), or Rh factor, is of particular concern

- A woman who is lacking Rh(D) (otherwise known as Rh-negative) may carry an Rh-positive fetus if the fetus inherited the D antigen from the father → maternal IgG antibodies to the D antigen may develop and cross the placenta, causing hemolysis of fetal blood cells

- Rh alloimmunization generally occurs by 1 of 2 mechanisms: (1) after incompatible blood transfusion or (2) after fetomaternal hemorrhage between a mother and an incompatible fetus

- Predispositions to **fetomaternal hemorrhage** include spontaneous or induced abortion, amniocentesis, chorionic villus sampling, abdominal trauma (eg, due to motor vehicle accidents or external version), placenta previa, abruptio placentae, fetal death, multiple pregnancy, manual removal of the placenta, and caesarean section

- As little as 0.1 mL of Rh-positive cells can cause sensitization

- 30% of Rh-negative persons never become sensitized (nonresponders) when given Rh-positive blood. ABO incompatibility also confers a protective effect

- **IgG is capable of crossing the placenta** and destroying fetal Rh-positive cells

- Hemolysis produces heme → converted to bilirubin, both of which are neurotoxic

Disease	Etiology, Prevalence, Risk Factors	Clinical Symptoms and Signs	Diagnostics	Therapy, Prognosis, and Health Maintenance
Rh-incompatibility Or **Rh isoimmunization**	**Rh-negative women without Rh antibodies** who has had fetal-to-maternal transfusion of Rh-positive fetal red cells Amniocentesis, chorionic villus sampling (CVS), spontaneous/threatened abortion, ectopic pregnancy, dilation and evacuation, placental abruption, antepartum hemorrhage, preeclampsia, C-section, manual removal of placental and external version	HX: previous infant with hemolytic disease of the newborn Elevated bilirubin levels Jaundice: yellow skin and discoloration of the eyes	1. IgM initially elevated • Fetal Rh (+) • **Mother: Rh (−)** • (+) for anti-D antibodies on **Indirect Coombs test** 2. U/S findings: **fetal hydrops** due to decreased hepatic protein production 3. **Direct Coombs test** on baby 4. **Kleihauer-Betke smear**: determines amount of fetal blood in maternal circulation, especially in fetomaternal hemorrhage	1. 300 μg **RhoGAM** administration at *28 wk* routinely and *within 72 h* of delivering an Rh-positive baby, following spontaneous or induced abortion, following antepartum hemorrhage, amniocentesis, or CVS • If the father is Rh (−), RhoGAM unnecessary, since fetus Rh (−) and not at risk • Administration given following amniocentesis at any gestational age • The protection afforded by standard RhoGAM is dose-dependent and Rh-sensitization may still occur 2. If too early, treat anemia via **transfusion into the umbilical vein** (intrauterine intravascular fetal transfusion), then deliver
Erythroblastosis fetalis (fetal hydrops) Hemolytic disease of the newborn, HDN, HDFN	When fetal red blood cell destruction far exceeds production and severe anemia occurs	1. Edema 2. Ascites Signs: 1. Heart failure 2. Pericardial effusion 3. Kernicterus: deposition in basal ganglia	1. U/S: pleural effusion, ascites, pericardial effusion, increased skin thickness, polyhydramnios, or increased placental thickness • Assess fetal MCA flow by Doppler: high peak velocity blood flow near circle of Willis 2. Hyperbilirubinemia	

- Once antibody screening (+) for alloimmunization → follow-up with antibody titers at intake, 20 weeks, then every 2 to 4 weeks

- History of prior alloimmunization → no antibody titers needed because amniocentesis indicated (fetus at risk if it contains D-antigen)

INTRAUTERINE GROWTH RESTRICTION

Disease	Etiology, Prevalence, Risk Factors	Clinical Symptoms and Signs	Diagnostics	Therapy, Prognosis, and Health Maintenance
Intrauterine growth restriction (IUGR)	Fetus: (chromosomal abnormalities, fetal gender, genetic inheritance, TORCH infection) Placenta: (abnormal implantation or insertion of the cord, preeclampsia, placental insufficiency) Mother (diabetes, systemic lupus erythematosus, or cyanotic heart disease; smoking; abnormal uterine anatomy; low pregnancy weight gain) Etiology never determined: 40%	1. Pattern of aberrant and reduced fetal growth that is identified by prenatal U/S examination	1. Toxoplasmosis and CMV studies—not necessary	

CHAPTER 51

Female Reproductive Infections

Refer to Family Medicine for In-Depth Coverage of the Following Topics:

Chlamydia and Gonoccocal Infections, p 182

Refer to Internal Medicine for In-Depth Coverage of the Following Topics:

Genital Herpes, p 272
Syphilis, p 269

Recommended Supplemental Topics:

OB/GYN

CHANDELIER SIGN

Also known as cervical motion tenderness or excitation; a sign found on pelvic examination suggestive of pelvic pathology, indicative of pelvic inflammatory disease (PID), ectopic pregnancy, and is used to rule out appendicitis.

- On bimanual exam, the patient unexpectedly jumps as if jumping to grab the proverbial chandelier

VAGINITIS

Disease	Etiology, Prevalence, Risk Factors	Clinical Symptoms and Signs	Diagnostics	Therapy, Prognosis, and Health Maintenance
Trichomonas (trichomoniasis) (Fig. 51-1A)	15% of all vaginitis Protozoa, *T. vaginalis*	1. Increased vaginal discharge and odor 2. Dysuria, frequency, dyspareunia 3. Vulvar irritation, itching Signs: 1. Diffuse, thin, yellow-green to gray, adherent **frothy** discharge in vagina 2. Malodorous, musty (amine odor) 3. Cervix–hyperemic mucosa, friable cervix, **strawberry cervix** (*petechiae*)	1. Wet mount (saline microscopy): **motile trichomonads** (60%-70% sensitive) 2. pH: 5-6.5 (basic)	1. **2 g metronidazole** PO **single** dose or (500 mg BID × 7 d) • No ETOH 48 h • Most males asymptomatic • **Treat partner** 2. Resistant: 2 g Flagyl daily 7 d or 2 g Tinidazole once
Trichuriasis (whipworm)	*Trichuris trichiura*, a nematode or roundworm MC in tropical climates RF: Poor hygiene Transmission: Via food or hands contaminated with soil Eggs are passed with the infected person's stool and are infective 15-30 d after; ingestion via contaminated hands or food occurs and eggs hatch into the small intestine, releasing larvae that mature in the colon (lifespan 1 y)	Most asymptomatic: 1. Loose stool +/− mucous or blood 2. Nocturnal stooling 3. Abdominal pain Signs: 1. Pica 2. Finger clubbing Associated: Secondary anemia, colitis, **rectal prolapse**	1. Stool examination for eggs • "Barrel shape" with smooth thick walls and hyaline plug at ends 2. Proctoscopy or colonoscopy: worms protruding from bowel 3. PCR	1. One of the following: • Mebendazole 100 mg PO BID × 3 d • Albendazole 400 mg PO × 3 d • Avoid both in first trimester of pregnancy • Ivermectin 200 µg/kg/d PO Health maintenance: 1. Adequate disposal of feces, good sanitation, good hygiene, wash vegetables and fruits 2. Only mebendazole can be used in lactating women Prognosis: 1. Reinfection common
Bacterial vaginosis (Fig. 51-2A)	**MCC of vaginitis (40%-50%)** Path: **Gardnerella**, *Mycoplasmas* RF: New sex partner, smoking, IUD, frequent douching, pregnancy Disruption of normal flora from hydrogen to non-hydrogen-peroxide–producing lactobacilli, allowing proliferation of anaerobic bacteria	Mostly asymptomatic: 1. Increased vaginal discharge 2. Dysuria, Frequency, Dyspareunia 3. Noticeable **fishy discharge** after menses or intercourse 4. No itching Signs: 1. Thin, ivory to **gray discharge** 2. Homogenous, adherent 3. Distinctive fishy odor	Amsel criteria: 3 of 4 1. Thin, gray, homogenous discharge 2. Positive *whiff* test (KOH = amine odor) 3. *Clue cells* on saline microscopy (wet mount, >20%) 4. Elevated pH > 4.5 (basic)	1. **Metronidazole 500 mg PO BID × 7 d** 2. OR 3. **Vaginal metronidazole** (MetroGel) 0.75% gel QHS × 5 d • Consider partner TX if recurrent 4. Increases risk for PID and premature delivery

Disease	Etiology, Prevalence, Risk Factors	Clinical Symptoms and Signs	Diagnostics	Therapy, Prognosis, and Health Maintenance
Atrophic vaginitis (Fig. 51-1B)	Postmenopausal women Thinning vaginal epithelium after menopause	1. Dyspareunia 2. Thin vaginal discharge (clear or serosanguineous) 3. Vaginal pruritus, burning, soreness Signs: 1. Atrophic vulvar changes: smooth, shiny, pale, dry, thin 2. Scattered vaginal petechiae 3. Thin clear or brown discharge (leukorrhea) Associated: urinary tract infection, urge incontinence	Clinical DX: 1. **Vaginal cytology: greater % of parabasal cells** (more atrophy) 2. Vaginal pH: 5-7	1. Water soluble lubricants 2. **Topical vaginal estrogens (Premarin)** or Estrace cream 3. Oral estrogen
Vulvovaginal **candidiasis** (VVC, candida vaginalis) Also known as a yeast infection (Fig. 51-2B)	Second MCC of vaginitis (20%-25%) Path: **C. albicans**, C. glabrata, C. tropicalis RF: High-dose OCP, diaphragm use, DM, recent ABX, pregnant, immune suppression, tight fitting clothing	1. Vulvar or vaginal **itching** and **burning**, external **dysuria** 2. Dyspareunia 3. Odorless thick **cottage cheese** curd-like discharge Signs: 1. Erythema of vulva and vagina 2. Excoriations from scratching	1. **Wet mount** (saline or 10% KOH): **budding yeast** (snowman) 2. Gram stain: pseudohyphae or tangles **(spaghetti and meatballs)** 3. Vaginal culture (+) for yeast 4. Microscopy only (+) in 50% 5. pH: <4.7 (acidic)	1. **Fluconazole** 150 mg PO once—repeat in 1 wk • Treat uncircumcised partners • Short-course topical Azole (1-3 d) for 80%-90% of patients 2. Recurrent—weekly topical/PO • 5% recurrence rate 3. Resistant—boric acid 600 mg gel capsules TID × 7 d

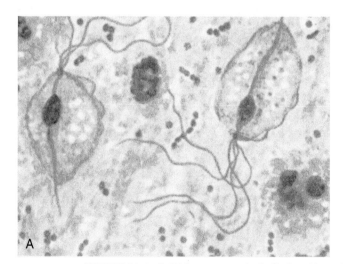
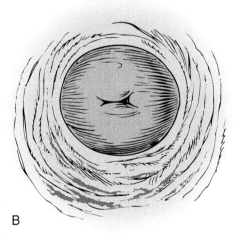

FIGURE 51-1. A, *Trichomonas vaginalis.* **B,** Atrophic vaginitis occurs when estrogen production is low after menopause, characterized by itching, burning, dryness, and painful urination. The vaginal mucosa may be pale, dry, or bleed easily. There may or may not be blood tinged discharge. (**A,** From Cornelissen CN. *Lippincott Illustrated Reviews Flash Cards: Microbiology.* Philadelphia: Wolters Kluwer Health; 2015. **B,** From Lewis P, Foley D. *Health Assessment in Nursing.* 2nd ed. Philadelphia: Lippincott Williams & Wilkins; 2003.)

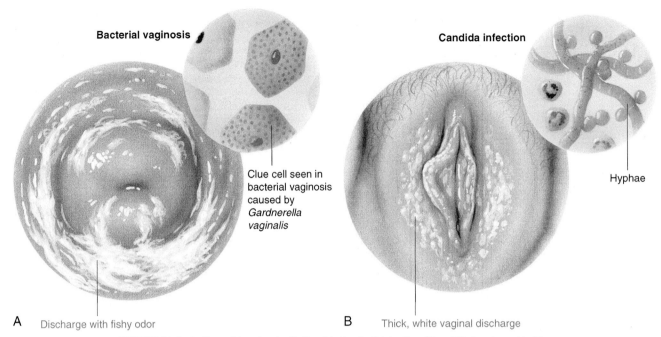

Bacterial vaginosis

Clue cell seen in bacterial vaginosis caused by *Gardnerella vaginalis*

A   Discharge with fishy odor

Candida infection

Hyphae

B   Thick, white vaginal discharge

FIGURE 51-2. **A**, Bacterial vaginosis. **B**, Candida (vaginal) infection. (**A** and **B**, Asset provided by Anatomical Chart Co.)

HUMAN PAPILLOMA VIRUS

- **Condyloma:** refers to an infection of the genitals
- **Condyloma acuminatum:** genital warts caused by HPV
- **Condyloma lata:** white lesions associated with secondary syphilis

Disease	Etiology, Prevalence, Risk Factors	Clinical Symptoms and Signs	Diagnostics	Therapy, Prognosis, and Health Maintenance
Human papillomavirus (genital warts)	MC: *Condylomata acuminatum* Low-risk types: 6, 11 (genital warts) Anogenital warts: most common viral STD in the US Incubation period: 3 wk-8 mo Causes nearly 100% of cervical cancers, most significant RF for cervical cancer	1. Most asymptomatic Signs: 1. **Flesh-colored, papillary exophytic lesions on genitalia**, including penis, vulva, scrotum, perineum, perianal skin 2. External warts - small bumps, or flat, verrucous, or pedunculated 3. Most common sites in women: vulva, perianal area, vagina 4. Most common sites in men: penis, scrotum	Clinical DX: 1. RPR/VDRL–r/o syphilis 2. HIV 3. HPV viral typing not recommended daily 4. Shave or punch biopsy confirms, if necessary • Uncertain diagnosis, poor response to therapy, atypical appearance, immunocompromised	1. Most resolve spontaneously–2 y • Treat to improve symptoms and remove warts 2. Podophyllin or trichloroacetic acid (TCA)–provider treat 3. **Podofilox** or maimed (Aldara) cream–patient treat 4. Surgery: cryotherapy, surgical excision, electrocautery, laser, intralesional interferon 5. Recurrence–often? 6. *Gardasil* (quadrivalent) 7. 6, 11 (warts) 8. 16, 18 (cervical CA) 9. For males and females 9-26 y/o

PELVIC INFLAMMATORY DISEASE

Disease	Etiology, Prevalence, Risk Factors	Clinical Symptoms and Signs	Diagnostics	Therapy, Prognosis, and Health Maintenance

Pelvic inflammatory disease (acute *salpingitis*)	Infection that ascends from the cervix or vagina to involve the endometrium and/or fallopian tubes
	MCC:
	N. gonorrhoeae, C. trachomatis, genital mycoplasmas (*M. hominis, U. urealyticum, M. genitalium*)
	RF:
	Presence of endocervical infection, bacterial vaginosis, history of salpingitis (PID), or recent vaginal douching, recent insertion of IUD, D&C or C-section
		1. **Mucopurulent malodorous vaginal discharge** (cervicitis)
		2. Midline abdominal pain
		3. Abnormal vaginal bleeding
		Progresses →
		4. **Bilateral lower abdominal and pelvic pain**
		• Dull, aching
		• May be absent
		• *Abnormal uterine bleeding* coincides with pain (40%)
		• Duration <3 wk
		5. **Nausea, vomiting**
		6. Urethritis (20%): dysuria
		7. Proctitis: anorectal pain, tenesmus, rectal discharge or bleeding
		8. Fever >38° C (33%)
		Signs:
		1. Speculum exam: yellow endocervical discharge, easily induced bleeding
		2. Bimanual exam:
		  • **Uterine or adnexal tenderness and swelling 50%)**
		  • **Cervical motion tenderness: by stretching the adnexae**
		3. Rebound, guarding
		4. Abdominal tenderness (if peritonitis develops)
			1. Labs
			• ESR elevated >15 mm/h(75%)
			• Leukocytosis (60%)
			• Serum β-hCG
			• NAATs: r/o GC/CT
			• Gram stain and culture of endocervical secretions
			2. U/S: enlarged fallopian tubes with fluid in cul-de-sac
			Rule:
			1. If cultures (+), r/o by laparoscopy or endometrial biopsy
			2. Laparoscopy: last line to r/o acute appendicitis, ectopic pregnancy, corpus luteum bleeding, and ovarian tumor (do if unilateral pain or mass)
			• Other indications: absence of lower genital tract infection, missed period, (+) pregnancy test, failed response to therapy
			3. Endometrial biopsy—r/o endometritis
			4. Complications/sequelae: Tuboovarian abscess, infertility, ectopic pregnancy, chronic pelvic pain, recurrent salpingitis
				1. *Outpatient*
				• IM **ceftriaxone** 250 mg once + PO **doxycycline** 100 mg BID × 14 d
				2. +/− PO Flagyl 500 mg BID × 14 d
				3. *Inpatient*
				• Consider hospitalization if
				  • Diagnosis uncertain, ectopic and appendicitis cannot be r/o
				  • Patient pregnant
				  • Pelvic abscess suspected
				  • Severely ill or nausea and vomiting preclude outpatient management
				  • HIV positive
				  • Unable to follow or tolerate outpatient regimen
				  • Failed to respond to outpatient therapy
				• **Doxycycline + IV cefotetan or cefoxitin** × 48 h until condition improves, then PO doxycycline 100 mg BID × 14 d
				• **Clindamycin + gentamicin daily**, if normal renal function, × 48 h until condition improves, then PO doxycycline 100 mg BID × 14 d

Fitz-Hugh-Curtis syndrome Perihepatitis	Pleuritic upper-abdominal pain and tenderness (RUQ) in 3%-10% of women with PID Chlamydial salpingitis	1. SX arise during or after onset of PID and may overshadow lower abdominal symptoms Signs: 1. RUQ tenderness 2. Adnexal tenderness and cervicitis	1. LFTs normal 2. RUQ U/S normal 3. Laparoscopy: "violin-string" adhesions over the liver	
Tuboovarian abscess				1. **Clindamycin** rather than doxycycline for continued therapy provides better anaerobic coverage 2. Surgery—drain abscess

OB/GYN

CHANCROID AND LYMPHOGRANULOMA VENEREUM

Disease	Etiology, Prevalence, Risk Factors	Clinical Symptoms and Signs	Diagnostics	Therapy, Prognosis, and Health Maintenance
Chancroid (Fig. 51-3A)	MC cause: Gram-negative *Haemophilus ducreyi* Age 15-19 y/o	1. **Painful** chancre • Starts as papule → pustule → ulcer within a few weeks 2. **Painful lymphadenopathy** (30%-60%) (Fig. 51-3B) • leads to bubo formation 3. Dysuria and dyspareunia in females Signs: 1. Multiple, painful, punched-out ulcers with undermined borders 2. +/− Abscess formation	1. Serologic testing for syphilis - RPR/VDRL 2. Culture and gram stain of fluctuant lymph node or ulcer for *H. ducreyi*	1. **1 g azithromycin** 2. Fluctuant inguinal lymph nodes should be incised and drained
Lymphogranuloma venereum (LGV) (Fig. 51-3C)	MCC: **Chlamydia trachomatis** Primary infection of **lymphatics and lymph nodes** RF: MSM (unprotected receptive anal intercourse), HIV, HCV	HX: proctitis with or without anal lesions: 1. First stage: *painless* genital ulcer, 3-12 d after infection 2. Second stage: 10-30 d later; unilateral lymphadenitis or lymphangitis with tender inguinal or femoral LAD 3. Enlarged nodes called buboes, which are painful Signs: 1. Tender lymphadenopathy at the femoral and inguinal lymph nodes, separated by a groove made by Poupart ligament ("sign of the groove")	1. Serologic testing for syphilis–RPR/VDRL	1. Drainage of buboes or abscesses by needle aspiration or incision 2. **Doxycycline 100 mg** PO **BID × 21 d**
Granuloma inguinale (donovanosis) (Fig. 51-3D)	Chronic ulcerative debilitating disease that affects the genitals Cause: Gram-negative, non-motile, *Klebsiella granulomatis* Affects people living in tropical and subtropical areas Transmission: Sexually, fecally? Incubation: 3 d-3 mo	1. Single or multiple papules or nodules develop and grow into a painless ulcer that may extend into the adjacent tissues and moist folds forming "kissing lesions" • MC: penis, scrotum, glans • MC (female): labia, perineum Signs: 1. Beefy red, easily bleeding, foul smelling ulcers with granulation tissue • Ulcers have a hypertrophic or verrucous border resembling condylomata, but may present as soft, red nodules that can ulcerate 2. May become necrotic and have copious gray, foul smelling exudate	1. Tissue biopsy or peripheral smear: intracellular Donovan bodies	1. Azithromycin (first line) × 3 wk 2. May add IV gentamicin 1 mg/kg q 8 h Complications: Relapse 6-18 mo after treatment, secondary bacterial infection, fistula, abscess formation

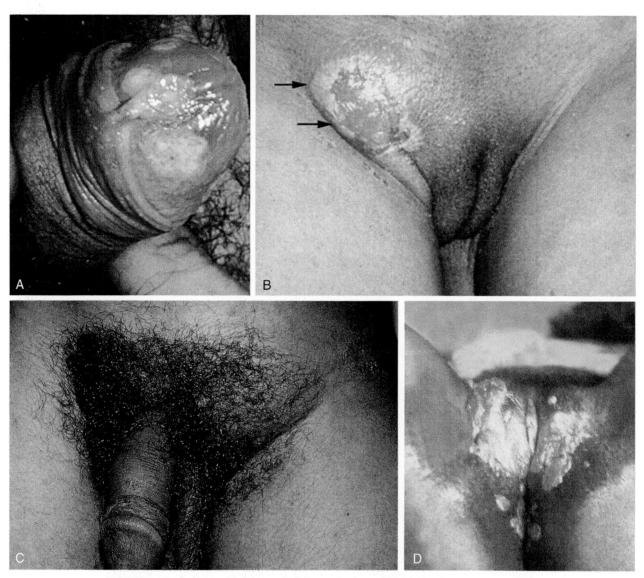

FIGURE 51-3. A, Chancroid of the penis. **B,** Inguinal buboes. **C,** Painful inguinal lymphadenopathy seen in lymphogranuloma venereum (LGV). **D,** Granuloma inguinale–characterized by a keratotic ulceration. (**A,** From Nath JL. *Using Medical Terminology,* 2nd ed. Wolters Kluwer; 2013. **B,** Courtesy of the Armed Forces Institute of Pathology. **C,** Image from Rubin E, Farber JL. *Pathology.* 3rd ed. Philadelphia: Lippincott Williams & Wilkins; 1999. **D,** From Schalock PC, Hsu JT, Arndt KA. *Lippincott's Primary Care Dermatology.* Philadelphia: Wolters Kluwer Health; 2011.)

OB/GYN

MOLLUSCUM CONTAGIOSUM, SCABIES, AND PEDICULOSIS PUBIS

Disease	Etiology, Prevalence, Risk Factors	Clinical Symptoms and Signs	Diagnostics	Therapy, Prognosis, and Health Maintenance
Molluscum contagiosum (Fig. 51-4A)	Poxvirus that causes a chronic localized infection **Humans are the only known host** Genotype 1 predominant (90% of cases) Affects <5% of children in the US RF: 1. Participation in contact sports 2. Immunodeficiency 3. Incubation: 1 wk-6 mo Transmission: • Direct skin-skin contact • Autoinoculation by scratching or touching a lesion • Fomite-spread on bath sponges or towels • Possibly swimming pool use • Sexually transmitted	1. Flesh-colored, dome-shaped papules 2. +/− itchy 3. Appears anywhere on the body *except* the palms and soles (MC: trunk, axillae, antecubital and popliteal fossa, crural folds) Signs: 1. 2-5 mm smooth, rounded, shiny papule with central umbilication 2. White to yellow amorphous structures 3. +/− Pruritus Complications: 1. Conjunctivitis, if on eyelid 2. Molluscum dermatitis	Clinical DX: **Biopsy** (confirms): reveals keratinocytes with eosinophilic cytoplasmic inclusion bodies (molluscum or Henderson-Paterson bodies)	1. Lesions resolve spontaneously in immunocompetent individuals within 2 mo; infection clears within 6-12 mo 2. Treat on case-by-case basis • Full skin examination first, otherwise autoinoculation may occur • Never use topical agents on oral mucosa or eyelids 3. First-line therapies • *Cryotherapy* • AE: scarring, temporary or permanent hypopigmentation, painful • *Curettage* • Discomfort, not suitable for all children, time consuming • Cantharidin • Must be applied by clinician • AE: burning, pain, erythema, itching, postinflammatory dyspigmentation • Podophyllotoxin (Podofilox 0.5%) • Antimitotic agent • AE: local erythema, burning, itching, inflammation, erosions Health maintenance: 1. Not necessary to remove children from daycare or school; lesions should be covered with clothing or watertight bandage 2. Avoid bathing child with others and do not share towels or sponges
Scabies (Fig. 51-4C)	Mite that burrows Caused by *Sarcoptes scabiei* Subspecies infecting cats and dogs distinct from those infecting humans Type-IV hypersensitivity to mite, mite feces (scybala), and mite eggs RF: • Crowded conditions • Winter > summer Transmission: Direct contact, including sexual	1. Severe itching, especially at night 2. Symptoms begin 3-6 wk after infestation unless previously infected (then 1-3 d after reinfestation) 3. Generalized swelling may occur Signs: 1. Erythematous papular lesions, often excoriated, tipped with hemorrhagic crusts 2. Located on wrists, between fingers, and in genital area • Flexor wrist area • Extensor elbow or knee area • Anterior and posterior axillary folds • Skin adjacent to nipples • Periumbilical areas, waist, male genitalia • Lower half of buttocks or adjacent thighs 3. Burrows are thin, gray-red, or brown	Clinical DX: 1. Skin scraping 2. Dermoscopy 3. Adhesive tape test Diagnostic criteria: 1. Widespread itching, worse at night, spares the head (except in infants and young children); out of proportion 2. Pruritic eruption with characteristics lesions and distribution 3. Other household members with similar symptoms	1. Topical **permethrin 5% cream** • Apply neck down and rinse after 8-14 h • Preferred in pregnancy 2. Oral ivermectin 200 µg/kg single dose • Not for pregnancy or lactating women or children <15 kg • First line for major outbreaks in nursing homes or other similar facilities • May be repeated after 1-2 wk Complications: 1. Secondary staph infections 2. Impetigo 3. Ecthyma 4. Paronychia 5. Furunculosis

Disease	Etiology, Prevalence, Risk Factors	Clinical Symptoms and Signs	Diagnostics	Therapy, Prognosis, and Health Maintenance
Pediculosis pubis (Fig. 51-4B)	Specifically infests humans *Phthirus pubis* Transmission: • Sexually transmitted • Fomites • Can extend beyond the pubic area to involve eye lashes • Life span of females: 3-4 wk; lays max of 3 eggs/d up to 26+ Incubation: 6-8 d Crawling lice die within 48 h of being removed from a host	1. Itching in the pubic area or axillae 2. Can affect any hair-bearing area, though scalp usually spared in most cases 3. +/− Inguinal lymphadenopathy Signs: 1. Live lice and nits attached to hair	Clinical DX: Microscopy: shows nits (louse eggs), confirmator	1. Topical **permethrin 1% cream** • Dry area completely before applying • Apply to all affected areas • Remove nits with fingernails, nit combs, or tweezers • Apply to area 10 min, then wash off 2. Pyrethrins with piperonyl butoxide • Apply to affected area and wash off after 10 min 3. If eyelashes are affected • Apply petroleum jelly or occlusive eye ointment for 8-10 d twice daily • Mechanically remove nits Health maintenance: 1. Abstain from sexual contact until reevaluated to rule out persistent infection 2. Treat all sexual contacts; nonsexual household contacts do not need to be treated if absent clinical findings 3. Wash bedding with hot water and dry with heat 4. Follow-up for reevaluation in 9-10 d, retreat if lice still present
Bartholin (vestibular) gland abscess (Fig. 51-4D)	MC complication of GC after PID; also caused by *Chlamydia trachomatis* Obstructed Bartholin duct (located in the vulva) that becomes infected Bartholin glands— Homologues of the bulbourethral glands in males Function: to secrete mucus to provide vaginal and vulvar lubrication Pathogens: • MRSA • **E. coli** (most common) • *N. gonorrhoeae* and *C. trachomatis*	1. Severe unilateral labial pain and swelling 2. +/− Purulent exudate from gland 3. Unable to walk, sit, or have sex Signs: 1. Absence of fever 2. No hemodynamic changes 3. Large, tender, soft, or fluctuant palpable Bartholin mass 4. Surrounding erythema (cellulitis) and edema (lymphangitis) Versus *Bartholin cyst*: 1. Painless 2. Asymptomatic or some discomfort during sex, sitting, or walking Signs: Soft, painless mass in posterior aspect of vaginal introitus	Clinical DX: 1. Biopsy—any age, if malignancy suspected (RF: 40+ years, solid mass, fixed, unresponsive or worsening) 2. Cultures for aerobic bacteria—NAAT testing	1. I&D with placement of a word catheter under local anesthesia • Insertion of inflatable bulb through stab incision × 4-6 wk • Silver nitrate ablation 2. Antibiotics for patients with risk factors or clinical signs of infection • Bactrim DS BID × 7 d (first line) • Augmentin + clindamycin × 7 d • 2nd or 3rd generation cephalosporin or FQ AND clindamycin or doxycycline 3. For spontaneous rupture, consider warm compresses or sitz baths 4. If infection present or advancing cellulitis, I&D with inpatient care and IV antibiotics • Treat underlying chlamydia or gonorrhea if present 5. Gland excision (definitive) Vs. Cyst 1. No intervention if asymptomatic 2. Age 40+ • I&D recommended with biopsy to r/o malignancy

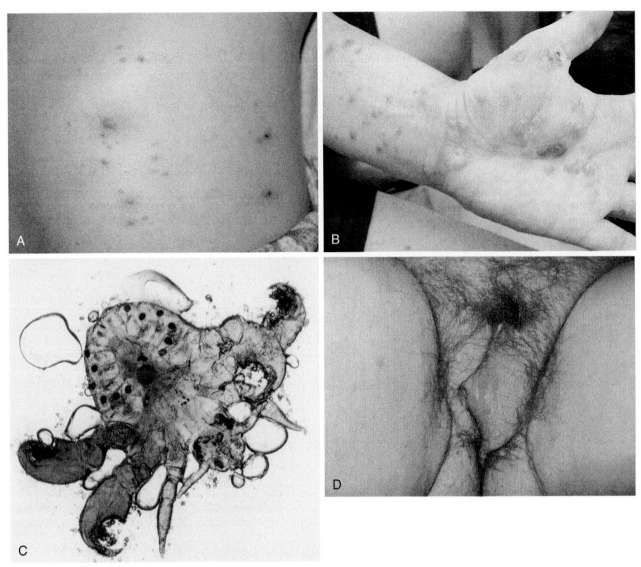

FIGURE 51-4. **A**, Molluscum contagiosum. **B**, Scabies. **C**, Pediculosis pubis on microscopy. **D**, Bartholin gland abscess. (**A**, From White AJ. *The Washington Manual of Pediatrics*. Philadelphia: Wolters Kluwer Health; 2017. **B**, From Anderson MK. *Foundations of Athletic Training*. Philadelphia: Wolters Kluwer Health; 2017. **C**, From Sweet RL, Gibbs RS. *Atlas of Infectious Diseases of the Female Genital Tract*. Philadelphia: Lippincott Williams & Wilkins; 2005. **D**, From Sherman S, Cico SJ, Nordquist E, et al. *Atlas of Clinical Emergency Medicine*. Philadelphia: Wolters Kluwer; 2016.)

CHAPTER 52

Female Reproductive Neoplasms

Breast Cancer—refer to Chapter 53, *Breast Disorders.*

Recommended Supplemental Topics:

Lichen Simplex Chronicus, p 497

Lichen Sclerosus, p 498

Vulvar Vestibulitis Syndrome, p 498

Breast Mass, p 499

OVARIAN NEOPLASMS

- Staging is surgical
- Debulking: benefit to removing some, not all of the tumor
- No effective screening tool, diagnosis does not affect overall survival rate

- Tumor markers are used to monitor, not diagnose
- 10% to 15% have family history of BRCA1 or BRCA2 mutation
- 5% to 10% have family history of ovarian cancer
- Most deadly of all gyn malignancies: 1.5% to 2.0% lifetime risk

Disease	Etiology, Prevalence, Risk Factors	Clinical Symptoms and Signs	Diagnostics	Therapy, Prognosis, and Health Maintenance
Ovarian neoplasms (ovarian cancer)	MC: Germ cell tumors (35%) Premenopausal: most likely benign adnexal masses (follicular cysts, endometriomas), small (~3 cm) **Postmenopausal: most likely *malignant*** (avg age: 63 y/o), (~10 cm) RF: 1. Nulliparity 2. White race 3. **Early menarche** 4. **Late menopause** (more ovulation cycles) 5. Family history 6. Inherited mutation (BRCA1/2 or Lynch)	HX: First-degree relative with breast or ovarian cancer Ascites: 1. **"*Bloating*"** (abdominal distension), early satiety, change in bowel habits 2. Evidence of **abdominal** or distant metastases Signs: 1. If >50, usually a **nodular** or **fixed solid pelvic mass** 2. Associated: Sister Mary Joseph nodule (metastatic implant in umbilicus)	1. U/S: blood flow within mass 2. Inhibin A and B (a) If <30: AFP, hCG, LDH (b) If 30-50: Ca-125, if FH (+) (c) If >50: CA-125, CA 19-9, +/− DEA 3. **CA-125**: >200 if premenopausal and <35 if *postmenopausal* *Note: >50% of stage I cancers will have a normal CA-125	**Simple cyst**—TX based on size and symptomatology Premenopausal: Functional—no TX or repeat TVS in 6-8 wk if symptomatic/persistent or large Postmenopausal: Benign—check CA-125 and repeat TVS, observe if no growth and normal CA-125; otherwise remove **Complex cyst** Premenopausal: Remove if symptomatic or persistent Postmenopausal: ALWAYS remove **Solid/predom-solid** Premenopausal: ALWAYS REMOVE Postmenopausal: ALWAYS REMOVE First-line chemo: IV **carboplatin** and **paclitaxel**

OB/GYN

Prognosis for Ovarian Cancer

>75% diagnosed with stage 3 or 4 (disease in upper abdomen) 75% will have complete response to surgery and chemo 75% will recur Recurrent ovarian cancer is incurable	5-y survival: Tumor **STAGE** is most important Stage 1: 90% Stage 2: 70% Stage 3/4: 25%	Protective factors: 1. Oral contraceptives (50% reduction) 2. Tubal ligation 3. BSO (bilateral salpingo-oophorectomy) 4. **Breastfeeding** 5. Chronic anovulation 6. Anything that reduces the number of ovulations: pregnancy, late menarche, early menopause

CERVICAL CARCINOMA AND CERVICAL DYSPLASIA

- Cervical cancer is the most common gynecologic malignancy in the world (third most common in the US, second most common cause of death from gyn malignancies)

- Graded based on extent of involvement of the epithelial layer but does not extend below the basement membrane (Fig. 52-1)

- Carcinoma in situ (CIS) represents abnormal cells involving the entire epithelium to the basement membrane

Disease	Etiology, Prevalence, Risk Factors	Clinical Symptoms and Signs	Diagnostics	Therapy, Prognosis, and Health Maintenance
Cervical carcinoma In cancer, the cells invade beyond the basement membrane. In microinvasive cancer, they invade less than 3 mm	Bimodal: 35-39, 60-64 RF: **HPV exposure,** early coitarche, multiple sex partners, a sex partner with multiple sex partners, history of HPV or other STDs, **immunosuppression,** *smoking,* low socioeconomic status, lack of regular Pap smears	1. Postcoital bleeding 2. Vaginal bleeding and discharge 3. Dyspareunia	1. Abnormal cytology, HPV (+) 2. Gross lesion	Stage 1: conservative, simple, or radical hysterectomy Stage 2 +: chemo +/− radiation 5-y survival— Stage 1: 85%-90% Stage 2: 65% Stage 3: 29% Stage 4: 21%
Cervical dysplasia MCC: **HPV (types 16** and 18) most common and carcinogenic **Type 18** most common with **adenocarcinoma** 100% of CIN and 90% of invasive lesions	Most transient, regress in 2 y Persistent HPV infection triggers HPV is not enough to cause cervical cancer by itself—requires *cofactors:* smoking, sex hormones, OCP (>5 y), dietary, immunosuppression (lupus), HIV RF: Old age, race (African American, Hispanic), low economic status, low education level Behavioral: increased # sexual partners, early coitus, SMOKING, long-term contraception use Gyn: multiparous, early parity, history of STD, lack of routine screening, immunosuppression			Indications for conization (LEEP or cold knife cone): 1. Unsatisfactory colposcopy, including inability to visualize the entire transformation zone 2. Positive endocervical curettage 3. Pap smear indicating adenocarcinoma in situ 4. Cervical biopsies that cannot rule out invasive cancer 5. Substantial discrepancy between Pap smear and biopsy results

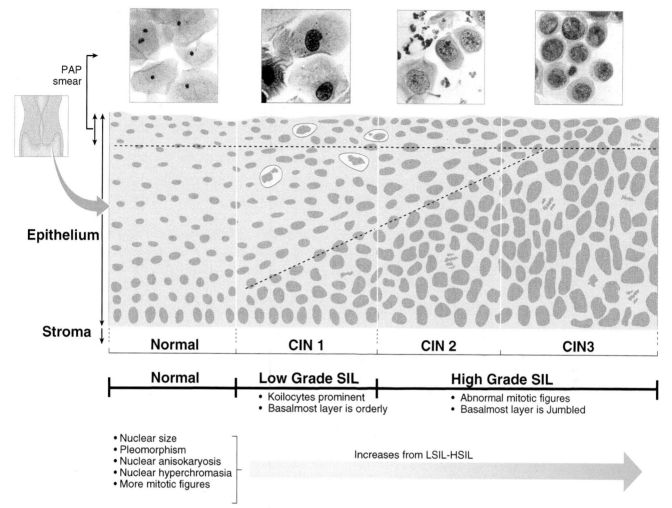

FIGURE 52-1. The Bethesda System for staging cervical cancer. The Bethesda System, which utilizes Pap smear results of the cervix, was introduced in 1988 and established in Bethesda, Maryland. It has since been revised in 1991 and 2001. Cytopathology is seen above. CIN 1 is the most common and benign form of cervical intraepithelial neoplasia (CIN). (From Strayer DS, Rubin E. *Rubin's Pathology*. Philadelphia: Wolters Kluwer Health; 2015.)

Cytology Results

Finding		Recommended Next Steps
ASC-US	Atypical squamous cells of undetermined significance	Repeat cytology at 6 and 12 mo → if both negative, return to routine screening If either (+) → colposcopy
AGC	Atypical glandular cells of undetermined significance	Colposcopy with biopsy of lesions
LSIL	Low-grade intraepithelial lesions	Colposcopy with biopsy of lesions
HSIL	High-grade intraepithelial lesions	Colposcopy with biopsy of lesions

- Colposcopy: diagnostic procedure that evaluates abnormal tissue of the cervix, vagina and vulva for lesion detection and staging

Biopsy Results/CIN Staging System

CIN I	Mild dysplasia		• Serial monitoring with colposcopy
CIN II	Moderate dysplasia		• Prophylactic hysterectomy
CIN III/stage 0	Carcinoma in situ (severe dysplasia)	Noninvasive "precancerous" lesion where tumor cells are present but have not penetrated the basement membrane and spread into local tissue	Must be removed due to high risk of invasive carcinoma transformation • LEEP (loop electrosurgical excision procedure): if margins are negative, follow-up in 1 y for repeat Pap • Positive margins: repeat Pap in 6 m +/− biopsy • Prophylactic hysterectomy

- Prophylactic hysterectomy with concomitant radiation and chemotherapy is recommended for patients with lesions <4 cm that are confined to the cervix or upper ⅔ of vagina
  - Usually for older women who do not plan to have children in the future

Screening for Cervical Cancer

Population	USPSTF	ACS/ASCCP/ASCP
Age <21	No screening	No screening
21-29	Cytology q 3 y	Cytology q 3 y
30-65	Cytology q 3 y OR Cytology + HPV test q 5 y	Cytology + HPV q 5 y (preferred) OR Cytology q 3 y (acceptable)
65+	Against screening, if prior adequate screening	Adequate screening + no HX of CIN2+ last 20 y = no screening Do not resume screening even if new sexual partner
Posthysterectomy	Against screening, if total* with removal of cervix, no HX of CIN 2 or 3 or cervical cancer *not subtotal	Against screening, if total with removal of cervix, no HX of CIN 2+ or cervical cancer Do not resume screening even if new sexual partner Evidence of prior negative screening not required
Vaccinated	Continue to be screened	Screening does not change based on vaccination status

ENDOMETRIAL CANCER

- AUB = abnormal uterine bleeding

Disease	Etiology, Prevalence, Risk Factors	Clinical Symptoms and Signs	Diagnostics	Therapy, Prognosis, and Health Maintenance
Endometrial cancer Type 1: endometrioid (75%) Type 2: serous, clear, mucinous	Most common gynecologic malignancy Mean age: 63 (most >50) RF: **H**ypertension **O**besity: greatest risk **N**ulliparity **D**iabetes **A**UB Unopposed estrogen use, old age, history of infertility, early menarche, late menopause, **Tamoxifen** use HRT without progesterone Chronic anovulation: PCOS Most common site of metastasis: **LUNGS**	1. **AUB** (#1): chronic anovulation, heavy or prolonged menses, intermenstrual spotting 2. **Peri- or postmenopausal (90%)** 3. **Bloating** 4. Early satiety 5. Changes in bowel or bladder function Other symptoms: abnormal vaginal discharge, lower abdominal discomfort Signs 1. Uterus enlargement	1. Sonogram 2. EMB, **ONLY IF SYMPTOMATIC OR RISK FACTORS** 3. Biopsy: if postmenopausal or premenopausal with RF 4. CXR–check for mets	**Hyperplasia WITHOUT atypia** (simple or complex): 1. Refer to gynecologist 2. Oral Progestin, Mirena 3. Hysterectomy **Hyperplasia WITH atypia (EIN):** 1. EMB with atypia → D&C 2. Hysterectomy 3. Progestins **Cancer:** 1. Surgery or radiation 2. Megace/Mirena IUD 75% diagnosed stage I Protective factors: 1. **SMOKING** 2. OCP use

OB/GYN

Treatment for Endometrial Cancer

Stage	Description	Mainstay Treatment	5-Year Survival
Ia	Tumor invades less than 1/2 of myometrium or endometrium	Surgical resection *only*: total hysterectomy with bilateral salpingo-oophorectomy with pelvic and paraaortic lymph node dissection	90%
Ib	Tumor invades >½ of myometrium	Surgery + radiation	
II	Tumor invades stromal connective tissue but confined to uterus	Surgery + radiation	
III	Tumor involves vagina, adnexa, with positive regional lymph nodes	Surgery + chemotherapy + radiation	50%
IV	Tumor invades bladder mucosa with distant metastasis	Surgery + chemotherapy + radiation	50%

VAGINAL/VULVAR NEOPLASMS

Disease	Etiology, Prevalence, Risk Factors	Clinical Symptoms and Signs	Diagnostics	Therapy, Prognosis, and Health Maintenance
Vaginal neoplasia	1%-2% of all gyn malignancies 80%-90% are *metastases* from: cervix, uterus, rectum, bladder (*CURB*) Most common: **Squamous cell carcinoma** Most common location: upper 1/3 of vagina, posterior to cervix RF: same as cervical cancer Multiple lifetime partners, early coitarche, current ***SMOKING, HPV 16 and 18*** (history of genital warts), CIN/VIN, history of radiation or DES exposure	<u>Asymptomatic (found after hysterectomy):</u> 1. **Vaginal bleeding**: postcoital or ***postmenopausal*** 2. Watery, blood tinged, malodorous discharge 3. Vaginal mass 4. Urinary SX: urgency, frequency, dysuria, hematuria 5. GI SX: constipation, melena <u>Signs</u>: • Speculum/pelvic exam • Palpable mass on posterior wall of upper vagina • Blood and malodorous discharge in vaginal vault • Ulcerative lesions	1. **Lugol solution:** turn's abnormal areas black 2. **Punch biopsy** • Squamous cell carcinoma 3. Colposcopy	1. Radiation and surgery • Laser ablation • WLE *Note:* If it extends to cervix or vulva, it is not vaginal
Vulvar neoplasia Most are **squamous cell carcinoma** (may arise in the setting of chronic irritation from lichen sclerosus)	4th most common (5%) Mean age: 65 <u>RF</u>: 1. Age 2. HPV infection (60%):#16 3. Coexisting or history of CIN or other invasive genital tract malignancy 4. **SMOKING** 5. ***Immuno suppression***: HIV, ***SLE***, chronic steroid use 6. Vulvar dystrophy (lichen sclerosis)	<u>HX: lichen sclerosus:</u> 1. Vulvar **itching** 2. Visible **lesions** on vulva <u>Less common:</u> Bleeding, pain, ulceration Dysuria <u>Signs</u>: Enlarged groin nodes	1. Histology: BIOPSY #1 pitfall is delayed biopsy 2. Vulvoscopy: **acetowhite lesions**	1. **Radical vulvectomy** and groin node dissection 2. If high risk → chemoradiation Progression of VIN 1 → VIN 2 → VIN 3 (<5% progress to invasive cancer)
Lichen simplex chronicus	Non-neoplastic disorder from chronic scratching and rubbing, damaging the skin, and leading to loss of protective barrier	1. Itch-scratch-itch cycle, susceptibility to infection 2. Severe vulvar itching, worse at night <u>Signs</u>: 1. Thick, lichenified, enlarge rugose labia with or without edema (localized or generalized)	Based on clinical history and vulvar biopsy	1. Short course of high-potency topical steroids 2. Antihistamines

OB/GYN

(continued)

(continued)

Disease	Etiology, Prevalence, Risk Factors	Clinical Symptoms and Signs	Diagnostics	Therapy, Prognosis, and Health Maintenance
Lichen sclerosus (Fig. 52-2)	Etiology: unknown, multifactorial	1. Involves scalp, nails, oral mucous membranes, and vulva 2. Mucocutaneous eruptions with remissions and flares 3. *Vulvar SX*: irritation, burning, itching, contact bleeding, pain, dyspareunia <u>Signs</u>: 1. Lacy, reticulated pattern of the labia and perineum, with or without scarring and erosions, oral lesions, alopecia, extragenital rashes 2. Skin appears thin, inelastic, and white with a ***"crinkled tissue paper"*** appearance		1. Multiple supportive therapies 2. Topical super potent corticosteroids
Vulvar vestibulitis syndrome	Inciting event undetermined Severe pain on vestibular touch or attempted vaginal entry, tenderness to pressure and erythema of various degrees	1. Abrupt onset of symptoms: sharp, burning, rawness sensation 2. **Pain with tampon insertion**, biking, wearing tight pants 3. Avoid intercourse because of marked introital dyspareunia <u>Signs</u>: 1. Exquisite vestibular tenderness 2. +/− focal/diffuse erythematous macules		1. TCAs 2. Pelvic floor rehabilitation 3. Biofeedback 4. Topical anesthetics 5. Surgery with vestibulectomy for unresponsive

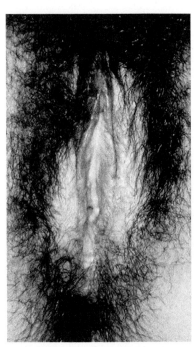

FIGURE 52-2. Lichen sclerosis. (From Snyder R, Dent N, Fowler W, et al. *Step-Up to Obstetrics and Gynecology*. Philadelphia: Lippincott Williams & Wilkins; 2014.)

CHAPTER **53**

Breast Disorders

Recommended Supplemental Topics:

Paget's Disease of the Breast, p 500

Breast Fibroadenoma, p 500

BREAST ABSCESS, BREAST FIBROADENOMA, FIBROCYSTIC DISEASE, MASTITIS

Breast Mass and Cancer

It is essential to understand the difference between in situ and invasive mammary carcinoma. Invasive carcinomas are composed of malignant epithelial cells that infiltrate the breast stromal tissues associated with a tendency for tumor metastasis to regional and distant sites. In situ carcinomas are confined inside the ductal-lobular system and are not capable of producing metastatic disease. In situ carcinomas give rise to invasive carcinomas. The process of invasion includes infiltration of tumor cells through the basement membrane surrounding ducts/lobules and loss of the myoepithelial cell layer.

The HER2-positive subtype comprises approximately 10% of invasive ductal carcinomas and is associated with aggressive biology. The typical HER2-positive subtype carcinoma is a grade 3 invasive ductal carcinoma showing loss of hormone receptor expression and HER2 gene amplification. All invasive breast carcinomas are tested for ER, PR, and HER2 overexpression/amplification. The main utility of these studies is to guide therapy for patients. Hormone receptor–positive status, particularly when strong, is associated with response to hormonal therapy, such as tamoxifen and aromatase inhibitors. Hormone receptor testing is currently evaluated using immunohistochemistry where nuclear staining is classified as positive. Hormone receptor status may also be evaluated using quantitative RT-PCR assays to quantify mRNA levels. Therapies target HER2-positive tumor cells using humanized monoclonal antibody (trastuzumab) against HER2 or tyrosine kinase inhibitors that interrupt the HER2 growth receptor pathway.

	Etiology	Presentation	Diagnostics	Treatment
Breast cancer	RF: Age, sex, first-degree relative, risk before menopause increased if BRCA1 or BRCA2 (+) Associated factors: nulliparity, early menarche, late menopause, postmenopausal ERT or radiation exposure, and advanced maternal age at first term birth All invasive lobular carcinomas and 2/3 of ductal carcinomas are estrogen-receptor positive (HER2 positive)	1. *Single*, *nontender*, firm, *immobile* mass; 45% occur in the **upper outer quadrant** and 25% under the nipple and areola Signs: 1. Early changes may appear with mammographic changes and **no palpable masses** 2. Rare: nipple discharge, retraction, dimpling, breast enlargement, shrinkage, skin thickening or peau d'orange, eczematous changes, breast pain, fixed mass, axillary node enlargement, ulcerations, arm edema, and palpable supraclavicular nodes	1. Any solid dominant breast mass on exam should be evaluated cytologically with • **FNA** or • histologically with **excisional biopsy** 2. Genetic testing for patients with strong family history 3. Axillary lymph node staging with **sentinel lymph node biopsy**	1. ***Tamoxifen***—used to treat women with estrogen receptor–positive disease and postmenopausal women 2. Adjuvant chemotherapy and hormonal manipulation benefits some 3. Lumpectomy with sentinel node biopsy preferred for early stage cancers Breast cancer **associated with higher risk of endometrial cancer** and vice-versa **Axillary lymph node status** is the most important *prognostic* factor for invasive carcinoma in the absence of distant metastasis

OB/GYN

(continued)

(continued)

	Etiology	Presentation	Diagnostics	Treatment
Paget disease of the breast	Uncommon Ductal carcinoma presenting as an eczematous lesions of the nipple Uncommon, 1% of all breast cancers	1. Eczematoid eruption and ulceration arising from the nipple and spreading to the areola • **Pain, itching, burning** 2. Superficial erosion or ulceration 3. Bloody discharge or nipple retraction <u>Signs</u>: 1. Scale, crust, and itching 2. **Palpable mass** (50%), 95% are invasive cancer infiltrating ducts • If no mass, noninvasive breast cancer or DCIS in 75%	1. Full-thickness biopsy: intraepithelial adenocarcinoma cells or Paget cells within the epidermis of the nipple Nests of tumor cells extending from DCIS within the ductal system into the nipple skin	1. Wide local excision 2. Breast conservation with whole breast radiation, if negative margins Most are high grade and show HER2 overexpression
Breast fibroadenoma (Fig. 53-1A)	Second most common benign breast disorder More common in African American women <u>MC</u>: 15-35 (*YOUNG*)	1. Round, **firm** (soft, rubbery) painless, freely movable, discrete, **mobile**, nontender 2. Hormonal relationship: cyclical size: grows in pregnancy, dissipates in postmenopausal women <u>Signs</u>: 1. Nontender 2. Unilateral 3. Mobile density 4. Smooth firm mass	1. New or growing lesions need evaluation • If <30: **U/S** +/– FNA • If >30: Mammogram 2. Excisional biopsy (if **<25**), if BRCA (+) mom	1. Decrease caffeine intake
Fibrocystic breast disease (Fig. 53-1B)	Most common benign breast condition <u>MC</u>: 30-50	Asymptomatic or **painful** and tender masses, bilateral pain, and size fluctuation during the menstrual cycle *MULTIPLE LESIONS*– distinguishes fibrocystic changes from carcinoma 1. Breast pain 2. Nipple discharge 3. *Lumpy and bumpy* prior to menses 4. Associated with <u>cyclic</u> mastalgia (hormonal response) <u>Signs</u>: 1. Diffusely TENDER 2. *Bilateral* 3. Mobile density 4. Thick, gray-green nipple discharge 5. Worse with caffeine intake	1. U/S +/– biopsy 2. FNA–diagnostic and therapeutic: strawberry-colored fluid	1. ***Support bra**, decrease caffeine intake*, vitamin E +/– primrose oil 2. Danazol <u>Health maintenance</u>: 1. Frequent nursing 8-12 × daily <u>Prognosis</u>: Increased risk of breast cancer when atypia is present

	Etiology	Presentation	Diagnostics	Treatment
Mastitis	MC in postpartum women Second to 4th week after delivery <u>MC pathogen:</u> *S. aureus*	1. Primarily in lactating women (associated with breastfeeding) 2. Significant **fever**, chills, and other flu-like symptoms 3. Acute onset 4. Responds to antibiotics <u>Signs:</u> 1. Decreased milk outflow 2. Redness, tender to touch 3. Firm mass, breast pain 4. **Unilateral** tenderness, heat	1. Culture of purulent material or milk (not routine)	1. Oral or IV antibiotics: dicloxacillin 250-500 mg PO q6h × 7-14 d (PEN allergic: erythromycin) 2. Cold compresses to reduce inflammation 3. NSAIDs and Tylenol for pain 4. CONTINUE TO BREAST FEED and EXPRESS MILK 5. If no response to antibiotics, pursue further workup (ie, biopsy, breast cancer workup)
Breast abscess	Especially during nursing <u>MC:</u> *S. aureus*	1. Redness 2. Tenderness 3. Induration	1. Incision and biopsy if severe or indurated—r/o inflammatory carcinoma	1. Bactrim 2. Clindamycin 3. Doxycycline

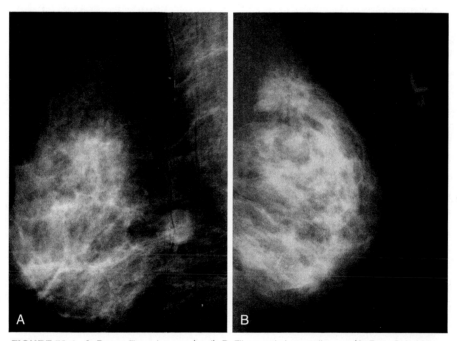

FIGURE 53-1. **A,** Breast fibroadenoma (oval). **B,** Fibrocystic breast disease. (**A,** From Sabel M. *Operative Techniques in Breast, Endocrine, and Oncologic Surgery.* Philadelphia: Wolters Kluwer Health; 2016. **B,** From Linn-Watson TA. *Radiographic Pathology.* Philadelphia: Wolters Kluwer Health; 2015.)

Breast Imaging Reporting and Data System

BIRADS is a scheme for putting the findings from mammography screening into a small number of well-defined categories.

OB/GYN

BIRADS	Assessment	Clinical Management
0	Incomplete	Need to review prior studies +/− complete additional imaging
1	Negative	Continue routine screening
2	Benign	
3	Probably benign	MMG 6 mo, then q 6-12 mo (1-2 y)
4	Suspicious abnormality	Biopsy—NEEDLE
5	Highly suspicious	Biopsy and TX
6	Known biopsy proven malignancy	Assure treatment is completed

Breast Cancer Screening Guidelines

	ACOG	American Cancer Society	USPSTF
Mammogram	Annually at 40 y/o (previously 1-2 y at 40, then annually at 50)	Annually at 40, continue while in good health	
SBE	All 20+	20+ (optional)	
CBE	20-30: 1-3 y 40+: annual	20-30: 2-3 y 40+: annual	
MRI	High risk: more frequent CBE, **annual MRI**, MMG before 40 *No MRI for average risk	MRI for high risk: BRCA carriers, 1st degree relative BRCA, h/o XRT (10-30 y/o) 40+: annual	<50: individual basis MMG: 50-74: biennial 75+: no screening

CBE, clinical breast exam; SBE, self breast exam.

- High risk is defined as >20% lifetime risk of breast cancer
- Women with strong family history (first or second-degree family member = mother, sister, daughter, grandmother, aunt, niece) with premenopausal breast cancer should initiate screening 5-10 years before the youngest age at diagnosis of breast cancer in a relative
- Patients with known BRCA mutations should begin screening at age 25 years with MRI imaging at 25 (then annually) and MMG at age 30 (then annually)—this may vary by source

CHAPTER 54
Labor & Delivery

Recommended Supplemental Topics:

DYSTOCIA

Disease	Etiology, Prevalence, Risk Factors	Clinical Symptoms and Signs	Diagnostics	Therapy, Prognosis, and Health Maintenance
Shoulder dystocia	Inability to deliver the shoulders after the head has delivered Incidence: 0.15%-1.7% of all vaginal deliveries <u>RF:</u> Fetal macrosomia, gestational or overt diabetes, history of shoulder dystocia in prior birth, prolonged second stage of labor, and instrumental (midpelvic) delivery	1. Any indication of macrosomia • Gentle downward pressure on the head fails to deliver the anterior shoulder from behind the pubic symphysis • Avoid continuing to apply downward pressure on the head to deliver to anterior shoulder → ineffective and can damage the brachial plexus 2. Attempt maneuvers Complications: Erb palsy (10%), postpartum hemorrhage and lacerations		1. Hyperflexion of the maternal hips **(McRoberts maneuver)** • Resolves in 42%, initial maneuver 2. Offer women a Cesarean delivery in future deliveries 3. Prevention: address history of shoulder dystocia macrosomia by estimated fetal weight (EFW), diabetes, prolonged second stage of labor, and instrumental delivery Previous history of dystocia places women at an increased risk of dystocia in future pregnancies

- **Cephalopelvic disproportion (CPD):** a term that describes obstructed labor resulting from a disparity in the fetal head size and maternal pelvis
- **Failure to progress:** lack of progressive cervical dilation or lack of fetal descent

Dystocia Maneuvers

- **McRoberts maneuver:** Hyperflexion of the maternal hips, flattening of the sacrum, and cephalad rotation of the symphysis pubis
  - If the shoulders are undelivered, suprapubic pressure is applied by an assistant to dislodge the anterior shoulder while gentle downward pressure on the head is applied
  - *Rubin maneuver:* Rotation of the fetal shoulders into the oblique position by placing two fingers against the posterior shoulder and pushing it around toward the fetal chest
  - *Wood maneuver:* Pushing the posterior shoulder around toward the fetal back in a corkscrew fashion
- **Barnum maneuver** (delivery of the posterior arm): insert hand posteriorly into hollow of the maternal sacrum and the posterior arm should be identified; apply pressure by the forefinger on the fetal antecubital fossa causing flexion of the fetal forearm. As the arm flexes across the chest, grasp the forearm and deliver the hand and forearm gently through the birth canal
- **Zavanelli maneuver** (last line): fetal head is replaced in anticipation of a cesarean delivery; a subcutaneous symphysiotomy is performed to allow disimpaction of the fetal shoulders

OB/GYN

FETAL DISTRESS (FIG. 54-1A-D)

- The **baseline fetal heart rate** is the approximate mean rate rounded to increments of 5 bpm during a 10-minute tracing segment
- In any 10-minute window, the minimum interpretable baseline duration must be at least 2 minutes

- *Magnesium sulfate* has been arguably associated with diminished beat-to-beat variability
- It is generally believed that **reduced baseline heart rate variability** is the single most reliable sign of fetal compromise

Pattern	Associated	Description
Sinusoidal	**Fetal anemia from Rh-alloimmunization**, fetal intracranial hemorrhage, severe fetal asphyxia, fetomaternal hemorrhage, twin-twin transfusion syndrome, or vasa previa	• Visually apparent, smooth, sine wave-line undulating pattern in FHR baseline with a cycle frequency of 3-5 per min, which persists for 20 min or more
Early decelerations	Normal head compression during uterine contractions (**active labor**)	• Visually apparent usually symmetrical gradual decrease and return of the FHR associated with a uterine contraction • A gradual FHR decrease is defined as from the onset to the FHR nadir of ≥30 s • The decrease in FHR is calculated from the onset to the nadir of the deceleration • The nadir of the deceleration occurs at the same time as the peak of the contraction • In most cases, the onset, nadir, and recovery of the deceleration are coincident with the beginning, peak, and ending of the contraction, respectively
Late decelerations	**Uteroplacental insufficiency**	• Visually apparent usually symmetrical gradual decrease and return of the FHR associated with a uterine contraction • A gradual FHR decrease is defined as from the onset to the FHR nadir of ≥30 s • The decrease in FHR is calculated from the onset to the nadir of the deceleration • The deceleration is delayed in timing, with the nadir of the deceleration occurring after the peak of the contraction • In most cases, the onset, nadir, and recovery of the deceleration occur after the beginning, peak, and ending of the contraction, respectively
Variable decelerations	**Umbilical cord compression** → fetal anoxia → death	• Visually apparent abrupt decrease in FHR • An abrupt FHR decrease is defined as from the onset to the FHR nadir of <30 s • The decrease in FHR is calculated from the onset to the nadir of the deceleration • The decrease in FHR is ≥15 bpm, lasting ≥15 s, and <2 min in duration • When variable decelerations are associated with uterine contraction, their onset, depth, and duration commonly vary with successive uterine contractions
Prolonged deceleration		• Visually apparent decrease in the FHR below the baseline • Decrease in FHR from the baseline that is ≥15 bpm, lasting ≥2 min but <10 min in duration • If a deceleration lasts ≥10 min, it is a baseline change
Acceleration		• A visually apparent abrupt increase (onset to peak in <30 s) in the FHR • At 32 wk and beyond, an acceleration has a peak of 15 bpm or more above baseline, with a duration of 15 s or more but less than 2 min from onset to return • Before 32 wk, an acceleration has a peak of 10 bpm or more above baseline, with a duration of ≥10 s but <2 min from onset to return • Prolonged acceleration lasts ≥2 min, but <10 min • If an acceleration lasts 10 min, it is a baseline change
Bradycardia	Epidurals, MgSO$_4$ Congenital heart block, placental abruption	• FHR baseline <110 bpm
Tachycardia	**Maternal fever from chorioamnionitis**, fetal compromise, cardiac arrhythmias, maternal administration of atropine or terbutaline	• FHR baselines >160 bpm

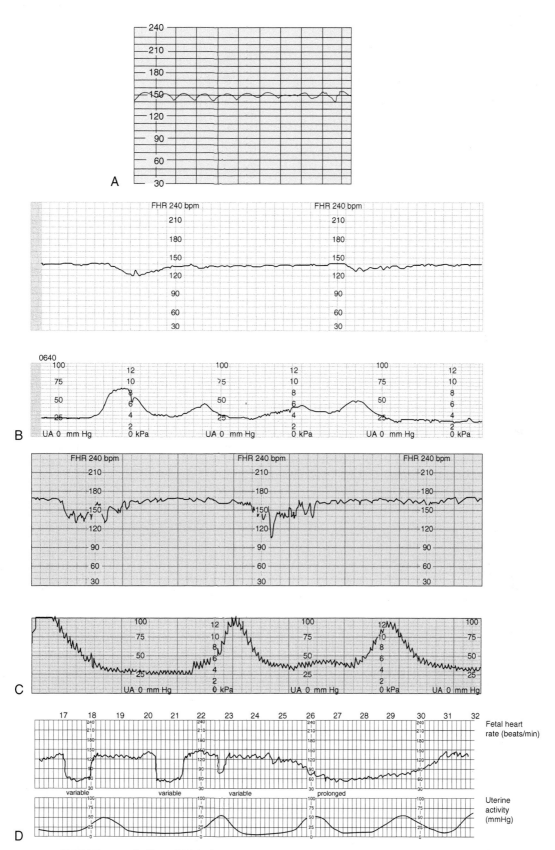

FIGURE 54-1. A, Sinusoidal fetal heart rate, associated with maternal hemorrhage and severe fetal anemia. **B**, Early decelerations (*above*) mirror the contraction (*below*). **C**, Late decelerations. Nadir of each deceleration occurs after the peak of each contraction. **D**, Variable and prolonged decelerations. Fetal heart rate (FHR) is seen *above*, note the large drop in both types of decelerations. (**A**, Modified from Beckmann CRB, Ling FW, Smith RP, et al. *Obstetrics and Gynecology*. 5th ed. Philadelphia: Lippincott Williams & Wilkins; 2006. **B**, Modified from Gabrielli A, Layon AJ, Yu M. *Civetta, Taylor & Kirby's Manual of Critical Care*. Philadelphia: Lippincott Williams & Wilkins, a Wolters Kluwer business; 2012. **C**, Modified from Pfeifer SM. *NMS Obstetrics and Gynecology*. 7th ed. Philadelphia: Lippincott Williams & Wilkins, a Wolters Kluwer business; 2012. **D**, Modified from Silbert-Flagg J, Pillitteri A. *Maternal & Child Health Nursing: Care of the Childbearing & Childrearing Family*. 8th ed. Philadelphia: Wolters Kluwer; 2018.)

PROLAPSED UMBILICAL CORD

- Compression of the umbilical cord compromises fetal circulation and, depending on the duration and intensity of compression, may lead to fetal hypoxia, brain damage, and death → considered an obstetric emergency

- Prolapse of the cord may follow amniotomy

Disease	Etiology, Prevalence, Risk Factors	Clinical Symptoms and Signs	Diagnostics	Therapy, Prognosis, and Health Maintenance
Prolapsed umbilical cord	Descent of the umbilical cord into the lower uterine segment, where it may lie adjacent to the presenting part (occult cord prolapse) or below the presenting part (overt cord prolapse)	Fetal complications: variable fetal heart rate decelerations during uterine contractions with prompt return of heart rate as contraction subsides; if compression is complete and prolonged, bradycardia occurs; hypoxia, metabolic acidosis, death Maternal complications: C-section, laceration during delivery		
Occult prolapse (Fig. 54-2A)	Umbilical cord cannot be palpated during a pelvic exam Unknown incidence, only detected by fetal heart rate changes characteristic of umbilical cord compression	1. Inferred only if fetal heart rate changes (variable decelerations, bradycardia or both) associated with intermittent compression of the umbilical cord		1. Immediate pelvic examination to rule out overt cord prolapse 2. Place patient in lateral Sims or Trendelenburg position to alleviate cord compression 3. If FHT return to normal, continue labor 4. Deliver O_2 to mother and monitor FHT continuously 5. Place intrauterine pressure catheter to instill fluid within the uterine cavity and decrease variable decelerations 6. Rapid caesarean section if compression persists
Funic (cord) presentation (Fig. 54-2B)	In funic presentation (prolapse of the cord below the level of the presenting part before ROM occurs), the cord can be palpated through the membranes	1. Pelvic exam—loops of cord are palpated through the membranes		1. Deliver by cesarean section prior to ROM • Hospitalize patient on bed rest in Sims or Trendelenburg position to reposition the cord within the uterine cavity
Overt cord prolapse (Fig. 54-2C)	Associated with **rupture of membranes** and displacement of the umbilical cord into the vagina, often through the introitus RF: Prematurity (<34 wk), abnormal presentation, occiput posterior position of the head, pelvic tumors, multiparity, placenta previa, low lying placenta, and cephalopelvic disproportion Cephalic: 0.5% Frank breech: 0.5% Complete breech: 5% Footling breech: 15% **Transverse lie: 20%**	1. Visualization of the cord protruding from the introitus or by palpating loops of cord in the vaginal canal	1. U/S at the onset of labor to determine lie and cord position 2. Continuous fetal heart rate monitoring 3. Avoid artificial rupture of membranes until presenting part is well applied to cervix 4. At spontaneous rupture, a prompt careful pelvic exam should rule out cord prolapse	1. Pelvic exam—determine effacement, dilation, station, strength, and frequency of pulsations within cord vessels 2. Place patient in knee-chest position and apply continuous upward pressure against presenting part to lift and maintain fetus away from prolapsed cord • May instill 400-700 mL saline into bladder to elevate presenting part • O_2 to mother 3. Reduction of prolapsed cord but should not delay CESAREAN delivery Mortality rate: 20%

OB/GYN

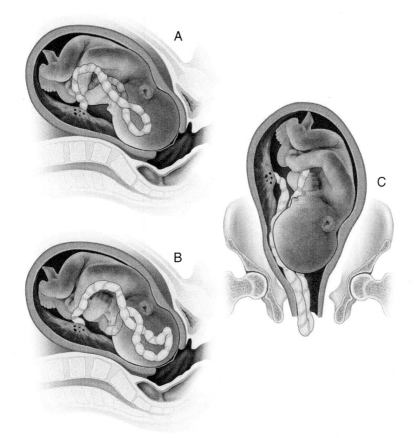

FIGURE 54-2. **A,** Occult prolapse. Prolapse of the umbilical cord within the uterus with the cord lying below or adjacent to the presenting part, but not beyond the presenting part, and may or may not be visible or palpated in the cervical os or vagina. **B,** Funic presentation. The presence of the umbilical cord in the funic position, prior to rupture of membranes, with the umbilical cord pointing toward the internal cervical os or lower uterine segment. **C,** Overt (Frank) cord prolapse–transverse lie. The umbilical cord descends following the rupture of the membranes, through the cervical os such that it lies outside the vagina. The cord is visible or palpable with the naked eye.

PREMATURE RUPTURE OF MEMBRANES, PRETERM LABOR

- **Nitrazine test**: performed to determine the nature of the fluid in the vagina during pregnancy when PROM is suspected
  - A drop of fluid from the vagina is placed on a paper strip containing nitrazine dye
  - The strip changes color based on the pH
  - Turns blue if pH > 6.0 = more likely to be ruptured
  - False-positives: blood-contaminated sample, infection present, high vaginal pH, semen present (recent intercourse)

- **Ferning**: detection of a *fernlike* pattern of cervical mucus when placed on a dry glass slide under low-power microscope; used to provide evidence of amniotic fluid to detect rupture of membranes and onset of labor
  - Due to the presence of sodium chloride in the mucus under estrogen effect
  - High levels of estrogen are present just before ovulation, making cervical mucus form a fernlike pattern as the crystallization of sodium chloride occurs

OB/GYN

Disease	Etiology, Prevalence, Risk Factors	Clinical Symptoms and Signs	Diagnostics	Therapy, Prognosis, and Health Maintenance
Premature rupture of membranes (PROM) (amniotic fluid leak, absence of active labor)	RF: **Genital tract infection** (bacterial vaginosis), smoking, **prior PPROM (2×)**, shortened cervical length, amniocentesis Rupture of membranes before the onset of active labor 10.7% of all pregnancies Important cause of PTL, prolapsed cord, placental abruption, and intrauterine infection The National Institutes of Health (NIH) consensus development panel recommends the use of steroids in PROM patients **before 32 wk** EGA in the absence of intra-amniotic infection	1. Term: >37 wk gestation (94%) 2. Sudden gush of fluid or continued leakage from vagina • Include color and consistency of fluid and presence of flecks of vernix or meconium, reduced size of uterus, and increased prominence of fetus to palpation Signs: 1. AVOID DIGITAL EXAM 2. Note: avoid introducing bacteria into the uterine cavity and **increasing the risk for chorioamnionitis**	3 **hallmark** findings differentiate PROM from things like vaginitis, increased vaginal secretions, and incontinence: 1. **Vaginal fluid for ferning** 2. **Nitrazine testing** of mucus swabbed from cervix • In absence of amniotic fluid, paper turns blue = alkaline pH 3. **Pooling**: collection of amniotic fluid in posterior fornix 4. CBC and U/A with culture 5. (+) **phosphatidyl glycerol** = indicates pulmonary maturity for patients 32-34 wk 6. AFI with U/S—may reveal oligohydramnios but does not confirm diagnosis	Delivery: 1. If chorioamnionitis present, patient should be **actively delivered vaginally** regardless of gestational age → induce labor if not already started 2. If no infection and term (>37 wk), manage expectantly or actively 3. If no infection and preterm (<37 wk), similar delivery to PTL 1. **Antibiotics and hydration**: prolongs latency period by 5-7 d and reduces the risk of amnionitis and neonatal sepsis • Start IV *ampicillin* 2 g q6h AND IV *erythromycin* 250 mg q6h • After 48 h, if still undelivered, switch to: PO amoxicillin 250 mg q8h AND PO erythromycin q8h • Continue × 7 d until patient delivered 2. Tocolysis—used to prolong the interval to delivery to gain time for steroids to be administered (risk of chorioamnionitis with tocolytics beyond 48 h)
Chorioamnionitis	Most common causes: mycoplasmas (MC: **Ureaplasma, Mycoplasma**), *E. coli*, GBS, anaerobes RF: 1. Longer duration of labor and ruptured membranes 2. Multiple digital vaginal exams 3. Cervical insufficiency 4. Nulliparity 5. Meconium stained amniotic fluid 6. Internal fetal/uterine monitoring 7. Prior chorio 8. Infections, ETOH, tobacco use	1. +/- PROM 2. Mat. Fever (100%) • Check every 4 h PLUS 1 or more of following signs: 1. **Uterine tenderness** - check every 4 h 2. Tachycardia • **Maternal** >100 bpm • **Fetal** >160 bpm 3. Foul smelling, purulent, amniotic fluid 4. Maternal **leukocytosis** (70-90%) • WBC >12,000 Fetal complications: Endomyometritis, **sepsis of the newborn**	1. Daily CBC w/diff 2. CRP not useful 3. U/A w/culture if uncertain etiology 4. Blood cultures only if septic 5. **Culture of amniotic fluid** (gold standard) • (+) gram stain, low glucose level, (+) culture, high WBC count, funisitis Differential: Physiologic discharge, bacterial vaginosis, passage of woman's mucus plug • Abruptio Placentae: can cause uterine tenderness + maternal tachycardia, but also has vaginal bleeding and absence of fever	Emergent delivery 1. Antibiotics • IV **Ampicillin** 2 g q 6 h PLUS • **Gentamicin** 5 mg/kg once daily • If C-section needed, add Clindamycin or Flagyl for anaerobic coverage • Opinion: Give until asymptomatic and afebrile x 48 h, no evidence to support this Prophylaxis: If ruptured membranes >18 h, give **ampicillin + gentamicin** Complications: 1. Dysfunctional labor (atony, PPH) 2. Infection/Sepsis

OB/GYN

Disease	Etiology, Prevalence, Risk Factors	Clinical Symptoms and Signs	Diagnostics	Therapy, Prognosis, and Health Maintenance
Preterm premature rupture of membranes (PPROM)	10%-15% of all pregnancies 1/3 of all preterm deliveries Preterm rupture of membranes before the onset of active labor			1. Augmentation of delivery • Vaginal suppositories of progesterone 2. Cerclage–if history of incompetent cervix 3. Weekly IM injections of 17 α-hydroxyprogesterone from 16 wk until 36-37 wk 4. No steroids after 32 wk! No study has shown that tocolytics improve fetal outcome in women with PPROM
Preterm uterine contractions		1. Uterine contractions without cervical change		1. Self-limited, resolves spontaneously, requires no intervention
Preterm labor (contractions with cervical changes)	MCC: Idiopathic (no cause identified) • Presence of regular uterine contractions leading to cervical change RF: PROM, history of preterm labor, multiple gestation, African American, intrauterine infection, Mullerian anomalies, smoking, substance abuse, bacteria vaginosis, limited access to prenatal care, short cervical length	1. **Labor after 20^{0/7} wk but before the 37^{0/7} wk** of pregnancy 2. Tocometer: **regular, rhythmic contractions** 5 min apart (frequent intervals) 3. Need not be painful to cause cervical changes and may manifest as abdominal tightening, lower back pain, or pelvic pressure Signs: 1. Cervix is long, closed 2. Cervical **dilation, effacement**, or both occur	1. TVUS: dilation and effacement change of at least 1 cm or cervix that is well effaced and dilated >2 cm on admission (diagnostic) 2. Continuous fetal monitoring with tocodynamometry 3. Labs: CBC, U/A with culture and sensitivity 4. **Fetal fibronectin** (fFN), if 24-35 wk–rules OUT preterm labor for 7-14 d but inconclusive if (+); can run between 22-34 wk Negative predictive value of 99.2% in symptomatic women, PPV of 16.7%, low sensitivity (do not use in asymptomatic women) fFN <50 ng/mL	1. Treat with **betamethasone**, if increased risk of delivering preterm from **24-34 wk** to increase pulmonary maturity 2. Hydration and observation **(expectant management)** 3. Tocolysis • Indications: dilation <5 cm • Goal: continue pregnancy 48 h after steroids but optimally beyond 34-36 wk • Success: <4-6 contractions/hr without cervical change • Stop if dilation reaches 5 cm Tocolysis: 1. **Terbutaline** and Ritodrine • AE: palpitations, tremors, nervousness, restlessness 2. **Mag-sulfate** • Inhibits calcium uptake into smooth muscle cells, reducing uterine contractility • Causes respiratory and cardiac depression • Monitor DTRs, RR, and fluid balance often 3. Nifedipine 50% have spontaneous resolution of uterine activity Bedrest has NOT been shown to reduce PT birth

- **Prevention of preterm birth**
  - If history of spontaneous PTB
    - Progestin: either vaginal suppository of progesterone or weekly IM injections of 17-alpha hydroxyprogesterone caproate at 16-20 weeks until 36-37 weeks can reduce the risk by 30%
    - Vaginal progesterone may reduce the risk if short cervix is found on TVUS

MALPRESENTATION

- Before 28 weeks, the fetus is small enough to rotate from cephalic to breech and back with ease, but as age and weight increase, the relative decrease in intrauterine volume makes changes more difficult

- Breech occurs when spontaneous version to cephalic presentation is prevented as term approaches or if labor occurs prematurely before version has taken place
- In multiple gestations, each fetus prevents the other from turning: 25% incidence of breech in first twin, 50% for second, and higher for additional fetuses
- In cases of Rh-negative-unsensitized woman, Rh-immune globulin (RhoGAM) should be given after external cephalic version to cover the calculated amount of fetomaternal hemorrhage

OB/GYN

Disease	Etiology, Prevalence, Risk Factors	Clinical Symptoms and Signs	Diagnostics	Therapy, Prognosis, and Health Maintenance

Breech presentation	Fetal pelvis or lower extremities engage the maternal pelvic inlet
	3%-4% of all pregnancies
	RF:
	Fibroids, oligohydramnios, polyhydramnios, uterine anomalies (bicornuate or septate uterus), pelvic tumors obstructing the canal, abnormal placentation, advanced multiparity, contracted maternal pelvis
		1. Clinical suspicion, palpation of fetal parts over maternal abdomen or by pelvic examination
		Signs:
		1. Leopold maneuvers to confirm breech presentation
		2. Pelvic exam
		  • Breech: soft, irregular
		  • Cephalic: round, firm, smooth
			1. U/S (confirms)—differentiate breech from cephalic presentations
			  • Determine presentation, attitude, size; multiple gestation; location of the placenta, and amniotic fluid volume
			2. Continuous electronic monitoring of baby
				1. Monitor closely for spontaneous version to cephalic presentation
				2. **External cephalic version**: manipulating the fetus through the abdominal wall from breech to cephalic presentation
				  • Indications: **singleton breech**, nonvertex second twin; women **36+ wk gestation**
				  • Contraindications: engagement of the presenting part, marked oligohydramnios, placenta previa, uterine anomalies, nuchal cord, multiple gestation, PROM, previous uterine surgery (myomectomy), IUGR
				  • Complications: placental abruption, uterine rupture, ROM with cord prolapse, amniotic fluid embolism, PTL, fetal distress, fetomaternal hemorrhage, fetal demise

Breech Presentations (Fig. 54-3)

Frank breech	50%-70%, pike position	1. Hips flexed 2. Knees extended bilaterally
Complete breech	5%-10%, cannonball position	1. Hips flexed 2. Knees flexed Complications: umbilical cord compression and prolapse (5%)
Footling or Incomplete	10%-30%	1. One or both hips extended below the level of the buttocks 2. Foot presenting Complications: umbilical cord compression and prolapse (15%)

OB/GYN

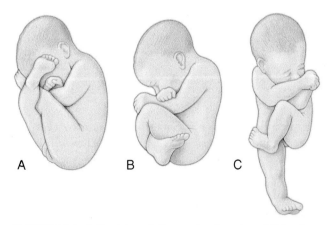

FIGURE 54-3. A, Frank breech, **B**, complete breech, and **C**, footling (incomplete) breech. (From Snyder R, Dent N, Fowler W, Ling F. *Step-Up to Obstetrics and Gynecology*. Philadelphia: Wolters Kluwer Health; 2015.)

Postpartum Care

POSTPARTUM HEMORRHAGE (FIG. 55-1)

- Most postpartum hemorrhage usually occurs during the immediate postpartum period (first hour of delivery), largely as a result of uterine relaxation, retained placental fragments, or unrepaired lacerations. Occult bleeding (eg, vaginal wall hematoma formation) may manifest as increasing pelvic pain

- Usual causes are uterine atony, retention of POCs, or uterine rupture after C-section

- Other causes: involution of placental site, vaginal tears, or bleeding from episiotomy

- Prevention: active management of third stage of labor (uterotonic drugs with or soon after delivery of the anterior shoulder, controlled cord traction, early cord clamping and cutting)

OB/GYN

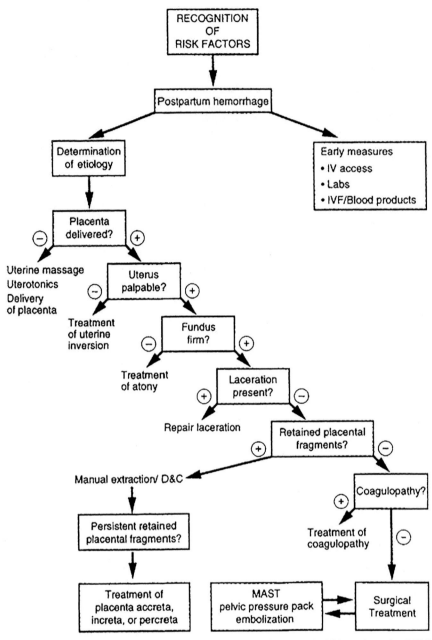

FIGURE 55-1. Management of postpartum hemorrhage. (From Evans AT, DeFranco E. *Manual of Obstetrics*. 8th ed. Philadelphia: Wolters Kluwer Health; 2014.)

Disease	Etiology, Prevalence, Risk Factors	Clinical Symptoms and Signs	Diagnostics	Therapy, Prognosis, and Health Maintenance
Postpartum hemorrhage (PPH)	RF: 1. Prolonged third stage of labor 2. Multiple delivery 3. Episiotomy 4. Fetal macrosomia 5. Prior history of PPH Most common cause of excessive blood loss in pregnancy	1. Patient returns to hospital a few days after delivery 2. **Brisk vaginal bleeding (>500 mL)** Signs: 1. Enlarged uterus or vaginal mass (inverted uterus) 2. Uterine bleeding with good tone and normal size 3. Hemorrhagic shock Complications: Uterine perforation, orthostatic hypotension, anemia, fatigue	CBC, coagulation studies (PT, PTT, platelet count), BUN, SCr, type and screen	Treat based on cause: 1. Insert fingers of one hand into vagina and compress the uterus against abdominal wall 2. IV **oxytocin (Pitocin)**, 10-40 units in 1 L normal saline for atony 3. Misoprostol (Cytotec) • More AE: shivering, pyrexia, diarrhea 4. Emergent OB/GYN consult 5. D&C (definitive)
Uterine atony	Myometrium cannot contract **Most common cause of postpartum hemorrhage (50%)** RF: Excessive manipulation of the uterus, general anesthesia, uterine overdistention (twins, polyhydramnios), prolonged labor, grand multiparity, oxytocin induction or augmentation of labor, previous hemorrhage in third stage, uterine infection, extravasation of myometrium, and intrinsic myometrial dysfunction	1. Brisk vaginal bleeding Signs: 1. Soft, boggy, enlarged uterus	Clinical DX	1. **Manual compression** of the uterus 2. IV **oxytocin**, 10-40 U in 1 L normal saline 3. Ergot alkaloids: **methylergonovine (Methergine)** (CI: HTN, preeclampsia), 1 dose every 2 h or every 20 min • AE: nausea, vomiting 4. Prostaglandin: **Hemabate or carboprost** (CI: asthma) • AE: Nausea, vomiting, diarrhea, HTN, headache, flush, pyrexia 5. B-lynch sutures: manually compresses uterus 6. Hysterectomy
Retention of products of conception	5%-10% of PPH Occurs in placenta accreta (multiple C-sections)	1. Retained placenta (failure to deliver within 30 min) Signs: 1. Uterine bleeding with good tone and normal size	1. Bedside U/S for localization: echogenic uterine mass	1. Inject umbilical vein with oxytocin 2. Remove manually or with ring forceps Uterine curettage
Obstetric lacerations	20% of PPH	1. Persistent bleeding (bright red) Signs: 1. Well contracted, firm, uterus		
Uterine rupture	0.6%-0.7% of vaginal births after C-section in women with low transverse or unknown uterine scar	1. Prior to delivery: **fetal bradycardia** 2. Tachycardia or late decelerations 3. Vaginal bleeding, abdominal tenderness Signs: 1. Maternal tachycardia 2. Circulatory collapse 3. Increasing abdominal girth		1. Surgical repair of defect or hysterectomy

OB/GYN

ENDOMETRITIS

Disease	Etiology, Prevalence, Risk Factors	Clinical Symptoms and Signs	Diagnostics	Therapy, Prognosis, and Health Maintenance
Endometritis	Infection of the endometrium	1. **Fever >38°C** (100.4°F) post C-section or vaginal delivery 2. Peritoneal pain 3. Vaginal discharge Signs: 1. Lower abdominal tenderness 2. Tachycardia and tachypnea 3. **Foul-smelling lochia** 4. **Uterine or fundal tenderness** 5. Fever	1. Gram stain: leukocytes and bacteria 2. CBC: leukocytosis 3. Urinalysis: may show moderate RBCs	1. **IV gentamicin** 2 mg/kg load, then 1.5 mg/kg IV q 8 h (Gram negative) *PLUS* 2. **IV clindamycin** 900 mg q 8 h (anaerobes) Severely ill 1. IV Cefoxitin 2 g q 6-8 h or IV meropenem 1 g q 8 h

PERINEAL LACERATION/EPISIOTOMY CARE

- **Episiotomy**: incision of the perineum (midline or mediolateral)
  - ACOG: recommends restricted use
  - Increased risk of 3rd to 4th degree lacerations (anterior) and fecal incontinence
  - Increased postop pain and slower healing
  - Indications: shoulder dystocia, breech, forceps, vacuum
- Routine episiotomy is unnecessary and is associated with increased maternal blood loss, increased risk of disruption of the anal sphincter (third-degree extension) and rectal mucosa (fourth-degree extension), and delay in the patient's resumption of sexual activity
- Immediately after delivery, cold compresses (usually ice) applied to the perineum decrease traumatic edema and discomfort. The perineal area should be gently cleansed with plain soap at least once or twice per day and after voiding or defecation. If the perineum is kept clean, healing should occur rapidly.
- Repair of vaginal lacerations should be performed using absorbable suture material, either 2-0 or 3-0
- Cold or iced sitz baths, rather than hot sitz baths, may provide additional perineal pain relief for some patients. The patient should be put in a lukewarm tub to which ice cubes are added for 20 to 30 minutes. The cold promotes pain relief by decreasing the excitability of nerve endings and slowing nerve conduction, and by promoting local vasoconstriction, which reduces edema, inhibits hematoma formation, and decreases muscle irritability and spasm.

- Episiotomy pain can be controlled with nonsteroidal anti-inflammatory agents, which appear to be superior to acetaminophen or propoxyphene.
- An episiotomy or repaired lacerations should be inspected daily

Characteristics	Midline	Mediolateral
Surgical repair	Easy	More difficult
Faulty healing	Rare	More common
Postop pain	Minimal	Common
Anatomical results after procedure	Excellent	Faulty
Blood loss	Less	More
Dyspareunia	Rare	Occasional
Extensions	Common	Rare

Obstetric Lacerations

- Management: run-locking stitches (continuous); rectal mucosa repair, then anal sphincter repair

First degree	Involves fourchette, **perineal skin**, vaginal mucous membrane
Second degree (most common)	Fascia and muscles of **perineal body**
Third degree	Extends to *external* anal sphincter
Fourth degree	Extends to rectal mucosa and includes internal anal sphincter RF: Midline episiotomy, mid/low forceps (operative delivery), nulliparity, second stage arrest of labor (pushing too long), persistent occiput posterior position, local anesthesia, Asian race

NORMAL PHYSIOLOGY CHANGES OF PUERPERIUM

- The **puerperium**: the time (about **6 weeks**) following delivery (postpartum) during which pregnancy-induced maternal, anatomical, and physiologic changes return to the nonpregnant state
- The uterus involutes progressively; after **5 to 7 days, it is firm and no longer tender**, extending midway between the symphysis and umbilicus.
- By **2 weeks**, the **uterus is no longer palpable abdominally**
- Typically, by **6 weeks**, the uterus returns to prepregnancy size

- Normal postpartum discharge
  - Begins as **lochia rubra**: blood, shreds of tissue, and decidua (serous, reddish-brown, lasts 3 to 4 days)
  - **Lochia serosa**: mucopurulent, pale, malodorous
  - **Lochia alba:** thick, mucoid, yellowish white (2nd to 3rd week)
  - Secretions cease by week 5 to 6 postpartum
- Cervix: gradually closes; external os converted to transverse slit
- Vagina: overdistended, smooth-walls return after 3rd week postpartum
- Ovulation occurs around 70 to 75 days (up to 6 months) after delivery; suppression of ovulation is due to high prolactin levels (up to 6 weeks)
- Menstruation returns as soon as 7 weeks (70%) in nonlactating women and as late as 36 months in lactating women
- Defer oral contraception until 6 weeks postpartum due to the risk of hypercoagulable state
- **Colostrum**, the premilk secretion, is a yellowish alkaline secretion that may be present in the last months of pregnancy and for the first 2 to 3 days after delivery. It has a higher specific gravity (1.040 to 1.060); a higher protein, vitamin A, immunoglobulin, sodium and chloride content; and a lower carbohydrate, potassium, and fat content than mature breast milk
- All classes of immunoglobulins are found in milk, but **IgA constitutes 90% of immunoglobulins in human colostrum and milk**

Pregnancy vs. Postpartum

Increased	• GFR increases by 50% during pregnancy but returns to normal by week 8 postpartum • Hematocrit (seen 3-7 d postpartum) • Red cell mass (25% during pregnancy, 15% postpartum) • **Leukocytosis** (occurs during labor, extending into early puerperium): increased percent of granulocytes • **Thrombocytosis** (decreases during first hour, then increases steadily over next 2 wk) • Lung volumes: TLC
Decreased	• Cholesterol and TG decrease within 24 h postpartum • Fibrinogen (initially, then returns to normal after 7-10 d) • Estrogen levels decline immediately after delivery and remain suppressed if lactating • FSH/LH (decrease first 10-12 d, then increase) • Total blood volume (normal by week 3 postpartum) • Iron level (normalizes by week 2) • Iron supplementation not necessary if Hct/Hgb is normal 5-7 d postpartum

OB/GYN

Disease	Etiology, Prevalence, Risk Factors	Clinical Symptoms and Signs	Diagnostics	Therapy, Prognosis, and Health Maintenance
Involution of the placental site	Complete obliteration of the vessels in the placental site *fails* to occur (should occur within 4-6 wk postpartum)	1. Persistent lochia 2. Brisk hemorrhagic episodes		1. Uterotonics • **Oxytocin** given after second stage of delivery and/or after placental delivery to prevent postpartum hemorrhage 2. Uterine curettage
Maternity blues	Occurs in 50%-70% of postpartum women Occurs in first few days postpartum, ceases after PP day 10	1. Tearfulness, anxiety, irritation, restlessness 2. Depression, feelings of inadequacy, elation, mood swings, confusion 3. Difficulty concentrating 4. Headache 5. Forgetfulness 6. Insomnia 7. Depersonalization 8. Negative feelings toward baby		1. Self-limiting: physical comfort and reassurance

CHAPTER 56

Structural Abnormalities

Recommended Supplemental Topics:

Bladder Fistula, p 518

Enterocele, p 520

CYSTOCELE, UTERINE PROLAPSE, RECTOCELE (FIG. 56-1A-C AND FIG. 56-3)

Disease	Etiology, Prevalence, Risk Factors	Clinical Symptoms and Signs	Diagnostics	Therapy, Prognosis, and Health Maintenance
Cystocele (bladder prolapse)	**Anterior vaginal prolapse** of the *posterior* bladder wall into the vagina, emerging from the introitus Pelvic floor injury during childbirth Etiology: • Genetics • Prior prolapse surgery • Occupational • Connective tissue disease RF: 1. Pregnancy 2. Vaginal delivery 3. *Parity* 4. Advanced age 5. Obesity 6. **Menopause** 7. DM 8. Race (Hispanic) More common than rectocele	1. **Vaginal bulge or fullness, pressure, heaviness:** • Feels like "sitting on a ball" • "Something is falling out" • Worse with valsalva • Better with recumbency 2. **Concurrent urinary incontinence** 3. **Incomplete emptying** → retention, straining to void (obstruction) 4. Frequency, urgency, retention Signs: 1. Pelvic exam: examine patient in *lithotomy* and **standing position** • Ask to valsalva or cough 2. Splinting: patient must push up bladder in order to void	1. **POP-Q** (pelvic organ prolapse quantification): quantifies the extent and location of defects 2. U/S or MRI 3. Additional testing: Q-tip test, voiding cystourethrogram (VCUG), cystometrogram	1. **Pessary fitting** • Ring pessary • Poor operative risk: vaginal pessary 2. **Anterior vaginal colporrhaphy**–surgical repair of vaginal wall • 52% recurrence rate 3. Tension-free vaginal tape procedure (TVT) 4. If asymptomatic, no intervention necessary Prophylaxis: 1. Kegel exercises: strengthen levator ani and perianal muscles 2. Estrogen therapy after menopause: maintains tone and vitality of tissue
Uterine prolapse	Loss of the normal ligamentous support for the uterus → cervix protrudes from the introitus Risk increases 50% **postmenopausal** RF: 1. Older, multigravid women 2. Any condition that increases intra-abdominal pressure increases the risk – obesity, chronic cough, constipation, repetitive lifting	1. **Vaginal fullness or mass** • SX worse after prolonged standing or late in the day and are relieved by lying down 2. **Lower abdominal aching** 3. **Low back pain** 4. Urinary incontinence 5. With moderate prolapse– patients describe a *falling out* sensation or a feeling of "**sitting on a ball**" Signs: 1. Pelvic exam: soft, reducible mass • **Examine** both resting and straining **in both supine and standing** positions Complications: Chronic decubitus ulceration of vaginal epithelium in procidentia	1. **POP-Q** (pelvic organ prolapse quantification): quantifies the extent and location of defects 2. Additional testing: Q-tip test, cystourethroscopy, cystometrogram, anoscopy, colonoscopy, anal manometry, or transanal U/S	1. **Conservative management:** weight reduction, smoking cessation, pelvic muscle exercises (Kegels) • Kegels are first line for low-grade prolapse; most effective in younger female w/childbirth 2. **Vaginal *pessary*** • Ring pessary • Doughnut for severe uterine prolapse • Best for older and postmenopausal women with straining to void and weakness or loss of tone 3. **Vaginal hysterectomy with sacrospinous ligament suspension (SSLS)** • For severe prolapse where majority of uterus exposed 4. Colpocleisis: vagina is surgically obliterated • For elderly women who are no longer sexually active Most accompanied by cystocele, rectocele, or enterocele

OB/GYN

(continued)

(continued)

Disease	Etiology, Prevalence, Risk Factors	Clinical Symptoms and Signs	Diagnostics	Therapy, Prognosis, and Health Maintenance
Rectocele (rectal prolapse)	Prolapse of the posterior vaginal wall and rectum; contents protrude into the vagina emerging from the introitus Associated: pelvic floor injury during childbirth	HX: prolonged, excessive use of laxatives or frequent enemas (constipation): 1. Introital **bulging** • Symptoms worse with standing or straining 2. **Concurrent fecal incontinence** • Loss of stool of flatus • Incomplete rectal evacuation 3. **Constipation** 4. Low back pain 5. Dyspareunia Signs: 1. Left decubitus position—for detection • Worse with valsalva Complications: Hemorrhoids	1. **POP-Q** (pelvic organ prolapse quantification): quantifies the extent and location of defects 2. Additional testing: anal manometry, transanal U/S, MRI, colonoscopy, defecography, EMG	1. Nonsurgical: use of medication to slow transit time • Bulking agents, laxatives, stool softeners • Biofeedback • Electrical stimulation therapy 2. **Posterior colporrhaphy**: repair of posterior fascial defects • Grafts, sphincteroplasty, repair of prolapse 3. Colpocleisis (closure) or colpectomy (removal) of the vagina, if not sexually active
Bladder fistula	A urinary fistula formed between the bladder and the vagina, also known as a vesicovaginal fistula RF: 1. History of preoperative radiation, endometriosis, pelvic inflammatory disease (PID), or previous pelvic surgery 2. 50% result from abdominal hysterectomy and vaginal hysterectomy	1. Painless and **continuous incontinence** 2. Occurs after pelvic surgery, pelvic radiation, or obstetric trauma • If after surgery, typically within 14 d postop	1. **Retrograde dye test:** Methylene blue or indigo carmine injected into bladder in retrograde fashion (+) if blue dye leaks out of vagina or if it stains a tampon inserted into the vagina 2. Cystourethroscopy and VCUG—used to quantify and locate the fistula(s) 3. IV pyelogram and retrograde pyelogram—used to localize fistula(s)	1. Surgery (first line) • Typically wait 3-6 mo before attempting to repair postsurgical fistulas 2. Antibiotics—to treat UTI 3. Estrogen—for postmenopausal women

OB/GYN

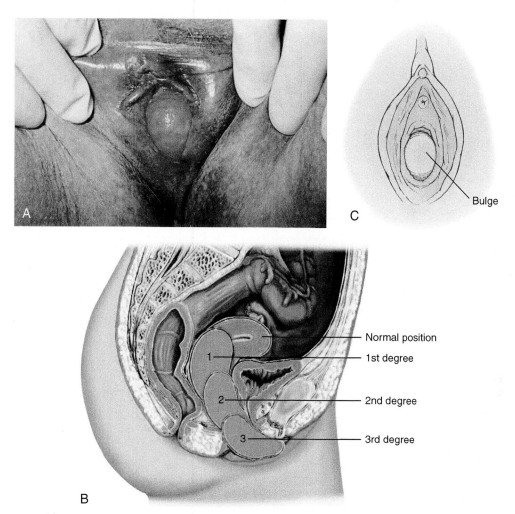

FIGURE 56-1. **A**, Cystocele. **B**, Uterine prolapse. First degree: mild prolapse—cervix remains in the vagina; second degree: moderate—cervix is at the vaginal introitus; third degree: severe—cervix and uterus are bulging out of vagina entirely. **C**, Rectocele. (**A**, © 1995 Science Photo Library/ CMSP. **B**, From Cohen BJ. *Medical Terminology*. Philadelphia: Wolters Kluwer Health; 2011. **C**, From Evans RJ, Brown YM, Evans MK. *Canadian Maternity, Newborn & Women's Health Nursing*. Philadelphia: Wolters Kluwer Health; 2015.)

Pessaries

- Contraindications: acute genital tract infections, adherent retropulsion of the uterus

- The patient should be examined 1 to 2 weeks after insertion to inspect for the presence of pressure and inflammatory or allergic reactions

- A repeat exam in 4 weeks can be done; then visits should be done at 3- to 6-month intervals to assess for continued proper fit and to evaluate for vaginal erosion and inflammation as a result of pessary use

- Vaginal pessaries are not curative of prolapse, but they may be used for months or years for palliation with proper supervision

Kegel Exercises

- These exercises are aimed to tighten and strengthen the pubococcygeus muscles

- Evidence strongly supports use the of Kegel exercises as first-line management in the treatment of urinary and fecal incontinence

OB/GYN

Disease	Etiology, Prevalence, Risk Factors	Clinical Symptoms and Signs	Diagnostics	Therapy, Prognosis, and Health Maintenance
Enterocele (Fig. 56)	Apical vaginal wall defect in which bowel is contained within the prolapsed segment; typically occurs in women post hysterectomy but can occur with uterus in situ			

OVARIAN TORSION

Disease	Etiology, Prevalence, Risk Factors	Clinical Symptoms and Signs	Diagnostics	Therapy, Prognosis, and Health Maintenance
Ovarian torsion	Associated with ovarian cysts or neoplasm in 94% Torsion of normal ovaries common in children	1. Sudden onset of unilateral lower quadrant pain 2. Nausea Signs: 1. Tenderness to palpation	1. WBC count: normal 2. β-hCG: negative 3. U/S: **ovarian mass**, free fluid in the pelvis 4. +/− Doppler U/S: check blood flow to ovaries (controversial) • Ovaries contain dual blood supply, so flow may still be present with torsion	1. **Rapid surgical exploration**

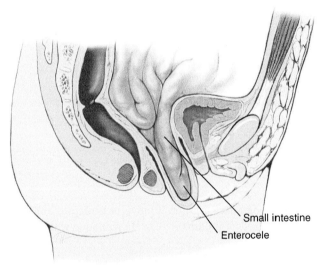

Small intestine

Enterocele

FIGURE 56-2. Enterocele with eversion. (Berek JS. *Berek & Novak's Gynecology*. 15th ed. Philadelphia: Lippincott Williams & Wikins; 2012.)

OB/GYN

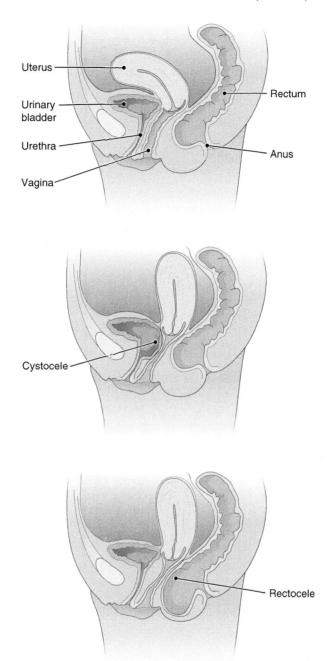

Uterus

Urinary
bladder

Urethra

Vagina

Rectum

Anus

Cystocele

Rectocele

FIGURE 56-3. Cystocele and rectocele. (From Weber JR. *Nurses' Handbook of Health Assessment.* Philadelphia: Wolters Kluwer Health; 2014.)

CHAPTER **57**

Miscellaneous

ENDOMETRIOSIS, OVARIAN CYST, LEIOMYOMA (FIBROIDS)

- The *stage* of endometriosis does not correlate with the *occurrence* or *severity* of pain symptoms
- For women attempting conception, selective COX-2 inhibitors (such as celecoxib, rofecoxib, and valdecoxib) should be avoided as NSAID therapy
- Fibroids are often described according to their location in the uterus
- **Leiomyomas (fibroids)**—are the most common indication for hysterectomy, accounting for 30% of hysterectomies in white women and over 50% of hysterectomies in black women
- **Serous cystadenomas**: larger than functional cysts and present with increasing abdominal girth
- **Mucinous cystadenomas**: multilocular, quite large
- **Dermoid tumors**: most common tumor found in women of all ages; solid components and appear on ultrasound, contain teeth, cartilage, bone, fat, and hair; median age is 30; 80% occur in reproductive years

OB/GYN

Disease	Etiology, Prevalence, Risk Factors	Clinical Symptoms and Signs	Diagnostics	Therapy, Prognosis, and Health Maintenance
Endometriosis Endometrial glands and stroma that occur *outside* the uterine cavity	HX: of PID/STD, laparoscopy for chronic pelvic pain or dysmenorrhea, infertility Present in 30% of *infertile* women MC: **25-35**, white Rare in young girls or postmenopausal women Estrogen-dependent, benign, inflammatory disease MC sites: *Ovaries*, anterior and posterior cul-de-sac, posterior broad ligaments, uterosacral ligaments, uterus, fallopian tubes, sigmoid colon, appendix, round ligament RF that increase risk: Nulliparity, prolonged endogenous estrogen (early menarche), late menopause, exposure to DES in utero, lower BMI, high consumption of trans unsaturated fat, outflow tract obstructions	"Missing work due to pain" 1. *Cyclical* pelvic pain, worsening • Sharp or dull, throbbing or burning 2. **Dysmenorrhea** • Dull or crampy pelvic pain starting 1-2 days before menses, persists throughout menses, can continue several days after 3. **Dyspareunia** 4. GI SX: **dyschezia**, hematochezia, *cramping*, constipation, diarrhea 5. Urinary SX: dysuria, hematuria, urgency, frequency Signs: 1. Uterus normal size, abdominal and lower • **Fixed uterus, retroflexed**, nonmobile in pelvis 2. **Palpable adnexal (or ovarian) mass** 3. Uterosacral ligament nodularity 4. Complications: Infertility	1. **Transvaginal U/S**: hypoechoic, vascular, and/or solid mass • Irregular margins, spiculated, infiltrates adjacent tissues • May also see ovarian cysts (endometriomas) • Most endometrial tissue cannot be seen on U/S with the exception of endometriomas 2. Definitive: **exploratory laparoscopy and biopsy**, although not required for treatment • **"Blue-black powder burn lesions"** • Raised flame-like patches, whitish opacifications, yellow-brown discolorations, translucent blebs, or reddish blue irregularly shaped islands 3. Serum CA 125 can be elevated (>35 U/mL); not routinely ordered	Mild–moderate: Does not cause regular absence from school/work, no evidence on U/S 1. **NSAIDs** for pelvic pain 2. Oral contraceptives (**OCPs**), **Depo, Mirena IUD** Severe: Regularly miss school/work, failed therapy, or recurrence 1. **GnRH Agonist (Leuprolide)** with OCPs 2. Laparoscopy–if failed medical treatment or planning pregnancy in future 3. *Definitive* treatment: **hysterectomy** + bilateral salpingo-oophorectomy • Persistent pain unresponsive to medical therapy, SX limiting function, or bladder lesions
Ovarian cysts (endometrioma) "chocolate cysts"	Ectopic endometrial tissue within the ovary bleeds and results in a hematoma surrounded by duplicated ovarian parenchyma **Endometrioma:** isolated collection of endometriosis involving an ovary	1. Asymptomatic masses OR 2. Pelvic pain 3. Menstrual delay (irregularity) 4. Urinary frequency 5. Constipation 6. Pelvic "heaviness" Signs: 1. Contains thick, brown, tarlike fluid: **"syruplike chocolate-colored material"**	1. *Pelvic U/S* (first line) 2. Pregnancy test, CBC 3. Check a CA-125 if concerning for ovarian cancer	Small, asymptomatic: 1. **Contraceptive hormones (OCP)**–prevent new cyst formation 2. Repeat U/S in 6-8 wk Large, symptomatic: 1. *Cystectomy*–if symptomatic (first line) • Follow with longterm OCPs to prevent recurrence 2. *Oophorectomy* (definitive)–for recurrent cysts, completed childbearing, postmenopausal or concerns for malignancy Complications: Hemoperitoneum (with rupture)
Follicular cysts	Usually multiple, occurring in BOTH ovaries Most are *functional*: result of failed ovulation			

OB/GYN

(continued)

(continued)

Disease	Etiology, Prevalence, Risk Factors	Clinical Symptoms and Signs	Diagnostics	Therapy, Prognosis, and Health Maintenance
Simple and complex follicular cysts	Result from failure of maturing follicles to ovulate and involute Cyst may continue to grow until it ruptures → tender and symptomatic at midcycle	1. Freely mobile pelvic or abdominal mass	1. Pelvic U/S • U/S: *Simple*, unilocular, smooth-walled cysts (reassurance) • U/S: *Complex*, multiloculated, with thick septations, papillae, or excrescences (worrisome) 2. Pregnancy test, CBC	1. Most regress spontaneously 2-8 wk • *Asymptomatic <6 cm* 2. Observe +/− OCPs 3. Aspiration • *Symptomatic >6 cm* 4. Cystectomy—if persistent, increased size, >4-6 cm, or SX
Ruptured ovarian cyst	Results in release of cyst fluid or blood that may irritate the peritoneal cavity RF: Vaginal intercourse, ovulation induction MC: Right ovary	1. **Mittelschmerz**: Abrupt onset severe pain in midmenstrual cycle • Unilateral lower abdominal pain • Severe, sharp, focal • Increased with sitting 2. **Immediately follows sexual intercourse or exercise** 3. Shoulder or upper abdominal pain Signs: 1. Unilateral lower quadrant tender to palpation 2. **Cullen sign** (periumbilical ecchymoses) 3. Adnexal mass +/− cervical motion tenderness	Clinical DX: 1. Serum or urine hCG—r/o ectopic pregnancy 2. CBC w/diff • Hct: low 3. Type and screen 4. Urine, cervical, blood tests for STIs or UTI 5. Pelvic U/S: adnexal mass and fluid in pelvis	**Laparoscopy** • Prevention of cyst rupture NOT an indication for surgery for asymptomatic cysts
Corpus luteum cysts Follicular cysts form midcycle followed by a corpus luteum	Rarely >4 cm Filled with blood FHX: Breast, ovarian, or nongyn cancer More likely to rupture in the luteal phase	1. Asymptomatic 2. Symptoms • GI SX—bloating, change in bowel habits, fixed pelvic mass, ascites • Pain • Fever • SX triggered by sexual intercourse Signs: 1. Adnexal mass, tenderness, nodularity	1. Pelvic U/S • Increased internal echoes	1. Observe: 2 wk-3 mo • Most involute spontaneously 2. OCP therapy 3. Immediate surgical intervention if anemia or hemodynamic instability 4. Increased risk of torsion due to increased ovarian size and weight
Tuboovarian abscess	Typically, a complication of pelvic inflammatory disease (PID) but can also be caused by other infectious sources, eg, diverticular disease, hemorrhagic cyst, especially if immunocompromised MC causes: *E. coli*, aerobic streptococci, *Bacteroides fragilis*, *Prevotella*, gonorrhoeae, *Chlamydia trachomatis*	1. Acute lower abdominal pain 2. Fever, chills 3. Vaginal discharge Signs: 1. Adnexal mass 2. Cervical motion tenderness 3. Uterine or adnexal tenderness	1. Pelvic U/S: complex multilocular mass that obliterates normal adnexal architecture 2. CBC: leukocytosis 3. GC/CT testing 4. Blood cultures 5. Pregnancy test	1. Immediate **laparotomy** if: • Hemodynamically unstable, peritoneal signs, acidotic 2. Antibiotics alone if: • Postmenopausal, <9 cm diameter, adequate response, hemodynamically stable • Cefoxitin or cefotetan + doxycycline +/− Clindamycin or metronidazole Complications: Abscess rupture, sepsis

OB/GYN

Disease	Etiology, Prevalence, Risk Factors	Clinical Symptoms and Signs	Diagnostics	Therapy, Prognosis, and Health Maintenance
Leiomyoma (fibroids) Estrogen and progesterone sensitive: grow during pregnancy and shrink after menopause	Most common **solid pelvic tumor** **Black** (20 s) > white (30-40 s) Benign, smooth muscle cell tumor of the myometrium RF: 1. Black (3×) 2. Early menarche (<10 y/o) 3. ETOH intake 4. (+) family history PF: Inc parity, long acting progestin only (Depo Provera), smoking	Mostly asymptomatic: 1. **Menorrhagia:** *excessive* and *prolonged* bleeding 2. **Pelvic pain/pressure:** • Bulk-related SX: *Voiding difficulties*, constipation, urethral compression (urinary urgency, frequency) • Sensation of pelvic *heaviness*/bearing down • Dyspareunia • Dysmenorrhea 3. **Infertility** Signs: 1. **Abdominal distention** 2. Bimanual exam: ***enlarged, mobile uterus*** with irregular contour Complications: Increased risk of miscarriage	1. **Pelvic U/S:** distinguishes fibroids from adnexal masses • First line, diagnostic • If SX or size increasing, proceed with additional workup • Also screen for hypothyroidism and anemia 2. Hysteroscopy—less accurate than U/S 3. MRI: size and location • Reserved for surgical planning and complicated procedures 4. Hysterosalpingogram (HSG): defines contour of endometrial cavity 5. EMB if >40 to r/o endometrial carcinoma	*Observation*, reassurance—if asymptomatic, small, or postmenopausal 1. Bimanual q 6 mo *Intervention*—large tumors, symptomatic, or unclear dx (uterine conservation) 2. **OCPs, POPs** (first line) 3. GnRH agonists (**Lupron**): most effective • AE: bone loss → osteoporosis 4. ***Myomectomy*** • Contraindications: pregnancy • Indications: AUB, bulk related SX, infertility, recurrent miscarriage 5. ***Hysterectomy*** (definitive tx) • Eliminates current SX and recurrence Not necessary to follow in pregnancy unless symptomatic—can cause soft tissue dystocia
Adenomyosis gland tissue grows during the menstrual cycle and, at menses, tries to slough but cannot escape the uterine muscle and flow out of the cervix as part of normal menses. This trapping of blood and tissue causes uterine pain in the form of monthly menstrual cramps	Endometrial glands and stroma embedded *within* the wall of the uterus (myometrium) Hypertrophy and hyperplasia of myometrium → globular uterus 20% of women Presents in 40s RF: parity and uterine surgeries (C-section)	Asymptomatic HX: tubal ligation: 1. ***Noncyclical*** pelvic pain • "Progressively worsening severe menstrual pain" regular menses • May occur during and after menses 2. **Menorrhagia:** very heavy flow 4. **Dysmenorrhea** • Differentiates from fibroids or sarcomas Signs: 1. *Enlarged*, globular uterus	1. CBC—Mildly anemic 2. MRI—most accurate 3. DX during hysterectomy (most)	1. NSAIDs for pain 2. GnRH agonists first line for pain but will recur after D/C therapy 3. ***Total hysterectomy*** (80% effective) • Difficult to excise

- Growth of fibroids stimulated by ESTROGEN – **GnRH agonists** inhibit endogenous estrogen production by suppressing the hypothalamic pituitary ovarian axis (40% to 60% reduction in size, 3 to 6 months)

- Initially increase release of gonadotropes → desensitize, downregulation → hypogonadotropic, hypogonadal "menopause"

OB/GYN

Surgical Treatments for Leiomyoma

Hysterectomy	• Indications
	  • women with acute hemorrhage who do not respond to other therapies
	  • women who have completed childbearing and have current or increased future risk of other diseases (cervical intraepithelial neoplasia, endometriosis, adenomyosis, endometrial hyperplasia, or increased risk of uterine or ovarian cancer) that would be eliminated or decreased by hysterectomy
	  • women who have failed prior minimally invasive therapy for leiomyomas
	  • women who have completed childbearing and have significant symptoms, multiple leiomyomas, and a desire for a definitive end to symptomatology
	• The main advantage of hysterectomy over other invasive interventions is that it eliminates both current symptoms and the chance of recurrent problems from leiomyomas
	• Definitive for fibroids, prolapse, or persistent bothersome endometriosis (do not plan future childbearing, failed both medical therapy and at least one conservative method)

Myomectomy	• Myomectomy is an option for women who have *not* completed childbearing or otherwise wish to retain their uterus • Although myomectomy is an effective therapy for menorrhagia and pelvic pressure, the disadvantage of this procedure is the *risk that more leiomyomas* will develop from new clones of abnormal myocytes
Endometrial ablation	• In women who have completed childbearing, endometrial ablation, either alone or in combination with hysteroscopic myomectomy, is an option for the management of bleeding abnormalities • Preserves the uterus and ovarian tissue but renders infertile • Since intramural and subserosal leiomyomas are not affected by this procedure, *bulk* or *pressure* symptoms are *unlikely to improve* • **First line** for *severe* endometriosis
Uterine artery embolization (UAE)	• Minimally invasive option for management of leiomyoma-related symptoms • Effective option for women who wish to preserve their uterus and are not interested in optimizing future fertility

SPOUSE OR PARTNER NEGLECT/ VIOLENCE

• Domestic violence screening at first prenatal visit, again at least once per trimester, again at postpartum visit

Disease	Etiology, Prevalence, Risk Factors	Clinical Symptoms and Signs	Diagnostics	Therapy, Prognosis, and Health Maintenance
Intimate partner violence (IPV)	Abusive behavior (physical, sexual, emotional) by a person in an intimate relationship with the victim F > M to be victims Goal of abuser: gain control over victim RF: Young (<35), pregnant; being single, divorced or separated; ETOH or drug abuse in victim or partner, smoking, low economic status	1. Explanation of injuries that do not fit with exam findings 2. Frequent visits to ED 3. Somatic complaints: headache, abdominal pain, fatigue Signs: 1. Vague during history 2. Minimal eye contact 3. Abuser in room answers all questions or declines to leave room 4. Injuries to central area of body, forearms 5. Bruises in various stages of healing	Screening tools: 1. HITS (Hurt, Insult, Threaten, Screamed at tool) 2. WAST (Women Abuse Screening Tool) 3. PVS (Partner Violence Screen) 4. AAS (Abuse Assessment Screen) 5. WEB (women's experience with battering) scale	1. Most important: Speak with patient alone 2. Document all history and findings carefully 3. USPSTF recommends screening women of childbearing age for IPV including domestic violence and refer women who screen (+) to intervention services • Interventions: leave abusive situation ensuring a safe place to go, counseling to assess risk of danger, create plan for safety

OB/GYN

SEXUAL ASSAULT

- Defined as any sex act done on a person who does not want it (includes rape but does not always indicate rape), which can occur when someone is passed out, drunk, or on drugs unable to make decisions for themselves
- Physical contact need not occur to be considered assault (eg, forced to watch sexual act)
- 1 in 3 women will be sexually assaulted in her lifetime, but 10% of rape victims are men
- Victims of assault should
  - Call a close friend or family member they trust
  - Call a doctor or nurse or go to the emergency room (or call the sexual assault hotline, 800-656-4673)
  - Not try to clean up before seeing a doctor or nurse
  - Find a counselor or someone to talk to about what happened
  - File a police report
  - Follow-up with a doctor or nurse in 1 to 2 weeks after
  - Ask about victim compensation services
  - Use a condom for at least 3 months after being raped to reduce the chance of spreading infection
  - Request emergency contraception up to 5 days after being raped if you are worried you might be pregnant (must be older than 17 to obtain without a prescription)

Disease	Etiology, Prevalence, Risk Factors	Clinical Symptoms and Signs	Diagnostics	Therapy, Prognosis, and Health Maintenance
In adults	MC: Women, age 16-24	1. Disturbances in sleep 2. Decreased appetite 3. Somatic symptoms (chronic pelvic pain, recurrent abdominal pain, chronic headache) 4. Depression 5. Suicidality 6. Anxiety 7. Decreased self-esteem or worth 8. Sexual dysfunction 9. Fragility of sense of masculinity and confusion about sexual orientation Signs: PTSD signs		1. Evaluate and collect evidence up to 24 h after assault 2. Report to authorities 3. Follow-up in 1-2 wk
In children		1. Nonspecific 2. Rectal or genital bleeding 3. STIs not acquired prenatally Signs: 1. Sexually explicit acting out 2. Signs of penetration 3. Inappropriate knowledge of sexual activity for development 4. Developmentally inappropriate play (asking to touch adult's genitals or asking adult to touch child's genitals) 5. Swelling or blue discoloration of the anus	1. Forensic evidence collection 2. Screen for STIs 3. Evaluate for pregnancy	1. Evaluate and collect evidence up to 24 h after assault 2. Report to CPS 3. Follow-up in 1-2 wk

OB/GYN

URINARY INCONTINENCE

Disease	Etiology, Prevalence, Risk Factors	Clinical Symptoms and Signs	Diagnostics	Therapy, Prognosis, and Health Maintenance
Urge incontinence (overactive bladder): detrusor overactivity (uninhibited bladder contractions) caused by irritation within the bladder or loss of inhibitory neurologic control of bladder contractions	Women 75+ (31%) Causes: cystitis, prostatitis, atrophic vaginitis, bladder diverticulum, pelvic radiation therapy Loss of neurologic control from stroke, dementia, spinal cord injury, Parkinson disease	1. Loss of urine preceded by a sudden and severe desire to pass urine • Loss of urine on way to toilet • Loss ranges from minimal to flooding 2. Contractions with change in body position (supine to upright) or with sensory stimulation (running water, hand washing, cold weather) 3. **Frequency** and **nocturia** common 4. **Urgency** w/o urinary loss (OAB)	1. Voiding diary: variable 2. Cough stress test: may show delayed leakage after cough 3. PVR: <50 mL 4. Check serum creatinine: elevated	• Pelvic floor muscle training (PFMT) • Scheduled voiding • Avoid diet triggers (ETOH, caffeine) <u>**Anticholinergics**</u>: Oxybutynin, Ditropan TCA: imipramine—helps with urgency symptoms Pseudoephedrine (a-block): improves urethral tone <u>Surgical</u>: Botox (may result in needing to self-cath); sacral neuromodulation
Stress incontinence: Sphincter weakness (urethral sphincter and/or pelvic floor weakness)	Primarily **F >30** <u>Causes</u>: May occur after childbirth in obese women	1. Loss of small amount of urine during physical inactivity or increased intra-abdominal pressure (**cough, sneeze, jump, lift, exercise**) • Can occur with minimal activity, such as walking or rising from a chair	1. Voiding diary: small volume leakage (5-10 cc) with activity 2. *Cough stress test* (+): leakage with coughing (most reliable) 3. PVR: <50 mL	Weight loss Pelvic floor exercises (Kegels): decreases urethral hypermobility Incontinence pessary Periurethral bulking **Retropubic urethropexy**, such as TVT (tension free vaginal tape) and other sling procedures—best 5-y success rates (due to hypermobility)
Overflow incontinence (urinary retention): overdistention of bladder caused by impaired detrusor contractility or bladder outlet obstruction	5% of patients with chronic incontinence <u>Causes</u>: Anticholinergic meds, pelvic organ prolapse, DM, multiple sclerosis, spinal cord injuries	1. **Dribbling** 2. Inability to empty bladder 3. Hesitancy 4. Urine loss without recognizable urge or sensation of fullness or pressure in lower abdomen	1. Voiding diary: varies 2. Cough stress test: no leakage 3. **Postvoid residual urine measurement: >200-300 mL**	Urethral bulking procedure
Functional incontinence: caused by environmental or physical barriers to toileting	Non-GU factors: cognitive or physical impairment resulting in patient's inability to void independently	History of severe dementia, physical frailty, or inability to ambulate, mental health disorder (depression)	1. Voiding diary: pattern in circumstances of incontinence 2. Cough stress test: no leakage 3. PVR: varies	

OB/GYN

INFERTILITY

Disease	Etiology, Prevalence, Risk Factors	Clinical Symptoms and Signs	Diagnostics	Therapy, Prognosis, and Health Maintenance
Infertility	<u>Ovary RF:</u> PCOS (most), h/o radiation, hypogonadotropic hypogonadism, ovarian failure Tubal RF: h/o pelvic infection (**pelvic inflammatory disease**), pelvic surgery, personal or family history of endometriosis <u>Uterine factor:</u> Asherman syndrome, structural abnormalities, history of D&C, recurrent miscarriage, IUD <u>Cervical factor:</u> Abnormal PAP, cervical infection <u>Male RF:</u> Illness with fever in last 70-90 d, viral (mumps) orchitis, chemotherapy, urogenital surgery, torsion, recent hot tub use, lubricant use, anabolic steroid use, chronic ETOH/smoking, marijuana	1. Inability to conceive after 1 year of unprotected sex	1. U/S, EMB, Pap smear, postcoital test, cervical cultures 2. Ovarian reserve testing, if >35, unexplained, or smoker 3. Ovulation testing (LH kit), BBT, midluteal progesterone (>3 ng/mL) 4. Hysterosalpingogram: tube patency 5. **Chromopertubation** (gold standard) 6. Hysterosonogram & pelvic U/S 7. Semen analysis (minimum values): *Volume > 1.5 mL* *Concentration > 15 million/mL* *pH > 7.2* *Viscosity < 2 cm* *Vitality > 58%* *Total Motility > 40%* *Morphology (normal forms) > 4%*	1. Ovarian stimulation with clomiphene citrate (**Clomid**) +/− intrauterine insemination 2. IVF if other treatments fail *Tubal infertility* • 12% after 1 episode of PID • 25% after 2 episodes of PID • 50% after 3 episodes of PID

PRACTICE QUESTIONS

1. A 62-year-old obese woman presents to the gynecologist complaining of painless vaginal bleeding for the past 10 months despite going through menopause 14 years ago. Her medical history is significant for hypertension, diabetes, breast cancer (currently on Tamoxifen), and a 40-pack year smoking history. Sonogram shows a thickened endometrial stripe, endometrial biopsy results are pending. Which of the following aspects of the patient's history contributes least to her suspected diagnosis?

   A. Tamoxifen-use

   B. Smoking

   C. Age

   D. Obesity

2. A 29-year-old G1 woman at 12 weeks comes to the clinic for scheduled prenatal testing. Both patient and father of baby have no personal or family history of chromosomal anomalies. Doppler shows good fetal heart tones. Which test is indicated to screen for trisomies 13, 18 and 21 as well as for Turner Syndrome?

   A. Chorionic villi sampling

   B. Amniocentesis

   C. Nuchal translucency screening test

   D. Nonstress test

3. A 26-year-old woman presents for follow-up of a palpable left breast lump found on breast exam 6 months ago. At the time of diagnosis, physical exam revealed a 1.5-cm diameter, well-circumscribed, firm, mobile mass that was nontender to palpation. Today the mass is 3 cm in diameter and has become painful. Ultrasound shows the mass to have uniform hypoechogenicity. What is the most appropriate therapy?

   A. Observation

   B. Fine needle aspiration

   C. Excision

   D. Mastectomy

4. A 21-year-old sexually active woman presents complaining of a genital lesion for the past 2 weeks. On physical exam, there is a painless ulcer with a raised, indurated margin and inguinal lymphadenopathy. Patient denies fever, chills, headache, abnormal gait, or dementia. What is the appropriate treatment?

   A. Penicillin G benzathine 2.4 million units IM once

   B. Penicillin G benzathine 2.4 million units IM once weekly for 3 weeks

   C. Aqueous penicillin G 4 million units IV every 4 hours for 14 days

   D. Doxycycline 100 mg twice daily for 14 days

OB/GYN

5. A 27-year-old G3P2002 woman at 36 weeks of gestation complains of abdominal pain and vaginal bleeding. She denies any history of trauma or leakage of fluid. Physical exam reveals a tender fundus and moderate amount of dark blood in vaginal vault. Cervix is not dilated. Fetal heart tones are in the 160 to 170 ranges. Which of the following is NOT a risk factor for the likely diagnosis?

    A. Advanced maternal age
    B. Cocaine use
    C. First pregnancy
    D. Smoking

6. The second stage of labor begins when the cervical os measures how many centimeters?

    A. 8
    B. 6
    C. 10
    D. 4

7. A 16-year-old girl complains of prolonged menstruation since her first period 6 months ago. She gets her cycle every 30 days, and experiences heavy bleeding for 10 days. She denies pain during her cycle. Bimanual pelvic exam reveals a normal sized cervix without any palpable masses. Transvaginal ultrasound is normal. What is the most likely diagnosis?

    A. Adenomyosis
    B. Endometriosis
    C. Dysfunctional uterine bleeding
    D. Leiomyoma

8. A 32-year-old woman had a spontaneous vaginal delivery with no complications. At one minute, the infant is crying, is pink at the trunk and has blue extremities, has a grimace on stimulation and is flexing arms and legs. Pulse is 96. What is the Apgar score?

    A. 5
    B. 6
    C. 7
    D. 4

9. A 14-year-old girl complains of painful menstruation. She reports crampy, intermittent lower abdominal pain a few days before the onset of menses that resolves within a day or two of menses. She has had irregular, heavy menses since menarche at 12 years old. Pelvic examination is unremarkable. What is the most likely diagnosis?

    A. Primary dysmenorrhea
    B. Secondary dysmenorrhea
    C. Pelvic inflammatory disease
    D. Adenomyosis

10. A 33-year-old G3P2002 woman presents at 36 weeks of gestation. She states she is feeling regular contractions. Vital signs are stable. Cervical exam shows no cervical os dilation. Fetal monitor shows a baseline of 120 with fetal HR accelerations increasing to 135 for 15 seconds. What is your next step in management?

    A. Administer oxytocin to induce labor.
    B. This is a nonreassuring fetal heart rate—change the position of the mother.
    C. Fetus is in distress; perform low transverse cesarean section.
    D. This is a reassuring fetal monitor. Continue regular cervical examinations.

11. A 26-year-old G2P1001 woman is at 29 weeks of gestation and arrives to the clinic for a routine prenatal visit. Her pregnancy has been complicated by persistent nausea and vomiting and back pain. She had a quad screen at 16 weeks that was normal. What would suggest that she has hyperemesis gravidarum?

    A. Less than 5% loss of prepregnancy weight
    B. Syncopal episodes
    C. Ketonuria
    D. Metabolic acidosis

12. A 26-year-old woman presents to the ER complaining of severe unilateral abdominal pain. Patient's LMP was 2 months ago but she started spotting last week. She also was treated for an STI in the past but she does not remember which one. Upon abdominal exam, patient has unilateral adnexal tenderness and the rest of exam is normal. Vital signs include temp 98.2°F, HR 110, BP 125/90, RR 18, pulse ox: 99% on room air. Urine pregnancy test is positive. Which diagnostic study is the best to determine diagnosis?

    A. CT abdomen/pelvis
    B. Transvaginal ultrasonography
    C. Repeat serum hCG levels in a week
    D. Blood type and Rh screen

13. A 31-year-old G2P1 woman presents to clinic at 26 weeks with no complaints. She has no history or family history of diabetes but was told her first baby was large for gestational age. Her 1-hour serum glucose was 160 a week ago and her 3-hour glucose tolerance test values from today are as follows:

    1 hour 200
    2 hour 170
    3 hour 35

    After 2 weeks of controlling her diet, she comes in with a fasting glucose reading of 145 and a 2-hour postprandial blood sugar measurement of 130. What is the most likely diagnosis and best treatment option at this time?

    A. Type II diabetes/insulin and continue diet and exercise
    B. Gestational diabetes/begin metformin and continue diet and exercise
    C. Neither type II nor gestational diabetes, but patient is at risk for type II diabetes after delivery and must initiate diet and exercise
    D. Gestational diabetes/begin insulin and continue diet and exercise

14. A 31-year-old woman complains of fishy smelling vaginal discharge for the past 3 days. On physical exam, a gray homogenous discharge is present. Wet mount shows clue cells. What is the most likely pathogen?

A. *Trichomonas vaginalis*

B. *Candida albicans*

C. *Chlamydia trachomatis*

D. *Gardnerella vaginalis*

15. A 28-year-old G2P1001 woman presents at 34 weeks' gestation and has had 6 contractions in the past hour. She denies pain or vaginal bleeding. Examination shows cervical os dilated at 2 cm. Nitrazine test is negative. What is the most likely diagnosis?

A. Premature rupture of membranes

B. Preterm labor

C. Abruption placentae

D. Braxton Hicks

16. A 33-year-old G2P1001 woman at 29 weeks of gestation presents complaining of feeling a gush of fluid from her vagina. Upon speculum examination, you visualize a pool of fluid in the vagina. What do you see under the microscope and what color does the nitrazine paper turn to suspect your diagnosis?

A. Ferning/blue

B. No ferning/blue

C. Ferning/red

D. No ferning/red

17. A 50-year-old woman presents complaining of amenorrhea for the past 10 months. She denies hot flashes, night sweats, and vaginal dryness. She wants to know if she is going through menopause. Which lab study would be elevated during menopause?

A. Estradiol

B. Progesterone

C. FSH

D. T4

18. A 28-year-old woman delivered a healthy baby via cesarean section and is postpartum 12 hours. She currently has no symptoms and no lacerations were found on vaginal exam. She had an estimated blood loss of 2500 cc and required a blood transfusion. What is her diagnosis?

A. Late postpartum hemorrhage

B. Early postpartum hemorrhage

C. Normal postpartum presentation

D. Endometritis

19. A 32-year-old woman postop day 5 from cesarean section without complications presents complaining of uterine tenderness. Vital signs are as follows: Temp: 102.1, HR 100, RR 16, Pulse O_2: 98% on room air. Labs show a WBC 30 000. Ultrasound did not show any products of conception. What is appropriate treatment for the diagnosis?

A. Antipyretics and follow-up in 2 days

B. Admit and administer IV gentamycin and clindamycin

C. Give PO clindamycin and discharge home with follow-up in 2 days

D. Perform dilation and curettage

20. A 58-year-old woman presents to her OBGYN complaining of right breast pain and itching for 4 weeks. Her PCP prescribed antibiotics for her a couple of weeks ago but symptoms remain unchanged. On physical exam, her right breast is red, swollen, and warm, without induration. The skin appears thickened with diffuse dimpling, similar to an orange peel. What is the most likely diagnosis?

A. Mastitis

B. Breast abscess

C. Inflammatory breast cancer

D. Fibroadenoma

21. A 25-year-old woman complains of malodorous vaginal discharge and dysuria for the past 4 days. On physical exam, a thin green frothy discharge is present, and there are punctate hemorrhages on the cervix. What is the most appropriate first step for diagnosis?

A. Wet mount

B. KOH prep

C. Tzank smear

D. Culture

22. A 28-year-old G1 woman at 10 weeks of gestational age presents with moderate vaginal bleeding for 2 days. Serum hCG is high for gestational age and transvaginal ultrasonography reveals multiple hyperechoic areas or "cluster of grapes" with no fetus. What is the diagnosis?

A. Ectopic pregnancy

B. Placenta previa

C. Hydatidiform mole

D. Abruptio placentae

23. A 30-year-old woman complains of cyclical breast pain, fatigue, bloating, depression, and angry outbursts associated with her last 4 menstrual cycles. During which phase of the menstrual cycle do these symptoms begin?

A. Follicular

B. Luteal

C. Ovulation

D. Entire menstrual cycle

24. A 32-year-old woman complains of breast pain and fever for the past 2 days. She has been breastfeeding since she gave birth 2 months ago. Three weeks ago, she was treated with antibiotics for left breast pain, erythema, and warmth. On physical exam, her there is a 3 cm diameter fluctuant, tender, red mass adjacent to the areola. What is the most likely diagnosis?

A. Mastitis

B. Breast abscess

C. Galactocele

D. Inflammatory breast cancer

25. A 72-year-old G3P3 postmenopausal woman presents with urinary incontinence for the past year. On speculum exam, the anterior vaginal wall is visible at the hymen during valsalva. Over the past 6 months, she has lost 10 pounds, improving her urinary symptoms a mild amount but not resolving them. What is the most appropriate therapy at this time?

A. Pessary
B. Hysterectomy
C. Colpocleisis
D. Anterior colporrhaphy

ANSWERS

1. History and Physical: Gyn Neoplasm. Answer B: Smoking is considered protective against endometrial cancer. More than 5 years of combined OCP use also decreases the incidence of endometrial carcinoma because progestin suppresses endometrial proliferation. A, Painless postmenopausal bleeding is associated with endometrial carcinoma. The main risk factor for endometrial carcinoma is unopposed estrogen exposure. Tamoxifen is a selective estrogen receptor modulator, which acts as an antagonist to estrogen in the breast but an agonist in the endometrium for postmenopausal women. C, Age is a risk factor for endometrial carcinoma. Mean age of diagnosis is 62. D, Obesity is a cause of excess endogenous estrogen because adipose tissue converts androstenedione to estrone. Other causes of excess estrogen include: chronic anovulation, early menarche, and late menopause, nulliparity, estrogen-secreting tumors, and postmenopausal estrogen therapy without progesterone (in women with a uterus).

2. Clinical Intervention: Prenatal Care. Answer C: NT testing is performed at 10 to 13 weeks and screens for trisomies 13, 18, 21, and for Turner syndrome. A, Chorionic villi sampling is performed between 10 and 13 weeks, but it is not indicated in this scenario. Indications include maternal age ≥35; previous child with chromosomal abnormality; patient, father of baby, or family history of chromosomal anomaly; abnormal first or second trimester maternal serum screening tests; two previous pregnancy losses, or an abnormal ultrasound. B, Amniocentesis is performed between 15 and 18 weeks of gestation for the same reasons as chorionic villi sampling and additionally for neural tube defect risks. D, Nonstress test involves an external Doppler monitor along with an external stress gauge for uterine contractions. It is used near term to monitor fetal well-being.

3. Clinical Intervention: Breast Fibroadenoma. Answer C: Excision is appropriate for benign fibroadenomas that are massively enlarging and symptomatic because of the possibility of malignancy. A, Benign fibroadenomas that are less than 2.5 cm and are not enlarging can be observed.

4. Clinical Therapeutics: Syphilis. Answer A: This is the treatment for early syphilis (primary syphilis, secondary syphilis, and early latent syphilis). B, This is the treatment for late syphilis (tertiary syphilis, and late latent syphilis). C, This is the treatment for neurosyphilis. D, This is an alternative treatment for penicillin allergic patients with early syphilis.

5. H&P: Placental Abruption. Answer C: Abruptio placentae is the premature separation of normally planted placenta after the 20th week gestation but before birth. It is the most common cause of third trimester bleeding and classically presents as painful vaginal bleeding. Risk factors for placental abruption are all of the above except: first pregnancy. The opposite is true—multigestation and multiparty are both risk factors. Other risk factors include: hypertension, trauma, decreased folic acid, uterine anomalies, and previous abruption.

6. Scientific Concepts: Normal Labor and Delivery. Answer C: The first stage of labor begins at the onset of true, regular contractions, and ends when the cervical os is fully dilated at 10 cm. The second stage of labor begins with the cervical os is fully dilated and ends with delivery of the infant.

7. Diagnosis: Dysfunctional Uterine Bleeding. Answer C: Dysfunctional uterine bleeding is irregular menstruation (duration, frequency, amount etc) without an organic cause. It is most common around menarche and perimenopause. Labs, physical exam, imaging will be unremarkable. Most common cause is chronic anovulation. A, Adenomyosis can present with menorrhagia, but bimanual exam would reveal a tender, symmetrically enlarged, globular uterus. B, Endometriosis typically presents with the triad of dysmenorrhea, pelvic pain, and dyspareunia. D, Fibroids most commonly present with menorrhagia, but pelvic exam would reveal a large, irregular, hard mass. US would show shadowing.

8. Scientific Concepts: APGAR Score. Answer B: Apgar score is 6 and calculated at 1 and 5 minutes upon delivery. See table.

APGAR	0	1	2
Skin color "**appearance**"	Blue or pale all over	Blue extremeties, pink body	No cyanosis, body and extremities pink
Pulse	Absent	<100 BPM	>100 BPM
Reflex "**grimace**"	No response to stimulation	Grimace on stimulation	Cry on stimulation
Activity	None	Arms and legs flexed	Active movement
Respiration	Absent	Slow, irregular	Good, crying

9. Diagnosis: Dysmenorrhea. Answer A: Primary dysmenorrhea is abdominal pain during menses in the absence of demonstrable disease. Primary dysmenorrhea is common in adolescents, with irregular or heavy menstrual flow. The pain is typically lower abdominal and described as crampy. B, Secondary dysmenorrhea is painful menstruation with identifiable cause. C, Pelvic inflammatory disease would present with exquisite pain during pelvic exam (chandelier sign). D, Adenomyosis on pelvic exam would reveal a tender, symmetrically enlarged, globular uterus.

10. Therapeutics: Normal Labor and Delivery. Answer D: This is a reassuring fetal monitor showing accelerations increasing 15 bpm for 15 seconds above baseline and is consistent with fetal well-being. Regular cervical examinations are necessary to check the progress of labor. A, Induction of labor is not warranted in this scenario. Mother is stable, and fetal monitor shows that the fetus is stable. Indications for the induction of labor include prolonged pregnancy, diabetes mellitus, Rh isoimmunization, preeclampsia, PROM, chronic hypertension, placental insufficiency, suspected IUGR. C, The fetal monitor does not show a distressed fetus. Late decelerations are defined as fetal heart rate dropping (B) during the second half of the contraction and are worrisome for uteroplacental insufficiency.

11. Diagnosis: Hyperemesis Gravidarum. Answer C: Hyperemesis gravidarum is a severe form of morning sickness in which women lose more than 5% of their prepregnancy weight and go into ketosis. With severe vomiting, a metabolic alkalosis would be expected. Syncopal episodes may occur secondary to dehydration but are not a part of the diagnosis. Treatment includes frequent small meals, antiemetics, such as phenergan and reglan. Acute management of hyperemesis gravidarum involves IV hydration, electrolyte repletion, and antiemetics. D, Metabolic alkalosis would be expected with severe vomiting not Acidosis.

12. Diagnostic Studies: Ectopic Pregnancy. Answer B: Transvaginal ultrasonography is diagnostic in 90% of cases of ectopic gestation. It may show adnexal mass or extrauterine pregnancy. A, CT is not recommended in pregnant women because of the ionizing radiation and must be avoided because other modalities without ionizing radiation, such as ultrasound are available. C, Serum hCG levels will be less than expected, and ectopic gestation should be suspected and confirmed with an ultrasound. Follow-up testing of serum hCG levels is crucial to exclude any remaining evidence of pregnancy. D, This is not diagnostic for an ectopic pregnancy. An Rh typing and antibody screening should be drawn if not previously done so and Rh-negative women with bleeding in pregnancy should be given Rh Immunoglobulin.

13. Diagnosis: Gestational Diabetes. Answer D: The patient has gestational diabetes proven by her glucose tolerance test. If the 1-hour serum glucose value is >130, a 3-hour gtt is performed. Two or more elevated values on the gtt give a diagnosis of gestational diabetes. 1 hour ≥180, 2 hours ≥155, 3 hours ≥140. If the patient has a fasting glucose measurement greater than 105 or a 2-hour postprandial blood sugar measurement greater than 120, Insulin is used because it does not cross the placenta. A, The patient in this scenario has no evidence of diabetes before pregnancy. B, The diagnosis is correct; however, the treatment option is incorrect. C, The patient has gestational diabetes.

14. Scientific Concepts: Bacterial Vaginosis. Answer D: *Gardnerella vaginalis* is the most common cause of bacterial vaginosis, characterized by fishy, gray homogenous vaginal discharge, clue cells on wet mount, and positive whiff test. A, Causes trichomoniasis, characterized by malodorous frothy discharge, wet mount will reveal motile trichomonads. B, Causes candidal vaginitis, characterized by cottage cheese discharge and vulvar pruritus, KOH prep will reveal budding yeast and hyphae. C, Causes chlamydia, the most common bacterial STD, characterized by purulent discharge.

15. Diagnosis: Preterm Labor. Answer B: Preterm labor is distinguished from Braxton Hicks contractions by changes in cervical dilation in response to the contractions. A, Nitrazine test is negative. C, Patient would have painful vaginal bleeding. D, Braxton Hicks contractions are generally painless uterine contractions with gradually increasing frequency. They occur during the last 4 to 8 weeks of pregnancy. They are not associated with cervical dilation.

16. Scientific Concepts: Premature Rupture of Membranes. Answer A: Premature rupture of membranes is suspected when patients describe a gush of fluid from the vagina and when a pool of fluid is seen on speculum exam. Ferning is seen when amniotic fluid is air dried on a microscopic slide. Nitrazine paper turns blue in the presence of amniotic fluid.

17. Diagnostic Studies: Menopause. Answer C: Elevated FSH is specific for menopause. A, Estradiol is low during menopause. B, Progesterone is low during menopause.

18. Diagnosis: Postpartum Hemorrhage. Answer B: Early PPH occurs less than 24 hours after delivery and is associated with abnormal involution of the placental site, cervical or vaginal lacerations, and retained portions of placenta. A, Late PPH occurs more than 24 hours after the delivery to 6 weeks postpartum and most commonly caused by subinvolution of uterus, retained products of conception, or endometritis. C, Blood loss requiring a transfusion or a 10% decrease in hematocrit between admission and postpartum period defines PPH. D, Endometritis does commonly occur after cesarean section; however, findings usually present 2 to 3 days postpartum and include fever (higher than 101°F) and uterine tenderness.

19. Clinical Therapeutics: Endometritis. Answer B: Patient most likely has endometritis. Classic presentation is fever, high WBC, uterine tenderness, and foul-smelling lochia. Patient needs to be admitted and administered IV antibiotics until afebrile for 24 hours. Clindamycin plus gentamycin is the first-line treatment. A, Highly suspect endometritis in this case, and patient must be admitted. C, Patient needs to be admitted and given IV antibiotics not PO. D, Dilation and Curettage is only performed if there are retained products of conception. The ultrasound in this case was negative for that.

20. Diagnosis: Inflammatory Breast Cancer. Answer C: Inflammatory breast cancer is considered in women with rapid onset of breast redness, swelling, warmth and peau d'orange (skin that resembles an orange peel). A, Mastitis is most common in breastfeeding women. Symptoms of redness, swelling, and pain would have resolved with antibiotic therapy. B, Breast abscesses will present with induration. D, Fibroadenomas present as painless, mobile masses in young women.

21. Diagnostic Studies: Trichomonas Vaginitis. Answer A: Microscopy will reveal motile trichomonads in patients with trichomonas vaginitis. B, KOH prep will reveal budding yeast and hyphae in patients with candidal vaginitis. C, Tzank smear is used to diagnose HSV. D, Culture is the gold standard for the diagnosis of trichomonas vaginitis, but it would not be the appropriate first diagnostic study.

22. Diagnosis: Molar Pregnancy. Answer C: Hydatiform mole or molar pregnancy is described. Molar pregnancies most commonly present with abnormal vaginal bleeding, uterine size greater than dates, hyperemesis gravidarum, or preeclampsia like symptoms. hCG levels are often greater than 100 000 mU/mL, and ultrasonography shows a characteristic "grapelike" vesicles or "snowstorm appearance" consistent with swelling of the chorionic villi. Initial treatment is suction curettage. A, Classic presentation for ectopic is unilateral adnexal pain, spotting, and tenderness on pelvic examination. hCG levels are less than expected for gestational age, and

transvaginal ultrasound will have no evidence of intra-uterine gestation. B, Placenta Previa will usually present with painless vaginal bleeding, but hCG levels will be consistent with gestational age. D, See C for explanation. Abruption placentae usually presents with painful vaginal bleeding.

23. History and Physical: Premenstrual Syndrome. Answer B: Premenstrual syndrome symptoms begin during the luteal phase (usually 5 days before the onset of menses) and resolve during the follicular phase (shortly after onset of menses). There is a one-week symptom-free period during the follicular phase, typically after menstrual flow has stopped. Affective symptoms (eg, depression, irritability, anxiety) and somatic symptoms (eg, breast pain, headache, bloating) must be present in at least 2 consecutive cycles for the diagnosis to be made.

24. Diagnosis: Breast Abscess. Answer B: Breast abscess, characterized by a red, painful, fluctuant breast mass, occurs most commonly during breastfeeding. Can occur concomitantly with mastitis or after mastitis, as in this example. A, Mastitis is characterized by unilateral breast pain, swelling, and erythema. Typically occurs in the first three months of breast feeding, caused by milk duct blockage. C, Galactoceles are milk retention cysts caused by a blocked milk duct. Also common during lactation. They are typically not painful. D, Inflammatory breast cancer is a rare form of breast cancer characterized by breast enlargement, pruritus, skin thickening, and warmth with a peau d'orange appearance (skin of an orange).

25. Clinical Intervention: Organ Prolapse. Answer A: Conservative therapy should be the initial therapy for anterior vaginal prolapse. B, Hysterectomy is a surgical option in the management of uterine prolapse. C, Colpocleisis is an option for treating pelvic organ prolapse in patients who are not surgical candidates and do not desire to be sexually active in the future. D, Anterior colporrhaphy is a treatment for anterior vaginal prolapse after the failure of nonsurgical management like pessary, estrogen, and Kegel exercises.

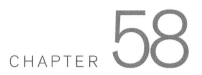
CHAPTER 58

Depressive and Mood Disorders

Recommended Supplemental Topics:

All of the conditions described in this chapter are currently updated with DSM-5 criteria

The fifth edition of the American Psychiatric Association's *Diagnostic and Statistical Manual (DSM-5)* utilizes specific criteria with which to objectively assess symptoms, rather than purely discrete diagnostic categories. For example, personality dimensions are more prominent than they were in *DSM-IV.* Nonetheless, the diagnosis is still based on a solid history and examination.

MAJOR DEPRESSIVE DISORDER AND PERSISTENT DEPRESSIVE DISORDER (DYSTHYMIA), DEPRESSION

- SIGECAPS = Sleep, Interest, Guilt, Energy, Concentration, Appetite, Psychomotor disturbance, Suicidal ideation
- Hypothyroidism—frequently associated with features of depression (depressed mood, memory impairment)
- Profound loss of pleasure in all enjoyable activities, early morning awakening, diurnal variation in mood (worse in morning)
- **Bereavement (grief)**—exhibit same signs/symptoms, but emphasis is on feelings of emptiness and loss, rather than anhedonia and loss of self-esteem; duration limited
- **Unipolar depressive disorders**—begin in early adulthood and recur episodically throughout lifetime

- Predictor of future risk—number of past episodes
- In minority of patients, severe depressive episodes progress to psychotic states
- **Seasonal affective disorder**—onset and remission of episodes at predictable times of the year
  - More common in women
  - Symptoms: Anergy, fatigue, weight gain, hypersomnia, episodic carbohydrate craving
- 40% of primary care patients with depression dropout of treatment and discontinue meds if symptomatic improvement is not noted within a month, unless additional support is provided
- Improved outcomes with (1) increased intensity and frequency of visits during first 4 to 6 weeks of treatment, (2) supplemental educational materials, (3) psychiatric consultation as indicated

- A previous response, or family history of positive response, to a specific antidepressant should be tried first
  - Otherwise, match patient's preference and medical history with the metabolic and side effect profile of the drug
- If a patient expresses minimal to no relief from a single antidepressant, it is **now suggested to augment with a second antidepressant and/or psychotherapy** (rather than switching to different antidepressants or switching from pharmacotherapy to psychotherapy)

- For patients who switch antidepressants, we suggest selecting a drug from a different class rather than within same class (ie, switch from an SSRI to an SNRI)
- If a patient expresses definite symptom relief that is not satisfactory and can tolerate a single or two antidepressants, consider adding another adjunctive medication and/or psychotherapy
- Adjuncts include: second-generation antipsychotics (aripiprazole, quetiapine, risperidone, olanzapine, in that order), lithium, and a second antidepressant from a different class

Major Depressive Disorder

Disease	Etiology, Prevalence, and Risk Factors	Clinical Symptoms and Signs	Diagnostics	Therapy, Prognosis, and Health Maintenance
Major depressive disorder (MDD) or unipolar major depression	One or more *major depressive* episodes Most common psychiatric disorder in general population (15% of general population) MDD is more frequent in families of bipolar individuals, but the reverse is not true Increases risk of developing CAD 66% present with somatic complaints (headache, back problems, chronic pain)	1. Syndrome with ≥**5 symptoms** lasting ≥**2 consecutive wk** • Depressed mood[a] nearly every day, most of the day (sad, indifference, apathy, empty, hopeless, tearful, irritable) • Loss in interests/pleasure[a] in activities, nearly every day • Appetite disturbance–significant weight loss when not dieting or weight gain; increased or decreased appetite • Sleep disturbance–insomnia or hypersomnia nearly every day • Psychomotor disturbance–restlessness or feeling slowed down • Fatigue–decreased energy, loss of self-esteem nearly every day • **Feelings of shame, *guilt*/worthlessness, hopelessness** • Impaired concentration/indecisiveness • Suicidal ideation–recurrent thoughts of death, suicidal ideation, or attempt • Abnormal self-perception 2. Not attributable to seasonal affective disorder, schizophrenia, schizophreniform disorder, delusional disorder 3. **Absence of manic or hypomanic episode** (differs from bipolar)	Clinical DX: 1. CBC, CMP, U/A, hCG, urine toxicology 2. Check TSH–10% have undetected thyroid dysfunction 3. Vitamin B_{12}, folate 4. EKG Screening: 1. PHQ-9 • Sens: 88% • Spec: 88% • Monitors response to treatment • Not accurate enough to definitively diagnose 2. PHQ-2 • Briefer, less accurate • Sens: 83% • Spec: 90% 3. **Beck Depression Inventory for Primary Care** • Sens: 97% • Spec: 99% • Available only by license; limited use in public domain	1. SSRI: first line • **Fluoxetine (Prozac)** • May interfere with hepatic metabolism of anticoagulants = increased anticoagulation 2. Bupropion (Wellbutrin) • Avoid in HTN patients • Good to avoid sexual dysfunction • Comorbid tobacco dependence tx 3. TCA–complicated or unresponsive cases; risk of death with overdose • Contraindicated in patients with BBB; can cause tachycardia in CHF patients • AE: Hyperglycemia and carbohydrate craving 4. MAOIs • Induce hypoglycemia and weight gain 5. **Psychotherapy**: insight oriented • Cognitive behavioral therapy and interpersonal therapy Health maintenance: 1. Most effective intervention for achieving remission and preventing relapse is medication, but combined treatment with psychotherapy improves outcome 2. Treat for 6-12 wk before deciding if medication effective 3. Improvement seen after 2 wk Prognosis: Increased risk of mortality compared to individuals without depression

Disease	Etiology, Prevalence, and Risk Factors	Clinical Symptoms and Signs	Diagnostics	Therapy, Prognosis, and Health Maintenance
Severe major depression		1. **7-9** depressive symptoms above that occur nearly every day, as indicated by score of 20+ points on PHQ-9	Clinical DX	1. **SNRIs**—have proven more efficacious than SSRIs for severe MDD 2. SSRI 3. Mirtazapine (Remeron) 4. Electroconvulsive therapy (ECT)

ªMUST include at least one of these.

Persistent Depressive Disorder (Dysthymia)

Disease	Etiology, Prevalence, and Risk Factors	Clinical Symptoms and Signs	Diagnostics	Therapy, Prognosis, and Health Maintenance
Dysthymia (persistent depressive disorder) DSM-5 consolidated dysthymic disorder and chronic major depression into persistent depressive disorder because there was little difference between dysthymic disorder and chronic major depression with regard to demographics, symptom patterns, treatment response, and family history	F: M (2:1), greater incidence with older age RF: first-degree relative Ongoing depressive symptoms that are less severe and/or less numerous Occur in 2% of general population Most potent stressors: death of a relative, assault, or severe marital or relationship problems	1. **Depressed mood** (dysphoria) lasting **2+ y** (chronic) and including **at least 2** of the following: *ACHESS* • **A**ppetite disturbance: decreased or increased • **C**oncentration/decision-making problems • **H**opelessness • **E**nergy (low) • **S**leep disturbance: hypersomnia, insomnia • **S**elf-esteem (low) 2. **No manic or hypomanic episodes** 3. Causes psychosocial **impairment** or distress 4. Never asymptomatic >2 mo 5. No MDD episodes during first 2 y Signs: 1. Many patients have a profile of pessimism, disinterest, and low self-esteem	Clinical Diagnosis	Pharmacotherapy plus psychotherapy recommended 1. Pharmacotherapy • **SSRI** • Bupropion 2. **Psychotherapy** • CBT • Interpersonal therapy

ADJUSTMENT DISORDER

- Maladaptive behavior in response to stress
- Adjustment disorders are entirely situational and resolve when the stressor resolves or when the individual adapts to the situation at hand
- May have symptoms that overlap with other disorders, such as anxiety symptoms

| Adjustment disorder | Precipitated by one or more stressors: exposure to actual or threatened death, combat/terrorist attack, natural disaster, serious accident; **can also be due to marital conflicts, a painful breakup, job loss, academic failure, or persistent painful illness with progressive disability**
RF:
Disadvantaged life circumstances result in higher rate of stressors and increase risk of adjustment disorder
F > M (2:1) | 1. The development of emotional or behavioral symptoms (low mood, tearfulness, hopelessness) in response to an identifiable stressor occurring **within 3 mo** of the **onset of the stressor**
2. These symptoms or behaviors are clinically significant, as evidenced by one or both of the following:
• *Marked distress* that is *out of proportion* to the severity or intensity of the stressor, taking into account the external context and the cultural factors that might influence symptom severity and presentation.
• *Significant impairment* in social, occupational, or other important areas of functioning (finances, going to school, divorce, illness)
3. The stress-related disturbance **does not meet the criteria for another mental disorder** and is not merely an exacerbation of a preexisting mental disorder (eg, MDD or another depressive disorder)
4. Symptoms do NOT represent normal bereavement
5. Once the stressor or its consequences have terminated, the symptoms *do not persist more* than an additional *6 mo*
Specifiers: with depressed mood, with **anxiety**, with mixed anxiety and depressed mood, with disturbance of conduct, with mixed disturbance of emotions and conduct, or unspecified | Symptoms can be short lived and resolve with time
1. **Antidepressants (first line)**
• SSRI (Zoloft, Paxil)
• SNRI
• Prazosin—for nightmares
2. Exposure therapy
Prognosis:
1. People diagnosed with adjustment disorder can be at higher risk of suicide
2. More vulnerable if they have personality disorder or organic impairment, loss of parent in infancy, or brought up by dysfunctional family
Comorbidities:
1. Depression
2. Anxiety |

ELECTROCONVULSIVE THERAPY (ECT)

Causes a generalized central nervous system seizure (peripheral convulsion is not necessary) by means of electric current. The key objective is to exceed the seizure threshold, which can be accomplished by a variety of means. The mechanism of action is not known, but it is thought to involve major neurotransmitter responses at the cell membrane. Electrical current insufficient to cause a seizure produces no therapeutic benefit.

- Most effective for severe depression (delusions and agitation, depression in elderly, nonresponsiveness to medications, extreme suicidality, mania, and psychoses during pregnancy)
- Most common side effects: memory disturbance and headache
- Most effective treatment of depression
- Most rapid response of all antidepressants
- No absolute contraindications exist
- Confusion and amnesia common, caution: can flip people into mania

Indications for Electroconvulsive Therapy (ECT)

- **First line–major depression with psychotic features**
- Catatonia
- Persistent suicidal intent
- Food refusal leading to nutritional compromise or dehydration
- Bipolar depression
- Mania
- Safe in pregnancy
- **≥3 episodes of major depression**
- 2 episodes of major depression PLUS 1 of the following:
  - Family history of recurrent depression or bipolar disorder
  - < 20 y/o at first episode
  - Severe or sudden depressive episode in last 3 y
  - Recurrence within 1 year of medication discontinuation
  - Major depression refractory to antidepressant medications
  - Previous (+) response to ECT
  - Severe symptoms (suicidal ideation or life-threatening behavior)

Increased Risk of Mortality with ECT

- Unstable or severe cardiovascular disease
  - Must have stable HTN before starting
  - Nitrates and BB should be continued
  - Delay in patients with decompensated HF or significant valvular disease
  - Okay for patients with pacemakers and AICDs
- Space occupying intracranial lesion with elevated intracranial pressure (ICP)
  - Safe as long as there is no evidence of elevated ICP
- Recurrent cerebral hemorrhage or stroke
- Bleeding or otherwise unstable vascular aneurysm
- Severe pulmonary condition
- ASA (American Society of Anesthesiologists) class 4 or 5

GRIEF AND BEREAVEMENT

- **Grief**: a natural response (thoughts, feelings, behaviors, physiologic response) to the death of a loved one (or bereavement)

- **Bereavement**: the situation in which someone who is close dies (not the reaction to the loss)
- **Mourning**: process of adapting to a loss and integrating grief

Disease	Etiology, Prevalence, and Risk Factors	Clinical Symptoms and Signs	Diagnostics	Therapy, Prognosis, and Health Maintenance
Normal (acute) grief and bereavement	Occurs in response to death of loved one or other meaningful losses Not a mental disorder, but includes symptoms that overlap	1. Intense focus on thoughts and memories of deceased 2. Sadness and yearning 3. Disbelief 4. Shock 5. Numbness 6. Loneliness 7. Crying	<u>Clinical DX:</u> 1. Begins within **2 mo** of loss 2. Lasts **< 2 mo**	1. Does **not** typically require treatment 2. Grief counseling or other psychotherapy <u>Prognosis:</u> 1. Adaptation to loss within 6-12 mo
Complicated (prolonged) grief disorder	Form of acute grief that is prolonged, intense, and disabling • Troubling thoughts • Dysfunctional behaviors • Dysregulated emotions • Serious psychosocial problems <u>RF:</u> **older** age (>61), **female**, low socioeconomic status, non-Caucasian race, **prior psychiatric history**, death of spouse, child, or young person; unexpected or violent death of loved one <u>Prevalence:</u> 2%-5% in general population Can occur in response to other nonbereavement losses: interpersonal loss (divorce), loss of pet, job, property, or community	1. Marked dysfunction in social and occupational domains 2. Bereavement for **6+ mo** 3. 1+ of the following • Separation distress: Persistent, intense *yearning or longing for person who died* • Inhibited exploration of the world: Frequent **preoccupying thoughts** *about deceased* • Frequent **intense feelings** of *loneliness* or that life is empty or meaningless without person who died • **Recurrent thoughts** that it is unfair or *unbearable to live without deceased*, or a recurrent urge to find or join deceased 4. 2+ of the following: • Frequent troubling rumination about circumstances or consequences of death • Includes guilt and self-blame • Traumatic distress: *Recurrent disbelief or inability to accept death* • Persistently **feeling** shocked, stunned, dazed, or numb since death • Anger or bitterness about death • Intense emotional or physiologic reactions (**insomnia**) to reminders of the loss • Marked change in **behavior** • Avoiding people, places or situations that remind one of loss • Wanting to see, touch, hear, or smell things to feel close to deceased	<u>Clinical DX:</u> 1. Brief Grief Questionnaire • If >4 = (+) 2. Interview to rule out or establish diagnosis	1. **Psychotherapy (CBT)–first line** • Prolonged exposure • Interpersonal psychotherapy • Motivational interviewing <u>Health maintenance:</u> 1. Outpatients—monitor every 1-4 wk <u>Prognosis:</u> 1. Can last between 10-16 y 2. Suicidal ideation and behavior occurs in 40%-60% <u>Comorbidities:</u> 1. MDD (50%) 2. PTSD (30%-50%) 3. GAD (20%) 4. Panic disorder (10%-20%)

BIPOLAR AND RELATED DISORDERS
Bipolar I and II Disorder and Cyclothymic Disorder

Bipolar disorder—characterized by unpredictable swings in mood from mania (or hypomania) to depression.

- **Mania**: expansive, euphoric mood with inflated self-esteem or grandiosity, decreased need for sleep, talkative, flight of ideas, distractibility, **increase in goal-directed activity (MC symptom)**, excessive involvement in high-risk fun activities
  - Frequently requires hospitalization
- **Severe mania**: patients are delusional and experience paranoid thinking indistinguishable from schizophrenia
- **Hypomania**: by definition, hypomania never necessitates hospitalization and is similar to mania, but less severe; sudden onset, progresses quickly over 1 to 2 days, resolves within several weeks

- **Major depression**: dysphoria, slowing in the pace of mental and physical activity (slow and soft speech, decreased output), minimal interest in pleasurable activities (sex), low energy, impaired memory and concentration; diminished appetite with weight loss or increased appetite and weight gain; agitation may occur (unable to sit still or wringing of hands), sleep disturbances, feelings of worthlessness and excessive guilt; suicidal thoughts and behavior; poor eye contact, poor hygiene, unkempt appearance; feelings of hopelessness or helplessness; rumination and indecisiveness; negative and nihilistic thoughts; somatic symptoms (pain), impaired psychosocial functioning
- **Psychosis**: delusions (false, fixed beliefs; may include grandiosity as well as persecutory, sexual, religious, or political themes) and hallucinations (typically auditory), disorganized thinking

Disease	Etiology, Prevalence, and Risk Factors	Clinical Symptoms and Signs	Diagnostics	Therapy, Prognosis, and Health Maintenance
Bipolar disorder	Mood disorder characterized by episodes of mania, hypomania, and major depression Pathogenesis unknown Prevalence: 1%-3% worldwide	1. Mood disorder at onset: • Major depression (54%) • Mania (22%) • Mixed (24%)	Clinical DX: 1. Psychiatric and medical history, mental status, and physical exam 2. Labs: TSH, CBC, CMP, urine toxicology 3. Mood disorder questionnaire • False-positive rate: 20% • Low sensitivity 4. PHQ-9 • Screens for major depression	Treatment as below: Comorbidities: alcohol and substance abuse, ADHD, eating disorders, anxiety disorders, personality disorders Prognosis: 1. 10%-15% die by suicide, recurrence of bipolar mood episodes increases risk of suicide attempts 2. More likely to perpetrate violence and be victimized by violence
Bipolar I	Mean onset: 18 y M = F	1. At least one **manic episode** (3+ symptoms for 7 d) 2. **Major depression** (not required) 3. **Hypomanic episodes**	Clinical DX	Treatment as below
Bipolar II	Mean onset: 20 y M = F More prevalent than bipolar I	1. At least **one hypomanic episode** (3+ symptoms for 4 d) 2. At least **one major depressive episode** (5+ symptoms for 2 wk) 3. *Absence* of manic episodes	Clinical DX	Treatment as below: Treatment with same medications as for bipolar I Prognosis: 5%-15% will suffer an episode of mania, requiring a diagnosis of bipolar I
Cyclothymia		1. Numerous *hypomanic* periods (**3+ symptoms for 4 d**) and *mild depressive periods* over ≥ **2 consecutive y** 2. No major depressive episodes or manic episodes during the first 2 y 3. Symptomatic at least 50% of time 4. Not symptom free for more than 2 mo 5. Causes significant distress or psychosocial impairment 6. Not substance/medication-induced, due to another medical condition, or better accounted for by another mental disorder	Clinical DX	Treatment as below

Mania	Hypomania
1. Abnormally and persistently *elevated, expansive, or irritable mood* lasting ≥ **7 d** (or requiring hospitalization) and including ≥ **3** (or 4 if irritable mood predominates) of the following: Remember **DIGFAST** • **D**istractibility • **I**mpulsivity/irresponsible: high-risk activities (spending, speeding, sex) • **G**randiosity • **F**light of ideas/Racing thoughts • **A**ctivity **increased = goal-directed activity** (sexual, occupational, religious, political) • **S**leep: *need* decreased • **T**alkativeness: pressured speech • Psychomotor agitation (restless, pacing, multiple conversations at once) 2. Impairs psychosocial functioning, **requires hospitalization**, or has accompanying psychotic features (hallucinations or delusions) 3. Symptoms not the result of substance or general medical condition	1. Abnormally and persistently *elevated, expansive, or irritable mood* lasting ≥ **4 d** (not requiring hospitalization) and including ≥ **3** (or 4 if irritable mood predominates) of the following: Remember **DIGFAST** • **D**istractibility • **I**mpulsivity/irresponsible: high-risk activities (spending, speeding, sex) • **G**randiosity • **F**light of ideas/Racing thoughts • **A**ctivity **increased = goal-directed activity** (sexual, occupational, religious, political) • **S**leep: *need* decreased • **T**alkativeness: pressured speech • Psychomotor agitation (restless, pacing, multiple conversations at once) 2. Impairs psychosocial functioning only mildly or improved, **does NOT require hospitalization**, and has no accompanying psychotic features (hallucinations or delusions) 3. Symptoms not the result of substance or general medical condition 4. May result from antidepressant therapy or ECT

	Treatment Options	Clinical Pearls

Acute Mania	1. **Lithium** (mainstay)
	 OR
	 2. Anticonvulsants
	    • **Valproic acid**
	 PLUS
	 3. Antipsychotics—adjunct to (1) or (2)
	    • Aripiprazole
	    • Haloperidol
	    • Olanzapine
	    • Quetiapine
	    • Risperidone
	 4. Benzodiazepines—for patients who cannot tolerate lithium, anticonvulsants, or antipsychotics; generally adjunct and limited to acute treatment
	    • Clonazepam
	    • Lorazepam
	 5. ECT—for refractory mania that does not respond to 4-6 medication combinations
	 6. Clozapine—for patients refractory to medication, decline ECT; adjunct to (1) or (2)
		1. Resolution of mood symptoms or improvement that only 1-2 symptoms of mild intensity persist
		 2. If psychosis is present, resolution is required for remission
		 3. The choice between lithium and valproic acid is based upon efficacy and tolerability

Hypomania	1. Monotherapy—first line
	    • **Risperidone**
	 OR
	    • **Olanzapine**
	 PLUS
	 2. Antipsychotics—adjunct
	    • Aripiprazole
	    • Quetiapine
	    • Ziprasidone
	 3. Anticonvulsants—adjunct
	    • Valproic Acid
	    • Carbamazepine
	 4. Lithium
		1. Absence of suicidal or homicidal ideation or behavior, aggressiveness, psychosis, and poor judgment
		 2. Consider past response to medications, past response of family members to medications, specific symptoms, adverse effects, comorbid illness, concurrent medications, and cost
		 3. If patient fails monotherapy within 2 wk of target dose or does not tolerate drug, discontinue medication over 1 wk and titrate a new medication
		 4. May combine antipsychotic with lithium or valproic acid if patient fails 3-5 monotherapy trials

Acute agitation	1. Antipsychotics (mainstay)
	    • Aripiprazole
	    • Haloperidol—first line
	    • Olanzapine
		1. Hospitalized patients should receive oral or IM medications as well as seclusion and restraints

Psychiatry

(continued)

(continued)

	Treatment Options	Clinical Pearls

Maintenance therapy	**Pharmacotherapy:**
	1. Treat acute mania (first line as above)
	2. Monotherapy
	  • **Lithium (first line)**
	  • Valproate (divalproex)
	  • Quetiapine–also great adjunct to lithium
	  • Lamotrigine
	3. Second Line Antipsychotics
	  • Aripiprazole
	  • Olanzapine
	  • Risperidone
	4. Third Line
	  • Carbamazepine
	  • Lurasidone
	  • Oxcarbazepine
	5. ECT
	Psychotherapy:
	1. **Group psychoeducation**–first line
	2. Cognitive behavioral therapy–adjunct
	3. Family therapy
		1. Haloperidol not used because it can cause movement disorders and may increase the risk of bipolar major depression
		2. Lithium has been widely studied and is efficacious for long-term treatment and may reduce the risk of suicide attempts and deaths
		3. Olanzapine is not used as first line for concerns of weight gain and diabetes
		4. Valproic acid is not prescribed to women of childbearing age due to teratogenicity and risk of polycystic ovarian syndrome
		5. Lithium and valproate reduce risk of relapse by 30%, lamotrigine reduces by 16%
		6. Adjunctive psychotherapy prevents relapses and improves medication compliance

Acute bipolar depression	1. Antidepressants
	  • Fluoxetine and olanzapine
	2. **Lithium**
	  • Takes 6-8 wk to take effect
	3. Anticonvulsants
	  • **Lamotrigine** (Lamictal)
	  • **Valproate** (Divalproex)
	4. Second-generation antipsychotics–the following can be used as monotherapy
	  • Quetiapine
	  • **Lurasidone** (Latuda)
	  • Olanzapine
	5. ECT
	  • For patients with suicidal ideations, psychosis, or depression during *pregnancy*
	6. Omega-3 fatty acids
		1. If monotherapy fails, add a second drug (atypical antipsychotic)
		2. Addition of antidepressants to lithium or valproate has not been effective
		3. Polytherapy–use of fluoxetine and olanzapine is frequently recommended
		4. Lamictal–first-line therapy for bipolar depression in pregnancy
		5. For pregnant women who cannot tolerate or do not respond to lamictal, quetiapine (Seroquel) is recommended

Psychotherapies and Psychoeducation in Bipolar Disorder

Group psychoeducation	1. Increases patient comprehension of disorder, alleviates stigma and guilt, and prevents learned helplessness 2. Replaces denial of illness with awareness, guilt with responsibility, and helplessness with proactive care
Cognitive behavioral therapy	1. Trains patients to recognize and change harmful thought patterns and behaviors 2. Cognitive therapy: attempts to modify automatic dysfunctional thoughts, beliefs, or attitudes 3. Behavioral therapy: focuses on modifying problematic behavioral responses to environmental stimuli or dysfunctional thoughts through techniques (stimulus control, exposure with response prevention) 4. Educates patients about bipolar disorder and teaches coping skills for psychosocial stressors 5. Also used to treat major depression, panic disorder, and bulimia nervosa
Family therapy	1. Addresses relationships between family members, behavioral change, communication, problem-solving skills, psychoeducation, or need to view family as a single system
Interpersonal and social rhythm therapy	1. Addresses interpersonal problems related to unresolved grief, interpersonal disputes, role transitions, and interpersonal deficits 2. Focuses on daily routines and sleep/wake cycles
Functional remediation	1. Addresses neurocognitive problems, such as memory, attention, and executive functioning, as well as functioning in interpersonal relationships, occupational functioning, finances, and leisure time

Other Therapies

Psychodynamic psychotherapy	1. Identifies and makes patients aware of patterns in relationships, unconscious meanings, conflicts, and desires that cause depression 2. Emphasizes understanding of unconscious conflict through transference, countertransference, defense mechanisms, and resistance
Motivational interviewing	1. Encourages patients to change maladaptive behaviors 2. Seeks to help patients recognize and make changes to behaviors, matching strategies to their stage of readiness to change 3. Key elements: expressing empathy, helping patient identify discrepancies between their problematic behaviors and broader personal values, expecting patient to resist change and accept it, enhance patient's self-efficacy 4. Used for weight reduction, substance use disorders, smoking cessation, and encourage adherence with complex medical treatments
Dialectical behavioral therapy	1. For patients with severe problems in emotional regulation, commonly patients with borderline personality disorder 2. Includes skills training, mindful practice, and close monitoring of and intervention in crises that may develop

Pharmacotherapy Principles

- SSRIs (fluoxetine, paroxetine, citalopram, escitalopram) = lower frequency of anticholinergic, sedating, and CV side effects, but greater incidence of GI complaints, sleep impairment, and sexual dysfunction
  - All SSRIs **impair sexual function**, resulting in diminished libido, impotence, or difficulty achieving orgasm
  - Akathisia (sense of restlessness, anxiety)—greater incidence in first week of treatment
- SNRIs (venlafaxine, desvenlafaxine, duloxetine, vilazodone)—linear dose–response curves
  - Possible increases in diastolic blood pressure, frequent daily dosing due to short half-life
- TCAs—cheap, well-defined dose–plasma relationships
  - Side effects: sedation, constipation, dry mouth, urinary hesitancy, blurred vision
  - Contraindicated in patients with serious CV risk factors
- MAOIs—highly effective in atypical depression, but risk of hypertensive crisis following intake of tyramine containing foods make them inappropriate as first-line agents
  - Side effects: orthostatic hypotension, weight gain, insomnia, sexual dysfunction
- Serotonin syndrome—hyperstimulation of brainstem 5-HT1A receptors
  - Do not use MAOIs in combination with SSRIs
  - Myoclonus, agitation, abdominal cramping, hyperpyrexia, hypertension, potentially death
- Bupropion—no anticholinergic, sedating, or orthostatic side effects and low incidence of sexual side effects
  - Stimulant like side effects may lower seizure threshold, short half-life requiring frequent dosing
- Electroconvulsive therapy—at least as effective as medication, but reserved for **pharmacotherapy-resistant cases** and delusional depressions
- Vagus nerve stimulation (VNS)—recently approved for treatment-resistant depression
- Regardless of treatment, **reevaluate after 2 months**

- Most show some degree of response, but treatment should be continued for at least 6 to 9 months to prevent relapse
  - In patients with 2+ episodes of depression, indefinite maintenance treatment should be considered
- Patient education is important—advice about stress reduction and cautions that alcohol may worsen depressive symptoms and impair drug response
- When clinical relief of symptoms is obtained, medication is continued for 12 months in the effective maintenance dosage, which is the dosage required in the acute stage. The full dosage should be continued indefinitely when the individual has a first episode before age 20 or after age 50, is over age 40 with two episodes, at least one episode after age 50, or has had three episodes at any age.
- Lithium—70% to 80% response rate in acute mania with beneficial effects in 1 to 2 weeks
  - Prophylactic effect in prevention of recurrent mania and recurrent depression
  - Patients should be monitored closely, since therapeutic blood levels are close to toxic levels
- Valproic acid—better for patients who experience rapid cycling or who present with a mixed or dysphoric mania

SUICIDE

- **Men over age 50** are more likely to *complete* a suicide because of their tendency to attempt suicide with more violent means (guns)
- Women make more attempts but are less likely to complete a suicide
- Suicide is 10× more prevalent in patients with schizophrenia than the general population with jumping from bridges the most common means of attempted suicide
- Increased suicide rate among age 15 to 35 and patients with cancer, respiratory illness, AIDS, and hemodialysis patients
- Having a gun in the home increases the likelihood of suicide 5-fold

- Positive associations: alcohol abuse, hopelessness, delusional thoughts, complete or nearly complete loss of interest in life or ability to experience pleasure
- RF: previous attempts, family history, medical or psychiatric illness, male sex, older age, contemplation of violent methods, humiliating social stressor, drug use, impulsiveness, or mood swings
- Reasons to hospitalize
  - History of impulsive behavior, poor social support, and/or suicidal plan
- Assess risk of suicide by direct questioning, as patients are reluctant to verbalize such thoughts without prompting
  - Suicide assessment using: Columbia-Suicide Severity Risk Scale
  - Measurement of mood facilitated by: Hamilton or Montgomery-Asberg rating scales or self-administered Patient Health Questionnaire-9 (PHQ-9)
- If specific plans are uncovered or if significant risk factors exist, refer to mental health specialist for immediate care

- Past history of suicide attempts, profound hopelessness, concurrent medical illness, substance abuse, social isolation
- If patient thinks about suicide >1 hour/d, consider them high risk
- The presence of anxiety, panic, or agitation significantly increases near-term suicide risk
  - 4%-5% of all depressed patients will commit suicide—most seek help within 1 month before deaths
- Formulate and institute a treatment plan or make adequate referral
  - National Suicide Prevention Lifeline, 1-800-273-8255
  - Remove guns and medications from household
  - No driving
- If starting patient on antidepressant, choose a drug with low toxicity to prevent likelihood of overdose
  - eg, never prescribe more than a 10-day supply of TCAs when suicide is a risk

CHAPTER 59

Anxiety, Trauma, and Stress-related Disorders

All of the following conditions are currently updated with DSM-5 criteria

The fifth edition of the American Psychiatric Association's *Diagnostic and Statistical Manual (DSM-5)* utilizes specific criteria with which to objectively assess symptoms, rather than purely discrete diagnostic categories. For example, personality dimensions are more prominent than they were in *DSM-IV*. Nonetheless, the diagnosis is still based on a solid history and examination.

GENERALIZED ANXIETY DISORDER

Anxiety

- Subjective sense of unease, dread, or foreboding
  - 15% to 20% of patients in the general population

Disease	Etiology, Prevalence, and Risk Factors	Clinical Symptoms and Signs	Diagnostics	Therapy, Prognosis, and Health Maintenance
Generalized anxiety disorder (GAD)	Onset before age 20 y HX: Childhood fears, social inhibition Prevalence: 5%-6%, increased if first-degree relatives with GAD F (2×) > M All anxiogenic agents work on the GABA-A receptor/chloride ion channel complex	DSM-5 criteria: 1. Chronic, excessive anxiety/worry about job performance, health, marital relations, social life • Duration **at least 6 mo** (usually lifetime), symptoms more days than not 2. Patient finds it difficult to control worry 3. **3 out of 6 symptoms** required • Restlessness, keyed up, on edge • Irritability • **Muscle tension** • Easily fatigued • Decreased concentration • Disturbed sleep: Insomnia or restless sleep 4. The anxiety, worry, or physical symptoms cause significant distress 5. Not attributable to physiologic effects of a substance 6. Not better explained by another mental disorder	Clinical DX: CBC, CMP, TSH, U/A, EKG, or urine or serum toxicology–rule out other possible causes	1. If New Diagnosis • SSRI/SNRI or CBT or both–first line • See Treatment Below Screening: 1. Generalized anxiety disorder (GAD-7) Prognosis: 1. If comorbid MDD–more severe and prolonged course of illness, greater impairment Comorbidities: 1. **Specific phobia** 2. **Social phobia** 3. Panic disorder 4. Major depression, dysthymia 5. Substance abuse common (alcohol and sedative or hypnotics) 6. PTSD 7. OCD

Treatment of Generalized Anxiety Disorder

	Treatment	Clinical Pearls

Generalized anxiety disorder	1. **SSRI or SNRI**–first line
	 • SSRI: Paroxetine, escitalopram, sertraline, citalopram
	  • AE: sexual dysfunction, GI upset (nausea, diarrhea), insomnia and withdrawal on discontinuation, weight gain, agitation, hyperactivation
	 • SNRI: Venlafaxine (extended release) and duloxetine
	  • AE: nausea, dizziness, insomnia, sedation, constipation, sweating; can also increase blood pressure
	2. **CBT**
	3. Buspirone (Buspar)
	 • Nonsedating, no tolerance or dependence, no interaction with BDZ receptors or alcohol, no abuse or disinhibition
	 • Second line adjunct or monotherapy
	 • TID dosing, fewer sexual AEs
	 • AE: insomnia, agitation, nausea
	4. Pregabalin (off-label)
	 • AE: sedation, dizziness
	5. Short-acting benzodiazepines (lorazepam, oxazepam, alprazolam)
	 • Adjunct or monotherapy, acute, maintenance, or long term
	 • Typically used in GAD during acute period before SSRI or SNRIs take effect, counteracting initial agitation
	 • Lowest dose possible, avoid "as needed" or large doses
	 • AE: rebound anxiety after short-term treatment, psychomotor impairment, amnesia, rebound anxiety, and insomnia with discontinuation
	 • Contraindicated in pregnancy
	6. Mirtazapine
	 • Monotherapy or adjunct
	 • AE: sedation, weight gain
	7. Antipsychotics
	 • Quetiapine
	  • AE: weight gain, elevated blood sugar and lipids, EPS, QT prolongation
	  • EKG prior to starting
	8. Long-acting benzos (diazepam, flurazepam, clonazepam)
	 • AE: sedation, impaired cognition, poor psychomotor performance
		1. Start low and go slow
		2. Time to onset is approximately 4 wk (**therapeutic: 4-6 wk**)
		3. If no response to first SSRI/SNRI, taper and start a different SSRI/SNRI
		4. If robust response, **continue for at least 12 mo**
		5. If relapse upon discontinuation, restart medication; if 2 relapses occur, consider ongoing maintenance treatment
		6. Agitation and insomnia can occur within days of starting SSRI/SNRI
		 • May start low-dose benzodiazepine, such as lorazepam 1-2 mg/d as adjunct
		7. Patients with chronic GAD, minimal depressive symptoms, and no history of substance use disorder are candidates for long-term low-dose benzos if antidepressants are ineffective or not tolerated

PANIC DISORDER

- History, physical and lab testing to rule out anxiety states from medical disorders—pheochromocytoma, thyrotoxicosis, hypoglycemia, irritable bowel syndrome
- Inducers of panic disorder—IV sodium lactate, yohimbine, CCK-4, CO_2
- Patients with panic disorder have a heightened sensitivity to somatic symptoms, which triggers increased arousal, setting off the panic attack
- Agents that block serotonin reuptake can prevent attacks

- **Panic attacks** (not a mental disorder) occur in 33% of individuals at some point in their life and represent a spontaneous, discrete episode of intense fear that begins abruptly and lasts several minutes to an hour
- **Agoraphobia**: anxiety about and/or avoidance of situations where help may not be available or where it may be difficult to leave the situation in the event of developing panic-like symptoms or other incapacitating or embarrassing symptoms. Examples include crowds, shopping malls, driving, public transportation, and being away from home; now diagnosed independently of panic disorder

Disease	Etiology, Prevalence, and Risk Factors	Clinical Symptoms and Signs	Diagnostics	Therapy, Prognosis, and Health Maintenance
Panic disorder	Lifetime prevalence: 2%-3% Genetic predisposition, altered autonomic responsivity, social learning Onset: usually late adolescence or early adulthood (mean: 24 y/o) F (2×): M First attack usually outside home, but may occur when waking from sleep	1. Episode of intense fear/discomfort 2. Begins abruptly (within 10 min), accelerates rapidly 3. Resolves over course of ~1 h 4. Requires at least *1 mo* of • Concern or worry about the attacks or their consequences (losing control, having a heart attack, going crazy) • Change in behavior related to attacks (avoidance of exercise or unfamiliar situation) 5. Recurrent (at least 2), *unexpected* panic attacks Signs: 1. Palpitations 2. Chest pain 3. Shortness of breath 4. Nausea, abdominal discomfort 5. Sweating, shaking, trembling, chills 6. Dizziness 7. Fear of dying, losing control, or going crazy 8. Paresthesias 9. Gastrointestinal distress 10. Depersonalization, derealization—feelings of unreality	Clinical DX: 1. CBC, TSH, CMP, EKG—rule out other causes 2. Echo 3. Coronary angiogram: normal 4. PFTs	1. **Antidepressants** • SSRI: fluoxetine, paroxetine, sertraline • SNRI: venlafaxine • Start at ⅓-½ usual dose • Take **8-12 wk to become effective** • Maintain for 1-2 y • MAOIs—benefit patients with comorbid atypical depression (hypersomnia, weight gain) 2. **Cognitive behavioral therapy** • Education about panic attacks • Relaxation training • Deep breathing Complications: 1. Anticipatory anxiety—patients try to predict attacks coming on • **Benzodiazepines** useful in early course of treatment and sporadically thereafter • Alprazolam, lorazepam, diazepam, or clonazepam Prognosis: 1. Higher likelihood of suicide attempts Health maintenance: 1. Panic Disorder Severity Scale (PDSS)—gold standard for monitoring changes in severity Comorbidities: 1. **Major depression** (75%) 2. **OCD** (25%) 3. **Agoraphobia** 4. GAD, social anxiety disorder, PTSD

POST-TRAUMATIC STRESS DISORDER (PTSD)

includes the requirement that the symptoms persist for at least 1 month.

- Has been reclassified from an anxiety disorder to a trauma and stressor-related disorder in the DSM-5. The DSM-5

Disease	Etiology, Prevalence, and Risk Factors	Clinical Symptoms and Signs	Diagnostics	Therapy, Prognosis, and Health Maintenance

Acute stress disorder	Prevalence of ASD depends on the trauma—20%-50% of people who experienced interpersonal trauma (assault, rape, witnessing a mass shooting) had ASD. Associated symptoms of detachment and loss of emotional responsivity; may feel depersonalized and unable to recall specifics of trauma	1. Exposure to **extreme traumatic events** (actual or threatened death, serious injury, or sexual violence)
		2. **9 or more symptoms**:
		  • Nightmares
		  • Intrusive memories
		  • Flashbacks
		  • Distress with cues
		  • Lack of positive emotions
		  • Disconnected
		  • Amnesia of event
		  • Avoiding thoughts/reminders
		  • Insomnia
		  • Irritability
		  • Concentration problems
		3. Duration: **3 d-1 mo** (occurs *shortly after* trauma)
		4. Actively avoid stimuli that precipitate recollections of the trauma and demonstrate increase in vigilance, arousal, and startle response
		5. Disturbance causes clinical distress
			<u>Clinical DX</u>:
			Begins 3 d and up to 1 mo after traumatic event (to differentiate from PTSD) = more acute
				1. Self-limited
				2. *Pharmacotherapy* **benzodiazepines + psychotherapy**

Post-traumatic stress disorder (PTSD)	Men: 61% experience trauma, of those, 8% develop PTSD (higher rates with combat: 20%)
	Women: 51% experience trauma, of those 20% develop PTSD
	<u>RF</u>:
	Past psychiatric history and personality characteristics of high neuroticism and extroversion
	Excessive release of norepinephrine in response to stress and increased noradrenergic activity
		1. Exposure to actual or threatened death, serious injury, or sexual violence
		  • Direct experience, witnessing in person, learning about events of a close family member/friend, experiencing repeated or extreme exposure to aversive details of events
		    • 1+ intrusion/re-experiencing symptoms
		    • 1+ persistent avoidance of associated stimuli
		    • 2+ negative alterations in cognitions/mood
		    • 2+ alterations in arousal and reactivity, feelings of isolation from close friends and family
		    • A, B, C, and D occur for more than *1 mo*
		2. Causes clinically-significant distress or impairment
		3. Not attributable to other physiologic effects of a substance or condition
		  • Anhedonia, poor concentration, and problem-solving skills
			<u>Clinical DX</u>:
			1. PTSD is a reaction that generally occurs far after trauma occurs
				1. **SSRIs (sertraline** and **paroxetine** have FDA approval for PTSD treatment)
				  • All reduce anxiety, symptoms of intrusion, and avoidance behaviors
				<u>Comorbid</u>:
				Alcoholism

PTSD Symptoms

- Remember: **PAIN**

At least 1 of the following: (**P**ersistent avoidance of associated stimuli)	At least 2 of the following (**A**lterations in arousal and reactivity)	At least 1: (**I**ntrusion and re-experiencing SX)	At least 2 of the following: (**N**egative alterations in cognition or mood)
• Avoiding memories, thoughts, or closely associated feelings • Avoiding external reminders (people, places, conversations, activities, objects, situations)	• Irritability and angry outbursts (little to no provoking)—verbal or physical aggression • Reckless/self-destructive behavior • Hypervigilance • Increased startle response • Concentration problems • Sleep disturbances (difficulty falling, staying asleep, or restless sleep)	• **Recurrent:** • Involuntary, intrusive *memories* • Distressing *dreams* • Dissociative reactions (*flashbacks*) • Psychological distress to cues • Physiological reactions to cues	• Amnesia of events • Negative beliefs–about self, others, or world • Distorted cognitions about cause or consequences of event–blames self or others • Negative emotional state (fear, horror, anger, guilt, shame) • Decreased interests in activities • Detachment or estrangement from others • Inability to experience positive emotions (happiness, satisfaction, love)

Other Treatment for PTSD

1. Other medications for PTSD:
   - Other antidepressants (SNRIs—venlafaxine), topiramate
   - Propranolol, opioids (morphine) for acute stress period
   - **Prazosin** for nightmares; other sleep aids
   - **Trazodone** for insomnia
   - No benefits seen with antipsychotics or benzodiazepines
   - Limited data to suggest any benefits from mood stabilizers
   - There are no controlled trials showing the usefulness of antihistamines or antidepressants for management of ASD
   - No data to support preventative pharmacological treatment
2. Psychotherapy:
   - **Trauma-focused cognitive behavioral therapy**—helps patient overcome avoidance behaviors and demoralization
   - **Exposure therapy**—helps master fear of recurrence of the truama
   - Stress inoculation training—for sexual trauma
   - **Eye movement desensitization and reprocessing**
   - Imagery rehearsal therapy, psychodynamic therapy, and PTSD education
   - Dialectical behavioral therapy, hypnosis (as adjunctives)
3. Other adjunct TX:
   - Patient education (eg, breathing retraining)
   - Social services
   - Vocational rehabilitation
   - Religious/spiritual support
   - Case management
   - Marriage/family counseling
4. Substance abuse treatment—seeking safety

PHOBIC DISORDERS

- Shyness: A nontechnical term referring to feelings of apprehension or awkwardness, and inhibited behavior when in proximity to other people. It does not generally imply psychopathology, but it is common among persons with social anxiety disorder
- Behavioral inhibition: A childhood temperament that has been operationally defined by researchers to refer to young children who manifest fear and withdrawal behavior when introduced to novel situations or unfamiliar persons

Disease	Etiology, Prevalence, and Risk Factors	Clinical Symptoms and Signs	Diagnostics	Therapy, Prognosis, and Health Maintenance
Phobic disorders	7%-9% of population F > M (2:1)	1. **Marked and persistent fear of objects or situations**—exposure causes immediate anxiety 2. Excessive fear of possible scrutiny, humiliation, or embarrassment in one or more social situations • **Exposure provokes anxiety** • Situation **avoided** or endured • **Recognized as unreasonable** 3. Patient avoids stimulus, which impairs occupational or social functioning 4. Panic attacks **triggered by stimulus** 5. Unlike other anxiety disorders, patients experience ***anxiety only in specific situation***	Clinical DX	1. Combination of medication and therapy • Anxiolytic antidepressants • Benzodiazepines
Social anxiety disorder (sad) (formerly general social phobia)	Prevalence: 5%-12% Mean onset: teens (though as early as 5 y/o) RF: 1. Female 2. (+) FH of SAD 3. Early childhood shyness or behaviorally inhibited temperament Examples include social interactions (eg, having a conversation, meeting unfamiliar people), being observed (eg, eating or drinking), and performing in front of others (eg, giving a speech) Specifiers: Performance only	1. Marked fear or anxiety about **one or more social situations** in which the individual is exposed to possible scrutiny by others 2. Fear that others will notice their irrational anxiety and experience anticipatory anxiety 3. Social situations always provoke fear or anxiety 4. Situations are avoided or endured with intense fear or anxiety 5. Out of proportion to actual threat posed by social situation 6. Persistent, **lasting 6+ mo** 7. Must cause impairment in functioning or marked distress 8. Not attributable to direct physiological effects of substances or medication 9. Not better explained by another mental disorder Signs: 1. Blushing 2. Sweating 3. Trembling 4. Palpitations	Clinical DX screening: 1. Mini Social Phobia Inventory • High sensitivity (89%) • High specificity (90%)	1. **Pharmacotherapy** • **Antidepressants: SSRI**/SNRIs (paroxetine, sertraline, venlafaxine) • MAOIs—for refractory cases • Benzodiazepines—used to reduce fearful avoidance, but not for chronic use 2. **CBT** • Teaches patient to identify negative thoughts associated with anxiety producing situations • Reduce fear of loss of control 3. **Desensitization therapy** • Patient encouraged to pursue and master gradual exposure to the anxiety producing stimuli 4. Performance only type • Preperformance β-blocker: **propranolol** 20-40 mg PO 2 h prior, atenolol • Benzodiazepines—as needed Comorbidities: 1. Avoidant personality disorder 2. Phobic disorders, other anxiety disorders 3. Affective disorders 4. Schizophrenia 5. Alcohol dependence 6. **Eating disorders**

(continued)

Psychiatry

(continued)

Disease	Etiology, Prevalence, and Risk Factors	Clinical Symptoms and Signs	Diagnostics	Therapy, Prognosis, and Health Maintenance
Specific phobias (formerly simple phobia)	Fear of a particular object or situation that leads to avoidance behavior Prevalence: 7%-12% RF: first-degree relatives <u>Five main specifiers:</u> 1. Animal: spiders, insects, dogs 2. Natural environment: heights, storms, water 3. Blood-injection-injury: needles, invasive medical procedures 4. Situation: airplane, elevators, enclosed spaces 5. Other: situations that may lead to choking or vomiting, loud sounds, or costumed characters	<u>DSM-5 criteria:</u> 1. Marked fear or anxiety about a specific object or situation (eg, flying, heights, animals, receiving an injection, seeing blood)[a] 2. The phobic object or situation almost always provokes immediate fear or anxiety 3. The phobic object or situation is actively avoided or endured with intense fear or anxiety 4. The fear or anxiety is out of proportion to the actual danger posed by the specific object or situation and to the sociocultural context 5. The fear, anxiety, or avoidance is persistent, typically lasting for **6 mo or more** 6. The fear, anxiety, or avoidance causes clinically significant distress or impairment in social, occupational, or other important areas of functioning 7. The disturbance is not better explained by the symptoms of another mental disorder	<u>Clinical diagnosis:</u> 1. Fear is excessive and out of proportion to situational demands 2. Cannot be alleviated with rational explanation 3. Is out of voluntary control 4. Leads to situational avoidance 5. Is maladaptive and persistent over time 6. Not age or stage-specific	1. **CBT** (first line): exposure therapy (systemic desensitization) 2. **Benzodiazepines** • Must have no hx of SUD • Lorazepam 0.5-2 mg 30 min before encounter 3. **SSRI** • If CBT unavailable or patient prefers medication • Used when there is sufficient time to attain therapeutic benefit, only when repeated exposure is anticipated • Sertraline or escitalopram <u>Comorbidities:</u> 1. **Other anxiety disorders** 2. Panic disorder with agoraphobia 3. GAD 4. MDD 5. Bipolar II 6. Alcohol dependence
Separation anxiety disorder	More prevalent in young children	1. Separation parent and child during sleep 2. Older children—separation of child from parent at school, sleepovers, camp 3. Must occur **>4 wk** for children 4. Leads to impairment or significant distress	Clinical DX	1. Cognitive behavioral therapy (CBT) 2. SSRI

[a]*Note*: In children, the fear or anxiety may be expressed by crying, tantrums, freezing, or clinging.

CHAPTER 60

Substance Abuse Disorders

All of the following conditions are currently updated with DSM-5 criteria

The fifth edition of the American Psychiatric Association's *Diagnostic and Statistical Manual (DSM-5)* utilizes specific criteria with which to objectively assess symptoms, rather than purely discrete diagnostic categories. For example, personality dimensions are more prominent than they were in *DSM-IV.* Nonetheless, the diagnosis is still based on a solid history and examination.

DISORDERS RELATED TO USE OF ALCOHOL, HALLUCINOGENS, OPIOIDS, STIMULANTS, SEDATIVES, HYPNOTICS, ANXIOLYTICS, CANNABIS, TOBACCO, AND INHALANTS

Screening for Drugs of Abuse

- The American Academy of Pediatrics (AAP) recommends screening adolescents using the CRAFFT screen for use of alcohol, tobacco, and other drugs annually beginning at 11 years of age. Two or more indicates a positive screen.
  - C—Have you ever ridden in a **Car** driven by someone (including yourself) who was high, drunk, or had been using drugs?
  - R—Have you ever used drugs or alcohol to **Relax?**
  - A—Do you ever use **Alone?**
  - F—Do you ever **Forget** things you did while using?
  - F—Do **Family** or **Friends** tell you to cut down?
  - T—Have you ever gotten into **Trouble** when using?
- The utility of urinalysis for the detection of drugs of abuse (DOA) varies depending on the pharmacokinetics as well as other factors, including the type of drug. For example, lipophilic (fat soluble) substances (barbiturates, THC, etc) remain in the urine for several days up to 1 to 2 months in chronic marijuana users, whereas water soluble drugs (such as ETOH, stimulants, and opioids) remain in the body for 24 to 48 hours. The sensitivity and specificity of hair analysis is considered as reliable as urinalysis and can predict drug use over longer periods.

Urine Detectability for Drugs of Abuse

Drug	Duration of Detectability in Urine	Drugs Causing False-positive Preliminary Urine Screens
Amphetamines	2-3 d	Ephedrine, pseudoephedrine, phenylephrine, selegiline, chlorpromazine, trazodone, bupropion, desipramine, amantadine, ranitidine
Cocaine	2-3 d	Topical anesthetics containing cocaine
Marijuana	1-7 d (light use), 1 mo with chronic moderate to heavy use	Ibuprofen, naproxen, dronabinol, efavirenz, hemp seed oil
Opiates	1-3 d	Rifampin, fluoroquinolones, poppy seeds, quinine in tonic water
Phencyclidine	7-14 d	Ketamine, dextromethorphan

From *Urine testing for drugs of abuse (addictive drugs). UpToDate.* 2018. https://www.uptodate.com/contents/image?imageKey=EM%2F58181&topicKey=PSYCH%2F7807&source=outline_link&search=drug%20testing&selectedTitle=2~150.

Psychiatry

Substance Abuse Disorders/Substance Use Disorder (SUD)

- The term substance abuse disorder (SUD) replaced the two DSM-IV diagnoses of substance abuse and substance dependence, now named by the type of substance involved (eg, Alcohol, cannabis, tobacco, etc) and specifying the severity

- Substance use disorder (SUD) is distinguished from substance use by the presence of psychological impairment and behaviors related to obtaining, using, or recovering from the substance

Disease	Etiology, Prevalence, and Risk Factors	Clinical Symptoms and Signs	Diagnostics	Therapy, Prognosis, and Health Maintenance
General substance use disorder (SUD)	RF: 1. (+) FH of SUD 2. Friends who have SUD 3. Romantic partner with SUD 4. Living in a community characterized by poverty, violence, and/or high alcohol and other drug availability Median onset: 15 y/o	DSM-5 criteria: 2 or more in 12 mo 1. Often used in larger amounts or over a longer period than was intended 2. Persistent desire or unsuccessful effort to cut down or control use 3. Spends a great deal of time obtaining, using, or recovering from effects 4. Craving or strong desire or urge to use 5. Recurrent use resulting in failure to fulfill major obligations at work, school, or home 6. Continued use despite having persistent or recurrent social or interpersonal problems caused or worsened by effects 7. Important social, occupational, or recreational activities given up or reduced due to use 8. Recurrent use in physically hazardous situations 9. Continued use despite knowledge of having a persistent or recurrent physical or psychological problem likely to have been caused or worsened by use 10. Tolerance 11. Withdrawal SX/Signs: 1. Significant weight loss or weight gain Signs: 1. Poor personal hygiene 2. Scars at injection sites ("track marks") 3. Atrophy of nasal mucosa, perforation of nasal septum 4. Slurred speech, unsteady gait, pinpoint pupils 5. Agitation or sedation 6. Tachycardia 7. Conjunctival injection, watery eyes 8. Diaphoresis 9. Runny nose	1. Clinical interview Severity based on criteria met: 1. Mild: 2-3 2. Mod: 4-5 3. Severe: 6+	Treatment varies by substance Prognosis: 1. Strong association with suicide, especially in adolescents Health maintenance: 1. To monitor progress, treatment attendance and urine drug screen results are a mainstay Comorbidities: 1. Depression 2. Bipolar disorder 3. Anxiety 4. PTSD 5. Eating disorders 6. Schizophrenia 7. ADHD 8. Personality disorders (borderline, ASPD)

Alcohol-Related Disorders

- Absorption of ethanol occurs primarily in the duodenum or small intestine (80%) and the stomach (20%)

- Flushing reaction: occurs in individuals homozygous for the gene coding for aldehyde dehydrogenase (ALDH2), which is responsible for breaking down acetaldehyde (a byproduct of alcohol metabolism)

- Binge drinking: consuming >5 alcoholic drinks on a single occasion

- All alcohol poisonings are associated with an increased osmolal gap

- An unhabituated drinker clears ethanol from the blood at a rate of 15 to 20 mg/dL per hour, whereas chronic abusers clear ethanol at a rate of 25 to 35 mg/dL

- Symptoms of withdrawal occur because ETOH is a CNS depressant and also enhances inhibitory tone (modulating GABA activity) and inhibits excitatory tone (glutamate binding to NMDA receptors)

- Alcoholic hallucinosis: (visual) hallucinations that develop within 12 to 24 hours of abstinence, resolve within 24 to 48 hours; patients aware they are hallucinating and distressed, no global clouding of the sensorium

- "Banana bag" (due to yellow color) contains thiamine, folate, and a multivitamin in isotonic saline with 5% dextrose; used in patients with alcohol withdrawal

Disease	Etiology, Prevalence, and Risk Factors	Clinical Symptoms and Signs	Diagnostics	Therapy, Prognosis, and Health Maintenance
"At-risk drinking"	Consumption of amount of alcohol that puts individual at risk for health consequences	1. 4+ drinks/d or 14 drinks/wk for men or 3+ drinks/d or 7 drinks/wk for women 2. Not severe enough to meet criteria for alcohol use disorder		
Alcohol use disorder (alcohol intoxication)	Problematic pattern of alcohol use leading to clinically significant distress or impairment M > F, more common in Native Americans MC age range: 18-29 y/o RF: 1. (+) FH in 50%-70% **Screening tests**: 1. **AUDIT** (Alcohol Use Disorder Identification Test)–BEST 2. CAGE • Ever felt you should **C**ut down on drinking? • Have people **A**nnoyed you by criticizing your drinking? • Felt **G**uilty about your drinking? • Ever had a drink first thing to steady nerves or get rid of hangover (**E**ye opener)?	1. **Slurred speech** 2. Incoordination 3. Disinhibited behavior 4. Impairment in attention or memory 5. Inappropriate sexual or aggressive behavior 6. Mood lability 7. Impaired judgment Signs: 1. Stupor or coma 2. Hypotension 3. Tachycardia 4. **Unsteady gait** 5. **Nystagmus** DSM-5 criteria: 1. Recurrent drinking resulting in failure to fulfill role obligations 2. Recurrent drinking in hazardous situations 3. Evidence of tolerance 4. Evidence of ETOH withdrawal or use of ETOH for relief or avoidance of withdrawal 5. Drinking in larger amounts over longer periods than intended 6. Persistent desire or unsuccessful attempts to stop or reduce drinking 7. Great deal of time spent obtaining, using, or recovering from ETOH 8. Important activities given up or reduced because of drinking 9. Continued drinking despite knowledge of physical or psychological problems 10. Alcohol craving	Acute (ED) setting: 1. Serum ethanol concentration 2. Basic chemistry 3. Serum glucose q 8 h Inpatient setting: 1. **Ethyl glucuronide testing (EtG)**– shows recent use of alcohol, but not AMOUNT of consumption 2. **GGT (gamma-glutamyl transpeptidase)**– most *sensitive* lab test to determine use of ETOH (shows heavy consumption) 3. **Carbohydrate deficient transferrin**–Most definitive marker (>60 mg/d) 4. **Macrocytosis**: Mean corpuscular volume >95 fL (men) and >100 fL (women) 5. **Elevated *LFTs*** • AST:ALT >2:1 6. Hypokalemia, hypomagnesemia, hypocalcemia, hypophosphatemia 7. Increased serum uric acid and triglycerides 8. **Pancytopenia** 9. Hypoglycemia 10. Lactic acidosis	Isolated, acute, mild: 1. Supportive Care & Observation • **Dextrose** infusion if hypoglycemic 2. For agitation, violence, uncooperativeness, give **benzos** or typical antipsychotics 3. For coma, to prevent Wernicke's encephalopathy • **Thiamine or B1** (100 mg) and folic acid (1 mg), prior to glucose infusion Moderate: 1. Treatment as Above 2. IV catheter insertion, IV fluids 3. Consider CT of head Severe (poisoning): 1. Frequent respiratory assessment • Intubation or mechanical ventilation 2. IV isotonic crystalloid 3. Activated charcoal and gastric lavage not helpful Prophylaxis: 1. Librium (**chlordiazepoxide**) 25-100 mg q 6 h × 1 d, then 25-50 mg every 6 h × 2 more days • For patients who have history of seizures, DT, or prolonged ETOH consumption who are minimally symptomatic or asymptomatic Bridge to maintenance: 1. **Naltrexone** 50 mg/d • Useful for 3-6 mo after quitting drinking, PO or IM (monthly) • Indications • Current, heavy use, ongoing risks from use • Motivated to reduce intake of ETOH • Prefer meds > CBT • No contraindications • MOA: blockade of mu-opioid receptor • CI: patients taking opioids, acute hepatitis, or liver failure • AE: Disulfiram reaction (vomiting with ETOH), nausea, headache, dizziness • Monitor: LFTs Health Maintenance: 1. Monitor GGT and carbohydrate deficient transferrin if elevated at beginning of treatment to track progress 2. Recommend AA meetings 3. Encourage abstinence Prognosis: 1. Majority of suicides and intrafamily homicides involve alcohol 2. Major factor in rapes and other assaults 3. Earlier onset associated with more rapid development of dependence and worse outcomes 4. Higher lifetime rate of suicide attempts (7%) Comorbidities: 1. Depression

Psychiatry

(continued)

(continued)

Disease	Etiology, Prevalence, and Risk Factors	Clinical Symptoms and Signs	Diagnostics	Therapy, Prognosis, and Health Maintenance

Alcohol with-drawal	Patients who suddenly stop or reduce alcohol intake
	Occurs 6-12 h after last drink or after reduction in drink-ing amounts, lasts up to 2-3 d
	Acute course (severe): CAN BE LIFE THREATENING
	Shorter course (mild): persists for weeks
		Within 6 h:
		1. **Insomnia**
		2. Confusion, **disorientation**
		3. Delusions
		4. Nausea, vomiting
		5. Sweating
		6. **Anxiety**
		7. Anorexia
		8. Headache
		Signs:
		1. Seizures or hallucinations
		  • **Visual hallucinations** and Delirium tremens
		2. **Tachycardia, hypertension,** palpitations
		3. Diaphoresis
		4. **Tremor**
		5. Agitation
		6. Death
		Associated: features of advanced liver disease (spider angiomata, pal-mar erythema, hepatic or splenic enlargement)
			Clinical DX:
			1. **CIWA-Ar:** Clinical Institute Withdrawal Assessment for Alcohol, revised; measures withdrawal severity
			  • <8: detoxifica-tion not needed
			  • 8-15: good can-didate for detox, if symptoms of DT
			  • >15: inpatient referral more appropriate
				Acute/detoxification:
				1. *Benzodiazepines*:
				  • Lorazepam (Ativan)
				  • *Diazepam* (Valium) 5-10 mg IV
				  • Chlordiazepoxide (Librium) 25-100 mg PO
				2. Phenobarbital
				3. Propofol
				Maintenance therapy:
				1. **Naltrexone** 50 mg/d
				  • Useful for 3-6 mo after quitting drinking, PO or IM (monthly)
				  • MOA: blockade of mu-opioid receptor
				  • CI: patients taking opioids, acute hepatitis, or liver failure
				  • AE: Disulfiram reaction (vomiting with ETOH), nausea, headache, dizziness
				  • Monitor: LFTs
				Health maintenance:
				1. Cut down 20%-30% per day
				2. Antipsychotics should NOT be used
				3. Monitor vital signs, fluid, and electrolyte levels
				Prognosis:
				1. Left untreated, seizures progress to delirium tremens in 33%

Delirium tre-mens	Alcohol withdrawal, cocaine addiction
	Onset within 72-96 h of last drink, lasts 1-5 d
	Occurs in 5% of patients with severe withdrawal from alcohol
	RF:
	1. HX of sustained drinking
	2. HX of previous DT
	3. Age >30
	4. Concurrent illness
	5. Significant ETOH withdrawal in presence of ele-vated ETOH level
		1. *Hallucinations*
		  • Visual or tactile
		2. *Disorientation*
		3. **Sweating**
		4. Fever
		5. Confusion
		6. **Tremor**
		7. Vomiting
		8. **Delirium**—only symptom that is always present
		Signs:
		1. **Severe Tachycardia, tachypnea**
		2. Hypertension
		3. Hyperthermia
		4. **Agitation**
		5. **Drenching sweats**
		6. **Fever**
		Associated:
		Seizure ("rum fits," 10%), cardiovascular abnormalities
			1. **Hypokalemia, hypomagnesemia,** hypophosphatemia, hypovolemia
			2. Increased arterial pH (respiratory alkalosis)
				1. Rule out comorbid illness
				2. Supportive care
				  • IV isotonic fluids, nutritional supplementation
				  • Place in quiet, protective environment
				3. Benzodiazepines for psychomotor control
				  • Lorazepam (Ativan) if severe, *diazepam* (Valium), or chlordiazepoxide (Librium)
				4. To prevent Wernicke encephalopathy
				  • **Thiamine** (100 mg) and folic acid (1 mg), prior to glucose infusion
				Prophylaxis:
				1. Librium (**chlordiazepoxide**) 25-100 mg q 6 h × 1 d, then 25-50 mg every 6 h × 2 more days
				  • For patients who have history of seizures, DT, or prolonged ETOH consumption who are minimally symptomatic or asymptomatic
				Prognosis:
				1. Mortality <5%, used to be 40%

- Serum levels are most accurate, but breath analysis is faster (will give lower ethanol concentrations compared to blood)
- Legal blood alcohol concentration in most of the US is 80 mg/dL (17 mmol/L)

- Clinical signs and symptoms may NOT correlate with the BAC depending on factors such as genetics; the type, amount, and rate of intake; frequency and pattern of use; history of use

BAC (%)	Clinical Signs/Symptoms
20-50 mg/dL	1. Diminished fine motor coordination
0.01%-0.10% 50-100 mg/dL	1. Euphoria 2. Mild deficits in cognition, attention, and coordination 3. Impaired judgment
0.10%-0.20% 100-150 mg/dL	1. Greater deficits in coordination, psychomotor skills 2. Decreased attention 3. Ataxia (impaired gait and balance) 4. Impaired judgment 5. Slurred speech 6. Mood variability
0.20%-0.30% 150-250 mg/dL	1. Lack of coordination 2. Incoherent thoughts 3. Confusion 4. Nausea and vomiting 5. Lethargy 6. Difficulty sitting upright without assistance
>0.30%	1. Stupor 2. Loss of consciousness 3. Coma (300 mg/dL) 4. Respiratory depression (400 mg/dL) 5. Death

A drink is defined by the CDC as 12 oz. of beer, 8 oz. of malt liquor, 5 oz. of wine, or 1.3 oz. or a "shot" of 80-proof distilled spirits of liquor.

- **Wernicke encephalopathy** triad: confusion, ataxia, and ophthalmoplegia (typically sixth nerve). Early recognition and treatment with thiamine can minimize damage.

- **Korsakoff psychosis**, sequelae of delirium tremens (and alcoholism) characterized by both anterograde and retrograde amnesia, with confabulation early in the course. Early recognition and treatment of the alcoholic with intravenous thiamine and B complex vitamins can minimize damage.

- Excessive alcohol consumption in men has been associated with faster cognitive decline compared with light to moderate alcohol consumption

- **Naltrexone** is an opiate antagonist that acts to lower relapse rates over the 3 to 6 months after cessation of drinking by lessening the pleasurable effects of alcohol. Naltrexone has been shown to be most effective when given during periods of drinking in combination with therapy that supports abstinence but accepts the fact that relapses occur. It is FDA-approved for maintenance therapy. It has also been shown to reduce alcohol craving when used as part of a comprehensive treatment program

- While the terms "opioids" and "narcotics" both refer to a group of drugs with actions that mimic those of morphine, the term "opioids" is used when discussing medications prescribed in a controlled manner by a clinician, and the term "narcotics" is used to connote illicit drug use.

Hallucinogen-Related Disorders

Disease	Etiology, Prevalence, and Risk Factors	Clinical Symptoms and Signs	Diagnostics	Therapy, Prognosis, and Health Maintenance
Hallucinogens, also known as psychedelics	Examples: LSD, Ecstasy, "bath salts," "angel dust," synthetic cannabinoids (K2 or "spice"), ketamine (special K, vitamin K) Rarely produce true hallucinations and instead distort body image, sensory perception, and time perception Consist of both natural and synthetic compounds Differential DX: alcohol or benzodiazepine withdrawal, anticholinergic poisoning, thyrotoxicosis, CNS infection, structural brain lesions, acute psychosis, hypoglycemia, hypoxia	1. Anxiety 2. **Nausea** and vomiting 3. Abdominal pain 4. Dizziness 5. Jaw tension or teeth grinding 6. Dry mouth Signs: 1. **Mydriasis** (miosis with angel dust) 2. **Tachycardia** 3. Nystagmus 4. Muscle tension 5. Ataxia 6. Bruxism 7. Agitation 8. Diaphoresis 9. Hypersalivation 10. Conjunctival injection Complications: 1. Hyperthermia 2. Hypertension 3. Seizures (rare) 4. Psychosis 5. Hyponatremia 6. Arrhythmias 7. Rhabdomyolysis 8. Paranoia	Clinical DX Acute/ED setting: 1. Rapid serum glucose 2. Chemistry 3. Creatine phosphokinase, to rule out rhabdomyolysis 4. EKG—rule out QT prolongation	1. Supportive care • Reassurance • Correct hypoxia, hypoglycemia, electrolyte abnormalities, and dehydration 2. Pharmacologic sedation and possibly physical restraints if staff are unable to calm patient 3. **Benzodiazepines** • Preferred agent to treat agitation and delirium • Reversible with flumazenil • Diazepam 5-10 mg PO or IV, Ativan 1-2 mg PO/IM/IV Health maintenance: 1. Gastric decontamination not necessary in most cases 2. Hallucinogens are rapidly absorbed and most adverse effects do not present until several hours after use 3. Monitor blood pressure and heart rate 4. Can be detected in urine for several days after use

Psychiatry

CNS Depressants

Opioids

Disease	Etiology, Prevalence, and Risk Factors	Clinical Symptoms and Signs	Diagnostics	Therapy, Prognosis, and Health Maintenance
Opioid intoxication	Examples: Heroin, morphine, codeine, buprenorphine, hydromorphone, meperidine, methadone, oxycodone, oxymorphone <u>RF:</u> 1. (+) FH in 23%-54%	1. Pruritus 2. **Euphoria**, apathy, or dysphoria 3. Nausea and/or vomiting 4. Psychomotor agitation 5. **Drowsiness** 6. Impairment in attention or memory 7. Slurred speech <u>Signs:</u> 　1. *Miosis* (pupil constriction) 　2. Respiratory depression **(decreased respiratory rate and tidal volume)** 　3. Hyporeflexia 　4. Hypothermia 　5. Dermal "track marks" 　6. Flushing 　7. Bradycardia 　8. **Hypotension** 　9. Decreased bowel sounds 　10. Depressed mental status <u>Associated:</u> 1. Pulmonary edema 2. Stupor or coma 3. Cardiovascular collapse 4. Death 5. Seizures 6. Delirium	<u>Clinical DX:</u> <u>Acute/ED setting:</u> 1. Rapid serum glucose 2. APAP level—if APAP overdose suspected 3. Serum CK—r/o rhabdomyolysis 4. Urine toxicology screens should NOT be routinely obtained 5. EKG—if intended self-harm or coexposure suspected 6. CXR—for patients with adventitious lung sounds or hypoxia	1. Supportive care 　• Tracheopharyngeal suctioning—aspirate and ventilate patient 　• Supplemental O_2 2. **IV *naloxone* (intranasal Narcan)**—acute overdose and intoxication 　• short acting opioid antagonist 　• Goal: adequate ventilation 　• If too much given, withdrawal will occur 　• Greater affinity for mu receptors <u>Prognosis:</u> Death often due to respiratory depression
Opioid withdrawal	Signs and symptoms begin 6-12 h after last dose of short acting opioid or 24-48 h after cessation of methadone Symptoms peak at 24-48 h of onset Symptoms may persist for days up to 2 wk More intense if shorter acting **Timeline of withdrawal** <u>12-16 h</u>: restless, anxiety, tremor, weakness, Nausea, vomiting, cramps, sweating <u>24 h</u>: coarse tremor, hyperreflexic <u>2-3 d (peak)</u>: convulsions (grand mal seizures) <u>4 d</u>: delirium, hallucinations, agitation, fever, exhaustion, CV collapse, psychomotor agitation	1. **Dysphoria**, restlessness 2. **Craving** for opioids 3. **Anxiety** 4. Salivation 5. Myalgias, arthralgias 6. Nausea, vomiting, abdominal cramping, **diarrhea**, anorexia 7. Restless sleep 8. Spontaneous orgasm or ejaculation <u>Signs:</u> 1. **Rhinorrhea** 2. **Yawning** 3. Lacrimation 4. **Diaphoresis** 5. *Mydriasis* (pupil dilation) 6. **Piloerection** 7. Tremor 8. Increased bowel sounds <u>Severe:</u> 1. Hypertension 2. Tachycardia 3. Tachypnea	<u>DX/screening:</u> 1. COWS (clinical opioid withdrawal scale)	<u>Acute therapy:</u> 1. Expectant management 2. Single dose of IM **Methadone** to relieve withdrawal symptoms without producing intoxication <u>Maintenance:</u> 1. **Methadone**—full agonist; *Preferred* drug of choice 　• First line in pregnancy 2. Buprenorphine—partial agonist (not for acute therapy) 3. Naltrexone—opioid antagonist 4. **Behavior modification program**—REQUIRED 5. Ultrarapid opioid detox (UROD)—antagonists administered while under general anesthesia; patient wakes up after sleeping through most difficult period of withdrawal 　• Risk of anesthesia, seizures, hemodynamic instability 　• Not routinely recommended

- Opioids are the desired treatment in most cases of withdrawal; however, when withdrawal is triggered by an antagonist (such as Naloxone), it may be difficult to give enough opioid to overcome the effects of the antagonist and rebound opioid intoxication could ensue

- The flip side of this is an individual who intentionally stopped using opioids to treat an addiction (such as methadone), either to harbor their own opioid supplies or sell them, in which case nonopioid adjuncts should be used to manage symptoms

Psychiatry

Opioid Agonists		Opioid Antagonists		Withdrawal Adjuncts	
Methadone	Buprenorphine	Naloxone (Narcan)	Naltrexone	Clonidine	Nausea and Vomiting
1. Long-acting full-opioid agonist with a 24-36-h half-life → treats muscle aches, cravings, and insomnia 2. Binds to and occupies μ-opioid receptors 3. Requires clinic-based treatment and daily in-clinic observed ingestion during initial treatment Indications: 1. Must be at least 18 y/o and physically dependent on opiates for at least 1 y (continuously or intermittently over several years) • Exceptions: pregnant women, recently released patients who were incarcerated or hospitalized, patients who have been on methadone within past 2 y 2. If <18, may be admitted to a methadone maintenance program if physical dependence present and two previous detox attempts 3. May be used for acute withdrawal up to 3 d, then must be in a withdrawal program; may never be unsupervised with use Adverse effects: 1. Constipation, drowsiness, excess sweating, peripheral edema 2. Reduced libido and erectile dysfunction 3. QTc prolongation at higher doses (baseline EKG recommended in patients with cardiac risk factors, then annually) 4. Chronic use may result in hyperalgesia Maintenance therapy: 1. If signs persist for more than 4-6 h, give another 10 mg q 4-6 h 2. Divide total amount by 2 and give amount q 12 3. Reduce total 24-h dose by 5-10 mg each day	1. Partial mu opioid agonist, used for long-term treatment of opioid dependence 2. Most commonly given sublingually and given with naloxone—prevents users from abusing drug by crushing tablets and dissolving for IV injection 3. Patient must be abstinent for a short period and have early symptoms of withdrawal before starting 4. Should be tapered gradually every 1-2 wk 5. Preferred over methadone for maintenance—better side effect profile Adverse effects: 1. Sedation 2. Headache 3. Nausea, constipation 4. Insomnia 5. Respiratory depression	1. Used for acute treatment of opioid intoxication, including respiratory depression 2. Given IN or IM 3. Pure opioid antagonist that competes and displaces opioids at opioid receptor sites	1. Started 6 d after last use of short acting opioids or 7-10 d after long acting—can cause immediate withdrawal symptoms 2. Optional for maintenance treatment to prevent relapse in opioid use disorder Adverse effects: 1. Nausea 2. Headache 3. Dizziness 4. Fatigue 5. Liver damage (rare)	1. Alleviates CV symptoms only (normal to elevated blood pressure) • Especially useful for patients who withdraw from opioid antagonists 2. α-2-adrenergic agonist that binds α-2 receptors and shares K^+ channels with opioids, blunting symptoms of withdrawal • Blocks release of norepinephrine 3. Can be given 0.1-0.3 mg PO 3-4 times daily as adjunct or alternative to methadone 4. Monitor blood pressure and heart rate • Monitor for hypotension, dry mouth, sedation, and constipation 5. May use benzodiazepines (diazepam) as supplement	1. Antiemetics • Promethazine 25 mg IM or IV (anticholinergic properties) • Loperamide 4 mg PO • Octreotide 50 µg SQ for diarrhea

CNS Stimulants

- **Amphetamines** → Release of stored **NE** and **dopamine** into the synaptic cleft and competitively inhibit MAO

- **Cocaine** → Inhibits reuptake of **NE** and **dopamine** leading to increased synaptic concentrations and psychomotor stimulation

Disease	Etiology, Prevalence, and Risk Factors	Clinical Symptoms and Signs	Diagnostics	Therapy, Prognosis, and Health Maintenance

Stimulant (cocaine) intoxication
Examples:
1. Amphetamines (speed), ice (smokable form)
2. Methylphenidate (Ritalin)
3. Dextroamphetamine
4. **Cocaine** (crack cocaine is a stronger and purer derivative)
	RF:
	1. (+) FH in 42%-79% for cocaine users
	Cocaine is an indirect sympathomimetic agent, which increases the availability of amines at adrenergic receptors by blocking their presynaptic reuptake; stimulates α-1, α-2, β-2, and β-2 adrenergic receptors through increased norepinephrine
	Euphoric properties derived from inhibition of serotonin reuptake
	Slows or blocks nerve conduction, acting as a local anesthetic by altering recovery of Na^+ channels = negative inotrope
	Methods:
	Inhalational, IV, intranasal, ingestion, anal
	Mostly urban men aged 15-35
	Appears in blood, urine, sweat, saliva, and breast milk; crosses the placenta and appears in meconium
	Faster administration: IV or inhaled (smoked) within 20-30 min up to 90 min
	Primarily eliminated in the URINE
	Cocaine-associated psychosis differs from acute schizophrenic psychosis by less thought disorder, bizarre delusions and fewer negative symptoms such as alogia and inattention
	More visual and tactile ("insects crawling under the skin" or "formication") hallucinations common
		1. Hyperarousal
		2. Sweating
		3. Improved performance on tasks of vigilance and alertness
		4. Sense of self-confidence, euphoria, and wellbeing
		5. Increased energy, decreased fatigue and need for sleep or appetite
		6. Sociability
		7. Nausea
		With increased dose or frequency:
		8. Delusions or hallucinations
		9. Weight loss
		10. Anxiety or depression
		11. Restlessness, agitation, tremor, dyskinesia, stereotypies
		Signs:
		1. **Hypertension**
		2. Tachycardia
		3. **Mydriasis** (pupil dilation)
		4. Diaphoresis
		5. Xerostomia
		6. Bruxism
		Complications:
		1. Accelerated atherosclerosis and LVH → MI → dilated cardiomyopathy; cardiac dysrhythmias
		2. Psychomotor agitation, seizures, coma, headache, ICH, CVA, focal neurologic signs
		3. Pneumothorax, pneumomediastinum, pneumopericardium; SOB due to "crack lung"; pulmonary infarction
		4. Perforated ulcers; ischemic colitis, intestinal infarction
		5. Rhabdomyolysis
		6. Acute angle closure glaucoma
		7. Abruptio placentae in pregnancy
		8. **Nasal septal perforation**
			Acute/ED setting:
			1. Bedside glucose
			2. Acetaminophen and salicylate levels
			3. EKG–r/o conduction system poisoning
			4. Pregnancy test for women of childbearing age
			1. **Benzoylecgonine** (BE)—major urinary metabolite of cocaine
			• Only detectable in blood for a few hours after use, but persists in urine up to 10 d or more
			• Detected in blood for 48 h
			2. Troponin—for chest pain
			3. CXR–r/o causes of chest pain
			4. CT head and possible LP–r/o ICH
			5. CK and urine myoglobin—may be elevated, r/o rhabdomyolysis
			6. CMP: hyperkalemia or hypocalcemia
			7. EKG–prolonged QRS complex
				1. Supportive care
				• Supplemental O_2 as needed
				• Intubation **without** succinylcholine
				  • Can prolong effects of cocaine and paralysis
				  • Can worsen hyperkalemia
				2. For severe, refractory, or symptomatic cocaine-induced hypertension
				• IV **phentolamine** must be given prior to β **blocker** use
				• Goal to rapidly lower diastolic pressure to 100-105 mm Hg in 2-6 h
				3. Hypotension treated with
				• 2-3 L rapidly infused isotonic saline
				• Direct acting vasopressors: NE or phenylephrine
				• If wide QRS on EKG, give hypertonic sodium bicarbonate
				4. Psychomotor agitation
				• Diazepam may be given after hypoglycemia and hypoxia have been ruled out
				5. GI decontamination
				• Activated charcoal 1 g/kg up to 50 g every 4 h as needed
				Health maintenance:
				1. β Blockers should **NOT be used alone** to treat cocaine-related CV complications; may create unopposed alpha-adrenergic stimulation (coronary vasoconstriction and end-organ ischemia)

Disease	Etiology, Prevalence, and Risk Factors	Clinical Symptoms and Signs	Diagnostics	Therapy, Prognosis, and Health Maintenance
Stimulant (cocaine) withdrawal	Cessation of heavy chronic cocaine use	1. Depression (dysphoria), anxiety 2. Fatigue 3. Difficulty Concentrating 4. Anhedonia: decreased ability to experience pleasure 5. Increased cocaine craving and appetite 6. Increased sleep and dreaming (REM sleep) 7. Musculoskeletal pain Initial "crash": 1. Psychomotor retardation 2. Severe depression 3. Suicidal ideation Signs: 1. Tremors 2. Chills 3. Involuntary motor movements 4. Bradycardia		

Sedatives, Hypnotics, and Anxiolytic Related Disorders

- Increase the affinity of GABA receptors for endogenous neurotransmitter (GABA)

Disease	Etiology, Prevalence, and Risk Factors	Clinical Symptoms and Signs	Diagnostics	Therapy, Prognosis, and Health Maintenance
BZD intoxication or overdose	Examples: Xanax, barbiturates, Ambien, rohypnol, roofies, benzodiazepines (BZD) Potentiate GABAs inhibitory actions by augmenting receptor binding (increase flow of chloride ions through GABA ion channel, causing postsynaptic hyperpolarization and decreased ability to initiate action potential) Most intentional ingestions of BZDs involve a coingestant, typically alcohol Inappropriate sexual or aggressive behavior, mood lability, impaired judgment	1. Slurred speech 2. Ataxia 3. Altered (MC: depressed) mental status 4. Stupor or coma Signs: 1. Unremarkable 2. Normal vital signs DX criteria: 1+ of following: 1. Slurred speech 2. Incoordination 3. Unsteady gait 4. Nystagmus 5. Impairment in cognition 6. Stupor/coma Associated: Agitation, anxiety, dizziness, insomnia, Muscle cramps, myoclonic contractions, high BP and HR	1. Rule out phenobarbital and ethanol intoxication by checking blood levels Acute/ED setting: 1. Bedside glucose 2. Acetaminophen and salicylate levels 3. EKG–r/o conduction system poisoning 4. Pregnancy test for women of childbearing age	Acute/ED setting: 1. Assessment of circulating, airway, and breathing • Endotracheal intubation if necessary • Supplemental O_2 2. Activated Charcoal is NOT recommended and provides NO benefit 3. Flumazenil (Romazicon) • Nonspecific competitive antagonist of BZD receptor • Good for reversing BZD-induced procedural sedation • In acute setting, can precipitate withdrawal seizures in patients with tolerance through chronic use or abuse • Risks can sometimes outweigh benefits • Dose is 0.2 mg IV over 30 s, repeated to max of 1 mg (0.01 mg/kg IV over 15 s for children) Health maintenance: 1. BZD are not detected in standard urine screenings for drugs of abuse Complications: Respiratory depression

Psychiatry

(continued)

Disease	Etiology, Prevalence, and Risk Factors	Clinical Symptoms and Signs	Diagnostics	Therapy, Prognosis, and Health Maintenance
BZD withdrawal	Abrupt or overly rapid reduction in BZD dose among chronic users Symptoms appear as early as 24-48 h after cessation up to 3 wk Most last 1-2 wk Decreased BZD activity results in decreased GABA receptor activity (less inhibition of excitatory neurotransmitters), which results in a pro-excitatory state Can be life threatening!	1. Tremors 2. Anxiety 3. Perceptual disturbances 4. Dysphoria 5. Psychosis 6. Seizures		1. Avoid withdrawal by gradually tapering BZD dose over several months 2. Use BZDs with long half-lives (diazepam or chlordiazepoxide)
GHB (gamma hydroxybutyrate) intoxication	Mostly white males Commonly used at club and dance venues, MSM Frequently used with MDMA, mephedrone, cocaine, alcohol, and methamphetamine Metabolite and precursor to GABA; direct agonist of GABA-B receptors resulting in neural inhibition Marketed to treat insomnia, anxiety, alcohol dependence, for body building, and narcolepsy with cataplexy	1. Confusion (**AMS**), dizziness, drowsiness 2. Agitation followed by somnolence 3. Psychomotor impairment 4. Impaired memory or amnesia 5. LOC and abrupt onset of coma (common) with spontaneous resolution 6. Ataxia; sudden loss of muscle control 7. Apnea, respiratory depression 8. Vomiting Signs: 1. Hypotension, bradycardia, bradypnea, hypothermia 2. Myoclonus or seizure-like effects 3. Nystagmus, dysconjugate gaze	Clinical DX: 1. Urine testing for GHB 2. Gas chromatography or mass spectrometry (GC/MS)—definitive • Requires 7-14 d to confirm • Detectable in blood for 4-6 h and urine 6-12 h Acute/ED setting: 1. Bedside glucose 2. Acetaminophen and salicylate levels 3. EKG—r/o conduction system poisoning 4. Pregnancy test for women of childbearing age 5. Check CK levels—r/o rhabdomyolysis	Acute/ED setting: 1. Assessment of circulating, airway, and breathing • Endotracheal intubation if necessary • Supplemental O_2 2. Activated Charcoal and gastric lavage are NOT recommended and provides NO benefit 3. No reversal agents or antidotes exist
GHB (gamma hydroxybutyrate) withdrawal	Frequent use is believed to lead to tolerance associated with down regulation of inhibitory GABA and GHB receptors; decreased consumption results in decreased neuro inhibition → unopposed excitatory neurotransmission	1. Rapid onset, within 1-6 h of cessation • Anxiety, confusion • Tremor—early sign • Sweating • Nausea, vomiting • **Insomnia** (common) • Occurs despite use of antipsychotics and benzodiazepines 2. Progresses to severe withdrawal in 24 h • Agitation • Hallucinations • Delusions • Delirium • Death Signs: 1. Tachycardia, hypertension, hyperthermia 2. Diaphoresis 3. Myoclonic jerks 4. Hypertonia 5. Cogwheel rigidity 6. Opisthotonos 7. Nystagmus Complications: Increased risk of sudden LOC, falls, and MVAs, seizures, Wernicke–Korsakoff disease, rhabdomyolysis, DIC	1. Elevated CK 2. Pulse oximetry and wave capnography	1. Supportive 2. Mild to moderate, without delirium • Inpatient detox • Diazepam, phenobarbital, pentobarbital, or propofol 3. Severe, with delirium • Larger doses of sedatives • ICU monitoring • Intubation and mechanical ventilation 4. Do NOT use haloperidol or other neuroleptic agents (ineffective and increase risk of adverse effects)

Cannabis (Marijuana)

Disease	Etiology, Prevalence, and Risk Factors	Clinical Symptoms and Signs	Diagnostics	Therapy, Prognosis, and Health Maintenance
Acute cannabis intoxication (use) Δ⁹-Tetrahydrocannabinol (THC) Slang terms used for cannabis include Aunt Mary, BC bud, blunt (cannabis within tobacco), boom, chronic, dope, gangster, ganja, grass, hash, herb, hydro, indo, joint (cannabis cigarette), kif, Mary Jane, mota, pot, reefer, roach, sinsemilla, skunk, smoke, weed, and yerba Synthetic cannabinoids have street or "brand" names that include synthetic weed, legal high, spice, K2, Blaze, RedX Dawn, Paradise, Demon, Black Magic, Spike, Mr. Nice Guy, Ninja, Zohai, Dream, Genie, Sence, Smoke, Skunk, Serenity, Yucatan, Fire, and Crazy Clown	17% start in adolescence (most age 12-17 y/o) Lower dependence, but doesn't mean less addiction Most commonly used illegal psychoactive substance worldwide RF: 1. (+) FH in 34%-78% 2. Young adults (18-25 y/o) 3. Male (2×) > female 4. Lower educational attainment Use disorder develops in 10% of regular users Effects occur within 10-20 min and last 2-3 h of smoking THC activates CB1 receptors in Dopaminergic mesolimbic circuit, resulting in increased release of presynaptic dopamine (mediates brain-reward system)	1. **Increased appetite** 2. Increased time perception, **decreased reaction time**; 3. **Impaired motor coordination** or judgment, concentration, and memory 4. **Euphoria, decreased anxiety** (may experience dysphoria and panic if first time user or history of anxiety) 5. **Increased sociability** (dysphoria may lead to social withdrawal) 6. Depression, cognitive impairment 7. Persistent pattern of use that results in clinically significant functional impairment in 2+ domains of life within 1 y • School work • Work function • Previously enjoyed social or recreational activities • Use in potentially hazardous situations (driving) Signs: 1. Tachycardia, hypertension, tachypnea 2. *Dilated* pupils (**mydriasis**) 3. Yellowing of fingertips 4. Odor on clothing 5. **Dry mouth** 6. Tachycardia 7. **Conjunctival injection** (red eye) 8. Nystagmus 9. Ataxia 10. Slurred speech Complications: Myocardial infarction	Clinical DX: 1. ***Urinalysis for THC*** • Urine detection periods span 4-6 d in short-term users and 20-50 d in long term users • Good for screening, but less helpful for acute diagnosis • More sensitive (more false positives): positive screens should be confirmed with additional testing • Reported with: dronabinol, efavirenz, PPIs, hemp seed oil, NSAIDs, baby wash products • Confirmed by at least 15 ng/mL (50 ng/mL standard) 2. Saliva, blood, and hair used as alternatives, sent for gas chromatography and mass spectrophotometry Acute/ED: 1. Urine toxicology 2. Rapid blood glucose 3. EKG for chest pain 4. CXR for difficulty breathing or pleuritic chest pain	Children: 1. Airway, breathing, circulation 2. Naloxone for opioid intoxication features 3. Midazolam or lorazepam for seizures 4. Lorazepam for dysphoria 5. Admit children with symptoms beyond 48 h, persistent vomiting, AMS, or excessive purposeless motor activity 6. Contact child abuse team if necessary Adolescents and adults: 1. Supportive care • Dimly lit room • Reassurance • Decreased stimulation • Lorazepam for anxiety 2. Treat underlying cause (asthma, pneumothorax), identify presence of other drug use 3. Activated charcoal NOT recommended for ingestion of cannabis 4. Admit for prolonged delirium or agitation requiring repeated use of antipsychotics or benzodiazepines Prognosis: 1. Diminished life satisfaction and achievement, addiction increases with potency 2. Associated with reduced IQ 3. Associated with death from MVAs 4. May be associated with development of schizophrenia 5. Small increased risk of MI and CVA 6. Associated with periodontal disease, hyperemesis syndrome, and lower sperm count
Cannabis withdrawal	50%-95% of heavy users Chronic use downregulates CB1 receptors Abstinence upregulates receptors in a few days, causing uncomfortable or distressing symptoms, which contributes to negative reinforcement and continued use	1. Insomnia or disturbing dreams 2. Irritability, anger, aggression 3. Nervousness, anxiety 4. Decreased appetite, **weight loss** 5. **Restlessness** 6. Depressed mood 7. **Abdominal pain**, *nausea*, vomiting 8. Fever, chills, headache Signs: 1. Shakiness/**tremors** 2. Diaphoresis		1. **Psychotherapy**—first line • CBT • Motivational enhancement therapy or interviewing (MET) Aim for sustained abstinence, but goal of moderation in use may be necessary to engage some patients in treatment process

Tobacco Use Disorder (Nicotine)

- May use free telephone quitline (1-800-QUIT-NOW) for follow up support and counseling

- One pack of cigarettes is ~20 cigarettes

Disease	Etiology, Prevalence, and Risk Factors	Clinical Symptoms and Signs	Diagnostics	Therapy, Prognosis, and Health Maintenance
Tobacco use disorder	Leading preventable cause of mortality Two-thirds of smokers say they want to quit and 50% report they tried to quit in the last year Dependence on nicotine: (1) determined by age of smoking initiation, (2) number of cigarettes smoked daily, (3) how soon after waking up a patient has first cigarette Nicotine dependence predicts the degree of difficulty patient will have in quitting and intensity of treatment required	Complications: lung cancer	5 As (assessment)—at every visit 1. Ask about smoking 2. Advise smokers to quit 3. Assess readiness to quit 4. Assist them with smoking cessation effort 5. Arrange follow up visits or contact	1. First line • **Varenicline** (Chantix)—best efficacy • **Bupropion SR** (Wellbutrin, Zyban) • Nicotine replacement therapy (NRT) • Recommended for inpatient use 2. Second line • Nortriptyline • Clonidine 3. **Cognitive behavioral therapy** • For every patient Prognosis: 1. Most relapses occur within the first 3 mo of quitting 2. 35%-40% relapse between 1-5 y after quitting Health maintenance: 1. Best success is with pharmacotherapy and psychotherapy 2. Recommend follow up after starting medication in 1-2 wk to monitor for adverse effects and provide reinforcement
Tobacco withdrawal	Development of cravings for cigarettes (nicotine) and symptoms in the absence of nicotine use Starts within first 3 d of smoking cessation and subside over 3-4 wk Common triggers for relapse: being around other smokers, drinking alcohol, smoking cues (drinking coffee), stressful situations	1. Increased appetite 2. Weight gain • 1-2 kg in first 2 wk, then 2-3 kg over next 4-5 mo 3. Mood changes (dysphoria, depression, anxiety) 4. Insomnia 5. Irritability 6. Difficulty concentrating 7. Anxiety 8. Restlessness		As above Prognosis: 1. Withdrawal symptoms peak 1-2 wk after quitting, but may continue for months

Nicotine Replacement Therapies (NRT)

1. Recommend combined use of long and short acting NRT as initial therapy

2. Dosing of products is based on number of cigarettes smoked daily and tapered as withdrawal symptoms subside

3. Safe to use in patients with stable cardiovascular disease, but limited information in use after acute coronary syndrome (ACS)

4. Okay for use in pregnancy (first or second line), preferred in breastfeeding women

5. Recommended for use in adolescents for smoking cessation

Long Acting	Short Acting	
Patch[a]	**Gum (Nicorette)[a]**	**Lozenges[a]**
1. Long acting, slow onset 2. Simple, continuous delivery of nicotine 3. Good compliance, but no control over nicotine dose 4. AE: skin irritation (MC), insomnia, vivid dreams	1. Short acting—used to control cravings and withdrawal symptoms in adjunct with long acting methods 2. MOA: released from chewing the gum, absorbed through oral mucosa 3. Peak levels in 20 min, available in multiple flavors 4. AE: mouth soreness or irritation (sore jaw), dyspepsia, nausea, vomiting, abdominal pain, constipation, hiccups, headache, excess salivation, mouth ulcers 5. Not good for people with TMJ, poor dentition or dentures	1. Short acting—used to control cravings and withdrawal symptoms in adjunct with long acting methods 2. Pharmacokinetics similar to gum 3. AE: mouth irritation or ulcers, abdominal pain, nausea, vomiting, headache, palpitations
Starting on quit day: 1. If >10 cigarettes/d, use highest dose (21 mg/d) × 6 wk, then 14 mg/d × 2 wk, then 7 mg/d × 2 wk 2. Apply new patch each morning to nonhairy skin site, remove and replace next morning 3. Rotate daily to avoid skin irritation 4. Remove at bedtime to avoid vivid dreams and insomnia, if experienced	1. 4 mg dose recommended for 25+ cigarette/d smokers 2. Chew the gum whenever an urge to smoke arises 3. One piece of gum every 1 ± 2 h × 6 wk, for 3 mo total duration 4. Avoid acidic beverages before and during use (coffee, carbonated beverages)—lowers oral pH causing nicotine to ionize and reducing nicotine absorption 5. Side effects related to vigorous chewing (excess nicotine release)	1. Resembles a "tic-tac," dissolves rapidly and delivers nicotine more rapidly 2. 4 mg dose for smokers who smoke within 30 min of waking up; 2 mg for all other smokers 3. Similar dosing schedule to gum, maximum 5 lozenges every 6 h or 20/d 4. Place in mouth and dissolves over 30 min, no chewing necessary

[a]Available without a prescription.

Chantix Versus Bupropion

	Chantix (Varenicline)	Bupropion (Zyban SR, Wellbutrin SR)
Class/MOA	1. Partial agonist at $\alpha_4\beta_2$ subunit of the nicotinic acetylcholine receptor • Binds to and produces **partial stimulation** of the $\alpha_4\beta_2$ nicotinic receptor, **reducing symptoms** of withdrawal • **Binds** to $\alpha_4\beta_2$ subunit **with high affinity**, *blocking* nicotine in tobacco smoke from binding to receptor, **reducing the reward** aspects of cigarette smoking 2. No liver metabolism, excreted by kidney (dose reduction in patients with renal insufficiency) 3. Safe for patients with COPD 4. Safe for adolescents (not first line, limited data)	1. Enhances central nervous system noradrenergic and dopaminergic release 2. Safe for use in patients with stable CVD or COPD 3. Good choice for patients concerned about post-cessation weight gain or with comorbid depression 4. Approved for use in pregnancy (first or second line) 5. Safe for adolescents (not first line, limited data)
Administration	1. Quit smoking 1 wk after starting medication (stable blood levels achieved) 2. 0.5 mg daily × 3 d, then 0.5 mg BID × 4 d, then 1 mg BID up to 12 wk 3. Risk of nausea minimized by taking with food and full glass of water, or by increasing dose 4. Abnormal dreams can be reduced by taking evening dose of Chantix earlier in the day, lowering the dose or skipping evening dose	1. Takes 5-7 d to reach steady-state blood levels 2. Start one week prior to quit-date 3. 150 mg/d × 3 d, 150 mg BID thereafter at least 12 wk
Safety	1. **Avoid in patients with current unstable psychiatric history or recent suicidal ideation** 2. Stop the medication if changes in behavior, hostility, agitation, depressed mood, suicidal ideation, and suicide attempts 3. May increase risk of adverse cardiovascular events if known CVD 4. May experience impairment in ability to drive or operative heavy machinery; may not be prescribed to pilots and air traffic controllers 5. AE: nausea, insomnia, abnormal dreams, visual disturbances, syncope, skin reaction	1. Reduces seizure threshold—**contraindicated** in patients with **seizure disorder** or predisposition to seizure and in patients with history of anorexia or bulimia 2. Avoid in patients with bipolar disorder 3. AE: insomnia, agitation, dry mouth, headache
Black box warning	Increased risk of suicide or self-injurious behavior—Removed in December 2016 based on RCT finding no difference in adverse neuropsychiatric events compared to nicotine patch or placebo in patients with coexisting psychiatric disorder	Increased risk of suicide or self-injurious behavior—removed in December 2016 based on RCT finding no difference in adverse neuropsychiatric events compared to nicotine patch or placebo in patients with coexisting psychiatric disorder

Psychiatry

Inhalant Related Disorders

Disease	Etiology, Prevalence, and Risk Factors	Clinical Symptoms and Signs	Diagnostics	Therapy, Prognosis, and Health Maintenance
Inhalant-use n-Hexane (glue sniffing) is a petroleum distillate and aliphatic hydrocarbon neurotoxin that causes giant axonal changes Volatile substances that are highly lipid soluble and readily absorbed across the pulmonary bed	M = F, mostly age 12-17 y/o Act as CNS depressants with alteration at the glutamate or GABA receptors MC: glue, shoe polish, **toluene** (30%); gasoline or lighter fluid (25%); nitrous oxide (25%) or "whippets"; spray paint (23%) Methods of use: Sniffing, huffing, "bagging" (highest concentration) First drugs of abuse by children and adolescents due to accessibility, low cost, and low risk of perceived use	1. **Euphoria** followed by lethargy 2. **Lightheadedness** 3. General state of intoxication 4. Impaired judgment and coordination 5. Effects last 15-45 min Signs: 1. Hypotension 2. Reflex tachycardia 3. Chemical odors on breath, skin, or clothes 4. "Glue-sniffer's rash": eczematoid dermatitis with erythema, inflammation, and pruritus in perioral area Complications: Permanent brain damage, cardiac dysfunction, liver toxicity, acute renal failure, death	Clinical DX	Treat as below Examples: solvents, glues, spray paints, coatings, silicones
Inhalant intoxication	Nitrous oxide toxicity: 1. Ataxia 2. Polyneuropathy 3. Psychosis	Acute: 1. Slurred speech 2. Ataxia 3. Disorientation 4. Headache 5. Hallucinations 6. Agitation 7. Violent behavior 8. Seizures Pulmonary: 1. Reactive airway, pneumothorax GI: 1. Nausea, vomiting, cramps Long term: 1. Peripheral neuropathy in hands/feet • Distal weakness • Muscle atrophy • Numbness Complications: Arrhythmias, myocarditis, MI	Clinical DX Acute/ED setting: 1. Rapid blood glucose 2. Pulse oximetry 3. Continuous EKG 4. Urine toxicology Other: 1. CT/MRI: loss of brain mass and white matter degeneration (toxic leukoencephalopathy) 2. EKG: QT prolongation 3. CBC: aplastic anemia, leukemia, multiple myeloma 4. CMP: hypokalemia, hypophosphatemia, elevated CK, metabolic acidosis 5. Urinalysis 6. Methemoglobin levels, if nitrite abuse suspected 7. VBG, if gasoline abuse suspected 8. CXR for hypoxemia, rales, or distress	Acute: 1. **Supplemental 100% O_2** by nonrebreather mask 2. Treat ventricular arrhythmias using PALS/ACLS guidelines • Amiodarone or Lidocaine preferred over Epinephrine 3. Treat underlying hypokalemia or methemoglobinemia, if present

61
Schizophrenia and Related Psychotic Disorders

Recommended Supplemental Topics:

Brief Psychotic Disorder, p 571

All of the following conditions are currently updated with DSM-5 criteria

The fifth edition of the American Psychiatric Association's *Diagnostic and Statistical Manual*

(DSM-5) utilizes specific criteria with which to objectively assess symptoms, rather than purely discrete diagnostic categories. For example, personality dimensions are more prominent than they were in *DSM-IV*. Nonetheless, the diagnosis is still based on a solid history and examination.

SCHIZOPHRENIA SPECTRUM DISORDERS

- **Schizophrenia**—most common of the psychotic disorders that are characterized by a loss of contact with reality

- **Symptoms of psychosis**
  - Hallucinations—the perception of a sensory process in the absence of an external source (auditory, visual, somatic, olfactory, or gustatory)
  - Delusions—fixed, false beliefs; can be bizarre or nonbizarre
  - Disorganized speech—reflect disruption in the organization of a person's thoughts (tangentiality and circumstantiality)
  - Disorganized behavior—patient with grossly disorganized behavior recognized by inability to complete daily, normative tasks (eg, Put on clothes, clean, etc)

Types of Delusions

Ideas or delusions of reference	Beliefs that random or neutral events are not random/neutral, but include the patient in a special way • Believing that occurrences on TV or radio are meant to deliver special messages to patient
Grandiose delusions	Form around the belief that the person has some special significance or power
Paranoid delusions	May prevent individual from cooperating with evaluation or treatment and may increase the likelihood of problems like homelessness as person goes "off the grid"
Nihilistic delusions	Uncommon, bizarre beliefs that one is dead or one's body is breaking down or that one does not exist
Erotomanic delusions	Person erroneously believes that they have a special relationship with someone

Psychiatry

Types of Disorganization

- Most commonly tangentiality or circumstantiality

Tangential speech	Patient becomes increasingly further off topic without appropriately answering question
Circumstantial speech	Patient eventually answers question, but in a markedly roundabout way
Derailment	Patient suddenly changes topic without any logic or segue
Neologisms	The creation of new, idiosyncratic words
Word Salad	Words thrown together without sensible meaning

Symptoms, Course, and Prognosis of Schizophrenia

Positive Symptoms	Course and Prognosis of Schizophrenia	

1. Hallucinations
2. Delusions
3. Bizarre behavior: Inappropriate, agitated
4. Disordered thought process: Tangential, incoherent, pressured
	1. Prodrome usually in adolescence
	  • "Weird" child
	  • Schizotypal characteristics
	2. Acute psychotic break (with/without stressor)
	3. First 5 y are prognostic
	4. Generally deterioration with each episode
	5. 20%-30% "somewhat normal" lives
	6. 40%-60% with severe impairment
	7. Support system can make a huge difference	

Negative Symptoms (5 As)	**Good Prognostic Factors**	**Poor Prognostic Factors**
1. Affective flattening 2. Alogia: poverty of speech (not interested in things or talk much) 3. Apathy/avolition: Indifference/lack of motivation 4. Anhedonia: Loss of interest in pleasurable activities 5. Impaired Attention	1. Late onset 2. Obvious precipitating event 3. Acute onset 4. Good premorbid functioning 5. Comorbid mood disorder or family history of mood disorders 6. Positive symptoms 7. Good support system	1. Young onset 2. Insidious onset 3. Social isolation 4. Negative symptoms (5 As) 5. Family history of schizophrenia 6. Hx of perinatal trauma 7. Recurrent relapses 8. Hx of assaultiveness (very likely to be victim of violence more than perpetrate it)

Negative Symptoms in Schizophrenia

Symptom Cluster	Negative Symptom	Manifestations
Diminished expression	Affective flattening	1. Unchanging facial expression 2. Little spontaneous movement 3. Little use of expressive gestures 4. Poor eye contact 5. Affective nonresponsivity 6. Lack of vocal inflections
	Alogia	1. Poverty of speech 2. Thought blocking 3. Increased latency of response
Avolition or apathy	Apathy	1. Poor grooming and hygiene 2. Failure of appropriate role responsibilities 3. Anergy
	Asociality or anhedonia	1. Failure to engage with peers socially 2. No interest in stimulating activities 3. Little interest in sex 4. Little to no intimacy with others

Subtypes of Schizophrenia

Paranoid	Disorganized	Catatonic	Undifferentiated
1. Dominated by relatively stable, often **paranoid, delusions, usually accompanied by hallucinations**, particularly of the auditory variety, and perceptual disturbances. 2. Disturbances of affect, volition, and speech, and catatonic symptoms are *not* prominent. Common SX: • Delusions of persecution, reference, exalted birth, special mission, bodily change, or jealousy; • Hallucinatory voices that threaten the patient or give commands, or auditory hallucinations without verbal form, such as whistling, humming, or laughing; • Hallucinations of smell or taste, or of sexual or other bodily sensations; visual hallucinations may occur but are rarely predominant Most common type	1. Behavior is disturbed & has no purpose 2. Marked by **disorganized speech, thinking, and behavior** on the patient's part, coupled with **flat or inappropriate emotional responses to a situation (affect)** 3. The patient may act silly or withdraw socially to an extreme extent SX: • Active behavior, but in an aimless and not constructive way • Bizarre and inappropriate emotional responses (laughter) • Difficulty feeling pleasure • Delusions • Grimacing • Lack of motivation • Hallucinations • Strange or silly behavior • Speech that makes no sense	1. Prominent motoric immobility OR 3. **Excessive, purposeless motor activity** SX: • **Negativism:** motiveless physical resistance to instruction or attempts to move the person • **Mutism:** refusal to speak in certain situations or to certain people • **Posturing:** assume & maintain some odd posture • **Catalepsy:** waxy flexibility (leave hand in the air after you placed it in the air) • **Echolalia:** echo anything you say • **Echopraxia:** echo any movements you do Treatment: Ativan	1. Patients in this category have the characteristic positive and negative symptoms of schizophrenia, but do not meet the specific criteria for the paranoid, disorganized, or catatonic subtypes. 2. Difficult diagnosis to make with any confidence because it depends on establishing the slowly progressive development of the characteristic "negative" symptoms of schizophrenia without any history of hallucinations, delusions, or other manifestations of an earlier psychotic episode, and with significant changes in personal behavior, manifest as a marked loss of interest, idleness, and social withdrawal.

- **Paranoia**—"a mind beside itself"
  - Designates people who show "fixed suspicions, persecutory delusions, dominant ideas, or grandiose trends logically elaborated and with due regard for reality once the false interpretation or premise has been accepted"
- In comparison to schizophrenia, these patients have good conduct, adequate emotional responses, and a coherent train of thought

SCHIZOPHRENIA

Disease	Etiology, Prevalence, and Risk Factors	Clinical Symptoms and Signs	Diagnostics	Therapy, Prognosis, and Health Maintenance

Schizophrenia	Onset before age 25, persists through life
	Peak: 18-25 in men
	Bimodal peak: 25-35, >50 in women
	M > F, men diagnosed earlier
	Lifetime prevalence: 1%
	RF:
	1. First degree relative (10×)
	2. Advanced paternal age at conception
	3. Urban living area
	4. Immigration
	5. Obstetrical complications
	6. Late winter or early spring birth
	Etiology:
	• Excess dopamine in the mesolimbic tract
	• Decreased dopamine in the prefrontal cortex
	• Hypofunction of the NMDA glutamate receptor
	• Dysfunctional GABAergic interneurons
	Most common hallucinations (**auditory**): threatening, obscene, accusatory, insulting
	Drugs that increase dopaminergic activity (cocaine, amphetamine)–increase positive symptoms
		DSM-5 criteria:
		1. **2+** of the following 5 characteristics present for significant portion of a **1-mo period**
		  • Delusions*
		  • Hallucinations*
		  • Disorganized speech*
		  • Disorganized or catatonic behavior
		  • Negative symptoms
		2. Impairment in one or more areas of functioning: work, interpersonal relationships, self-care, academics
		3. Continuous signs for **at least 6 mo** (must include 1 mo of symptoms in A-E), including prodromal and residual symptoms
		4. Rule out schizoaffective and mood disorder with psychotic features
		  • No concurrent MDD, mania, or mixed episodes
		  • If mood episodes in (a) have occurred, they have been brief relative to total duration of active/residual periods
		5. Disturbance not due to direct physiologic effects of substance or other medical condition
		6. If autistic or other pervasive developmental disorder, schizophrenia only diagnosed if prominent delusions or hallucinations for at least 1 mo
			Clinical DX of exclusion:
			• Major distinguishing feature: psychotic symptoms occur in absence of prominent mood symptoms
			• At least 2 of the 5 criteria must include delusions, hallucinations, or disorganized speech
			• Must specify presence of catatonia
			• Must rate severity of criteria in A-E
			• 5 subtypes as above
				1. **Atypical antipsychotics** (first line)
				  • Risperidone (Risperdal)
				  • Olanzapine (Zyprexa)
				  • Quetiapine
				  • Ziprasidone
				  • Clozapine
				Comorbidities:
				1. Metabolic: **Diabetes**, HLD, HTN
				2. Substance abuse is common (>50%) with 90% dependent on nicotine
				3. Mood and anxiety symptoms common; higher rate than general population
				Prognosis:
				1. See table above for prognostic factors
				2. MCC of death: suicide (20%-50% attempt)
				3. Better for females, men more likely to be impaired by negative symptoms
				Health maintenance:
				1. Resolution of psychotic symptoms occurs over several days up to 4-6 wk with medication
				2. Resist the urge to change medication or dose prematurely
				3. Explain risks of sedation, restlessness, postural hypotension, etc before starting medication

* Must include at least 1 of these criterion: delusions, hallucinations, or disorganized speech.

- Clozapine—effective in the treatment of 30% of psychoses resistant to other antipsychotics and is effective in decreasing suicidality in patients with schizophrenia

Treatment of Schizophrenia

Pretreatment assessment	1. Evaluate: BMI, waist circumference, heart rate, BP, and extrapyramidal symptoms (EPS) 2. CBC, electrolytes, fasting glucose, lipid profile, liver, renal and thyroid function tests 3. WBC count with differential for patients on Clozapine 4. EKG for patients with cardiac history of treatment with Clozapine, Thioridazine, Iloperidone, or Ziprasidone
Acute therapy	1. **Antipsychotics** (first line)—reduce positive symptoms • Consider AE of various medications: weight gain, EPS, sedation 2. Clozapine—most effective for patients who do not respond to other antipsychotics • AE: risk for agranulocytosis • Recommend slow taper over 1-2 wk due to withdrawal movement disorders and cholinergic rebound 3. Okay to switch antipsychotics when poor response is related to side effects 4. Add second antipsychotic when response to initial antipsychotic is suboptimal
Acute agitation	1. Treatment guided by cause • Extrapyramidal symptoms (akathisia)—benzodiazepines (lorazepam) • Substance use • Psychosis—antipsychotics +/− benzodiazepines • IM haloperidol, olanzapine, aripiprazole, and ziprasidone with benztropine or Benadryl to reduce risk of EPS (dystonias) • PO risperidone or olanzapine • ODT risperidone, olanzapine, aripiprazole • Common combination: 5 mg haloperidol, 2 mg lorazepam, 1 mg benztropine for severe agitation
First-episode psychosis	1. Antipsychotics recommended other than clozapine and olanzapine • Low doses because at high risk for EPS symptoms • 1-3 mg risperidone or 10 mg aripiprazole daily
Maintenance therapy	1. Continue antipsychotics indefinitely, even if remission achieved from first psychotic episode 2. Use lowest effective therapeutic dose

Treating the Side Effects of Schizophrenia

Akathisia	1. β **Blockers** (propranolol) • First line for antipsychotic induced akathisia 2. Benzotropine 3. Benzodiazepines
Parkinsonian syndrome	1. Benztropine (first line) 2. Amantadine—for patients who do not tolerate benztropine or experience anticholinergic effects
Dystonia	1. IM or IV benztropine 2. IM or IV benadryl
Tardive dyskinesia	1. Avoid treatment with antipsychotics 2. Metoclopramide—should not be used continuously >12 wk
Metabolic syndrome	1. Change antipsychotics 2. Diet and exercise counseling 3. Behavioral intervention 4. Symptomatic treatment with statins, hypertensives, etc 5. Metformin use for weight gain
Prolactin elevation	1. Change to a different antipsychotic

DELUSIONAL DISORDER (FIG. 61-1)

Disease	Etiology, Prevalence, and Risk Factors	Clinical Symptoms and Signs	Diagnostics	Therapy, Prognosis, and Health Maintenance
Delusional (paranoid) **disorder**	A persistent delusion that is not part of any other mental disorder, specifically, criteria for schizophrenia have not been met EXCEPTION: patient with olfactory or tactile hallucinations consistent with the delusion, but no auditory hallucinations Prevalence: 0.2% M = F Mean onset: 35-45 y/o RF: 1. (+) **FH paranoid personality disorder** 2. Sensory impairment Subtypes: 1. Persecutory (48%) 2. Jealous (11%) 3. Mixed (11%) 4. Somatic (5%) 5. NOS (23%)	DSM-5 criteria: 1. Presence of **1+ delusions** with duration of **at least 1 mo** 2. Criteria for schizophrenia have *never* been met 3. Apart from impact of delusions or its ramifications, functioning not impaired, behavior not bizarre or odd • This means they could occur in real life (being followed, poisoned, infected, loved at a distance, deceived by a spouse, or having a disease) 4. If manic or depressive episodes have occurred, these have been brief relative to duration of delusional periods 5. Not attributable to other physiological effects of substance or other mental disorder Signs: 1. Alert, oriented, memory and attention within normal limits 2. Insight and judgment impaired	Clinical DX: • Absence of other positive symptoms of psychosis (except hallucinations that are part of delusional theme) • Absence of functional impairment	1. Pharmcotherapy • **Antipsychotics** (first line) • Recommended: Aripiprazole or ziprasidone 2. Cognitive behavioral therapy (CBT) for patients who cannot tolerate medication or refuse it • Supportive psychotherapy as adjunct 3. Treat comorbidities Comorbidities: 1. **Depression** 2. Anxiety Prognosis: 1. In 2/3 of cases, the disorder is lifelong

Subtypes of Delusional Disorder

Erotomanic	Grandiose	Jealous	Persecutory	Somatic	Unspecified
1. Believes that another person is secretly in love with them 2. Person may be famous or have some kind of higher status, usually not in their social circle and not attainable 3. May attempt to communicate or meet them in person 4. Can lead to stalking in some cases	1. Believes they have special prominence or talent, unusual fame, or major achievements 2. Mood disturbance and behaviors of mania not present	1. Believes that spouse or lover is unfaithful and finds "evidence" to support the delusion 2. Accuses lover 3. Relentlessly tries to substantiate the offense 4. Can lead to aggressive, threatening, or violent behavior, including homicide or suicide	1. Preoccupied by delusion that they are being persecuted, conspired against, or potentially harmed 2. Their actions are consistent with these concerns 3. May resort to court system and violence to right the "wrongs" directed at them	1. Believes that something awful is wrong with their body • Ill with undiagnosed disease • Infested with parasites or insects (delusional parasitosis) • Parts of body are misshapen, ugly, or emanate foul odor 2. Travel from doctor to doctor, specialist to specialist, disappointed by failure to detect and diagnose the problem	1. Cannot be clearly determined or not described by others

BRIEF PSYCHOTIC DISORDER

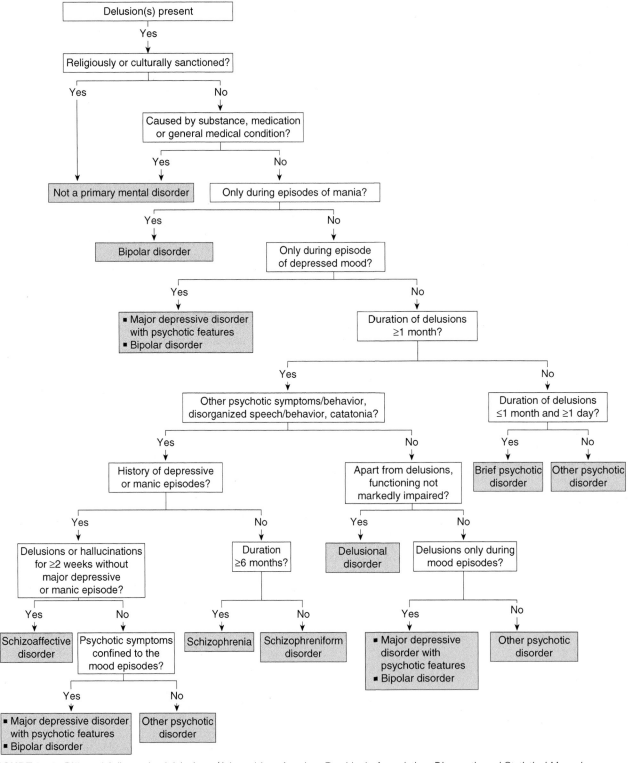

FIGURE 61-1. Differential diagnosis of delusions. (Adapted from American Psychiatric Association. *Diagnostic and Statistical Manual of Mental Disorders: DSM-5.* 5th ed. Washington, DC: American Psychiatric Association; 2013. https://www.uptodate.com/contents/image?imageKey=PSYCH%2F100456&topicKey=PSYCH%2F17193&search=delusions&source=outline_link&selectedTitle=1~150.)

Disease	Etiology, Prevalence, and Risk Factors	Clinical Symptoms and Signs	Diagnostics	Therapy, Prognosis, and Health Maintenance
Brief psychotic disorder	Rare, low incidence Cause is unknown F >>> M Mean onset: varies (usually late teens, early 20s) Usually in **response to a stressful life event**, but can occur without marked stressor, and can occur postpartum (within 4 wk of delivery) Presence of 1+ psychotic symptoms with a sudden onset and full remission within 1 mo	1. Presence of 1+ of the following • Delusions • Hallucinations • Disorganized speech • Grossly disorganized or catatonic behavior 2. Lasts at least *1 d* but no longer than *1 mo* 3. Eventual full return to premorbid level of functioning 4. Absence of symptoms of mood disorder or psychosis from substance use/withdrawal	Clinical DX: • Distinguish from schizophreniform disorder and schizophrenia by symptom duration • Lack of negative symptoms • Confusion during early course of illness	1. **Antipsychotics** • Risperdal • Switch to another antipsychotic if no response • Monitor for side effects and symptoms of disorder 2. Benzodiazepines • Clonazepam • Effective for agitation 3. Supportive psychotherapy Prognosis: 1. Maintenance treatment for at least 5 y with meds indefinitely

SCHIZOAFFECTIVE DISORDER AND SCHIZOPHRENIFORM DISORDER

Disease	Etiology, Prevalence, and Risk Factors	Clinical Symptoms and Signs	Diagnostics	Therapy, Prognosis, and Health Maintenance
Schizoaffective disorder	Primary psychotic disorder (psychosis underlying everything) PLUS mood symptoms intermittently (there *most of the time*) Same time frame for schizophrenia SX	1. SX of schizophrenia with superimposed symptoms of • Major *depression* and/or • *Mania*—precede or develop with psychotic manifestations 2. Psychotic episode lasts at **least 2 or more wk** in *absence* of any mood symptoms	Clinical DX: **Differentiate from bipolar I disorder:** *psychosis can/does occur in absence of mood episodes*, while in bipolar I, psychosis occurs only with mania or major depression	1. Manic: Lithium or carbamazepine 2. Depression: SSRI 3. Psychosis: antipsychotic Prognosis: 1. Outcome better than schizophrenia, but worse than mood disorders
Schizophreniform disorder		1. Psychotic symptoms present at least *1 mo* but no longer than *6 mo* 2. 2+ types of psychotic symptoms present for significant portion of 1 mo period if left untreated 3. Negative symptoms constitute one of the characteristic types of symptoms present 4. No impairment in social or occupational functioning	Clinical DX: • Distinguish from brief psychotic disorder and schizophrenia by symptom duration • <6 mo	1. Treatment as for schizophrenia

CHAPTER 62

Conduct, Developmental, Impulse and Attention-related Disorders

Recommended Supplemental Topics:

Impulse Control, p 575
Disruptive Mood Regulation Disorder (DMDD), p 575
Neurodevelopmental Disorders, p 576

All of the following conditions are currently updated with DSM-5 criteria

The fifth edition of the American Psychiatric Association's *Diagnostic and Statistical Manual*

(DSM-5) utilizes specific criteria with which to objectively assess symptoms, rather than purely discrete diagnostic categories. For example, personality dimensions are more prominent than they were in *DSM-IV.* Nonetheless, the diagnosis is still based on a solid history and examination.

ATTENTION-DEFICIT/HYPERACTIVITY DISORDER

- **Inattention** manifests as wandering off task, lacking persistence, having difficulty sustaining focus, and being disorganized and is not due to defiance or lack of comprehension
- **Hyperactivity** refers to excessive motor activity (such as a child running about) when it is not appropriate, or excessive fidgeting, tapping, or talkativeness. In adults, hyperactivity may manifest as extreme restlessness or wearing others out with their activity

- **Impulsivity** refers to hasty actions that occur in the moment without forethought and that have high potential for harm to the individual (eg, darting into the street without looking). Impulsivity may reflect a desire for immediate rewards or an inability to delay gratification. Impulsive behaviors may manifest as social intrusiveness (eg, interrupting others excessively) and/or as making important decisions without consideration of long-term consequences (eg, taking a job without adequate information)
- Gold standard for diagnosis: (1) **Autism Diagnostic Observation System** (ADOS) and (2) the Autism Diagnostic Interview

Disease	Etiology, Prevalence, and Risk Factors	Clinical Symptoms and Signs	Therapy, Prognosis, and Health Maintenance

Attention-deficit hyperactivity disorder (ADHD)	Begins in childhood
	Associated:
	ODD (50%), conduct disorder (25%), specific learning disorder
	5% of children, 2.5% of adults
	<u>RF:</u>
	VLBW (<1500 g, 2-3× risk), smoking during pregnancy, first degree relative
	M (2×) >F
		<u>History:</u>
		May include child abuse, neglect, multiple foster placements, lead exposure, encephalitis, alcohol exposure in utero
		1. Several *inattentive* or *hyperactive-impulsive* symptoms present **PRIOR to age 12**
		  • Motoric hyperactivity present in preschool
		  • Inattention more prominent in elementary
		  • Hyperactivity less common in adolescence
		  • Adulthood: impulsivity remains problematic
		2. Several symptoms present in 2 or more settings (home, school, work; with friends or relatives)
		3. Symptoms interfere with or reduce quality of social, academic, or occupational function
		4. Do not occur exclusively during course of schizophrenia or another psychotic/mental disorder
			See treatment below
			Increased risk of suicide attempt (when comorbid mood, conduct, or substance use disorders)

Inattention		1. Six or more of the following for at least 6 mo (at least 5 for age 17+)
		  • Fails to give close attention to detail or makes careless mistakes in schoolwork, at work, or during other activities
		  • Difficulty sustaining attention in tasks or play activities (remaining focused during lectures, conversations, or length reading)
		  • Does not seem to listen when spoken to directly (seems elsewhere, even in absence of obvious distraction)
		  • Does not follow through on instructions; fails to finish homework, chores, or duties in workplace (starts, but loses focus and easily sidetracked)
		  • Difficulty organizing tasks and activities (managing sequential tasks, keeping materials and belongings in order; messy, disorganized work; poor time management; fails to meet deadlines)
		  • Avoids, dislikes, or is reluctant to engage in tasks that require sustained mental effort (schoolwork, homework, preparing reports, completing forms, reviewing lengthy papers)
		  • Often loses things necessary for tasks or activities (school materials, pencils, books, tools, wallets, paperwork, eyeglasses, mobile phones)
		  • Often distracted by extraneous stimuli
		  • Forgetful in daily activities (doing chores, running errands)
			See treatment below

Hyperactivity and impulsivity		1. Six or more of the following symptoms for at least 6 mo:
		  • Often fidgets or taps hands/feet or squirms in seat
		  • Leaves seat in situations when remaining seated is expected
		  • Runs about or climbs in situations where inappropriate
		  • Often unable to play or engage in leisure activities quietly
		  • Often "on the go," acting as if "driven by a motor" (unable to be still for extended period of time)
		  • Talks excessively
		  • Blurts out answers before question has been completed (completes people's sentences)
		  • Difficulty waiting for his/her turn in line
		  • Interrupts or intrudes on others (butts into conversations, games, activities; starts using other people's things without asking or permission)
			See treatment below

ADHD Therapies

Stimulants	1. Most commonly prescribed
	2. Sympathomimetic drugs that increase intrasynaptic catecholamines (dopamine) by inhibiting the presynaptic reuptake mechanism and releasing presynaptic catecholamines
		1. **Methylphenidate** (Ritalin, Concerta, Metadate)
		  • Blocks the dopamine transporter protein
		  • Short acting, onset 30-60 min (peak 1-2 h, lasts 2-5 h)
		  • Extended release AE: headaches and moodiness
		  • Short-term AE: reduced appetite, insomnia, edginess, GI upset
		  • **Growth retardation, psychosis**
		Dexmethylphenidate (Focalin-XR)
		2. **Amphetamine** (Dexedrine, Adderall)
		  • Release dopamine stores and cytoplasmic dopamine directly into the synaptic cleft
		  • Intermediate acting, onset 60 min (lasts 6-8 h)
		Lisdexamfetamine (Vyvanse): prodrug converted to dextroamphetamine

Nonstimulants	1. Second line if difficulty with adverse effects, comorbid (Tourette or seizure), concerns about stimulant abuse, or parental choice	1. Atomoxetine (Strattera): NE reuptake inhibitor; antidepressant
		  • No growth suppression, tics, or insomnia
		  • AE: nausea, vomiting, weight loss, sleep problems
		  • Black Box Warning: liver damage (D/C if jaundice), risk of suicide

Antidepressants	1. Control abnormal behavior and improve cognitive impairment	1. Tricyclic antidepressants
		  • AE: tachycardia
		2. Bupropion (Wellbutrin)
		  • Block reuptake of norepinephrine
		  • Avoid in patients with seizure hx or eating disorders
		3. Atomoxetine
		4. SSRIs—not useful for ADHD

Antihypertensive	1. Alpha-adrenergic agonists
	2. Treat ADHD, as well as tics, aggression, and sleep disturbance
	3. Good for angry outbursts and aggression
	4. More effective for **hyperactivity and impulsivity** than attention
		Clonidine (Catapres), timed-release clonidine (KAPVAY)
		  • Can reduce motor tics, headaches, jitteriness
		  • AE: hypotension, sedation
		Guanfacine (Tenex), ER guanfacine (INTUNIV)
		  • Longer acting, less sedating than Clonidine
		  • No effects on growth or appetite

Modafinil	1. Antinarcoleptic agent	AE: SJS

CONDUCT DISORDER AND OPPOSITIONAL DEFIANT DISORDER

Disease	Etiology, Prevalence, and Risk Factors	Clinical Symptoms and Signs	Therapy, Prognosis, and Health Maintenance

Conduct disorder	Mostly **male**
	2%-10% prevalence
	Comorbidities: ADHD, ODD, learning disorders
	90% of children with conduct disorder have had ODD
		1. Patient violates basic rights of others or major age-appropriate societal norms/rules
		2. At least 3 of the 15 criteria in past 12 mo with at least 1 criterion in past 6 mo
		  • **Aggression to people and *animals***
		    • *Bullies*, threatens, intimidates others
		    • Initiates physical fights
		    • Used a weapon that causes serious harm to others
		    • Physically cruel to people or animals
		    • Stolen while confronting a victim (mugging, armed robbery, extortion, purse snatching)
		    • Forced someone into sexual activity
		  • **Destruction of property**
		    • Engaged in fire-setting with intention of causing damage
		    • Deliberately destroyed others' property
		  • **Deceitfulness or theft**
		    • Broken into house, building, car
		    • Lies to obtain goods or favors or to avoid obligations
		    • Stolen items of nontrivial value without confronting victim (shoplifting without breaking and entering, forgery)
		  • **Serious violations of rules**
		    • Stays out at night despite parental prohibitions (before age 13)
		    • Runs away from home overnight at least 2× while living in home or once without returning for lengthy period
		    • Truant from school
			1. Early intervention programs
			2. Pharmacotherapy
			  • **Methylphenidate**: reduces defiance, oppositionalism, aggression, and mood changes (age 5-8)
			  • Divalproex: reduces hyperarousal, anger, and aggression in incarcerated adolescents
			Prognosis:
			1. Most develop **antisocial personality disorder (ASPD)**

Disease	Etiology, Prevalence, and Risk Factors	Clinical Symptoms and Signs	Therapy, Prognosis, and Health Maintenance

Oppositional defiant disorder (ODD)	Precursor to Conduct Disorder
	Prevalence: 1%-11%
	M > F
	Average age onset: 6 y
	<u>Comorbidities:</u>
	Anxiety, depression, substance use disorder
		1. Pattern of angry/irritable mood, argumentative or defiant behavior, or vindictiveness lasting at least *6 mo* with at least 4 symptoms
		• **Angry or irritable mood**
		  • *Loses temper, touchy or easily annoyed, angry and resentful*
		• **Argumentative and defiant behavior**
		  • Argues with authority figures
		  • Actively defies rules or refuses to comply with requests
		  • *Deliberately annoys others*
		  • Blames others for his or her mistakes
		• **Spiteful or vindictive** at least twice during past 6 mo
			1. Children <12, **effective parenting**
			  • Positive attention with praise and reinforcement of desirable behavior
			  • Ignore inappropriate behavior
			  • Give clear, brief commands, reduce task complexity, eliminate competing influences
			2. **Family therapy** if >18
			<u>Prognosis:</u>
			25% will develop conduct disorder

Impulse-control		1. Includes compulsive buying, kleptomania, pathological gambling, trichotillomania, skin picking disorders, and onychophagia (nail biting)	
Disruptive mood regulation disorder (DMDD)		1. **Chronic, severe, persistent irritability** accompanied by severe temper outbursts at least 3× per week that are out of proportion to provocation and inconsistent with developmental level 2. Duration for at least 1 y (no interruption longer than 3 mo) 3. Onset by age 10 (not before age 6 or after 18) 4. No symptoms of hyperarousal	1. Stimulants +/− clonidine 2. Depakote for mood dysregulation 3. Risperdal for aggression 4. CBT for children

AUTISM SPECTRUM DISORDER

- Autism spectrum disorder encompasses disorders previously referred to as early infantile autism, childhood autism, Kanner's autism, high-functioning autism, atypical autism, pervasive developmental disorder not otherwise specified, childhood disintegrative disorder, and Asperger's disorder

- An early feature of autism spectrum disorder is impaired joint attention as manifested by a lack of pointing, showing, or bringing objects to share interest with others, or failure to follow someone's pointing or eye gaze

- First symptoms of autism spectrum disorder frequently involve delayed language development, often accompanied by lack of social interest or unusual social interactions (eg, pulling individuals by the hand without any attempt to look at them), odd play patterns (eg, carrying toys around but never playing with them), and unusual communication patterns (eg, knowing the alphabet but not responding to own name).

Disease	Etiology, Prevalence, and Risk Factors	Clinical Symptoms and Signs	Therapy, Prognosis, and Health Maintenance
Autism spectrum disorder	1% of general population RF: Advanced parental age, low birth weight, fetal exposure to Valproate, 15% have known genetic mutation **Males (4×)** > females, African American Associated: anxiety, depression, mental retardation	Symptoms—typically observed during second year of life, but may be seen <12 mo 1. Persistent deficits in social communication and interaction • **Deficits in social-emotional reciprocity** (back-forth conversation, sharing of interests, emotions, affect; failure to initiate or respond to social interactions) • Deficits in **nonverbal communicative behaviors** (abnormalities in eye contact and body language or understanding of gestures → total lack of facial expression, nonverbal communication) • Deficits in **developing, maintaining, and understanding relationships** (adjusting behavior to suit social contexts, **sharing imaginative play,** or making friends, no interest in peers) 2. **Restricted, repetitive patterns of behavior, interests, activities:** 2 of following • Stereotyped or repetitive motor movements, use of objects, or speech (motor stereotypies, lining up toys or flipping objects, echolalia) • Insistence on sameness, inflexible adherence to routines, or ritualized patterns of nonverbal or verbal behavior (extreme distress at small changes, difficulties with transitions, rigid thinking patterns, greeting rituals, need to take same route or eat same food everyday) • Highly restricted, fixated interests that are abnormal in intensity or focus (strong attachment to or preoccupation with unusual objects) • Hyper or hyporeactivity to sensory input or unusual interest in sensory aspects of environment (indifference to pain/temperature, excessive smelling or touching of objects, visual fascination with lights or movement, adverse response to specific sounds or textures) 3. Symptoms present in early childhood 4. Cause significant impairment in social, occupational, or other areas of functioning 5. Not better explained by intellectual disability Signs: 1. Motor deficits—odd gait, clumsiness, abnormal motor signs (walking on tiptoes) 2. Self-injury—head banging, biting the wrist 3. Disruptive or challenging behaviors Complications: Seizures	1. Educational and Behavioral intervention • Focus on speech and language therapy • Communication skills and vocabulary 2. Medication • **Abilify, Risperdal** • SSRIs 3. Psychotherapy • Limited therapy 4. Good prognosis: functional language by age 5 5. Poor prognostic factors: epilepsy as comorbidity (more intellectual disability and low verbal ability)

NEURODEVELOPMENTAL DISORDERS

Intellectual Disability

- The term intellectual disability (ID), commonly used in Europe, is now becoming preferred to the previous one, mental retardation (MR), although both are still used interchangeably

- Requires impairment in (1) intellectual functioning, (2) adaptive functioning, and (3) onset before age 18 (usually refers to children >5)

  - Adaptive behavior must affect at least 1 of 3 domains: conceptual, social, and practical
    - Conceptual: language, reading, writing (literacy); money, time, number concepts; reasoning; memory; self-direction; judgment.

    - Social: interpersonal social communication, empathy, ability to relate to peers as friends, social problem-solving; social responsibility, self-esteem, gullibility, ability to follow rules and avoid being victimized
    - Practical: personal care or daily living activities (eating, dressing, mobility, toileting); following a routine schedule, using a phone, managing money, preparing meals, occupational skills

- Intellectual functioning can impact general mental capacity including learning, reasoning, abstract thinking, problem solving skills, and judgment. This usually corresponds to an intelligence quotient (IQ) 2 standard deviations below the mean

- Overall, ID affects approximately 1% of patients nationwide, highest in school aged children and males

- Risk factors: AMA, low maternal education level

- Causes: mostly genetic abnormalities, but metabolic disorders, neurologic abnormalities (epilepsy, structural brain defect), congenital anomalies

- Most common cause: chromosomal aberrations (most common being Down syndrome, or trisomy 21)

- 15% to 30% of ID patients have visual impairment and 18% have hearing impairment

- The severity of ID is currently defined according to the level of support needed to address impaired adaptive functioning in one or more settings (eg, school, home, work)

Disease	Etiology, Prevalence, and Risk Factors	Clinical Symptoms and Signs	Diagnostics	Therapy, Prognosis, and Health Maintenance
Mild	Represents 85% of affected ID individuals Previously defined as an IQ between 50 and 55-70	1. Parental concern for • language delay • immature behavior and play • immature self-help skills 2. Child fails to meet expected developmental milestones during screening and surveillance	Clinical DX: 1. Adaptive functioning • Vineland Adaptive Behavior Scale III 2. IQ <65-75 • No longer used as sole clinical or legal decision maker • Does not determine severity	Comorbid: Depression, anxiety, PTSD Screening: 1. Chromosomal microarray analysis (CMA)—first line 2. Whole exome sequencing (WES) 3. Karyotype analysis—for suspected aneuploidy 4. Metabolic testing—for patients with seizures, developmental regression, FTT, abnormal neurological exam
Moderate	Previously defined as an IQ between 35-40 and 50-55			
Severe	Previously defined as an IQ between 20-25 and 35-40	1. Presents with language delay		
Profound	Previously defined as an IQ less than 20-25			

Screening Tools for ID

Ages and Stages Questionnaire (ASQ)-3	Age specific questions about child, completed by parents in 10-15 min Screens children age 1 mo-5.5 y
Bayley Infant Neurodevelopmental Screener (BINS)	Screens children age 3-24 mo Takes 10-15 min
Brigance Early Childhood Screens-III	Screens children from infancy through 5 y Takes 10-15 min
Infant-Toddler Checklist	Screens children 6-24 mo of age
Parents' Evaluation of Developmental Status (PEDS)	Brief screening of children from infancy to 8 y/o

Global Developmental Delay

- Describes intellectual and adaptive impairment in children <5 years old, based on failure to meet developmental milestones on time in several areas of functioning

Chromosomal Aberrations

Mutation	Syndrome	Development
MECP2 Mutation	Rett syndrome	• Females • Normal development 6-18 mo, then loss of speech and purposeful hand use, stereotypic hand movements, gait abnormalities • Mod to severe ID
FMR1 mutation: • Abnormal expansion mutation of a CGG triplet repeat (>200)	Fragile X syndrome	• Most common X-linked disorder • M (2×): F • Macrocephaly, large ears, enlarged testes, perseverative speech, poor eye contact • Mod to severe ID
Trisomy 21	Down syndrome	• G banded karyotype analysis recommended

CHAPTER **63**

Personality Disorders

All of the following conditions are currently updated with DSM-5 criteria

The fifth edition of the American Psychiatric Association's *Diagnostic and Statistical Manual (DSM-5)* utilizes specific criteria with which to objectively assess symptoms, rather than purely discrete diagnostic categories. For example, personality dimensions are more prominent than they were in *DSM-IV*. Nonetheless, the diagnosis is still based on a solid history and examination.

PERSONALITY DISORDERS

- Personality disorder: enduring patterns of inner experience and behavior that are inflexible and pervasive and cause clinically significant distress or impairment in social, occupational, or other areas of functioning
- First-line treatment: **psychotherapy**
- Benzodiazepines should be avoided in patients with personality disorders when possible. Selective serotonin reuptake inhibitors (SSRIs) may reduce irritability, but higher than average doses may be needed. Antipsychotic drugs may also decrease irritability and aggression; they are typically used in personality disorders at doses lower than those used for in psychotic disorders.
- Patients with personality disorders are at increased risk for adverse outcomes related to physical trauma, suicide, substance use disorders, and concurrent other mental disorders

Disease	Etiology, Prevalence, and Risk Factors	Clinical Symptoms and Signs	Therapy, Prognosis, and Health Maintenance
1. Different (Weird)			
Paranoid	<u>MC</u>: Men, first-degree relative of schizophrenic Hostile, argumentative, hypervigilant	1. **Distrust and suspiciousness** of others → motives interpreted as malevolent; **4+ of following:** • Suspects, without sufficient basis, that others are exploiting, harming, or deceiving them • Preoccupied with **unjustified doubts about the loyalty or trustworthiness** of friends or associates • Reluctant to confide in others because of unwarranted fear that the information will be used maliciously against him/her • Reads hidden demeaning or threatening meanings into benign remarks or events • Persistently **bears grudges** (unforgiving of insults, injuries, or slights) • Perceives attacks on his/her character or reputation that are not apparent to others and is quick to react angrily or to counterattack • Has recurrent **suspicions**, without justification, **regarding fidelity of spouse** or sexual partner = JEALOUSY	**Psychotherapy**: Avoid confrontation—counterproductive and reinforces their beliefs

Disease	Etiology, Prevalence, and Risk Factors	Clinical Symptoms and Signs	Therapy, Prognosis, and Health Maintenance
Schizoid	Loner without seeming need for much human relatedness MC: Men, first degree relative of schizophrenic eg, Night watchmen without many friends	1. **Detachment** from social relationships and restricted range of expressive of emotions in interpersonal settings; 4+ of the following: • Neither desires nor enjoys close relationships, including being part of a family • Almost always chooses **solitary activities** • Has **little interest in sexual experiences** • Takes pleasure in few activities • **Lacks close friends** or confidants other than first degree relatives • Appears indifferent to the praise or criticism of others • Shows **emotional coldness**, detachment, or flat affect Signs: 1. May have constricted affect, seem distant, anhedonia 2. **Flat affect, emotionally blunted**	Individual **psychotherapy**, NOT group
Schizotypal Now listed as a schizophrenia-spectrum disorder, while retaining its classification as a personality disorder	Genetic relationship to schizophrenia? Regarded as "Odd or eccentric" Fascinated by unusual ideas, but unlike patients with delusions, willing to consider alternatives if facts are presented 3% prevalence MC: First-degree relative of schizophrenic	1. **Social and interpersonal deficits** marked by acute discomfort with, and reduced capacity for, close relationships as well as by cognitive or perceptual distortions and eccentricities of behavior; 5+ of the following: • **Ideas of reference** (excluding delusions of reference) • **Odd beliefs or magical thinking** that influences behavior and is inconsistent with subcultural norms (superstitious, belief in clairvoyance, telepathy, "sixth sense") • Unusual perceptual experiences, including bodily illusions • **Odd thinking and speech** (vague, circumstantial, metaphorical, overelaborate, or stereotyped) • Suspiciousness or paranoid ideation • **Behavior or appearance that is odd, eccentric, or peculiar or unkempt** • **Lack of close friends** or confidants other than first-degree relatives • **Excessive social anxiety** that does not diminish with familiarity → paranoid fears, not negative judgements about self 2. Do not have delusions or hallucinations Signs: 1. Paranoid ideas (but not frank delusions) 2. **Inappropriate, constricted affect** 3. Speech: circumstantial, metaphorical, vague Ideas of reference 4. Laugh inappropriately while discussing their problems 5. Talk to themselves in public, gesture for no reason	Psychotherapy: Not motivated to seek treatment Comorbidities: Anxiety disorder, MDD

(continued)

(continued)

Disease	Etiology, Prevalence, and Risk Factors	Clinical Symptoms and Signs	Therapy, Prognosis, and Health Maintenance
2. Action Oriented (Wild)			
Borderline	Hostile/angry Dependent/child-like behavior RF: Childhood history of abuse or parental neglect Mostly female RF: First-degree relative (5×)	1. **Instability** in personal relationships, self-image, and affective regulation 2. Marked **impulsivity** that is potentially **self-damaging**, inappropriate, intense anger or control of anger, recurrent suicidal attempts, gestures or threats, and identity disturbances • Frantic efforts to **avoid real or imagined abandonment** • Unstable and intense interpersonal relationships (extremes of idealization and devaluation) • Identity disturbance: markedly and persistently unstable self-image or sense of self • **Impulsivity** in at least 2 areas that are self-damaging (spending, sex, substance abuse, reckless driving, binge eating) • Recurrent suicidal behavior, gestures, threats, or self-mutilating behavior • **Affective instability** due to a marked reactivity of mood (intense episodic dysphoria, irritability, or anxiety lasting a few hours and only rarely more than a few days) • **Chronic feelings of emptiness** • Inappropriate, intense anger or difficulty controlling anger (recurrent physical fights, constant anger, temper) • Transient, stress related paranoid ideation Signs: 1. Idealize versus devalue: overvalue some and devalue others depending on their perception of others' intentions, interest, and level of caring 2. Countertransference: stirrup strong feelings to rescue/take care of others 3. Splitting: see others (and themselves) as wholly good or totally bad 4. Self-harm: cutting 5. Chronic dysphoria common—desperate dependence on others caused by inability to tolerate being alone	1. **Psychotherapy** (DBT) 2. SSRI Comorbidity: **Mood disorder**
Narcissistic	Mostly males, <1% Described as: arrogant, envious, exploitative	• Pattern of grandiosity (in fantasy or behavior), need for admiration and lack of empathy; 5+ of following: • **Grandiose** sense of self-importance (exaggerates talents, achievements, expects to be recognized as superior without commensurate achievements) • Preoccupied with fantasies of unlimited success, power, brilliance, beauty, or ideal love • Believes that he or she is special and unique and can only be understood by, or should associate with, other special or high-status people (or institutions) • Requires **excessive admiration** • **Sense of entitlement** (unreasonable expectations of favorable treatment) • Interpersonally **exploitative** (takes advantage of others to achieve his/her own ends) • **Lacks empathy**: unwilling to recognize or identify with feelings and needs of others • **Envious** of others or believes that others are envious of him/her • Shows **arrogant**, haughty behaviors or attitudes	1. **Psychotherapy** 2. Lithium: use if mood swings are prominent 3. Antidepressants: use if comorbid depression

Disease	Etiology, Prevalence, and Risk Factors	Clinical Symptoms and Signs	Therapy, Prognosis, and Health Maintenance
Histrionic	Dramatic Strong affect Sexualization/flirtatious Vague/over inclusive: overfamiliar in history giving Mostly female, prevalence 2%-3%	1. *Excessive emotionality* and attention seeking; 5+ of following: • Uncomfortable in situations where he/she is not center of attention • Interaction with others characterized by **inappropriate sexually seductive or provocative behavior** • Rapidly shifting and shallow expression of emotions • Uses physical appearance to draw attention to self (attention seeker) • Has a style of speech that is excessively impressionistic and lacking in detail • Shows self-dramatization, *theatricality*, and **exaggerated expression of emotion** • Suggestible (easily influenced by others) • **Considers relationships to be more intimate than actually are**	Psychotherapy
Antisocial (ASPD)	Strong genetic component ASPD: criminal activity, fights with weapons, history of rape/assault M:F (3:1) RF: First-degree relative with ASPD Fail in roles requiring fidelity (spouse), honesty (employee), or reliability (parent)	1. Disregard for and violation of rights of others, *occurring since age 15*; 3+ of following: • **Failure to conform to social norms** with respect to lawful behaviors (arrested) • Deceitfulness: lying, use of aliases, or conning others for personal profit or pleasure • Impulsivity or failure to plan ahead • Irritability and aggressiveness (physical fights, assaults) • Reckless disregard for safety of self/others • Consistent irresponsibility: repeated failure to sustain consistent work behavior or honor financial obligations • *Lack of remorse or empathy*: being indifferent to or rationalizing having hurt, mistreated, or stolen from another	1. Perform CAGE questionnaire for alcoholism 2. Inpatient self-help groups 3. Psychotropics Anticonvulsants, lithium, BB Prognosis: Often have ODD that then develops into conduct disorder and onto ASDP later in life
3. Anxiety Prone (Worried)			
Avoidant	Self-depreciating Fear of getting hurt Moody—apologize a lot	1. Social inhibition, feelings of inadequacy, and hypersensitivity to negative evaluation; 4+ of following: • Avoids occupational activities that involve significant interpersonal contact because of *fears of criticism, disapproval, or rejection* • Unwilling to get involved with people unless certain of being liked • Shows *restraint within intimate relationships* because of fear of being shamed or ridiculed • **Preoccupied with being criticized or rejected in social situations** • Inhibited in new interpersonal situations because of *feelings of inadequacy* • Views self as **socially inept, personally unappealing, or inferior to others** • Unusually reluctant to take personal risks or engage in any new activities because may prove embarrassing Signs: 1. Timid, social awkwardness 2. Apologetic demeanor—hate to bother others, guilty	1. Individual or group *psychotherapy* 2. β-Blockers 3. If social phobia—SSRI Comorbidities: Depression, anxiety, **substance abuse** (ETOH)

(continued)

(continued)

Disease	Etiology, Prevalence, and Risk Factors	Clinical Symptoms and Signs	Therapy, Prognosis, and Health Maintenance
Dependent	Mostly women RF: childhood illness or separation anxiety disorder	1. **Excessive need to be taken care of** that leads to submissive and clinging behavior and fears of separation; 5+ of following • Has **difficulty making everyday decisions** without an excessive amount of advice and reassurance from others • Needs others to assume responsibility for areas of his/her life • Has difficulty expressing disagreement with others because of fear of loss of support or approval • Difficulty initiating projects or doing things on his/her own (*lack of self confidence* in judgment or abilities, rather than lack of motivation or energy) • **Goes to excessive lengths to obtain nurturance and support from others,** to point of volunteering to do things that are unpleasant • Feels **uncomfortable or helpless** when alone because of exaggerated fears of being unable to care for him/herself • **Urgently seeks another relationship** as a source of care and support when close relationship ends • Unrealistically preoccupied with fears of being left to care for him/herself	1. **Psychotherapy:** insight oriented 2. Frequent, short visits that are not crisis-driven 3. Allow them to keep aspects of "sick role" without needing to escalate Associated: Increased risk for mood and anxiety disorders
Obsessive compulsive personality disorder (OCPD)	Mostly males (2:1) <u>RF:</u> First-degree relative Differentiate from OCD (egodystonic) "I should" phrase—captures overly high standards, drive, perfectionism, rigidity, and devotion	1. Preoccupation with orderliness 2. **Perfectionism,** and mental and interpersonal control, at the expense of flexibility, openness, and efficiency; 4+ of following • Preoccupied with details, rules, lists, order, organization, or schedules to extent that major point of activity is lost • Perfectionism *interferes with task completion* (strict standards not met, unable to complete) • Excessively devoted to work and productivity to exclusion of leisure activities and friendships • Over conscientious, scrupulous, and inflexible about matters of morality, ethics, or values • Unable to discard worn-out or worthless objects when they have no sentimental value • Reluctant to delegate tasks or to work with others unless they submit exactly to his/her way • Adopts a miserly spending style toward both self and others; money viewed as something to be hoarded for future catastrophes • Shows *rigidity and stubbornness* <u>Signs:</u> 1. Orderly, scheduled, regular—hate spontaneity 2. Denies feelings 3. Meticulous, effortful	1. *High-dose SSRIs* or clomipramine (serotonergic TCA) 2. FDA approved: Fluvoxamine, paroxetine, sertraline, fluoxetine

BODY DYSMORPHIC DISORDER

• In adults with BDD, fluoxetine protects against worsening of suicidality more than placebo, and suicidality decreases with other SSRIs

• If relevant, discuss the likelihood that cosmetic treatment will not help

• Involve family members: Family members often bring patients with BDD for treatment, and can support the patient and encourage adherence with the treatment plan

• Monitor depression with the self-report Patient Health Questionnaire—Nine Item (PHQ-9)

• Cognitive behavioral therapy techniques that are helpful: psychoeducation, motivational interviewing, goal setting, cognitive restructuring, *exposure* to avoided situations, prevention of rituals, perceptual retraining when looking in a mirror, advanced cognitive strategies, daily homework, relapse prevention

Disease	Etiology, Prevalence, and Risk Factors	Clinical Symptoms and Signs	Therapy, Prognosis, and Health Maintenance
Body dysmorphic disorder	F > M Specifier—with muscle dysmorphobia • Almost always male	1. Preoccupation with at least one nonexistent or slight defect in physical appearance (thinks about it **>1 h/d**) 2. At some point, concerns about appearance lead to repetitive behaviors (mirror checking, excessive grooming, skin picking) or mental acts (comparing one's appearance to others) 3. Clinically significant stress or psychosocial impairment that results from appearance concerns 4. Preoccupations not better explained by eating disorder	1. **SSRIs or clomipramine** • Fluoxetine or escitalopram • Decrease obsessive preoccupations, compulsive behaviors, and functional impairment 2. Cognitive behavioral therapy Comorbidities: Unipolar **major depression** or social anxiety disorder, bipolar disorder, substance use disorder

OBSESSIVE-COMPULSIVE DISORDER

• **Obsessive-compulsive disorder (OCD)** was classified as an anxiety disorder in the *DSM-IV* and is now a part of a separate category of Obsessive-Compulsive Disorder and Related Disorders in *DSM-5*. The new category includes such disorders as trichotillomania and compulsive gambling in addition to OCD.

Disease	Etiology, Prevalence, and Risk Factors	Clinical Symptoms and Signs	Therapy, Prognosis, and Health Maintenance
Obsessive-compulsive disorder (OCD)	Mostly males (2:1) RF: First-degree relative Comorbidities: **Depression** (most common), other anxiety disorders, eating disorders, tics Lifetime prevalence of 2%-3% worldwide Onset in early adulthood, but childhood onset is not rare	Onset is gradual with waxing and waning course 1. **Fears of contamination and germs** (common), **handwashing, counting behaviors, and having to check and recheck** such actions as whether door is locked 2. Activities take up >1 h/d 3. Undertaken to relieve anxiety triggered by core fear 4. Want to control their feelings and emotions of others Signs: 1. Chafed and reddened hands, patchy hair loss (*trichotillomania*)	1. **Pharmacotherapy** • *High-dose SSRIs or clomipramine* • FDA approved SSRIs (adults): Fluvoxamine, fluoxetine paroxetine, sertraline • FDA approved (children): Fluvoxamine • Treatment-resistant cases: add buspirone or neuroleptic or benzodiazepine • Deep brain stimulation 2. **Behavior therapy** • *Systemic desensitization*: Gradually increase exposure to stressful situations • *CBT*: Maintain diary to clarify stressors • Homework that substitute new activities for compulsions Only 50%-60% benefit from medication only Prognosis: 40% of patients will experience remission as adults

• Trichotillomania—hair pulling
• Excoriation disorder—skin picking
• Onychophagia—nail biting

CHAPTER 64

Somatic and Conversion Disorders

Recommended Supplemental Topics:

Somatization Disorder, p 585
Malingering, p 586

All of the following conditions are currently updated with DSM-5 criteria

The fifth edition of the American Psychiatric Association's *Diagnostic and Statistical Manual (DSM-5)* utilizes specific criteria with which to objectively assess symptoms, rather than purely discrete diagnostic categories. For example, personality dimensions are more prominent than they were in *DSM-IV*. Nonetheless, the diagnosis is still based on a solid history and examination.

Please note: The DSM-5 **does not use the term somatization** and has eliminated the category of diagnoses called "somatoform disorders" (illnesses with physical symptoms that were not explained by a general medical condition). This was because it is difficult to prove that a symptom is **not** caused by a general medical condition and many of the somatoform disorders lacked validity due to insufficient evidence for a discrete set of characteristics, an unpredictable course of illness, and arbitrary exclusion criteria.

SOMATIC SYMPTOM DISORDER

Disease	Etiology, Prevalence, and Risk Factors	Clinical Symptoms and Signs	Diagnostics	Therapy, Prognosis, and Health Maintenance
Somatic symptom disorder	Distressing somatic symptoms: abnormal thoughts, feelings, and/or behaviors Multiple somatic symptoms (pain common) Chronic courses with significant disability F > M 75% of patients previously diagnosed with hypochondriasis	1. At **least 1** somatic symptom that is distressing or causing impairment (psychological distress): • Disproportionate and persistent thoughts about seriousness of symptoms • Persistently high anxiety about symptoms or general health • Excessive devotion of time/energy to symptoms or health concerns 2. Although specific somatic symptom may change, disorder is persistent (**>6 mo**)	<u>Clinical DX:</u> 1. Screening 2. Somatic Symptom Scale-8 3. Somatic Symptom Disorder-B Criteria Scale 4. Somatic Symptoms Experiences Questionnaire	1. General principles • Regularly scheduled visits with *one* PCP • Become familiar and learn their typical from new symptoms • Minimize redundant workup, referrals, etc • Minimize polypharmacy • Ask about psychosocial support, stressors • Empathy & support • **Encourage graduated exercise program** 2. Pharmacotherapy • Dual action agents (5-HT and NE): *TCA* • SSRI/SNRIs 3. Psychotherapy • *CBT* • Other: family therapy, psychoeducation, supportive therapy, stress management, psychodynamic psychotherapy 4. Other interventions • Hypnosis <u>Health maintenance:</u> 1. Management of symptoms, no cure 2. Avoid premature psychiatric referral 3. Educate about mind-body duality 4. Noninvasive, non-narcotic treatment whenever possible <u>Comorbidities:</u> 1. Major depression 2. Panic disorder
Somatization disorder "Stress headache" "Abdominal upset" before an exam "Pseudoseizure"	Psychological distress manifests as physical symptoms Common <u>RF:</u> 1. Female 2. Fewer years of education 3. Minority ethnic status 4. Low socioeconomic status Mind-body disconnect: brain senses or creates a physical problem (psychological paralysis)	<u>DSM-IV criteria:</u> 1. 4+ unexplained physical symptoms in men and 6+ unexplained physical symptoms in women 2. Pain, often related to gastrointestinal and sexual dysfunction, and pseudoneurological symptoms 3. Symptoms NOT consciously or intentionally produced, NOT imaginary	<u>Clinical DX:</u> Lab testing should be judicious when evaluating current and new physical symptoms	1. Frequent, regular, short-visits, brief physical examinations to assess somatic complaints 2. Limit diagnostic evaluations 3. Communication, multidisciplinary approach: physical medicine + rehab, psychiatry, or psychology <u>Health maintenance:</u> 1. Do not tell them they need a psychiatrist 2. Inform them that their diagnosis is treatable (mood and anxiety disorders) 3. Acknowledge physical and emotional suffering, emphasizing that their symptoms are real and not in their head <u>Comorbidities:</u> 1. **Depression** 2. Anxiety 3. Personality disorders • Avoidance • Paranoia • Self-defeating • OCPD

Psychiatry

(continued)

Disease	Etiology, Prevalence, and Risk Factors	Clinical Symptoms and Signs	Diagnostics	Therapy, Prognosis, and Health Maintenance
Factitious disorder (imposed on self) eg, Feces in veins, bleed themselves, induce hypoglycemia (insulin), put blood in urine, wound healing problems, excoriations, infection, GI ailments	Rare; intentionally faking symptoms **in order to assume the sick role or the role of the patient**, even in the absence of external gain Most common falsified symptoms: abdominal pain, joint pain, chest pain, coagulopathy, diarrhea, hematuria, hypercortisolism, hyperthyroidism, hypoglycemia, infections, seizures, skin wounds that do not heal, vomiting, weakness Most frequent psychiatric factitious symptoms: bereavement, depression, psychosis, suicidal ideation **Munchausen by proxy syndrome** (most severe case): caregiver causes harm to child for child to be sick (child abuse)	1. Symptoms physical, but can mimic psychiatric illness 2. Symptoms intentionally induced or produced 3. Goal is NOT to dupe doctor or for external incentives, but to assume a "sick" role 4. No obvious external benefits (financial gain, avoiding work or criminal prosecution)	1. Medical records from prior episodes 2. Video monitor or 1:1 sitter 3. Collateral contacts—information provided by family and friends DSM-5 criteria: 1. Falsifying physical or psychological signs or symptoms, or induction of injury or disease associated with identified deception 2. Presents themselves to others as ill, impaired, or injured 3. The deceptive behavior is evident in the absence of obvious external rewards 4. Behavior not better explained by another mental disorder, such as delusional disorder or psychotic disorder	1. General approach • One clinician should oversee patient management • Consult psychiatry • Inform all members of team about diagnosis and plan • Assess suicide risk • Monitor patient to prevent self-injurious behaviors • Treat comorbid psychiatric disorders • Maintain awareness of countertransference (clinician's feelings and thoughts about patient) 2. *Psychotherapy* (standard) Prognosis: Poor; infrequent recovery
Malingering	Intentionally faking or exaggerating symptoms **for an obvious external benefit** (money, housing, medication, child custody, avoiding work or criminal prosecution) *Behavior*—Not a psychiatric disorder Goal: External incentives	1. Intentional production or feigning of physical or psychological signs and symptoms for external gain (financial, occupational, or legal) 2. Symptoms intentionally induced or produced 3. Patient will flee or argue rather than confess if confronted Signs: 1. Marked discrepancy between history and MSE (appears calm while reporting distressing symptoms) 2. Discrepancy between claimed distress and objective findings (reports depression; jokes with staff, eats every meal and sleeps throughout night) 3. Use of technical medical terms to describe symptoms 4. Conditional threats ("I'll kill myself if you don't admit me") 5. Eagerly or dramatically describing symptoms 6. History notable for multiple inconsistencies and vague responses 7. Demanding specific medications 8. Nonadherence with diagnostic evaluation or treatment	The only way to establish diagnosis is by video monitoring, 1:1 sitter, if the patient acknowledges deliberately producing the symptoms, or if other evidence demonstrates major consistency between what is reported and what is observed	As above Comorbidities: Most have antisocial personality d/o

Disease	Etiology, Prevalence, and Risk Factors	Clinical Symptoms and Signs	Diagnostics	Therapy, Prognosis, and Health Maintenance
Conversion disorder (functional neurological symptom disorder)	Etiology: psychological F > M La belle indifference: indifference about symptoms (paralyzed legs) Symptoms of altered voluntary motor or sensory function that cause substantial distress or psychosocial impairment	1. Occurs after an ACUTE stressor 2. Onset of symptoms or deficits mimicking neurological or medical illness 3. Motor and/or sensory symptoms incompatible with neurological or medical disease: paralysis, blindness, mutism, seizures, hemianesthesia, ataxia	Clinical DX: 1. Positive clinical findings that indicate the symptom is congruent with anatomy, physiology, or known diseases; or the symptom is inconsistent at different times	1. **_Education_** about diagnosis (first line) • State symptoms are real and taken seriously • Elicit how patients conceptualize their symptoms • Give diagnostic label and discuss how it was made • Explain patient does not have neurologic disease • Emphasize symptoms are potentially reversible • Reassure patients that understanding diagnosis leads to improvement • Get family involved • Describe self-help techniques • Acknowledge prior unhelpful therapies 2. Second Line • **_CBT_** • Physical therapy 3. Third line for refractory patients • Pharmacotherapy: antidepressants— **_SSRI_** • Hypnosis • Psychodynamic therapy • Inpatient treatment 4. Other interventions • Biofeedback • Family therapy • Group therapy Prognosis: 1. 5% missed diagnoses 2. Most resolve in days-weeks with recurrence during stressful times (25%)
Illness anxiety disorder (IAD) (hypochondriasis)	Preoccupation with having or acquiring a specific illness Anxiety about health status: excessive health-related behavior and avoidant behaviors M = F Onset: early adulthood, rarely after age 50 DDx: OCD—hypochondriacs limit their obsessions to their body	DSM-5 criteria: 1. At **least 6 mo** 2. **Preoccupation with having or acquiring a serious, undiagnosed illness despite appropriate medical evaluation and reassurance** 3. Somatic symptoms are mild or nonexistent at most 4. Substantial anxiety about health and a low threshold for becoming alarmed about one's health 5. Either excessive behaviors related to health (eg, Repeatedly checking oneself for signs of illness) or maladaptive avoidance of situations or activities (eg, exercise) that are thought to provoke health threats 6. Not better explained by other mental disorders	Clinical DX: Negative physical examination and laboratory testing	1. Primary principles • Schedule regular follow ups with PCP • Acknowledge health fears • Evaluate and treat diagnosable medical diseases/illnesses • Limit diagnostic testing and referrals • Provide reassurance that serious medical illness has been ruled out • Treat comorbid psychiatric disorders • Explicitly make functional improvement the goal of treatment 2. Psychotherapy • **_CBT_**—first line 3. Pharmacotherapy • **_SSRIs_**/SNRIs • First line for IAD + comorbid anxiety or depression

Psychiatry

CHAPTER 65

Feeding or Eating Disorders

Recommended Supplemental Topics:

Refeeding Syndrome, p 593

All of the following conditions are currently updated with DSM-5 criteria

The fifth edition of the American Psychiatric Association's *Diagnostic and Statistical Manual*

(DSM-5) utilizes specific criteria with which to objectively assess symptoms, rather than purely discrete diagnostic categories. For example, personality dimensions are more prominent than they were in *DSM-IV*. Nonetheless, the diagnosis is still based on a solid history and examination.

SCREENING FOR EATING DISORDERS

- The **SCOFF**, which is clinician administered, is recommended to identify patients with eating disorders to determine if further evaluation is necessary
  - Do you make yourself **S**ick because you feel uncomfortably full?
  - Do you worry you have lose **C**ontrol over how much you eat?
  - Have you recently lost more than **O**ne stone (14 lbs. Or 6.35 kg) in a 3-month period?
  - Do you believe yourself to be **F**at when others say you are too thin?
  - Would you say that **F**ood dominates your life?
  - Answering "Yes" to two-plus questions has sensitivity of 100% and specificity of 87.5% for diagnosis of eating disorder

- Eating Attitudes Test (EAT) is one of the most widely used self-reporting eating disorder instruments
  - Accuracy is 90%

ANOREXIA NERVOSA

- Anorexia is a misnomer, because patients retain their appetite
- Minimally normal weight: 18.5 kg/m^2
- Diagnostic criteria: weight loss to 85% of required body weight
- Mild: BMI 17 to 18.49 mg/m^2; mod: 16 to 16.99; severe: 15 to 15.99; extreme: <15

Psychiatry

Disease	Etiology, Prevalence, and Risk Factors	Clinical Symptoms and Signs	Diagnostics	Therapy, Prognosis, and Health Maintenance
Anorexia nervosa	MC: **F, 14-21 y/o** F:M (3:1) Prevalence: 0.6% RF: Female gender, child sexual abuse, OCD, childhood/parental obesity, substance abuse, rigid perfectionist, professions that emphasize thinness, athletes (gymnasts, runners, skaters, rowers, wrestlers), **homosexual men** Median onset: 18 y/o Basic principle is that starvation induces protein and fat catabolism → loss of cellular volume and atrophy in kidneys, brain, heart, liver, intestines, and muscles	DSM-5 criteria: 1. Persistent **restriction of energy intake** leading to low body weight in context of age, developmental trajectory, and physical health 2. Intense **fear of gaining weight** or becoming fat, or persistent behavior that prevents weight gain • Interferes with weight gain even though low weight 3. Distorted perception of body weight and shape, undue influence of weight and shape on self-worth, or denial of the medical seriousness of one's low body weight Amenorrhea no longer required for diagnosing AN 1. Palpitations 2. Dizziness 3. Weakness 4. Exertional fatigue 5. Cold intolerance 6. Amenorrhea • May precede anorexia in 20% 7. Abdominal pain or bloating 8. Early satiety 9. Constipation 10. Swelling of feet Signs: 1. Bradycardia (<60) 2. Orthostatic hypotension • <90/50 3. BMI <17.5 4. Emaciation • Body weight <70% ideal body weight 5. Hypothermia 6. Hypoactive bowel sounds 7. Brittle hair and hair loss 8. Xerosis (dry, scaly skin) 9. Lanugo hair growth 10. Abdominal distention 11. Other: brittle nails, pressure sores, yellow skin (palms), cyanotic and cold hands/feet, ankle or periorbital edema, heart murmur (MVP)	Clinical DX: 1. EKG (for BMI <14) • Increased PR interval • First-degree heart block • ST-T wave abnormalities • QT prolongation 2. CBC • **Anemia (83%)** • **Leukopenia (79%)** • **Thrombocytopenia (25%)** 3. Electrolytes • **Hypokalemia** • **Hypomagnesemia** • Hypophosphatemia • **Hyponatremia**, • Cr: low • Cl⁻, Zn, Thiamine, BUN, serum albumin and prealbumin 4. LFTs • Bilirubin, Alk-Phos,, AST/ALT: **elevated** 5. Thyroid: T3/T4: **low** 6. FSH/LH: **low** 7. Cholesterol: **high (50%)** 8. Serum glucose: hypoglycemia 9. INR 10. Vitamin D 11. Pregnancy test 12. Testosterone in males 13. Echo or CT scan—rule out SMA syndrome 14. If amenorrheic >9 mo, consider DEXA 15. MRI—For cognitive impairment	1. **Psychotherapy** (first line) • CBT • Psychodynamic psychotherapy • Motivational interviewing • Family therapy • Specialist supportive clinical management • Cognitive remediation therapy 2. **Nutritional rehabilitation** 3. Pharmacotherapy • Avoid Bupropion: higher incidence of seizures in eating disorders • Avoid drugs that impact cardiac function: antipsychotics and antidepressants (TCA) Comorbidities: 1. Depression 2. Anxiety 3. **OCD** (most common personality d/o) 4. Body dysmorphic disorder 5. PTSD 6. Substance use disorders 7. Disruptive, impulse control, conduct disorders Health maintenance: 1. Many comorbid disorders resolve with weight restoration 2. Following remission, patient should be reassessed for comorbidities 3. Weigh patient at each visit with as little clothing as appropriate and after voiding 4. For patients who remain ill with AN, repeat DEXA every 2 y and repeat EKG only if cardiac symptoms persist despite weight restoration 5. Follow up within 3 d after any discharge to check for refeeding syndrome, especially in first few weeks after weight restoration 6. Initially, weekly to monthly PCP visit to check phosphate, electrolytes and LFTs and monitor weight gain Prognosis: 1. ETOH use associated with increased mortality 2. 50% fully recover 3. 34% cross over to bulimia nervosa, then 50% of those people will cross back over to AN 4. Risk factors for developing complications include degree of weight loss and chronicity
Restricting-type	Based on the symptoms of the previous 3 mo	1. Dieting, fasting, or excessive exercise 2. Absence of recurrent binge eating or purging		

(continued)

(continued)

Disease	Etiology, Prevalence, and Risk Factors	Clinical Symptoms and Signs	Diagnostics	Therapy, Prognosis, and Health Maintenance
Binge-eating type	Based on the symptoms of the previous 3 mo	1. Recurrent (once/week or more) episodes of binge-eating (eating any amount of food that is larger than most people would eat under similar circumstances) OR 2. Purging (self-induced vomiting, misuse of laxatives, diuretics, or enemas)		

Indications for Hospitalization

Anorexia Nervosa	Bulimia

1. Unstable vital signs
  • Orthostatic increase in pulse (>20 bpm) or decrease in systolic BP (>20 mm Hg)
  • Bradycardia (**HR < 40**) and hypotension or lightheadedness
  • Hypothermia (core temp <35°C or 95°F)
2. Cardiac dysrhythmia (eg, QTc > 0.499 ms) or any rhythm other than sinus bradycardia
3. Weight <70% ideal body weight or BMI <15 kg/m², especially if rapid weight loss
4. Marked dehydration
5. Acute complication of malnourishment: syncope, seizures, cardiac failure, liver failure, pancreatitis, hypoglycemia, or electrolyte disturbance
6. Moderate to severe refeeding syndrome:
  • Marked edema
  • Serum phosphorus <2 mg/dL
7. Poor response as outpatient	

Complications of Anorexia and Bulimia

- Medical complications account for 50% of deaths in AN
- Treatment for each includes nutritional replenishment
- Most are reversible with weight gain
- Most are managed as inpatients or in residential care facilities, though the majority can be effectively handled in the outpatient setting if the patient's weight is >70% ideal body weight or BMI > 15 kg/m²

Anorexia	Bulimia
Constitutional (whole body) 1. Cachexia and low BMI 2. Arrested growth 3. Hypothermia	1. Dental erosion

Cardiovascular
1. **EKG changes**
  • Increased PR interval
  • First-degree heart block
  • ST-T wave abnormalities
2. Arrhythmia, leading to sudden death
3. Bradycardia
4. Hypotension
5. Acrocyanosis
6. Myocardial atrophy
7. **Mitral valve prolapse**
8. Pericardial Effusion
	1. EKG changes
	  • Increased PR interval
	  • Increased p-wave amplitude
	  • Depressed ST segment
	  • QT prolongation
	  • Wide QRS
	2. Arrhythmia: SVT, ventricular ectopic rhythm, Torsade de pointes
	3. Hypotension and orthostasis
	4. Sinus tachycardia
	5. Edema

Anorexia	Bulimia

Gynecologic and reproductive
1. **Functional hypothalamic amenorrhea** in postmenarchal females
  • LH/FSH: both low
  • Estrogen: low
2. Unplanned pregnancy and neonatal complications
  • Recommend vitamin D and calcium supplementation, diet enriched in phosphate and protein
  • Greater risk of complications: miscarriage, premature birth, small head circumference, low birth weight
	1. Menstrual irregularity
	  • Impaired fertility
	  • Spotty and scanty periods
	  • Oligomenorrhea
	  • Amenorrhea

Endocrine 1. **Osteoporosis** and pathologic stress fractures 2. **Euthyroid sick syndrome** 3. **Hypercortisolemia** 4. **Hypoglycemia** 5. Neurologic diabetes insipidus 6. Poor diabetes control	1. Type I and II diabetes mellitus 2. Osteopenia and osteoporosis

Gastrointestinal
1. Gastroparesis: delayed emptying
  • Bloating (gas, distension)
2. **Constipation**
3. Gastric dilatation
4. Increased colonic transit time
5. Hepatitis
6. Superior mesenteric artery syndrome
7. **Diarrhea**
	1. Gastric dilatation
	2. **Parotid and submandibular (salivary) gland hypertrophy**
	  • Hot packs
	  • NSAIDs
	  • Sucking on hard, tart candy
	  • Oral pilocarpine
	3. Laryngopharyngeal reflux
	4. Loss of gag reflex
	5. Esophageal dysmotility
	6. **Abdominal pain and bloating**
	7. Heme stained emesis
	8. Mallory-Weiss syndrome
	9. Esophageal rupture (Boerhaave syndrome)
	10. GERD
	11. Barrett's esophagus
	12. **Diarrhea**, malabsorption
	13. Steatorrhea
	14. Protein losing gastroenteropathy
	15. Hypokalemic ileus
	16. Colonic dysmotility
	17. **Constipation**
	18. Irritable bowel syndrome
	19. Melanosis coli
	20. Cathartic colon
	21. Rectal prolapse
	22. **Pancreatitis**

Renal and electrolytes 1. Decreased GFR 2. Renal calculi 3. Impaired concentration of urine 4. Dehydration 5. **Hypokalemia** 6. **Hypomagnesemia** 7. Hypovolemic nephropathy	1. Dehydration 2. **Hypokalemia** 3. Hypochloremia 4. Hyponatremia 5. Metabolic alkalosis 6. **Hypomagnesemia** 7. Hypophosphatemia
Pulmonary 1. Pulmonary muscle wasting 2. Decreased pulmonary capacity 3. Respiratory failure 4. Spontaneous pneumothorax and pneumomediastinum 5. Enlargement of peripheral lung units without alveolar septa destruction	

Psychiatry

(continued)

(continued)

Anorexia	Bulimia
Hematologic 1. **Anemia** 2. **Leukopenia** 3. **Thrombocytopenia**	
Neurologic 1. Brain atrophy • Cerebral atrophy (decreased gray and white matter) • Enlarged ventricles 2. Cognitive impairment 3. Peripheral neuropathy 4. Seizures 5. Korsakoff syndrome • Anterograde and retrograde amnesia	
Dermatologic 1. Xerosis (dry skin)–back/arms 2. Lanugo hair (fine, downy, dark hair)–back, abdomen, forearms 3. Telogen effluvium (hair loss) 4. Carotenoderma (yellowing) 5. Scars for self-injurious behavior (cuts and burns) 6. Acne 7. Seborrheic dermatitis (MC scalp) 8. Acrocyanosis 9. Striae distensae–do not resolve with weight gain	1. Russell sign: scarring or calluses on dorsum of hand 2. Xerosis 3. Poor skin turgor 4. Petechiae 5. Telogen effluvium 6. Acne 7. Self-injurious behavior (cuts, burns)
Muscular 1. Muscle wasting	1. Ipecac induced myopathy
Miscellaneous 1. Wernicke encephalopathy–caused by thiamine (B_1) deficiency • Global confusion • Oculomotor dysfunction • Gait ataxia	1. Adrenal insufficiency (Addison's disease) 2. Celiac disease 3. Psoriasis 4. Vitamin B_{12} deficiency

Treatment of Complications

Disease	Etiology, Prevalence, and Risk Factors	Clinical Symptoms and Signs	Diagnostics	Therapy, Prognosis, and Health Maintenance
Gastroparesis		1. Bloating 2. Abdominal distention 3. Flatulence		1. Liquid food supplements should comprise 50% of calories for first 1-2 wk of refeeding 2. Divide daily caloric intake into 3 small meals and 2-3 snacks/d 3. Avoid legumes, excessive fiber, and bran products 4. Metoclopramide–stimulates stomach contraction and hastens emptying 5. Macrolide–adjunct • Erythromycin or Azithromycin Health maintenance: 1. Gastroparesis and dilation will resolve within 4-6 wk of weight restoration
Constipation		1. Infrequent and small bowel movements 2. Abdominal pain 3. Worsens with bulking, fiber containing laxatives or stimulant laxatives		1. Increase water intake (6-8 glasses per day) 2. Avoid high doses of fiber 3. Polyethylene glycol powder 4. Lactulose

Disease	Etiology, Prevalence, and Risk Factors	Clinical Symptoms and Signs	Diagnostics	Therapy, Prognosis, and Health Maintenance
Refeeding syndrome	The clinical complications that occur as a result of fluid and electrolyte shifts during refeeding too rapidly and/or aggressively for weight restoration in malnourished patients RF: 1. Patients who weigh <70% ideal body weight or BMI <15-16 2. High amount of weight loss during current episode 3. Patients who lose weight rapidly 4. Low baseline phosphate, K, or Mg prior to refeeding 5. Little to no intake previous 5-10 d before refeeding Potentially fatal	Marked by: 1. Congestive heart failure symptoms 2. SOB 3. Weakness 4. Diarrhea 5. Tremors, paresthesias Signs: 1. A normal heart rate may be indicative of cardiac compromise (>70) 2. Hypertension, hypotension 3. Peripheral edema 4. Delirium 5. Encephalopathy 6. Gait ataxia Complications: 1. Rhabdomyolysis 2. Seizures 3. Hemolysis	Marked by: 1. **_Hypophosphatemia_** (hallmark) 2. Hypokalemia 3. Vitamin (thiamine) deficiency 4. CK: abnormally high 5. LFTs: elevated	1. Correct electrolyte abnormalities 2. Treat cardiovascular and pulmonary complications 3. Nutritional replenishment after electrolyte abnormalities corrected Prevention: 1. Restore weight with initial caloric intake above resting energy expenditure 2. Avoid rapid increase in caloric intake 3. Closely monitor clinical signs and symptoms Health maintenance: 1. Highest risk during first 2 wk of replenishment Prognosis: Most fatalities occur from cardiac complications

REFEEDING SYNDROME

- During periods of starvation and anorexia nervosa, stores of phosphate are depleted. When nutritional replenishment commences and the body receives carbohydrates, glucose promotes the release of insulin triggering the cellular uptake of phosphate (potassium and magnesium). Insulin also causes cells to produce other previously depleted molecules requiring phosphate (such as ATP), further decreasing stores. Tissue hypoxia results from a lack of phosphorylated intermediates, causing myocardial dysfunction and respiratory failure from lack of diaphragmatic contraction.

- Vitamin deficiencies exist from starvation and are worsened with the onset of anabolic processes accompanying refeeding.

- Volume overload results from an increase in insulin secretion with carbohydrate load during refeeding, which increases sodium reabsorption and retention, then fluid retention.

BULIMIA NERVOSA

Disease	Etiology, Prevalence, and Risk Factors	Clinical Symptoms and Signs	Diagnostics	Therapy, Prognosis, and Health Maintenance
Bulimia nervosa	Prevalence: 1.0% F:M (3:1) Median onset: 18 y/o Normal to slightly over-weight patients Restriction model sequence: 1. Caloric restriction 2. Binge eating 3. MC: **Self-induced vomiting** RF: Childhood trauma (eg, sexual abuse)	DSM-5 criteria: 1. Recurrent episodes of *binge eating*: • Eating in short amount (2 h) of time, more than average • Lack of control of overeating (what or how much) 2. ***Compensatory behavior*** to prevent weight gain: vomiting, *laxative use*, diuretics, *fasting* or *excessive exercise* 3. Both 1 and 2 occur at least ***1×/wk for 3 mo*** 4. Excessive concern about body weight and shape 5. Lethargy 6. Irregular menses 7. Abdominal pain 8. Bloating 9. Constipation Signs: 1. Tachycardia 2. Hypotension (<90 mm Hg systolic) 3. Xerosis 4. Parotid gland swelling (sialadenosis) 5. Erosion of dental enamel 6. Other: hair loss, edema, subconjunctival hemor-rhage, epistaxis 7. **(+) Russell sign**: scar-ring or calluses on knuck-les or back of hand due to self-induced vomiting Associated: impulse of com-pulsive nonsuicidal self-injury (skin cutting, picking, or burning with lit cigarette)	Clinical DX: 1. Serum albumin: normal or low 2. Serum electrolytes • **Hypokalemia**, with metabolic alkalosis if loss is significant • Hypochloremia • Hyponatremia 3. BUN/Cr 4. CBC w/diff 5. LFTs 6. U/A 7. In severely ill: • EKG • Depressed ST segment • QT prolongation • Wide QRS • Increased p-wave amplitude • Increased PR interval • Calcium, Mg, Phos • **Hypomagnesemia** • Hypophosphatemia 8. LH/FSH, prolactin, B-hCG for persistent amenorrhea 9. Check stool or urine for bisacodyl, emodin, aloe-emodin, and rhein if suspected laxative abuse 10. Check serum amylase for pancreatitis and frac-tionated for salivary gland isozyme	1. **Psychotherapy** • CBT 2. **Nutritional rehabilitation** 3. **Pharmacotherapy** • May be used alone or in combination with (1) and (3) • ***Antidepressants*–** Fluoxetine (first line) • Other SSRIs • TCAs/MAOIs Health maintenance: 1. Pharmacotherapy alone is less efficacious than psychotherapy alone, but is reasonable if psycho-therapy unavailable 2. Antidepressants may increase risk of suicidality in young adults 3. Maintenance pharma-cotherapy × 6-12 mo beyond remission Prognosis: 1. 50% fully recover 2. 30% will relapse within 6 mo following remission 3. Increased risk of suicidality Comorbidities: 1. **Personality disorder** (MC: borderline) 2. Anxiety disorders 3. Body dysmorphic disorder 4. PTSD 5. Substance use disorders

CHAPTER 66

Paraphilias and Sexual Dysfunctions

Recommended Supplemental Topics:

All of the following conditions are currently updated with DSM-5 criteria

The fifth edition of the American Psychiatric Association's *Diagnostic and Statistical Manual (DSM-5)* utilizes specific criteria with which to objectively assess symptoms, rather than purely discrete diagnostic categories. For example, personality dimensions are more prominent than they were in *DSM-IV.* Nonetheless, the diagnosis is still based on a solid history and examination.

PARAPHILIC DISORDERS: EXHIBITIONISTIC, FETISHISTIC, PEDOPHILIC, SEXUAL MASOCHISM, VOYEURISTIC

- **Paraphilic disorder:** "a paraphilia that is currently causing distress or impairment to the individual or a paraphilia whose satisfaction has entailed personal harm, or risk of harm, to others"

- Sexual urges and behaviors that are intense, enduring, arousing that involve (nonhuman objects, suffering or humiliation, children, or nonconsenting persons)

- First-line treatment: **Cognitive behavioral therapy (CBT)**

Disease	Etiology, Prevalence, and Risk Factors	Clinical Symptoms and Signs	Therapy, Prognosis, and Health Maintenance
Exhibitionistic disorder	2%-4% male Onset before 18 y, directed at females	1. Exposure of genitals to unsuspecting person or manifestation of urges to do so +/– masturbation or shock value, hope observer will become aroused or join 2. Period of at least 6 mo	Prognosis: 25% receive treatment
Fetishistic disorder	Does not include items for cross dressing or vibrators M > F MC foci: Feet, footwear, socks, and female undergarments	1. Involves use of nonliving objects (women's underpants, bras, stockings, shoes, boots) or focus on nongenital body parts +/– Masturbation while holding, rubbing, or smelling item 2. Trouble becoming aroused without item 3. Must have significant distress or psychosocial role impairment for DX	Prognosis: 1. 2% receive treatment

(continued)

Psychiatry

(continued)

Disease	Etiology, Prevalence, and Risk Factors	Clinical Symptoms and Signs	Therapy, Prognosis, and Health Maintenance
Pedophilic disorder	3%-5% M RF: Child porn?	1. Intense, recurrent, sexually arousing fantasies, urges, or behaviors involving a prepubescent child or children (<13 y/o) for at least 6 mo 2. DX if acted on or marked distress 3. Must be at least age 16 y and at least 5 y older than child	Prognosis: 45% receive treatment, but do not initiate it
Sexual masochism disorder	2% M > 1% F Done with a consenting partner	1. Intense sexually arousing fantasies, urges, or behaviors involving act of being humiliated, beaten, bound, or made to suffer (restraint, blindfolding, paddling, spanking, whipping, beating, electrical shocks, cutting, piercing, and being urinated or defecated on) 2. Typically consenting, nondistressing, and nonpathological 3. Specifier: +/− asphyxiophilia 6+ mo	Prognosis: 3% receive treatment
Voyeuristic disorder	M (12%) > F (4%) Onset in adolescence DX at age 18	1. Fantasy or actual viewing of unsuspecting and nonconsenting people who are naked, disrobing, or engaging in sexual activity 2. Period of at least 6 mo	Prognosis: 12% receive treatment

FEMALE SEXUAL INTEREST/AROUSAL DISORDER AND MALE HYPOACTIVE SEXUAL DESIRE DISORDER

Disease	Etiology, Prevalence, and Risk Factors	Clinical Symptoms and Signs	Therapy, Prognosis, and Health Maintenance
Female sexual *interest/arousal* disorder	Arousal: vaginal lubrication (not clitoral engorgement) Female failure to lubricate	1. **Lack of sexual interest/arousal:** no interest, erotic thoughts or fantasies, initiation, or responsiveness 2. Reduced interest/arousal in response to external cues (written, verbal, visual) 3. Absent genital/nongenital sensations 4. At least 6 mo, significant distress	1. Sex therapy 2. CBT: effective as sildenafil, avoid performance anxiety 3. Lubrication 4. PDE inhibitors 5. Venous ligation, position change 6. EROS clitoral therapy device
Male hypoactive sexual *desire* disorder	Age related: after age 50	1. No sexual/erotic thoughts or fantasies/desire for sexual activity for at **least 6 mo,** significant clinical distress	1. Early therapy: • Psychotherapy • Behavioral or exposure therapy 2. Late: Precoital benzodiazepine 3. Treat underlying depression or hypogonadism (testosterone)
Male erectile disorder (dysfunction)	Anxiety 40+: vascular disease, smoking, inactivity, depression	1. Marked difficulty in obtaining or maintaining erection during or to completion, decrease in rigidity for 6 mo, significant distress	1. Stop smoking, no ETOH or drugs, healthy diet, exercise 2. PDE-5 inhibitors 3. Vacuum pump, rings intraurethral alprostadil

DISORDERS OF ORGASM

Disease	Etiology, Prevalence, and Risk Factors	Clinical Symptoms and Signs	Therapy, Prognosis, and Health Maintenance
Female orgasmic disorder (anorgasmia)	Etiology: MAOI, TCA, SSRI, spinal cord injury, MS, or radiation	1. Marked delay in, frequency of, or absence of orgasm or reduced intensity for 6 mo, significant distress	1. CBT, psychotherapy 2. PDE-5 inhibitors
Genitopelvic pain or penetration	Female only MC: **Vaginismus** (vaginal muscle spasm) Gynecological problems Dyspareunia: pain with sex	1. Persistent/recurrent difficulty with vaginal penetration, vulvovaginal or pelvic pain, anxiety of pain, tensing/tightening of floor muscles 2. Minimum 6 mo, significant distress	1. **Desensitization** with graduated dilators then penetration with small dilators 2. CBT and sex therapy
Delayed ejaculation	MC: **Fear of impregnation**, anxiety, or hostility Idiosyncratic masturbatory pattern, interpersonal stress Associated with: DM, MS	Delay, infrequency, or absence in ejaculation for 6+ mo	CBT, psychotherapy Refrain from sexual activities Switch buproprion or buspirone for SSRI
Premature ejaculation		Within 60 s after penetration for at least 6 mo on almost/all occasions, significant distress	**Stop-start treatment** Frenulum squeeze technique: Pinch base or corona of penis SSRI: **Paroxetine**

FROTTEURISTIC DISORDER, SEXUAL SADISM, AND TRANSVESTIC DISORDER

Disease	Etiology, Prevalence, and Risk Factors	Clinical Symptoms and Signs	Therapy, Prognosis, and Health Maintenance
Frotteuristic disorder	<30% adult males Crowded areas (bus, subway, hall, sidewalk)	1. Touching and rubbing against another nonconsenting person or fantasies to do so 2. A single act cannot diagnose 3. Period of at least 6 mo	
Sexual sadism disorder	2%-30% Subcategories: necrophilia, sadistic and lust murders, sadistic rape	1. Real acts (not simulated) of psychological or physical suffering of another individual 2. A disorder when involving nonconsenting person 3. Controlling or dominating (restraint, blindfolding, paddling, spanking, whipping, pinching, beating, burning, electrical shocks, rape, cutting, stabbing, strangulation, torture, mutilation, killing)	Prognosis: 3% receive treatment
Transvestic disorder	A type of fetish	1. Involves cross-dressing producing sexual arousal (arousal to garments, materials, fabrics) 2. Autogynephilia: if accompanied by images of female	Prognosis: 3% receive treatment

Psychiatry

PRACTICE QUESTIONS

1. Which of the following is a common adverse effect of mirtazapine (Remeron)?
   A. Decreased libido
   B. Sedation
   C. Diarrhea
   D. Hypertension

2. A 22-year-old male is brought to your clinic by his girlfriend. She is concerned about him because for the past 2 months he has had thoughts that the CIA is spying on him and that they implanted a device in his body that is now controlling him. He admits that he often hears voices that are commanding in nature. Which of the following is the most likely diagnosis?
   A. Schizophrenia
   B. Schizoaffective disorder
   C. Schizophreniform disorder
   D. Schizoid personality disorder

3. For which of the following conditions would flumazenil (Romazicon) be the treatment of choice?
   A. Alcohol withdrawal
   B. Opioid overdose
   C. Organophosphate poisoning
   D. Benzodiazepine overdose

4. A 57-year-old war veteran with history of post-traumatic stress disorder has been on Sertraline (Zoloft) for the past 6 months. Most his symptoms are well controlled but he continues to have trouble sleeping at night. Which of the following medication classes would be an appropriate addition to help with his sleep?
   A. Tricyclic antidepressant
   B. Benzodiazepine
   C. Monoamine oxidase inhibitor
   D. α-adrenergic receptor blocker

5. A 30-year-old man is brought into the ED via EMS by his brother. His brother states that he has been very rude and angry lately and "has not been acting normally." Over the past week he spent $100 000 on lottery tickets. He hasn't slept in 3 days and he can't seem to sit still. Which of the following would you expect to be an additional finding during the interview?
   A. Pressured speech
   B. Decreased appetite over the past week
   C. Auditory hallucinations
   D. Ideas of reference

6. Which receptor does methadone act on in the treatment of opioid withdrawal?
   A. GABA
   B. Dopamine
   C. Mu
   D. 5HT

7. A 30-year-old male has an intense fear of flying in an airplane. He reports that when he boards an airplane he gets very anxious that the plane will crash. As a result, he departs the plane before it takes off. He recently got promoted at work and his new position will require frequent travel. Which of the following is the most appropriate intervention?
   A. Insight-oriented therapy
   B. β-Blocker
   C. Electroconvulsive therapy
   D. Exposure therapy

8. A 14-year-old male has recently been in juvenile detention for setting fire to his neighbor's garage. In the past he was expelled from school for bringing knives onto the school campus and getting into numerous fights with other students. Most recently, he has been roaming the streets at night and slashing the tires of cars parked on the street. As this patient grows up, which of the following is the most at risk for developing?
   A. Antisocial personality disorder
   B. Oppositional defiant disorder
   C. Schizophrenia
   D. Borderline personality disorder

9. A 36-year-old female presents with a 3-week history of difficulty sleeping, poor concentration, and decreased energy. She reports that she does not feel like doing her normal activities. Her husband has been concerned about her because she has not been eating and she has no interest in working in her garden, which she normally enjoys. Which of the following is the most likely diagnosis?
   A. Major depressive disorder
   B. Bipolar disorder
   C. Dysthymia
   D. Generalized anxiety disorder

10. A 30-year-old female with history of schizophrenia is currently being treated with risperidone (Risperdal). Which of the following should you monitor for during your regular follow up appointments?
    A. Risperidone levels
    B. Involuntary movements of the lips or tongue
    C. Urinalysis
    D. Electrocardiogram

11. Which of the following patients is at highest risk of completing suicide?
    A. 54-year-old woman that is married with two children
    B. 20-year-old college student
    C. 70-year-old man with diabetes and coronary artery disease
    D. Teenage girl

12. A 20-year-old female presents to your clinic with a 3-week history of fatigue, poor appetite, and depressed mood. Which of the following diagnostic tests would be most appropriate in the evaluation of this patient?

    A. EEG
    B. EKG
    C. TSH
    D. Cortisol levels

13. A 15-year-old female with a history of substance abuse was recently diagnosed with attention-deficit/hyperactivity disorder. Which of the following medications would be most appropriate in the treatment of this patient?

    A. Dexmethylphenidate (Focalin)
    B. Fluoxetine (Prozac)
    C. Atomoxetine (Strattera)
    D. Lorazepam (Ativan)

14. A 40-year-old female presents to your clinic for decreased energy, inability to sleep at night, irritability, and difficulty concentrating at work. She states that this has been going on since she was a teenager but that she cannot handle it anymore. Which of the following additional findings would she most likely have?

    A. Mydriasis
    B. Muscle tension
    C. Tremor
    D. Hyperthermia

15. A 17-year-old female presents to your clinic for help with weight loss. The patient states that she has been running at least 6 miles per day but is still not happy with the way she looks. She reports that her LMP was 4 months ago. On exam, the patient appears thin and is bradycardic. Her BMI is 16. Which of the following additional findings are you most likely to appreciate on exam?

    A. Dry skin
    B. Hypertension
    C. Coarse hair
    D. Hyperthermia

16. A 21-year-old female college student presents to the emergency department for chest tightness, racing heartbeat, and shortness of breath that started 10 minutes ago while she was about to take her biology midterm. She reports that she is beginning to feel better, but she is worried that there is something wrong with her heart. On physical exam, she is mildly tachycardic. Which of the following diagnostic tests would be most appropriate to evaluate this patient?

    A. EKG
    B. CBC
    C. EEG
    D. Blood cultures

17. A 30-year-old female presents to your clinic requesting a referral to a new plastic surgeon. The patient has had two nasal reconstructive surgeries in the past. She is insistent that her prior surgeon did a bad job and states that her "big nose" causes her to spend hours per day in front of the mirror. On physical exam, you are unable to appreciate any abnormalities of her nose and it appears normal in size. Which of the following is the most appropriate intervention for this patient?

    A. Refer her to a different plastic surgeon
    B. Begin SSRI treatment
    C. Schedule her for electroconvulsive therapy
    D. Begin treatment with lithium

18. When following up with a 32-year-old patient diagnosed with social anxiety disorder, which of the following screening tests would be appropriate?

    A. Mini-Mental State Examination
    B. Montreal Cognitive Assessment
    C. CAGE questionnaire
    D. Clinical Institute Withdrawal Assessment

19. A 37-year-old male expresses that over the past year he has had the urge to expose his genitals to women who work in his office. The patient has not yet acted on these thoughts but is seeking help to diminish the urges that he has experienced. Which of the following medications classes would be appropriate for this patient?

    A. Benzodiazepine
    B. Selective serotonin reuptake inhibitor
    C. Atypical antipsychotic
    D. Tricyclic antidepressant

20. A 65-year-old female with end-stage breast cancer presents to the emergency department via EMS for trouble breathing and altered mental status. She is on fentanyl for management of her pain and her dose was increased yesterday. On physical exam, you note pinpoint pupils and diminished breath sounds bilaterally with rales in the lower lung fields. Her respiratory rate is 6 per minute. Which is the most appropriate next step in the management of this patient?

    A. Administer methadone
    B. Obtain urine toxicology screen
    C. Administer naloxone (Narcan)
    D. Apply ice packs

21. A 40-year-old male has presented to your clinic 20 times in the past 6 months. He states that he "just knows there is something wrong" with him. He spends hours per day worrying that he has prostate cancer because his father was diagnosed with it last year. All of his laboratory studies have come back negative and he has had two rounds of prostate biopsies performed that showed no signs of cancer. In which of the following situations would it be appropriate to start this patient on SSRI treatment?

    A. The patient recently started attending cognitive behavioral therapy
    B. The patient has comorbid panic disorder
    C. The patient should be started on an SSRI now if he has no contraindications
    D. The patient is responding to psychotherapy

22. Which of the following theories regarding neurotransmitters is the most widely accepted for the pathogenesis of schizophrenia?

    A. Decreased serotonin
    B. Increased dopamine
    C. Increased acetylcholine
    D. Increased norepinephrine

23. Which of the following laboratory abnormalities could be expected in a patient with bulimia nervosa without laxative use?

    A. Hyperkalemia
    B. Decreased urine specific gravity
    C. Metabolic alkalosis
    D. Hyperchloremia

24. A 43-year-old school teacher is admitted to the hospital for a nonhealing wound after a hysterectomy 5 months ago. On exploration of the wound there is surrounding erythema and tenderness. There are no signs of abscess or fistula formation. During her hospital stay, you notice that every time you enter her room, there is a new bouquet of flowers from one of her students. She frequently states that "it is nice to be taken care of." When her wound culture results return, it showed different organisms including anaerobic bacteria consistent with the normal flora present in stool. On further review of her electronic medical record, you note that the patient has presented to the emergency department 17 times in the past 5 months and left against medical advice each time after she was told that they could clean out her wound and send her home with antibiotics. Which of the following is the most appropriate long-term management for this patient?

    A. Psychotherapy
    B. Selective serotonin reuptake inhibitor
    C. Lithium
    D. Confront the patient and discharge her with antibiotics

25. A 34-year-old female presents to your clinic for her yearly physical. When she is checking in at the receptionist desk, she begins telling everyone in the waiting room that it has been "the worst week" of her life because her cat died, the coffee shop she frequently goes to give her the wrong drink, and her boyfriend of 2 weeks broke up with her. She begins to cry in front of the waiting room full of people. When she realizes that her heavily applied makeup is smudged on her face, she immediately stops crying and pulls out a compact mirror to fix it. Which of the following is the most likely diagnosis?

    A. Narcissistic personality disorder
    B. Borderline personality disorder
    C. Dependent personality disorder
    D. Histrionic personality disorder

ANSWERS

1. Clinical Therapeutics: Depression. Answer B: The most common adverse effects of mirtazapine are sedation, weight gain, constipation, and orthostasis. A, Mirtazapine does not cause sexual dysfunction unlike many of the other antidepressant medications. C, Mirtazapine does not commonly cause diarrhea; it is more likely to cause constipation. D, Mirtazapine is not known to cause hypertension.

2. Diagnosis: Schizophreniform Disorder. Answer C: The patient is having delusions and hallucinations which are consistent with a schizophrenia spectrum disorder. These symptoms have been going on for a time period of 2 months so it is considered schizophreniform disorder. A, The patient cannot yet be diagnosed with schizophrenia because the total duration of symptoms is less than 6 months. B, Schizoaffective disorder has a mood component in addition to the psychotic symptoms. D, Schizoid personality disorder is characterized by a long-term lack of interest in social relationships and desire for a solitary lifestyle.

3. Clinical Therapeutics: Benzodiazepine Intoxication. Answer D: Flumazenil is used to reverse the sedative effects in benzodiazepine overdose. However, it should be used with caution because it can precipitate withdrawal symptoms. A, The treatment of choice in alcohol withdrawal would be a benzodiazepine along with thiamine and glucose. B, The treatment of choice in opioid intoxication would be naloxone. C, The treatment of choice in organophosphate poisoning would be an anticholinergic agent.

4. Clinical Therapeutics: Post-traumatic Stress Disorder. Answer D: α-Adrenergic receptor blockers, such as Prazosin, have been shown to decrease nightmares and improve sleep in patients with PTSD. They can also safely be used in patients taking an SSRI. A, TCAs have

not shown to be effective in the treatment of PTSD. B, Benzodiazepines are used to treat hyper-arousal and anxiety seen in PTSD. They are not commonly used to help with sleep. C, MAOIs should not be administered along with SSRIs due to the risk of serotonin syndrome.

5. History and Physical: Bipolar Disorder. Answer A: The patient's history is consistent with bipolar disorder. Bipolar disorder is manifested by grandiosity, irritability, distractibility, flight of ideas, pressured speech, decreased need for sleep, high-risk behaviors, and impulsivity. B, Decreased appetite is not a symptom of bipolar disorder, it is more associated with depression. C, Patients with bipolar disorder do not often have auditory hallucinations. This is more common in schizophrenia and other psychotic disorders. D, Ideas of reference is a form of delusional thinking often seen with schizophrenia.

6. Scientific Concepts: Opioid Use. Answer C: Methadone is a long-acting mu-opioid receptor agonist.

7. Clinical Intervention: Specific Phobia. Answer D: Exposure based cognitive behavioral therapy is the most appropriate treatment for specific phobia. This form of therapy exposes the patient to their phobia in incremental steps. A, Insight-oriented therapy helps patients understand the reasons for their fear and would not likely help abate his symptoms. B, β-blockers can be used in performance anxiety, but is not the best choice in treating other specific phobias. C, ECT is not indicated for the treatment of anxiety disorders.

8. Health Maintenance: Conduct Disorder. Answer A: It is estimated that 25% of girls and 50% of boys with conduct disorder will develop antisocial personality disorder. Patients with conduct disorder have an increased risk of comorbid ADHD and learning disorders. B, ODD is often a precursor to conduct disorder so it is likely that the patient has a prior diagnosis of ODD. C, Patients with conduct disorder are not at increased risk for schizophrenia. D, Patients with conduct disorder are more at risk for developing antisocial personality disorder than borderline personality disorder.

9. Diagnosis: Major Depressive Disorder. Answer A: Major depressive disorder is characterized by at least 2 weeks of 5 symptoms including depressed mood, sleep disturbance, decreased interests, feelings of guilt or worthlessness, decreased energy, poor concentration, poor appetite, psychomotor disturbance, and suicidal thoughts.

10. Health Maintenance: Schizophrenia. Answer B: Involuntary movements of the lips or tongue would be consistent with tardive dyskinesia, a side effect of antipsychotic medications. This should be monitored for every 6 to 12 months. A, It is not necessary to monitory drug levels of risperidone. C, It is not necessary to routinely monitor urine for patients on risperidone. It would only be necessary to obtain a urinalysis if a patient complains of genitourinary symptoms. D, Although antipsychotic medications can cause cardiovascular arrhythmias and EKG changes, it is not necessary to monitor this with serial EKGs unless patients are symptomatic.

11. History and Physical: Suicide. Answer C: Patients with comorbid medical illness have an increased risk of suicide. Additionally, males complete suicide 3 times more often than females. A, Marriage and having children are protective factors that decrease the risk of suicide. B, Adolescents and young adults (D) attempt suicide more often than older adults however, they are less likely to complete suicide.

12. Diagnostic Studies: Depression. Answer C: Hypothyroidism is a medical cause of depressive symptoms and it is therefore important to check TSH levels to rule out hypothyroidism as an organic cause for the patient's symptoms.

13. Clinical Therapeutics: Attention-Deficit/Hyperactivity Disorder. Answer C: Atomoxetine is an appropriate treatment of ADHD in patients with a personal or family history of substance abuse. A, Stimulant medications such as methylphenidate, amphetamine, and Dexmethylphenidate have a potential for abuse and should be avoided in patients with a history of substance abuse. B, SSRIs are not used in the treatment of ADHD. D, Benzodiazepines like lorazepam are not used in the treatment of ADHD.

14. History and Physical: Generalized Anxiety Disorder. Answer B: Muscle tension and headaches with pain in the neck and shoulders are common for patients with generalized anxiety disorder. C, Tremor and hyperthermia (D) are not common findings associated with generalized anxiety disorder. A, Mydriasis would be more likely with a substance-related disorder, particularly with stimulant use.

15. History and Physical: Anorexia Nervosa. Answer A: Anorexia nervosa is associated with the following physical exam findings: dry skin, hypothermia, hypercarotenemia, lanugo, swelling of the parotid and submandibular glands, peripheral edema, and thinning hair.

16. Diagnostic Studies: Panic Disorder. Answer A: EKG would be appropriate for a patient presenting with symptoms that could be due to panic disorder. An EKG would help you assess for an arrhythmia as a cause of the patient's symptoms.

17. Clinical Therapeutics: Body Dysmorphic Disorder. Answer B: This patient is exhibiting characteristics of body dysmorphic disorder. She is preoccupied with the physical appearance of her nose which has led to repetitive behaviors of spending hours in front of the mirror. The first-line treatment for body dysmorphic disorder is SSRIs or clomipramine as well as cognitive behavioral therapy. A, Additional surgeries for this patient would not be helpful. C, Electroconvulsive therapy is reserved for treatment resistant body dysmorphic disorder. D, Lithium is not used for first-line treatment of body dysmorphic disorder.

18. Health Maintenance: Anxiety Disorders. Answer C: Patients with social anxiety disorder are at high risk for comorbid alcohol dependence. A CAGE questionnaire would be appropriate to screen for alcohol abuse. A, The Mini-Mental State Examination (MMSE) is a screening test for cognitive impairment in elderly patients. B, The Montreal Cognitive Assessment (MoCA) is a screening test for cognitive impairment in elderly patients. D, Clinical Institute Withdrawal Assessment (CIWA) protocol would be appropriate if the patient were exhibiting symptoms of alcohol withdrawal.

19. Clinical Therapeutics: Exhibitionistic Disorder. Answer B: SSRI treatment is useful in patients with exhibitionistic disorder because it treats impulse-control problems and additionally has sexual side effects that decrease libido. Other medications used include lithium, anti-androgens, and mood stabilizers.

20. Clinical Therapeutics: Opioid Intoxication. Answer C: Naloxone is a short-acting opioid antagonist that helps restore ventilation, therefore would be an appropriate treatment for this patient. A, Administration of an additional opioid agent would be harmful for the patient. B, This would not be helpful in the management of this patient since it is known that she has been taking an opioid. D, Patients with opioid intoxication often experience hypothermia so cooling the patient would not be appropriate.

21. Clinical Therapeutics: Illness Anxiety Disorder. Answer B: SSRI treatment is first line for patients with illness anxiety disorder plus a comorbid anxiety or depressive disorder. A, First-line treatment of illness anxiety disorder is cognitive behavioral therapy. If the patient declines CBT or does not show improvement with it, SSRI treatment may be necessary. C, The first-line treatment of illness anxiety disorder is cognitive behavioral therapy provided that the patient does not have a comorbid anxiety or depressive disorder. D, If the patient is responding to psychotherapy, an SSRI is not necessary at this time.

22. Scientific Concepts: Schizophrenia. Answer B: Medications that block dopamine receptors result in a decrease in positive psychotic symptoms, leading to the widely accepted hypothesis that increased dopamine levels in the mesolimbic tract cause positive symptoms.

23. Diagnostic Studies: Bulimia Nervosa. Answer C: Patients with bulimia nervosa often exhibit hypochloremic metabolic alkalosis on laboratory evaluation due to self-induced vomiting behaviors. A, Due to behaviors of self-induced vomiting, bulimia is often associated with hypokalemia. B, Patients with bulimia nervosa are often dehydrated so their urine specific gravity would be elevated. D, Hypochloremia is more common in bulimia nervosa due to self-induced vomiting behaviors.

24. Clinical Intervention: Factitious Disorder. Answer A: This patient is expressing characteristics of factitious disorder. It appears that she enjoys assuming a sick role and she is contaminating her wound in order to continue to assume this role. Psychotherapy is the standard treatment of factitious disorder. B, SSRIs are used in the treatment of factitious disorder if the patient has comorbid depression or anxiety disorders. C, Lithium is not used in the management of factitious disorder. D, This patient requires psychotherapeutic treatment. She would likely seek medical attention elsewhere if she was simply discharged with an antibiotic regimen again.

25. Diagnosis: Histrionic Personality Disorder. Answer D: Histrionic patients are attention seeking, overexaggerating, overly familiar, and often sexually provocative in their behavior and/or appearance. A, Narcissistic patients have a sense of special entitlement and are often grandiose and envious. B, Borderline patients have an unstable self-image, unstable relationships, and exhibit impulsive and self-harming behavior. They will go to great lengths to avoid abandonment and often idealize some people and devalue others. They are not as attention-seeking and overexaggerating as the patient in this scenario. C, Patients with dependent personality disorder have difficulty making decisions without reassurance of others. They require others to take responsibility for areas in their life and feel uncomfortable when they are alone.

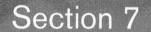

CHAPTER 67

Preoperative Care

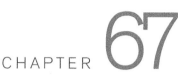

Refer to Internal Medicine ⚕ for In-depth Coverage of the Following Topics:
Diabetes Mellitus, p 231

Refer to ⚕ for the Following Topics:
Substance Use Disorder, see Substance Abuse Disorders, p 552
Tobacco Use/Dependence, see Substance Abuse Disorders p 562

RISK ASSESSMENT

- **Pain**—Remember: OPQRST
  - **Onset**: sudden or gradual
  - **Precipitant**: fatty foods, movement, etc
  - **Quality**: sharp, dull, cramps
  - **Radiation**: to back or shoulder
  - **Stop**: any relief?
  - **Temporal**: duration, frequency, crescendo-decrescendo, etc
- **Allergies**
  - Egg—do not use propofol
  - Shellfish—do not use IV iodinated contrast
- *Cardiac disease*—eg, History of MI, unstable angina, valvular disease, hypertension, arrhythmias, and heart failure
  - If previous infarction, there is a 5% to 10% risk of postoperative MI
  - If current unstable angina—avoid elective surgeries
  - If Stage III HTN—control prior to surgery
  - If history of rheumatic heart disease—provide prophylactic antibiotic therapy
  - Send patient to cardiologist for clearance to have stress test or Echo if any concerns
    - Start with **12-lead EKG**
    - **Noninvasive stress testing** before *noncardiac* operations is indicated in patients with:
      - active cardiac conditions (eg, unstable angina, recent MI, significant arrhythmias, or severe valvular disease)

      - patients who require vascular operations and have clinical risk factors and poor functional capacity (see below)
  - **Coronary revascularization** before *noncardiac* operations in patients with:
    - significant left main coronary artery stenosis
    - stable angina with three-vessel coronary disease
    - stable angina with two-vessel disease
    - significant proximal left anterior descending coronary artery stenosis with either an ejection fraction <50% or ischemia on noninvasive testing
    - high-risk unstable angina or non–ST-segment elevation MI, or acute ST-elevation MI
- *Pulmonary disease*—History of asthma, COPD
  - Established risk factors for postoperative pulmonary complications (PPC)
    - Advanced age
    - Elevated ASA class
    - Congestive heart failure
    - Functional dependence
    - Known chronic obstructive pulmonary disease
    - Others: malnutrition, alcohol abuse, and altered mental status
    - Sleep apnea is an independent risk factor for PPC
  - Smoking cessation also confers favorable effects on wound healing. Therefore, patients should be encouraged to **stop smoking at least 1 month before operations**, ideally with programmatic support through

formal counseling programs and possibly smoking cessation aids such as varenicline or transdermal nicotine
- Asthma should be well controlled
- Postoperative pulmonary complications: hypoxia, atelectasis, pneumonia
- Aggressive postoperative pain management to promote early ambulation
- Incentive spirometry—inspiratory muscle training, deep inspiration, coughing, and good oral hygiene
- *Metabolic disease*— eg, History of diabetes, adrenal insufficiency
  - Blood glucose is elevated preoperatively in DM patients—especially if physical trauma is present with emotional and physiologic stress
    - Elevated postoperative blood glucose levels in diabetic patients translate to progressively greater chances of SSIs (surgical site infection) following cardiac operations, as well as a greater likelihood of postoperative infections and prolonged hospital stays in patients with noncardiac operations
    - The relative risk of an SSI seems to incrementally increase in a linear pattern with the degree of hyperglycemia, with levels greater than 140 mg/dL being the sole predictor of SSI
    - Intravenous insulin is best for perioperative glucose control due to its rapid onset of action, short half-life, and immediate availability (as opposed to subcutaneous absorption)
  - Check for symptomatic or asymptomatic heart disease with DM
  - Perioperative hyperglycemia should be treated with IV short acting insulin or SQ sliding scale insulin

- Glycemic control
  - Normal: 90 to 100 mg/dL, preferred; control with IV insulin
  - Moderate control: 120 to 200 mg/dL
- Postoperative monitoring for:
  - Hyperglycemia or hypoglycemia
  - Infection
  - Poor healing and wound issues
  - CVD: double the risk for men, quadruple the risk for women
- Obesity—contrary to popular belief, this is not a risk factor for most major adverse postoperative outcomes, except pulmonary embolism
- *Hematologic disease*— eg, History of clotting disorders, anticoagulant use

Functional Capacity

Excellent (activities requiring >7 METs)	1. Carry 24 lbs. up 8 steps 2. Carry objects that weigh 80 lb. 3. Outdoor work (shovel snow, spade soil) 4. Recreation (ski, basketball, squash, handball, jog or walk 5 mph)
Moderate (>4 but <7 METs)	1. Sexual intercourse without stopping 2. Walk at 4 mph on level ground 3. Outdoor work (garden, rake, pull weeds) 4. Recreation (roller skate, dance)
Poor (<4 METs)	1. Shower or dress without stopping, make the bed, dust, or wash dishes 2. Walk at 2.5 mph on level ground 3. Outdoor work (eg, clean windows) 4. Recreation (golf or bowl)

MET, metabolic equivalent.

American College of Chest Physicians (ACCP) Risk Stratification for Perioperative Thromboembolism

Risk Category	Mechanical Heart Valve	Atrial Fibrillation	Venous Thromboembolism
High (>10%/y risk of ATE or >10%/mo risk of VTE)	Any mechanical mitral valve Other aortic valve Recent (<6 mo) stroke or TIA	CHADs2 score of 5-6 Recent (<3 mo) stroke or TIA Rheumatic valvular disease	Recent (<3 mo) VTE Severe thrombophilia
Moderate (4%-10%/y risk of ATE or 4%-10%/mo risk of VTE)	Bileaflet aortic valve and 1 of the following: 1. Atrial fibrillation 2. Prior stroke or TIA, hypertension, diabetes, heart failure, age >75	CHADs2 score of 3-4	VTE within past 3-12 mo Recurrent VTE Nonsevere thrombophilic conditions Active malignancy
Low (<4%/y risk of ATE or <2%/mo risk of VTE)	Bileaflet aortic valve without atrial fibrillation and no other risk factors for stroke	CHADs2 score of 0-2 (and no prior stroke or TIA)	Single VTE within past 12 mo and no other RF

- Extended (4-week) course of LMWH in patients undergoing resections of abdominal or pelvic malignancies
- Heparin prophylaxis = 4% to 5% chance of wound hematoma, 2% to 3% mucosal bleeding, 1% to 2% risk reoperation

Risk Category	Intervention	Clinical Pearls
High (>10%/y risk of ATE or >10%/mo risk of VTE)	Bridging anticoagulation with therapeutic dose SQ heparin or IV enoxaparin sodium (Lovenox) 1. IPC + LMWH (Lovenox) or Low-dose SQ heparin	If patient already on warfarin → hold 1 wk prior, place on Lovenox, and remain on Lovenox 1 wk postop before returning to warfarin

Risk Category	Intervention	Clinical Pearls
Moderate (4%-10%/y risk of ATE or 4%-10%/mo risk of VTE)	Bridging anticoagulation with 1. Therapeutic dose SQ heparin or 2. Therapeutic dose IV Lovenox or 3. Intermittent pneumatic compression devices	
Low (<4%/y risk of ATE or <2%/mo risk of VTE)	Mechanical prophylaxis with intermittent pneumatic compression (IPC) devices	Bridging anticoagulation with low-dose heparin or no bridging
Very Low	Early ambulation alone	

- **Renal disease**
  - Dialysis-dependent CKD—risk of complications (postop hyperkalemia, pneumonia, fluid overload, bleeding) significantly increased
    - Patients should undergo dialysis within 24 hours before surgery and electrolytes should be monitored immediately before and during postop period
  - Monitor weight, I&Os, and renal function
- **Hepatic disease**
  - Liver disease complications: hemorrhage, infection, renal failure, encephalopathy, and substantial mortality rate
  - Elevated LFTs after major surgery is common; transient, not associated with hepatic dysfunction
  - When elective, attempt to reduce severity of ascites, encephalopathy, and coagulopathy preoperatively
    - Ascites—leads to wound dehiscence or hernias
    - Hepatic encephalopathy—worsened by sedatives and analgesics
    - Coagulopathy—give patients vitamin K +/− plasma transfusion
  - Postoperatively
    - Check platelet number and function—increased bleeding risk with low platelets
    - Check for electrolyte disturbances—especially hypernatremia
    - Risk for upper GI hemorrhage—esophageal or gastric varices
    - Alcoholics—malnutrition potential for vitamin deficiency → be aggressive with refeeding to prevent abnormalities in glucose metabolism and cardiac arrhythmia
      - Alcoholic withdrawal (1 to 5 days, peak at 3 days), prevent with benzodiazepines
- **Tobacco use or dependence**
  - Can decrease functional capacity and increase risk of bleeding, infections, and wound dehiscence
  - Hernia recurrence rate increases with tobacco use
- **Substance abuse**
  - In general, patients should be advised to refrain from taking illicit drugs for at least a couple of weeks before an operation
  - Similarly, a history of heavy alcohol consumption raises the possibility of a postoperative withdrawal syndrome, which can be associated with significant morbidity and even death

- Ideally, patients should cease drinking alcohol for at least one week before an operation
- **Chronic steroid use**
  - Preoperative use—Increased risk of postoperative complications
    - Infection, superficial or deep
    - Dehiscence
    - Mortality
    - Poor wound healing
    - Staple line leaks (rare)
  - Inadequate amounts of perioperative steroids can result in an Addisonian crisis, with hemodynamic instability and even death
  - The need for perioperative "stress" steroid administration is a function of the duration of steroid therapy and the degree of the physiologic stress imposed by the operation
  - Supplemental corticosteroids should definitely be administered for established primary or secondary adrenal insufficiency, for a current regimen of more than the daily equivalent of 20 mg of prednisone, or for those with a history of chronic steroid usage and a Cushingoid appearance
  - Perioperative steroids should be considered if the current regimen is 5 to 20 mg of prednisone for 3 weeks or longer, for a history of more than a 3-week course of at least 20 mg of prednisone during the past year, for chronic usage of oral and rectal steroid therapy for inflammatory bowel disease, or for a significant history of chronic topical steroid usage (>2 g daily) on large areas of affected skin
  - Excessive amounts of steroids can have adverse consequences, including increased rates of SSIs, so hydrocortisone should not be indiscriminately prescribed.
  - Glucose levels should be monitored

Medications

- Antidepressants
  - MAOI → D/C 2 weeks prior
  - SSRI → D/C 3 weeks prior, especially if high risk surgeries
  - TCA, Depakote, lithium, buspirone, benzodiazepines, antipsychotics → continue up to and including day of surgery

- Blood thinners
  - Aspirin, warfarin, clopidogrel → D/C 7 days prior (increases bleeding time)
    - Preoperative aspirin usage should continue among patients at moderate to high risk for coronary artery disease
    - Thienopyridines or P2Y12 receptor blockers (ticlopidine or clopidogrel)—when used for long-term CVA prophylaxis, discontinue 7 to 10 days prior to surgery
    - Elective operations with a **significant risk of bleeding should be delayed 12 months before the discontinuation of the thienopyridine in the presence of a drug-eluting stent, at least 4 to 6 weeks for bare-metal stents, and 4 weeks after balloon angioplasty**. Therefore, if a patient requires percutaneous coronary artery intervention prior to noncardiac surgery, bare-metal stents or balloon angioplasty should be employed rather than drug-eluting stents.
    - Even when thienopyridines are withheld, aspirin should be continued, and the thienopyridine is to be resumed as soon as possible after the operation. In circumstances such as cardiovascular surgery, the dual antiplatelet agents are continued throughout the perioperative course to minimize the likelihood of vascular thrombosis.
    - Oral anticoagulants should be stopped 3 to 5 days before surgery; heparin may be administered until 6 hours before operation
  - Heparin → resume 36 to 48 hours postop (increases bleeding time) along with oral anticoagulation
- COX-2 (impairs renal function) → hold 2 to 3 days
  - eg: celecoxib (Celebrex), rofecoxib (Vioxx), valdecoxib (Bextra)
- Diabetes medications (oral)
  - All oral DM II meds, continue insulin → hold 1 day prior
- Estrogen (OCP, ERT, SERMs) → D/C 4 to 6 weeks prior due to increased risk of postop DVT

Others

- All hypertension and cardiac meds → continue or risk of perioperative MI
  - Includes statins, β blockers, α_2 agonists, CCB
  - ACE inhibitors and ARBS—hold night before surgery unless for HF and if baseline blood pressure is adequately controlled
  - Diuretics—hold morning dose prior to surgery
- GI medications
  - H2 blockers, PPIs—continue unchanged including day of surgery
- Pulmonary medications
  - Inhaled bronchodilators, leukotriene inhibitors—continue including day of surgery
  - Theophylline—discontinue evening before surgery
- D/C all herbs and vitamins including
  - Echinacea, fish oil, vitamin E, garlic, ginger, ginkgo, glucosamine, St. John's wort, valerian

Preoperative and Follow-up Labs

	CBC	Basic Chemistries	INR or PT	PTT	Liver Chemistries	Urinalysis	EKG	CXR	Urine Pregnancy Test
Cardiac disease (MI, CHF), pacemaker/AICD, coronary stents	x						x		
Pulmonary disease (COPD, active asthma)	x						x	x	
End-stage renal disease on dialysis	x	x					x		
Renal insufficiency	x	x							
Liver disease	x	x	x		x				
Hypertension							x		
Diabetes		x					x		
Vascular disease	x						x		
Symptoms of urinary tract infection						x			
Chemotherapy	x	x							
Diuretics		x							
Anticoagulants			x	x					
Major operation (eg, cardiac, thoracic, vascular, or abdominal)	x	x					x	x	
Menstruating women									x

- Normal lab results obtained **within 4 months** of elective operation do not need repeating
- Baseline
  - Hgb—recommended for all patients 65+ undergoing major surgery and for younger patients undergoing major surgery with increased risk of blood loss
  - CBC (Hgb)—especially if surgery with increased risk of blood loss, renal insufficiency, diabetes, anemia, malignancy, cardiac disease, and pregnancy
  - BMP
    - Electrolytes—especially if risk of loss of fluids or electrolytes, long-term diuretic use, diabetes, intractable vomiting, or elderly
    - Creatinine—especially if history or PE finding of chronic disease (diabetes, hypertension, cardiovascular disease, renal disease, hepatic disease)
  - Blood glucose—routine measurement is not recommended for healthy patients and does not influence perioperative outcomes
  - Liver function tests—not routinely recommended
- PT/aPTT/platelet count—not routinely recommended
- Urinalysis—not routinely recommended unless UTI symptoms, history of chronic urinary tract disease, and urologic procedures
- Pregnancy test—for all reproductive-aged women prior to surgery
- CXR—rarely indicated, but especially for intrathoracic procedures, signs/symptoms of known pulmonary disease, new respiratory symptoms, or suspected congestive heart failure
- EKG—men older than 40, women older than 50, history of CAD, hypertension, or diabetes; thoracic, intraperitoneal, aortic, or emergent surgery
- PFTs (spirometry)—pulmonary procedures, history of chronic smoking with COPD or SOB, suspected lung disease
- Prealbumin (NL: 18 to 35)
  - If concerned about nutritional compromise
  - If low—greater complication risk, longer healing time, higher risk of infection; patient needs to be admitted and placed on TPN 7 days prior

American Society of Anesthesiologists (ASA) Classification System

- Determines degree of perioperative risk for patients

Classification	Preoperative Health Status	Example
ASA 1	Normal healthy patient	No organic, physiologic, or psychiatric disturbance; excludes the very young and very old; healthy with good exercise tolerance
ASA 2	Patients with mild systemic disease	No functional limitations; has a well-controlled disease of one body system; controlled hypertension or diabetes without systemic effects, cigarette smoking without chronic obstructive pulmonary disease (COPD); mild obesity, pregnancy
ASA 3	Patients with severe systemic disease	Some functional limitation; has a controlled disease of more than one body system or one major system; no immediate danger of death; controlled congestive heart failure (CHF), stable angina, former heart attack, **poorly controlled hypertension**, morbid obesity, chronic renal failure; bronchospastic disease with intermittent symptoms
ASA 4	Patients with severe systemic disease that is a constant threat to life	Has at least one severe disease that is poorly controlled or at end-stage; possible risk of death; unstable angina, symptomatic COPD, symptomatic CHF, hepatorenal failure
ASA 5	Moribund patients who are not expected to survive without the operation	Not expected to survive >24 h without surgery; imminent risk of death; multiorgan failure, sepsis syndrome with hemodynamic instability, hypothermia, poorly controlled coagulopathy
ASA 6	Declared brain-dead patient whose organs are being removed for donor purposes	

Preoperative Antibiotics

Examples	Pathogens	First-line Antibiotics
Cardiac surgeries Coronary artery bypass, cardiac device insertion procedures (eg, pacemaker implantation), placement of ventricular assist devices	*Staphylococcus aureus, S. epidermidis*	One of the following: 1. Cefazolin 2. Cefuroxime 3. Vancomycin 4. Clindamycin
Gastroduodenal surgery Procedures involving entry into lumen of gastrointestinal tract	Enteric gram-negative bacilli, gram-positive cocci	1. Cefazolin

Biliary Tract Surgery (Including Pancreatic Procedures)

Examples	Pathogens	First-line Antibiotics
Open procedure or laparoscopic procedure	Enteric gram-negative bacilli, enterococci, clostridia	One of the following: 1. Cefazolin 2. Cefotetan 3. Cefoxitin 4. Ampicillin-Sulbactam
Laparoscopic procedure	N/A	None
Appendectomy	Enteric gram-negative bacilli, anaerobes, enterococci	**Flagyl** plus One of the following: 1. Cefoxitin 2. Cefotetan 3. Cefazolin

Small Intestine Surgery

Examples	Pathogens	First-line Antibiotics
Nonobstructed	Enteric gram-negative bacilli, gram-positive cocci	1. Cefazolin
Obstructed	Enteric gram-negative bacilli, anaerobes, enterococci	**Flagyl** plus One of the following: 1. Cefoxitin 2. Cefotetan 3. Cefazolin

Hernia Repair

Pathogens	First-line Antibiotics
Aerobic gram-positive organisms	1. Cefazolin

Colorectal Surgery

Pathogens	First-line Antibiotics
Enteric gram-negative bacilli, anaerobes, enterococci	**Flagyl** plus One of the following four: 1. Cefoxitin 2. Cefotetan 3. Cefazolin or 4. Oral neomycin + erythromycin base or Flagyl

Genitourinary Surgery

Examples	Pathogens	First-line Antibiotics
Cystoscopy	Enteric gram-negative bacilli, enterococci	Choose one of the following: 1. Ciprofloxacin (better for high risk or invasive procedures) 2. Bactrim

OB/GYN Surgery

Examples	Pathogens	First-line Antibiotics

Hysterectomy (abdominal, vaginal, laparoscopic, or robotic)
Urogynecology procedures including those involving mesh
		Choose one of the following:
		1. Cefazolin
		2. Cefoxitin
		3. Cefotetan
		Alternative options:
		1. Ampicillin-sulbactam
		2. Clindamycin or vancomycin with one of the following:
		  • Gentamicin
		  • Aztreonam
		  • Fluoroquinolone
		3. Flagyl plus one of the following:
		  • Gentamicin
		  • Fluoroquinolone

Examples	Pathogens	First-line Antibiotics
Cesarean section		1. Cefazolin
Abortion, surgical		1. Doxycycline
Hysterosalpingogram or chromotubation		1. Doxycycline
Laparoscopy (diagnostic, tubal sterilization, operative except for hysterectomy) **Other transcervical procedures:** **Hysteroscopy (diagnostic or operative, including hysteroscopic sterilization)** **Intrauterine device insertion** **Endometrial biopsy**		None

Head and Neck Surgeries

Examples	Pathogens	First-line Antibiotics
Clean surgeries	N/A	None
Clean with placement of prosthesis (excludes tympanostomy tubes)	*Staphylococcus aureus, S. epidermidis,* streptococci	Choose one of the following: 1. Cefazolin 2. Cefuroxime 3. Vancomycin 4. Clindamycin
Clean-contaminated	Anaerobes, enteric gram-negative bacilli, *S. aureus*	Choose one of the following: 1. Cefazolin + Flagyl 2. Cefuroxime + Flagyl 3. Ampicillin-sulbactam 4. Clindamycin

Neurosurgery

Examples	Pathogens	First-line Antibiotics
Elective craniotomy **Cerebrospinal fluid shunting procedures** **Implantation of intrathecal pumps**	*Staphylococcus aureus, S. epidermidis*	Choose one of the following: 1. Cefazolin 2. Vancomycin 3. Clindamycin

Orthopedic Surgery

Examples	Pathogens	First-line Antibiotics
Clean operation involving hand, knee, or foot with no implantation of foreign material	*N/A*	None
Spinal procedures **Hip fracture** **Internal fixation** **Total joint replacement**	*Staphylococcus aureus, S. epidermidis*	Choose one of the following: 1. Cefazolin 2. Vancomycin 3. Clindamycin

Thoracic (Noncardiac) Surgery

Examples	Pathogens	First-line Antibiotics
Thoracic (noncardiac) procedures: lobectomy, pneumonectomy, lung resection, thoracotomy	*Staphylococcus aureus, S. epidermidis,* streptococci, enteric gram-negative bacilli	Choose one of the following: 1. Cefazolin 2. Vancomycin 3. Clindamycin 4. Ampicillin-sulbactam

General Surgery

Vascular Surgery

Examples	Pathogens	First-line Antibiotics
Arterial surgery involving a prosthesis, the abdominal aorta, or a groin incision	*Staphylococcus aureus, S. epidermidis*, enteric gram-negative bacilli	Choose one of the following: 1. Cefazolin 2. Vancomycin 3. Clindamycin
Lower extremity amputation for ischemia	*S. aureus, S. epidermidis*, enteric gram-negative bacilli, clostridia	Choose one of the following: 1. Cefazolin 2. Vancomycin 3. Clindamycin

Percutaneous Procedures

Examples	Pathogens	First-line Antibiotics
Angiography, angioplasty, thrombolysis, arterial closure device placement, stent placement **Superficial venous insufficiency treatment** **IVC filter placement** **Tunneled central venous access**	*Staphylococcus aureus, S. epidermidis*	None 1. Cefazolin used if high risk: immunocompromised, chemotherapy patients, or history of catheter infection 2. For penicillin allergy: Vancomycin or clindamycin
Endograft placement	*S. aureus, S. epidermidis*	1. Cefazolin 2. For penicillin allergy: Vancomycin or clindamycin

Breast Surgery

Examples	Pathogens	First-line Antibiotics
Reduction mammoplasty **Mammoplasty** **Lumpectomy** **Mastectomy** **Axillary node dissection**	*N/A*	None
Breast cancer procedures	*Staphylococcus aureus, S. epidermidis*, streptococci	Choose one of the following: 1. Cefazolin 2. Vancomycin 3. Clindamycin

CHAPTER 68

Postoperative Care

For In-depth Coverage Refer to the Following Topics:

Pernicious Anemia, see chapter 76, p 652

Disseminated Intravascular Coagulation, see chapter 76, p 652

Carotid Artery Stenosis, see chapter 73, p 641

Supplemental Material:

Fluid/Volume Disorders (Volume Overload/Depletion), see Appendix E: Volume Disorders, p 702

Electrolyte Disorders, see Hypocalcemia in Appendix D: Electrolyte and Fluid Disorders, p 699

Acid Base Disorders, see Appendix C, p 683

THE IMMEDIATE POSTOPERATIVE PHASE (POSTANESTHETIC PHASE)

- Primary causes of early complications and death: acute pulmonary, cardiovascular, and fluid derangements
- Patient may be discharged from the PACU (post-anesthesia care unit) after 1 to 3 hours once they have returned to baseline

Postanesthesia Care Unit (PACU) Discharge Requirements
Vital signs
2 = BP + pulse within 20% preop baseline
1 = BP + pulse within 20%-40% preop baseline
0 = BP + pulse >40% preop baseline
Activity
2 = Steady gait, no dizziness, or meets preop level
1 = Requires assistance
0 = Unable to ambulate
Nausea and vomiting
2 = Minimal/treated with PO medication
1 = Moderate/treated with parenteral medication
0 = Severe/continuous despite treatment
Pain
Controlled with oral analgesics and acceptable to patient:
2 = Yes
1 = No
Surgical bleeding
2 = Minimal/no dressing changes
1 = Moderate/up to two dressing changes required
0 = Severe/more than three dressing changes required
Score ≥9 for discharge

Reprinted from Benumof JL, Dagg R, Benumof R. Critical hemoglobin desaturation will occur before return to an unparalyzed state following 1 mg/kg intravenous succinylcholine. *Anesthesiology*. 1997;87:979, with permission.

- If a patient requires ventilatory or circulatory support, they are transferred to an ICU
- **Postop monitoring**
  - Monitor vital signs frequently until stable, then regularly until discharged from recovery room
    - Continuous EKG indicated for most patients
  - Central venous pressure (CVP) should be recorded periodically, especially if large blood loss or fluid shift
    - Swan-Ganz catheter is indicated to measure pulmonary artery wedge pressure
  - Fluid balance—including all fluid administered as well as blood loss and UOP during procedure; also, include any fluid loss from drains and stomas
    - Notify surgeon if patient has not voided within 6 to 8 hours after operation (or after Foley removal, if placed)
  - Respiratory care—mechanical ventilation, supplemental O2 by mask or nasal prongs, intubation with tracheal suctioning, or other respiratory therapy; non-intubated patients should be instructed how to cough

and do deep breathing exercises (or incentive spirometry) to prevent atelectasis
  - Deep breathing exercises: slow, deep inspiration followed by a breath hold of 2 to 5 seconds and slow exhalation; in theory, this opens collapsed alveoli, reducing atelectasis, promoting secretion removal, and restoring lung volume
  - Incentive spirometry (IS) measures the amount of air inhaled
- Bed position and mobilization—most patients should be **turned side to side every 30 minutes** until conscious and then hourly for first 8 to 12 hours to minimize atelectasis
  - Early ambulation to reduce venous stasis, upright position increases diaphragmatic contraction
  - Pneumatic stockings (SCDs) to prevent venous stasis
  - Special safety considerations for fall risk (red socks, bed rails), one-on-one monitoring, assisted transferring
  - Knee and heel supports to reduce back pain and tension from immobility
- Diet—nothing by mouth (NPO) for patients at risk for emesis or aspiration until GI function has returned (usually within 4 days), but can tolerate liquids shortly after
- IV fluids and electrolytes—maintenance, operative losses, replacement of GI losses from drains, fistulas, and stomas
- Drain instructions—type, pressure of suction, irrigation fluid and frequency, skin exit site care, support during ambulation, showering; monitor output
- Medications—antibiotics, analgesics, gastric acid suppression, DVT prophylaxis, sedatives
  - Antipyretics, laxatives, and stool softeners used as indicated
  - Nausea and vomiting prophylaxis
- Postop Labs—CBC, CMP, CXR, LFTs or renal function panels
- **"Postoperative" check**
  - If patient remains in the hospital beyond 4 to 6 hours, they must be evaluated by a medical provider
    - Review subjective status and any objective changes during that period and assess whether postop orders are appropriate or adequate

INTERMEDIATE PHASE (HOSPITALIZATION PERIOD)

Complete recovery from anesthesia, lasting the rest of the hospital stay.

- Patient becomes self-sufficient, recovering most basic of functions
- Wound care—fills with an inflammatory exudate within hours after surgery
  - Epidermal cells at the edges divide and migrate across the wound surface with deeper structures closing after 48 hours (sterile dressings provide protection)

- Aseptic technique should be used during first 24 hours to remove dressing and handle wound healing
- Dressings over closed wounds should be removed by day 3 or 4; if dry, do not reapply; remove dressings earlier if wet or placed in contaminated setting (soaked dressings increase bacterial contamination), patient has fever or increasing wound pain
- Culture and gram-stain any drainage from wounds
- Vacuum dressings should be placed in 24 to 72 hours
- **Remove sutures and staples on day 5**, replace with tape; sutures that cross creases (groin, popliteal), incisions under tension, hand incisions, and debilitated patients → leave in at least 2 weeks, or remove if signs of infection
- Showering—patient may **shower or bathe by day 7**
- Drains—used to prevent unwanted pus, blood, or serum from accumulating and to evacuate air from the pleural cavity to re-expand lungs
  - External portion must be handled with aseptic technique and must be removed as soon as it is no longer needed
  - Small risk of retrograde infection of the peritoneal cavity
  - Jackson-Pratt (JP) and Blake drains are "closed" and connected to suction: preferred to open drains
    - Open drains (Penrose) predispose patient to contamination
- GI tract care
  - Following laparotomy, **peristalsis temporarily decreases and returns to small intestine in 24 hours, right colon by 48 hours, left colon by 72 hours**
  - Opioids may interfere with motility and should be limited in patients with slow gastric emptying
  - Gastrostomy and jejunostomy tubes should be connected to suction or dependent drainage for 24 hours postop; **feeding started on postop day 2 even if motility is not normalized**; do not remove before 3rd postop week; crush and flush any pills put through
  - Patient may resume normal diet as soon as anesthesia effects have resolved

- Pulmonary care
  - Initially postop: decreased vital capacity and functional residual capacity; increased risk for pulmonary edema
    - Vital capacity—decreases to 40% of preop values within 1 to 4 hours of surgery, remains there for 12 to 14 hours and slowly increases to 60% to 70% normal by 7 days, returning to baseline the next week
    - FRC is close to preop level after surgery, but decreases to 70% preop values after 24 hours, remaining depressed for several days, then returning to normal by day 10
    - Accentuated changes in obese, smokers, and patients with preexisting lung disease—**reduced FEV1 → higher risk of infection due to inability to clear secretions**
  - Pain is thought to be one of the main causes of shallow breathing postoperatively, but pain reduction does not restore pulmonary function → affected by factors such as obesity, abdominal distention and factors that limit diaphragmatic excursion
  - Minimize atelectasis by utilizing deep inspiration and coughing
    - Use an incentive spirometer (IS) to facilitate periodic hyperinflation
    - Early mobilization
    - Encouragement to take deep breaths (especially standing)
  - **Postop pulmonary edema**—caused by elevated hydrostatic pressures (LVF, fluid overload, decreased oncotic pressure) or increased capillary permeability, or both. Manage IV fluids and treat heart failure and signs of sepsis.
  - Offer pneumococcal or influenza vaccine prior to surgery in patients at risk (see sections on these individual vaccinations for indications)
  - Preexisting pulmonary disease—hydrate to avoid hypo- or hypervolemia (hyperventilation and labored breathing causes dehydration), dry secretions, thick sputum → use epidural blocks in patients with COPD which relieves pain and permits respiratory muscle function

Disease	Etiology, Prevalence, and Risk Factors	Clinical Symptoms and Signs	Diagnostics	Therapy, Prognosis, and Health Maintenance
Early postop respiratory failure	Major operations (chest, abdomen), severe trauma, preexisting lung disease	1. Onset over short period (minutes to 1-2 h) 2. No evidence of precipitating cause Signs: 1. Tachypnea: 25-30 breaths/min 2. Low tidal volume <4 mL/kg 3. Low cardiac output	1. High PCO_2 >45 mm Hg 2. Low PO_2 <60 mm Hg	1. Endotracheal intubation 2. Ventilatory support 3. Determine cause—atelectasis, pneumonia, pneumothorax
Late postop respiratory failure	Triggers: pulmonary embolism, abdominal distention, opioid overdose	1. Develops beyond 48 h postop 2. Same as above	Same as above	Same as above

MECHANICAL COMPLICATIONS

• Occur as direct result of technical failure from procedure or operation

Disease	Etiology, Prevalence, and Risk Factors	Clinical Symptoms and Signs	Diagnostics	Therapy, Prognosis, and Health Maintenance
Hematoma Collection of blood and clot in wound caused by inadequate hemostasis	Much higher risk in patients on systemic anticoagulation and preexisting coagulopathies, aspirin, low-dose heparin, vigorous coughing, or arterial hypertension postop. Dangerous on thyroid, parathyroid or carotid artery because it may expand rapidly and compromise the airway	1. Elevation and discoloration of wound edges 2. Discomfort 3. Swelling 4. Blood leaking between sutures		1. Evacuation of the clot under sterile conditions 2. Ligation 3. Reclosure of the wound
Hemoperitoneum (Fig. 68-1)	<u>RF:</u> Dilution of hemostatic factors after massive blood loss, mismatched transfusion, administration of heparin. Bleeding is the most common cause of shock in first 24 h after surgery	1. Manifests within 24 h postop as intravascular hypovolemia • Tachycardia • Hypotension • Decreased UOP • Peripheral vasoconstriction • Increased abdominal girth • Intraabdominal hypertension • Abdominal compartment syndrome	1. Hct changes within 4-6 h	1. Reoperation: Stop bleeding, evacuate clots, rinse peritoneal cavity with saline solution <u>Prognosis:</u> Rapidly evolving, life threatening
Seroma (Fig. 68-2)	Delay healing time, increase risk of wound infection. Fluid collection in the wound other than pus or blood following operations that involve elevation of skin flaps and transection of numerous lymphatic channels (eg, mastectomy, groin operations)			1. Evacuate using needle aspiration, unless of the groin, which you should leave to resorb spontaneously since risks of infection and disruption of vascular structures are greater than benefit 2. If persistent → explore wound in OR and oversew draining sites

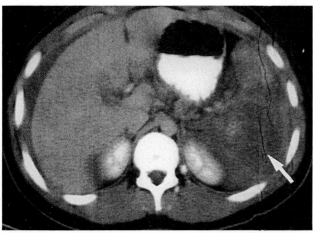

FIGURE 68-1. Massive hemoperitoneum on CT (splenic rupture shown by *arrow*). (From Fleisher GR, Ludwig S, Henretig FM, Ruddy RM, Silverman BK. *Textbook of Pediatric Emergency Medicine.* Philadelphia: Wolters Kluwer Health; 2005.)

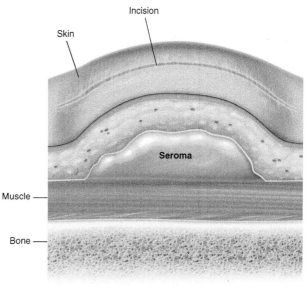

FIGURE 68-2. Seroma.

- **Wound dehiscence**—partial or total disruption of any or all layers of the operative wound (1% to 3% of all abdominal procedures)
  - **Evisceration**: rupture of all layers of the abdominal wall and extrusion of abdominal viscera
  - Systemic factors: 5% of patients >60, more common in patients with DM, uremia, immunosuppression, jaundice, sepsis, hypoalbuminemia, cancer, obesity, and chronic steroid use
  - Local factors: **inadequate closure**, increased intraabdominal pressure, deficient wound healing, <u>not</u> influenced by the type of incision
    - **Closure (most important)**
    - Intraabdominal pressure
    - Poor wound healing

POSTOPERATIVE FEVER

- The timing of fever onset after surgery is one of the most important factors in prioritizing your differential diagnosis
  - Immediate—onset in the OR or within hours after surgery complete
    - Medication or blood product exposure during preop, surgery, or immediately postop (PACU)
      - Presenting sign: hypotension and sometimes rash
    - Trauma suffered prior or as part of surgery
    - Infections present prior to surgery
  - Acute—onset within first week after surgery (see 5 Ws right)

- Subacute—onset from 1 to 4 weeks postop
  - SSI—common cause >1 week after surgery
  - Central venous catheters
  - Antibiotic-associated diarrhea
  - Febrile drug reactions (β lactams, sulfa products, H2 blockers, procainamide, phenytoin, heparin)
- Delayed—onset more than 1 month after
  - Mostly due to infection (viral), including CMV, hepatitis viruses, HIV, and parasitic infections (though rare)
- Infectious origin likely if 3+ present
  - Preoperative trauma
  - ASA class 2+
  - Fever after POD #2
  - Initial temperature elevation >38.6°C
  - Postop WBC >10 k/L
  - Postop serum BUN 15 mg/dL+
- **5 Ws (order of likely postoperative fever etiology) in the acute period**
  - Wind (POD 1 to 2): pneumonia, aspiration, PE, atelectasis
  - Water (POD 3 to 5): UTI (indwelling catheter, Foley); more common with GU procedures and chronic indwelling catheters
  - **Walking (POD 4 to 6): DVT or PE**
  - Wound (POD 5 to 7, though typically 1 week after): surgical site infection (SSI)
  - Wonder drugs (POD 7+): drug fever, infection from lines, reaction to blood products

Disease	Etiology, Prevalence, and Risk Factors	Clinical Symptoms and Signs	Diagnostics	Therapy, Prognosis, and Health Maintenance
Atelectasis *Obstruction* by secretions (COPD), intubation or anesthesia *Nonobstructive* causes: closure of bronchioles (<1 mm)	**Most common postop complication** (25% of abdominal surgeries) RF: Elderly, overweight, smokers, respiratory disease Fever **within 48 h** after surgery Caused by decreased lung tissue compliance, impaired regional ventilation, retained airway secretions, and/or postop pain interfering with breathing and coughing	1. Fever (unknown origin) 2. **Increased work of breathing** Signs: 1. Elevation of diaphragm 2. Scattered rales 3. Decreased breath sounds in area 4. Dullness to percussion 5. Tachypnea 6. Tachycardia 7. **Hypoxemia**	1. V/P mismatch 2. CXR–abnormal findings dependent on location	1. Chest percussion, coughing, nasotracheal suction–fever decreases with reexpansion of the lung 2. Bronchodilators and mucolytics via nebulizer for COPD 3. Trial of CPAP if hypoxemia and increased respiratory effort Prevention: Early ambulation, frequent changes in position, cough encouragement, incentive spirometry Prognosis: If atelectasis persists beyond 72 h, pneumonia will likely occur

Disease	Etiology, Prevalence, and Risk Factors	Clinical Symptoms and Signs	Diagnostics	Therapy, Prognosis, and Health Maintenance
Pneumonia	Tends to occur within 5 d postop Highest risk: peritoneal infection, prolonged ventilatory support RF: Atelectasis, aspiration, copious secretions Caused by **S. aureus** and **gram-negative bacilli** (>50%): *E. coli, Pseudomonas, Klebsiella*	1. Fever 2. Increased secretions Signs: 1. Tachypnea 2. Physical changes suggestive of pulmonary consolidation 3. Hypercapnia	1. CXR: localized parenchymal consolidation 2. CBC: leukocytosis or leukopenia 3. Sputum must be obtained by endotracheal suctioning	1. Clear secretions 2. Empiric antibiotics No changes in incidence with: pain control or prophylactic antibiotics Prevention: Early ambulation, frequent changes in position, cough encouragement, incentive spirometry Prognosis: Mortality: 20%-40%
Phlebitis	Inflammation at entry site due to needle or catheter insertion **MCC of fever after postop day#3** Most common in lower extremity veins	1. Swelling Signs: 1. Erythema 2. Tenderness 3. Edema 4. Induration		1. Remove catheters at earliest signs Prevention: Aseptic technique during insertion, frequent change of tubing (48-72 h), rotation of insertion sites (q 4 d) Use silastic catheters (least reactive), and hypertonic solutions in veins with substantial flow
Suppurative phlebitis	MC bug: *Staphylococcus* Presence of infected thrombus around indwelling catheter	Signs: 1. Local signs of inflammation + pus from venipuncture site 2. High fever	1. (+) Blood cultures	1. Excise affected vein 2. Extend incision proximally to first open collateral 3. Leave wound open

Pulmonary edema	Postop *cardiogenic edema*: occurs within 36 h when fluid retention exceeds 67 mL/kg/d
	RF:
	Preexisting heart disease and over administration of IVF
	MCC postop *noncardiogenic edema*: negative pressure pulmonary edema (laryngospasm, upper airway obstruction following extubation)
	RF:
	Obesity, short neck, OSA, acromegaly
		1. Rapid onset SOB at rest
		2. Pink, frothy sputum
		Signs:
		1. Crackles, wheezing
		2. S3 gallop
		3. Elevated JVP
		4. Peripheral edema
		5. Tachypnea
		6. Tachycardia
		7. Severe hypoxemia
		Complications:
		1. Pulmonary hemorrhage
		2. Frank hemoptysis
			1. CXR
			  • If cardiogenic–enlarged cardiac silhouette, vascular redistribution, interstitial thickening, **perihilar alveolar infiltrates**
			  • Noncardiogenic–normal heart size, uniform alveolar infiltrates
			2. Echo–identifies systolic and diastolic dysfunction and valvular lesions
			3. EKG: ST elevation and evolving Q waves suggest AMI
			4. BNP: elevated, supports heart failure
			5. Swan-Ganz catheter: high PCWP pressure (cardiogenic) vs. normal (noncardiogenic)
				1. Treat underlying cause
				2. Oxygenation and ventilation
				  • Mechanical ventilation with adequate O_2 delivery: nasal/face mask, intubation
				  • Positive end-expiratory pressure (PEEP)
				3. Reduce preload
				  • Loop diuretics: furosemide
				  • Nitrates
				  • Morphine
				  • ACE inhibitors

(continued)

General Surgery

(continued)

Disease	Etiology, Prevalence, and Risk Factors	Clinical Symptoms and Signs	Diagnostics	Therapy, Prognosis, and Health Maintenance

Postop urinary retention (POUR)	Inability to void postoperatively following anesthesia
	Incidence: 5%-70%, varies widely
	RF:
	• Patient factors: old age, male gender, history of preexisting urinary retention, neurologic disease, prior pelvic surgery
	• Procedural: anorectal surgery, joint arthroplasty, hernia repair, incontinence surgery
	• Anesthetic: excessive fluid administration, medications (opioids, anticholinergics, BB), prolonged anesthesia, type of anesthesia
		1. Bladder fullness
		2. Lower abdominal discomfort
			1. Bladder ultrasound (preferred, confirms)
			2. Catheterization
				1. If unable to void 4 h after surgery and 600+ mL detected on U/S
				  • one-time bladder catheterization
				  • if volume drained >400 mL, leave catheter in place
				  • remove before discharge
				Prophylactic catheterization for operations 3+ h or high IVF volumes

Postop urinary tract infections	RF: Preexisting contamination of UT, urinary retention, instrumentation	Signs/SX of cystitis: 1. Dysuria 2. Mild fever Signs/SX of pyelonephritis: 1. High fever 2. Flank tenderness 3. Ileus	1. Examine urine and obtain culture	1. Adequate hydration, proper drainage of bladder, and antibiotics

Treatment of Pneumonia

	Pathogens	First Line	At Risk for Pseudomonas
Inpatient, non-ICU	*S. pneumoniae, Legionella, H. influenzae, Enterobacteriaceae, S. aureus, Pseudomonas*	1. **Respiratory FQ**: IV levofloxacin 750 mg daily OR 2. IV ciprofloxacin 400 mg q 8-12 h	1. IV Macrolide PLUS IV β lactam (HD Ampicillin 1-2 g q 4-6 h or Cefotaxime 1-2 g q 4-12 h or Ceftriaxone 1-2 g q 12-24 h)

Hospitalized or ICU patients
Duration: 5 d minimum or until patient afebrile × 48-72 h
	ICU: *S. pneumoniae, Legionella, H. influenzae, Enterobacteriaceae, S. aureus, Pseudomonas*	1. Azithromycin or respiratory FQ (moxifloxacin, **levofloxacin**)
		PLUS
		2. Antipneumococcal β-lactam: **cefotaxime**, ceftriaxone, Unasyn
		β-lactam allergy:
		1. FQ
		PLUS
		2. Aztreonam 1-2 g q 6-12 h
			1. Antipneumococcal and antipseudomonal B-lactam: **Zosyn**, cefepime, imipenem or meropenem
			PLUS
			2. Ciprofloxacin or **levofloxacin**
			OR
			  • Antipneumococcal B-lactam (cefotaxime, ceftriaxone, Unasyn)
			PLUS
			  • Aminoglycoside (gentamicin, tobramycin, amikacin)
			PLUS
			  • Azithromycin or respiratory FQ
			If at risk for MSSA
			1. Add vancomycin or linezolid 600 mg BID

		Low risk for MDR pathogens	High risk for MDR pathogens

	Pathogens	First Line	At Risk for Pseudomonas
Nosocomial acquired pneumonia, also known as hospital acquired pneumonia (HAP)		One of the following: 1. Ceftriaxone 1-2 g IV q 12-24 h 2. Moxifloxacin 400 mg PO or IV 3. Levofloxacin 750 mg PO or IV 4. Ciprofloxacin 400 mg IV q 8-12 h 5. Unasyn 1.5-3 g IV q 6 h 6. Zosyn 3.375-4 g IV q 6 h 7. Ertapenem 1 g IV daily	One agent from each: 1. Antipseudomonal • Cefepime 1-2 g IV BID or ceftazidime 1-2 g IV q 8 h • Imipenem 0.5-1 g IV q 6-8 h or meropenem 1 g IV q 8 h • Zosyn 3.375-4.5 g IV q 6 h • PCN allergy: Aztreonam 1-2 g IV q 6-12 h 2. Second antipseudomonal • Levofloxacin 750 mg IV daily OR ciprofloxacin 400 mg IV q 8-12 h • IV gentamicin, tobramycin, amikacin 3. MRSA coverage • IV vancomycin • Linezolid

DEEP VENOUS THROMBOSIS, VENOUS THROMBOEMBOLISM (VTE), PULMONARY EMBOLISM (PE) FIG. 68-3

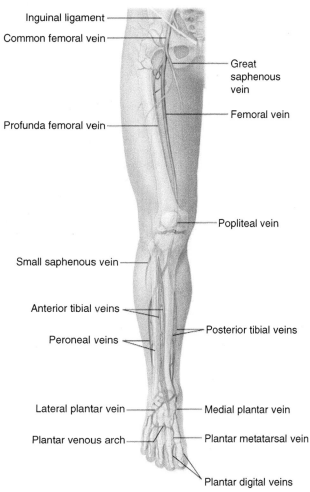

FIGURE 68-3. Major venous system of the lower extremity. (From Kupinski AM. *The Vascular System*. Philadelphia: Wolters Kluwer Health; 2018.)

Disease	Etiology, Prevalence, and Risk Factors	Clinical Symptoms and Signs	Diagnostics	Therapy, Prognosis, and Health Maintenance
Venous thromboembolism (VTE)	Virchow's triad: hypercoagulable state, stasis, vessel damage Trauma patients, cancer operations, dissection of pelvis Nonmodifiable RF: Thrombophilia, prior VTE, CHF, chronic lung disease, paralytic stroke, malignancy, SCI, age >40, varicosities Modifiable RF: Type of surgery, mechanical ventilation, major trauma, central lines, chemotherapy, HRT, pregnancy, immobility, obesity			Prevention: 1. Lovenox, SCDs, and early ambulation 2. IVC filters for patients with contraindications to anticoagulation or refractory cases Complications: Pulmonary hypertension and pulmonary embolism

Deep vein thrombosis (DVT)
Symptomatic DVT: presence of symptoms leading to radiographic diagnosis
Asymptomatic DVT: incidental finding in patient without symptoms
Unprovoked DVT: implies no identifiable provoking event (ex hospitalization, surgery, ERT, reduced mobility)
	25% of postoperative patients will develop a DVT without prophylaxis
	Aspirin is not supported as single agent for prophylaxis
	RF:
	1. History of immobilization or prolonged hospitalization
	2. Recent surgery or trauma
	3. Obesity
	4. Previous VTE
	5. Malignancy
	6. OCP or HRT use
	7. Pregnancy or postpartum
	8. Age >65
	9. Stroke with hemiplegia or immobility
	10. Family history of VTE
	11. HF or IBD
	Proximal DVT: located in popliteal, femoral, or iliac veins
	Isolated distal DVT: no proximal component; located below the knee, confined to calf veins (peroneal, posterior, anterior tibial, muscular veins)
		1. Lower extremity (calf) swelling
		2. Unilateral or bilateral leg, pain
		3. Warmth
		Signs:
		1. Hypoxia
		2. HR >100
		3. Erythema
		4. Pitting edema
		5. Dilated superficial veins
		6. Tenderness
		7. Warmth
		8. Local inguinal mass
		9. Larger calf diameter (if unilateral)
		10. Homan's sign—calf pain with passive dorsiflexion is unreliable
			1. CBC, chemistry, LFTs, coagulation studies
			2. Measure pretest probability (PTP) using Wells criteria above
			3. D-dimer in patients with low suspicion
			• NL is <500 ng/mL
			• Positive is >500 ng/mL
			• Useful to rule out DVT
			4. Compression ultrasonography with Doppler (preferred)
			• Treat if
			  • Proximal DVT identified
			  • Distal DVT identified and patient meets criteria for treatment of Distal DVT
			• Primary evaluation for patients with prior DVT
				1. Anticoagulation
				• For patients with first DVT (provoked or unprovoked)—anticoagulate for minimum 3 mon
				• The need to anticoagulate indefinitely is based on risk of recurrence, occupation, life expectancy, burden of therapy, etc
				2. IVC filter
				• When risk of bleeding outweighs risk of VTE
				• CI to anticoagulation: active bleeding or diathesis, platelet count <50 k/uL, high-risk bleeding surgery or procedure, major trauma, history of ICH
				3. Malignancy
				• For patients with cancer, treat with LMWH for initial and long-term management unless CI or renal insufficiency (CrCl < 30)
				4. Pregnancy
				• Adjusted dose SQ LMWH for initial and long-term management
				• D/C 24 h prior to predicted delivery; neuraxial anesthesia use increases risk for spinal hematoma
				• Temporary IVC filter can be placed in patients with prior VTE
				• Restart heparin (SQ LMWH, IV UFH, or SQ UVH) 12 h after c section or 6 h after vaginal
				5. Thrombectomy
				• For patients with massive iliofemoral DVT or who fail therapeutic anticoagulation
				• For pregnant women whom risk of life threatening PE is high
				Prevention
				1. Early ambulation
				2. Compression stockings × 2 y, start after anticoagulation initiated

Disease	Etiology, Prevalence, and Risk Factors	Clinical Symptoms and Signs	Diagnostics	Therapy, Prognosis, and Health Maintenance
Pulmonary embolism	Obstruction of pulmonary artery or one of its branches by material (thrombus, tumor, air, or fat) that originated elsewhere in the body MC site: Deep veins of lower extremity above the knee (iliofemoral) Upper extremity (rare) is found in IVDU RF: Age >60, malignancy, prior history, hypercoagulable states (factor 5 Leiden, protein C/S deficiency, antithrombin III deficiency), prolonged immobilization or bed rest, long-distance travel, cardiac disease (CHF), obesity, nephrotic syndrome, major surgery (pelvic), major trauma, pregnancy, estrogen use (OCP) Virchow's triad: hypercoagulable state, venous stasis, endothelial injury	Mostly asymptomatic 1. Dyspnea (MC) • Typically, rapid onset within seconds to minutes 2. Pleuritic chest pain 3. Cough 4. Orthopnea 5. Calf or thigh pain and/or swelling 6. Wheezing 7. Syncope (large PE) 8. Hemoptysis (rare) Signs: 1. Tachypnea 2. Rales 3. Tachycardia 4. S4 5. Increased P2 6. Shock with rapid circulatory collapse 7. Calf or thigh swelling, erythema, edema, tenderness, palpable cords 8. JVD 9. Others: low-grade fever, decreased breath sounds, dullness to percussion	Screening 1. CXR–normal, +/– atelectasis or pleural effusion • Hampton's Hump • Westermark's sign 2. D-dimer–if low clinical suspicion, do first (sensitive) 3. EKG: S1Q3T3 (though MC seen are ST and T-wave changes) 1. Helical CT w/ contrast–intraluminal filling defects in central, segmental, or lobular pulmonary arteries with clinical suspicion 2. Doppler U/S of lower extremity–helpful when (+), useless when negative, perform if pt w/renal insufficiency 3. V/Q scan: normal scan r/o PE, treat if high probability 4. Increased (widened) A-a gradient: PAO_2-PaO_2 due to VQ mismatch 5. (+) CT Pulmonary angiogram (gold standard), invasive 6. ABG–respiratory alkalosis, low PaO_2 and $PaCO_2$ (hypocapnia), pH high *A-a gradient = alveolar-arterial gradient for O_2	Prevention: 1. Early ambulation 2. Elastic graduated compression stockings Prognosis: 1. Recurrence common • 2% at 2 wk • 6% at 3 mon • 30% at 10 y 2. ~10% mortality when diagnosed and treated, 30% if undiagnosed and untreated *Complications* in patients with PE who survive initial event: recurrent PE or pulmonary HTN (2/3)
Surgical site infection (SSI)	RF: Systemic factors (DM, immunosuppression, obesity, smoking, malnutrition, previous radiation), local factors (surgical wound classification and techniques)	Clinical DX 1. Pain 2. Warmth 3. Erythema 4. Drainage through incision		1. Primary source control 2. Antibiotic prophylaxis Prevention: 1. Skin preparation 2. Maintain sterility 3. Judicious use of cautery 4. Respect dissection planes 5. Approximate tissue neatly 6. Administer preoperative antibiotics

Anticoagulation for DVT and PE

Proximal DVT (All Patients, Even if Asymptomatic) Risk of Complications is Higher, Especially Embolization and Death	Distal DVT (Select Patients)	Pulmonary Embolism
1. First 10 days—Choose one of the following: • LMWH + warfarin • **Low-dose UFH (Lovenox) 5000 U SQ BID** • LMWH, then dabigatran or edoxaban • Rivaroxaban or apixaban monotherapy 2. 10 d to 3 mon: Long-term anticoagulation • warfarin 3. **Thrombin inhibitors** (preferred): Dabigatran 4. **Direct factor Xa inhibitors** (preferred): Rivaroxaban, apixaban, edoxaban 5. SQ LMWH (Lovenox) • LMWH (Lovenox 30 mg BID or 40 mg qd) • Lovenox 5000 units SQ TID for high risk (bridge with therapeutic dose) 6. Fondaparinux • Fondaparinux 2.5 mg qd for moderate risk	1. Treat symptomatic patients if bleeding risk is low 2. Asymptomatic patients with • Unprovoked DVT • D-dimer >500 mg/mL • Extensive thrombosis (>5 cm length, >7 mm diameter) in multiple veins • Thrombosis close to proximal veins • Persistent or irreversible risk factors (active malignancy) • Prior DVT/PE • Prolonged immobility • Inpatient status	Hemodynamically unstable—systolic <90 mm Hg for 15 min or longer or clear evidence of shock (8% of patients) 1. IV fluids, vasopressors, O2 supplementation, stabilize airway 2. Immediate anticoagulation with **unfractionated heparin** 3. Prompt CT pulmonary angiogram (CTPA) 4. If patient is unconscious or requires high doses of pressors for resuscitation, consider: **thrombolytics** • Contraindications: intracranial neoplasm, recent (<2 mon) intracranial or spinal surgery/trauma, history of hemorrhagic stroke, active bleeding or diathesis, or nonhemorrhagic stroke within last 3 mon • tPA (Alteplase)—natural enzyme that binds to fibrin, increasing affinity for plasminogen, enhancing plasminogen activation 5. Embolectomy—if thrombolysis contraindicated or unsuccessful Hemodynamically stable (most patients) 1. Nonpregnant • General: IV fluids, O$_2$ supplementation • Empiric anticoagulation while awaiting diagnostic test results 2. Pregnant • Adjusted dose SQ LMWH (initial and long term) Contraindications to anticoagulation, recurrent DVT/PE, or high bleeding risk 1. IVC filter placement Anticoagulant options 1. UFH one bolus + continuous infusion × 5-10 d (**PTT goal: 1.5-2.5**) OR 2. Oral warfarin + heparin day 1, INR 2-3 Menstruation, epistaxis, and minor hemoptysis are NOT contraindications to anticoagulation

Factors Influencing Anticoagulation Selection

Cancer; liver disease and coagulopathy; pregnancy or pregnancy risk	LMWH aNot for use in patients with renal insufficiency who need rapid onset anticoagulation
Renal disease and CrCl < 30 mL/min, poor compliance	VKA
Coronary artery disease	VKA, rivaroxaban, apixaban, or edoxaban
Dyspepsia or history of GI bleed	VKA, apixaban
Thrombolytic therapy use	UFH infusion aPreferred in patients who are hemodynamically unstable in anticipation of need for thrombolytics or embolectomy

aDirect thrombin inhibitors and factor XA inhibitors should not be used for hemodynamically unstable patients.

WOUND INFECTIONS

- RF: surgical technique, limit wound contamination, blood loss, duration of operation, local trauma, and ischemia
- Antibiotics—administered **within 1-hour period before incision** for clean operations and all clean-contaminated and dirty operations
- Give in adequate doses, redose at appropriate intervals, and D/C as soon as appropriate (within 24 hours)
- Infuse about every 2 half-lives during operation (q4h cefazolin)
- Standard: **Cefazolin 1 to 2 gm**
  - PCN allergy: Vancomycin or clindamycin
  - MRSA (+): Vancomycin
- Wound perfusion and oxygenation are essential to minimize the likelihood of SSIs. Intravascular blood volume is what provides end-organ perfusion and delivery of oxygen to the surgical site. The maintenance of perioperative body temperature has strong effects on wound O$_2$ tension levels and can reduce the incidence of SSIs. The **application of warming blankets immediately prior to the operation** may support the patient's temperature in the OR, especially for high-risk operations such as **bowel resections** that often involve a prolonged interval of positioning and preparation when a broad surface area is exposed to room air.
- **Mupirocin nasal ointment application** and **chlorhexidine soap showers** prior to surgery have reduced the incidence of SSIs among patients colonized with methicillin-sensitive *S. aureus* (MSSA)
- **Hypoalbuminemia** (albumin <3.0 mg/dL) is an independent risk factor for the development of SSIs, with a fivefold

increased incidence versus patients with normal albumin levels

- **Wound dehiscence**—partial or total disruption of any or all layers of the operative wound; unaffected by the type of incision; most commonly occurs during postop days 5 to 8
  - Risk factors:
    - Inadequate closure—most important factor
      - Most that dehisce do so because sutures tear through fascia
      - Prevention: perform neat incision, avoid devitalization of the fascial edges, place, and tie sutures correctly, select appropriate suture material
      - Place sutures **2 to 3 cm from wound edge and 1 cm apart**
      - Often the result of placing too few stitches and placing them too close to the edge of the fascia
    - Increased intraabdominal pressure
    - Poor wound healing—normally you will find a "healing ridge" (palpable thickening or swelling extending about 0.5 cm on each side of incision), but this may not be present in cases of wound dehiscence
  - The first sign of intraabdominal sepsis is discharge of serosanguineous fluid from the wound or sudden evisceration
  - Patient may describe a "popping sensation" associated with severe coughing or retching
- **Evisceration**—rupture of all layers of the abdominal wall and extrusion of the abdominal viscera

- Anastomotic leaks
  - Risk factors: age, malnutrition, vitamin deficiencies, and comorbidities (DM, smoking, IBD, previous chemotherapy, anemia)
  - Clinical signs: pain, fever, peritonitis; drainage of purulent, bilious, or fecal material
  - XR: fluid and gas-containing collections tracking to an anastomosis
  - Management: depends on clinical status, time since operation, and location/severity
    - Bowel rest, observation, antibiotics, and percutaneous drainage of abscess
    - Operative: open drainage, proximal diversion, and revision of anastomosis

Types of Wound Closure

- **Primary intention**: wound edges are reapproximated within hours of initial injury. Wound must be acute and clean. There is an increased risk of infection if you attempt to primarily close a wound that is contaminated or has been open for a long period of time.

- **Secondary intention**: wounds that are left open close via granulation tissue formation, wound contracture, and reepithelialization

- **Tertiary intention** (delayed primary closure): wounds that are left open and temporarily treated with local wound care are closed surgically when suitable for closure (clean, absent of infection), which accelerates healing and reduces formation of scar tissue

Classification of Operative Wounds

Clean (OR, clinician, or patient's skin)	1. Elective, nonemergent, nontraumatic, primarily closed
	2. No acute inflammation; no break in technique
	3. Respiratory, GI, biliary, GU tract not entered
	4. <12 h old eg, Inguinal hernia repair, aortic graft, thyroidectomy, mastectomy
		Risk: <2%
		1. **Cefazolin 2 g**
		  • Aseptic technique, anesthesia
		  • Hemostasis
		  • Debridement
		  • Irrigation
		  • Closure

Clean-contaminated (endogenous colonization)	1. Urgent or emergency case that is otherwise clean 2. Elective opening of respiratory, GI biliary, GU tract with minimal spillage (appendectomy) not encountering infected urine or bile 3. Minor technique break eg, Elective colon, stomach resection, gastric tube, common bile duct exploration	Risk: <10% 1. **Cefazolin + Flagyl**
Contaminated (gross contamination)	1. Nonpurulent inflammation; gross spillage from GI tract; entry into biliary or GU tract in the presence of infected bile or urine 2. Major break in technique 3. Penetrating trauma <4-h old 4. Chronic open wounds to be grafted or converted eg, Traumatic wounds w/soil or particulate matter	Risk: 20% 1. Second-generation cephalosporins (cefotetan or cefoxitin) may be superior 2. β-lactam allergy: Clindamycin or vancomycin 3. For colorectal patients: mechanical bowel cleanse and oral erythromycin and neomycin
Dirty (established infection)	1. Purulent inflammation (abscess) 2. Preoperative perforation of respiratory, GI, biliary, or GU tract 3. Penetrating trauma >4 h old eg, Abscess, resection of infarcted bowel	Risk: 40% 1. Should receive a booster injection of tetanus toxoid if last booster was >5 y ago 2. If unclear immunization history or those who never received any: tetanus IG and toxoid booster at same time in different injection sites

General Surgery

FLUID OR VOLUME DISORDERS (VOLUME OVERLOAD OR DEPLETION)

- ~1% suffer reduced kidney function postop
- Risk higher during cardiac procedures = 10% to 30% with AKI
- Maintain good intravascular volume to reduce risk, avoid NSAIDs and IV contrast should be minimized or avoided
- Blood transfusions may be necessary before operations, especially in the setting of active hemorrhage or profound anemia
- Maintenance fluids
  - Daily maintenance for sensible and insensible loss in adult = 1500 to 2500 mL depending on age, gender, weight, BSA
  - Multiply patient weight (kg) × 30 = fluid over 24 hours
  - Increased requirements for fever, hyperventilation, and increased catabolism
- IV fluid replacement for short period (most)
  - Do not have to measure electrolytes postop, unless extra fluid loss, sepsis, preexisting electrolyte abnormalities, or renal insufficiency
  - Get accurate records of intake and output, weigh patient before and after
- General rule: 2000 to 2500 mL of 5% dextrose in normal saline or lactated Ringer's solution delivered daily
  - Do not add potassium during first 24 hours because K⁺ is already increased during surgery (stress) with increased aldosterone activity
  - Otherwise, 20 mEq of potassium added to each liter, only if good urine output
  - With exception of urine, body fluids are isosmolar
  - If external losses >1500 mL/d, electrolyte concentrations should be measured periodically and fluids compensated
  - Reevaluate IV fluid orders every 24 hours or more often if indicated
  - Replace postoperative ionized serum calcium in patients with thyroidectomy or parathyroidectomy
- **Indications for urinary catheter placement:** (1) anticipating long procedure, (2) performing urologic or low pelvic surgery, (3) need to monitor fluid balance

GASTROINTESTINAL DISORDERS

Disease	Etiology, Prevalence, and Risk Factors	Clinical Symptoms and Signs	Diagnostics	Therapy, Prognosis, and Health Maintenance
Postoperative ileus	Refers to obstipation and intolerance of oral intake after abdominal or nonabdominal surgery RF: 1. Prolonged abdominal or pelvic surgery 2. Lower GI surgery 3. Open surgery 4. Delayed nutrition or NG placement 5. Intraabdominal inflammation 6. Postoperative complications 7. Increased BMI 8. Anesthesia 9. Electrolyte imbalance 10. Narcotic use Motility returns hours to days postop • Small bowel: hours after • Colon: up to 2-3 d	1. Constipation (day 5) 2. Lack of flatus/BM 3. Abdominal distention 4. Bloating and gas 5. Nausea or vomiting 6. Inability to tolerate PO diet Signs: 1. Absent bowel sounds 2. Diffuse abdominal tenderness 3. +/– distention	1. CBC 2. Electrolytes • **Hypokalemia** (hyperpolarizes the resting membrane potential, decreasing nerve stimulation of GI tract) 3. BUN 4. LFTs 5. Amylase and lipase Imaging: 1. Abdominal XR: air in the colon and rectum, with no transition zone or free air (distinguishes from SBO) 2. **CT scan with gastrografin**—Must exclude mechanical obstruction	1. NPO 2. IV Fluid replacement, correct electrolytes 3. r/o SBO Prevention: 1. Limited opioid use 2. Early ambulation 3. Dietary supplements Health maintenance: 1. Follow-up imaging within 48-72 h if not improved or worsening
Adhesions	Common cause of SBO following surgery Most common cause of SBO in US	Hyperactive bowel sounds (tinkling)		

Disease	Etiology, Prevalence, and Risk Factors	Clinical Symptoms and Signs	Diagnostics	Therapy, Prognosis, and Health Maintenance
Small bowel obstruction	**MCC:** **Adhesions or hernias,** cancer, IBD, volvulus, intussusception RF: >2 abdominal surgeries	1. Abdominal pain 2. Distention 3. Vomiting of partially digested food 4. Obstipation Signs: 1. Dehydration + electrolyte imbalance 2. High pitched bowel sounds, come in rushes → silent bowls	1. KUB: air–fluid levels, multiple dilated bowel loops	1. NPO, nasogastric suction, IV fluids, monitoring Partial obstruction in hemo-stable patient → IV hydration and NG decompression 2. Pain management
Pseudomembranous colitis	*Clostridium difficile* Occurs secondary to **treatment with antibiotics** Mostly elderly hospitalized patients Relies on secretion of toxins A (enterotoxin) and B (cytotoxin) Occurs after use of broad spectrum penicillins, cephalosporins, and FQ Disruption of normal colonic flora Presents 2 d after initiation up to 2 wk after cessation	1. Mild **watery foul-smelling diarrhea** (>3 but <20 stools/d) 2. **Fever** (30%-50%), but lack of fever does not rule it out 3. Abdominal pain 4. Generalized constitutional symptoms	1. **PCR Identification** of *C. difficile* toxin or *C. difficile* toxin gene in stool—if patient has clinically significant diarrhea • Toxin B is clinically important 2. Culture from stool sample or rectal swab—for patients with ileus and suspected C. difficile infection • Most sensitive method, but cannot distinguish toxin producing strains from nontoxin producing 3. X-ray: severe inflammation of inner lining of bowel CBC: **Leukocytosis**	1. IV metronidazole OR 2. PO vancomycin (this is the only use for oral vancomycin) Prevention: • Strict hand washing • Enteric precautions • Minimize antibiotic use Complications: Bowel perforation, toxic megacolon
Constipation	Causes: anesthesia, ileus, pain, and narcotics	1. Abdominal pain and distention		1. Stool softener, fiber 2. Fluids
Acute peritonitis	Intraabdominal infection secondary to ruptured viscus Bacteria: aerobes and anaerobes	1. Acute abdominal pain 2. Fever Signs: 1. Guarding 2. Rigidity	1. CBC: leukocytosis 2. CXR and KUB show free air 3. CT scan if abscess suspected	Surgical exploration and repair 1. Peritoneal lavage or drainage 2. Drainage of wound/abscess 3. Broad spectrum antibiotics

POSTOPERATIVE PAIN

- The physiology of postoperative pain involves **transmission of pain impulses via splanchnic** (not vagal) **afferent fibers** to the central nervous system, where they initiate spinal, brainstem, and cortical reflexes

  - Spinal responses result from stimulation of neurons in the anterior horn, resulting in skeletal muscle spasm, vasospasm, and gastrointestinal ileus
  - Brain stem responses to pain include alterations in ventilation, blood pressure, and endocrine function
  - Cortical responses include voluntary movements and psychologic changes, such as fear and apprehension.

- These emotional responses facilitate nociceptive spinal transmission, lower the threshold for pain perception, and perpetuate the pain experience

- Pain following thoracic and upper abdominal operations, for example, causes voluntary and involuntary splinting of thoracic and abdominal muscles and the diaphragm. The patient may be reluctant to breathe deeply, promoting atelectasis. The limitation in motion due to pain predisposes to venous stasis, thrombosis, and embolism. Release of catecholamines and other stress hormones by postoperative pain causes vasospasm and hypertension, which may in turn lead to complications such as stroke, myocardial infarction, and bleeding. Prevention of postoperative pain is thus important for reasons other than the pain itself.

- Effective pain control may improve the outcome of major operations.
- **Opioids are the mainstay of therapy for postoperative pain.** Their analgesic effect is via two mechanisms: (1) A direct effect on opioid receptors, (2) Stimulation of a descending brain stem system that contributes to pain inhibition

- Opioids administered intramuscularly, while convenient, result in wide variations in plasma concentrations
- Frequently, the dose of opioid prescribed or administered is too small and too infrequent to alleviate all pain. When opioid usage is limited to temporary treatment of postoperative pain, drug addiction is extremely rare.

CHAPTER **69**

Gastrointestinal and Nutrition

General Surgery

ABDOMINAL PAIN

	RUQ	Epigastric	LUQ	Periumbilical	RLQ	Suprapubic	LLQ
Colonic	Colitis, diverticulitis			Early appendicitis	Appendicitis, colitis, diverticulitis, IBD, IBS	Appendicitis, colitis, diverticulitis, IBD, IBS	colitis, diverticulitis, IBD, IBS
Biliary	Cholecystitis, cholelithiasis, cholangitis	Cholecystitis, cholelithiasis, cholangitis					
Hepatic	Abscess, hepatitis, mass						
Pulm	Pneumonia, embolus						
Cardiac		MI, pericarditis	Angina, MI, pericarditis				
Vascular		Aortic dissection, mesenteric ischemia	Aortic dissection, mesenteric ischemia	Aortic dissection, mesenteric ischemia			
Pancreatic		Mass, pancreatitis	Mass, pancreatitis				
Renal	Nephrolithiasis, pyelonephritis		Nephrolithiasis, pyelonephritis		Nephrolithiasis, pyelonephritis	Nephrolithiasis, pyelonephritis, cystitis	Nephrolithiasis, pyelonephritis
Gastric		Esophagitis, gastritis, PUD	Esophagitis, gastritis, PUD	Esophagitis, gastritis, PUD, small bowel mass, obstruction			
GYN					Ectopic, fibroids, ovarian mass, torsion, PID Endometriosis	Ectopic, fibroids, ovarian mass, torsion, PID Endometriosis	Ectopic, fibroids, ovarian mass, torsion, PID Endometriosis
Primary test of choice	U/S	CT			CT with contrast	U/S	CT with oral and IV contrast

CONSTIPATION, OBSTIPATION, AND CHANGE IN BOWEL HABITS

- **Obstipation**: severe or complete constipation

SMALL BOWEL CARCINOMA (CARCINOID TUMORS)

- Barium esophagogram is obtained as the first study to evaluate the dysphagia
- Endoscopy with biopsy establishes the diagnosis

COLORECTAL CANCER (CRC)

Disease	Etiology, Prevalence, and Risk Factors	Clinical Symptoms and Signs	Diagnostics	Therapy, Prognosis, and Health Maintenance
Hereditary Nonpolyposis CRC: Without Adenomatous Polyps				
Lynch syndrome I (site-specific CRC)	**Autosomal dominant** Early onset CRC Absence of antecedent multiple polyposis		1. **Amsterdam criteria** "3-2-1" rule: 3 affected members, 2 generations, 1 under age 50 2. **Bethesda criteria**: developed to identify individuals with CRC who should undergo tumor testing for microsatellite instability (MSI)	
Lynch syndrome II (cancer family syndrome)	All features of Lynch 1 plus increased number and early occurrence of other cancers • Brain • Skin • Stomach, *CRC* • Pancreas • Biliary tract • Ovary, endometrium, Breast	1. SX of colorectal cancer • GI bleed, abdominal pain, change in bowel habits 2. Extracolonic manifestations: **endometrial cancer** (MC)	1. Amsterdam I criteria • 3+ relatives with histologically verified Lynch syndrome (one must be first degree relative) • Lynch syndrome associated cancers involving at least 2 generations • 1+ cancer diagnosed before age 50	
Rectal cancer	20%-30% of all CRCs	• Hematochezia (most common) • Tenesmus: constantly feel like you have to go • Rectal mass; feeling of incomplete evacuation of stool		

PANCREATIC PSEUDOCYST

Disease	Etiology, Prevalence, and Risk Factors	Clinical Symptoms and Signs	Diagnostics	Therapy, Prognosis, and Health Maintenance
Pancreatic pseudocyst	Patients with chronic pancreatitis from alcohol usage or gallstones are at risk 10% occur after acute pancreatitis Collection of fluid surrounded by granulation tissue If it communicates with the pancreatic ductal system, it can contain digestive enzymes; does not contain epithelial lining (not cystic lesion of the pancreas)	1. Persistent abdominal pain, anorexia, or **abdominal mass after pancreatitis** 2. Jaundice or sepsis from infection (rare) Physical exam: 1. Tender abdomen 2. **Palpable abdominal mass** 3. Peritoneal signs suggesting rupture 4. Fever 5. Scleral icterus 6. **Pleural effusion (common)**	1. **CT scan** (standard) 2. ERCP–not for diagnosis, but useful for drainage Labs: 1. Serum amylase and lipase: elevated, limited use 2. Serum bilirubin and LFTs: elevated, limited use 3. Cyst fluid analysis: CEA, CEA-125, fluid viscosity, amylase (all low)	1. Supportive care only–MOST 2. Drainage for–complications, symptoms, possible malignancy • **Percutaneous catheter drainage** (preferred) • ERCP • Surgical drainage (standard) 10% become infected, but can also rupture causing peritonitis or death Poor prognostic factors: size of cyst and duration of presence Outpatient monitoring: if stents placed, monitor with serial CT scans to observe resolution

ANORECTAL ABSCESS

- Goodsall's Rule:
  - All fistula tracts with external openings within 3 cm of the anal verge and posterior to a line drawn through the ischial spines travel in a curvilinear fashion to the posterior midline.
  - All tracks with external openings anterior to this line enter the anal canal in a radial fashion

- Complex fistulas: Extrasphincteric or high fistulas proximal to dentate line; women with anterior fistulas; fistulas with multiple tracts; recurrent fistulas; fistulas related to IBD, TB, HIV, or radiation treatment; history of anal incontinence; rectovaginal fistulas

- Parks described four types of anorectal fistulas (see Fig. 3-3) that originate from cryptoglandular infections. Fistulas can have a complicated anatomy with one or more extensions and accessory tracts. The original Parks' classification did not include a superficial fistula tract.

- **Type 1** is an intersphincteric fistula that travels along the intersphincteric plane.
- **Type 2** is a transsphincteric fistula that encompasses a portion of the internal and external sphincter.
- **Type 3** is a suprasphincteric fistula that encompasses the entire sphincter apparatus.
- **Type 4** is an extrasphincteric fistula that extends from a primary opening in the rectum, encompasses the entire sphincter apparatus, and opens onto the skin overlying the buttock

HEMORRHOIDS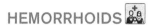

BARIATRIC SURGERY

		BMI (kg/m²)	Indications
Class I	Obesity	>30-34.9	
Class II	Severe obesity	**>35-39.9**	Surgical intervention if severe weight related conditions: diabetes, hypertension, debilitating osteoarthritis, sleep apnea
Class III	Morbid obesity	>40 or greater	Surgical intervention with or without comorbidities

- Complications of obesity: OSA, hypertension, CAD, non-alcoholic fatty liver disease, adult-onset diabetes mellitus, pseudotumor cerebri
- Unfavorable prognostic elements (for surgery) include BMI ≥50 kg/m², male sex, hypertension, PE risks (eg, presence of a VTE event, prior inferior vena cava filter placement, history of right heart failure or pulmonary hypertension, findings of venous stasis disease), and age ≥45 years
- Bariatric surgeons typically enforce a preoperative regimen of weight reduction before proceeding with surgery to enhance outcomes and to assure the patient's commitment to the process
- Contraindications
  - Patients with unstable angina, end-stage pulmonary disease, or cirrhosis
  - Unstable psychological disease: uncontrolled schizophrenia or bipolar, recent suicide attempt, current eating disorder
  - Chronic steroid use

- Chronic NSAID use (tramadol, Tylenol)
- Preoperative evaluation
  - Testing: EKG, CMP, CBC
  - Psychology clearance
  - PCP clearance if medical issues not severe enough to warrant specialist
  - Cardiology clearance: age 60+, history of cardiac disease, hypertension, or diabetes age 50+
  - Severe GERD or hiatal hernia history—upper GI or EGD
  - History of GI bleed or colonic issues—colonoscopy
  - Specialist clearances for individuals with significant disease
- Perioperative diet
  - Fasting: 2 weeks before surgery, high protein shakes, 1 sensible meal
  - Phase I: day before to 2 weeks postop; full liquid diet (protein shakes and zero calorie beverages)
  - Phase II: 2 to 5 weeks postop; full liquids and 1 cup soft foods
  - Phase III: 4 to 6 weeks postop; solid foods

	Mechanism	Indications	Adverse Effects or Complications	Follow-up and Prognosis
Roux-en-Y gastric bypass (RYGB)	**Restrictive and malabsorptive** procedure involving bypass of most of the stomach, entire duodenum, and 100-150 cm of small intestine Pouch is restrictive, causing fullness Roux limb: limits amount of absorption	BMI >35	Dumping syndrome	Mortality: 1/500
Vertical sleeve gastrectomy (VSG)	**Restrictive** and hormonal Reduces stomach to <25% of original volume by resection of a large portion along greater curvature including entire fundus Ghrelin made in fundus → decreased with removal	BMI >35	Lack of hunger 1-2 y Barium swallow	70% estimated weight loss at 2 y Hospital stay: 2 nights Return to work: 3 wk Mortality: 1/2000
Adjustable gastric banding (ABG), lap-band	Restrictive	BMI >30-35 with comorbid conditions, but insurance does not cover this Ideal: Volume eater, no sweets, no liquid calories Trains you to eat and chew slower	Regurgitation Must see annually for upper GI (barium swallow) checking for band slippage, **prolapse,** and dilation	Less operative risk, but less average weight loss Must repair hiatal hernias before Hospital stay: 1 night Return to work: 1-2 wk

Short-term Complications

- Nausea and vomiting (most common, 30% to 40%)
- Dehydration
- Wound infections
- Pulmonary embolism/DVT
- **Anastomotic leak** (sleeve and bypass): tachycardia, tachypnea, fever, pain, leukocytosis
  - Persistent leaks require conversion from sleeve to RYGB

Long-term Complications

- Vitamin deficiencies (bypass): iron, folate, B12, thiamine, calcium, vitamin D (check annually)
- Ventral hernia formation (open approach)
- Pouch ulcer (10% after RYGB)—PPI therapy and smoking cessation, no NSAIDs
- Internal hernia formation through mesenteric defects with risk of bowel compromise is delayed complication after RYGB, especially in patients with good weight loss → colicky abdominal pain
- Small bowel obstruction from adhesions
- Lap band slippage → nausea, vomiting for up to 4 months
- Erosion
- Pouch and esophageal dilation
- Prolapse
- Port complication
- Reoperation

Postop Care and Complications

- Avoid NSAIDs, steroids, and smoking = increased risk of erosions and leaks

Benefits

- Remission of type 2 diabetes
- Reduces inflammatory mediators (angiotensinogen, transforming growth factor, tumor necrosis factor, interleukin-6) which may lead to development of diabetes, hypertension, dyslipidemia, and thromboembolic events
- Most decrease in Ghrelin levels with sleeve gastrectomy, some gastric bypass, but not in lap bands
  - Ghrelin responsible for increased appetite

Nonsurgical Management

- Behavioral modification—limited efficacy and sustainability
- Pharmacotherapy for weight loss is better than diet alone as many will regain weight and hunger will return
- Bariatric surgery has the best cost-benefit ratio and is considered weight loss treatment of choice by NIH for patients with severe obesity (class II or higher)

Sibutramine (Meridia)	Blocks presynaptic uptake of NE and serotonin Anorexia effect on CNS
Orlistat (Xenical)	Inhibits pancreatic lipase and 30% of fat absorption
Phentermine (Adipex)	Appetite suppressant Tend to regain weight within 1 y if patient stops medication

Disease	Etiology, Prevalence, and Risk Factors	Clinical Symptoms and Signs	Diagnostics	Therapy, Prognosis, and Health Maintenance
Dumping syndrome	Late complication of post-gastrectomy patients Sugars → rapid fluid shifts	1. **Abdominal cramping, diarrhea**—shortly after meals (especially meals high in sugar) 2. **Nausea**, vomiting 3. **Palpitations** 4. Lightheadedness 5. **Diaphoresis**		Health maintenance: 1. Check vitamin D, B$_{12}$, and folate annually

HERNIAS

- A **reducible hernia** is one in which the contents of the sac return to the abdomen spontaneously or with manual pressure when the patient is recumbent.
- An **irreducible (incarcerated) hernia** is one whose contents cannot be returned to the abdomen, usually because they are trapped by a narrow neck. The term "incarceration" does not imply obstruction, inflammation, or ischemia of the herniated organs, though incarceration is necessary for obstruction or strangulation to occur.
- Compromise to the blood supply of the contents of the sac (eg, omentum or intestine) results in a **strangulated hernia**, in which gangrene of the contents of the sac has occurred

- The **Hesselbach triangle** is bounded by the inguinal ligament, the inferior epigastric vessels, and the lateral border of the rectus muscle
- Nerves and vasculature
  - Iliohypogastric nerve (T12, L1) emerges from lateral edge of psoas muscle and travels inside external oblique, emerging medial to external inguinal ring to innervate suprapubic skin
  - **Ilioinguinal nerve** (L1) parallels iliohypogastric nerve—travels on surface of spermatic cord to innervate base of penis (mons pubis), scrotum (labia majora), and medial thigh—most frequently injured in anterior open inguinal repairs

- **Genitofemoral** (L1, L2) and **lateral femoral cutaneous nerves** (L2, L3) travel on and lateral to psoas muscle and provide sensation to scrotum and anteromedial thigh and to lateral thigh, respectively → subject to injury during laparoscopic repairs
- Femoral nerve (L2 to L4) travels from lateral edge of psoas, extends lateral to femoral vessels
- External iliac artery—travels along medial aspect of psoas muscle beneath inguinal ligament, gives off inferior epigastric artery, bordering medial side of internal inguinal ring
- Risk factors
  - Marked obesity, abdominal strain from heavy exercise or lifting, cough, constipation with straining at stool, and prostatism with straining on micturition
  - Other RF: cirrhosis with ascites, pregnancy, chronic ambulatory peritoneal dialysis, enlarged pelvic organs or tumors

Types of Hernia Repair

- Bassini repair—most widely used method
  - Conjoined tendon is approximated to the Poupart ligament and spermatic cord remains in its normal anatomic position under the external oblique aponeurosis

- Halsted repair—places external oblique underneath the cord, but otherwise same as Bassini
- Lotheissen-McVay—brings conjoined tendon farther posteriorly and inferiorly to the Cooper ligament; effective for femoral hernia
- The most widely used technique is that of Lichtenstein, an open mesh repair that allows an early return to normal activities and a low complication and recurrence rate.
- Long-term hernia recurrence is equivalent with open and laparoscopic mesh repairs at approximately 4%
- Specific indications for laparoscopic procedures: repair of recurrent hernias after anterior open repairs, repair of bilateral hernias simultaneously, and repair in patients who must return to work particularly quickly

Recommendations for Hiatal Hernia Repairs by the SAGES (Society of American Gastrointestinal and Endoscopic Surgeons)

- In absence of reflux disease, repair of type I hernia is unnecessary
- All symptomatic paraesophageal hernias (types II-IV) should be repaired, especially in presence of acute obstructive symptoms or volvulus
- The laparoscopic approach is as effective as the open approach; mesh is preferred to reduce recurrence rates

CHAPTER **70**

Cardiology

General Surgery

DYSPNEA ON EXERTION

- **Dyspnea** (per American Thoracic Society): "a term used to characterize a subjective experience of breathing discomfort that is comprised of qualitatively distinct sensations that vary in intensity. The experience derives from interactions among multiple physiological, psychological, social, and environmental factors, and may induce secondary physiological and behavioral responses."

- The peripheral chemoreceptors, located in the carotid bodies and aortic arch, sense changes in the partial pressure of oxygen in arterial blood and are also stimulated by acidosis and hypercapnia. The central chemoreceptors, located in the medulla, respond to changes in pH and arterial tension of carbon dioxide ($PaCO_2$).

- Clues to the need for an urgent evaluation include heart rate >120 beats/minute, respiratory rate >30 breaths/minute, pulse oxygen saturation (SpO_2) <90%, use of accessory respiratory muscles, difficulty speaking in full sentences, stridor, asymmetric breath sounds or percussion, diffuse crackles, diaphoresis, and cyanosis

Cardiovascular Causes	Respiratory Causes
1. Acute myocardial infarction 2. Heart failure 3. Cardiac tamponade	1. Bronchospasm 2. Pulmonary embolism 3. Pneumothorax 4. Pulmonary infection 5. Upper airway obstruction

History and Physical Examination in the Emergent Setting

History	Physical
1. PMH: new or recurrent, preexisting conditions, medication list 2. Events leading up to episode (recent symptoms), triggers (medication noncompliance or diet noncompliance, exposure to cold or allergen, onset after eating a particular food, new onset cough, recent surgery or immobilization, trauma 3. Prior intubation 4. Time course (sudden or insidious) 5. Severity 6. Associated: chest pain, trauma, fever, hemoptysis, sputum, cough 7. Tobacco or drug use 8. Psychiatric conditions	<u>Danger signs:</u> 1. Depressed mental status 2. Inability to maintain respiratory effort 3. Cyanosis 4. Tachypnea 5. Tripod position 6. Diaphoresis 7. Use of accessory muscles 8. Stridor or wheezing <u>Severe respiratory distress:</u> 1. Retractions 2. Fragmented speech 3. Inability to lie supine 4. Profound diaphoresis 5. Agitation or other AMS <u>Other:</u> 1. Peripheral edema 2. Heart murmur 3. Pulsus paradoxus Crackles, augmented breath sounds

Workup in the Emergent Setting for Acute Dyspnea

1. EKG and CXR

2. Ancillary testing: cardiac biomarkers, ultrasound, BNP, D-dimer, ABG/VBG, CO2 monitoring, chest CT or VQ Scan, Peak flow and PFTs

Management

1. Oxygen provided

2. Establish IV access and obtain blood for measurements

3. EKG and pulse oximetry monitoring

4. Airway management

5. Establish most likely cause of dyspnea and initiate further treatment

CHAPTER **71**

Endocrinology

 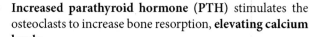
TREMORS

- DDx: Hyperthyroidism, thyrotoxicosis

FATIGUE

Difficulty or inability to initiate activity and is a perception of generalized weakness. See chapter 47.

- Other definitions: easy fatigability (or reduced capacity to maintain activity)
- Associated with: concentration and memory difficulties, emotional fatigue/stability

PALPITATIONS

- DDx: Hyperthyroidism, Pheochromocytoma

HEAT AND COLD INTOLERANCE

- Heat Intolerance DDx: hyperthyroidism
- Cold Intolerance DDx: myxedema (hypothyroidism)

HYPERPARATHYROIDISM

- **Increased parathyroid hormone (PTH)** stimulates the osteoclasts to increase bone resorption, **elevating calcium levels**
  - Works in the kidney to increase calcium reabsorption
  - Increases renal excretion of phosphorous
  - Hematocrit unaffected by parathyroid hormone
  - Causes a proximal renal tubular acidosis (a **hyperchloremic metabolic acidosis**), increasing bicarbonate loss

- **High calcium levels**
  - **Suppresses PTH** secretion (be aware that a normal PTH level is 'abnormal' in the setting of high calcium levels)
  - Can cause **nephrogenic diabetes insipidus** as the renal tubule becomes unresponsive to the action of ADH
  - Asymptomatic patients with primary hyperparathyroidism have defects in their ability to concentrate urine
- **Indications for surgery in asymptomatic patients with primary hyperparathyroidism:**
  - Markedly elevated serum calcium (*above 12.0 mg/dL*)
  - History of life-threatening hypercalcemia
  - Reduced creatinine clearance (below 30% for age-matched normals)
  - *Nephrolithiasis*
  - Markedly elevated 24-hour urinary calcium excretion (above 400 mg)
  - Reduced bone mass as measured by direct measurement (more than 2 standard deviations below age-matched normals)
- **Surgery should be strongly considered in the following circumstances**: (1) the patient desires surgery; (2) meticulous, long-term follow-ups are unlikely; (3) coexistent illness complicates management; and (4) the patient is young (younger than age 50 years)
- Most (80%) hyperparathyroidism cases are caused by a single adenoma and removal of the offending gland is curative
  - When hyperplasia is identified, most surgeons remove 3.5 glands, marking the remaining portion of gland so it can be identified if necessary in the future

General Surgery

- After **parathyroidectomy**, patients should be watched closely for **72 hours for signs of hypocalcemia.**
  - Nervousness, tingling, and a positive Chvostek or Trousseau sign may indicate hypocalcemia, which should be confirmed by total or **ionized serum calcium levels (more reliable)**

- Only supplement if total calcium <8 mg/dL
- Persistent hypocalcemia—give 1000 to 1200 mg daily
- Complications of thyroid or parathyroid surgery include recurrent laryngeal nerve (RLN) injury, which manifests as hoarseness of voice (if unilateral) or airway obstruction (if bilateral), hypoparathyroidism, and neck hematoma

HYPERTHYROIDISM

THYROID NODULES AND CANCER

Disease	Etiology, Prevalence, and Risk Factors	Clinical Symptoms and Signs	Diagnostics	Therapy, Prognosis, and Health Maintenance
Postoperative hypoparathyroidism	Results after total thyroidectomy, thyroid lobectomy, and some parathyroid surgeries	1. Extremity paresthesias 2. Progressive severe muscle cramps	1. Hypocalcemia	1. PO calcium

ADRENAL CARCINOMA AND ADRENAL INSUFFICIENCY

- **Hyperpigmentation** is most pronounced in skin areas exposed to increased friction or shear stress and is increased by sunlight

- **Hyponatremia** is primarily caused by mineralocorticoid deficiency but can also occur in secondary adrenal insufficiency due to diminished inhibition of antidiuretic hormone (ADH) release by cortisol, resulting in mild syndrome of inappropriate secretion of antidiuretic hormone (SIADH)

Disease	Etiology, Prevalence, and Risk Factors	Clinical Symptoms and Signs	Diagnostics	Therapy, Prognosis, and Health Maintenance
Adrenal carcinoma	Rare Excess production of steroids and adrenal androgen precursors	1. Cushing syndrome-like presentation 2. Virilization	1. CT with contrast 2. FNA not indicated	1. Early detection and complete surgical removal (adrenalectomy) 2. Adjuvant treatment with mitotane (especially if >8 cm, vascular invasion or Ki67 index >10%) 3. Steroid replacement 4. Metastasis: liver and lung

PHEOCHROMOCYTOMA

ACROMEGALY

MULTIPLE ENDOCRINE NEOPLASIA (MEN)

- Inherited condition: propensity to develop multiple endocrine tumors

- Autosomal dominant inheritance with incomplete penetrance
- MEN2: Suspect in any patients with medullary thyroid carcinoma or pheochromocytoma, especially when it occurs at young age (<35 years), are multicentric, or when more than 1 family member affected

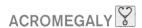

Disease	Etiology, Prevalence, and Risk Factors	Clinical Symptoms and Signs	Diagnostics	Therapy, Prognosis, and Health Maintenance
MEN type I (Wermer syndrome)	Rare, autosomal dominant disorder with the 3P characteristics below M:F is 1:1, most show characteristics by age 40-50 y 3 Ps: Characteristics: 1. **Parathyroid** hyperplasia (90%): nephrolithiasis, secondary to hyper-parathyroidism; initial manifestation in most patients 2. **Pancreatic** islet cell tumors (66%)—greatest risk of malignant transformation 3. Anterior **pituitary** tumors (66%)—bilateral temporal hemianopsia MC type: Lactotroph Prevalence: 0.002%	1. Nephrolithiasis 2. Amenorrhea 3. Galactorrhea 4. Growth abnormalities 5. Cushingoid changes 6. Headache 7. Vision changes 8. Erectile dysfunction 9. Peptic ulcer disease 10. Diarrhea 11. Neuroglycopenic or sympathoadrenal symptoms from hypoglycemia Associated: 1. Gastrinomas (ZES), which cause peptic ulcer disease; MC found in duodenum 2. Thymic or bronchial carcinoid tumors 3. Enterochromaffin cell-like gastric tumors 4. Adrenocortical adenomas 5. Lipomas 6. Angiofibromas 7. Angiomyolipomas 8. Spinal cord ependymomas	Clinical DX: 1. Requires at least 2+ primary MEN1 tumor types 2. If (+) family history of MEN1, requires at least 1+ MEN1 tumor types Labs: 1. Hypercalcemia—most detected incidentally 2. PTH elevated 3. Prolactin—check to r/o pituitary adenoma	1. Parathyroidectomy • Indications: symptomatic Hypercalcemia, nephrolithiasis, evidence of bone disease • Subtotal (3.5 gland) parathyroidectomy 2. Zollinger Ellison Syndrome • PPI therapy • Duodenal pancreatic surgery 3. MEN1 and insulinomas • Local excision of tumors found in head of pancreas with distal subtotal pancreatectomy Health maintenance: No data to show benefit in screening family members of patients (+) for MEN1
Classical MEN type 2A	M = F Rare, most common MEN2 variant 100% penetrance Characteristics: 1. **Medullary thyroid carcinoma (100%)** = thyroid adenomas 2. Pheochromocytoma (40%) 3. Primary hyperparathyroidism (50%)	1. Medullary thyroid cancer • solitary thyroid nodule • cervical lymphadenopathy 2. Pheochromocytoma • Attacks (paroxysms) of anxiety, headache, diaphoresis, palpitations, tachycardia 3. Primary HPT • Mild, asymptomatic • Kidney stones, symptomatic hypercalcemia, bone loss, major hypercalciuria Associated: 1. Hirschsprung Disease 2. Cutaneous lichen amyloidosis	Clinical DX: 1. Suspect in any patient with • Medullary thyroid cancer **OR** • Pheochromocytoma 2. Young age <35 3. Multicentric 4. Affected family member Labs: 1. Abnormally high or Normal PTH in setting of Hypercalcemia (Serum calcium) 2. Plasma fractionated metanephrines—r/o pheochromocytoma • If (+), measure serum calcitonin and obtain thyroid and neck ultrasound—r/o thyroid carcinoma 3. *RET* mutation genetic analysis	1. **Total thyroidectomy**—as early as the neonatal period • Serial monitoring of serum calcitonin and CEA • Thyroid hormone therapy to maintain euthyroidism • Prophylactic central lymph node dissection 2. **Bilateral or unilateral adrenalectomy** for pheochromocytoma 3. Hyperparathyroidism • If asymptomatic, defer surgery • Supportive measures and monitoring for hypercalcemia, renal impairment, and bone loss every 1-2 y • If symptomatic • Parathyroid surgery with resection of visibly enlarged glands only is recommended Health maintenance: 1. **Screen for pheochromocytoma** in all patients with medullary thyroid cancer; **if found, remove BEFORE thyroidectomy** 2. If screening tests for pheochromocytoma negative, evaluate annually 3. If serum calcium normal, measure annually

(continued)

General Surgery

(continued)

Disease	Etiology, Prevalence, and Risk Factors	Clinical Symptoms and Signs	Diagnostics	Therapy, Prognosis, and Health Maintenance
MEN type 2B	Occurs in 8%-15% of all MEN2 patients Autosomal dominant Characteristics: 1. Mucosal neuromas (100%): nasopharynx, oropharynx, larynx, conjunctiva 2. **Medullary thyroid carcinoma (85%)** 3. Marfanoid body habitus 4. Pheochromocytoma (50%)	1. Chronic constipation 2. Mucosal neuromas of the lips and tongue 3. Intestinal ganglioneuromas 4. Developmental abnormalities 5. Kyphoscoliosis or lordosis 6. Joint laxity 7. Marfanoid habitus 8. Myelinated corneal nerves Associated 1. Megacolon	Clinical DX as above Diagnostic studies as above	As above 1. **Total thyroidectomy**—as early as the neonatal period • Often NOT curative Prognosis: Onset at earlier age than MEN2A and more aggressive course than MEN2A

CHAPTER 72

Dermatology

Refer to Family Medicine for In-depth Coverage of the Following Topics:

Cellulitis, p 156

Drug Eruptions, see Erythema Multiforme, Stevens Johnson Syndrome, Toxic Epidermal Necrolysis, p 132

Urticaria, p 132

Pressure Ulcers, p 164

Basal Cell Carcinoma, p 145

Melanoma/Malignant Melanoma, see Melanoma, p 146

Refer to Pediatrics for In-depth Coverage of the Following Topics:

Burns, See Pediatrics, p 189

Recommended Supplemental Topics:

Erysipelas, p 157

Acute Paronychia, p 151

Methicillin-resistant *Staphylococcus aureus*, see Burns below, p 637

Pseudomonas Burn Infection, see Burns below, p 637

RASH AND REDNESS (ERYTHEMA)

- Difficult to diagnose, especially if generalized; it is easier to generate a broad differential diagnosis to guide diagnostic studies and rule out as many diseases as possible to eliminate unnecessary workup and to prevent delay in effective treatment

- Decide whether to observe and treat empirically, perform diagnostic testing, or refer to dermatology for workup

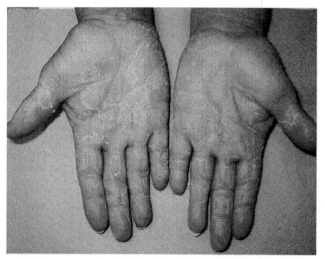

FIGURE 72-1. Contact dermatitis. Note the scaling of this irritant contact dermatitis seen in a health care worker. (Image provided by Stedman's.)

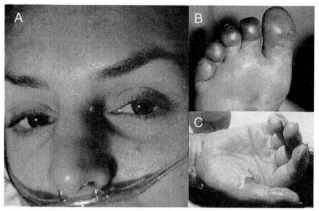

FIGURE 72-2. Toxic shock syndrome. **A.** Appearance of the rash associated with staphylococcal toxic shock syndrome (TSS). **B.** Gangrenous toes associated with prolonged hypotension in TSS. **C.** Desquamation of the skin that occurs during the resolution of TSS. (From Engleberg NC, Dermody T, DiRita V. *Schaechter's Mechanisms of Microbial Disease*. Philadelphia: Wolters Kluwer Health; 2013.)

Disease	Etiology, Prevalence, and Risk Factors	Clinical Symptoms and Signs	Diagnostics	Therapy, Prognosis, and Health Maintenance
Contact dermatitis (Fig. 72-1)	**Irritant:** Nonimmune modulated skin irritation caused by skin injury, direct cytotoxic effects, or cutaneous inflammation from contact with irritant **Allergic:** *Type IV, T-cell mediated, delayed hypersensitivity* reaction from foreign substance <u>MC:</u> Poison ivy, nickel, fragrances	1. Not painful, but **red** and itchy 2. Onset after contact with irritant or allergen 3. Distribution patterns from irritant or allergen <u>Signs:</u> 1. **Scaly** occurring on thin areas of skin (flexural surfaces, eyelids, face, anogenital region) 2. Acute = Erythema, vesicles, and bullae 3. Chronic = lichenification with cracks and fissures	1. Determine if problem resolves with removal of substance	1. Localized = mid- or high-potency topical steroids (triamcinolone 0.1%/Kenalog or clobetasol 0.05%) If >20% of BSA, systemic steroids recommended with resolution in 12-24 h 5-7 days of prednisone 0.5-1 mg/kg/day
Drug exposure or eruption	See next page			
Urticaria	See next page			

(continued)

(continued)

Disease	Etiology, Prevalence, and Risk Factors	Clinical Symptoms and Signs	Diagnostics	Therapy, Prognosis, and Health Maintenance
Staphylococcal toxic shock syndrome (TSS) (Fig. 72-2)	Result of capillary leak and tissue damage from release of inflammatory cytokines induced by group A streptococcus (GAS) *Staphylococcus aureus* strains produce exotoxins, though isolation not necessary for diagnosis Caused by toxic shock syndrome toxin-1 (TSST-1) 50% of cases are menstrual related (tampon use) *Nonmenstrual* cases are associated with **surgical** or cesarean section **wound infections, breast augmentation, septorhinoplasty,** hysterectomy, **osteomyelitis,** liposuction, bunionectomy, bone pinning, **burns,** Onset of surgical cases: **within 2 d** postop up to 65 d postop May occur with deep seated infections (osteomyelitis) or bacteremia	Preceding: pain and site of minor trauma (bruise, strained muscle, sprained ankle) 1. Fever 2. Flu-like symptoms: Chills, malaise, myalgias, fatigue 3. Abdominal pain, vomiting, severe watery diarrhea 4. Dizziness or syncope 5. **Rash** 6. Sore throat Signs: 1. Fever >38.9°C (102°F) 2. Hypotension 3. Diffuse macular erythroderma 4. Desquamation (may be delayed onset) of palms or soles 5. Decreased UOP 6. Severe watery diarrhea 7. Cyanosis 8. Peripheral edema 9. Neurologic: somnolence, confusion, irritability, agitation, hallucinations Complications: 1. Irreversible respiratory failure 2. Coagulation defects 3. Cardiac arrhythmias 4. Cardiomyopathy	1. Pelvic exam with speculum—r/o foreign material in vaginal canal and remove 2. CK: 2 × ULN 3. BUN or SCr >2× ULN 4. U/A: pyuria (>5 WBC/HPF) in absence of UTI 5. Bilirubin or AST/ALT >2× ULN 6. CBC: platelets <100k/uL, mild leukocytosis with left shift 7. Blood and CSF cultures 8. Serologic tests for RMSF, leptospirosis, measles DX: 1. Fever >38.9°C 2. Hypotension 3. Diffuse erythema 4. Desquamation (may be delayed onset) 5. Involvement of at least 3 organ systems • Renal dysfunction • Coagulopathy • Liver dysfunction • ARDS • Macular rash • Soft tissue necrosis (necrotizing fasciitis, myositis, gangrene)	1. Supportive care 2. IVF Replacement • May required 10-20 L/d due to intractable hypotension and diffuse capillary leak • May utilize pressors if needed 3. **Debridement**—In surgical patients, infected wounds may not appear infected due to a decreased inflammatory response, but should be investigated 4. Antibiotics • IV **clindamycin** every 8 h (empiric) 5. PLUS **vancomycin** × 2 wk minimum • If MSSA (+), Clindamycin PLUS Oxacillin or Nafcillin • If MRSA (+), Clindamycin PLUS Vancomycin or Linezolid Health maintenance: Nasal cultures; if positive, treat with topic mupirocin for prophylaxis Prognosis: Death-associated TSS occurs within first days of admission, but occurs as late as 2 wk after admission

DISCHARGE

- Depending on location and onset after surgery, a wide differential must be considered, which includes the following:
- Paronychia
- Pressure or decubitus ulcers—see below

CELLULITIS

Disease	Etiology, Prevalence, and Risk Factors	Clinical Symptoms and Signs	Diagnostics	Therapy, Prognosis, and Health Maintenance
Necrotizing fasciitis	Affects young, healthy patients RF: Increased age, immunocompromised, chronic illness, alcoholism, and IV drug use Arises at sites of recent tattoos Pathogens: **Group A B-hemolytic strep** Pathophysiology not fully understood, but bacteria produce enzymes that degrade fascia and allow rapid proliferation of bacteria → local thrombosis, progressive ischemia, liquefaction necrosis, superficial gangrene	1. Early (stage 1): painful at first then swelling, **erythema,** warmth, tenderness, resembles cellulitis • Constitutional sx: high fever, toxicity 2. Stage 2: **Induration worsens, bullae develop** 3. Stage 3: skin color becomes purple, frank cutaneous gangrene • No longer tender, nonpainful	1. XR: subcutaneous air caused by gas-forming organisms within the fascia	1. **Urgent irrigation and debridement** 2. Antibiotics • PCN G 3. Adjunctive therapies: hyperbaric oxygen

Disease	Etiology, Prevalence, and Risk Factors	Clinical Symptoms and Signs	Diagnostics	Therapy, Prognosis, and Health Maintenance
Type I necrotizing fasciitis	Mix of facultative and anaerobic microbes Cause: Delivery into SQ tissue after surgery, trauma, bowel perforation, IV drug abuse Most common form (90%), most often in diabetics or immunocompromised Bacteroides–suspect in diabetics	1. Crepitus often develops	1. Open surgical exploration with direct visualization and palpation of necrotic fascia: grayish, nonbleeding, foul smelling discharge	1. Urgent debridement 2. Antibiotics • PCN G 3. Adjunctive therapies: hyperbaric oxygen
Gangrenous cellulitis	Pathogens: **Clostridium perfringens** → large spore forming gram (+) bacilli	Necrotic ulcer at site of abdominal or thoracic lesions or fistulous tracts • Inadequately debrided wounds, needle stick, or surgery • Insidious onset, within 1-2 wk of procedure		1. Urgent debridement 2. Antibiotics • PCN G 3. Adjunctive therapies: hyperbaric oxygen

BURNS

- Most common species in burn-wound infections: *Pseudomonas aeruginosa* and Methicillin-resistant *Staphylococcus aureus* (most common)
- **Zone of coagulation**: most severely burned portion and is typically in the center of the wound; likely needs excision and grafting
- **Zone of stasis**: peripheral to the zone of coagulation with variable degrees of vasoconstriction and resultant ischemia, much like a second-degree burn
- **Zone of hyperemia**, which heals with minimal to no scarring and is most like a superficial or first-degree burn

- Appropriate resuscitation and wound care may help prevent conversion to a deeper wound, but infection or suboptimal perfusion may result in an increase in burn depth
- Burn wounds evolve over the 48 to 72 hours after injury
- One of the most effective ways **to determine burn depth** is **full-thickness biopsy**, but this has several limitations
  - The procedure painful and potentially scarring
  - Accurate interpretation of the histopathology requires a specialized pathologist and may have slow turnaround times
- **Prognosis** is directly related to the extent of injury both **size and depth**

SQUAMOUS CELL CARCINOMA AND MELANOMA

Disease	Etiology, Prevalence, and Risk Factors	Clinical Symptoms and Signs	Diagnostics	Therapy, Prognosis, and Health Maintenance
Squamous cell carcinoma	Higher mortality and metastasis Second most common skin cancer RF: Sunlight exposure, actinic keratosis, chronic skin damage, immunosuppressive therapy	Pink, red, or skin colored papule, plaque, or nodule Well-circumscribed with **central ulceration and crust** Exophytic, indurated, friable No overlying telangiectasia Vary in appearance	1. If **deep shave biopsy (+)** → Complete excisional removal	1. **Complete excisional removal** 4-mm margin: for low-risk tumors <2 cm 6-mm margin: for large tumors, high risk, extension into SQ and high-risk locations (ear, lip, scalp, eyelid, nose) Higher likelihood of metastasis, but slower than melanoma 95% cure rate if completely excised Poor prognosis if lymph node involvement or thickness >6 mm

- **Mohs surgery indications**
  - Lesions larger than 2 cm
  - Lesions with ill-defined clinical borders
  - Lesions with aggressive histologic subtypes
- Recurrent lesions
- Lesions on or near the eye, nose, ear, mouth, hair-bearing scalp
- Chronic ulcers

CHAPTER 73

Neurology and Neurosurgery

Refer to Family Medicine 👥 for In-depth Coverage of the Following Topics:

Change in Vision or Speech, refer to Senile Cataract, Amaurosis Fugax, Retinal Detachment, Retinal Vascular Occlusion, Age-related Macular Degeneration, p 93

Refer to Internal Medicine 🩺 for In-depth Coverage of the Following Topics:

Motor and/or Sensory Loss, refer to Multiple Sclerosis, Guillain-Barre, p 245

Refer to Emergency Medicine for In-depth Coverage of the Following Topics:

Motor and/or Sensory Loss, refer to Spinal Cord Injury, p 415

Change in Vision or Speech, refer to Temporal Arteritis 🩺, p 252

Subarachnoid Hemorrhage, p 410

Acute Epidural and Subdural Hematoma, p 414

Recommended Supplemental Topics:

Autonomic Dysreflexia, p 642

Peroneal Nerve Palsy, p 639

MOTOR AND/OR SENSORY LOSS 🩺

- Refer to amyotrophic lateral sclerosis, upper and lower motor neuron disorders, spinal cord injury, multiple sclerosis, Guillain-Barre

- The approach to any patient with sensory loss is localizing the lesion using information from both your history and your physical examination

Disease	Etiology, Prevalence, and Risk Factors	Clinical Symptoms and Signs	Diagnostics	Therapy, Prognosis, and Health Maintenance

Upper motor neuron lesion	Degeneration of frontal motor neurons located in the motor strip (Brodman area 4) and their axons traversing the corona radiata, internal capsule, cerebral peduncles, pontine base, medullary pyramids, and the lateral corticospinal tracts of the spinal cord	1. **Weakness** with slowness, incoordination, stiffness
		  • Poor dexterity
		2. **Hyperreflexia**
		  • Ankle clonus
		3. **Spasticity**
		  • Spastic gait with poor balance and leg flexor spasms		

Disease	Etiology, Prevalence, and Risk Factors	Clinical Symptoms and Signs	Diagnostics	Therapy, Prognosis, and Health Maintenance

Lower motor neuron lesion	Degeneration of lower motor neurons in the brainstem and spinal cord producing muscle denervation	1. **Weakness**
		  • Hand: Difficulty manipulating small objects (buttons, zippers, coins) and writing
		  • Proximal arm: Difficulty bathing, dressing, grooming, eating
		  • Foot/ankle: Tripping, slapping gait, falling
		  • Proximal leg: Cannot arise from chair, climb stairs, or get up off floor
		  • Upper face: Incomplete eye closure
		2. **Atrophy** (amyotrophic)
		3. **Fasciculations**
		4. **Muscle cramps**		

Amyotrophic lateral sclerosis (Lou Gehrig's disease)	Amyotrophy with the pathological finding of lateral sclerosis
	65-70 y/o: M > F
	peak: 70-80 s, but can occur in 20 s
	Sporadic
	Only 10% familial
		1. Asymmetric limb weakness (80%)
		  • Upper extremity onset: **hand weakness,** but may begin in **shoulder girdle**
		  • Lower extremity: weakness of foot dorsiflexion (**foot drop**)
		2. *Bulbar symptoms*: dysarthria, dysphagia
		  • Coughing, choking
		  • Increased masseter tone and difficulty opening mouth (trismus)
		  • Laryngospasm
		3. **Autonomic symptoms**: constipation, urgency without incontinence, excessive sweating
		  • Early satiety, bloating
		4. Parkinsonism and supranuclear gaze palsy
		  • Facial masking, tremor, bradykinesia, postural instability
		5. Sensory (20%-30%): tingling
		6. Respiratory: muscle weakness, generalized weakness
		7. Weight loss
			<u>DX: Clinical</u>
			1. Upper and lower MN signs and symptoms
			2. Progressive spread
			EMG: fibrillations, positive sharp waves
			Electrodiagnostics: decreased motor conduction velocity
			MRI (preferred) to r/o other causes
			Unilateral arm onset (MC) → contralateral arm → ipsilateral leg → contralateral leg → bulbar muscles
			Unilateral leg → contralateral leg → ipsilateral arm → contralateral arm → bulbar muscles
				1. **Riluzole** 50 mg BID
				AE: asthenia, dizziness, GI upset, elevated LFTs
				MCC death: progressive respiratory failure
				<u>Complications:</u>
				Aspiration
				Median survival: 3-5 y

Peroneal nerve palsy	Caused by lateral knee trauma (lateral collateral ligament) and injury of the common peroneal or superficial peroneal nerve Develops in 35% of PLC injuries	1. Paresthesias in the distribution of the peroneal nerve 2. Prolonged foot drop <u>Signs:</u> 1. Assess sensation and lower extremity strength (dorsiflexion, eversion) 2. Observe patient's gait and look for a foot drop	1. **EMG/NCS**–helps to differentiate from an L5 root lesion (denervation in L5 muscles outside of the peroneal territory) and peroneal nerve palsy (focal slowing in peroneal nerve at fibular head)	1. Ice, compression, analgesics × 48-72 h <u>Health maintenance:</u> Ice (or cryotherapy) should only be applied intermittently for treatment, generally for no longer than 15 min every 2 h to prevent foot drop

- **Mononeuropathy**: refers to pathology affecting an individual peripheral nerve, which are diagnosed clinically based on signs and symptoms
  - Also consider carpal tunnel syndrome (numbness/tingling in median nerve distribution)
- **Radiculopathy**: refers to pathology affecting the nerve root, which is expressed by signs and symptoms in a corresponding dermatome

- **Hypoesthesia**: decreased ability to perceive pain, temperature, touch, or vibration
- **Anesthesia**: complete inability to perceive pain, temperature, touch, or vibration
- **Hypoalgesia**: decreased sensitivity to painful stimuli
- **Analgesia**: complete insensitivity to painful stimuli

General Surgery

VASCULAR DISORDERS (CAROTID DISEASE) (FIG. 73-1)

- In most individuals, the right common carotid artery (CCA) originates from the innominate (brachiocephalic) artery, which is typically the first branch off the aortic arch, and the left CCA arises as the second branch off the arch

- The CCA bifurcates into the internal carotid artery (ICA) and the external carotid artery at the level of the C4 to C5 intervertebral space

- The ICA continues superiorly and gives rise to its first major branch, the ophthalmic artery, in the subarachnoid space

- The ICA then bifurcates into the anterior and middle cerebral arteries. The ICA is divided into the prepetrous, petrous, cavernous, and supraclinoid segments

DEGREES OF STENOSIS AND HELPFUL INDICATIONS AND DEFINITIONS

- Mild stenosis <50%, moderate stenosis = 50% to 69%, severe stenosis >70%

- **Carotid artery stenting (CAS)** indications: symptomatic patients at average or low risk of complications associated with endovascular intervention when the diameter of the lumen of internal carotid artery is reduced by **>70%** by noninvasive imaging or >50% by catheter-based imaging with corroboration

  - Consider patient age: >70 years (**CEA > CAS**) and CAS for younger patients (less risk for periprocedural stroke, MI, or death, long term risk of stroke)

  - May be chosen if neck anatomy is surgically unfavorable or if comorbidities make patient high risk

- **Carotid endarterectomy (CEA):** symptomatic patients with average or low risk and >5 years life expectancy

  - Perform within 2 weeks of ischemic event

- Routine long-term follow-up imaging of extracranial carotid circulation not recommended

- Hyperperfusion syndrome is a potentially deadly complication from CAS or CEA

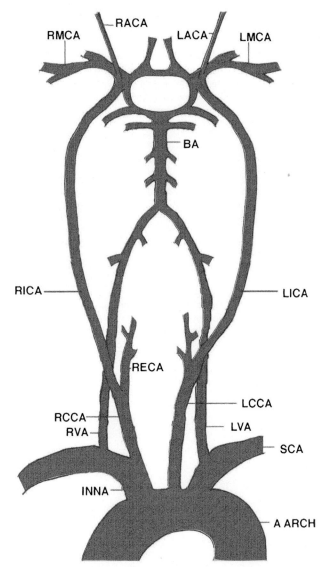

FIGURE 73-1. Normal intracranial anatomy. A, Arch (aortic arch); BA, basilar artery; INNA, innominate artery; LACA, left anterior cerebral artery; LCCA, left common carotid artery; LICA, left internal carotid artery; LMCA, left middle cerebral artery; LVA, left vertebral artery; RACA, right anterior cerebral artery; RCCA, right common carotid artery; RECA, right external carotid artery; RICA, right internal carotid artery; RMCA, right middle cerebral artery; RVA, right vertebral artery; SCA, subclavian artery. (From Sanders RC. *Clinical Sonography: A Practical Guide.* Philadelphia: Wolters Kluwer Health; 2016.)

Disease	Etiology, Prevalence, and Risk Factors	Clinical Symptoms and Signs	Diagnostics	Therapy, Prognosis, and Health Maintenance
Carotid artery stenosis	Extracranial internal carotid artery stenosis >80% +/– symptoms of ischemia *Asymptomatic*–refers to presence of narrowing of the ICA in individuals without a history of recent ipsilateral ischemic stroke or TIA *Symptomatic*–refers to neurologic symptoms caused by TIA or ischemic stroke in the carotid artery territory and ipsilateral to significant carotid atherosclerotic pathology	<u>Symptoms of *ischemia*</u>: 1. Partial or complete blindness in one eye and absent pupillary light response 2. Contralateral homonymous hemianopsia, hemiparesis, hemisensory loss 3. Left hemisphere–aphasia 4. Right hemisphere–left visuospatial neglect, constructional apraxia, dysprosody 5. Unilateral limb shaking, transient loss of monocular vision upon exposure to bright light 6. Does *NOT* cause vertigo, lightheadedness, or syncope <u>Signs</u>: 1. Carotid bruit 2. Funduscopic exam: arterial occlusion or ischemic damage to retina	1. **Cerebral angiography** (gold standard) • Permits use of entire carotid system, provides info about tandem atherosclerotic disease, plaque morphology, and collateral circulation • Identifies people who would benefit from endarterectomy (CEA) 2. **Carotid duplex ultrasound** • Noninvasive, but hairline residual lumens can be missed and can overestimate degree of stenosis 3. **Magnetic resonance angiography** (MRA) neck • Less accurate for detecting moderate stenosis, more expensive, time consuming, patient must lie still, renal insufficiency can be an issue 4. CT angiography (CTA) • Impaired renal function is a relative contraindication since contrast bolus must be given (DM/CHF)	See treatment of asymptomatic and symptomatic CAS

Treatment of Carotid Stenosis

Asymptomatic bruits
1. Start daily **antiplatelet therapy**, statin therapy, manage diabetes, treat hypertension, and healthy lifestyle (limit ETOH consumption, weight control, aerobic physical activity, Mediterranean diet)
2. **Carotid endarterectomy (CEA): >80% stenosis**, recurrent TIAs on medical therapy (preferred)
   • If patient has life expectancy of >5 y
3. Duplex ultrasonography - repeat annually to assess progression or regression of disease and response to therapeutic intervention if stenosis >50%
4. Carotid artery stenting (CAS) only for high-risk patients
   • Unlikely to benefit if: severe comorbidity, prior ipsilateral stroke, total occlusion of ICA

Symptomatic bruits–Manifested as recent TIA or ischemic stroke and ipsilateral CAS
1. *Anticoagulation (warfarin)*
2. Carotid endarterectomy (CEA) indicated for
   • Severe stenosis (70%-99%) → CEA recommended
   • Mod stenosis (50%-69%) → CEA recommended
   • Mild stenosis (<50%) → no indication for CEA or carotid angioplasty with stenting
   • Consider AGE: If >70, CEA may be associated with better outcome compared to CAS; for younger patients, CAS = CEA in terms of periprocedural complications
3. CAS is indicated as an alternative to CEA for symptomatic patients at average or low risk of complications when diameter of lumen of ICA is reduced by >70% by noninvasive imaging, or >50% by catheter angiography, or >50% by noninvasive imaging with corroboration
4. High risk: progression of asymptomatic CAS, detection of embolism, plaque burden and morphology, reduced cerebrovascular reserve, silent embolic infarcts

EPIDURAL AND SUBDURAL HEMATOMA

Disease	Etiology, Prevalence, and Risk Factors	Clinical Symptoms and Signs	Diagnostics	Therapy, Prognosis, and Health Maintenance
Acute epidural hematoma	Classic: "talk and die" Collection of blood between dura and bones of the skull MCC: Trauma MC affects temporoparietal region, 2/2 laceration of **middle meningeal artery**	<u>Progressive symptoms</u>: 1. History of trauma with overlying skull fracture 2. **Brief loss of consciousness** 3. Return to alertness (**lucid interval**) 4. **Headache, vomiting**, lethargy, hemiparesis → coma (20%) <u>Signs</u>: Associated hematoma	1. Noncontrast CT: **lens-shaped** (lenticular, biconvex) extra-axial collection of blood that does not cross suture lines (differentiates it from subdural)	1. Urgent neurosurgery consult 2. If evidence of herniation (pupil dilation or contralateral hemiparesis) → burr hole ipsilateral to trauma 3. Decrease ICP <u>Complications</u>: Herniation

General Surgery

(continued)

(continued)

Acute subdural hematoma	<u>MCC:</u> Trauma <u>Other RF:</u> Alcoholism, seizures, coagulopathies Collection of blood between the dura and arachnoid mater; source is bridging veins	<u>Nonspecific, nonlocalizing symptoms, or absent, stable, or rapidly progressive;</u> 1. Headache 2. Confusion 3. Depressed level of consciousness 4. +/– seizures <u>Signs:</u> 1. Hemiparesis–contralateral to lesion (60%) 2. Ipsilateral pupillary dilation (75%)	1. CT scan–hyperdense **crescent-shaped** (biconcave) extra-axial collection of blood, rarely crosses the falx or tentorium • Subacute lesions (2-3 wk): isodense	1. Immediate hospitalization 2. Emergent neurosurgery consult 3. Unstable patients with rapidly worsening neurologic deficits → treat for increased ICP

AUTONOMIC DYSREFLEXIA

• Splanchnic outflow conveying sympathetic fibers to the lower body exits at the T8 region. Patients with lesions above T8 are prone to autonomic dysreflexia

Disease	Etiology, Prevalence, and Risk Factors	Clinical Symptoms and Signs	Diagnostics	Therapy, Prognosis, and Health Maintenance
Autonomic dysreflexia	Most common precipitating cause: plugged catheter <u>Others:</u> Calculi, infection of urinary system, pelvic autonomic afferent activity (overdistended bowel or bladder, erection), somatic afferent activity (ejaculation, spasm of lower extremities), fecal impaction, pressure sores	1. Bouts of **hypertension**: dramatic elevations in systolic or diastolic BP, increased pulse pressure • Can be life-threatening • Dizziness • **Sweating** • **Headaches**–severe <u>Signs:</u> 1. Bradycardia 2. Piloerection	Clinical DX	1. Immediate catheterization 2. If unresponsive to treatment of causative agent → PO nifedipine 20 mg 3. Electroejaculation 4. Transurethral sphincterotomy and peripheral rhizotomy

74

Urology and Renal

Refer to Family Medicine 👥 for In-depth Coverage of the Following Topics:

Refer to Internal Medicine 🩺 for In-depth Coverage of the Following Topics:

EDEMA

Disease	Etiology, Prevalence, and Risk Factors	Clinical Symptoms and Signs	Diagnostics	Therapy, Prognosis, and Health Maintenance
Edema	Lower extremity: either increased venous or lymphatic pressures, decreased intravascular oncotic pressure, increased capillary leak or infection/local injury MCC: Chronic venous insufficiency Common complication of DVT	1. MC symptom: **Sensation of "heavy legs"** 2. Itching 3. Pain Signs: 1. Hyperpigmentation, stasis dermatitis 2. Lipodermatosclerosis (thick, brawny skin), atrophie blanche (small depigmented macules) 3. Measure size of calves 10 cm below tibial tuberosity 4. Check for tenderness and pitting 5. **Ulcer located over medial malleolus** (hallmark finding)	1. If low suspicion—D-dimer indicated 2. Use Wells criteria rule out DVT or go to step 3 3. Color duplex ultrasound, as well as ABI 4. Urine dipstick to rule out nephrotic syndrome 5. SCr to check kidney function	1. Treat underlying cause 2. If chronic venous insufficiency without volume overload, avoid diuretics • May enhance sodium retention through increased secretion of renin and angiotensin → AKI and oliguria 3. Supportive care • Leg elevation above heart × 30 mins TID and during sleep • Compression stockings • Ambulatory exercise

- Other causes of lower extremity edema: cellulitis, musculoskeletal related disorders (Baker cyst rupture, diabetic myonecrosis, gastrocnemius rupture or tear), lipoedema, heart failure, lymphedema, cirrhosis, **nephrotic syndrome**, medication side effects (CCB, minoxidil, pioglitazone), left common iliac vein compression, and prolonged airline flights (>10 hours)

ORTHOSTATIC HYPOTENSION

- Inability to maintain cerebral flow when standing or sitting upright, with resultant hypotension, dizziness, or syncope

Disease	Etiology, Prevalence, and Risk Factors	Clinical Symptoms and Signs	Diagnostics	Therapy, Prognosis, and Health Maintenance
Orthostatic hypotension	Volume depletion, medication, autonomic dysfunction Cerebral hypoperfusion and syncope in standing position Primary: Shy-Drager syndrome, Parkinson, rare dysautonomias Secondary: DM, anemia, amyloidosis, MS, HIV Medications that commonly cause OH—diuretics, antihypertensives (ACE inhibitors, BB, CCB), and ethanol	1. 20 mm Hg+ decline in systolic BP or 10 mm Hg+ decline in diastolic BP on assuming an upright posture 2. Precipitating factors: micturition, cough, exertion 3. Premonitory symptoms: aura 4. Associated symptoms: palpitations, chest pain, headache 5. Activity: at rest or with exercise 6. Position: standing, sitting, changing position 7. Injury, incontinence, rapid recovery vs. postictal state	1. EKG 2. Toxicology screens and medication levels 3. If cardiac history • Echo: r/o aortic stenosis, HCM • Stress Testing: helpful if exertional symptoms • Holter monitor: r/o bradyarrhythmias • Head Up Tilt-Table Testing: (+) if syncope or presyncope occurs • Electrophysiology study (EPS): r/o ventricular tachyarrhythmias	Treat the cause 1. SVTs: BB, K+/Na+ channel blockers, CCB 2. Neurocardiogenic and situational: • Avoid precipitants • Ephedrine, midorine • Metoprolol, pindolol • Scopalamine

URINARY RETENTION

- The most common cause of urinary retention postoperatively is general anesthesia
- Obstructive causes: urethral stricture, bladder calculi or neoplasm, foreign body
- Neurogenic causes: Multiple sclerosis, Parkinson disease, CVA, postoperative retention
- Traumatic causes: Urethral, bladder, or spinal cord injury
- Extraurinary: Fecal impaction, AAA, rectal or retroperitoneal mass
- Infectious: Local abscess, cystitis, genital herpes, zoster

Disease	Etiology, Prevalence, and Risk Factors	Clinical Symptoms and Signs	Diagnostics	Therapy, Prognosis, and Health Maintenance
Acute urinary retention	Inability to void in the presence of a full bladder RF: Male gender, prostatic enlargement; epidural, spinal or prolonged anesthesia; antihistamine and narcotic use; pelvic and perineal procedures M > F	1. Suprapubic discomfort with urgency and inability to void 2. Unable to void within 8 h after surgery or 8 h after catheter removal 3. **Painful** 4. Vomiting Signs: 1. Palpable bladder on exam 2. Hypotension, bradycardia, cardiac dysrhythmias Complication: Infection, ischemia, long-term bladder dysfunction	1. Bladder ultrasound: 500 mL urine 2. Postvoid residual: 500 mL or greater 3. Urine culture 4. CBC if suspected infection	1. Immediate sterile catheterization • Place for 24 h, then void trial 2. Identify and treat underlying cause
Chronic urinary retention		1. Painless 2. Develops gradually 3. Frequent urination of small amounts or overflow incontinence: sensation of fullness Signs: 1. Suprapubic dullness 2. Rounded midline mass	1. Postvoid residual bladder volume by catheterization or ultrasound 2. Abdominal US or CT indicated to identify suspected masses, stones, or hydronephrosis	As above
Detrusor (bladder) sphincter dyssynergia	Consequence of neurological pathology: SCI or multiple sclerosis Urethral sphincter muscle dyssynergically contracts during voiding causing the flow to be interrupted and bladder pressure to arise Obstructive cause	1. Daytime and nighttime wetting 2. Urinary retention 3. History of UTI/Bladder infections Associated: Constipation and encopresis	1. Postvoid residual urine volume (PVR) >150 mL	1. Botulinum A toxin injections 2. Surgical incision of bladder neck • Can result in incontinence

WILMS TUMOR

Disease	Etiology, Prevalence, and Risk Factors	Clinical Symptoms and Signs	Diagnostics	Therapy, Prognosis, and Health Maintenance
Wilms tumor	Most common primary malignant tumor of the kidney in children Peak: Age 3 97% are sporadic	1. Asymptomatic mass • Flank or upper abdomen • Discovered while dressing or bathing 2. Hypertension, hematuria, obstipation, weight loss	1. Abdominal and chest CT • Characterize the mass, identify mets, look at opposite kidney 2. Abdominal US to evaluate renal vein and vena cava	1. **Surgery**—complete removal • Radical **nephroureterectomy** if unilateral • If bilateral, biopsy both and start chemotherapy after nephron-sparing procedure 2. Chemotherapy 97% 4-y survival rate

CHRONIC RENAL FAILURE (SHUNTS AND ABSCESS) (FIG. 74-1)

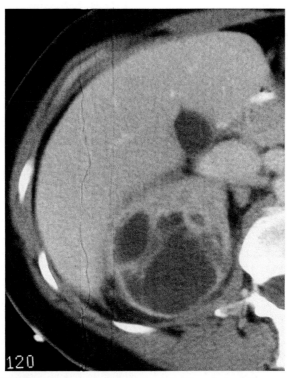

FIGURE 74-1. Acute renal abscess. Note the cavity is multiloculated. The abscess itself has thick walls, septations, and internal fluid density. (From Dunnick NR, Newhouse JH, Cohan RH, Maturen KE. *Genitourinary Radiology*. Philadelphia: Wolters Kluwer Health; 2018.)

Disease	Etiology, Prevalence, and Risk Factors	Clinical Symptoms and Signs	Diagnostics	Therapy, Prognosis, and Health Maintenance
Renal abscess	Most occur secondary to chronic nonspecific infection of the kidney, often complicated by stone formation RF: hemodialysis patients, IVDU, DM	1. Abrupt onset • High **fever** • General malaise • SX can last for >2 wk 2. **Flank or abdominal pain** 3. Chills 4. Dysuria Signs: 1. CVAT 2. Palpable flank mass	1. *Renal ultrasound*: range from anechoic mass within or displacing the kidney to echogenic fluid collection with normal echogenic fat within Gerota's fascia 2. *CT scan*: enlarged kidney with focal hypoattenuation (early) → mass with rim of contrast enhancement "ring sign"; thickening of Gerota's fascia, stranding of the perinephric fat, or obliteration of surrounding tissue planes 3. U/A w/culture: WBC 4. Blood cultures	1. Percutaneous drainage and irrigation with antibiotic solutions • Empiric: 2 ABX • Ampicillin or vancomycin PLUS • Aminoglycoside or third generation cephalosporin • Drain under CT or ultrasound guidance after 48 h • Culture fluid 2. If multilocular, surgical drainage and **heminephrectomy** may be necessary
Perinephric abscess	Abscess between the renal capsule and perirenal fascia Results from *rupture* of intrarenal abscess into perinephric space MCC: *E. coli* Associated: renal or ureteral calculi	1. Similar findings to renal abscess 2. Pleural effusion on affected side Signs: 1. Psoas sign (+)	1. Abdominal XR: obliteration of psoas muscle shadow 2. IV urogram: poor concentration of contrast medium, hydronephrosis 3. **CT scan** (required for diagnosis)	1. Prompt drainage of abscess 2. Systemic antibiotics with anaerobic coverage 3. Open surgical drainage if percutaneous unsuccessful

CHAPTER 75

Pulmonology

Refer to Family Medicine 👪 for In-depth Coverage of the Following Topics:

Pneumonia, p 24
Lung Carcinoma, p 30
Tuberculosis, p 28

Refer to Internal Medicine 🩺 for In-depth Coverage of the Following Topics:

Solitary Pulmonary Nodule, p 212

Refer to Emergency Medicine ✳ for In-depth Coverage of the Following Topics:

Shortness of Breath, p 384
Hemoptysis, p 386
Pleural Effusion, p 391
Pneumothorax, p 397 ✳

WEIGHT LOSS

- From a pulmonary standpoint, the differential diagnosis includes: pulmonary neoplasm, pneumonia, tuberculosis, and bronchiectasis

Disease	Etiology, Prevalence, and Risk Factors	Clinical Symptoms and Signs	Diagnostics	Therapy, Prognosis, and Health Maintenance
Bronchiectasis	Causes: **cystic fibrosis** (most common, 50%), infection, immunodeficiency, airway obstruction Infection with airway obstruction or impaired defense/drainage precipitates disease	1. Chronic cough with large amounts of mucopurulent, **foul smelling sputum** 2. Dyspnea (SOB) 3. Hemoptysis–mild, self-limited 4. Recurrent or persistent pneumonia 5. +/– weight loss Signs: 1. Crackles at the lung bases	1. **High-resolution CT** (gold standard) 2. PFTs (obstructive pattern) 3. CXR (abnormal, nonspecific) 4. Other labs: CBC (anemia)	1. Antibiotics–acute exacerbations 2. Bronchial hygiene–fluids, chest physiotherapy, inhaled bronchodilators

TUBERCULOSIS 👪

FATIGUE

Difficulty or inability to initiate activity and is a perception of generalized weakness.

- Other definitions: easy fatigability (or reduced capacity to maintain activity)
- Associated with: concentration and memory difficulties, emotional fatigue/stability

PLEURAL EFFUSION (POSTOPERATIVE)

- Defined as excess quantity of fluid in the pleural space
- Accumulation occurs when formation of pleural fluid exceeds pleural fluid absorption. Normally, fluid enters the pleural space from the capillaries in the parietal pleura and is removed via the lymphatics in the parietal pleura.

- A pleural effusion may develop when there is excess pleural fluid formation (from the interstitial spaces of the lung, the parietal pleura, or the peritoneal cavity) or when there is decreased fluid removal by the lymphatics

- Thoracentesis: Percutaneous procedure in which a needle is inserted into the pleural space and pleural fluid is removed

- Diagnostics: Chest ultrasound has replaced lateral decubitus CXR in evaluation of suspected pleural effusions, and guides thoracentesis

- Differentiate between transudative and exudative: The primary reason for making this differentiation is that additional diagnostic procedures are indicated with exudative effusions to define the cause of the local disease

Indications for Thoracentesis	Contraindications for Thoracentesis	When Thoracentesis is Not Needed
• New finding of a pleural effusion • Pleural effusion in setting of heart failure with atypical features • Regression of symptoms in first days of diuretic therapy • Unilateral effusion • Presence of fever or chest pain	• Therapeutic anticoagulation or bleeding diathesis • PT and PTT greater than twice midpoint of normal range • Platelet count <50 k platelets/mm³ • SCr >6 mg/dL • Small effusions with <1 cm distance from pleural fluid line to chest wall on decubitus CXR • Patients receiving positive pressure mechanical ventilation • Active skin infection at point of needle insertion	• Small amount of pleural fluid • Clear clinical diagnosis (eg, viral pleurisy) • Obvious clinical heart failure without atypical features

Potential Complications of Thoracentesis

- Pain at the puncture site
- Bleeding (hematoma, hemothorax, hemoperitoneum)
- Pneumothorax (MC complication)
- Empyema
- Soft tissue infection
- Spleen or liver rupture
- Vasovagal events
- Seeding the needle tract with tumor
- Adverse reaction to anesthetic or topic antiseptic solution

- Atypical features: bilateral effusions of marked disparate sizes, pleurisy, fever or other clinical features suggesting infection, absence of cardiomegaly on CXR, ultrasound or CT findings suggestive of cause other than heart failure, echocardiogram inconsistent with HF, BNP levels inconsistent with HF, alveolar-arterial O2 gradient larger than expected for HF, does not resolve with HF therapy

Indications for Thoracostomy

- Gram (+) stain of pleural fluid, (+) pleural fluid culture, pus
- → Remove when <100 mL fluid drains in 24 h

- **Diagnostic thoracentesis**: refers to removal of a small volume of pleural fluid for analysis
- **Therapeutic thoracentesis**: refers to removal of large volume of pleural fluid for relief of symptoms, but remove no more than 1.5 L per procedure
- **Video-assisted thoracoscopic surgery (VATS)** may be required to lyse extensive intrapleural adhesions

Pleural Fluid Analysis

- Commonly ordered tests: cell count and cell differential, pH, protein, lactate dehydrogenase (LDH), and glucose

- Other studies: amylase, cholesterol, triglycerides, BNP, adenosine deaminase, gram and acid-fast bacillus (AFB) stain, bacterial and AFB culture, and cytology
- If 1+ exudative criteria are met and the patient is clinically thought to have a condition producing a transudative effusion, measure the difference between protein levels in pleural fluid vs. serum
- If a patient has an exudative pleural effusion, the following tests on the pleural fluid should be obtained: description of the appearance of the fluid, glucose level, cell count and differential, microbiologic studies, and cytology
- **Light's criteria**—helps you differentiate between a transudative and exudative pleural effusion; not enough to formulate a diagnosis by itself

- **Pleural fluid [protein]:serum [protein] ratio >than 0.5 (less protein in the blood)**
- **Pleural fluid [LDH]:serum [LDH] > than 0.6 (less LDH in the blood)**
- Pleural fluid [LDH] > than ⅔ ULN serum [LDH]
- Exudate if any 1 of the above criteria is met, otherwise usually transudate

	MOA	Examples	Findings	
Transudates Imbalance of pressure in vessels Mnemonic: Transudate is transparent (no proteins)	1. Increase in *hydrostatic pressure* of pleural membrane microvessel 2. Decrease in serum *colloid osmotic pressure* (eg, nephrotic syndrome)	1. MCC: **left ventricular heart failure** and cirrhosis 2. Nephrotic syndrome 3. Cirrhosis 4. Hepatic hydrothorax 5. **Pulmonary embolism** 6. Hypothyroidism 7. Peritoneal dialysis 8. Hypoalbuminemia 9. **Atelectasis**	1. Bilateral inspiratory crackles 2. Low pleural fluid concentrations of plasma protein (albumin), LDH, cholesterol • Absolute **total protein <3 g/dL** • Can be elevated in HF or tuberculous pleural effusions • Serum: pleural fluid albumin gradient >1.2 g/dL • NT-proBNP elevated (supports HF) • Pleural pH: 7.4-7.55	Treatment varies based on etiology as below

(continued)

	MOA	Examples	Findings	
Exudates Injury and inflammation Mnemonic: Exudate exudes proteins	1. Increased *permeability* of microvessels in pleural membranes, can be due to pleural inflammation in neoplasia 2. Fibrin deposits limit outflow rate via lymphatics 3. *Increased protein* and other biomarkers	1. MCC: **parapneumonic effusion** (40%-50% of bacterial pneumonias) 2. **Pneumonia** 3. **Empyema** 4. **Malignancy** 5. **Pulmonary embolism** 6. Connective tissue disease 7. Pancreatitis 8. Tuberculous pleurisy 9. Esophageal rupture 10. Drug reaction *Thoracic empyema*: overt pus in pleural space; end result of complicated exam findings	1. Pleural fluid LDH >1000 IU/L (found in empyema) 2. Pleural fluid:serum LDH >1.0 and pleural fluid:serum protein <0.5 found in PCP Pneumonia or malignancy 3. Pleural cholesterol >45 mg/dL 4. Pleural pH: 7.3-7.45 5. Nucleated cell count >5 k/uL	Treatment varies based on etiology 1. Uncomplicated parapneumonic effusion: exudative, free-flowing effusion developing with infectious pneumonia → treat pneumonia, requires **thoracentesis** 2. Complicated parapneumonic effusion: requires pleural space drainage for resolution → intrapleural adhesions, loculated fluids, trapped lung

Postoperative Effusion (Differential Diagnosis)

Disease	Etiology, Prevalence, and Risk Factors	Clinical Symptoms and Signs	Diagnostics	Therapy, Prognosis, and Health Maintenance
Hepatic hydrothorax	5%-10% patients with cirrhosis and portal HTN Trans-diaphragmatic movement of abdominal ascitic fluid from peritoneal compartment to pleural space via diaphragmatic openings	1. Ascites 2. Jaundice	1. LFT abnormalities 2. Diagnostic thoracentesis (can be therapeutic as well) 3. Confirm with radionuclide scan	1. **Sodium restriction, diuresis** Refractory hepatic hydrothorax (10%) 1. Transjugular intrahepatic portosystemic shunt (TIPS)—decreases portal venous pressure and rate of ascites formation
Parapneumonic effusion	Effusions that form in the pleural space adjacent to bacterial pneumonia Anaerobic organisms common, but also *S. aureus* and gram-negative bacilli (*Klebsiella pneumoniae*) Found in 40% of bacterial pneumonias Uncomplicated: Most effusions are sterile; forms when interstitial lung fluid moves across visceral pleural membrane with influx of neutrophils into pleural space; effusion forms when resorptive capacity of pleural space is exceeded Complicated: Bacterial invasion of the pleural space with invasion and lysis of neutrophils; lysis of neutrophils causes increased LDH Empyema: Develops from bacterial infection of pleural fluid with pus formation	1. Cough 2. **Fever** 3. **Pleuritic chest pain** 4. Dyspnea 5. Sputum production 6. With empyema patients report a longer duration of fever and malaise (days) Signs: 1. **Decreased fremitus** 2. **Decreased breath sounds** 3. No egophony, fine/coarse crackles 4. Dullness to percussion (not useful)	1. Imaging • CXR: pleural-based opacity • Ultrasonography • Chest CT with contrast: thickening of visceral or parietal pleura = empyema 2. **Diagnostic thoracentesis** if: • Free-flowing, layers >25 mm on lateral decubitus or CT • Loculated • Thickened parietal pleura on CT scan 3. Pleural fluid analysis • Drain if: pH<7.2, glucose <60 mg/dL • Obtain: stains and cultures, cell count, chemistry (total protein, LDH, glucose), pH	1. Empiric therapy = anaerobic coverage • Clindamycin • β-lactams + Augmentin, Unasyn, or Zosyn • Carbapenems: imipenem, meropenem, ertapenem 2. If gram-negative suspected • Second or third generation cephalosporin + Flagyl 3. Complicated effusions or empyema—Drainage + above • **Thoracostomy** (chest tube) under CT or ultrasound guidance • Least invasive • Preferred to drain multiloculated empyemas • Lysis of adhesions • Decortication 4. Video-assisted thoracoscopic surgery (VATS) for debridement and drainage Health maintenance: Obtain serial CXR or ultrasounds to assess improvement Prognosis: Radiographic improvement may take weeks-months

Serum albumin ascites gradient is used for finding out the cause of ascites.

- **SAAG = albumin in serum—albumin in ascitic fluid**
- If SAAG >1.1, it is portal hypertension.
- If SAAG <1.1, it could be cancer, nephrotic syndrome, tuberculosis, etc (Fig. 75-1).

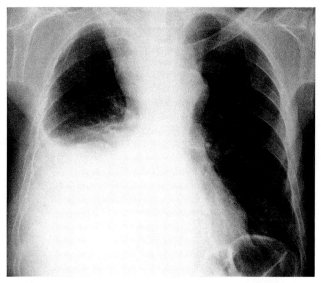

FIGURE 75-1. Pleural effusion. (From Webb WR, Higgins CB. *Thoracic Imaging*. Philadelphia: Wolters Kluwer Health; 2017.)

Disease	Etiology, Prevalence, and Risk Factors	Clinical Symptoms and Signs	Diagnostics	Therapy, Prognosis, and Health Maintenance
Pleural effusion	Common after upper abdominal operations Highest risk: patients with free peritoneal fluid and postop atelectasis May suggest subdiaphragmatic inflammation (subphrenic abscess, acute pancreatitis) Abnormal collection of fluid in pleural space resulting from excess fluid production, decreased absorption, or both Typically detected by physical exam or thoracic imaging studies	1. Dyspnea (MC) 2. **Cough**—mild, nonproductive 3. Chest pain—mild to severe, sharp, and stabbing, worse with deep inspiration, localized or referred to ipsilateral shoulder 4. Other SX: increasing lower extremity edema, orthopnea, PND NO physical exam findings if <300 mL, otherwise: 1. Dullness to percussion 2. Decreased tactile fremitus 3. Egophony changes in superior aspect 4. Decreased breath sounds 5. Asymmetrical chest expansion 6. Mediastinal shift away from the effusion if >1000 mL 7. Pleural friction rub	1. Diagnostic thoracentesis—to determine nature of effusion (transudate vs. exudate) and identify potential causes	1. Spontaneous resolution—If not compromising airway function, leave alone 2. If suspicious for infection, sample by needle aspiration 3. If respiratory compromise, drain with thoracostomy tube 4. Indications for urgent drainage: • frank purulent fluid, • pleural fluid pH <7, • loculated effusions, • bacteria on gram stain or culture

POSTOPERATIVE PNEUMOTHORAX

Disease	Etiology, Prevalence, and Risk Factors	Clinical Symptoms and Signs	Diagnostics	Therapy, Prognosis, and Health Maintenance
Pneumothorax (PTX)	Follows insertion of subclavian catheter or positive-pressure ventilation, or injured pleura (nephrectomy, adrenalectomy) Air in the pleural space • Spontaneous: • Primary (simple)—without underlying disease (healthy), spontaneous rupture of subpleural blebs, **MC in tall, lean men**, 50% recurrence in 2 y • Secondary (complicated)— underlying lung disease (MC: COPD), asthma, ILD, neoplasm, CF, TB, life-threatening • Traumatic—iatrogenic	1. **Ipsilateral chest pain**, sudden onset 2. **Dyspnea** 3. Cough 1. **Decreased/ absent tactile fremitus** 2. Mediastinal shift toward affected side 3. **Decreased breath sounds** over affected side 4. **Hyperresonance**	1. CXR—confirms dx, **visceral-pleural line**	Primary (Spontaneous) 1. Small and asymptomatic: observe 10 days +/− small chest tube 2. Large +/− symptoms: O2 with chest tube 3. Secondary—chest tube drainage 4. Repeat CXR daily until resolved
Pulmonary aspiration	Aspiration of oropharyngeal and gastric contents High RF: pregnant, intestinal obstruction, trauma victims, thoracic or abdominal surgery, tracheostomy Basal segments affected most	1. Tachypnea 2. Rales 3. Hypoxia within hours 4. Less common: cyanosis, wheezing, apnea, hypovolemia		1. Preoperative fasting, proper positioning of patient, careful intubation 2. H2 or PPI before anesthesia if high risk Prognosis: Death rate is 50%
Atelectasis	Most common complication postop (25% of abdominal surgeries) RF: Elderly, overweight, smokers, respiratory disease **Fever within 48 h** (before POD 2) *Obstruction* by secretions (COPD), intubation or anesthesia *Nonobstructive* causes: closure of bronchioles (<1 mm)	1. Fever (unknown origin) 2. Tachypnea 3. Tachycardia Signs: 1. Elevation of diaphragm 2. Scattered rales 3. Decreased breath sounds in area 4. Dullness to percussion	1. V/P mismatch 2. CXR—abnormal findings dependent on location	1. Chest percussion, coughing, nasotracheal suction— fever decreases with reexpansion of the lung 2. Bronchodilators and mucolytics via nebulizer for COPD Prevention: Early ambulation, frequent changes in position, cough encouragement, incentive spirometry Prognosis: If atelectasis persists beyond 72 h, pneumonia will likely occur

POSTOPERATIVE PNEUMONIA

Disease	Etiology, Prevalence, and Risk Factors	Clinical Symptoms and Signs	Diagnostics	Therapy, Prognosis, and Health Maintenance
Community acquired pneumonia (pneumococcal pneumonia)– **Immuno competent**	Most common complication leading to mortality after surgery Highest RF: Peritoneal infection, prolonged ventilatory support RF: Atelectasis, aspiration, copious secretions Caused by gram-negative bacilli (>50%): E. Coli, Pseudomonas, Klebsiella	1. Acute or sub-acute onset of **fever** 2. Gradual onset **cough** with or without sputum production 3. **Shortness of breath** on exertion 4. Other: sweats, chills, rigors, chest discomfort, pleurisy, hemoptysis, fatigue, myalgias, anorexia, headache, abdominal pain Signs: 1. Fever or hypothermia 2. Tachypnea 3. Tachycardia 4. O$_2$ desaturation 5. Inspiratory crackles and *bronchial* breath sounds 6. Dullness to percussion	Imaging: 1. CXR: patchy airspace opacities to **lobar consolidation with air bronchograms** to diffuse alveolar or interstitial opacities • Not necessary in outpatient because empiric therapy is effective • Recommended if unusual presentation, history, or inpatient • Clearing of opacities can take 6 wk or longer! 2. CT chest • More sensitive and specific Labs: 1. Sputum gram stain and sensitivity • Not sensitive or specific for *S. pneumoniae* 2. Urinary Ag test for *S. pneumoniae* and *Legionella* • As sensitive/specific as gram stain, readily available 3. Rapid Ag test for flu • Sensitive, not specific 4. Preantibiotic **sputum and blood cultures** • 2 sticks at separate sites 5. CBC and CMP, LFTs, bilirubin 6. ABG in hypoxemic patients 7. HIV testing in at-risk patients 8. Procalcitonin–released by bacterial toxins and inhibited by viral infections	See *Family Medicine* section for treatment Prophylaxis: 1. Pneumovax 23 2. Prevnar 13 • Ind: Age 65+ and immunocompromised give both, or any chronic illness with increased risk of CAP • Immunocompromised patients at high-risk should get single revaccination of 23 6-y after first, regardless of age • Immunocompetent and 65+ get second dose of 23 if first received vaccine 6+ y ago (<65) 3. Influenza Ind: age 65+, residents of LTCF, pulmonary or CV disease, chronic metabolic disorder, or health care worker

CHAPTER 76

Hematology

Refer to Emergency Medicine for In-depth Coverage of the Following Topics:

Easy Bruising/Bleeding, see HIT, ITP, TTP, HUS, Hemophilia, DIC, and vWF, p 440
Fatigue, p 441

Refer to Internal Medicine for In-depth Coverage of the Following Topics:

Anemia, p 75

Recommended Supplemental Material:

Disseminated Intravascular Coagulation, p 652
Pernicious Anemia, see Vitamin B$_{12}$ Deficiency, p 652
Lymphoma, see Int Med, p 281
Blood Cell Morphology and Life Cycle, see Int Med, p 274

EASY BRUISING AND BLEEDING

Disease	Etiology, Prevalence, and Risk Factors	Clinical Symptoms and Signs	Diagnostics	Therapy, Prognosis, and Health Maintenance
Disseminated intravascular coagulation (DIC)	Generalized activation of coagulation cascade → widespread **fibrin formation** (antithrombin + protein C) → **consumption of platelets and clotting factors** → microthrombosis → increased fibrinolysis Causes: Infection, mechanical tissue injury, malignancy, pregnancy **Consumptive coagulopathy**—consumption of clotting factors 5 and 8, protein C, and low platelets Hereditary and acquired factors tip balance in favor of clotting → thrombophilic vs. hypercoagulable state	1. Generalized **hemorrhage (bleeding)** • Petechiae and ecchymoses → GI bleed, GU bleed, surgical wound, mucocutaneous or venipuncture site bleed 2. Mental status changes 3. Focal ischemia or gangrene 4. Oliguria 5. Renal cortical necrosis 6. ARDS	1. **Thrombocytopenia** 2. FDP/**D-dimer:** increased (specific) 3. **Fibrinogen:** decreased (consumed) 4. PT/PTT: **prolonged** 5. Protein C: decreased	1. **Supportive care** and manage underlying disease • IVF, RBCs, inotropic agents 2. Replete platelets or clotting factors *if going into surgery* • Fibrinogen repletion with cryoprecipitate • Platelet concentrates to replace platelets • **FFP** to replace coagulation factors • *Vitamin K and Folate* 3. Anticoagulation—only if DIC shifted toward hypercoagulability • Heparin Complications: Thrombosis, organ failure, purpura fulminans, **sepsis**, bacteremia

ANEMIA

Disease	Etiology, Prevalence, and Risk Factors	Clinical Symptoms and Signs	Diagnostics	Therapy, Prognosis, and Health Maintenance
Vitamin B$_{12}$ deficiency (pernicious anemia)	**Autoimmune** destruction of fundic parietal cells → atrophic gastritis → lack of intrinsic factor production (required for absorption in small intestines) Cofactor for 2 enzymatic reactions required for DNA synthesis, brain/nervous system function, formation of RBC Causes/RF: Chronic alcoholism, vegetarian, celiac diseases, Crohn disease, **gastric bypass surgery** (gastrectomy, blind loop syndrome, resection), Parasites MCC: **Pernicious anemia** (lack of intrinsic factor)	1. Anemia: weakness, fatigue, bruising/gum bleeding, **sore tongue** (unique) 2. Neuropsychiatric manifestations: peripheral neuropathy, balance probs, depression, dementia → can be irreversible if untreated 3. *Glossitis*: beefy red tongue Signs: Loss of vibratory and fine touch	1. B$_{12}$ level: decreased, can be false (+) with folate deficiency 2. Homocysteine: *increased* 3. **Methylmalonic acid (MMA):** increased 4. Hypersegmented neutrophils 5. Endoscopy with biopsy	1. Lifelong IM B$_{12}$: 1-3 µg/d (animal products, fortified cereal) for pernicious anemia • IV **Cyanocobalamin 1 mg** IM daily × 7 d, then weekly × 4 wk, then monthly for life 2. PO B$_{12}$ 1-2 mg PO daily for vegans and bariatric surgery Years to deplete stores

PRACTICE QUESTIONS

1. A 55-year-old male with coronary artery disease and hypertension presents for preoperative evaluation of cholecystectomy. Patient is followed closely by cardiology, with normal stress test 1 year ago. What is the recommended screening for this patient prior to surgery?

   A. Electrocardiogram

   B. Treadmill stress test

   C. 24-hour ambulatory monitoring

   D. Echocardiogram

2. A 30-year-old female presents to the emergency department complaining of heavy menstrual bleeding. She is concerned that she is "losing too much blood." On further questioning, she notes a lifelong history of easy bruising and intermittent nose bleeds. Hgb/Hct, PT, aPTT, BT, platelet count, factor VIII, and factor IX are within normal limits. What is the most likely etiology of the patient's bleeding?

   A. Hemophilia A

   B. von Willebrand disease

   C. Disseminated intravascular coagulation

   D. Idiopathic thrombocytopenic purpura

3. Which laboratory study has a high sensitivity for diagnosis of acute pancreatitis, rises in the first 4 to 8 hours of acute onset, peaks around 24 hours and normalizes within 2 weeks?

   A. Lipase

   B. Amylase

   C. Red blood cell count

   D. Hemoglobin

4. A 70-year-old patient presents with complaints of sudden loss of vision in the right eye. He reports that one moment he could see perfectly and all the sudden he had a "black curtain" fall over his right visual field. What element of his previous medical history may have caused his symptoms?

   A. Atrial fibrillation

   B. Hyperthyroidism

   C. Anemia

   D. Myocardial infarction

5. Which of the following studies is used to diagnose suspected *H. pylori*?

   A. Urea breath test

   B. Upper GI series

   C. Secretin

   D. Abdominal ultrasound

6. A 45-year-old male presents with painless hematuria for the past month, which is confirmed with positive red blood cells on urinalysis. What is the gold standard diagnostic study for the suspected diagnosis?

   A. Urine culture

   B. Pelvic ultrasound

   C. CT scan abdomen and pelvis

   D. Cystoscopy with biopsy

7. A 72-year-old female with a history of atrial fibrillation presents with acute onset of diffuse mild to moderate abdominal pain. On exam, the pain is out of proportion to the patient's presentation. What is the definitive diagnostic study of choice?

   A. CT angiography

   B. MRI

   C. Abdominal ultrasound

   D. Exploratory laparotomy

8. Which of the following is a common etiology of an indirect inguinal hernia?

   A. Appendicitis

   B. Congenital defects in the anterior abdominal wall

   C. Nissen fundoplication surgery

   D. Increased abdominal pressure

9. A 57-year-old male postop day 4 after laparoscopic cholecystectomy is being evaluated on morning rounds. He complains of cough and generalized malaise. Temperature is 102°F, HR 104, 122 BP/84, RR 25. The patient is ill-appearing, diaphoretic and is found to have crackles in the base of his right lung. Chest x-ray reveals small right lower lobe consolidation. Diagnostic thoracentesis is performed with pleural fluid protein to serum protein ratio greater than 0.5. What is the most probable cause of the patient's presentation?

   A. Pneumonia

   B. Congestive heart failure

   C. Cirrhosis

   D. Bronchitis

10. A patient presents with an expanding red, painful and swollen area on the left thigh. Patient has also experienced associated fever and chills. On exam, the area is tender, but without fluctuance. What is the first line treatment for the suspected infection?

    A. Vancomycin

    B. Dicloxacillin

    C. Zosyn

    D. Nitrofurantoin

11. What symptom differentiates small bowel obstruction from paralytic ileus?

    A. Abdominal pain

    B. Nausea and vomiting

    C. Diarrhea

    D. Obstipation

12. A 60-year-old male with a previous medical history of atrial fibrillation and atherosclerosis presents with left leg pain. The patient complains of left lower leg pain, worse with ambulation and on palpation. On exam, the patient has severely diminished dorsalis pedis and posterior tibialis pulses on the left, the foot and half of the lower leg are pale, cooler than the rest of the leg and cap refill is about 5 seconds. The patient also notes that during the exam, he cannot feel anything below his left knee. What is the most likely etiology?

    A. Cauda equina

    B. Acute arterial emboli

    C. Sciatica

    D. Acute venous thrombus

13. A patient is being evaluated for persistent epigastric abdominal pain. Upper endoscopy reveals peptic ulcers and is confirmed to have *H. pylori*. The patient denies use of NSAIDs, tobacco, or alcohol. What is the recommended treatment to initiate at this time?

    A. Long-term proton pump inhibitor therapy

    B. Clarithromycin, amoxicillin, and PPI for 14 days minimum

    C. Ranitidine

    D. Low-fat diet

14. Which of the following diagnostic studies should be used in a patient that presents with episodic headache, tachycardia, and sweating refractory to over the counter medications?

    A. 24-hour urine metanephrines
    B. CBC
    C. Urine culture
    D. Bone marrow biopsy

15. A 14-year-old male presents with 24-hour history of severe abdominal pain, fever, nausea, and vomiting. On abdominal exam, the patient has right lower quadrant tenderness, with involuntary guarding and positive McBurney's point tenderness. White blood cell count, neutrophils, and C-reactive protein are elevated. What is the most appropriate treatment at this time?

    A. Watchful waiting
    B. Antibiotics
    C. Interventional radiology guided incision and drainage
    D. Appendectomy

16. Which nonsurgical treatment of Graves disease causes permanent resolution of hyperthyroidism, but also in turn results in permanent hypothyroidism, requiring lifelong thyroid hormone replacement?

    A. Atenolol
    B. PTU
    C. Methimazole
    D. Radioiodine

17. In a patient with no previous medical history, but family history of colorectal cancer in their mother, who was diagnosed at age 40, what is the recommended screening?

    A. Colonoscopy at 40 years old
    B. Fecal occult blood testing beginning at 40 years old
    C. Colonoscopy at 30 years old
    D. Colonoscopy at 35 years old

18. A 32-year-old male presents with right-sided weakness and slurred speech that began approximately 30 minutes prior to arrival to the ED. Noncontrast CT scan is negative for intracranial hemorrhage. The patient would like the most aggressive treatment at this time. Past medical and surgical history of hypercholesterolemia. Which of the following is the treatment of choice at this time?

    A. Lovenox
    B. Alteplase
    C. Atorvastatin
    D. Aspirin

19. A 44-year-old obese female presents with complaints of right upper quadrant pain, with associated nausea and vomiting. Symptoms are worse with eating. With deep palpation in the right upper quadrant, the patient inspires deeply and rapidly and experiences pain. What is the preferred initial study to confirm the suspected diagnosis?

    A. Abdominal x-ray
    B. HIDA scan
    C. MRI
    D. Right upper quadrant ultrasound

20. What is advised of postoperative patients to prevent atelectasis?

    A. Bed rest
    B. Frequent urination
    C. Incentive spirometry
    D. Sequential compression devices

21. A patient presents complaining of 12-hour history of fever, nausea, vomiting, and abdominal pain. The abdominal pain originally started centrally and has now localized to the right lower abdomen. On exam, the patient has rebound tenderness, guarding and pain on palpation of the right lower quadrant. What is the most likely cause?

    A. Cholecystitis
    B. Gastroesophageal reflux
    C. Appendicitis
    D. Pancreatitis

22. Which of the following lab findings are indicative of hypoparathyroidism?

    A. Low PTH, low calcium, low phosphate
    B. Low PTH, low calcium, high phosphate
    C. Low PTH, high calcium, high phosphate
    D. Low PTH, high calcium, low phosphate

23. A 45-year-old female presents with abdominal pain, nausea, vomiting, diarrhea, diaphoresis, and lightheadedness. Her heart rate is currently 120 bpm. Previous medical and surgical history includes morbid obesity, hyperlipidemia, hypertension and gastric bypass surgery performed 8 months ago. The patient states that this episode is similar to many prior episodes in the past 2 months, which typically occur 10 to 15 minutes after eating a meal with a lot of carbohydrates. What is the most likely etiology?

    A. Viral gastroenteritis
    B. Dumping syndrome
    C. Gastroesophageal reflux
    D. Celiac sprue

24. A 47-year-old female with atherosclerosis presents with chest pain radiating into the left side of her jaw, with associated nausea. EKG reveals ST elevation. The patient is given aspirin, morphine, and nitroglycerin and is put on oxygen. She is then sent to the cath-lab where she is found to have multivessel disease, including the left main coronary artery. What is the proper intervention at this time?

    A. Observation and morphine
    B. tPA administration
    C. Percutaneous coronary intervention (PCI)
    D. Coronary artery bypass graft (CABG)

25. A 68-year-old female presents with recent anal pain and small amounts of bright red bleeding, worse with bowel movements. The patient has no previous medical history, other than recent constipation. What is the most likely etiology?

A. Anal fissure
B. Internal hemorrhoids
C. Colon polyps
D. Crohn disease

ANSWERS

1. Diagnostic Studies: Cardiac Risk Evaluation in Noncardiac Surgery. Answer A: A, At this time, an electrocardiogram is the recommended screening. The other methods are not recommended unless they are needed aside from the surgery.

2. Diagnosis: Von Willebrand Disease. Answer B: Easy bruising, heavy menstrual bleeding, nosebleeds, and other mucosal bleeding are common in von Willebrand disease. This is further supported by laboratory findings. Additional lab findings suggestive of vwd are decreased von Willebrand factor antigen and decreased von Willebrand factor: Ristocetin cofactor activity. A, Hemophilia A and B typically present with large joint hemarthroses and hematomas and have prolonged aptt, but normal PT, bleeding time and platelet counts. C, DIC presents with bleeding and shock and has increased PT and aptt, decreased platelet count and peripheral smear shows schistocytes. D, ITP presentation can vary from few symptoms to mild bruising (petechiae and purpura), to severe bleeding and has normal PT, aptt, and decreased platelet count.

3. Scientific Concepts: Acute Pancreatitis. Answer A: Lipase is highly sensitive and specific for the diagnosis of acute pancreatitis. It rises within 4 to 8 hours and peaks at 24 hours, with normal levels within 8 to 14 days. B, Amylase elevation is also indicative of acute pancreatitis. Rise occurs within 6 to 12 hours and returns to normal within 3 to 5 days. C-D, Patients with acute pancreatitis may have elevation of wbcs and hematocrit (a result of hemoconcentration due to third spacing).

4. H&P: Retinal Artery Occlusion. Answer A: This presentation is suggestive of retinal artery occlusion, which is commonly caused by either carotid artery atherosclerosis or cardiogenic source, often atrial fibrillation.

5. Diagnostic Studies: *H. pylori*. Answer D: Abdominal ultrasound is not indicated for the diagnosis of *H. pylori*. A, In cases of suspected *H. pylori* that do not require endoscopy, urea breath test or stool antigen is the tests of choice. B, Upper GI series is not indicated for the diagnosis of *H. pylori*. C, Secretin is used to test for gastrin secreting tumors or Zollinger-Ellison syndrome.

6. Diagnostic Studies: Bladder Cancer. Answer A: Urine culture is indicated for suspected infection, which would be more likely with fever, dysuria, and lower abdominal discomfort. D, Painless hematuria is the most common presentation of bladder cancer. The gold standard for staging is cystoscopy with biopsy. Ultrasound (B) and CT scan (C) are not considered gold standards for bladder cancer.

7. Diagnostic Studies: Mesenteric Arterial Embolism. Answer A: The presentation of older patient with atrial fibrillation and abdominal pain is classic for mesenteric arterial embolism. The definitive diagnostic test of choice is CT angiography.

8. Scientific Concepts: Inguinal Hernia. Answer D: Increased abdominal pressure is a common cause of acquired indirect inguinal hernia. A, Not a cause. B, This is a common cause of congenital umbilical hernia. C, Surgery may cause hernias but is not a common cause of indirect inguinal hernia.

9. Diagnosis: Pneumonia. Answer A: Clinical presentation is indicative of pneumonia, and pleural fluid analysis meets Light's criteria for an exudative pleural effusion (see below). CHF and cirrhosis are causes of transudative pleural effusion.

> **Light's Criteria** - diagnostically differentiates between a transudative and exudative pleural effusion.
> - Pleural fluid [protein]: serum [protein] ratio >0.5 (less protein in the blood)
> - Pleural fluid [LDH]: serum [LDH] > 0.6 (less LDH in the blood)
> - Pleural fluid [LDH] > 2/3 ULN serum [LDH]
>
> **Exudate if any 1 of the above criteria is met, otherwise usually transudate.**

10. Clinical Therapeutics: Cellulitis. Answer B: Dicloxacillin and other oral penicillinase-resistant penicillin antibiotics are the treatment of choice for cellulitis. A, Vancomycin and Zosyn (C) are intravenous antibiotics used to initially treat severe infections and bacteremia. Zosyn does not have coverage for MRSA, VRE, or atypicals, but does cover MSSA and other gram positives (streptococci) and gram negatives (including *Pseudomonas*). Vancomycin covers MRSA, MSSA, but does not cover gram negatives or anaerobes. They would not be first line for the treatment of cellulitis. D, Nitrofurantoin is commonly used to treat utis but is not indicated for the treatment of cellulitis.

11. Scientific Concepts: Obstipation. Answer D: Obstipation, or the inability to pass stool or gas, is a differentiation symptom between small bowel obstruction and paralytic ileus. A, Abdominal pain and (B) nausea and vomiting are common presenting symptoms of both small bowel obstruction and paralytic ileus. C, Diarrhea is not a presenting symptom of either small bowel obstruction or paralytic ileus.

12. Diagnosis: Acute Arterial Emboli. Answer B: This is typical of acute arterial emboli. The presentation is known as the 6 Ps: pain, pallor, pulselessness, poikilothermia, paresthesias, and paralysis. A, Cauda equina typically presents with numbness and weakness proximally, with associated saddle anesthesia. C, Sciatica often presents as shooting pains into the buttocks with radiation down the back of the leg, often exacerbated by certain positions. D, Acute venous thrombus, often known as DVT when in the extremities, presents with leg swelling and pain, but in a patient with warm and erythematous leg and intact distal pulses.

13. Clinical Therapeutics: *H. pylori*. Answer B: This is the suggested regimen to eradicate *H. pylori*, and thus the PUD. A, Long-term therapy with ppis is indicated in refractory PUD. C, Ranitidine is an H2 blocker and is not indicated in the treatment of *H. pylori* PUD. D, While low-fat diet may help to avoid exacerbations of PUD, it is not the desired treatment.

14. Diagnostic Studies: Pheochromocytoma. Answer A: Episodic headache, sweating, and tachycardia are a classic triad in patients with pheochromocytoma. The diagnostic study of choice is 24-hour urine metanephrines (or catecholamines depending on institution).

15. Clinical Intervention: Appendicitis. Answer D: This presentation is suggestive of early appendicitis (1 to 2 days), with clinical findings suggestive for severe infection and potential for rupture. The most appropriate treatment at this time is appendectomy, which may be preceded by imaging. A, Watchful waiting is not indicated in the setting of acute early appendicitis. B, While antibiotics may be utilized to treat the patient, surgery is still necessary. C, IR-guided incision and drainage are not indicated in setting of acute early appendicitis.

16. Clinical Therapeutics: Graves Disease. Answer D: Radioiodine causes permanent resolution of hyperthyroidism, but also causes permanent hypothyroidism which requires thyroid hormone supplementation. A, Atenolol is a β blocker and is used to treat the symptoms of hyperthyroidism but does not treat the underlying Graves disease. B, PTU and methimazole (C) are thionamides, which have the possibility of causing permanent remission, but it is not guaranteed.

17. Health Maintenance: Colorectal Cancer. Answer C: The recommended screening for colorectal cancer in a patient with a first-degree family member who was diagnosed with colorectal cancer at age less than 60 years is at 40 years of age, or 10 years before the youngest relatives' diagnosis. In this case, the patient's relative was diagnosed at 40, so 10 years prior would be to screen them at age 30.

18. Clinical Intervention: Intracranial Hemorrhage. Answer B: Alteplase (tpa) would be the most appropriate treatment at this time based on patient presentation and preferences. Inclusion criteria for the administration of tpa are: clinical diagnosis of ischemic stroke (ruled out hemorrhagic stroke), onset of symptoms <4.5 hours prior to treatment administration, and age >18. Absolute contraindications to thrombolytic therapy include a previous hemorrhagic stroke, a stroke within 1 year, a known intracranial neoplasm, active internal bleeding, a suspected aortic dissection. Relative contraindications include controlled hypertension, use of anticoagulation, and active peptic ulcer disease. A, Lovenox and aspirin (D) are not the treatment of choice in this setting. C, Atorvastatin is a medication used to treat high cholesterol. This may be started upon discharge but is not indicated for acute treatment.

19. Diagnostic Studies: Acute Cholecystitis. Answer D: Acute cholecystitis is common in middle-aged obese females, presenting with right upper quadrant abdominal pain, nausea, and vomiting worse with food, as well as positive Murphy's sign. Initial diagnostic study of choice is an ultrasound, as it is the least invasive, yet highly sensitive. Signs suggestive of cholecystitis include gallbladder wall thickening and sonographic Murphy's sign. A, Abdominal x-ray is not a preferred method of diagnosis. B, HIDA scan is used to diagnose acute cholecystitis but is not the initial study of choice. C, MRI is not indicated.

20. Health Maintenance: Atelectasis. Answer C: Incentive spirometry is used to prevent atelectasis, as well as early ambulation. A, Bed rest and frequent urination (B) are not indicated to prevent atelectasis. D, Sequential compression devices are used to prevent deep vein thrombosis

21. Diagnosis: Appendicitis. Answer C: This is the typical presentation for appendicitis. A, Abdominal pain associated with cholecystitis is often located in the right upper quadrant. B, Pain associated with gastroesophageal reflux is often located in the epigastric area. D, Pancreatitis is often associated with epigastric pain with radiation to the right upper quadrant.

22. Scientific Concepts: Hypoparathyroidism. Answer B: Hypoparathyroidism is underproduction of PTH due to decreased function of the parathyroid glands. This can be due to removal or trauma to the parathyroid glands, autoimmune dysfunction, hemochromatosis, or magnesium deficiency. The parathyroid glands contain chief cells which sense serum levels of calcium. Normally, PTH stimulates calcium release from the bones, as calcium is required for muscle and nerve function. Low levels of PTH cause hypocalcemia, as there is no longer positive feedback on calcium release and PTH normally acts on several organs to increase calcium levels, such as absorption in the bowel and bone resorption. PTH also reduces calcium excretion from the kidneys. PTH normally inhibits the proximal tubular transport of phosphate from the lumen to the interstitium, which means when there is excess PTH, hypophosphatemia occurs (more phosphate is excreted). The exact opposite occurs with hypoparathyroidism—phosphate remains elevated in the serum.

23. Diagnosis: Dumping Syndrome. Answer B: This presentation is characteristic of dumping syndrome. The high carb content causes rapid fluid shifts from plasma into the bowel, resulting in hypotension and sympathetic response, including abdominal pain, nausea, vomiting, diarrhea, tachycardia, diaphoresis, and lightheadedness. A, Gastroenteritis often presents in this manner, in the setting of multiple prior episodes triggered by high carbohydrate content meals in a post-gastric bypass patient. Dumping syndrome is more likely. C, Gastroesophageal reflux may cause episodes of abdominal pain, nausea and vomiting after meals, but is not often associated with sympathetic response. D, While patients with celiac sprue may present similarly in response to carbohydrates, although less likely, these episodes began acutely after gastric bypass surgery.

24. Clinical Therapeutics: STEMI. Answer D: In the setting of a stable patient with left main coronary artery disease or severe multivessel (>3 vessels) disease, CABG is the preferred method of treatment. A, This is not indicated in acute ST elevation in myocardial infarction. B, tpa is not indicated in this setting. C, PCI is indicated in <3 vessel disease and not involving the left main coronary artery.

25. Diagnosis: Anal Fissure. Answer A: This is a typical presentation of anal fissure. On exam, may see a laceration, most commonly located in the posterior anal midline. B, Internal hemorrhoids often present with painless rectal bleeding. C, Colon polyps do not typically present with pain. D, Crohn disease does not typically present with rectal pain or bleeding.

General Surgery

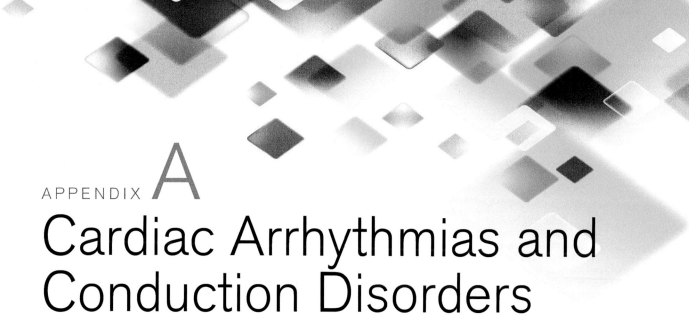

Cardiac Arrhythmias and Conduction Disorders

- Atrial fibrillation—Most common chronic arrhythmia, incidence and prevalence increase with age → decreases CO and is the most common cause of embolic cerebrovascular accidents; called the "holiday heart" when caused by excessive ETOH use or withdrawal

- Paroxysmal supraventricular tachycardia (PSVT)—Most common paroxysmal tachycardia and usually occurs in people with structural heart problems; described as "racing heart"

Disease	Etiology, Prevalence, Risk Factors	Clinical Symptoms and Signs	Diagnostics	Therapy, Prognosis, and Health Maintenance
Premature atrial contractions (PACs)	Adrenergic stress, drugs, ETOH, tobacco, electrolyte imbalance, ischemia, infection Originates in atria instead of sinus node	1. Asymptomatic or palpitations	1. Routine EKG: early P waves differing in morphology from normal sinus P wave, normal QRS complex 2. Holter monitor	1. Observation 2. **β-Blockers** if SX
Supraventricular arrhythmias		1. Palpitations 2. Angina 3. Fatigue 4. HF symptoms <u>Unstable:</u> 1. Chest pain 2. Dyspnea 3. AMS 4. Hypotension	1. Routine EKG 2. If significant bradycardia or tachyarrhythmia—monitor continuously	1. Stable—amiodarone or lidocaine 2. Unstable—synchronized cardioversion
PSVT (paroxysmal supraventricular tachycardia)	**AV node reentrant tachycardia: 2 pathways** in AV node, so reentrant circuit is within AV node • MCC of SVT • Initiated or terminated by PACs <u>Causes:</u> Digoxin toxicity, IHD, excessive caffeine or ETOH intake	1. "Racing heart"	1. Routine EKG: narrow, complex tachycardia, **no discernable P waves** because circuit short and conduction rapid; impulses exit and activate atria/vent simultaneously	1. Stable: • **Valsalva maneuver,** bearing down, cough, breath holding, carotid sinus massage • Med—**Adenosine IV** push <u>Prevention:</u> • **Digoxin** • Radiofrequency catheter ablation

(continued)

(continued)

Disease	Etiology, Prevalence, Risk Factors	Clinical Symptoms and Signs	Diagnostics	Therapy, Prognosis, and Health Maintenance
Atrial fibrillation	Irregularly irregular rhythm **Atrial rate > 400 bpm**, but most impulses blocked by AV node, so ventricular rate 75-175 At high risk for VTE and hemodynamic compromise if underlying heart disease Multiple foci in atria firing continuously in chaotic pattern MCC: **Hyperthyroidism and mitral stenosis**	1. Fatigue 2. Exertional dyspnea Signs: Uncontrolled—rapid ventricular response	1. Routine EKG: **irregularly irregular rhythm**; irregular R-R intervals and excessive rapid series of tiny, erratic spikes on EKG with wavy baseline, **no identifiable P waves** • Narrow-complex, absence of discernable P waves	1. If **stable** • **Rate control**: 60-100, β-blockers preferred • Nondihydropyridine CCB • **Cardioversion** to sinus rhythm (first A-fib, worsening, or hemo-unstable) • **Anticoagulation** to prevent CVA • If present >48 h, anticoag with warfarin for *3 wk before and 4 wk after* cardioversion, **INR 2-3** • May obtain TEE → IV heparin and cardioversion within 24 h 2. **Unstable** (decompensated HF, hypotension, uncontrolled angina): **cardioversion 200 J** 3. Chronic A-Fib • Rate control: BB • Anticoagulation: not for young (<60) 4. New onset—rate control • **CCB or BB**: diltiazem or metoprolol • Anticoagulants: IV Hep or LMWH
Atrial Flutter	**Saw-tooth pattern**, most likely in inferior leads (II, III, aVF) MCC: **heart failure** Also, COPD, rheumatic fever, or ASD, initiation of anti-arrhythmics, thyrotoxicosis, obesity, OSA, sinus sick syndrome, pericarditis, PE, s/p cardiac surgery, s/p ablation One irritable automaticity focus in atria fires **250-350 bpm**, giving rise to atrial contractions; ventricular rate of about 150 bpm in patients not taking AV node blockers	1. Palpitations 2. Lightheadedness 3. Fatigue 4. SOB (mild) 5. Less common: chest pain, anxiety, presyncope/syncope Signs: 1. Hypotension 2. Tachycardia 3. Diaphoresis 4. Evidence of CHF Complications: increased risk of atrial thrombus formation → embolization	1. Routine **EKG**: saw-tooth baseline, QRS complex appearing every 2nd or 3rd "tooth" • P waves absent • Best seen in inferior leads: II, III, aVF • 2:1 conduction across AV node so ventricular rate = ½ flutter rate in absence of AV node dysfunction 2. Echocardiogram (**TEE** preferred): obtain in all patients to evaluate size of atria, size/function of ventricles, and to r/o pericardial or Valvular disease or LVH 3. Labs: lytes, LFT's, BUN/Cr, TFTs 4. Other testing: Exercise testing, Holter Monitor	**Stable** 1. Watchful waiting if hemo-stable: can spontaneously revert to NSR 2. Rate control: **BB or (NDP) CCB** a. Esmolol, Verapamil, Diltiazem b. Digoxin + BB, if concurrent HF or hypotension 3. Drug refractory cases: ablation of AV node, pacemaker implantation Definitive: 1. Radiofrequency catheter ablation (definitive) 2. If not readily available, can use synchronized direct current or IV ibutilide Acute A-Flutter: 1. IV Amiodarone to lower rate quicker Health Maintenance: 1. Anticoagulants after rate control to decrease embolization • Depends on risk factors (CHADS2), but generally DTI or Factor Xa inhibit. Complications: AMI, dizziness or syncope, heart failure, embolization of clot

Disease	Etiology, Prevalence, Risk Factors	Clinical Symptoms and Signs	Diagnostics	Therapy, Prognosis, and Health Maintenance
Ventricular arrhythmias	Complication of acute MI and dilated CM	1. Sustained or unsustained 2. Stable vs unstable 3. May present without a pulse		
Premature ventricular contraction (PVC)	Benign Occurs with ischemia or electrolyte disturbances Occurs in patients with or without structural heart disease: hypoxia, electrolyte imbalance, stimulants, caffeine, meds, heart disease 50% of men with Holter monitor Fires on its own from focus in ventricle and spreads to other ventricle Slower conduction = wide QRS	1. Asymptomatic or palpitations 2. If low CO → syncope, dizziness, sudden death	1. Routine EKG: wide, bizarre QRS complexes followed by compensatory pause → p wave unseen because it is "buried" within QRS complex 2. Holter monitor	1. Observation! 2. **BB or CCB** if symptomatic, otherwise untreated 3. Patients with frequent, repetitive PVCs and underlying cardiac disease—increased risk for sudden death due to V-fib → electrophysiologic study
Ventricular tachycardia: originates below bundle of His	V-tach: 3+ consecutive ventricular premature beats, rate **100-250 bpm** *Sustained*: persists in the absence of intervention, **lasts longer than 30 seconds**, almost always symptomatic • Hypotension, life-threatening → V-fib **"Wide QRS tachycardia"**	1. Palpitations 2. Dyspnea 3. Light-headedness 4. Angina 5. Syncope or near-syncope • Sudden cardiac death • Cardiogenic shock • "Cannon A" waves in the neck and S1 varying in intensity *Nonsustained*: brief, self-limited, asymptomatic If CAD/LV dysfunction → risk factor for sudden death	1. Routine EKG: **wide, bizarre QRS** complexes • Monomorphic–all QRS are identical • Polymorphic: QRS are all different	Does not respond to vagal maneuvers or adenosine 1. **Treat reversible causes** 2. *Sustained VT*– • Stable = IV **amiodarone** • Unstable = synchronous DC cardioversion → **IV amiodarone** • Eventual **ICD placement** 3. *Nonsustained VT*– • No heart disease or asymptomatic → no treatment • Heart disease, recent MI, LVD → electrophysiology study 4. Post-MI: poor prognosis
Ventricular fibrillation	MCC: **ischemic heart disease** QT prolonging meds If develops within 48 h of MI, good long-term prognosis and chronic amiodarone not needed If not → prophylactic amiodarone or ICD needed Multiple foci in ventricles fire rapidly, leading to chaotic quivering of ventricles = no cardiac output	1. Sudden **unconsciousness** and death, early morning 2. Cannot measure BP; absent heart sounds and pulse	1. Routine EKG: no atrial P wave or QRS complexes	1. Severe hypotension or LOC → **synchronized cardioversion** 2. Pulseless V-tach: immediate **defibrillation** and **CPR** 3. If continued → **1 mg IV bolus epinephrine**, then q 3-5 min Defibrillate q 30-60 s 4. Refractory V-fib: IV amiodarone, followed by shock 5. If cardioversion successful: continuous IV infusion of the effective drug, implantable ICD
Prolonged QT syndrome	Congenital or acquired	1. Recurrent syncope 2. Death	1. Routine EKG: QT 0.5-0.7 s Ventricular arrhythmias	1. Treat electrolyte abnormalities and D/C drugs that prolong QT

(continued)

(continued)

Disease	Etiology, Prevalence, Risk Factors	Clinical Symptoms and Signs	Diagnostics	Therapy, Prognosis, and Health Maintenance
Torsades de pointes (turning of the points): rapid polymorphic VT	V-tach, QRS complex twists around the baseline Dangerous: Can lead to V-fib Factors that prolong QT: congenital, TCAs, anticholinergics, electrolyte abnormalities, ischemia	Occurs spontaneously	1. EKG: continuously changing axis 2. Hypokalemia 3. **Hypomagnesemia**	1. **IV magnesium**, correct electrolyte abnormality 2. Remove offending drugs 3. Isoproterenol infusion and overdrive pacing after initial therapy 4. Recurrent—permanent pacemaker
Sinus bradycardia	Sinus rate <60 bpm	1. Asymptomatic 2. Fatigue 3. Inability to exercise 4. Angina 5. Syncope	1. Routine EKG: normal PR interval	1. Most do not require treatment 2. May trial **atropine** if severely symptomatic
Sinus tachycardia	Sinus rate >100 bpm	1. Palpitations	1. Routine EKG: normal PR interval	
Sick sinus syndrome: persistent spontaneous sinus bradycardia (Fig. A-1)	Abnormality of cardiac impulse formation that may be caused by an intrinsic disease of sinus node that makes it unable to pace-make or by extrinsic causes MC: **Elderly** May occur in **heart surgery** patients Caused by scarring of heart's conduction system	1. Worse with: digitalis, CCB, BB, sympatholytic agents, anti-arrhythmic drugs, aerosol propellant abuse 2. Nonspecific: fatigue, irritability, memory loss, light-headedness, palpitations 3. Most asymptomatic *Syncope, presyncope, palpitations, dizziness, confusion, HF, palpitations, decreased exercise tolerance*	1. Routine EKG: **sinus bradycardia**, sinus arrest, sinoatrial block, alternating patterns of bradycardia and tachycardia, **loss of P waves** 2. Holter monitoring—two 24-h periods; must last for at least 1 min 3. Exercise stress test	1. *Symptomatic—atrial or dual-chamber* **permanent pacemaker** • Provides effective relief of symptoms • Lowers incidence of atrial fibrillation, thromboembolic events, heart failure, and mortality • Digitalis can cause bradyarrhythmias in SSS Complications: Myocardial perforation, pneumothorax, wound hematoma, venous thrombosis, pacemaker lead failure, infection
Wolff-Parkinson-White (WPW) syndrome	A **narrow**-complex SVT	1. Chest pain • Sudden onset • Without exertion • Lasts 10-20 min • Can describe as chest heaviness • Resolves spontaneously • Recurrent episodes 2. **Palpitations** and SOB 3. Light-headedness, chest pain lasting longer 4. Syncope Signs: Tachycardic, hypertensive, cool, diaphoretic	1. CBC, CMP, LFT, TSH, drug screen 2. Routine EKG: **delta waves, short PR interval**, wide QRS	*Terminating acute episodes* 1. Vagal maneuvers 2. AV blockade: IV adenosine 6-12 mg • **Radiofrequency catheter ablation** (preferred) • Anti-arrhythmics to slow accessory conduction • AV node blocking drugs • Avoid in acute setting Avoid: CCB (verapamil), digoxin → both increase ventricular rates
First-degree heart block: delay in AV node	All atrial beats conducted to ventricles, but **PR interval greater than 0.21 s** Benign	1. Asymptomatic 2. Higher blocks: weakness, fatigue, light-headedness, syncope	1. Routine EKG: prolonged PRI with a QRS following each P wave	1. None

Disease	Etiology, Prevalence, Risk Factors	Clinical Symptoms and Signs	Diagnostics	Therapy, Prognosis, and Health Maintenance
Second degree type 1 (wenckebach): site within AV node	Not all atrial beats conducted to ventricles Abnormal conduction in AV node Can occur in **normal subjects or athletes** with no underlying cardiac pathology Reversible causes: 1. Pathologic: MI, Myopathy (amyloidosis, sarcoidosis), myocarditis (Lyme), endocarditis with abscess formation, hyperkalemia, hypervagotonia 2. Iatrogenic: AV node blockers, s/p cardiac surgery or s/p catheter ablation, s/p AV implant	Asymptomatic OR 1. Symptoms of hypoperfusion: a. Fatigue b. Lightheadedness c. Syncope or presyncope d. Angina 2. Heart Failure Signs: 1. Bradycardia 2. Diaphoresis 3. Crackles, JVD, peripheral edema	EKG: 1. Progressive ≥lengthening of PR with shortening of RR interval 2. Eventual dropped beat *Signs of hemodynamic instability: hypotension, AMS, signs of shock, ongoing ischemic chest pain, evidence of acute pulmonary edema	1. Unstable* a. If symptomatic and hemo-unstable - IV Atropine 0.5 mg, every 3-5 minutes up to 3 mg b. **Transcutaneous pacing** (temporary) c. If the patient remains unstable or has HF - IV Dobutamine d. Transvenous pacing e. Follow algorithm below 2. Stable - Evaluate for reversible causes a. No cause/symptoms = no treatment b. No cause, symptomatic • Temporary trans. pacing • **Permanent Pacemaker** (PPM) (definitive) c. Treat reversible cause if identified and if AV block persists, place PPM
Second degree type 2 (mobitz): site of block within His-purkinje system	Not all atrial beats conducted to ventricles Due to a block within His bundle Rarely seen in patients without underlying heart disease Reversible causes: Same as for 2nd Degree Type I above, MC: AMI with ischemia of AV node, AV node blockers (digoxin, BB, CCB)	Most are symptomatic: 1. Fatigue 2. Dyspnea 3. Syncope or presyncope 4. Sudden cardiac arrest Signs: 1. Bradycardia 2. Pale 3. Diaphoretic 4. Crackles, JVD, peripheral edema	EKG: 1. Intermittently nonconducted atrial beats 2. Fixed PR interval with occasional dropped beats	Same treatment algorithm as above for 2nd Degree Type I 1. If stable, no urgent therapy required, however, Mobitz Type II is unstable by nature and frequently progresses to 3rd degree heart block a. Transcutaneous pacing – recommended b. If AMI is source, revascularization recommended c. Remove any offending agents, if any d. If Lyme carditis or electrolyte/TFT abnormality, pacemaker not necessary e. If no reversible cause identified, dual chamber (AV) **permanent pacemaker** (definitive) recommended even if asymptomatic
Third degree heart block (complete): Due to lesion distal to his bundle	Complete dissociation between atria and ventricles Vent rate: 25-40 bpm A/V dissociation Reversible causes: Same as for 2nd Degree Type I and II above, MC: idiopathic (>50%)	Same as above for 2nd degree heart blocks: 1. Fatigue 2. Dyspnea 3. Cardiac Death Signs: 1. Bradycardia 2. Pale 3. Diaphoretic 4. Crackles, JVD, peripheral edema	EKG: 1. Dissociation between the electrical activity of atrium and ventricle (P wave does not correlate at all with QRS wave)	Same treatment algorithm as above for 2nd Degree Type I 1. Atropine (as above) 2. Temporary transthoracic or transvenous pacing • Dobutamine (as above) 3. **Permanent pacing** if no reversible cause identified or if heart block does not resolve

CARDIOVERSION VERSUS DEFIBRILLATION

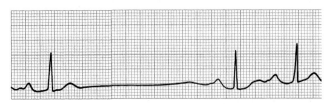

FIGURE A-1. EKG findings in a patient with sinus sick syndrome. This may include bradycardia-tachycardia syndrome, sinus arrest for >3 seconds, sinus arrhythmia, or sinus bradycardia. (From Young V, Kormos W, Chick D. *Blueprints Medicine*. 6th ed. Philadelphia: Wolters Kluwer; 2016.)

- Couplet: 2 successive PVCs
- Bigeminy: sinus beat followed by PVC
- Trigeminy: 2 sinus beats followed by PVC

		Indications
Cardiac pacemakers	1. Delivers direct electrical stimulation to heart when heart's natural pacemaker is unable to do so • Permanent—long term • Transcutaneous or transvenous—use external pulse generator that the patient secures to waist with straps	• **Sinus node dysfunction, also known as sinus sick syndrome (MC):** with symptomatic bradycardia, HR <40 bpm, minimal symptoms with HR <30, • Symptomatic heart block (Mobitz type II and complete) • Symptomatic bradyarrhythmias • Tachyarrhythmias
Cardioversion	• Delivery of shock that is in synchrony with the QRS complex • Purpose is to terminate dysrhythmias (PSVT, VT) • An electrical shock during T wave can cause V-fib	A-fib, atrial flutter VT with a pulse SVT
Defibrillation	• Delivery of a shock not in synchrony with QRS complex • Purpose is to convert dysrhythmia to normal sinus rhythm	VT **without** a pulse V-fib
Automatic implantable defibrillator	Device that is surgically placed: when it detects a lethal dysrhythmia, it delivers a shock to defibrillate Delivers a set number of shocks until the dysrhythmia is terminated	VT not controlled by medical therapy V-fib
Pharmacologic cardioversion	IV ibutilide, procainamide, flecainide, sotalol, amiodarone	If electric cardioversion fails

Heart Murmurs and Valvular Heart Disease

MITRAL VALVE PROLAPSE

- Primary MVP: degenerative disease in the absence of identifiable connective tissue disease, sporadic, or familial

- Secondary MVP: associated with an identifiable disorder, such as Marfan syndrome, infective endocarditis, acute rheumatic fever

- Echocardiography is indicated for patients with a family history of MVP

Disease	Etiology, Prevalence, Risk Factors	Clinical Symptoms and Signs	Diagnostics	Therapy, Prognosis, and Health Maintenance
Mitral valve prolapse Other names: click-murmur syndrome, Barlow disease, myxomatous mitral valve disease, floppy mitral valve	Common cause of mitral regurgitation Prevalence: 2.4% Currently defined using *definitions of imaging:* billowing of any portion of the mitral valve leaflets >2 mm above the annual pane in a long axis view (parasternal or apical three-chamber) Physiology: Abnormal systolic displacement of one or both leaflets into the left atrium due to a disruption or elongation of leaflets, chordae, or papillary muscles • Decreased left ventricular volume (decreased venous return) results in earlier prolapse and click heard earlier in systole, closer to S1 • Increased left ventricular volume (increased chamber size and venous return) results in delayed prolapse, click heard later in systole "Click" is caused by prolapse of leaflets into left atrium and tensing of mitral valve apparatus	1. Nonspecific • *Chest pain* (MC) • Atypical or nonanginal • Mild or disabling and recurrent • Palpitations • MC: dyspnea • Panic/anxiety • Exercise intolerance • Dizziness or syncope • Numbness or tingling • Skeletal abnormalities Signs: 1. Pectus excavatum 2. Narrow AP chest diameter 3. Scoliosis 4. Loss of kyphosis in thoracic spine 5. **Mid-systolic click** followed by a mid-to-**late systolic murmur** and loud S2 1. Grade: N/A 2. Quality: N/A 3. Systolic 4. Heard best: precordium (anterior) or apex (posterior) 5. Radiation: axilla and back 6. Earlier click: sitting, standing from seated position, handgrip, Valsalva 7. Later click: *squatting* from seated or standing position 8. Associated: • Tricuspid valve abnormality in 40%-50%	1. **TTE**: >2 mm of leaflet displacement above the plane of the mitral annulus in the long axis view (diagnostic) 2. TEE is especially helpful for diagnostic accuracy if undergoing surgical and percutaneous repair	1. Reassurance about benign nature 2. Lifestyle modifications • Aerobic exercise • Avoid stimulants (caffeine), alcohol, and undue fatigue • Reduce stressors 3. Do not treat chest pain with β-blockers—ineffective 4. Treat underlying anxiety, panic disorder, or depression Health maintenance: 1. ADA no longer recommends prophylactic antibiotics for MVP 2. Repeat routine imaging • Stage B (progressive) with mild regurgitation: every 3-5 y • Stage B with moderate regurgitation: every 1-2 y • Stage C1 (asymptomatic severe mitral regurgitation without evidence of LVD): every 6-12 mo Complications: 1. Leads to mitral regurgitation 2. Predisposed to **infective endocarditis** 3. Heart failure 4. TIA or CVA • Aspirin recommended in unexplained TIA with no atrial thrombi 5. Atrial fibrillation with severe mitral regurgitation or embolic events • Treat with warfarin, goal INR 2.5 (range: 2-3) 6. Sudden cardiac death (SCD)

MID-SYSTOLIC MURMURS

Disease	Etiology, Prevalence, Risk Factors	Clinical Symptoms and Signs	Diagnostics	Therapy, Prognosis, and Health Maintenance
Hypertrophic cardiomyopathy (HCM)	Prevalence: 1:500 (0.2%) Most: **autosomal dominant trait**, 60%-70% caused by mutation in sarcomere gene; (+) family history Left ventricular hypertrophy leading to LV outflow obstruction, diastolic dysfunction, myocardial ischemia, and mitral regurgitation MC presentation: **Heart failure with resultant DOE** (90% of symptomatic patients) MC location: increased wall thickness in basal anterior septum in continuity with anterior free wall **Crescendo-decrescendo** murmur Differentiate from aortic stenosis by having patient perform routine maneuvers and position changes	Infants: 1. Lethargy 2. Rapid breathing 3. Difficulty feeding Signs: 1. S4 2. **Systolic murmur** 3. Left ventricular lift 4. **Bisferious pulse** (carotid pulse with 2 upstrokes) 5. Prominent "a" wave in neck veins 1. Grade: varies 2. Quality: harsh 3. Systolic 4. Heard best: 4thLICS (**LLSB**) and apex 5. Radiation: axilla, base 6. Louder: squatting, sitting, or supine → standing; **Valsalva**; NTG administration (decreases LV volume) 7. Quieter: standing → sitting or squatting; **handgrip**; passive elevation of legs 8. Associated: palpable/**loud S4,** LV heave	1. EKG (first line): **LVH with RAE**; left axis deviation • Most sensitive 2. TTE: unexplained **LV wall thickness >15 mm** (diagnostic); systolic anterior motion (SAM) of mitral valve or hyperdynamic LV 3. Exercise *stress testing:* test for ischemia and arrhythmias 4. Cardiac MR (CMR) imaging 5. Cardiac catheterization 6. Genetic testing	1. Asymptomatic–close observation, no therapy indicated 2. Negative inotropic monotherapy • β-Blockers: nadolol Or • Nondihydropyridine CCB: verapamil • ± adjunctive disopyramide • Slow HR, allowing ventricle to fill and prolonging diastole–improves dyspnea and chest pain 3. Surgery indications: • Reserved for patients with NYHA class III/IV despite maximum tolerated drug therapy • Recurrent syncope • LVOT gradient >50 mm Hg at rest or with exercise • Options: surgical myectomy and non-surgical septal ablation Health maintenance: 1. Prohibit strenuous activities 2. If (+), test siblings every year between ages 12 and 18, then every 5 y 3. First-degree family members of the affected individual should be tested for inheritance: H&P, EKG, TTE; no genetic screening unless definite HCM-mutation identified 4. Endocarditis prophylaxis **not** recommended Prognosis: 1. Annual mortality rate: 1% or less per year 2. Increased risk of death from sickle cell disease, HF, stroke 3. Death rate varies with age of the patient at diagnosis: younger the patient, higher the risk 4. In HCM patients with A-fib: increased risk of VTE → warfarin recommended long term, INR 2-3

Aortic stenosis	Most common cause of left ventricular outflow obstruction: 1. Diastolic dysfunction with an increase in LV filling pressure with exercise 2. Inability of LV to increase CO during exercise <ins>MC presentation:</ins> **Elderly with syncopal episodes** "Severe AS": AS with a maximum aortic transvalvular velocity >4 m/s with an aortic valve area <1 cm² <ins>Etiology:</ins> • Congenital • Calcific disease of a trileaflet valve **or congenital bicuspid aortic valve** (MC in the United States, MCC in children with AS) • Rheumatic valve disease (MC worldwide)	1. ***Dyspnea on exertion*** (MC) or decreased exercise tolerance 2. Exertional dizziness (presyncope) or syncope 3. Exertional angina 4. Symptoms of heart failure 5. Syncope 6. Angina <ins>Signs:</ins> 1. Carotid pulse • "Parvus and tardus" (small/weak, rises slowly) • ± thrill or coarse vibration (shuddering) 2. Palpable S4 1. Grade: varies (1-4) 2. Quality: **harsh**, loud 3. Systolic 4. Heard best: second right ICS (base of heart, aortic region) 5. Radiation: **carotids** 6. Louder: N/A 7. Quieter: N/A 8. Associated • If severe: brisk upward deflection **of carotids** • Paradoxically split S2 • **Crescendo-decrescendo** *harsh* "systolic ejection" click • 80% have concurrent aortic regurgitation	<ins>In acute setting:</ins> 1. CXR–r/o heart failure and other causes of SOB • Typically, normal in AS • May see dilatation of ascending aorta <ins>Otherwise:</ins> 1. EKG: Left ventricular hypertrophy (nonspecific), increased voltage of QRS complex, ST-T wave changes, ± left atrial hypertrophy • Used to detect concurrent atrial fibrillation or coronary disease 2. **TTE** (diagnostic) • Thick and calcified aortic leaflets 3. Exercise (stress) testing–used to verify asymptomatic severe AS • Do not perform in symptomatic severe AS 4. Cardiac catheterization–recommended if noninvasive evaluation is nondiagnostic and clinical suspicion high 5. Coronary angiography • Indicated before valve intervention in patients with angina, objective ischemia, decreased LV systolic function, history of CAD or coronary RF (men >40 y/o or postmenopausal women)	<ins>Asymptomatic AS:</ins> 1. No proven therapies to delay progression 2. Statin therapy not recommended for *prevention* of AS *progression* 3. Treat HTN and monitor/titrate carefully 4. Treat *CAD risk factors*, including statin therapy for primary or secondary prevention <ins>Symptomatic AS:</ins> 1. Prompt valve replacement • Surgical aortic valve replacement (SAVR)–see section "SAVR Versus TAVI" • Transcatheter aortic valve implantation (TAVI) • Percutaneous aortic balloon dilation • Only used as a bridge to TAVI or SAVR in patients with severe symptomatic AS 2. Supportive, if surgery must be delayed • Mild physical activity • Management of cardiovascular risk factors (hyperlipidemia) • Control atrial fibrillation with digoxin and/or β-blockers • Manage HTN • Control HF (diuretic + ACEI) 3. Patients with CAD and AS (>70% reduction in luminal diameter in major arteries or >50% reduction in left main) • Coronary artery bypass grafting (CABG) • Percutaneous coronary intervention (PCI) <ins>Prognosis for symptomatic AS:</ins> 1. Mortality increases after development of cardiac symptoms 2. Pulmonary hypertension commonly occurs <ins>Health maintenance:</ins> 1. Serial echo every: • Stage B (mild): 3-5 y • Stage B (mod): 1-2 y • Stage C1: 6-12 mo, unless change in symptoms/signs or worsening cardiac status <ins>Complications:</ins> 1. Atrial fibrillation (5%-6% of adults) • RF: older age, severe AS, LV hypertrophy, LV systolic dysfunction 2. Sudden cardiac death (incidence 1%) 3. Infective endocarditis • Antibiotic prophylaxis no longer recommended for undergoing dental or other invasive procedures, unless high risk • High risk: previous IE or prosthetic heart valves 4. Increased risk of bleeding, including chronic GI bleeding due to angiodysplasia (AVM) → simply put, due to acquired von Willebrand syndrome
Aortic stenosis (children)	>75% of affected children are males	1. Asymptomatic 2. Symptomatic • Heart failure (10%) at 2-6 mo <ins>Signs:</ins> 1. Tachypnea 2. Poor feeding 3. Growth failure 4. Hepatomegaly 5. Peripheral edema	1. 2D Echo with Doppler 2. EKG–limited utility • LV hypertrophy, inverted T wave 3. CXR–cardiomegaly 4. Cardiac catheterization– if diagnosis uncertain • Balloon valvotomy can be performed concurrently	1. IV prostaglandin E1 (Alprostadil) to open or maintain patency of ductus arteriosus 2. Percutaneous balloon aortic valvuloplasty (PBAV; definitive) preferred 3. Valvotomy 4. Valve replacement (reserved for adults with severe AS) • May be used in children with congenital AS who develop severe AR following BAV • Mechanical valves preferred

Bicuspid aortic valve (BAV)	Most common congenital heart lesion Prevalence: 0.5%-2%	1. Grade varies
		2. Constant
		3. Early systolic ejection click
		4. Heard best: apex
		5. No radiation
		6. Louder: N/A
		7. Quieter: N/A
		8. Associated: aortic stenosis, aortic regurgitation
			1. **Echocardiography**—needed for differentiation of normal physiologic split of S1
			2. CMRI or CTA
				1. Medical therapy
				  • If BAV and AS: treat HTN and monitor diastolic BP
				  • If AR and HTN: long-term vasodilators (ACEI, ARB, DHP-CCB)
				2. Balloon valvuloplasty
				  • For children and select young adults
				3. Surgery
				  • For severe AS with symptoms of LV systolic dysfunction (LVEF <50%), symptomatic AR, or severe AR
				Health maintenance:
				1. Recommend EKG screening in first-degree relatives

Indications for Aortic Valve Replacement for Aortic Stenosis

- Based on symptom status, severity of aortic stenosis, left ventricular ejection fraction, and whether other cardiac surgery is indicated
- Recommended valve replacement
  - *Promptly* for patients with severe high-gradient AS with symptoms (based on history or exercise testing)
  - Asymptomatic patients with severe AS and LVEF <50%
  - Severe AS when undergoing other cardiac surgery
- May not be recommended if:
  - Comorbid conditions, including malignancy
  - High-risk patients (may be candidate for TAVI)
  - Refusal by patient

SAVR Versus TAVI

- Society of Thoracic Surgeons Predicted Risk of Mortality (STS-PROM) used to determine risk of mortality and morbidity
- Must have life expectancy of >1 year, and quality of life must be likely to improve with either treatment to be a candidate
- Must not have comorbidities that would preclude an expected benefit from correction of AS

	SAVR	TAVI

Indications	1. Symptomatic severe AS
	  • Low surgical risk (score <4)
	  • Intermediate surgical risk (score 4-8), only if transfemoral TAVI not feasible
		1. Symptomatic severe AS
		  • High surgical risk (score >8)
		  • Intermediate surgical risk (score 4-8)—preferred
		  • Extreme surgical risk or absolute contraindication to SAVR

Contraindications	1. Extreme surgical risk 2. Porcelain aorta, hostile chest (radiation damage or complications from prior surgeries making sternotomy or thoracotomy dangerous)	1. Life expectancy <1 y owing to noncardiac comorbidities 2. Unlikely improvement in QOL owing to comorbidities 3. Severe other valve disease only treatable by surgery

Severity of Aortic Valve Replacement

Stage	Description and Symptoms	Valve Anatomy		Hemodynamics		LVEF
		Calcium	Mobility	Key Criteria	Additional Measures	
A	At risk (asymptomatic)	+	Normal	Aortic V_{max} <2 m/s	–	Normal
B	Progressive (asymptomatic)	++	↓ to ↓↓	Mild AS: aortic V_{max} 2.0-2.9 m/s or mean ΔP <20 mm Hg Moderate AS: Aortic V_{max} 3.0-3.9 m/s or mean ΔP 20-39 mm Hg	–	Normal
C1	Asymptomatic severe AS with normal LVEF	+++	↓↓↓	Aortic V_{max} ≥4 m/s or mean ΔP 40 mm Hg (severe) Aortic V_{max} ≥5 m/s or mean ΔP ≥60 mm Hg (severe)	AVA typically ≤1 cm² (or AVAi ≤0.6 cm²/m²	Normal
C2	Asymptomatic severe AS with low LVEF	+++	↓↓↓	Aortic V_{max} ≥4 m/s or mean ΔP 40 mm Hg (severe)	AVA typically ≤1 cm² (or AVAi ≤0.6 cm²/m²	<50%
D1	Symptomatic severe high-gradient AS	++++	↓↓↓↓	Aortic V_{max} ≥4 m/s or mean ΔP 40 mm Hg (severe)	AVA typically ≤1 cm² (or AVAi ≤0.6 cm²/m² but may be larger with mixed AS/AR	Normal or ↓

(continued)

(continued)

Stage	Description and Symptoms	Valve Anatomy		Hemodynamics		LVEF
		Calcium	Mobility	Key Criteria	Additional Measures	
D2	Symptomatic severe low-gradient AS with low LVEF	++++	↓↓↓	Resting AVA ≤1 cm² with aortic V_{max} <4 m/s or mean ΔP <40 mm Hg	Dobutamine stress shows AVA ≤1 cm² with V_{max} ≥4 m/s at any flow rate	<50%
D3	Symptomatic severe low-gradient AS with normal LVEF	++++	↓↓↓	AVA ≤1 cm² with aortic V_{max} <4 m/s or mean ΔP <40 mm Hg Measured when the patient is normotensive (systolic BP <140 mm Hg)	Indexed AVA ≤0.6 cm²/m² **and** stroke volume index <35 mL/m²	Normal

Reproduced from Otto CM, Nishimura RA. New ACC/AHA valve guidelines: aligning definitions of aortic stenosis severity with treatment recommendations. *Heart*. 2014;100:902. Copyright © 2014 BMJ Publishing Group Ltd and British Cardiovascular Society. All rights reserved.

Choice of Valve Replacement

- EKG performed every 6 to 12 months in children with mechanical valves and every 3 to 6 months with bioprosthetic valves

- Replacement of the aortic valve by a pulmonary autograft (the Ross procedure), when performed by an experienced surgeon, may be considered in young patients when VKA anticoagulation is contraindicated or undesirable

Bioprosthesis	Mechanical Prosthesis
• Any age, if long-term anticoagulant therapy contraindicated, cannot be managed appropriately, or not desired • Reasonable in patients 60-70 y/o • High failure rate in children and young adults (20% within 3 y)	• For AR or MR in patients <60 y of age with no contraindication to long-term anticoagulation • Reasonable in patients 60-70 y/o • Preferred for long-term durability, even though they require systemic anticoagulation

FUNCTIONAL AND INNOCENT MURMURS

- One-third to three-fourths of children have innocent murmurs present between ages 1 and 14 years, most commonly innocent Still murmur

Disease	Etiology, Prevalence, Risk Factors	Clinical Symptoms and Signs	Diagnostics	Therapy, Prognosis, and Health Maintenance
Peripheral pulmonary stenosis	Occurs in early infancy as pulmonary vascular resistance decreases Turbulent flow in proximal pulmonary arteries Common functional murmur	1. Grade 1-2 2. Medium to high pitch 3. Mid-systolic ejection murmur 4. Heard best at upper LSB or RSB 5. Radiates to axilla and back		1. Spontaneously resolves by age 6-12 mo
Innocent (Still) murmur	Most common murmur of childhood (2-7 y of age)	1. Grade: 1-2 2. **Vibratory** or **musical** quality; **short, high-pitched** 3. Systolic murmur 4. Heard best: LLSB or between LLSB and apex 5. Minimal radiation 6. Louder: squatting, **supine**, *anxiety*, ***fever***, **anemia, sinus tachycardia** 7. Quieter: squat → stand, Valsalva, ***sitting***, **inspiration**		1. Resolves spontaneously by early adolescence if not sooner

Disease	Etiology, Prevalence, Risk Factors	Clinical Symptoms and Signs	Diagnostics	Therapy, Prognosis, and Health Maintenance
Cervical venous hum (Fig. B-1)	Common innocent murmur in children Alteration of intensity with movement is key in distinguishing from PDA Right-sided, changes with position, local compression	1. Grade varies 2. Continuous 3. Venous hum 4. LUSB or ***RUSB***, infraclavicular or supraclavicular regions 5. No radiation 6. **<u>Louder</u>**: sitting with head extended 7. **<u>Quieter</u>**: rotation or flexion of head or applying light pressure over jugular vein while sitting; supine		

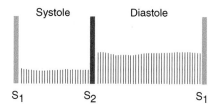

FIGURE B-1. Cervical venous hum during systole and diastole.

HOLOSYSTOLIC MURMURS

Disease	Etiology, Prevalence, Risk Factors	Clinical Symptoms and Signs	Diagnostics	Therapy, Prognosis, and Health Maintenance

Acute mitral regurgitation	Etiology:
	• Ruptured mitral chordae tendineae from MVP, infective endocarditis, or trauma, acute rheumatic fever
	• Papillary muscle rupture due to AMI, trauma, or displacement
	• LV outflow obstruction (HCM), Takotsubo CM
	MOA:
	Increased LA volume → high LA pressure → pulmonary edema; despite increased HR, fall in CO can result in cardiogenic shock
		1. Sudden onset, rapid progression of pulmonary edema, hypotension, and cardiogenic shock
		  • SOB
		  • Dyspnea on exertion
		  • Fatigue
		  • Weakness
		Signs:
		1. Hypotension
		2. Pallor
		3. Diaphoresis
		4. Thready pulses
		5. JVD
		6. Crackles
		7. S3 (common)
		
		1. Grade: 3-4
		2. Quality: soft, low pitched
		3. Holo**systolic**
		4. Heard best: LSB, base
		5. Radiation: **axilla** → posterior left thorax
		6. Louder: leg raising, lying down, isometric handgrip, squatting
		7. Quieter: ***Valsalva*** or standing
		8. Associated: **widely split S2**, mid or late systolic murmur (with MVP), mid-systolic click (with MVP)
			1. EKG: AMI, LVH, P-mitral
			2. CXR: symmetric pulmonary edema
			3. TTE (confirmatory): normal LA and LV size, hyperdynamic systolic function
			4. Cardiac catheter (coronary angiography)
			  • Recommended before elective valve surgery in patients with angina, ischemia, chronic severe secondary MR, decreased LVEF, hx of CAD or risk factors
				1. Medical therapy
				  • Support patient until dx officially made
				    • IV nitroprusside
				2. Surgery (definitive)
				  • Promptly recommended
				  • Valve repair
				Prognosis:
				1. Mortality rate with surgery is 50%

Chronic mitral regurgitation	Etiology:
	1. Primary (organic MR): degenerative mitral valve disease **(mitral valve prolapse = MCC)**, rheumatic heart disease (first 2 decades of life), infective endocarditis, trauma, drug use, valve cleft, mitral annular calcification, papillary muscle rupture
	2. Secondary (functional MR): caused by another cardiac disease **(CHD**, dilated cardiomyopathy, HCM)
	Retrograde blood flow and volume overload of the left atrium
	Differentiate from other murmurs: does not vary with respiration, louder with LV volume increase (HF, increased venous return or arterial pressure), decreased with reduced venous return
		1. Mild-mod: asymptomatic
		2. **Exertional *dyspnea***
		3. **Fatigue**
		4. Paroxysmal or persistent atrial fibrillation
		5. Heart failure SX
		  • Weakness
		  • Fatigue
		  • Exercise intolerance
		Signs:
		1. HF signs
		  • Pulmonary edema (crackles)
		2. **S3 gallop**
		3. Palpable thrill
		4. Murmur as below
		5. Grade: 3-4
		6. Quality: **High pitched, blowing**
		7. Holo**systolic**
		8. Heard best: **apex**
		9. Radiation: **axilla** → posterior left thorax
		10. Louder: leg raising, lying down, isometric handgrip, squatting
		11. Quieter: **_Valsalva_** or standing
		12. Associated: **widely split S2**, mid or late systolic murmur (with MVP), mid-systolic click (with MVP)
			1. EKG: left axis deviation or LVH, P-mitrale
			2. CXR: cardiomegaly
			3. TTE (confirmatory): increased LA size, decreased ejection fraction
			4. TEE if TTE nondiagnostic or suboptimal
			5. CMRI
			6. Cardiac cath
			7. Coronary angiography
			  • For patients with suspected CAD
			8. Stress testing
			Complications:
			Atrial fibrillation (stroke, embolization)
				1. Medical therapy
				  • For HF and HTN
				    • LVEF <60%, not candidates for surgery: treat as heart failure
				  • ACEI, BB, aldosterone antagonist, diuretics
				2. Surgery (gold standard)
				  • MV repair ≫ replacement
				3. For A-fib
				  • DC cardioversion
				  • Anti-arrhythmics
				Health maintenance:
				1. Routine monitoring with TTE every:
				  • 3-5 y: mild MR
				  • 1-2 y: mod MR
				  • 6-12 mo: severe
				2. Endocarditis prophylaxis not recommended
				3. Long-term prophylaxis against rheumatic fever recommended
				Prognosis:
				1. Correlation between the MR grade and regurgitant severity with primary mitral valve disease

Disease	Etiology, Prevalence, Risk Factors	Clinical Symptoms and Signs	Diagnostics	Therapy, Prognosis, and Health Maintenance
Ventricular septal defect (VSD)	Results in L-to-R shunt **Most common congenital anomaly;** occurs in 50% of all patients with CHD MC location: **perimembranous** (just beneath aortic valve, behind septal leaflet of tricuspid valve) Causes: • **Down syndrome** DiGeorge • FAS • Diabetes **Size** and type of VSD determine characteristics	*Acyanotic* or *cyanotic* based on **size** Neonatal: 1. Isolated systolic murmur 2. HF symptoms/signs: tachypnea, increased WOB, poor weight gain, FTT, diaphoresis with feeding Small: Asymptomatic Mod-large: 1. DOE 2. Recurrent URI 3. HF symptoms 4. FTT, poor weight gain Signs: 1. Tachypnea 2. Increased WOB 3. Rales, grunts, retractions 4. Diaphoresis 5. Pallor 6. Hepatomegaly 1. Grade: 2-3, grade 4 if thrill present 2. Quality: harsh, high pitched, or **blowing** 3. Holo**systolic** 4. Heard best: LLSB (third to fourth LICS) 5. Radiation: diffuse 6. Louder: **isometric handgrip** 7. Quieter: Valsalva 8. Other descriptors: thrill (first to second LICS), apical S3, diastolic rumble (if large, at apex) 9. Associated: pulmonary HTN and **Eisenmenger syndrome** → cyanosis + bidirectional shunt	Clinical DX: 1. EKG: LVH and RVH (**biventricular hypertrophy**) 2. CXR: cardiomegaly, increased pulmonary vascularity; enlarged LA, LV, and pulmonary artery 3. **TTE** (confirmatory): location/size of defect, direction of flow 4. Cath (rarely utilized): assesses need for closure (Qp:Qs) or perioperative management planning Complications: Endocarditis, aortic regurgitation, subaortic stenosis, right ventricular outflow tract obstruction, atrial shunting	1. Asymptomatic and small: delay treatment, 75% **close spontaneously in first 2 y of life** 2. HF symptoms: • Nutritional support: >150 kcal/kg/d • Diuretics (mainstay): PO or IV **furosemide** 1-2 mg/kg BID-TID 3. Surgical repair • **Direct patch closure** via median sternotomy • Transcatheter closure (Amplatzer muscular closure) Surgical indications: • Persistent SX despite maximal medical therapy • Mod to large defect with pulmonary HTN • Qp:Qs > 2:1, asymptomatic • Double-chambered RV Prognosis: 1. If surgery not performed in first year of life, increased risk for irreversible pulmonary vascular disease, especially in children with Down syndrome Health maintenance: 1. All immunizations up-to-date, including pneumococcal and flu; RSV prophylaxis if <1 y with VSD and HF 2. Monitor growth and development 3. Monitor for SX of heart failure 4. No endocarditis ABX prophylaxis recommended except: • Device closure or surgical ligation with prosthetics, first 6 mo after • Device closure or ligation and residual defect at site of repair

DIASTOLIC (ARMS) MURMURS

Disease	Etiology, Prevalence, Risk Factors	Clinical Symptoms and Signs	Diagnostics	Therapy, Prognosis, and Health Maintenance

Acute aortic regurgitation (aortic insufficiency)
Classic: younger patient with h/o Marfan syndrome
	Etiology:
	1. **Endocarditis** (MC)
	2. **Aortic dissection**
	3. Rupture of a congenitally fenestrated cusp
	4. Traumatic rupture of valve leaflets
	5. Iatrogenic
	6. Regurgitant flow fills a small ventricle that has not had time to dilate, causing acute/rapid increase in LV diastolic pressure and a fall in forward CO
	7. LV stroke volume increased
	*Location of murmur varies with cause:
	
	1. Valvular disease: heard at LSB
	2. Aortic root diseases: RSB and apex
		1. Symptoms of endocarditis or aortic dissection
		 • Chest or back pain
		Signs:
		1. Cardiovascular collapse
		 • Hypotension
		 • Pallor
		 • Diaphoresis
		 • Cyanosis
		 • Weak, thready, rapid pulse
		2. Pulmonary edema
		3. Signs of endocarditis or aortic dissection
		 • Unequal BP in left and right arms
		  1. Grade: varies
		  2. Quality: low pitch
		  3. *Diastolic*
		  4. Heard best: **left sternal border** (third to fourth ICS) or RSB and apex*
		  5. Radiation: none
		  6. Louder: sitting up, leaning forward, holding breath in end-expiration; **squatting**
		  7. Quieter: **Valsalva**
		  8. Other descriptors:
		  9. Associated:
		   • Soft or absent S1
		   • Soft S2, loud P2
		   • S3 present, S4 not
		   • Rumbling sound at apex (Austin Flint murmur)
			1. EKG–nonspecific ST-T wave changes
			2. CXR
			 • Normal sized left atrium and ventricle
			 • Evidence of HF and pulmonary edema
			3. TTE (diagnostic, confirms)
			4. TEE–more accurate
				1. **Medical emergency**
				 • Left ventricle unable to adapt to rapid increase in end diastolic volume due to regurgitant blood
				 • Emergent aortic valve replacement or repair
				2. If delayed, stabilize in ICU
				 • Nitroprusside
				 • Dobutamine
				3. Intra-aortic balloon pump contraindicated
				4. For aortic dissection
				 • β-Blockers with caution
				  • HR target: <60 before vasodilators
				 • If hypertensive, vasodilator therapy
				 • Emergent surgery (definitive)
				5. Treat endocarditis with antibiotics
				Complications:
				Cardiogenic shock

Chronic aortic regurgitation	Volume overload of the left ventricle gradually increases LV size maintaining forward cardiac output, despite regurgitant flow LV diastolic pressures remain normal Etiology: • MCC: aortic root dilation • Congenital bicuspid valve • Calcific valve disease • Rheumatic heart disease	1. Asymptomatic 2. Exertional dyspnea 3. Angina 4. Symptoms of HF • Orthopnea • Paroxysmal nocturnal dyspnea Signs: Pulmonary edema Signs: 1. Arterial pulse findings as below 2. Early diastolic murmur 3. Wide pulse pressure 4. **High** pitched, *blowing,* or rumbling holodiastolic **decrescendo-crescendo** ("V")	As above	1. Asymptomatic • Long-term vasodilator therapy with HTN and AR • ACEI > nifedipine

Disease	Etiology, Prevalence, Risk Factors	Clinical Symptoms and Signs	Diagnostics	Therapy, Prognosis, and Health Maintenance
Mitral stenosis	Etiology: • **Rheumatic fever** (MC) • Annular calcification • Congenital stenosis Presentation: Hemoptysis, presents in 30-40s Causes blood flow obstruction from the LA to LV, increasing pressure in LA, pulmonary vasculature, and right heart Leads to pulmonary hypertension and right-sided heart failure → high LA pressures = high pulmonary vasculature and right heart pressures 1. **Loud first heart sound**: wide closing excursion of leaflets 2. **Prominent P2 of second heart sound (split S2)**: elevated pulmonary artery pressures 3. **Opening snap**: sudden tensing of leaflets after they have completed their opening excursion 4. **Mid-diastolic rumble**–increased flow across stenotic MV during atrial contraction	1. Exertional **dyspnea** (MC) 2. Decreased exercise tolerance 3. Hemoptysis 4. Chest pain 5. Fatigue 6. Hoarseness 7. Orthopnea 8. Paroxysmal nocturnal dyspnea Signs: 1. Ascites 2. Lower extremity edema 3. Increased JVP 4. Hepatomegaly 5. RV heave 6. Palpable S2 7. Crackles (pulmonary edema) 1. Grade: varies 2. Quality: **low pitched** 3. **Diastolic rumble** 4. Heard best: apex and left sternal border 5. Radiation: little to none 6. Louder: left lateral decubitus with held **expiration**, lying supine and lifting legs 7. Quieter: **inspiration**, amyl nitrate, Valsalva, standing after squatting 8. Associated: • Preceding opening snap	1. EKG • May show atrial fibrillation • Nonspecific: left atrial hypertrophy (p-mitrale) 2. CXR–only recommended for evaluation of HF symptoms 3. **TTE** (diagnostic) • Rheumatic changes: thick mitral leaflets and doming (commissure fusion) 4. Stress testing • Used when there is a discrepancy between resting echo and clinical symptoms 5. Cardiac catheterization and angiography • Used if echo nondiagnostic or conflicts with clinical findings	1. Symptomatic treatment • Vascular congestion– loop diuretics and dietary salt restriction • HR and SOB control–β-blockers 2. Atrial fibrillation • Hemo-stable: BB, CCB, or digoxin • Anticoagulation • Hemo-unstable: immediate cardioversion 3. **Percutaneous balloon valvotomy** 4. Surgery • For patients with congenital MS Health maintenance: 1. Follow up H&P annually 2. TTE–frequency based on severity; annually or every 3-5 y (if worse) Prophylaxis: 1. Anticoagulation (vitamin K antagonist) with target INR: 2.5 • For: atrial fibrillation, prior embolic event, or left atrial thrombus 2. If *rheumatic* MS give antibiotic prophylaxis to prevent rheumatic fever • Penicillin, ampicillin, amoxicillin, clindamycin, macrolides, cephalosporins 3. No prophylaxis for bacterial endocarditis Complications: 1. CVA 2. Thromboembolic events 3. Infective endocarditis 4. Atrial fibrillation

Arterial Pulse Findings

- **Corrigan pulse**—A "water hammer" or "collapsing" pulse is characterized by a rapidly swelling and falling arterial pulse. This finding is generally best appreciated by palpation of the radial or brachial arteries (exaggerated by raising the arm) or the carotid pulses.

- **Traube sign**—A pistol shot pulse (systolic and diastolic sounds) heard over the femoral arteries.

- **Duroziez sign**—A systolic and diastolic bruit heard when the femoral artery is partially compressed.

- **Hill sign**—Popliteal cuff systolic pressure exceeding brachial pressure by more than 20 mm Hg with the patient in the recumbent position.

- **Austin Flint murmur**: Retrograde blood across aorta mixes with anterograde blood from left atrium causing a low pitched, mid-to-late diastolic rumble, heard at the apex.

Increasing Venous Return	Decreasing Venous Return
• Lying down supine, lifting legs up	• Amyl nitrate • Valsalva maneuver • Standing after squatting

Indications for Intervention for Mitral Stenosis

Percutaneous Mitral Balloon Valvotomy (PMBV)	Surgery (Repair, Commissurotomy, Valve Replacement)
1. Symptomatic patients with severe MS in patients with favorable valve morphology, absence of left atrial thrombus, and absence of moderate to severe mitral regurgitation (MR) 2. Asymptomatic with very severe MS, favorable valve morphology, absence of moderate to severe MR, and no left atrial thrombus	1. Severely symptomatic patients (NYHA class III or IV) with severe MS who are not high risk for surgery and who are not candidates for or who have failed PMBV 2. Concomitant surgery for patients undergoing other cardiac surgeries 3. Severe symptomatic patients (NYHA class II to IV) with severe MS who are candidates for PMB but are undergoing cardiopulmonary bypass for other indications

Severe MS: mitral valve area <1.5 cm^2, stage D.

VALVULAR HEART DISEASE (FIG. B-2)

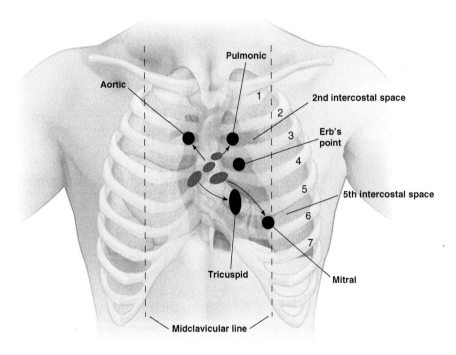

FIGURE B-2. Auscultative heart sounds.

Cyanotic Defects

Disease	Etiology, Prevalence, Risk Factors	Clinical Symptoms and Signs	Diagnostics	Therapy, Prognosis, and Health Maintenance
Tetralogy of Fallot	R-to-L shunt "Blue baby syndrome" 7%-10% of children M = F Most common cyanotic CHD 10% of all CHD Anatomic features: 1. **VSD** 2. **Overriding aorta** 3. **Pulmonic/subpulmonic stenosis** 4. **Right ventricular hypertrophy** Crescendo-decrescendo murmur primarily due to right ventricular outflow obstruction (not VSD)	1. Exertional dyspnea Signs: Cyanosis • Worse with age "Tet-spells" or "hypercyanotic spells" 1. Irritability or agitation 2. Tachypnea 3. Cyanosis worse with exertion (feeding or intense crying) • Prominent in nail beds and lips 1. Grade: varies 2. Quality: **harsh** 3. Holo**systolic ejection** 4. Heard best: LUSB 5. Radiation: ***back*** (posteriorly) 6. Louder: acidosis, stress, infection, exercise, beta-adrenergic agonists, dehydration, closure of the Ductus Arteriosus, posture 7. Quieter: squatting (increases SVR) 8. Other descriptors: N/A 9. Associated: click with single loud S2; palpable R ventricular lift; systolic thrill at LSB	1. EKG: RAD, RVH 2. CXR: **boot-shaped heart** • Triad: "egg on a string," increased pulmonary congestion, mild cardiomegaly 3. TTE (confirmatory) 4. Cardiac catheter	1. Neonates with SX: • **IV PGE-1 (Alprostadil)** • Prevents ductal closure, allowing pulmonary flow until surgical repair Tet Spells: 1. Place patient in **knee-chest position** • Increases SVR → moves blood from RV to pulmonary circ 2. **Supplemental O$_2$** 3. IV morphine 0.1 mg/kg/dose + IV fluid bolus 4. IV Propranolol 0.1 mg/kg/dose 5. Emergency surgical repair Heart failure: 1. Medical therapy • Digoxin • Furosemide 2. Surgery • Palliative shunts • Medically refractory tet spells with severe RV obstruction; premature • **Intracardiac repair** by 1 year of age Prognosis: 1. An associated PDA increases survival because it allows for mixing of oxygenated and deoxygenated blood Health maintenance: 1. Endocarditis ABX prophylaxis for <u>all</u> patients with unrepaired cyanotic CHD 2. Pregnancy not recommended in unrepaired TOF

Noncyanotic Defects (Mnemonic: All Ventricles Provide Circulation)

Disease	Etiology, Prevalence, Risk Factors	Clinical Symptoms and Signs	Diagnostics	Therapy, Prognosis, and Health Maintenance

Atrial septal defect (ASD) (Fig. B-3A)	Hole in atrial septum or patent foramen ovale (opening between R and L atrium)
	 Increased flow across pulmonary valve owing to right ventricular volume overload from L-to-R atrial shunting
	 Ostium secundum (75%): openings without a tissue flap
	 10% incidence
	 Often undetected until adulthood, very subtle findings
	 Crescendo-decrescendo murmur
		1. *Acyanotic*
		  • Mostly asymptomatic until 30 y/o
		 Infants/children:
		 1. HX recurrent URI
		 2. **Failure to thrive**
		 3. Exertional dyspnea
		 Adults/adolescents:
		 1. **Exertional dyspnea**
		 2. **Fatigue**
		 3. Palpitations
		 4. Syncope
		 5. MC presenting symptom: **atrial arrhythmias**
		
		 1. Grade: 1-2
		 2. Quality: soft
		 3. Mid-**systolic ejection murmur**
		 4. Heard best: **LUSB** (pulmonic area, second LICS)
		 5. Radiation: none
		 6. Louder: N/A
		 7. Quieter: N/A
		 8. Other descriptors: **fixed, widely split S2** (unchanged with inspiration, may be only finding) due to increased RV volume and delayed closure of pulmonic valve; **early mid-systolic rumble**
		 9. Associated: loud S1
			Prenatal period:
			 1. Ultrasound: can diagnose in fetus at 18-22 wk gestation
			  • Must be confirmed by postnatal echo
			 Clinical DX:
			 1. EKG: normal or RAD ± RVH (**incomplete RBBB**)
			 2. CXR: dilation of right atrium, ventricle, and pulmonary arteries; **cardiomegaly**
			 3. TTE (*confirmatory*): determines defect size and position
			 4. MRI—measures ventricular volumes, *pulmonary and systemic flow (Qp/Qs)*
			 5. Cardiac cath (gold standard to measure Qp/Qs)
				1. Small (<6 mm diameter): **40%-80% close spontaneously** by 2 y; most by 5 y
				 2. Moderate (6-8 mm) and large (>8 mm): *percutaneous closure*, median sternotomy, or thoracotomy
				 3. Indications for repair:
				  • (Qp/Qs) > 2:1
				  • Pericardial or Dacron patch used
				  • Complications: pericardial effusion, pleural effusion, arrhythmias, bleeding, PTX, wound infection
				 Prognosis:
				 1. No definitive evidence that ASD closure is beneficial
				 2. Repair closures success: 88%-98%
				 Health maintenance:
				 1. No antibiotic prophylaxis with isolated ASD unless:
				  • Repaired ASD with prosthetic material or device—ABX first 6 mo after repair
				  • Repaired ASD with residual defect at site or adjacent
				  • Prophylaxis for respiratory and dental procedures only
				 Complications:
				 Embolic stroke, atrial arrhythmias

Disease	Etiology, Prevalence, Risk Factors	Clinical Symptoms and Signs	Diagnostics	Therapy, Prognosis, and Health Maintenance
Ventricular septal defect (VSD)	Results in L-to-R shunt **Most common congenital anomaly,** occurs in 50% of all patients with CHD <u>MC location:</u> **Perimembranous** (just beneath aortic valve, behind septal leaflet of tricuspid valve) <u>Causes:</u> 1. **Down syndrome** DiGeorge 2. FAS 3. Diabetes ***Size*** and type of VSD determine characteristics	*Acyanotic* or *cyanotic* based on ***size*** <u>Neonatal:</u> 1. Isolated systolic murmur 2. HF symptoms/signs: tachypnea, increased WOB, poor weight gain, FTT, diaphoresis with feeding <u>Small:</u> 1. Asymptomatic <u>Mod-large:</u> 1. DOE 2. Recurrent URI 3. HF symptoms 4. FTT, poor weight gain <u>Signs:</u> 1. Tachypnea 2. Increased WOB 3. Rales, grunts, retractions 4. Diaphoresis 5. Pallor 6. Hepatomegaly 1. Grade: 2-3, grade 4 if thrill present 2. Quality: harsh, high pitched, or **blowing** 3. Holo**systolic** 4. Heard best: LLSB (third to fourth LICS) 5. Radiation: diffuse 6. Louder: **isometric handgrip** 7. Quieter: Valsalva 8. Other descriptors: thrill (first to second LICS), apical S3, diastolic rumble (if large, at apex) 9. Associated: pulmonary HTN and **Eisenmenger syndrome** → cyanosis + bidirectional shunt	<u>Clinical DX:</u> 1. EKG: LVH and RVH (**biventricular hypertrophy**) 2. CXR: cardiomegaly, increased pulmonary vascularity; enlarged LA, LV, and pulmonary artery 3. ***TTE*** (confirmatory): location/size of defect, direction of flow 4. Cath (rarely utilized): assesses need for closure (Qp:Qs) or perioperative management planning <u>Complications:</u> Endocarditis, aortic regurgitation, subaortic stenosis, right ventricular outflow tract obstruction, atrial shunting	1. <u>Asymptomatic and small:</u> Delay treatment, 75% **close spontaneously in first 2 y of life** 2. <u>HF symptoms:</u> • Nutritional support: >150 kcal/kg/d • Diuretics (mainstay): PO or IV **furosemide** 1-2 mg/kg BID-TID 3. Surgical repair • **Direct patch closure** via median sternotomy • Transcatheter closure (amplatzer muscular closure) <u>Surgical indications:</u> • Persistent SX despite maximal medical therapy • Mod to large defect with pulmonary HTN • Qp:Qs > 2:1, asymptomatic • Double-chambered RV <u>Prognosis:</u> 1. If surgery not performed in the first year of life, increased risk for irreversible pulmonary vascular disease, especially in children with Down syndrome <u>Health maintenance:</u> 1. All immunizations up-to-date, including pneumococcal and flu; RSV prophylaxis if <1 y with VSD and HF 2. Monitor growth and development 3. Monitor for SX of heart failure 4. No endocarditis ABX prophylaxis recommended except: • Device closure or surgical ligation with prosthetics, first 6 mo after • Device closure or ligation and residual defect at site of repair

(continued)

(continued)

Disease	Etiology, Prevalence, Risk Factors	Clinical Symptoms and Signs	Diagnostics	Therapy, Prognosis, and Health Maintenance
Patent ductus arteriosus (PDA) Normally, the ductus arteriosus (DA) connects the main pulmonary artery and the aorta during development, diverting blood away from the lungs; it is kept open by low arterial O_2 and circulating PGE2 produced by the placenta After birth, the DA normally constricts and obliterates after 10-15 h as arterial O_2 increases and PGE2 decreases turning into the ligamentum arteriosum after 2-3 wk	RF: 1. *Prematurity*, perinatal distress, or hypoxia (decreased PVR sooner) → delays closure 2. Rubella 3. Birth at high altitude 12%-15% of significant congenital heart disease F > M (2:1) In PDA the DA fails to completely close postnatally Differentiate from other continuous murmurs based on location and quality Crescendo-decrescendo murmur	Infant/child: 1. *Acyanotic*–asymptomatic unless pulmonary HTN or LVF results 2. Poor feeding, weight loss 3. Frequent URIs or pulmonary congestion Infant/child signs: 1. Heart failure • FTT • Poor feeding • Respiratory distress • Sweating 2. SOB 3. Easy fatigability 1. Grade: 2-4 2. Quality: **continuous, rough, machinery** 3. Late *systolic* 4. Heard best: LUSB (2nd LICS) 5. Radiation: *precordium* 6. Louder: N/A 7. Quieter: increased pulmonary pressure 8. Other descriptors: **associated LV thrill,** multiple clicks throughout murmur, ± S3 → apical diastolic rumble Associated: **Wide pulse pressure,** bounding peripheral pulses	1. EKG: **BVH, LAE** 2. CXR: prominent aortic knob along LUSB; cardiomegaly, increased pulmonary vasculature; enlarged LV and LA 3. **TTE** (confirmatory): (+) ductus arteriosus, retrograde flow in the pulmonary artery 4. Cardiac catheter: P-HTN 5. MRI Small: Qp/ Qs < 1.5-1 Mod: Qp/Qs between 1.5 and 2.2-1 Large: Qp/ Qs > 2.2-1	1. **PGE or COX *inhibitor*** • NSAIDs: • **IV indomethacin** • Or • **IV ibuprofen** • For *premature* infants • Ineffective in term neonates and older children 2. Medical management for infants with HF: • Digoxin and diuretics; stabilize until candidates for device or surgical ligation • If asymptomatic, observation until large enough for surgery 3. Surgery • For term neonates and older infants >5 kg • Repair before age 1 y • Surgical ligation (VATS) • Preferred if preterm • **Percutaneous occlusion** (preferred) • Term infants <5 kg with large PDAs who have failed COX inhibitors, adolescents, adults 4. Surgical Repair of PDA Indications: • Significant L-to-R shunting • Left-sided volume overload • Reversible PAH • hx of endocarditis Health maintenance: 1. No endocarditis prophylaxis required *except* • Eisenmenger syndrome • Device closure or surgical ligation with prosthetics, first 6 mo after • Device closure or ligation and residual defect at site of repair 2. If left untreated, follow up every 3-5 y (adults) or every 6-12 mo (children) Prognosis: 1. 60% of untreated patients die by age 60 y 2. Usually closes **48 h after birth** (90% of full term infants) 3. Clinical manifestations determined by degree of L-to-R shunting, dependent on size and length of PDA and difference between pulmonary and systemic vascular resistances Complications: Short life, endocarditis, CHF, PHTN

Disease	Etiology, Prevalence, Risk Factors	Clinical Symptoms and Signs	Diagnostics	Therapy, Prognosis, and Health Maintenance

Coarctation of the aorta (CoA) (Fig. B-3B)	4%-6% of all congenital heart defects
	M > F (3:1)
	MC:
	Ligamentum arteriosum 98% juxtaductal
	Associated:
	Turner syndrome (5%-15% of girls with CoA), diabetes, **bicuspid aortic valve (70%)**
	Discrete or long segment narrowing adjacent to left subclavian; systemic collaterals develop
	Malformation originating in left side of heart (proximal to distal), **narrowing of descending thoracic aorta** from transverse arch to iliac bifurcation
		1. *Acyanotic* **or** cyanotic (if severe or large PDA)
		Infants:
		1. HF symptoms or shock
		2. FTT
		3. Poor feeding
		Signs:
		1. Pale
		2. Irritable
		3. Diaphoretic
		4. Dyspneic
		5. Absent femoral pulses
		6. HM
		Young children:
		1. HTN
		2. New murmur
		3. Underdeveloped lower extremities
		Signs:
		1. Hypertension in upper extremities than lower extremities
		  • **Systolic pressure gradient >10 mm Hg between right arm and leg**
		2. *Weak/absent or delayed femoral* pulse
		
		1. Grade varies
		2. Quality: Continuous
		3. **Systolic ejection click** over left infraclavicular region
		4. Heard best: **back** between the scapulae
		5. Radiation: LUSB and left scapula
		6. Louder: none
		7. Quieter: none
		8. Other descriptors: N/A
		9. Associated: S4 gallop
		Complications:
		Dissection, aortic rupture, HTN, CHF, endocarditis, stroke
			Clinical Diagnosis:
			1. EKG: **LVH**
			2. CXR: *cardiomegaly* ± pulmonary vascular markings, **rib notching**
			3. Echo (confirmatory): reduced and delayed systolic amplitude with persistent flow during diastole; **discrete area of narrowing within lumen of proximal descending thoracic aorta**
			4. CV MRI/CT: defines location and severity
			  • Recommended in all adults with CoA
			5. Cardiac catheter:
			6. Barium swallow (not routinely performed): reverse **"three" or "E" sign**
			7. CTA (gold standard): **"three sign"** due to coarctation site with proximal and distal dilations
			8. Genetic testing—in females with CoA, test for Turner Syndrome
			9. Associated (adults): headache, epistaxis, heart failure, aortic dissection
				Infants—at risk for HR and death when ductus arteriosus closes
				1. Continuous IV **PGE-1 (alprostadil)** to maintain patent ductus arteriosus until surgery
				2. Dopamine and/or dobutamine to increase contractility in HF
				3. Supportive care—correct MA, hypoglycemia, respiratory failure, anemia
				4. Once stabilized→
				End-to-end anastomosis
				Or
				Balloon angioplasty
				  • Indicated: child 4 mo-5 y (preferred)
				Adults:
				1. Indication for **stent placement**:
				  • Coarctation gradient >20 mm Hg or <20 with anatomic imaging of severe narrowing and radiologic evidence of increased collateral flow
				Prognosis:
				1. Unoperated mean survival rate of adults: 35 y
				2. Perioperative mortality <1%
				Complications:
				Recoarctation (especially in infants/children), aneurysm formation, femoral occlusion

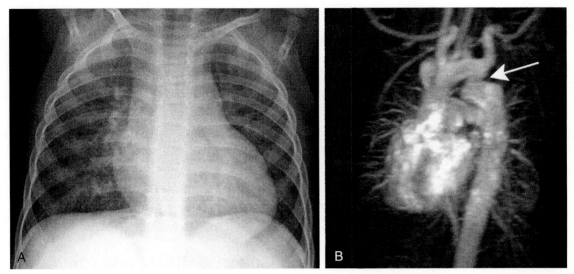

FIGURE B-3. **A**, Cardiomegaly seen with atrial septal defect on X-ray. **B**, Coarctation of the aorta on CT. Arrow shows the "three sign" due to coarctation site with proximal and distal dilations (**A**, From Kline-Tilford A, Haut C. *Lippincott Certification Review: Pediatric Acute Care Nurse Practitioner.* 1st ed. Philadelphia: Wolters Kluwer; 2016. **B**, From Shirkhoda A. *Variants and Pitfalls in Body Imaging.* 2nd ed. Philadelphia: Wolters Kluwer; 2011.)

EISENMENGER SYNDROME

Seen with PDA, VSD, TOF (± ASD)

1. Pulmonary HTN (rise in pulmonary artery pressures, PVR ≫ SVR), RV pressure overload, and RV hypertrophy; flow reverses and patients become cyanotic

- L-to-R (acyanotic) → R-to-L (cyanotic, hypoxemia)
- Generally irreversible, but serious problem that can result in death as early as 30s

Nonselective COX Inhibitors for PDA Treatment

	Indomethacin	Ibuprofen
Adverse effects	Increased risk of bleeding, renal insufficiency, NEC, spontaneous intestinal perforation, kernicterus	Kernicterus
Contraindications	• Proven or suspected infection, untreated • Active bleeding • Thrombocytopenia ± coagulation defects • NEC (necrotizing enterocolitis) • Impaired renal function • CHD	
Dosing	0.1-0.2 mg/kg/dose every 12-24 h × 3	10 mg/kg → 5 mg/kg every 24 h
MOA	Inhibit prostaglandin synthetase by blocking COX sites	

MURMUR GRADING

Grade 1—Very faint; may not hear throughout. Need to be "tuned in"

Grade 2—Quiet but heard immediately

Grade 3—Moderately loud

Grade 4—Loud w/ palpable thrill

Grade 5—Very loud w/ thrill. May be heard w/ stethoscope partly off chest

Grade 6—Very loud w/ thrill. May be heard w/ stethoscope entirely off the chest

Acid-Base Disorders

ARTERIAL BLOOD GASES

- **Acidosis**: a process or disorder that increases H^+ or decreases HCO_3^-
  - pH <7.35
- **Alkalosis**: a process or disorder that decreases H^+ or increases HCO_3^-
  - pH >7.45
- **$PaCO_2$** (arterial partial pressure of CO_2) aka pCO_2
  - pCO_2 (normal range): 45 to 35 mm Hg
  - pCO_2 > 45: acidotic
  - pCO_2 < 35: alkalotic
- **HCO_3^-** (bicarbonate anions in blood): 22 to 26 mEq/L
  - HCO_3^- < 22: acidotic
  - HCO_3^- > 26: alkalotic
- **PaO_2** (partial pressure of O_2 in blood) aka pO_2
  - pO_2: 80 to 100 (well oxygenated)
  - pO_2: 60 to 80 (moderately oxygenated)
  - pO_2: <60 (poorly oxygenated)

Base Deficit or Excess

A measure of the metabolic component of an acid base disorder (equation normalizes the CO_2)

- −2.4 to +2.3 mEq
- Base deficit (excess acid): possibly metabolic acidosis
- Base excess: may indicate metabolic alkalosis

The Bicarbonate Buffering System

- Balances carbonic acid (H_2CO_3), bicarbonate ion (HCO_3^-), and carbon dioxide (CO_2) in order to maintain pH in the blood and duodenum. Catalyzed by carbonic anhydrase, CO_2 reacts with water (H_2O) to form carbonic acid (H_2CO_3), which rapidly dissociates, forming hydrogen ions (H^+, present as hydronium ion, H_3O^+) and bicarbonate ion (HCO_3^-):

$$CO_2 + H_2O \rightleftarrows H_2CO_3 \rightleftarrows HCO_3^- + H_3O^+$$

Lungs control the level of pCO_2 in the blood with compensation occurring in minutes-hours. Arterial chemoreceptors increase or decrease ventilation based on pH, pO_2, and pCO_2.

- Hypoventilation = increase in pCO_2 = increased H^+ (acidifies blood)
- Hyperventilation = decrease in pCO_2 = decreased H^+ (alkalinizes blood)

Compensation for a pH of 7.25 (Fig. C-1)

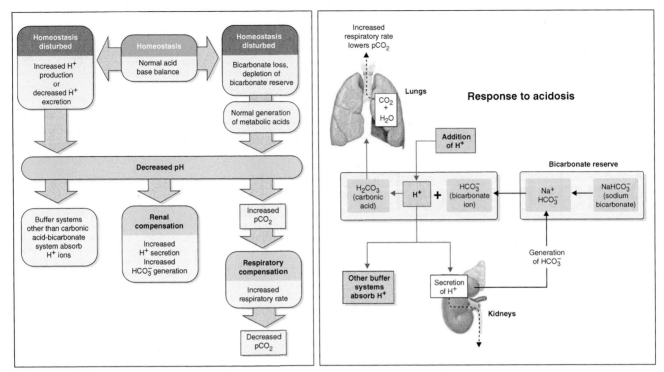

FIGURE C-1. Acidosis homeostasis. This diagram illustrates the response of the kidneys and the lungs to alkalosis. When homeostasis is disturbed (from decreased respiratory rate or increased bicarbonate), the relative increase in bicarbonate results in renal secretion of bicarbonate and generation of hydrogen ions to buffer the pH. This increased pH subsequently increases breathing rate to increase the amount of exhaled CO_2 in an attempt to equilibrate the existing alkalosis.

The kidneys control the level of HCO_3^- (bicarbonate) in the blood, compensating for changes within 1 to 2 days by reabsorbing HCO_3^- anions, forming titratable acids (H^+ formation), and retaining and excreting ammonium (NH_4) and hydrogen ions (H^+).

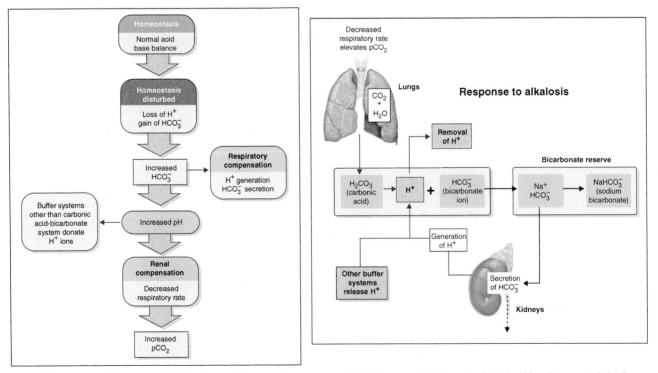

FIGURE C-2. Alkalosis homeostasis. This diagram illustrates the response of the kidneys and the lungs to alkalosis. When homeostasis is disturbed (from decreased respiratory rate or increased bicarbonate), the relative increase in bicarbonate results in renal secretion of bicarbonate and generation of hydrogen ions to buffer the pH. This increased pH subsequently increases breathing rate to increase the amount of exhaled CO_2 in an attempt to equilibrate the existing alkalosis.

Compensation for a pH of 7.5 (Fig. C-2)
Remember R-O-M-E

1. **Respiratory = Opposite**—in respiratory alkalosis and acidosis, the pH and CO_2 values will be higher or lower than normal but will be oriented in different directions (ie, one is "up," other is "down")
   - Respiratory alkalosis = high pH and low CO_2
   - Respiratory acidosis = low pH and high CO_2

2. **Metabolic = Equal**—in metabolic acidosis and alkalosis, the pH and CO_2 values will be oriented in the same direction (either both high or both low)
   - Metabolic alkalosis = high pH and high HCO_3^-
   - Metabolic acidosis = low pH and low HCO_3^-

Primary Disorder	Compensation	Causes
Metabolic acidosis(decreased HCO_3^- or increase in acid) pH <7.35	Decrease CO_2 (respiratory—increase breathing)	1. Increased endogenous acids: lactic acid, keto-acid, salicylates, D- or L-lactate 2. Ingested toxins (exogenous acids): ethylene glycol, methanol 3. Decreased excretion (renal) of H^+: type 1 renal tubular acidosis (RTA) or uremia 4. Renal loss of HCO_3^- in type 2 renal tubular acidosis (RTA) 5. Diarrhea
Metabolic alkalosis (increased HCO_3^- retention)	Increase CO_2 (respiratory—decrease breathing)	1. To determine cause, obtain urine chloride 2. 2 types • Saline sensitive • Saline resistant
Respiratory acidosis (increased CO_2 >45) Acute or chronic	Increase HCO_3^- (metabolic—renal bicarbonate retention)	1. Hypoventilation 2. CNS depression 3. Airway obstruction 4. Chronic: sleep apnea, COPD, neuromuscular disease, restrictive lung disease
Respiratory alkalosis (decreased CO_2)	Decrease HCO_3^- (metabolic—renal bicarbonate excretion)	1. Hyperventilation 2. Anxiety 3. Stroke 4. Subarachnoid hemorrhage 5. Aspirin ingestion 6. Fever/sepsis 7. Liver disease with high ammonia level

- Compensation can be described as:
  - Full compensation: pH brought back to normal by buffering from opposite system
  - Partial compensation: pH improving but not back to normal owing to another mixed acid-base disorder
  - Uncompensated: pH abnormal, no compensation occurring

Serum Chemistry Normal Ranges

Use this table as a reference to determine what type of acid/base disorder is present. Remember to check whether the labs show blood gas values or a serum chemistry below. This will affect how the disorder and direct intervention are interpreted.

Sodium (Na⁺)	**135-147 mEq/L**
Chloride (Cl⁻)	**98-106 mEq/L**
Potassium (K⁺)	3.5-5.5 mEq/L
CO_2	**22-30 mEq/L** **If low, acidosis** **If high, alkalosis**

Anion Gap

- If metabolic acidosis is present (low CO_2 on chemistry) or pH is below 7.35 on ABG, then calculate anion gap!
- If high anion gap, obtain **osmolar gap** (shown below)
  - **Osmolar gap** = $OSM_{Measured} - OSM_{Calc}$
  - $OSM_{Calc} = 2 \times [Na^+] + [glucose]/18 + [BUN]/2.8$
- **Osmolality (OSM)**: total solute concentration in blood (sodium, glucose, mannitol/diuretics, sorbitol, urea, ethylene glycol, methanol, isopropanol/rubbing alcohol)
- Why do we measure osmolar gap? Patients present comatose or with significant mental status changes and it will help us obtain a better understanding of what might be the cause when they are unable to dictate history or symptoms. Substances causing acidosis need to be corrected or removed.

Calculating Anion Gap Using Serum Chemistry

- **Anion gap** $(\Delta) = [Na^+] - [Cl^- + CO_2]$
- Normal range for anion gap (A/G): 8 to 16 mEq

Causes of Anion Gap Metabolic Acidosis (GOLD MARK)

- If high, check that the increase in anion gap equals the decrease in HCO_3^- (1:1, for lactic acidosis—divide Δ A/G by 1.5), otherwise it is a mixed disorder
- **G**—Glycols (ethylene glycol [antifreeze], propylene glycol [solvent of IV lorazepam], phenobarbital, phenytoin, etomidate)
- **O**—Oxoproline (chronic acetaminophen)
- **L**—Lactate (hypoperfusion, shock, sepsis)
- **D**—Lactate (short small bowel syndrome, Crohn disease, weight loss, surgery)
- **M**—Methanol (wood alcohol ingestion), metformin
- **A**—Aspirin
- **R**—Renal failure
- **K**—Ketoacidosis

Intervention for Causes of Anion Gap Metabolic Acidosis

Lactate	Correct underlying cause, hypoperfusion, sepsis
Alcohol	Correct hypoperfusion, administer thiamine, folate
Salicylates	Administer bicarbonate, dialysis if severe
Ethylene glycol	Administer fomepizole; perform dialysis
Methanol	Administer fomepizole; perform dialysis
Isopropyl (rubbing alcohol)	Increases OSM gap, but not anion gap

Nonanion Gap Metabolic Acidosis

- To determine the cause of a nonanion gap metabolic acidosis (NAGMA), obtain a **urine anion gap** (UAG) = $(Na - Cl^- + K^+)$
- If (+) UAG = renal loss of bicarbonate (type 2 RTA)
- If (−) UAG = GI loss (diarrhea, pancreatic fistula)
- HCO_3^- is replaced by Cl^-, so expect to see hyperchloremic NAGMA

METABOLIC ALKALOSIS

Urine Chloride <10 mEq (Saline Responsive)	Urine Chloride >10 mEq (Saline Resistant)
1. Volume depletion 2. GI losses: vomiting, chronic diarrhea, NG tube suction 3. **Cystic fibrosis** 4. Diuretics	1. Hyperaldosteronism: HTN, severe K^+ depletion (hypokalemia) 2. **Cushing syndrome** 3. CHF/cirrhosis with high diuretic use 4. Renal failure

Easy ABG Analysis

1. Alkalemia or acidemia? pH >7.45 or <7.35, respectively.

2. Determine the PRIMARY disorder. (Respiratory or metabolic?)
   - Apply the ROME Criteria
     - DiffeREnt directions = REspiratory
       - High pH/Low CO_2 = Respiratory acidosis
       - Low pH/High CO_2 = Respiratory alkalosis
   - SaME direction = MEtabolic
     - High pH/high HCO_3^- = Metabolic alkalosis
     - Low pH/low HCO_3^- = Metabolic acidosis

3. Metabolic disorders—Is the disorder fully compensated, uncompensated, or partially compensated? Check compensation with **ABG**. Calculate the **predicted pCO_2** and compare.
   - If the pH is normal, and HCO_3^-/CO_2 are "opposite" one another (one up, one down), then it is fully compensated

- If the pH is abnormal, and HCO_3^-/CO_2 are normal, then the disorder is uncompensated
- If **metabolic acidosis**
  - How to use serum chemistry to calculate anion gap
    - $A/G = Na - [Cl^- + CO_2]$
    - Normal A/G: 12 ± 2
    - "Delta-delta rule"—If you have an AGMA, does the change in A/G equal the change in bicarbonate?
      - If measured HCO_3^- is greater than the increase in A/G, then you have a concomitant metabolic alkalosis
      - If measured HCO_3^- is lesser than the increase in A/G, then you have a concomitant non-anion gap metabolic acidosis (NAGMA)
  - **Expected pCO_2** $= [1.5 \times HCO_3^-] + 8 \ (\pm 2 \ mm)$
  - If measured PCO_2 higher than predicted = combined respiratory acidosis
  - If measured PCO_2 lower than predicted = combined respiratory alkalosis
- If metabolic alkalosis—use **urine chloride** to determine if saline resistant/responsive

- **Expected pCO_2** $= 40 + 0.7 \times$ [measured HCO_3^- − normal HCO_3^-] (± 5 mm)
  - Normal $HCO_3^- = 24$
- If measured PCO_2 higher than predicted = combined respiratory acidosis
- If measured PCO_2 lower than predicted = combined respiratory alkalosis
- If urine Cl^- <10 = saline responsive, if >10 = saline resistant
- If NAGMA—obtain urinary A/G
  - (+) = RTA (renal tubular acidosis)
  - (−) = GI causes

4. If respiratory alkalosis/acidosis, identify cause and correct!
- Respiratory acidosis
  - Acute: increase in $HCO_3^- \times 1$: 10 mm pCO_2
  - Chronic: increase in $HCO_3^- \times 3.5$: 10 mm pCO_2
- Respiratory alkalosis
  - Acute: increase in $HCO_3^- \times 2$: 10 mm pCO_2
  - Chronic: increase in $HCO_3^- \times 5$: 10 mm pCO_2

Electrolyte and Fluid Disorders

POTASSIUM HOMEOSTASIS AND DISORDERS

- Principal cation of intracellular fluid (ICF), normal: 120 to 150 mEq/L

  - Extracellular fluid (ECF): 3.5 to 5.0 mEq/L
  - Normal cell function (monocytes, neurons) requires maintenance of ECF [K^+] within a narrow range

- Short-term potassium regulation occurs via transmembrane shifts, whereas long-term maintenance is regulated by excretion

- **Acidosis** limits intracellular shift—K^+ leaks out of cells as H^+ enters (hyperkalemia)

- **Renal dysfunction limits excretion of K^+**

- Internal balance—**insulin** and **catecholamines** regulate K^+ distribution between intracellular and extracellular compartments

  - Postprandial rise in insulin concentration (primarily due to elevated glucose concentrations) moves K^+ and glucose into intracellular compartment where 98% of total body K^+ resides

- Transcellular gradient managed by active K^+ transport and Na-K-ATPase pumps

- Increased splanchnic K^+ concentration stimulates pancreatic insulin secretion → stimulates K^+ uptake by the liver and muscle returning K^+ to normal

- Intake: **dietary** (50 to 150 mEq/d), IV KCl, hyperalimentation, drugs, blood products

  - *Note*: a **high salt intake** will expand ECF volume, inhibiting renin and aldosterone levels → **increases** delivery and **excretion of Na^+**; conversely, a low Na^+ concentration contracts the ECF, stimulating renin and aldosterone → reduces distal CD Na^+ delivery and excretion

- Renal **reabsorption: most in proximal tubule** (65% filtered), thick ascending limb (25%), cortical and medullary collecting ducts (10%)

- Potassium **excretion: collecting duct** (90% to 95% of dietary intake) → most excreted in the urine

- Aldosterone—stimulates K^+ secretion by binding intracellular receptors in the collecting duct, activating a transcriptional regulator, increasing synthesis of aldosterone-induced protein (AIP), which increases the number of open K^+/Na^+ channels, excreting more K^+

Etiology of Hyperkalemia and Hypokalemia

Hyperkalemia	Hypokalemia
1. Decreased renal excretion (MC): acute/CKD, decreased distal tubular flow (**volume depleted**, CHF, cirrhosis, ACE/ARB, NSAID), mineralocorticoid deficiency (**adrenal insufficiency**, diabetes), distal tube dysfunction (AIN, K⁺ diuretics) 2. Cell leak/transcellular shift—**respiratory acidosis**, rhabdomyolysis, tumor lysis (chemotherapy), transfusion reaction or severe hemolytic anemia, hemolysis from large hematoma, extensive burns, ischemia/necrosis 3. High-K⁺ intake (rare) 4. **Insulin deficiency**, elevated [glucose] (**hyperglycemia**), diabetic ketoacidosis 5. Drugs: succinylcholine	1. Hyperadrenergic states: ETOH withdrawal, hyperthyroidism, B-sympathomimetics (tocolytic terbutaline), theophylline poisoning, hypothermia 2. Increased renal excretion: **diuretics**, mineralocorticoid excess (cortisol acts on aldosterone receptors), salt-wasting nephropathy, hypomagnesemia, postdiuretic phase of ATN, amphotericin B, primary hyperaldosteronism 3. Intracellular shift—**metabolic alkalosis**, cell proliferation, **insulin excess**, B-adrenergic activity, osmotic diuresis (uncontrolled DM), RTA type I and II 4. Inadequate intake: alcoholism and malnutrition (refeeding after prolonged starvation) 5. Extrarenal losses—vomiting, **diarrhea, laxatives**, NG tube, metabolic alkalosis 6. Cutaneous losses—sweating, severe burns

- Causes no shift: metabolic acidosis (lactic and ketoacidosis)
- The clinical manifestations of an abnormal plasma [K⁺] vary greatly and depend on
  - its magnitude
  - acuity of onset
  - the relative contributions of K⁺ shift versus change in total body K⁺
  - coexisting abnormalities that either potentiate or blunt the [K⁺] effects, including underlying heart disease, drugs (digoxin, anti-arrhythmic agents), hypocalcemia or hypercalcemia, cardiac pacing devices, and others
- An acute K⁺ shift into or from the intracellular space alters intracellular [K⁺] only minimally because it is quantitatively so large; about 3000 mEq or 98% of total body K⁺ is within cells. However, the effect on the extracellular concentration can be dramatic because the total quantity of K⁺ outside of cells is only about 60 mEq

- In contrast, states of chronic K⁺ depletion reduce both intracellular and extracellular K levels and have a much smaller effect
  - Example: A dialysis patient with a chronically elevated [K⁺] who presents with a [K⁺] of 6.5 mEq/L and minimal EKG effects may not require urgent intervention. However, a diabetic patient with chronic kidney disease who develops acute hyperglycemia and a rapid [K⁺] rise to 6.5 mEq/L may manifest major EKG changes, which mandate quick action
- Comorbid illness such as **coronary heart disease** will amplify the clinical importance of dyskalemia by increasing the risk of serious arrhythmia
- Coexisting hyperkalemia and hypocalcemia is a particularly pernicious combination and is common in patients with severe kidney failure

Disease	Etiology, Prevalence, Risk Factors	Clinical Symptoms and Signs	Diagnostics	Therapy, Prognosis, and Health Maintenance

Hyperkalemia
Reduces resting potential across myocyte membrane → the cell becomes less negative, more sensitive to excitation
Following depolarization, the cell is unable to adequately repolarize and becomes unexcitable
	• Cell lysis
	• Acidosis
	• Aldosterone insufficiency
	• ACE inhibitors, ARBs
	• Aldosterone antagonists
	• Hyporeninemic **hypoaldosteronism:** Reduced collecting duct Na⁺ delivery with low aldosterone activity
	MCC:
	Acute or **chronic renal failure**
	Pseudohyperkalemia:
	  repeated fist clenching during phlebotomy, hemolysis due to traumatic venipuncture, delayed processing of specimen, K⁺ release from WBCs during severe leukocytosis or from platelets with extreme thrombocytosis, prolonged tourniquet application
		1. Fatigue, myalgia
		2. **Muscle weakness** (lower extremity)
		  • Ascending paralysis, hypoventilation, respiratory failure
		3. **Flaccid paralysis**
		4. Muscle cramps
		5. Paresthesias
		Signs:
		1. Hyporeflexia
			1. Serum [K⁺]:
			  >5.0 mEq/L
			2. EKG changes: **tall peaked T** and flat P waves, QRS widening, ventricular fibrillation and asystole
				Prevention:
				1. Review medications, diet, OTC drugs (NSAIDs)
				2. Use of aldosterone antagonists in patients with CHF (taking ACEI or ARB + BB)
				See *Acute Treatment* table

Hypokalemia				
Hypokalemia Increases resting potential across myocyte membrane → cell becomes more negative, less sensitive to excitation	• Cell proliferation (leukemia) • Alkalosis • **Primary *hyperaldosteronism*:** increased CD Na$^+$ delivery with high aldosterone levels • Secondary hyperaldosteronism • Insulin MCC: Thiazide or loop diuretics, vomiting/ NG suction, diarrhea (laxatives) Reduction of total body K$^+$ stores	1. Profound acute **flaccid muscle paralysis** • Proximal limbs, sparing ocular and respiratory • Develops after exercise or ingestion of lots of carbohydrates 2. Weakness, muscle cramps, fatigue Signs: 1. DTRs–absent Complications: 1. Paralytic ileus, rhabdomyolysis 2. CV: **arrhythmias** (elderly, digoxin), digitalis toxicity 3. Endocrine: glucose intolerance, interstitial change 4. Renal: vasopressin resistance, increased ammonia generation (encephalopathy), **metabolic alkalosis**, nephrogenic DI, renal cysts 5. Structural: cystic or interstitial changes	1. Serum [K$^+$]: **<3.5 mEq/L** • Hypophosphatemia • Hypomagnesemia 2. 24-h urine K$^+$-excretion: less than 20-30 mEq/d 3. EKG changes: **flat or inverted T waves**, prominent U waves, ST depression	1. Exogenous K$^+$ salts • Replenish PO route: K$^+$-rich foods (dried fruit, nuts, bananas, oranges, tomatoes, spinach, potatoes, meat) • See PO and IV treatment table 2. β-Blockers: propranolol Prevention: 1. Avoid the use of thiazide and loop diuretics in combination

Treatment of Hyperkalemia and Hypokalemia

Hyperkalemia	Hypokalemia
If EKG changes or [K$^+$] > 6-6.5 mEq/L–treat quickly to reverse effects 1. Translocating K$^+$ into cells • IV **Ca^{2+} gluconate** (10 L of 10% solution) or Ca^{2+} chloride to **reverse effect on cardiac cells** • Rapid onset 1-3 min, lasts 30-60 min • Only if EKG changes • B$_2$ agonist–redistributes into cells • Increases uptake by muscle/liver by activating B$_2$ receptor • Neb-Albuterol 10-20 mg in 4 mL NS • Onset 30 min, lasts 2-6 h • Decreases K$^+$ by 0.5-1.0 mEq/L • Sodium bicarbonate–helps if acidotic • Intracellular movement of K$^+$, less effective in acute, not effective for ESRD with acidosis • Excessiveness causes Na$^+$ retention and hypernatremia • Avoid in CHF and volume overloaded patients 2. Increasing K$^+$ excretion • **Insulin and glucose**–redistributes into cells • Increases uptake by muscle/liver by activating insulin receptor • 10 U regular insulin + 50 mL of D50 • Onset 10-20 min lasts 4-6 h • Decreases K$^+$ by 0.5-1.2 mEq/L • Loop diuretics–short-term and acute TX • Reduces total body K$^+$ • Higher dose if low GFR, may combine loop and HCTZ to increase urinary excretion • Mineralocorticoids–reduces total body K$^+$, if chronic • Fludrocortisone 0.1-0.3 mg/d • Cation exchange resins (**Kayexalate**)–exchanges Na$^+$ for K$^+$ in colon • Add sorbitol PO to prevent constipation • 30-50 g in D50, retain 30-60 min, q 6 h PRN • More effective for chronic therapy • Side effects: colonic necrosis • RRT (renal replacement therapy)–preferred when rapid removal necessary (CVVHD, continuous venovenous hemodialysis) • Recommended for acute or chronic severe kidney failure	1. Rapid drop to <2.5 mEq/L requires urgent treatment • High-risk patients (CHF, digoxin, MI, arrhythmias)–keep level >4 mEq/L • Cirrhotic patients have increased ammoniagenesis with hypokalemia–**keep >4 mEq/L** • KCl is the most appropriate and effective replacement for K$^+$ deficits associated with metabolic alkalosis • Alkalinizing K$^+$ salts (KHCO$_3$, K-citrate, K-acetate, K-gluconate) are best for hypokalemia associated with metabolic acidosis, such as RTA, or chronic diarrhea 2. IV [K$^+$]–only for SX patients and **who cannot tolerate PO**; faster with PO; use central lines for high K concentrations • A parenteral fluid **KCl concentration of 20-40 mEq/L is** generally well tolerated • KCl concentrations of 60 mEq/L and greater are painful and may induce peripheral vein necrosis • When IV administration of a large volume of fluid is contraindicated, K$^+$ concentrations of up to 200 mEq/L (20 mEq in 100 mL of isotonic saline) may be given via a central vein, but the administration rate should not exceed 10-20 mEq/h • The choice of intravenous fluid must also be considered, because **dextrose will increase insulin and shift K$^+$ into cells**, thereby potentially worsening hypokalemia 3. PO K$^+$–each gram of salt substitute 10-13 mEq of K$^+$ • All forms of oral K$^+$ well absorbed, liquid is cheaper In general: • Plasma [K$^+$] between 3-3.5 = 200-400 mEq deficit • Plasma [K$^+$] between 2-3.0 = 400-800 mEq deficit

FLUID BALANCE (FIG. D-1)

- The extracellular water composes 20% of the total body weight and is divided between plasma (5% of body weight) and interstitial fluid (15% of body weight). Intracellular water makes up approximately 40% of an individual's total body weight

- The **intracellular** fluid compartment is composed primarily of the cations K^+ and magnesium, and the anions, phosphate and sulfate, and proteins

- Although the movement of ions and proteins between the various fluid compartments is restricted, water is freely diffusible

- Sodium, however, is confined to the **ECF** compartment, and because of its osmotic and electrical properties, it remains associated with water. Therefore, Na^+-containing fluids are distributed throughout the ECF and add to the volume of both the intravascular and interstitial spaces. Although the administration of Na^+-containing fluids expands the intravascular volume, it also expands the interstitial space by approximately three times as much as the plasma

- The osmolality of the intracellular and extracellular fluids is maintained between 290 and 310 mOsm in each compartment

- Daily water losses include 800 to 1200 mL in urine, 250 mL in stool, and 600 mL in insensible losses. Insensible losses of water occur through both the skin (75%) and lungs (25%) and can be increased by factors such as fever, hypermetabolism, and hyperventilation

- The **most common cause of volume deficit** in surgical patients is a **loss of GI fluids** from nasogastric suction, vomiting, diarrhea, or enterocutaneous fistula

- Osmoreceptors are specialized sensors that detect even small changes in fluid osmolality and drive changes in thirst and diuresis through the kidneys

- Baroreceptors also modulate volume in response to changes in pressure and circulating volume through specialized pressure sensors located in the aortic arch and carotid sinuses

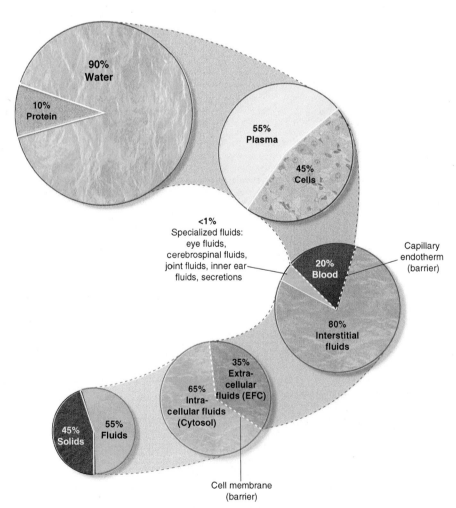

FIGURE D-1. The body's composition is made up of 45% solids and 55% fluids. It is then further broken down as above. For example, fluids of the body include 65% intracellular fluids and 35% extracellular fluids, so on and so forth.

INTRAVENOUS FLUID BASICS (FIG D-2)

- **Bolus therapy**: large doses of IV fluids for volume replacement (1 L 0.9 NaCl over 1 hour)
- **Maintenance therapy**: small amounts of fluid to cover metabolic demands and insensible losses (IV D5 and 0.225% NaCl + 20 mEq KCl at 60 mL/h)

3% NaCl (hypertonic saline, osmolality 3× human plasma)

- Indications: severely symptomatic **hypo**natremia (ICU patients)
- Calculate Na-deficit (mEq Na as 3%) = {Na desired – Na measured} × TBW
  - *Eg,* (135 – 119) × 0.5 (70) = 560 mEq Na

- Na-deficit (mEq Na as 3%) = 513
- 560/513 = 1.08 (1 L given)
- Never correct to normal, only increase [Na$^+$] by 6 to 8 mEq over 8 hours to improve symptoms and avoid cerebral edema

Isotonic fluids: 0.9% NSS and lactated Ringer's; osmolality close to human plasma

- Indications: volume expansion, dehydration, shock, burns

Hypotonic fluids: 0.45% saline (500 mL NaCl, 500 mL water); osmolality is half human plasma

- Indications: volume depleted patient (low BP) with **hypernatremia**
- NaCl expands volume and water corrects hyper natremia

Solution	Glucose	Osm	Na	Cl	Use
D5W "hypotonic"	50 g	252	0	0	Free water
0.45% "half normal" "hypotonic"	0	154	77	77	Free water and NaCl
0.9% (most used) "isotonic"	0	308	154	154	Volume replacement No free water
Lactated Ringer's "isotonic"	0	272	139	109 + lactate, Ca, K$^+$	Volume replacement
3% NaCl "hypertonic"	0	1026	513	513	Severe hyponatremia

	D5W	0.45% NSS	0.9% NSS
Plasma [Na]	↓↓	↓	Unchanged
ECF volume	↑	↑	↑↑↑↑↑

FIGURE D-2. Basics of IV fluid therapy.

D5W (dextrose 5% and water, 1000 mL water, 50 g glucose)

- Indications:
  - Provide free water in patient with **severe hyper**natremia (hypertonic hypernatremia)
  - Keep vein open (KVO) in patients to avoid fluid overload (does not provide unwanted NaCl to avoid fluid overload)
  - Contraindicated: diabetics owing to hyperglycemia

Why add K+ to maintenance IV fluids in patients with normal K+ levels?

- Increased delivery of Na$^+$ to the collecting tubule increases [K$^+$] excretion rate by increasing the amount of Na$^+$ presented for exchange with K$^+$
- IV saline infusions cause K$^+$ excretion

Hyper- and Hyponatremia Rules

1. Symptoms are related to the **rate of change in Na$^+$**, not the absolute value

2. Hypo/hypernatremia = disorders of **free water** balance (too much or not enough water)

3. Hypo/hypervolemia= **Na$^+$** control problem
   Total body water (TBW) comprises:

- 65% intracellular fluid volume (ICFV) and 35% extracellular fluid (ECFV)
  - ECFV = 80% interstitial fluid + 20% blood (intravascular fluid)
- **TBW women** = 0.5 × body weight (kg)
- **TBW men** = 0.6 × body weight (kg)
  Osmolality$_{Calculated}$ = [2 × Na$^+$] + [Gluc]/18 + [BUN]/2.8
- Osmolar gap = OSM$_{Measured}$ – OSM$_{Calculated}$
- Dehydration = cell shrinkage
- Volume depletion = decrease in extracellular fluid volume (ECFV)
- Normal Na$^+$ level: 135 to 145 mEq/L

HYPERNATREMIA AND HYPONATREMIA (FIGS. D-3 AND D-4)

- Serum glucose also should be measured; serum Na^+ falls by 1.4 mM for every 100-mg/dL increase in glucose, owing to glucose-induced H_2O efflux from cells

- Plasma osmolality estimate (pOsm) = $2 \times [Na^+]$ (approximately)
- Na^+ deficit = $0.6 \times$ body weight $\times$ (target $[Na^+]$ − starting $[Na^+]$)

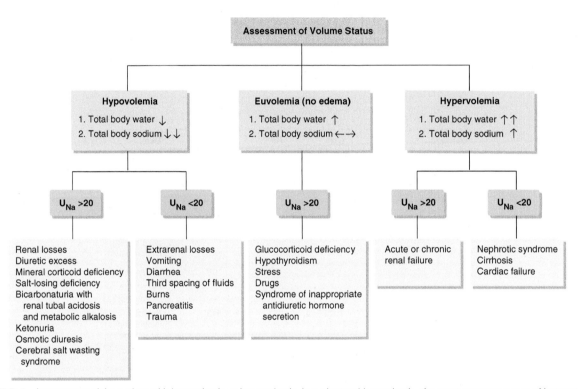

FIGURE D-3. Assessment of the patient with hypovolemia or hypervolemia. In patients with euvolemia, the most common cause of hyponatremia is due to SIADH. Hypovolemic hyponatremia is typically due to extrarenal sodium losses (vomiting, diarrhea).

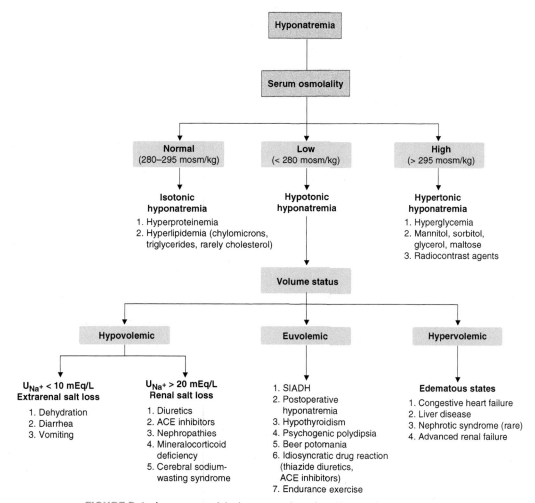

FIGURE D-4. Assessment of the hyponatremic patient. U_{Na^+} = urinary sodium level.

Disease	Etiology, Prevalence, Risk Factors	Clinical Symptoms and Signs	Diagnostics	Therapy, Prognosis, and Health Maintenance
Hypernatremia	Most common in elderly owing to inadequate water intake and loss		1. **Na > 145 mEq/L** 2. • Calculate free water deficit = TBW × {[Na] measured − [Na] desired}/[Na]desired • Eg, 0.6 × 70 − (170 − 160)/160 = 2.6 L over 18 h • Add insensible losses = 0.5 L × 24 h = 0.37 × 18 h • IV fluids necessary: 2.6 L + 0.37 L = 0.3 L/18 h • 0.3 L/18 h = 166 mL/h = IV D5W at 166 mL/h	1. Acute hypernatremia—occurs within <48 h, correct rapidly • Hypotonic saline solutions (0.45% NSS) 2. Chronic hypernatremia—correct slowly over 48-72 h
Hypodipsic hypernatremia Deficient intake due to deprivation: due to lack of thirst (hypodipsia)	Destruction of the osmoreceptors in anterior hypothalamus that regulate thirst <u>MCC:</u> Primary hyperaldosteronism Chronic or recurrent hypertonic dehydration	Muscle weakness, pain <u>Signs:</u> Tachycardia, hypotension <u>Complications:</u> Rhabdomyolysis, obtundation, coma	1. Azotemia, hyperuricemia, hypokalemia—secondary to hyperaldosteronism 2. Hyperglycemia, hyperlipidemia, AKI	1. Administer H_2O orally if alert and cooperative 2. IV 0.45% NSS or 5% dextrose and water if not A&O 3. MRI of brain once rehydrated

(continued)

(continued)

Disease	Etiology, Prevalence, Risk Factors	Clinical Symptoms and Signs	Diagnostics	Therapy, Prognosis, and Health Maintenance
Diabetes insipidus Excretion of a large volume of dilute urine (osmolality <250 mOsmol/kg)		1. **Polyuria**: urinary frequency, enuresis 2. **Nocturia**—may disturb sleep and cause day-time fatigue or somnolence 3. **Polydipsia**—increase in fluid intake	1. Plasma Na^+ concentration: high (>142), **hypernatremia** (only occurs if the patient has thirst defect or no access to water) 2. 24-h urine collection: >50 mL/kg/d Urine osmolality: low (<300) 3. **Water restriction test** (confirmatory)—differentiates central DI from primary polydipsia 4. Administer exogenous ADH once plasma osm reaches 295-300 or plasma Na^+ 145+ • Increase of >50% indicates pituitary DI	
Central DI (neurohypophyseal, neurogenic) Deficient secretion of ADH resulting in variable degree of polyuria *"The sodium is high, in central DI"*	**Idiopathic** (50%), possibly autoimmune injury to ADH-producing cells, but also, pituitary surgery, trauma, hypoxia, or ischemia **Most common type**	1. **Polyuria** (5-10 L in 24 h) • Abrupt • Excretion of dilute colorless urine 2. Polydipsia 3. Nocturia	1. Plasma Na^+ concentration: high (**hypernatremia**) Plasma osmolality: 280-310 (high) 2. Urine osmolality: <150 mOsm/L (low), low specific gravity 3. **Water restriction and desmopressin test**: *increase in urine osmolality* by >300 4. ADH: **low** (takes forever to get results)	1. **Desmopressin** (DDAVP) • Acts at V2 receptors to increase urine concentration and decrease urine flow • Via nasal spray, PO, or injection 2. **Chlorpropamide**—increases ADH secretion and enhances effect of ADH (retain H_2O)
Nephrogenic DI Normal ADH secretion, but varying renal resistance to water-retaining effect	Children: X-linked Acquired from drug exposure: **chronic lithium use**, amphotericin B, metabolic conditions (hypercalcemia, hypokalemia), or renal damage	1. Polyuria • Gradual 2. Nocturia	1. Plasma Na^+ concentration: high (**hypernatremia**) Plasma osmolality: 280-310 (high) 2. Urine osmolality 3. **Water restriction and desmopressin test**: will not increase urine osmolality 4. ADH: **NL to high**	1. High dose of DDAVP 2. **Thiazide diuretics**—±amiloride with **low Na^+ diet** and indomethacin • Increase proximal H_2O reabsorption, decrease distal solute delivery → decrease polyuria • AE: hypokalemia, gastric irritation
Hyponatremia	Excess of total body water in relation to Na^+ Primarily a disorder of H_2O homeostasis	1. Nausea, vomiting 2. Confusion, lethargy, disorientation 3. Weakness, cramps 4. Severe → seizures, coma, death <u>Signs:</u> 1. Decreased DTRs <u>Complications:</u> **Central pontine myelinolysis**—occurs if you correct too quickly	1. Serum osmolality **[Na^+] < 135 mmol/L** • Symptomatic <120 2. Serum glucose	1. Presence, absence, or severity of symptoms determines urgency of therapy 2. Hyponatremia >48 h (chronic) puts the patient at risk for osmotic demyelination syndrome (CPM) • Corrected by >10-12 mM in first 24 h or >18 mM in first 48 h 3. Response to hypertonic saline or vasopressin antagonists requires frequent monitoring of Na^+ (q 2-4 h)
Acute symptomatic hyponatremia				1. Hypertonic saline • Increase [Na^+] by 1-2 mM/h to 4-6 mM 2. Monitor every 2-4 h 3. Administer O_2 and vent support 4. IV loop diuretics to treat pulmonary edema and increase free H_2O excretion

Disease	Etiology, Prevalence, Risk Factors	Clinical Symptoms and Signs	Diagnostics	Therapy, Prognosis, and Health Maintenance
Hypertonic hyponatremia	Hyperglycemia: high concentration of osmotically active solutes in the ECF with net water out of ICF into ECF, diluting [Na$^+$] and increasing plasma osmolarity		1. Serum osmolality–pOsm > 295	
Pseudohyponatremia (isotonic)	Due to hyperlipidemia, hyperproteinemia, hyperglycemia Increased levels of protein/lipids cause a factitious lower Na$^+$ value (even though [Na] and osmolarity are normal)		1. Serum osmolality • pOsm 275-295	
Syndrome of inappropriate ADH secretion (**SIADH, hyponatremia due to inappropriate antidiuresis**)	Excess water retention → expands, dilutes body fluids; exceeds insensible and urinary losses Etiology: pulmonary (pneumonia, TB, effusion, CNS (tumor, SAH, meningitis), neoplasm (SCC of lung), medications (SSRI, TCA, nicotine, vincristine, cyclophosphamide)	1. Asymptomatic 2. Water intoxication • Headache • Confusion • Anorexia • Nausea, vomiting • Coma, convulsions 3. Weight gain	1. Hypotonic hyponatremia • pOsm < 275 2. Urine Osm > 100 3. Euvolemic (no ECF depletion)	Acute: 1. Treat underlying disorder • Most self-limited and remit spontaneously in 2-3 k • Raise plasma osm and/or plasma [Na$^+$] by 1%/h • Infuse hypertonic saline at 0.05 mL/kg body weight/min 2. **Vasopressin antagonists** • Vaptan, conivaptan • Blocks ADH effect, increases UOP Chronic: 1. Water restriction: <1 L/d 2. Oral vaptan, tolvaptan 3. Coadministration of loop diuretics
Primary polydipsia (psychogenic, water intoxication): secondary insufficiency of ADH due to physiologic inhibition of ADH secretion by excess water intake	Middle-aged women, patients with psychiatric illness, carbamazepine, thiazide diuretics	1. Polyuria–appropriate response to increased H$_2$O intake • Gradual	1. Plasma Na$^+$ concentration: low (<137), **hyponatremia** 2. Plasma osmolality: 255-280 (NL) 3. Urine osmolality: low	1. Do not treat with antidiuretics–eliminating polyuria does not eliminate urge to drink 2. Patient education
Central pontine myelinolysis (CPM)	Osmotic shift of water out of cells → brain swells Herniation, permanent neurologic deficits, myelinolysis	1. Lethargy, coma, spontaneous cerebral bleeding 2. Ataxia Signs: 1. Quadriparesis 2. Abnormal EOM		

All three forms of hyponatremia share an exaggerated, "nonosmotic" increase in circulating AVP, in the setting of reduced serum osmolality

Hypotonic: pOsm < 275		
Hypovolemic Hyponatremia	**Euvolemic Hyponatremia**	**Hypervolemic Hyponatremia**
• Primary adrenal insufficiency, hypoaldosteronism, diuretics, osmotic diuresis • Renal causes: vomiting, diuretics, RTA, AIN, CKD • Extrarenal: vomiting, diarrhea, NG tube suction, enteric fistula, sweating, adrenal insufficiency, burns, peritonitis Increased AVP → retention of free H_2O → hyponatremia	• **SIADH** (most common) • Hypothyroidism, medications, porphyria • Water intoxication (**psychogenic polydipsia**) • Secondary adrenal insufficiency	• Edematous disorders: CHF, hepatic cirrhosis, nephrotic syndrome • Renal failure • Effective circulating volume is decreased due to specific factors (cardiac dysfunction, peripheral vasodilation in cirrhosis, hypoalbuminemia in nephrotic syndrome) • Volume overloaded, inability to excrete H_2O
1. Urine $[Na^+]$ <20 mEq/L (GI and integumentary losses) 2. Urine $[Na^+]$ >20 mEq/L: renal losses, diuretics, osmotic diuresis	1. Urine $[Na^+]$ >20 mEq/L: SIADH, drugs, stress, hypothyroidism	1. Urine $[Na^+]$ <20 mEq/L: nephrotic syndrome, cirrhosis, cardiac failure 2. Urine $[Na^+]$ >20 mEq/L: acute or chronic renal failure

1. Volume administration
  • **Isotonic crystalloid** (0.9% NaCl)
  • Hypotonic fluids (0.45% NSS)
	1. Treat underlying disorder
	2. Water restriction: <1 L/d
	3. Vasopressin antagonists
	4. Coadministration of loop diuretics
		1. Treat underlying disorder (afterload reduction in HF, large volume paracentesis in cirrhosis, immunomodulatory therapy in nephrotic syndrome)
		2. Na^+ restriction
		3. Diuretic therapy ± water restriction
		  • Mildly symptomatic or asymptomatic = **water restriction**
		  • Critical hyponatremia = ICU admission + **hypertonic saline** (3% NaCl), correct slow (0.5-1 mEq/h) to avoid osmotic demyelination syndrome

DIURETICS

- Block Na^+ reabsorption (Na^+ loss from body)
- Na^+ is major cation in ECFV, so Na^+ loss = decrease in ECFV

	Mechanism of Action	Examples
Loop diuretics	Blocks Na^+ reabsorption at thick ascending loop of Henle (20%-30% of Na^+-reabs) Powerful diuretic Na^+ loss = H_2O loss **ECFV decreased,** but Na^+/H_2O concentration maintained	Furosemide (Lasix) Torsemide Bumetanide (Bumex) Ethacrynic acid
Thiazide diuretics	Blocks Na^+ reabsorption at distal convoluted tubule (DCT, 5%-10% Na-reabs) **Na^+ loss > H_2O loss** Retention of H_2O lowers ECFV = **hyponatremia** Increases urine output	Hydrochlorothiazide Chlorothiazide (Diuril) Chlorthalidone Metolazone
K^+-sparing diuretics	Competes with aldosterone for mineralocorticoid receptors at late distal tubule and collecting duct K^+ reabsorption + Na^+ secretion = **hyperkalemia, hyponatremia**	Spironolactone (Aldactone) Eplerenone

OSMOTIC DEMYELINATION SYNDROME

- Water enters the cell to obtain osmotic equilibrium, and cells swell causing cerebral edema
- Rapid overcorrection can cause water to shift **out of cells**, causing cell shrinkage, and causing permanent neurologic damage
- High risk for intracranial bleeding!

CALCIUM HOMEOSTASIS: HYPOCALCEMIA AND HYPERCALCEMIA

- Calcium has important effects on myocyte depolarization

- Hypocalcemia reduces the depolarization threshold potential and renders the cardiac myocyte more excitable
- Conversely, hypercalcemia reduces membrane excitability by increasing the depolarization threshold
- **Most Ca^{2+} is bound to protein (albumin), so the total Ca^{2+} concentration fluctuates with protein concentration**
- Free ionized Ca^{2+} (physiologically active) is under tight control by PTH and independent of albumin levels
- Increased pH increases the binding of Ca^{2+} to albumin → alkalemia, total Ca^{2+} is normal but ionized Ca^{2+} is low → signs/symptoms of hypocalcemia

Etiology of Hypocalcemia and Hypercalcemia

Hypocalcemia	Hypercalcemia

• **Hypoparathyroidism** (most common)
• Acute pancreatitis: deposition of Ca^{2+} lowers serum Ca^{2+}
• **Renal insufficiency**: decreased vitamin D production
  • Vitamin D deficiency
• Hyperphosphatemia: PO_4 precipitates with Ca^{2+} resulting in calcium phosphate deposition
• Pseudohypoparathyroidism–autosomal recessive causing end organ resistance to PTH
• Hypomagnesemia
• Malabsorption–short bowel syndrome
• Blood transfusion–Ca^{2+} binds citrate
• Hypoalbuminemia
• DiGeorge syndrome
	• Endocrinopathies
	  • **Hyperparathyroidism**–increased Ca^{2+}, low PO_4
	  • Renal failure–usually results in hypocalcemia, but sometimes secondary hyperparathyroidism elevates PTH levels to cause hypercalcemia
	  • Paget disease of the bone–due to osteoclast resorption
	  • Acromegaly, Addison disease
	• Malignancies
	  • Bone mets
	  • Multiple myeloma
	• Pharmacologic
	  • Vitamin D intoxication
	  • Milk-alkali syndrome: hypercalcemia, alkalosis, and renal impairment due to excessive intake of Ca^{2+} and antacids
	  • Drugs–thiazide diuretics, lithium
	• Sarcoidosis: increased GI absorption
	• Familial hypocalciuric hypercalcemia

Disease	Etiology, Prevalence, Risk Factors	Clinical Symptoms and Signs	Diagnostics	Therapy, Prognosis, and Health Maintenance
Hypocalcemia	Increased neuromuscular irritability Associated: Rickets and osteomalacia, basal ganglia calcifications	Asymptomatic: 1. **Numbness/tingling:** circumoral in fingers, toes, face (periorbital, tip of nose) 2. Tetany 3. Grand mal seizures Signs: 1. Hyperactive DTRs 2. **Chvostek sign**–tapping a facial nerve leads to a contraction (twitching) of facial muscles 3. **Trousseau sign**–inflate BP cuff to a pressure higher than the patient's systolic BP × 3 min → elicits carpal spasms	1. EKG: arrhythmias, QT prolongation 2. BUN/Cr, Mg, albumin, ionized Ca^{2+} 3. Amylase, lipase, LFTs 4. Serum PO_4: high in renal insufficiency and hypoparathyroidism 5. PTH **Hypoparathyroidism = low** **Vitamin D deficiency = high** Pseudohypoparathyroidism = very high	1. If symptomatic → **IV Ca^{2+} gluconate** Long term = **oral $CaCO_3$ and vitamin D** 2. PTH deficiency → replace with vitamin D (calcitriol) + high oral Ca^{2+} intake, thiazide diuretics lower urinary Ca^{2+} and prevent urolithiasis 3. **Correct hypomagnesemia**: very difficult to correct Ca^{2+} if you do not correct magnesium first

(continued)

(continued)

| Hypercalcemia | | Children:
1. **Hypotonicity**
2. **Muscle weakness**
3. Apathy, mood swings, bizarre behavior
4. Nausea, vomiting, abdominal pain
Signs:
1. Hyperextensibility of joints
2. Hypertension, bradycardia
3. Cardiac anomalies, short QT interval, intractable peptic ulcer, pancreatitis (adults)
4. **Decreased DTRs** | 1. Draw same labs as for hypocalcemia
• **Serum Ca^{2+} >11 mg/dL** (>13 mg/dL severe)
• Ca^{2+} high, PTH low
2. Slit lamp examination: **band keratopathy**–deposits in cornea or conjunctiva
3. Radioimmunoassay of PTH: high in primary PT, low in occult malignancy
4. Radioimmunoassay of PTH-related protein: high in malignancy
5. Bone scan or bone surgery → lytic lesions
6. Urinary cAMP: elevated in primary PTH | • Increased urinary excretion
1. **Vigorous hydration (IV normal saline)–first step**
2. **Loop diuretics (Lasix)**–forced Ca^{2+} diuresis with diuretic (furosemide 1 mg/kg q 6 h)
• Inhibit bone resorption in patients with malignancy
  • Bisphosphonates
  • Calcitonin
• Give steroids if vitamin D related and multiple myeloma
• Hemodialysis for renal failure |

Complications of Hypercalcemia

1. **Stones**: nephrolithiasis, nephrocalcinosis

2. **Bones**: bone aches/pains, **osteitis fibrosa cystica** (brown tumors)

3. **Grunts and groans**: muscle pain and weakness, pancreatitis, PUD, gout, constipation

4. **Psychiatric overtones**: depression, fatigue, anorexia, sleep disturbances, anxiety, lethargy

5. Other findings: polydipsia, polyuria, HTN, weight loss, short QT

	Plasma Ca^{2+}	Plasma PO_4	Bone Resorption	Kidney	Gut
PTH	↑	↓	↑	↑ Ca^{2+} reabsorption ↓ PO_4 reabsorption	Activation of vitamin D
Calcitonin	↓	↓	↓	↓Ca^{2+} reabsorption ↑ PO_4 reabsorption	↓ postprandial Ca^{2+} absorption
Vitamin D	↑	↑	↑	↑ Ca^{2+} resorption ↓ PO_4 reabsorption	↑ Ca^{2+} resorption ↑ PO_4 reabsorption

Volume Disorders

- Remember the **60-40-20** rule
  - TBW (total body water) is 60% of body weight (50% for women)
  - ICF is 40% of body weight
  - ECF is 20% of body weight
    - Interstitial fluid is 15% and plasma is 5%
- Normal urine output for an adult is 0.5 to 1.0 mL/kg/h
  - *Example*: A 70-kg man (154 lb) should be urinating about 840 to 1680 mL/day

CLINICAL PICTURE:

- Patients with sepsis, burns, fever, or open wounds have higher insensible losses

- For each degree of atmospheric temperature >37°C, the body loses 100 mL/day
- Patients with liver failure, nephrotic syndrome, or any condition causing hypoalbuminemia third-space fluid out of vasculature and may be total body hypervolemic but intravascularly depleted
- Patients with CHF may have either pulmonary edema or anasarca, depending on which ventricle is involved
- Patients with ESRD are prone to hypervolemia

ETIOLOGY OF HYPOVOLEMIA AND HYPERVOLEMIA

Hypovolemia	Hypervolemia
• **GI losses**: vomiting, diarrhea, NG suction, fistula drainage • **Third spacing**: ascites, effusions, bowel obstruction, crush injuries, burns • Inadequate intake • Polyuria (eg, DKA) • Sepsis, intra-abdominal or retroperitoneal inflammation • Trauma, open wounds, sequestration of fluid into soft tissue injuries • Insensible losses—evaporative losses **through the skin** (75%) and the respiratory tract (25%)	• Iatrogenic (parenteral overhydration) • Fluid retaining states: CHF, nephrotic syndrome, cirrhosis, ESR, hypoalbuminemia

HYPOVOLEMIA AND HYPERVOLEMIA

Disease	Etiology, Prevalence, Risk Factors	Clinical Symptoms and Signs	Diagnostics	Therapy, Prognosis, and Health Maintenance

Hypovolemia	Decrease in ECF volume (see previous table for etiology)	HX: blood loss, GI loss, excess sweating, diuretics
		1. Polyuria, polydipsia, polyphagia (diabetes)
		2. Thirst, salt craving
		3. Desire to drink pickle juice or ingest salty foods (inherited salt wasting)
		4. **Weakness**, LOC
		5. MS changes, **sleepy**, apathetic
		Signs:
		1. **Tachycardia, postural hypotension**
		2. JVD not visible
		3. Dry mucous membranes (tongue) and decreased skin turgor
		4. Hypothermia, pale extremities
		5. Oliguria
			1. Measure serum Na^+, K^+, Cl^-, HCO_3^-
			  • High Na^+
			  • Increased hematocrit (3% for each liter lost)
			2. Metabolic alkalosis
			3. BUN: Cr >20:1
			4. FeNa: <1% (prerenal azotemia)
			5. Pulmonary artery catheter (Swan-Ganz) to measure CVP (definitive): decreased CVP, PCWP, pulse pressure
				See treatment table
				Complications:
				1. Uremia
				2. ATN
				3. Shock
				4. Coma

Hypervolemia	(See previous table for etiology)	1. **Weight gain** 2. **Peripheral edema** (pedal or sacral), ascites Signs: 1. **Jugular venous distention** 2. Pulmonary edema (**pulmonary rales**)	1. Pulmonary artery catheter (Swan-Ganz) to measure CVP (definitive): elevated CVP and PCWP 2. Low hematocrit or hypoalbuminemia	See treatment table

Treatment of Hypovolemia and Hypervolemia

Hypovolemia	Hypervolemia

1. Correct volume deficit
  • Bolus to achieve euvolemia, **begin with isotonic solution (NS or lactated ringers)**
  • Monitor HR, BP, UOP, and weight
  • Maintain UOP at 0.5-1.0 mL/kg/h
  • Replace blood loss with crystalloid at 3:1 ratio
Note: using albumin does not improve effectiveness
2. Maintenance fluid
  • D5/NS solution with 20 mEq KCl/L (most common)
	1. Fluid restriction
	2. Judicious use of diuretics
	3. Monitor urine output and daily weights, consider Swan-Ganz catheter

Calculating Maintenance Fluids

- **100/50/20 Rule**
  - 100 mL/kg for first 10 kg, 50 mL/kg for next 10 kg, 20 mL/kg for every 1 kg over 20
  - Divide total by 24 for hourly rate
  - *Example*: 70-kg man: $100 \times 10 = 1000$; $50 \times 10 = 500$; 20×50 kg = 1000. Total = 2500
    - Divide 2500/24 hours = 104 mL/h

- Crystalloid administration
  - 50 to 100 mL/h greater than ongoing losses or repeated 500-mL boluses every 30 minutes (except if bleeding → give blood products to increase Hct up to 35%)
  - Maintain CVP of 8 to 12 mm Hg to improve outcomes

Contraceptive Methods

CONTRACEPTION WHILE BREASTFEEDING

Progestin-only contraception may be initiated at 6 weeks postpartum for those exclusively breastfeeding or at 3 weeks if not exclusively. Copper-containing intrauterine contraception in breastfeeding women has a category 1 or 2 rating, that is, the advantages consistently outweigh the risks. Because progestin-only oral contraceptives have little effect on lactation, they are also preferred by some for use up to 6 months in women who are exclusively breastfeeding. Combination hormonal contraception may begin at 6 weeks following delivery if breastfeeding is well established and the infant's nutritional status is surveilled. This may be initiated as early as 4 weeks after delivery if compliance with later-scheduled postpartum follow-up is a concern and if venous thrombo-embolism (VTE) risks are absent.

	Advantages	Reversible	Disadvantages	Side Effects
Barrier methods: condoms, diaphragms, cervical caps	• Easy access, cheap • Protection against STIs: decreased risk of HIV, gonorrhea, nongonococcal urethritis, herpes	Yes	• Highly dependent on adherence and proper use • Natural membrane condoms less effective than latex • Petroleum-based lubricants can degrade condoms and decrease efficacy for preventing HIV	• Rare reports of toxic shock syndrome with the diaphragm and contraceptive sponge
Sterilization	• **Reduces risk of ovarian cancer** by limiting upward migration of potential carcinogens • Most commonly used method • Examples: hysterectomy, BSO, tubal ligation, vasectomy	No Permanent and irreversible	• 1.85% risk of pregnancy, with 30% risk of ectopic pregnancy • Azoospermia may be delayed 2-6 mo postvasectomy and other forms of contraception must be used until 2 sperm-free ejaculations provide proof of sterility	• Regret of undergoing tubal ligation • Menstrual irregularity: decreased duration and volume of flow, less dysmenorrhea, increased cycle irregularity • Ectopic pregnancy (high with electrocoagulation method) • Functional ovarian cysts

(continued)

(continued)

	Advantages	Reversible	Disadvantages	Side Effects
Intrauterine devices (IUDs)	• High level of efficacy in the absence of systemic metabolic effects • Ongoing motivation not required • No increased rate of pelvic infection and infertility as with earlier devices • Mirena: good for women with menorrhagia • Skyla: good for 3 y • Mirena: good for 5 y • ParaGuard: good for 10 y	Yes	• Not for use in women at high risk for bacterial STI in last 3-6 mo • May not be effective in women with uterine leiomyomas because they alter the size or shape of uterine cavity	• ParaGuard: **increased menstrual blood flow, dysmenorrhea** • Mirena: more frequent **spotting** up to 6 mo after placement or **amenorrhea** (lighter, absent), 30% by 2 y and 60% by 12 y • Expulsion (5%) during first year, likely during first month • Uterine perforation (0.1%) • Not associated with an increased risk of pelvic infection for low-risk patients
Implanon	• Up to 3 y of contraception	Yes	• Not for use in women who cannot tolerate unpredictable and irregular bleeding	• Causes **irregular bleeding** that does not normalize over time
OCPs	• **Increased bone density** • Reduced menstrual blood loss and anemia • Low risk of ectopic pregnancy and hirsutism progression • Improved dysmenorrhea from endometriosis • Improved acne • Fewer premenstrual complaints • **Decreased risk of ovarian and endometrial cancer**, and various benign breast diseases • Prevention of atherogenesis • Decreased activity of RA and incidence and severity of acute salpingitis	Yes	• Highly user-dependent; effectiveness is dependent upon woman's compliance with taking a daily pill • Increased risk of thromboembolic event, contraindicated with hypercoagulable state (eg, smoking >35 y/o, h/o VTE) • Contraindicated in ER/PR positive breast cancer	• Breakthrough bleeding, amenorrhea, breast tenderness, weight gain • Increased risk of cardiovascular disease (MI, stroke, VTE): breakthrough bleeding and amenorrhea depends on the type of OCP

LONG-ACTING REVERSIBLE CONTRACEPTIVES

Prevent pregnancy through primarily spermicidal effect caused by a sterile inflammatory reaction induced by presence of a foreign body in the uterine cavity (copper) or by the release of progestins (Mirena).

- Screen women at high risk for STIs before IUD insertion

- For women who develop infection with IUD already in place, do not remove device, but treat as STI

- If a tubo-ovarian abscess forms, start IV antibiotics and remove device immediately

- IUDs can be placed immediately after uterine evacuation, after first or second trimester abortions

- Typically inserted at the end of normal menstruation, when cervix is softer and dilated, insertion may be easier and early pregnancy can be excluded

	MOA	Indications and Duration	Contraindications
Copper-containing (**ParaGuard** T 380A)	• Local inflammatory response induced in uterus leads to lysosomal activation (spermicidal)	Good for 10 y	1. Pregnancy or suspicion of **pregnancy** 2. Abnormalities of the uterus resulting in distortion of the uterine cavity (eg, **fibroids**) 3. **Acute pelvic inflammatory disease**, or current behavior suggesting a high risk for pelvic inflammatory disease 4. Postpartum endometritis or postabortal endometritis in the past 3 mo 5. Known or suspected uterine or cervical malignancy 6. Genital bleeding of unknown etiology 7. Mucopurulent cervicitis 8. Wilson disease 9. Allergy to any component of ParaGard 10. A previously placed IUD that has not been removed
Progestin-releasing IUD (**Mirena**–levonorgestrel-releasing intrauterine system) = LNG-IUS 20 mg/d release of levonorgestrel	• Progestin renders endometrium atrophic • Stimulates cervical mucus thickening, **blocking sperm penetration into uterus** • Decreases tubal motility that thereby prevents ovum and sperm union • May inhibit ovulation (not proven)	Good for 5 y following insertion	1. Pregnancy or suspicion of **pregnancy** 2. Congenital or acquired uterine anomaly if it distorts the uterine cavity (eg, **fibroids**) 3. Acute **pelvic inflammatory disease** (PID) or history 4. Postpartum endometritis or infected abortion in the past 3 mo 5. Known or suspected uterine or cervical neoplasia or abnormal Pap smear 6. Genital bleeding of unknown etiology 7. Untreated acute cervicitis or vaginitis or other lower genital tract infections 8. Acute liver disease or liver tumor (benign or malignant) 9. Increased susceptibility to pelvic infection 10. A previously placed IUD that has not been removed 11. Hypersensitivity to any component of Mirena 12. Known or suspected carcinoma of the breast 13. Prior ectopic pregnancy
Implanon single rod system (subdermal implant system, Organon, Nexplanon) 68 mg of progestin (etonogestrel)	• Progestin continuously suppresses ovulation • Increases cervical mucus viscosity • Endometrial atrophy	Contraception for up to 3 y	1. Pregnancy 2. Thrombosis or VTE 3. Benign or malignant hepatic tumors, active liver disease 4. Undiagnosed abnormal genital bleeding 5. Breast cancer

ORAL CONTRACEPTIVE PILLS, PATCHES, RINGS, AND INJECTIONS

- Highly user-dependent; effectiveness is dependent upon woman's compliance with taking a daily pill, changing transdermal patches or rings, or presenting for an injection
- Made from synthetic estrogen (ethinyl estradiol or mestranol) and progestins (norethindrone, desogestrel, gestodene, drospirenone, levonorgestrel)
  - Most androgenic = levonorgestrel
  - Least androgenic = desogestrel, gestodene, drospirenone
- Current doses of EE range from 10 to 50 µg; lower doses decrease side effects and associated risks
- Lo Loestrin Fe = only 10 µg of ethinyl estradiol
- Progestin dose can be constant throughout the cycle (monophasic) or varied (biphasic or triphasic)
- Progestins lower serum free testosterone levels and lowers 5-α-reductase (converts testosterone to active dihydrotestosterone) → decreasing androgen-related conditions (acne)
- The lowest acceptable dose is governed by the ability to prevent unacceptable breakthrough bleeding
- Start on first day of menstrual cycle and use additional contraceptive method for 1 week
- Some women have concern that amenorrhea may be a sign of pregnancy or that it may affect future fertility—reassure them that continuous progestins maintain a healthy endometrium

COMBINED HORMONAL CONTRACEPTIVES

	MOA	Indications and Duration	Contraindications	Adverse Effects
Oral contraceptive pills (OCPs)	• Inhibits ovulation by suppression of hypothalamic gonadotropin-releasing factors • Prevents pituitary secretion of FSH and LH • Estrogens suppress FSH release and stabilize the endometrium, preventing menorrhagia (heavy bleeding) • Progestins inhibit ovulation by suppressing LH, thickening cervical mucus, and rendering endometrium unfavorable for implantation	• Taken 3 out of every 4 wk each month	1. Pregnancy 2. Uncontrolled **hypertension** 3. **Smokers older than 35 y** 4. **Diabetes** with vascular involvement 5. Thrombogenic heart arrhythmias 6. Thrombogenic cardiac valvulopathies 7. Cerebrovascular or coronary artery disease 8. **Migraines** with aura 9. Thrombophlebitis or thromboembolic disorders 10. **History of VTE** 11. Undiagnosed abnormal genital bleeding 12. Known or suspected **breast carcinoma** 13. Cholestatic jaundice of pregnancy or jaundice with pill use 14. Hepatic adenomas or carcinomas, or active liver disease with abnormal liver function 15. Carcinoma of the endometrium or other known or suspected estrogen-dependent neoplasia	• Breakthrough bleeding, **amenorrhea**, breast tenderness, **weight gain** • Increased risk of cardiovascular disease (MI, stroke, VTE)
Yaz (drospirenone)	• Antiandrogenic and antimineralocorticoid activity: potassium retention	• Premenstrual dysphoric disorder (PMDD) • Premenstrual syndrome • Moderate acne vulgaris	• Renal or adrenal insufficiency • Hepatic dysfunction	• Hyperkalemia
Ortho Evra (transdermal patch) 150 μg progestin, norelgestromin 20 ug of EE	• Estrogens suppress FSH release and stabilize the endometrium, preventing menorrhagia (breakthrough bleeding) • Progestins inhibit ovulation by suppressing LH, thickening cervical mucus, and rendering endometrium unfavorable for implantation	• Weekly contraceptive patch applied to buttocks, upper outer arm, lower abdomen, or upper torso • New patch each week × 3 wk, 1 wk patch-free	• Increased risk of VTE	• Skin reactions • Dysmenorrhea • Breast tenderness • Breakthrough bleeding in first 2 cycles • Decreased efficacy in women >90 kg
NuvaRing 15 μg EE and 120 μg of progestin, etonogestrel	• Estrogens suppress FSH release and stabilize the endometrium, preventing menorrhagia (breakthrough bleeding) • Progestins inhibit ovulation by suppressing LH, thickening cervical mucus, and rendering endometrium unfavorable for implantation	• Monthly vaginal ring • Rings should be kept refrigerated, shelf life 4 mo • Inserted within 5 d after onset of menses • Left in for 3 wk • Removed for 1 wk to allow withdrawal bleeding • New ring inserted • Can be removed for coitus and replaced in 3 h		• Breakthrough bleeding (uncommon) • 20% of women and 35% of men report feeling the ring during intercourse

	MOA	Indications and Duration	Contraindications	Adverse Effects
Seasonale (continuous CHC)		• 3 mo preparation with 84 d of active drug and 7 d of placebo		• Loss of menstrual normalcy (less frequent, lighter, unpredictable) • Amenorrhea (8%-63%) • Less headache, fatigue, bloating, dysmenorrhea compared with other OCPs

PROGESTIN-ONLY PRODUCTS

- When used in combination with breastfeeding, POPs are nearly 100% effective for up to 6 months after delivery

	MOA	Indications and Duration	Contraindications	Adverse Effects
Progestin-only pill (POPs) or *minipills*	• Progestins **inhibit ovulation** by suppressing LH, ***thicken cervical mucus***, and render endometrium unfavorable for implantation	• Good for women at increased risk of CVD (hypertension) • Great for women with a history of thrombosis or migraine headaches or smokers older than 35 y • Suitable for lactating women • Reduced risk of ovarian and endometrial cancer • Taken daily at the same time to be effective	• Women with unexplained uterine bleeding • Breast cancer • Hepatic neoplasms, active or severe liver disease • Pregnancy	• Higher incidence of irregular bleeding: amenorrhea, intermenstrual bleeding, prolonged periods of menorrhagia • Higher pregnancy rate
Depo-Provera (DMPA) • 150 mg IM • 104 mg SQ • Slower absorption with SQ, so IM = SQ	Inhibits ovulation and causes changes in endometrium and cervical mucus that result in decreased implantation and sperm transport	• Intramuscular injection given every 90 d • Given within first 5 d after menses onset • No backup contraception necessary • Does not suppress lactation • Good for women for whom an estrogen-containing contraceptive is contraindicated (migraine exacerbation, sickle cell anemia, fibroids) • Decreased risk of ovarian and endometrial cancers	• Women with unexplained uterine bleeding • Breast cancer • Severe liver disease • Pregnancy • Active or history of VTE	• Irregular bleeding, amenorrhea • **Weight gain** • Breast tenderness • Depression? • Increased (possible) risk of cervical carcinoma in situ • Return of fertility delayed up to 12-18 mo • Should not be used longer than 2 y unless other BCM are inadequate owing to risk of decreased bone mineral density (mostly seen in long-term users)

- A pregnancy test is not necessary before the use of oral methods, but pregnancy should be excluded before IUD insertion

POSTCOITAL CONTRACEPTION

1. Copper IUD insertion—maximum of 5 days after with 99% to 100% efficacy by spermicidal effect

2. Oral antiprogestins (ulipristal acetate, 30 mg single dose) or mifepristone 600 mg single dose—prevent by delaying or preventing ovulation, administered within 72 hours but up to 120 hours after intercourse with 98% to 99% efficacy

3. Levonorgestrel (1.5 mg single dose) delays or prevents ovulation and not effective after ovulation; taken within 72 hours of unprotected intercourse with efficacy between 60% to 94%

OBESITY AND CONTRACEPTION

Intrauterine contraception may be *more effective* than oral or transdermal methods for obese women. The WHO guidelines provide no restrictions (class 1) for the use of intrauterine contraception, DMPA, and progestin-only pills for obese women (BMI ≥ 30) in the absence of coexistent medical problems, whereas methods that include estrogen (pill, patch, ring) are considered class 2 (advantages generally outweigh theoretical or proven risks) owing to the increased risk of thromboembolic disease. There are no restrictions to the use of any contraceptive methods following restrictive bariatric surgery procedures, but both combined and progestin-only pills are relatively less effective following procedures associated with malabsorption.

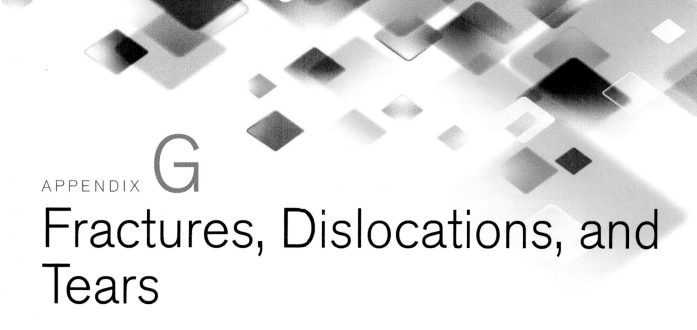

APPENDIX G

Fractures, Dislocations, and Tears

SPINE

Disease	Etiology, Prevalence, Risk Factors	Clinical Symptoms and Signs	Diagnostics	Therapy, Prognosis, and Health Maintenance

Herniated disc (lumbar disc)	Most common: **L5-S1,** L4-L5, L3-L4, L2-L3, L1-L2
	Major cause of severe and chronic or recurrent low back and leg pain
	Mostly 30-40
	Sudden movement causes the weakened and frayed nucleus pulposus to prolapse and protrude through the annulus where they impinge on one or more nerve roots and cause sciatica or radicular pain
		1. Pain referral (**sciatica**)
		  • Mid-gluteal sciatica; posterior thigh; posterolateral leg; lateral foot, heel, or toes
		  • Mild to aching discomfort to severe knife-like stabbing, **radiating down leg**, superimposed on intense ache
		2. **Stiff or unnatural posture**
		3. Some combination:
		  • Weakness
		    • Plantar flexor and hamstring weakness
		  • Reflex change
		    • Absent or diminished ankle jerk
		  • Paresthesias
		<u>Signs:</u>
		1. Pain with straight leg raise and tenderness over lumbosacral joint and sciatic notch
		2. Discomfort walking on heels
		3. Drop foot (L5) and weakness with plantar flexion (S1)
			1. **Straight leg raise** with healthy leg (Lasegue maneuver): flexion at the hip, extension at the knee
			  • Produces sciatic pain on contralateral side
			2. **MRI of lumbar spine:** herniated nucleus pulposus
			  • Not needed unless persistent pain for weeks
			3. CT with myelography
				1. Most comfortable lying supine with legs flexed at knees and hips, shoulders raised on billows
				2. Analgesics—**NSAIDs or opioids** for a few days
				  • Repeated epidural injections of steroids with unconfirmed efficacy
				3. Surgical decompression—emergent if:
				  • Bilateral sensorimotor loss
				  • Sphincteric paralysis

Vertebral compression fracture	Most common in elderly (>60) with osteoporosis Thoracic spine: wedge compression fracture Lumbar: compression or burst fracture	1. Axial pain localized to fractured level 2. **Dowager hump:** loss of height, patient's "back becomes rounded" 3. No neurologic dysfunction and no radiation of pain	1. X-ray 2. CT scan 3. DEXA (dual energy X-ray absorptiometry): most useful	Key: Prevention of osteoporosis 1. HRT if no history of breast cancer, VTE, or endometrial disease 2. Calcitonin therapy if HRT contraindicated 3. Bisphosphonates (alendronate) prevent osteoclastic resorption of bone 4. Surgery (anterior decompression and fusion) for neurologic deficits or significant compression

(continued)

(continued)

Disease	Etiology, Prevalence, Risk Factors	Clinical Symptoms and Signs	Diagnostics	Therapy, Prognosis, and Health Maintenance
Spondylolysis (includes lumbar stenosis) (Fig. G-1)	Congenital and probably genetic bony defect in the **pars interarticularis** (the segment at the junction of pedicle and lamina) of the lower lumbar vertebrae Most common cause of persistent low back pain in adolescents, associated with sports-related injuries Mostly children: 5-7 y/o Spondylolysis: affects cervical spine (C5-C6) caused by degenerative disc disease → nerve root irritation and canal narrowing	Cervical: 1. Neck, shoulder pain and spasms 2. Fatigue, sleep disturbance 3. Radicular pain or muscle weakness Lumbar: 1. Sensorimotor impairment and pain worse with standing and walking or exercising • **Unilateral** low back aching pain • **Worse with *hyperextension*** and twisting • **Better with flexion**	Straight leg raise (<10% positive) 1. X-ray: formation of osteophytes and disc narrowing → facet joints and joints of Luschka affected • **"Scotty dog" view** shows defect in lumbar region 2. CT scan, postmyelographic CT 3. Bone scan	1. Rest, isometric abdominal exercises, pelvic tilt, flexion exercises, NSAIDs, weight reduction 2. Lumbar epidural injections for symptomatic relief 3. Decompression and fusion for compressive symptoms and decreased QOL 1. Cervical collar, traction, PT, analgesics 2. ACDF in advanced disease
Spondylolisthesis (Fig. G-2)	Anterior displacement of one vertebral body in relation to the adjacent one Older adults MCC: Degenerative arthritis of the spine In the usual bilateral form, small fractures at the **pars interarticularis** allow the vertebral body, pedicles, and superior articular facets to *move anteriorly*, leaving the posterior elements behind	1. Dull, aching pain 2. Neurologic symptoms more common • Paresthesias and numbness, feeling of weakness in extremity • Fingers or referred pain to shoulder • Radiation down leg to buttocks or posterior thigh	1. Palpation of spinous processes: "step off" forward displacement of spinous process and exaggerated lordosis 2. Meyerding system to stage	Try conservative treatment above 1. Refer to surgery if failure to respond (grade II or higher)
Costochondritis	Tietze syndrome: <40, M = F Age >40, mostly F	1. Anterior chest pain • Sudden or gradual • Sharply localized or radiates to arms or shoulders • Worse with sneezing, cough, deep inspiration, or twisting • Brief and darting • Persistent dull ache 2. Reproduced with palpation Tietze syndrome 1+ joints are swollen, red, and tender	1. X-ray 2. Bone scan 3. Vitamin D level 4. Biopsy	1. Analgesics, anti-inflammatories 2. Local steroid injections

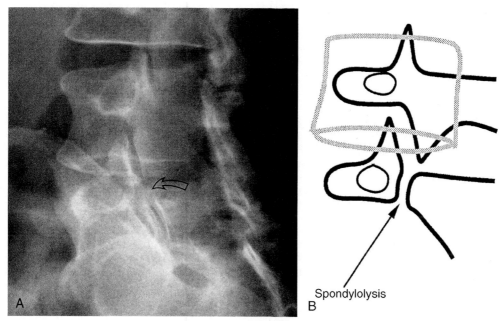

FIGURE G-1. Spondylolysis: fracture of the pars interarticularis. (From Brant W, Helms C. *Brant and Helms Solution*. Philadelphia: Wolters Kluwer; 2007.)

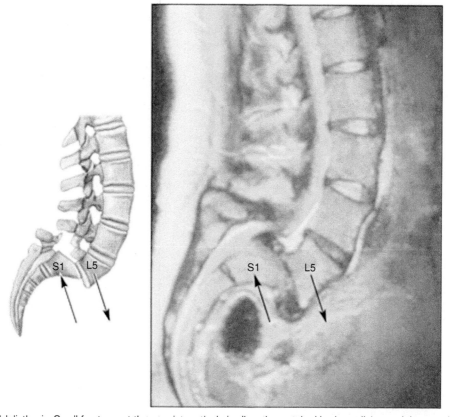

FIGURE G-2. Spondylolisthesis. Small fractures at the pars interarticularis allow the vertebral body, pedicles, and the superior articular facets to move anteriorly. (From Werner R. *Massage Therapist's Guide to Pathology*. 5th ed. Philadelphia: Wolters Kluwer; 2013.)

FRACTURES OF THE SHOULDER, FOREARM/WRIST/HAND, HIP, KNEE, ANKLE/FOOT

Types of Fractures

- Transverse—right angle to axis of the bone
- Spiral—bone has twister appearance; torsion

- Oblique (fracture line between horizontal and vertical)
- Comminuted (splintered or crushed)
- Segmental (double)
- Incomplete—line of fracture does not continue through to the other side of the bone

- Torus (buckle) fractures—one side of cortex buckles as a result of compression (FOOSH); differ by mechanism of injury and buckle on both sides; 6 weeks in cast

- Greenstick fracture—occurs in long bones when bowing causes a break in one side of cortex; angulation of fracture <15°; long arm or leg cast × 4 to 6 weeks; fractures with angulation >15° need referral

ELBOW AND FOREARM

Disease	Etiology, Prevalence, Risk Factors	Clinical Symptoms and Signs	Diagnostics	Therapy, Prognosis, and Health Maintenance
Nursemaid's elbow (radial head subluxation)	Mechanism of injury: fall onto dorsiflexed hand Most common fracture of elbow in adults **Nursemaid's elbow**—subluxation of the radial head in children is caused by excessive longitudinal traction • MC before age 4 y • Radial head slips anteriorly	1. Arm pain, crying with any movement 2. Holding arm at side, motionless 3. Refuses to move arm, forearm, or wrist Signs: 1. Forearm extended and in pronation 2. No edema, deformity, or erythema 3. Distal pulses and capillary refill normal	AP and lateral XR of elbow • Displacement of posterior fat pad implies hemarthrosis • r/o fracture in children	1. Subluxations can be reduced • Hold the affected arm above the wrist and just below the elbow • Place the thumb of the proximal hand over the radial head, while fully supinating and flexing the forearm • Apply direct posterior pressure
Radial head fracture (Fig. G-3A)	33% of all elbow fractures Mechanism: FOOSH with pronated forearm or with elbow slightly flexed, direct blow to lateral elbow	1. Elbow pain, swelling and pain on movement of the forearm Signs: 1. Elbow tender to palpation over radial head, just distal to lateral epicondyle Complications: loss of elbow motion	1. AP and lateral XR • Elbow joint effusion (sail sign and/or posterior fat pad) 2. **Mason classification** • Type I: nondisplaced, no mechanical obstruction to movement • Type II: displaced >2 mm or angulation >30° • Type III: comminuted • Type IV: associated elbow dislocation	1. Type 1: no ortho referral • Posterior splint or sling for up to 1 wk 2. Type II-IV: ortho referral required Health maintenance: 1. Follow-up XR in 2 wk 2. Elbow movement ASAP 3. Normal function by 2-3 mo
Cubital tunnel syndrome (Fig. G-3B)	Ulnar nerve entrapment at the elbow Second most common after carpal tunnel	1. Neuropathy in small and ring fingers: numbness, tingling, aching, burning, shooting, or stabbing pain • Worse with elbow flexion or resting on work surface 2. Allodynia: normal touch is painful 3. Weakness Signs: 1. Tenderness over ulnar nerve 2. Elbow flexion sign: **full elbow flexion × 60 s** (wrists straight) worsens sx 3. Abnormal sensory examination 4. Weakness and atrophy of interossei or thumb adductor muscles	1. **(+) Tinel sign:** percussion of ulnar nerve at the elbow produces discomfort and paresthesia 2. **Wartenberg sign:** patients have difficulty placing the hand in pocket because small finger gets stuck outside • Unopposed abductor digiti quinti muscle 3. **Froment sign:** inability of thumb to oppose index finger • Ask the patient to hold a piece of paper between the thumb and index finger • If you can pull the paper away or the thumb flexes at IP joint to compensate for weakness = (+) 4. Nerve conduction studies of ulnar nerve	1. Activity modification: avoid elbow flexion of 90° or more 2. Nighttime elbow splints—**maintain elbow in 45 degrees of flexion** 3. Surgical decompression: medial epicondylectomy

Disease	Etiology, Prevalence, Risk Factors	Clinical Symptoms and Signs	Diagnostics	Therapy, Prognosis, and Health Maintenance
Radial tunnel syndrome	Radial nerve compressed in radial tunnel (proximal radius) Usually occurs in combination with lateral epicondylitis	1. Pain over midportion of the mobile wad (brachioradialis, extensor carpi radialis longus, extensor carpi radialis brevis) 2. Pain with resisted forearm supination	1. Long-finger extension test: worse with extension of the wrist and fingers, while the long finger is passively flexed by the examiner	1. Avoid forceful extension of the wrist and fingers 2. Splint the wrist in dorsiflexion while forearm is immobilized in supination 3. Surgical decompression of radial nerve
Golfer elbow (medial epicondylitis)	Due to repetitive resisted motions of wrist flexion and pronation	1. Pain over medial side of the elbow due to repeated **wrist flexion and pronation** • Radiates into the forearm Signs: 1. Tenderness distal to medial epicondyle 2. Pain reproduced by resisting wrist flexion and pronation with elbow extended	XR: normal	1. Conservative • Rest, ice, NSAIDs, friction massage 2. Splint 3. Steroid injections 4. Surgical release of flexor muscle at its origin Health maintenance: 1. Rest at least 1 mo 2. Start physical therapy once pain subsides
Tennis elbow (lateral epicondylitis) (Fig. G-3C)	Tendon tears and necrosis at the attachment of the extensor carpi radialis brevis to the lateral humeral epicondyle and the extensor carpi radialis longus origin along the supracondylar line Related more to fibrosis and degenerative changes than acute inflammation Mechanism: Overuse, hitting backhand with elbow flexed	1. Pain after work or 5 **d supination** against resistance • Tennis, pulling weeds, carrying suitcases, using a screwdriver • Worse with shaking hands, opening doors, steering wheel 2. Pain radiates into the dorsal aspect of the forearm • Occurs at night and rest Signs: 1. Local tenderness 2. Pain at distal third of humerus 3. Weakness with grasp	Clinical DX: 1. Cozen test: extend the elbow, extend the patient's wrist against resistance 2. MRI to r/o intra-articular pathology	1. **Rest and NSAIDs** 2. **Ice and friction massage** 3. If severe—place in sling or splint at 90° of flexion 4. If localized, inject steroid • Rest arm × 1 mo, avoid aggravating activities • AE: fat necrosis, skin atrophy, loss of pigmentation 5. Surgical release of extensor aponeurosis Health maintenance: 1. Once asymptomatic, begin rehab with isometric and concentric exercises 2. Avoid forceful pinching or gripping, especially with wrist extension
Supracondylar humerus fractures	Mechanism of injury: FOOSH with hyperextension of the elbow	1. Pain with minimal swelling Complications: Volkmann ischemic contractures, injury to all 3 nerves, varus (gunstock) or valgus deformities of the elbow	Full neovascular examination—attention to brachial artery injuries looking for Volkmann ischemic contracture AP and lateral views In children, obtain comparative views	1. Closed reduction in or with posterior splint application for displaced fractures in children 2. ORIF for adults
Maisonneuve fracture	Combination of **oblique proximal fibular fracture**, disruption of interosseous membrane and tibiofibular ligament distally, and a **medial malleolar fracture** or tear of the deltoid ligament Produced by an external rotational force applied to the foot	Ankle pain Signs: 1. Tenderness at medial and anterolateral ankle joint 2. Tenderness at proximal fibula		1. Sugar-tong splint 2. Surgery (most)

WRIST/HAND

Disease	Etiology, Prevalence, Risk Factors	Clinical Symptoms and Signs	Diagnostics	Therapy, Prognosis, and Health Maintenance
Colles' (distal radius) fracture "Dinner-fork deformity" (Fig. G-3D)	Most common injury of the wrist Mechanism of injury: fall onto a dorsiflexed hand (FOOSH)	1. Pain 2. Swelling 3. Palmar paresthesias from compression of median nerve Signs: 1. Swelling 2. Tenderness at distal forearm Complications: Median nerve compression, tendon damage, ulnar nerve contusion or compression, acute compartment syndrome	1. AP and lateral XR • Dorsal displacement of the distal fragment • **Dorsal angulation** of the distal intact radius with radial shortening	1. Cast immobilization in most after reduction • **Volar or sugar-tong splint** 2. *Definitive* treatment depends on the patient and fracture • Good bone density and nondisplaced: **functional brace** • Minimally displaced or osteopenia: **cast** • Any cast or splint should not obstruct motion of the elbow, MCP, or fingers 3. Referral to ortho if unstable for internal fixation Health maintenance: 1. Fracture at greatest risk of displacement during first 3 wk 2. Reassess at weekly intervals with XR × 3 wk • Remove cast at 6-8 wk → brace • Callus should be seen at 8-12 wk follow-up
Smith's fracture (reverse Colles' fracture) "Garden spade or silver fork deformity"	Break of the distal end of the radius Results from a blow or fall on the hyperflexed hand Results from a blow or fall onto a hyperflexed wrist	1. Similar to Colles'	1. AP and Lateral XR • **Volar displacement of the distal fragment** • **Volar angulation** of the distal intact radius with radial shortening and comminuted	1. Similar to Colles' • During reduction, pressure is applied in the opposite direction
Carpal tunnel syndrome (mononeuropathy)	Numbness and tingling and/or pain in median nerve distribution F > M (3:1) RF: Obesity, female, comorbidity (DM, **pregnancy [third trimester]**, RA, hypothyroid), genetics, aromatase inhibitor use 65% bilateral Severe cases: Clumsiness, "difficulty holding objects, turning keys or doorknobs, buttoning clothing, or opening jar lids"	1. **Pain** • Involvement of the first 3 digits and radial half of the fourth digit • Worse at night and awaken the patient from sleep • Better by shaking or wringing hands or placing them under warm water 2. **Paresthesias** • May radiate proximally into the forearm or above the elbow to shoulder • Provoked by flexion or extension of the wrist or raising arms (driving, reading, typing, holding phone) 3. **Weakness** (less commonly) Signs: 1. Weakness of thumb adduction and opposition 2. Thenar atrophy	Clinical DX: 1. **Phalen maneuver:** flex the wrist with elbow in full extension (backs of hands against one another to provide hyperflexion) • Positive if pain and/or paresthesia in median innervated fingers within 1 min of wrist flexion 2. Tinel test—percussion over proximal portion of carpal tunnel • Positive if pain and/or paresthesia • Less sensitive than Phalen sign (50%) 3. Wrist compression test: pressure over median nerve provokes symptoms in 30 s 4. **Nerve conduction study (NCS) with EMG** (confirms) • Excludes polyneuropathy, plexopathy, and radiculopathy • Delayed distal latencies and slowed conduction velocity	1. Mild (nonsurgical) • **Nocturnal wrist splinting** in neutral position × 1 mo • **Steroid injections** of methylprednisolone 40 mg, no more than 1 per wrist q 6 mo • Oral steroids of 20 mg prednisone daily 10-14 d • PT/OT or yoga 2. Moderate-severe • Electrodiagnostic studies (first) • Surgical decompression *Note:* Should resolve postpartum in pregnancy

Disease	Etiology, Prevalence, Risk Factors	Clinical Symptoms and Signs	Diagnostics	Therapy, Prognosis, and Health Maintenance
Boxer fracture (Fig. G-3E)	Fracture of the metacarpal neck of the fourth or fifth finger Cause: Punch to another's mouth, direct blow to the hand or fall Also known as street fighter's fracture	1. Loss of prominence of knuckle with tenderness and pain Signs: 1. Decreased grip strength 2. Local tenderness and swelling Complications: Decreased ROM	1. AP and lateral XR 2. Oblique pronated XR of the fourth and fifth metacarpals • Dorsal angulation due to interosseous muscle pull	1. Fractures with 25°-30° of angulation: • Closed reduction with application of **ulnar gutter × 3-4 k** 2. Surgical management Health maintenance: 1. Continue casting until symptomatic resolution and clinical healing 2. 2 wk postcasting XR
DeQuervain tenosynovitis	Inflammation of abductor pollicis longus and extensor pollicis brevis Cause: repetitive twisting of wrist	1. Pain upon grasping with thumb: pinching Signs: 1. Swelling and tenderness over radial styloid process	1. **Finkelstein sign (+):** patient's thumb placed in the palm and close fingers over it; wrist ulnar deviated resulting in pain over tendon sheath	1. Forearm-based **thumb spica splint** 2. NSAIDs 3. Steroid injections
Gamekeeper's thumb (skier's thumb) (Fig. G-3F)	Sprain or tear of the **ulnar collateral ligament** of the thumb from forcible radial deviation History of sprained thumb or fall on the hand	1. Pain over ulnar border of the MCP joint Signs: 1. **Increased** ligamentous **laxity** of the UCL 2. Instability of the MCP and weakness of pinch • Check radial deviation in **full extension and 30° of flexion** 3. Tenderness over the MCP joint 4. Stener lesion	1. XR of thumb–r/o avulsion fracture	1. Immobilization with a **thumb spica** cast × 6 wk for partial rupture • Must wear at all times except for skin care • Avoid any radial deviation when off 2. Surgical repair for complete rupture
Trigger finger or trigger thumb (flexor tenosynovitis) (Fig. G-3G)	Stenosing flexor tenosynovitis History of repetitive strain More common in diabetic patients	1. Pain referred to the PIP joint 2. Catching or snapping with forceful flexion • Finger becomes locked in flexed position • Worse in morning Signs: 1. Tenderness over proximal tendon pulley at the MCP joint		1. Long-acting steroid injection into flexor sheath • Insert proximal palmar crease for the index finger • Insert at distal palmar crease for middle, ring, small fingers 2. Surgical release of A1 pulley if refractory to steroids
Scaphoid (navicular) fracture (Fig. G-3H)	Most commonly fractured carpal bone Caused by forceful hyperextension of the wrist due to FOOSH with wrist dorsiflexed and radially deviated A scaphoid fracture is stable *unless* there is 1. Displacement >1 mm 2. Scapholunate angulation >60° 3. Radiolunate angulation >15°	1. Painful wrist over anatomic snuffbox 2. Paresthesias of the affected hand 3. Swelling Signs: 1. Tenderness over anatomic snuffbox 2. Swelling over the region 3. Pain with radial deviation and axial compression of thumb Complications: Nonunion of fracture, development of AVN (ground glass appearance of proximal pole or increased bone density)	1. **AP, lateral**, and scaphoid views (PA view in ulnar deviation) 2. Bone scan or MRI	*Nondisplaced or minimally displaced (<1 mm)* 1. Short-arm **thumb spica cast** used for nondisplaced fractures 2. Refer to orthopedic surgeon • If displacement >1 mm, ORIF required Health maintenance: 1. 2 wk follow-up AP, lateral, oblique XR 2. Rehab 3-6 mo

(continued)

(continued)

Disease	Etiology, Prevalence, Risk Factors	Clinical Symptoms and Signs	Diagnostics	Therapy, Prognosis, and Health Maintenance
Mallet finger, "baseball" or "drop" finger (Fig. G-4)	Traumatic disruption of the terminal slip of **extensor tendon at the DIP** caused by direct blow to the tip of the finger → sudden forceful flexion of distal phalanx Most common closed tendon injury of the finger <u>MC:</u> Middle-aged men <u>MC:</u> Middle finger	1. Pain over the dorsum of the DIP joint • Swelling, ecchymosis, deformity 2. **Inability to extend the DIP joint fully** (flexed DIP at rest); hold the PIP in full extension and test active extension at the DIP • Should be able to perform passively • Assess neurovascular function	1. XR AP, lateral, oblique—all mallet finger deformities • May see avulsion or volar (palmar) subluxation of distal phalanx	1. Splinting with immobilization of the DIP joint in **full extension** or slight hyperextension • **Stack (mallet) splint × 6-8 wk** • Follow-up q 1-2 wk <u>Indications for referral:</u> Inability to achieve full passive extension of the DIP, full laceration of extensor tendon, volar subluxation of distal phalanx, fracture of >30% of joint surface
Boutonniere deformity (buttonhole) (Fig. G-5A)	Commonly seen in rheumatoid arthritis patients or forceful flexion of the PIP joint during full extension The **central slip** of extensor hood on the dorsal surface of middle phalanx disrupted by laceration or closed rupture or elongated by synovitis of the PIP joint	1. Hyperextension of the DIP joint 2. Persistent flexion of the PIP joint		1. **Splint the PIP joint alone in extension × 3-6 wk**
Swan neck deformity (Fig. G-5B)	Result of contracture of intrinsic hand muscles secondary to systemic diseases, such as rheumatoid arthritis and SLE	1. Hyperextension of the PIP 2. Flexion of the DIP and MCP joints		1. Splint
Dupuytren contracture (Fig. G-5C)	Nodular thickening on palmar surface of the hand affecting preexisting palmar fascia (MCP joint) Most common in 40-60 y/o men <u>MC involved:</u> Ring and pinky	1. Early—subcutaneous, nonmobile nodules felt at the palm 2. Late—palpable subcutaneous cords felt, extending into digits causing puckering of the overlying skin <u>Signs:</u> 1. Fixed contractures of MP and PIP joints 2. Cannot lay the hand flat on table		1. Asymptomatic—observe 2. **Fasciotomy** • Indications: fixed contracture of >30° at MCP or any degree of flexion contracture at PIP <u>Complications:</u> Hematoma <u>Health maintenance:</u> Quit smoking, drinking, and avoid high levels of physical work

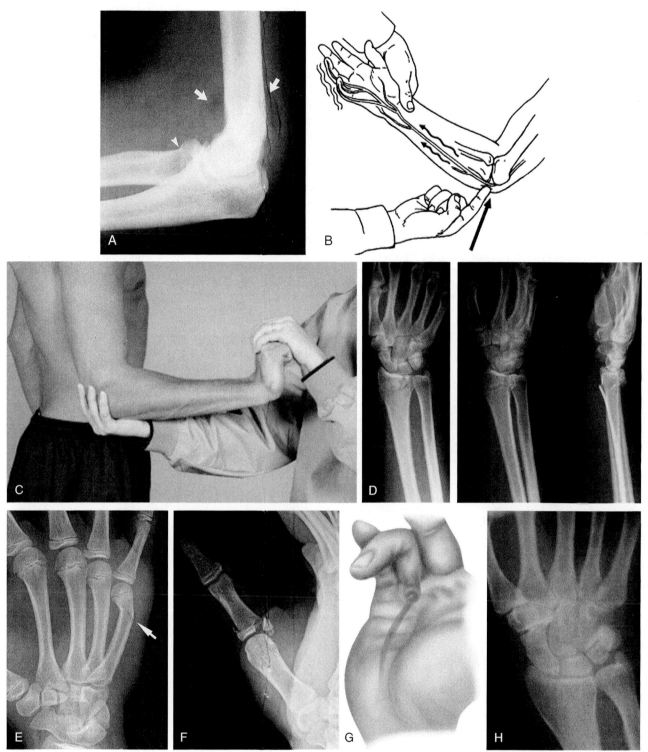

FIGURE G-3. A, Radial head fracture on X-ray. Note the anterior and posterior fat-pads, of which the posterior fat pad is a more reliable marker of fracture. Arrows in (A) note areas of radiolucency projecting away from the distal humeral shaft referring to the anterior and posterior fat pads and the arrowhead denotes the fracture of the radial neck B, Tinel Sign. This tests ulnar nerve entrapment, indicative of cubital tunnel syndrome. C, Cozen test. Resisted extension and radial deviation of the wrist tests for extensor tendinitis. D, Colles' Fracture showing a "dinner-fork" deformity. Dorsal displacement of the distal fragment with dorsal angulation of the distal radius. E, Boxer's fracture. Fracture of the metacarpal neck of the fourth or fifth digit (*arrow*). F, Gamekeeper's thumb. Sprain or tear of the ulnar collateral ligament of the thumb. G, Trigger finger. Stenosing flexor tenosynovitis. H, Scaphoid (navicular) fracture. Soft tissue swelling on the lateral aspect of the scaphoid often presents as the hallmark "scaphoid fat pad sign." (A, From Terry R. Yochum, Lindsay J. *Rowe, Yochum And Rowe's Essentials of Skeletal Radiology.* 3rd ed. Philadelphia: Lippincott Williams & Wilkins; 2004; B, From Palmer M, Epler M. *Fundamentals of Musculoskeletal Assessment Techniques.* 2nd ed. Philadelphia: Lippincott Williams & Wilkins; 1999; C, From Anderson M. *Foundations of Athletic Training.* 5th ed. Philadelphia: Lippincott Williams & Wilkins; 2013; D, From Shah K. *Procedimientos básicos en medicina de urgencias.* 2nd ed. Philadelphia: Wolters Kluwer; 2017; E, From Siegel M, Coley B. *Core Curriculum: Pediatric Imaging.* Philadelphia: Wolters Kluwer; 2006; F, From Flynn J, Skaggs D, Waters P. *Rockwood and Wilkins' Fractures in Children.* 8th ed. Philadelphia: Wolters Kluwer; 2015; G, From Bickley LS, Szilagyi P. *Bates' Guide to Physical Examination and History Taking.* 8th ed. Philadelphia, PA: Lippincott Williams & Wilkins; 2003; H, From Bucholz RW, Heckman JD. *Rockwood & Green's Fractures in Adults.* 5th ed. Lippincott Williams & Wilkins; 2001.)

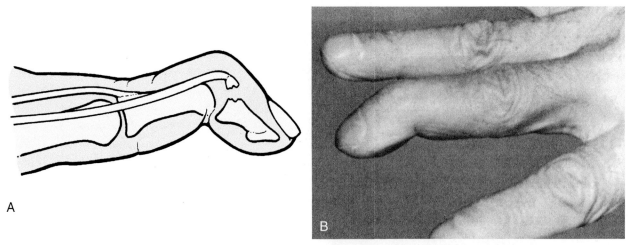

FIGURE G-4. Mallet finger. A, Traumatic disruption of the terminal slip of extensor tendon at the DIP. B, A direct blow to the tip of the finger causes inability to fully extend the DIP joint, leaving the DIP joint flexed at rest. (A, From *Stedman's Medical Dictionary. 28th ed. Philadelphia: Wolters Kluwer; 2006; B, From Salter R. Textbook of Disorders and Injuries of the Musculoskeletal System. 3rd ed. Philadelphia*Stedman's Medical Dictionary. 28th ed. Philadelphia: Stedman's Medical Dictionary. 28th ed. Philadelphia:Wolters Kluwer; 1999.)

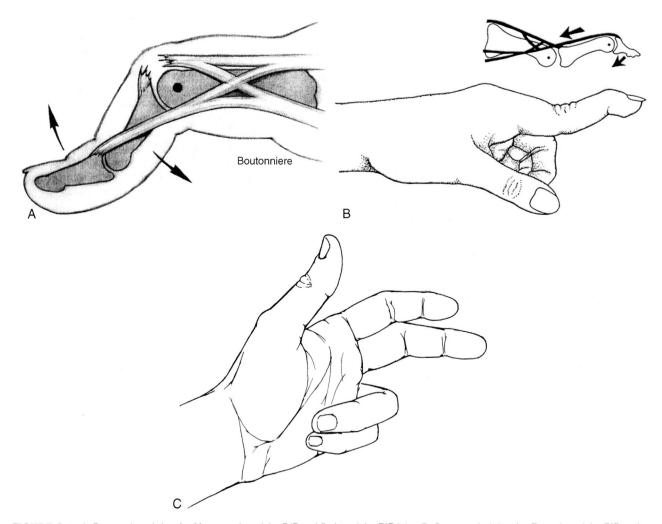

FIGURE G-5. A, Boutonniere deformity. Hypertension of the DIP and flexion of the PIP joint. B, Swan neck deformity. Extension of the PIP and flexion of the PIP and MCP joints. C, Dupuytren contracture. Contractures of the MP and PIP joints. (A, From Thorne C, Bartlett S, Beasley R, Aston S, Gurtner G, Spear S. *Grabb and Smith's Plastic Surgery.* 6th ed. Philadelphia: Wolters Kluwer; 2007; B, From Rayan G, Akelman E. *Hand.* 4th ed. Philadelphia: Wolters Kluwer; 2012; C, From Oatis CA. *Kinesiology - The Mechanics and Pathomechanics of Human Movement.* Baltimore: Lippincott Williams & Wilkins; 2004.)

Shoulder

Disease	Etiology, Prevalence, Risk Factors	Clinical Symptoms and Signs	Diagnostics	Therapy, Prognosis, and Health Maintenance
AC joint separation/ sprain	Fall onto the tip of the shoulder (superior aspect of the acromion) Causes: Fall, direct trauma Common in ice hockey and football Stability across the AC joint is provided by conoid and trapezoid ligaments	1. Pain over AC joint 2. Ecchymosis Signs: 1. Decreased rotator cuff strength 2. Pain lifting arm • Tender to palpation over the AC joint while arm adducted 3. Distal end of clavicle prominent	1. Allman/Rockwood classification: classifies according to degree of ligamentous disruption 2. **AP and axillary lateral views**	1. Type I-II: sling, NSAIDs, RTP × 4 wk 2. Type III: possible operation 3. Type IV-VI: evaluate for operative repair
Type I	Stretching of the AC ligament	1. Diagnosis made based on point tenderness over the AC ligament, history, and mechanism of injury	1. XR: normal	1. Rest, ice, analgesics, simple sling
Type II	Tear of the AC ligaments and stretching of the coracoclavicular ligaments		1. XR: 0%-50% displacement at the AC joint 2. No increase in coracoclavicular interval	1. Rest, ice, analgesics, simple sling
Type III	Complete disruption of the AC and coracoclavicular ligaments		1. XR: displacement at the AC joint 2. Clavicle will appear to be displaced superiorly 50%-100% its width compared with NL	1. Nonoperative • Sling 2. Operative • Ortho consult
Type IV	Complete disruption of the AC and coracoclavicular ligaments			1. Operative
Type V				1. Operative
Type VI				1. Operative
Clavicle fracture (Fig. G-6)	Common: 2%-5% of all fractures in adults MC location: Middle third Mechanism of injury: FOOSH or direct blow to shoulder or clavicle	HX: significant injury (fall or direct blow) 1. Pain involving affected shoulder 2. Arm supported by contralateral extremity • Holds in **adduction and internal rotation**, avoiding any motion Signs: 1. Deformity, **skin tenting** 2. Tender to palpation over site 3. Grinding sensation with arm raised	1. **AP view**–difficult to view 2. CT: fracture at medial end of clavicle	1. Children–figure-of-eight **sling × 4-6 wk** • Shoulder ROM after 2-3 wk 2. Adults–**sling × 6 wk** 3. Surgical reduction • Nonunion, open fractures, fractures that compromise airway or vascularity Health maintenance: 1. Avoid overhead activity • May return to activity when painless, healed on XR, full ROM, and near-normal strength 2. 2-wk follow-up XR • D/C once clinically and radiographically healed 3. Resume noncontact sports at 6 wk, contact sports at 4 mo 4. Callus should form between 4 and 6 wk Complications: Injury to subclavian vessels or brachial plexus, nonunion (if 100% displaced)
Scapula fracture	High-energy trauma: MVA, fall from significant height	1. Pain and tenderness at back of shoulder Signs: 1. Holding arm securely by side 2. Abrasion, ecchymosis over back of shoulder 3. Tender to palpation over acromion	1. XR: axillary, AP shoulder and chest, lateral 2. CT for poorly visualized fractures or if glenoid involved	1. Sling, ROM after 1 wk 10% mortality due to MOI

(continued)

(continued)

Disease	Etiology, Prevalence, Risk Factors	Clinical Symptoms and Signs	Diagnostics	Therapy, Prognosis, and Health Maintenance

Rotator cuff tear	MC tear: supraspinatus	HX: tear on contralateral side
		1. Painful tearing or popping sensation
		  • Painful with overhead activity
		  • Pain at rest or at night
		2. Weakness overhead with lifting away from the body
		Signs:
		1. Supraspinatus or external rotation weakness
		  • No active elevation past 90° of flexion
		  • Weakness to external rotation
		2. (+) impingement signs
		3. Popeye muscle
			1. MR arthrography with contrast
			2. Shrug sign (+)
			3. **Supraspinatus isolation test** (empty can test): downward resistance is applied to the arm after the shoulder is abducted to 90° and forward flexed 30° and the straight arm is rotated so that the thumb is pointing to the ground. Weakness, when compared with the opposite side, indicates disruption of the supraspinatus tendon
			4. **Hawkins-Kennedy test**: the arm is passively flexed forward to 90° and the elbow is flexed to 90°. When the examiner internally rotates the shoulder, pain indicates impingement of the supraspinatus tendon
				1. Rest, NSAIDs
				2. PT: pendulum exercises (flex at waist, relax shoulder girdle, dangle arm in pendulum-like fashion)
				3. Subacromial injections
				4. Surgery
				  • Full thickness tears

Frozen shoulder (adhesive capsulitis)	Age: 40-70 y/o, F > M Nondominant extremity	1. Sedentary occupation 2. Restricted shoulder motion without previous major injury or surgery Signs: 1. Global stiffness 2. Motion is painful, especially at extremes	1. XR: normal cartilaginous surfaces and periarticular surfaces • Decreased capsular space	1. NSAIDs, stretching, moist heat 2. Steroid injections 1-2 y for full ROM
(Proximal) humerus head fracture	Most in older patients with osteoporosis F:M (2:1) MC: Surgical neck	HX: fall or prior rotator cuff injury 1. Pain, swelling, tenderness in greater tuberosity 2. Ecchymosis does not appear until after 24-48 h 3. Patient holds extremity against chest wall Complication: **Axillary artery injury** (forearm and hand appear pale)	1. XR: AP, lateral, and "Y" views 2. Neer classification—classify fracture	1. Closed reduction with sling and swath (Velpeau sling) • 3-4 wk 2. Early mobilization to prevent frozen shoulder 3. ORIF for displaced fractures
Humeral shaft fractures	Mechanism of injury: **MVA, FOOSH,** penetrating injuries (gunshot wounds)	1. Pain, swelling, deformity, shortening 2. Radial nerve injury Complication: **Radial nerve injury** (weakness in wrist or finger extension, numbness in dorsal web space)	1. XR: AP and lateral views including elbow and shoulder	1. Coaptation splint, followed by hanging cast, Sarmiento brace, or operative repair Complications: Radial nerve injury
Thoracic outlet syndrome	F, 20-50 y/o Cause: Congenital anomaly, extra fibromuscular band in TO, fibrosis of scalene muscles Compression of **subclavian artery**, vein, lower trunk (C8, T1) of brachial plexus	1. Aching pain and paresthesias (neck to fingers) 2. Intermittent swelling and discoloration of arm Signs: Bruit	1. EAST (elevated arm stress test): abduct arms 90°, open and close fists for 3 min = (+) if symptoms reproduced 2. XR: r/o apical lung tumor, infection, visualize ribs/spine 3. C spine MRI: if symptoms of disc rupture or spondylosis	1. Physical therapy 2. NSAIDs or muscle relaxants

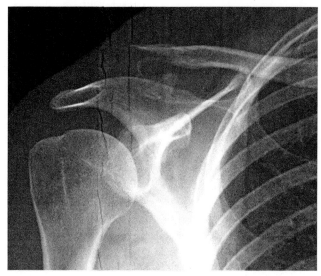

FIGURE G-6. Clavicle fracture. (From Burkhart S. *The Cowboy's Conundrum: Complex and Advanced Cases in Shoulder Arthroscopy.* 1st ed. Philadelphia: Wolters Kluwer; 2018.)

HIP

Disease	Etiology, Prevalence, Risk Factors	Clinical Symptoms and Signs	Diagnostics	Therapy, Prognosis, and Health Maintenance

Femur (hip) fractures (Fig. G-7)	Most occur secondary to serious trauma, but can be due to low-energy injuries associated with old age, osteoporosis, or bone cancer	1. Significant hematoma
		2. Pain
		  • Can be referred to thigh or knee
		Signs:
		1. Affected side—externally rotated, shortened, abducted
		2. Significant blood loss
		3. Absent or diminished pulses
		4. Progressive neurologic signs
			1. Radiographs of pelvis, hip, and knee—r/o hip dislocation	Initial—stabilize and evaluate for life-threatening injuries
				1. 2 large-bore IV lines
				2. Hold in place with Hare traction splint
				3. Open fracture = orthopedic emergency
				  • Tetanus prophylaxis
				  • Antibiotics
				  • Irrigation and debridement
				1. Neck—percutaneous screws or hemiarthroplasty
				2. Shaft—intramedullary rods or plates
				3. Intertrochanteric—sliding hip screw fixation or long gamma nail

KNEE

Disease	Etiology, Prevalence, Risk Factors	Clinical Symptoms and Signs	Diagnostics	Therapy, Prognosis, and Health Maintenance

Osgood-Schlatter disease (osteochondritis of tibial tubercle) Inflammation of tibial tubercle apophysis	**MC: adolescents (boys 9-14 y/o), rapid growth spurt**
	Most commonly **very active or "overuse"** syndrome
	Caused by repetitive strain and chronic avulsion of apophysis of tibial tubercle
	RF:
	Sports involving running, cutting, or jumping
	DDX:
	Jumper's knee (Sinding-Larsen-Johansson): apophysis at inferior pole of patella gets inflamed
		1. Anterior knee pain
		  • Gradually increases over time → impairs activity
		  • Worse: direct pressure (kneeling), running, squatting, jumping, climbing stairs, walking uphill
		  • Relieved: rest
		  • 25%-50% bilateral
		2. Visible and palpable prominence of tibial tubercle
		1. Tenderness and soft tissue or bony prominence over tibial tubercle
		2. Pain reproduced by:
		  • Extending knee against resistance
		  • Stressing quads
		  • Squat with knee fully flexed
		3. Straight leg raise is painless
			Clinical DX:
			1. X-ray (not necessary)
			  • Soft tissue swelling anterior to tibial tubercle
			2. MRI for staging
				1. Conservative TX:
				  • Ice 20-30 min BID
				  • Anti-inflammatories (NSAID)
				  • Physical therapy: quadriceps and hamstring stretching
				  • **Continue activity**
				  • Protective pad over tubercle
				2. Surgery
				  • For patients who fail to respond to conservative TX
				Prognosis:
				1. Waxes and wanes over 6-18 mo
				2. Subsides completely by 14-18 y of age
				Complications:
				Avulsion fracture (rare), genu recurvatum (rare), persistent prominent tubercle, persistent pain

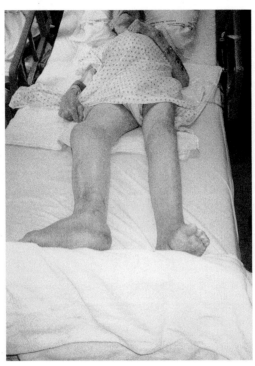

FIGURE G-7. Hip fracture. Note the affected right leg is externally rotated, shortened, and abducted. (From Dale B, Katherine W. *Atlas of Adult Physical Diagnosis*. Philadelphia: Lippincott Williams & Wilkins; 2006.)

ANKLE AND FOOT

Disease	Etiology, Prevalence, Risk Factors	Clinical Symptoms and Signs	Diagnostics	Therapy, Prognosis, and Health Maintenance
Jones fracture (dancer's fracture) (Fig. G-8)	Transverse fracture of the base of the fifth metatarsal Mechanism: Ankle in **plantar flexion** and **inverted** with large adduction force applied to forefoot High incidence of delayed healing and nonunion	1. Pain and swelling on the outside of the foot at the base of the little toe 2. Difficulty walking Complications: delayed union and nonunion		1. **Non–weight bearing immobilization** and **posterior splint × 6-8 wk** 2. If healing present at 6-8 wk → immobilization with fracture brace • ROM and gradual weight bearing 3. If no healing present → surgery or continued cast • Intramedullary screw fixation or bone grafting
Avulsion of base of 5th metatarsal (MT) (Fig. G-9)	Results from sudden foot inversion	1. Pain and swelling at the lateral aspect of midfoot 2. Difficulty walking Signs: 1. Swelling 2. Decreased ROM 3. Tenderness over lateral aspect of midfoot	1. XR: diaphyseal fracture of the fifth MT base	1. Hard-soled shoe or walking cast × 2-3 wk • Can bear weight as tolerated
Lisfranc injury (midfoot fracture dislocation) (Fig. G-10)	Lisfranc joint = tarsometatarsal joint that connects the midfoot to forefoot Lisfranc ligament connects second metatarsal base to medial cuneiform High-energy mechanisms	1. Severe midfoot pain Signs: 1. Inability to bear weight 2. Swelling	1. Dorsoplantar (DP), oblique, lateral XR: • Lateral subluxation of second MT base in relationship to middle cuneiform • First and third MT bases have migrated laterally • Lateral view: superior subluxation in relation to cuneiform bones	1. Orthopedic referral 2. Closed reduction can be attempted 3. Most need surgery

Disease	Etiology, Prevalence, Risk Factors	Clinical Symptoms and Signs	Diagnostics	Therapy, Prognosis, and Health Maintenance
Plantar fasciitis	Common in runners and overweight patients Caused by microscopic tears in plantar fascia at calcaneal origin Peak: 40-60s RF: Obesity, pes planus (flat-foot), pes cavus (high arched foot), prolonged standing, walking on hard surfaces, faulty shoes	1. Patients will complain of pain with first few steps in AM or following inactivity during day • Lessens with weight-bearing activity • Worse with walking barefoot or up stairs 2. Heel pain at night Signs: 1. Pain at inferior heel 2. Inflexible Achilles tendon	1. Plain XR normal, but may reveal calcaneal fracture or bone spur 2. MRI: calcifications of plantar fascia	1. Conservative treatment × 6-12 mo • Physical therapy for stretching plantar fascia and Achilles tendon • Heel pads • Arch supports • Massage of area with tennis ball 2. Steroid injections used with caution due to risk of rupture of plantar fascia 3. Fasciotomy for cases that fail 6-12 mo of conservative treatment
Morton neuroma	Perineural fibrosis of the common digital nerve as it passes between the metatarsal heads MC: Between 3rd-4th toes	1. "Walking on a marble" • Feels like there is a pebble in shoe • Worse with high heels or tight, restrictive shoes 2. Dysesthesias		1. Conservative • Wear low-heeled, well-cushioned shoes with wide toe box • Metatarsal pads 2. Lidocaine and corticosteroid injection proximal to metatarsal head 3. Surgical excision if persistent or recurrent
Hallux valgus (bunion, metatarsus adductovarus, hallux abducto valgus)	Subluxation of the first MTP joint → first metatarsal head medial prominence and lateral deviation of proximal phalanx on first metatarsal Prevalence: 2%-50% F RF: Flatfoot, family history ligamentous laxity Associated: Concurrent gout	1. Laterally deviated hallux, erythema, edema • Often bilateral 2. Hypermobility 3. Flatfoot deformity 4. Pain under second MT head 5. Overlapped second digit 6. Hammer toe deformity Signs: 1. Tenderness on medial eminence at first MTP joint 2. Pain through first MTP joint ROM 3. Decreased ankle dorsiflexion and first MTP ROM	1. Weight bearing XRs in dorsoplantar, lateral, and medial oblique • Lateral deviation of hallux • Medial deviation of the first MT bone • Lateral: dorsal spur formation of first MTP joint, hammer-toe • First MTP joint narrowing, osteophyte formation, subchondral cysts, sclerosis	1. Conservative • Change shoes to wider toe box • Place toe spacer in first interdigital space • Pad the she to limit shearing force • Custom made orthoses • Rest, NSAIDs, ice • Physical therapy 2. Surgery • Exostectomy: for patients with no joint pain, but extraarticular "bump" pain • Osteotomy: realigns bony structure • Arthrodesis: in severe cases 3. 2-6 wk of non−weight bearing)

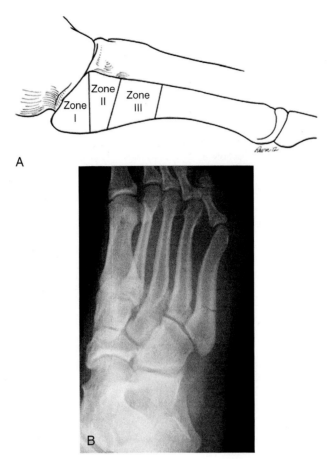

FIGURE G-8. Jones' fracture. A, Fractures of the 5th Metatarsal Classification. B, Fracture at the base of the fifth metatarsal occurring in zone II, also known as the vascular watershed area, where blood is supplied by metaphyseal vessels and diaphyseal nutrient arteries. There is an increased risk for nonunion in this area. (A, From Kitaoka H. *Master Techniques in Orthopaedic Surgery: The Foot and Ankle*. 3rd ed. Philadelphia: Wolters Kluwer; 2014; B, From Wiesel S. *Operative Techniques in Orthopaedic Surgery*. Vol 4. Philadelphia: Wolters Kluwer; 2011.)

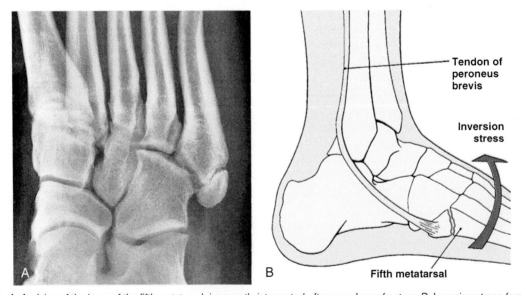

FIGURE G-9. A, Avulsion of the base of the fifth metatarsal, incorrectly interpreted often as a Jones fracture. B, Inversion-stress forces on the peroneus brevis tendon causes an avulsion fracture. (From Greenspan A. *Orthopedic Imaging*. 6th ed. Philadelphia: Wolters Kluwer; 2015.)

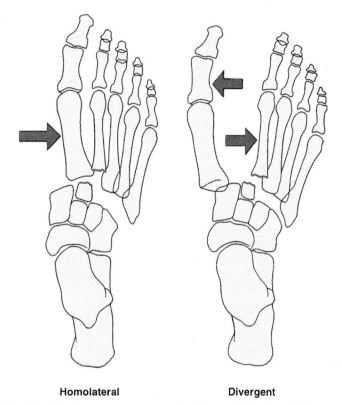

Homolateral   **Divergent**

FIGURE G-10. Lisfranc fracture dislocation (also known as tarsometatarsal dislocation). The first to fifth metatarsal (MT) joints dislocate laterally in the homolateral Lisfranc fracture, whereas in divergent form, the first metatarsal is medially dislocated. Both are associated with fracture of the base of the second MT. (From Greenspan A. *Orthopedic Imaging*. 6th ed. Philadelphia: Wolters Kluwer; 2015.)

Salter-Harris Fracture Classification (Fig. G-11)

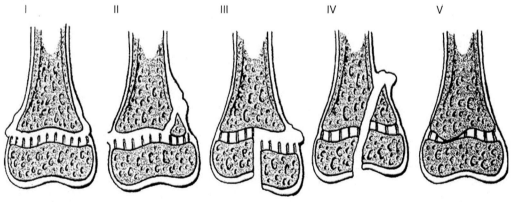

I   II   III   IV   V

FIGURE G-11. Salter-Harris fracture classification. I, Transverse fracture through the physis (growth plate). II, Fracture through the metaphysis and physis (most common). III, Fracture through the physis and epiphysis, sparing the metaphysis. IV, Fracture through the distal metaphysis, epiphysis, and the physis. V, Compression fracture of the physis. (From O'Connell C, Zarbock S. *Comprehensive Review for the Certification and Recertification Examinations for Physician Assistants*. 4th ed. Philadelphia: Wolters Kluwer; 2011.)

DISLOCATIONS

- Dislocation—total loss of congruity occurring between the articular surfaces of the joint

- Most common sites: anterior shoulder, posterior hip, posterior elbow

Disease	Etiology, Prevalence, Risk Factors	Clinical Symptoms and Signs	Diagnostics	Therapy, Prognosis, and Health Maintenance
Shoulder dislocation	Anterior > posterior	1. Fall on outstretched arm in abduction and extension (MCC) 2. Supporting affected arm with other arm 3. Loss of shoulder contour with elbow pointing outward (anterior)	1. AP view of shoulder and transthoracic "Y" view	1. Reduction and immobilization • Sling and swath (Velpeau sling) • If <40, begin therapy after 3 wk • If >40, begin after 1 wk
Anterior shoulder dislocation	MC: Traumatic **Radial head**	"Shoulder slips out" when abducted and externally rotated	1. Apprehension test: place hand behind the head 2. XR: AP and axillary 3. MRI: if 40+ and history of traumatic dislocation	Surgery required
Hip dislocations	MC: Posterior dislocations			
Posterior hip dislocation	MVA due to seat position and high angle of hip flexion	Signs: Shortened, adducted, and internally rotated	AP and lateral X-ray views: required for diagnosis	Closed reduction—if acetabulum not fractured
Anterior hip dislocation	Less common Sports—where leg extended and externally rotated at trauma	Signs: 1. Flexed, abducted, and externally rotated 2. Fractures rarely involved	AP and lateral X-ray views: required for diagnosis	Closed reduction—if acetabulum not fractured
Slipped capital femoral epiphysis (SCFE)	**Adolescent, obese males** Age: **11-13** y (obese males, hypothyroid) RF: Endocrine disorders, obesity, coxa profunda, femoral or acetabular retroversion Femoral epiphysis **always: posterior** and some **medially** relative to femoral neck Slipping of femoral head off neck at physis—**displacement of proximal femoral epiphysis** due to disruption of growth plate Chronic SCFE is MC presentation: >3 wk of vague symptoms, no preceding trauma	1. **Painful limp** and referred **pain to thigh/medial knee** • Acute onset • Minor trauma • Nonradiating • Dull • Aching pain 2. **Inability to walk** • Stable—child able to bear weight on affected extremity • **Unstable**—unable to bear weight (most) 3. Bilateral in 20%-40% Signs: 1. **Limitation of internal rotation** and abduction of the hip 2. Intense pain with passive motion 3. Affected limb abducts and externally rotates with passive flexion from extended position 4. Standing on the affected leg (**Trendelenburg test**) causes pelvic tilt	1. **X-rays** (diagnostic): bilateral AP and frog-leg-lateral • **Displacement of femoral head and rotation of femoral neck anteriorly** • Widening of proximal femoral physis • Metaphyseal remodeling ± joint effusion • "Ice cream slipping off cone"	1. If acute, make patient **non-weight bearing on crutches** and immediate orthopedic referral 2. **Percutaneous pinning** across epiphysis • Screw fixation Prognosis: 1. Determined by degree of slippage • Mild: <30 • Moderate: 30-50 • Severe: >50° 2. Increased rate of AVN with inability to bear weight 3. Increased risk of osteoarthritis Complications: Arthrofibrosis leading to frozen joint with thickened contracted capsule, femoroacetabular impingement, **AVN of femoral head**
Legg-Calve-Perthes (LCP) disease	M:F (4:1) 3-12 y (**MC: 5-7**) Etiology: Undefined, 10% familial Idiopathic osteonecrosis of the proximal femoral head of the femur	1. **Painless limp** 2. Persistent **hip pain** 3. Insidious onset 4. Bilateral in 10%-20% Signs: 1. **Limited hip ROM** and thigh atrophy	Clinical DX: 1. X-ray: can be negative initially, then collapse seen in femoral head • Necrosis with effusion • Joint space widening • Periarticular swelling • Negative aspiration 2. MRI: marrow changes	Based on % of collapse: 1. Mild: **only observation** needed • Protection of the joint by minimizing impact • No bracing required • Non-weight bearing • Referral to ortho 2. Advanced: **surgical osteotomy** or abduction bracing—correct subluxation Prognosis: 1. Better if age <6-8; more time permitted for femoral remodeling

KNEE

Disease	Etiology, Prevalence, Risk Factors	Clinical Symptoms and Signs	Diagnostics	Therapy, Prognosis, and Health Maintenance
Patella dislocation	Usually a lateral dislocation MC: F, 20s	HX: valgus force and external rotation of tibia applied to flexed leg 1. Pain 2. Swelling 3. Patella shifted laterally • Reduction with knee extension Signs: 1. Tenderness over medial border of patella 2. Apprehension Test with **knee flexed and patella pushed laterally** 3. Patella alta (high riding patella): measure the length of patellar tendon and divide by the length of patella (>1.2 ULN) 4. Q-angle: NL is 10° 5. Genu recurvatum: general hypermobility	XR: osteochondral fragment	Immobilization in cylinder cast × 6 wk → rehab, arthroscopy ± repair, surgical repair of torn retinaculum
Knee dislocation	Classified by the direction of tibial displacement relative to femur Anterior more common, occurs after high-energy hyperextension injury	1. Painful 2. Visually striking 3. Absent effusion Signs: Knee grossly unstable Complications: **Popliteal artery injury**, common peroneal nerve injury	1. XR	1. If arterial injury not detected and repaired within 8 h, amputation may be necessary 2. May spontaneously reduce 3. Early reduction, immobilization • Flex the hip 20°, apply longitudinal traction on leg while keeping one hand on tibia and simultaneously lifting the femur back into position • Posterior splint with the knee in 20° of flexion 4. Emergent orthopedic referral

ANKLE (FIGS. G-12 AND G-13)

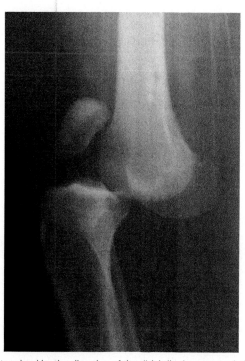

FIGURE G-12. Anterior knee dislocation. Determined by the direction of the tibial displacement relative to the femur. (From Sherman S, Ross C, Nordquist E, Wang E, Cico S. *Atlas of Clinical Emergency Medicine.* Philadelphia: Wolters Kluwer; 2016.)

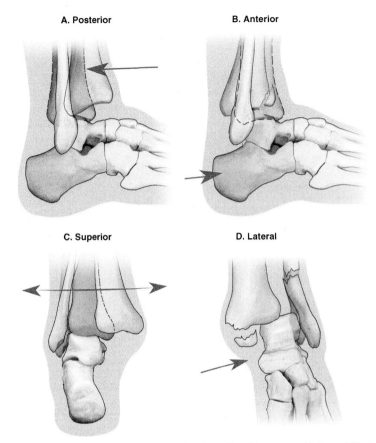

FIGURE G-13. Ankle dislocation. (Redrawn from Raukar NP, Raukar GJ, Savitt DL. *Chapter 11. McGraw-Hill global educa-tion holdings.* In: *The Atlas of Emergency Medicine.* 3rd ed. LLC. http://accessemergencymedicine.mhmedical.com/content.aspx?bookid=351&sectionid=39619710&jumpsectionID=39621806.)

Disease	Etiology, Prevalence, Risk Factors	Clinical Symptoms and Signs	Diagnostics	Therapy, Prognosis, and Health Maintenance
Ankle dislocation	Require forces of great magnitude Associated: Malleoli fracture MC: Posterior and lateral dislocations	Posterior: 1. Locked in plantar flexion with anterior tibia palpable 2. Shortened foot, swollen ankle Anterior: 1. Dorsiflexed foot and elongated Lateral: 1. Entire foot displaced laterally	1. Lateral XR: overlap of talus and calcaneus 2. AP mortise XR: intact mortise	1. Reduce emergently, even if open • Apply gentle traction to food with one hand cupping the heel and other on dorsal aspect of foot while assistant applies countertraction 2. Often require ORIF • 50% open, requiring surgical debridement first

- Subluxation—less serious loss of congruity or less than a complete dislocation

CONGENITAL DEFORMITIES

Disease	Etiology, Prevalence, Risk Factors	Clinical Symptoms and Signs	Diagnostics	Therapy, Prognosis, and Health Maintenance
Genu valgum (knock-knee)	MCC: Osteoarthritic narrowing of lateral knee compartment Most dramatic at 3-6 y/o	1. Legs deviate away from midline, often bilaterally		1. Gradual remodeling spontaneously 2. Reassurance that condition is benign
Genu varum (bowleg)	MCC: Medial knee compartment osteoarthritis Before to age 3 y	1. Legs deviate toward midline, knees are further apart than normal when medial malleoli are together		If >3 y/o, may require further evaluation or treatment

Disease	Etiology, Prevalence, Risk Factors	Clinical Symptoms and Signs	Diagnostics	Therapy, Prognosis, and Health Maintenance
Metatarsus adductus	(Fig. G-14)	1. Femur and tibia normal 2. Hip examination normal		Resolves by 1 y/o
Femoral anteversion	"Pigeon toed gait" (Fig. G-15)	1. Patella internally rotated 2. Internal rotation of the hip exceeds external rotation		Resolves by 9-10 y/o
Developmental dysplasia of the hip (DDH)	<u>RF:</u> (+) family history, ligament laxity, breech presentation, female gender, large fetal size, first-born status <u>MC:</u> Left hip, 1%-3% of newborns	1. Unequal thigh folds 2. Shortening of leg 3. Painless limp and/or lurch to the affected side <u>Signs:</u> 1. Both hips are flexed 90° and then slowly abducted from the midline, one hip at a time. With gentle pressure, an attempt is made to lift the greater trochanter forward 2. Ortolani sign: a feeling of slipping as the head relocates is a sign of instability 3. Barlow sign: When the joint is more stable, the deformity must be provoked by applying slight pressure with the thumb on the medial side of the thigh as the thigh is adducted, thus slipping the hip posteriorly and eliciting a palpable clunk as the hip dislocates 4. Galeazzi sign: knees are at unequal heights when the hips and knees are flexed, the dislocated hip will be on the side with the lower knee 5. Trendelenburg sign: child stands on the affected leg and the dip of the pelvis is evident on the opposite side due to weakness of gluteus medius	1. Careful physical examination at birth and repeated evaluation at each well-child visit until the child walks • Limited hip abduction of less than 60° while the knee is in 90° of flexion (most sensitive) 2. **U/S**: useful for diagnosis, but false positives before 8-10 wk of age, expensive, and training required for interpretation 3. X-rays after first 6 wk of life	1. If corrected in the first few weeks of life—reversible • Spontaneous correction by 2-6 wk 2. **Pavlik harness**—maintains reduction by keeping hips externally rotated 3. Closed reduction with arthrogram w/ hip spica cast *Note:* Use of double/triple diapers is ineffective Most important and severe complication: AVN of capital femoral epiphysis—due to forced abduction or reduction

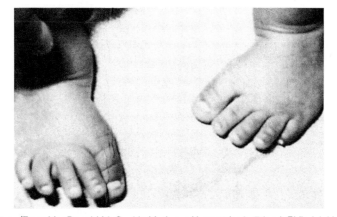

FIGURE G-14. Metatarsus adductus. (From MacDonald M, Seshia M. *Avery Neonatología.* 7th ed. Philadelphia: Wolters Kluwer; 2017.)

Normal   **Femoral anteversion**

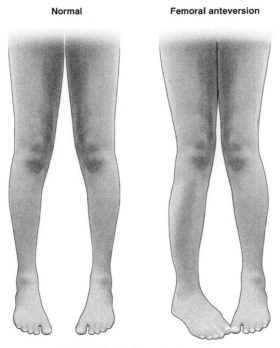

FIGURE G-15. Femoral anteversion.

SOFT TISSUE INJURIES

- Ottawa knee rules are less sensitive in children; use Pittsburgh rules to determine whether or not to obtain radiographs
- MRI is 95% and 90% accurate in identifying ACL tears and meniscal injuries, respectively
- Pain with varus or valgus stress is more suggestive of ligament damage than a meniscus tear
- The MCL is the primary static stabilizer against valgus stress at the knee
- The LCL is the primary static stabilizer against varus stress at the knee
- The ACL is the primary static stabilizer of the knee against anterior translation of the tibia with respect to the femur
- The PCL is the primary static stabilizer of the knee against posterior translation of the tibia with respect to the femur
- WB, NWB = weight bearing or non–weight bearing
- Ligament injuries are graded as follows:
  - Grade 1: stretching of the ligament with no detectable instability
  - Grade 2: further stretching of the ligament with detectable instability, but with the fibers in continuity
  - Grade 3: complete disruption of the ligament.

Ligaments of the knee, anterior view

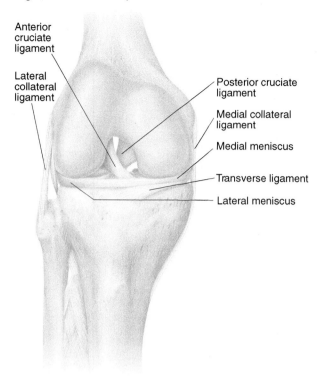

Anterior cruciate ligament

Lateral collateral ligament

Posterior cruciate ligament

Medial collateral ligament

Medial meniscus

Transverse ligament

Lateral meniscus

FIGURE G-16. Key knee anatomy. (From Anatomical Chart Company. *Hip and Knee Inflammations Anatomical Chart.* 2nd ed. Philadelphia: Wolters Kluwer; 2008.)

Disease	Etiology, Prevalence, Risk Factors	Clinical Symptoms and Signs	Diagnostics	Therapy, Prognosis, and Health Maintenance

Meniscal tear	<u>Acute:</u>
	Twisting injury on weight-bearing knee
	Chronic: degenerative tears, mechanical grinding of osteophytes on meniscus
	Late teens, peak (30-40)
	<u>MC:</u>
	Medial meniscus
	<u>HX:</u>
	1. Foot planted with femur rotated internally with valgus stress (medial) or
	2. Femur rotated externally with varus stress (lateral)
	1. Most acute tears (younger patient) are vertical longitudinal or oblique tears
	2. Complex and degenerative tears (older patient)
		HX: axial loading with rotation or HX of osteoarthritis
		1. **Pain** (variable)
		• Event followed by **insidious pain and swelling** over 24 h
		• Worse with twisting or pivoting
		• Mechanical SX: "tearing" or "popping" sensation: popping, **locking, catching,** or "knee giving out"; cannot extend fully
		2. **Effusion** (common)—patient will complain of **stiffness**
		<u>Signs:</u>
		1. **Joint line tenderness** (sensitive, nonspecific)
		2. Abnormal ROM: loss of smooth passive motion or full extension
		• Locking, instability
		3. Inability to squat or kneel; can bear weight
		4. **Joint effusion**
			1. **McMurray maneuver:** catching, pop, or click at joint line
			2. Flexion McMurray: pain over posteromedial joint line
			3. Apley grind test: pain at either joint line
			4. Thessaly test: shows pain
			<u>Imaging:</u>
			1. X-ray of the knee: degeneration, calcification
			2. **MRI**—most sensitive (confirm)
				1. Rest, ice for 15 min every 4-6 h, elevate, crutches, patellar restraining brace
				2. Steroid injection—only useful if the patient has OA complicated by meniscal tear
				3. Surgery if mechanical symptoms present
				• Arthroscopy
				• If small <15 mm: heals spontaneously
				• Repair larger tears
				  • Partial meniscectomy: short recovery
				  • Repair rather than meniscectomy (especially in young)
				<u>Health maintenance:</u>
				1. Tears that occur centrally have a longer healing rate
				2. Return to full function may be expected in 6-8 wk
				3. High-risk of OA if meniscectomy at young age

(continued)

(continued)

Disease	Etiology, Prevalence, Risk Factors	Clinical Symptoms and Signs	Diagnostics	Therapy, Prognosis, and Health Maintenance

Anterior cruciate ligament (ACL) tear (Fig. G-17)	Occur with sudden deceleration with a rotational maneuver, usually without contact; OR contact injury with valgus force to extended knee
	F > M
	<u>Associated:</u>
	High incidence of **lateral meniscal tears**
		<u>HX:</u>
		Hyperextension and/or valgus force to knee by direct blow
		1. "**Pop**" reported by patient
		2. Knee swelling within 4-12 h of injury
		<u>Signs:</u>
		1. Unable to fully bear weight (instability), knee giving out with twisting activities
			1. **Lachman test**
			  • Most sensitive for diagnosis
			2. Anterior drawer test
			3. Pivot shift test: helps evaluate rotational instability
			<u>Imaging:</u>
			1. XR: normal
			2. MRI (confirms)
				1. Supportive
				  • Pain relief with Tylenol ± NSAID
				  • Limit ROM, place in long leg brace
				  • Obtain XR if indicated
				  • Consider MRI
				2. Refer to ortho
				  • Surgical repair once full ROM obtained
				  • Double-bundle reconstruction
				  • RTA in 4-6 mo
				  • Physical therapy

Lateral collateral ligament (LCL) injuries	"Knee buckling" into hyperextension with normal gait
	<u>Associated:</u>
	Peroneal nerve injury (12%-29%)
		1. HX: valgus/varus stress to extended knee
		2. Pain over the lateral aspect of the knee joint
		3. Hemarthrosis
		<u>Signs:</u>
		1. Able to bear weight without instability or locking
		2. Laxity with **varus** stress testing with knee at 30° of flexion
		3. Tenderness along lateral joint line
		4. Neurovascular examination: r/o peroneal nerve injury
		5. **Dial test**: most useful to evaluate for posterolateral instability
			1. XR: normal or fibular head avulsions, patellar dislocation, loose bodies; lateral joint space narrowing with osteophytes and subchondral sclerosis
			2. MRI: abnormal
				1. Supportive
				  • Pain relief with Tylenol ± NSAID
				  • Limit ROM, place in long leg brace
				  • Obtain XR if indicated
				  • Consider MRI
				2. Refer to ortho
				  • All start early PT
				  • Grade I: 2-4 wk immobilization → quad strengthening
				  • Grade II: brace blocking last 20° of flexion, WBAT
				  • Grade III: surgery
				<u>Health maintenance:</u>
				1. Limit weight bearing after surgery for 6 wk, brace for at least 3 wk

Medial collateral ligament (MCL) injuries	MCL is primary restraint to valgus stress, attached to medial meniscus at the joint line
	Forced abduction of the leg at the knee
	Associated: tear of medial meniscus and **rupture of the ACL** (look for immediate swelling)
		1. HX twisting injury or direct blow at knee with valgus strain
		2. Pain over medial aspect of knee joint
		3. Joint effusion if severe
		<u>Signs:</u>
		1. **Medial joint line tenderness**
		2. Patellar apprehension test
		  • Check for patellar dislocation
		3. Laxity to **valgus** stress at 30° of flexion
			1. XR: not helpful unless made with valgus stress applied
			2. MRI–r/o concomitant meniscal injury (confirms)
				1. Supportive
				  • Pain relief with Tylenol ± NSAID
				  • Limit ROM, place in a long leg brace
				  • Obtain XR if indicated
				  • Consider MRI
				2. Refer to ortho
				  • All start early PT
				  • Grade I: WBAT, early amb
				  • Grade II: **brace** blocking last 20° of flexion, WBAT
				  • Grade III: hinged brace, initial NWB, advance WB over 4 wk

Posterior cruciate ligament (PCL) tear	Most common mechanism of injury: direct blow to **anterior tibia with knee flexed** or fall to ground with foot plantar flexed
	<u>Associated:</u>
	Posterolateral corner (meniscus) tear (60%)
		1. Knee **pain**
		  • Biggest complaint
		2. Swelling
		3. Stiffness
		<u>Signs:</u>
		1. Abrasions or ecchymosis around proximal anterior tibia
		2. Ecchymosis in popliteal fossa
		3. Instability
			1. **Posterior drawer test**
			2. Posterior sag (Godfrey) test
			3. Reverse pivot test
			<u>Imaging:</u>
			MRI
				1. Nonsurgical
				  • Obtain full quad strength
				  • Grade I/II: early motion, WBAT
				  • Grade III: keep knee immobilized in extension
				  • Surgery to prevent osteoarthritis or instability
				<u>Health maintenance:</u>
				1. Bracing is ineffective
				2. Minimum 3 mo rehab before return to play

- Thessaly test: have the patient hold your hand and stand on one leg with knee flexed to 20°, then the patient will internally and externally rotate his or her knee

  - Pain or locking/catching sensation = (+) test, 90% sensitive, 96% specific

- *McMurray test*: repeated passive flexion and extension of knee; painful click in early or mid-extension of the knee = meniscal tear

- Grasp patient's heel with one hand and place fingers and thumb of the other hand along joint line; passively flex knee and internally rotate tibia; extend the knee while maintaining internal rotation; passively flex the knee while externally rotating

- Sensitivity: 50%, specificity 60% to 97%

- *Apley test*: With the patient prone with the affected knee flexed 90°, stabilize thigh with a knee or hand; press patient's heel toward the floor while internally and externally rotating the foot; pain = (+) test
  - Sensitivity: 38% to 41%
- *Lachman test*: Knee flexed at 20°, stabilizing the distal femur with one hand, and pulling forward on the proximal tibia with the other hand
- *Anterior drawer test*: With the patient supine and the knee flexed to 90° (hip flexed to about 45°), the foot is restrained by sitting on it and the examiner's hands are placed around the proximal tibia. Then, while the hamstrings are felt to relax and the tibia is pulled forward, the displacement and the end point are evaluated.
- *Pivot shift (Losee) test*: a valgus and internal rotation force is applied to the tibia; starting at 45° of flexion, the lateral tibial plateau is reduced. Extending the knee causes the lateral plateau to subluxate anteriorly with a thud at about 20° of flexion. It reduces quietly at full extension
- *Posterior drawer test*: The posterior drawer test evaluates the integrity of the PCL. It is performed with posterior pressure on the proximal tibia with the knee flexed at 90°
- *Posterior sag (Godfrey) test*: This test involves flexing the knee and hip and noting the posterior pull of gravity creating posterior "sag" of the tibia on the femur
- *Dial test*: externally rotate each tibia and note the angle subtended between the thigh and the foot. The dial test is performed at 30 and 90° of flexion with a significant difference being an angle of 5° or greater than the contralateral leg. Injury to the posterolateral capsule alone is confirmed with greater external rotation at 30°, an isolated PCL at 90°, and to both structures when there is greater rotation at 30 and 90° compared with the uninjured leg

Obtain X-ray for:

Ottawa Knee Rules Sensitive	Pittsburg Knee Rules Greater Specificity
1. Age >55 2. Tenderness to head of fibula 3. Isolated tenderness to patella 4. Inability to flex knee to 90° 5. Inability to bear weight for 4 steps both immediately and in examination room regardless of limp	1. Recent fall or blunt trauma 2. Age <12 y or >50 y 3. Unable to take 4 unaided steps

Arthroscopy Indications

- Acute hemarthrosis, meniscus injuries, loose bodies, selected tibial plateau fractures, patellar chondromalacia, chronic synovitis, knee instability, recurrent effusions, chondral, and osteochondral fractures

Knee Joint Effusion

- *Joint aspiration*—all patients with knee effusion not associated with acute trauma, and when infection cannot be ruled out
- *Bursal aspiration*—distinguishes bursitis due to trauma, crystal deposition disease (gout), or infection

Achilles Tendon Rupture

- *Thompson test*: The patient should be placed in a prone position, the knee and ankle flexed to 90°, and the gastrocnemius muscle should be grasped and squeezed. If the Achilles tendon is even partially intact, then the foot will plantar flex; if completely ruptured, there will be no movement of the foot

Disease	Etiology, Prevalence, Risk Factors	Clinical Symptoms and Signs	Diagnostics	Therapy, Prognosis, and Health Maintenance

Achilles tendon rupture	Most common in middle-aged male athletes
	Can also occur with steroid injections and FQ use
		1. May hear or feel a pop
		2. Pain, edema, ecchymosis
		Signs:
		1. Weakness when pushing off foot
		2. ±plantar flexion
		3. **Thompson test** (diagnostic): plantar flexion or no movement of the foot
			1. XR lateral	1. Conservative
				  • Immobilize in plantar flexion
				  • Non–weight bearing
				  • RICE
				2. Surgery if complete rupture
				25% diagnosed as ankle sprains

SPRAINS AND STRAINS

- **Strain**—injury to the bone-tendon unit at the myotendinous junction or the muscle itself
- **Sprain**—involves collagenous tissue, such as ligaments or tendons
  - 90% of ankle injuries result from inversion and plantar flexion

Disease	Etiology, Prevalence, Risk Factors	Clinical Symptoms and Signs	Diagnostics	Therapy, Prognosis, and Health Maintenance
Acute low back strain	Minor, self-limiting injuries that are usually associated with lifting heavy loads when the back is in a mechanically disadvantaged position, a fall, prolonged uncomfortable postures such as in air travel or car rides, or sudden unexpected motion (car accident)	Signs: 1. Paraspinal muscle spasms		1. Short duration of bed rest, apply ice (acute) 2. Heat and massage 3. NSAIDs during first few days 4. Muscle relaxants (cyclobenzaprine, carisoprodol, metaxalone, and diazepams) 5. Weight bearing resumed
Ankle sprain/ strain	One of most common sports-related injuries; 85% from inversion injury Mostly involves lateral ligaments (**anterior talofibular ligament, ATL**)	1. Hear a "pop" 2. Ecchymosis and tenderness of lateral ankle	1. XR to r/o fracture, especially if unable to bear weight or tenderness to palpation over the bone • Often not required to guide management	1. If able to bear weight–RICE first • Compressive wrapping, icing • Early mobilization • Supervised PT: isometric exercises • Once 90% strength, active isotonic (eccentric and concentric) as well as isokinetic exercise 2. If unable to bear weight • Crutches 48-72 h, brace for support • Posterior splint 3. Refer to physical therapy • Up to 3-4 mo for full recovery

Disease	Etiology, Prevalence, Risk Factors	Clinical Symptoms and Signs	Diagnostics	Therapy, Prognosis, and Health Maintenance
Nerve root irritation		Pain originating in back Radiates down leg	XR of spine in nontraumatic low back pain (required) Red flags: **Fever, weight loss, morning stiffness, history of IV or steroid use, trauma, history of cancer, saddle anesthesia, loss of anal sphincter tone, major motor weakness** CT: Demonstrates bony stenosis and lateral nerve root entrapment MRI: Identifies cord pathology, neural tumors, stenosis, herniated discs, infections	1. **Short-term relative rest** (max 2 d) with support under the knees and neck • NSAIDs or analgesics 2. Progressive ambulation to normal activities may follow if pain has subsided 3. Fitness program: postural exercises (McKenzie exercises for disc derangement) 4. If no improvement × 6 wk → bone scan, CT, MRI, or EMG 5. Surgical intervention if treatment fails (5%)
Musculoskeletal		Localized area of point tenderness		
Sciatica	Pain in the distribution of the sciatic nerve	Pain felt in the buttock, posterior thigh, and posterolateral aspect of the leg around lateral malleolus to dorsum of foot and entire sole		
Sacroiliac joint		Unilateral low back and buttock pain Worse with standing in one position		
Spinal stenosis		Pain in the elderly Increased with walking Relieved by leaning forward		

The Ottawa Ankle Rules
• Tenderness over the lateral or medial malleolus • Inability to bear weight for 4 steps both immediately postinjury and in the ED

ANKYLOSING SPONDYLITIS

Inflammatory disorder of unknown cause that affects the axial skeleton; peripheral joints and extraarticular structures also frequently involved.

- Synovitis and myxoid marrow (early) → pannus and subchondral granulation tissue

- Eroded margins are replaced by fibrocartilage regeneration → ossification

- Inflammatory granulation tissue in paravertebral connective tissue at junction of annulus fibrosus and vertebral bone → syndesmophyte → bridges adjacent vertebral bodies

Etiology, Prevalence, Risk Factors	Clinical Symptoms and Signs	Diagnostics	Therapy, Prognosis, and Health Maintenance
20-30s M:F (2-3:1) HLA-B27 (+) in 90%	Must have for >3 mo (chronic) with 4+ of the following: age <40, insidious onset, improvement with exercise, no improvement with rest, pain at night with improvement upon getting up 1. **Sacroiliitis** (earliest)–dull pain, insidious onset, felt deep in *lower* lumbar or gluteal region • Low back morning stiffness (hours) that improves with activity and returns following inactivity • Becomes persistent and bilateral • Nocturnal exacerbation forces patient to rise and move around 2. Bony tenderness • Common sites: costosternal junctions, spinous processes, iliac crests, greater trochanters, ischial tuberosities, tibial tubercles, heels 3. Hip and shoulder (root joint) arthritis 4. Neck pain and stiffness from cervical spine involvement (30%) 5. Loss of spinal mobility • Limitation of anterior and lateral flexion and extension of lumbar spine Extraarticular manifestation: Preceding acute anterior uveitis (40%)–unilateral eye pain, photophobia, increased lacrimation	Schober test–measures lumbar spine flexion **HLA-B27** (+) ESR/CRP high Alk-PHOS: high Serum IgA: high XR: "**bamboo spine**," "squaring," or "barreling"	1. **NSAIDs** (first line) Complications: Spinal fracture

BURSITIS/TENDINITIS

- Aspirate bursa if concerned for infection: cell count, Gram stain, bacterial culture, and crystals

  - **WBC > 20k with PMN predominance** is suspicious for bacterial infection (most commonly *Staphylococcus aureus*)

- Assess adjacent joint effusion, which can also be septic
- Start empiric antibiotics for mild presentation (*Staph/Strep*) and vancomycin if ill-appearing × 1 to 4 weeks
- Serial aspirations every 1 to 3 days until sterile or no reaccumulation of fluid

Disease	Etiology, Prevalence, Risk Factors	Clinical Symptoms and Signs	Diagnostics	Therapy, Prognosis, and Health Maintenance
Bursitis	Inflammatory disorder of the bursa (thin-walled sac lined with synovial fluid) Caused by trauma or overuse Common sites: Subacromial, subdeltoid, trochanteric, ischial, iliopsoas, olecranon, prepatellar, suprapatellar	1. Pain, swelling, tenderness for weeks		1. Prevent precipitating factors 2. Rest, heat, time 3. NSAIDs 4. Steroid injections only if no infection exists 5. Antibiotics if unclear cause (*S. aureus* and *Strep* spp.) • Obtain bursal aspiration
Pes anserine bursitis Pes anserine is made up of the gracilis, sartorius and the semitendinosus, which meet at the medial tibia below the knee joint and above the MCL and medial femoral condyle	Anterior medial knee pain Common: Obese women with OA of the knee, runners, various overuse syndromes	1. Anterior pain below the joint line 2. Focal swelling over the bursa 3. Increased tenderness to palpation		
Prepatellar bursitis (housemaid's knee, nun's knee, carpet layer's knee) (Fig. G-18)	Pain anterior to patella Inflamed through repetitive kneeling on hard surfaces	1. Pain is mild with restricted ROM from swelling 2. Presents as effusion over lower pole of patella 3. Tender to palpation with bursal margins palpable		

(continued)

(continued)

Disease	Etiology, Prevalence, Risk Factors	Clinical Symptoms and Signs	Diagnostics	Therapy, Prognosis, and Health Maintenance
Olecranon bursitis	Caused by acute injury or repetitive trauma to olecranon bursa Less frequently caused by break in the skin, leading to septic cause (*S. aureus*)	1. Swelling over olecranon process (MC finding) • Mildly painful (acute) or painless (chronic) 2. ROM preserved	No imaging indicated unless significant history of trauma or fracture suspected	1. Avoid continued trauma to elbow and ace wrap for compression 2. **NSAIDs** and **warm compresses** 3. Surgical removal of the bursa reserved for septic bursal sacs that are nonresponsive to conservative management
Tendinitis and tenosynovitis	Common causes: overuse injuries, arthritides Commonly appears at: rotator cuff, supraspinatus, biceps, flexor carpi ulnaris, flexor carpi radialis, flexor digitorum, patella, hip adductor, Achilles	1. Commonly occur together, causing pain with movement 2. Swelling 3. Impaired function 4. May resolve over several weeks, but recurrence is common		1. **Rest, ice, stretching** 2. **NSAIDs** + steroid injection + anesthesia alongside tendon • Avoid intratendon injection due to rupture 3. Excise scar tissue and necrotic debris
Subacromial or *bicipital* (shoulder) *tendinitis*	Produced by friction on the tendon of the *long* head of the biceps as it passes through bicipital groove	1. Anterior shoulder pain • Radiates down biceps into forearm • Worse with overhead activity Signs: 1. Limited abduction and external rotation 2. Bicipital groove tender to palpation	1. Yergason supination sign (+): **pain with resisted supination of forearm with elbow at 90°**	1. Young—repair surgically 2. Older—Surgery not necessary owing to little to no pain
Achilles tendinitis	Pain attributed to inflammation and degeneration of the Achilles tendon and attachment to calcaneus Common in runners and patients who suddenly increase their activity level, or people who improperly stretch or train	1. Gradual onset of pain during activity or after activity is complete 2. Pain on posterior calf, 2-6 cm above insertion of Achilles tendon 3. Tenderness over posterior calf above calcaneus • Pain on passive dorsiflexion and resisted plantar flexion 4. Ankle ROM and strength = normal Thompson test: r/o tendon rupture	XR: Soft-tissue shadow and calcifications along tendon and insertion MRI: Hypertrophy of Achilles tendon to r/o rupture	1. NSAIDs 2. Physical therapy for stretching and strength exercises If left untreated, may progress to rupture of Achilles tendon

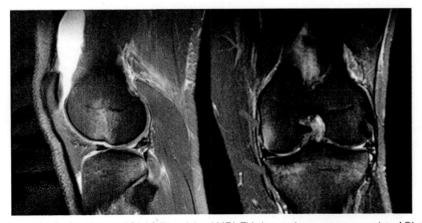

FIGURE G-17. ACL tear on sagittal (*left*) and coronal (*right*) T2-weighted MRI. This image demonstrates complete ACL tear with bony contusion of the medial femoral condyles and medial tibial plateau (*arrows*). (From Egol K. *The Orthopaedic Manual: From the Office to the OR.* 1st ed. Philadelphia: Wolters Kluwer; 2018.)

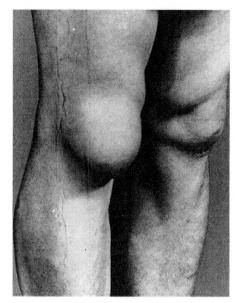

FIGURE G-18. Extreme case of prepatellar bursitis (also known as housemaid's knee) of the right knee. (From Salter R. *Textbook of Disorders and Injuries of the Musculoskeletal System.* 3rd ed. Philadelphia: Wolters Kluwer; 1999.)

- Tendinitis—inflammation of the tendon
- Tenosynovitis—inflammation of the enclosed tendon sheath

CONNECTIVE TISSUE DISORDERS

Disease	Etiology, Prevalence, Risk Factors	Clinical Symptoms and Signs	Diagnostics	Therapy, Prognosis, and Health Maintenance
Osteogenesis imperfecta	(+) family history Mutation in one of two genes for type I collagen Association: Aortic regurgitation, floppy mitral valves, mitral incompetence, fragility of large vessels 4 types of varying severity	1. Brittle bones 2. Progressive hearing loss • Begins in 20s (50% over age 30) • Conductive, sensorineural or both Signs: 1. Blue sclerae 2. Dentinogenesis imperfecta • Enamel is normal, but teeth can be amber, yellow-brown, or translucent bluish gray	Clinical DX: 1. Fractures, blue sclerae, dentinogenesis imperfecta, or family history 2. XR: decreased bone density, mottled appearance 3. Bone microscopy	1. Mild—little treatment after fractures decrease after puberty 2. Pregnancy—women require attention during pregnancy and after menopause 3. Children severely affected • Physical therapy, surgical management Health maintenance: 1. Stapedectomy for hearing loss 2. Bisphosphonates and physical therapy to prevent fractures
Ehlers-Danlos syndrome **Type I:** severe form **Type II:** mild form of skin and joint issues Type III: more joint hypermobility Type IV: vascular type (more skin changes) Type V: X-linked, similar to type II Type VI: ocular-scoliotic type Type VIIA/B: marked joint hypermobility Type VIII: periodontotic type	Hyperextensible skin and hypermobile joints caused by a defect in collagen genes 0.02% incidence, more common in African Americans Associated: pes planus, scoliosis Type I: *mitral valve prolapse*, hernias	1. Joint hypermobility 2. Hyperextensible skin Signs: 1. Skin—**thin, velvety, hyperextensible**, easily scarred • "Cigarette paper" scars • Easily bruisable • Hyperpigmentation over bony prominences 2. Laxity and hypermobility of joints	Clinical DX: 1. DNA sequencing 2. Evaluate for bleeding disorders	1. Surgical repair and tightening of joint ligaments Health maintenance: Limit physical activity to avoid dislocations

(continued)

(continued)

Disease	Etiology, Prevalence, Risk Factors	Clinical Symptoms and Signs	Diagnostics	Therapy, Prognosis, and Health Maintenance
Marfan syndrome	0.02%-0.03% incidence Autosomal dominant Mutations in fibrillin-1 gene (*FBN1*) Associated: **Mitral valve prolapse** → mitral valve regurgitation (25%) Spontaneous pneumothorax Inguinal and incisional hernias	1. Long, thin extremities, loose joints • Tall 2. Reduced vision due to dislocation of lenses: **ectopia lentis** • Upward displacement of lenses → cataracts • Elongated, myopic 3. **Aortic aneurysms** Signs: 1. **Arachnodactyly**: fingers and hands are long and slender, "spider-like" 2. Chest deformities: pectus excavatum, pectus carinatum, asymmetry 3. Scoliosis, kyphosis 4. High arched palate 5. High pedal arches (pes cavus) 6. Striae over shoulders and buttocks Complications: Dilation of aorta → aortic regurgitation, dissection of aorta, aortic aneurysms • Worse with pregnancy and stress	1. CT or MRI examination of lumbosacral area: • Enlargement of neural canal • Thinning of pedicles and laminae • Widening of foramina • Anterior meningocele (dural ectasia) 2. Slit lamp examination 3. Echocardiogram 4. Plasma amino acid analysis—r/o homocystinuria Ghent criteria—at least 4 abnormalities: 1. Ectopia lentis 2. Dilation of ascending aorta ± dissection 3. Dural ectasia 4. Blood relative who meets same criteria ± DNA diagnosis	1. Propranolol or β-adrenergic antagonists • Lowers BP, delays and prevents aortic dilation 2. Surgery • Correct aorta, aortic valve, mitral valve Health maintenance: 1. Increased by physical exertion, emotional stress, pregnancy 2. Scoliosis is progressive • Treated if >20°: bracing • Treated if >45°: surgery 3. Dislocated lenses require surgical removal

Psychiatry Medication Guide

Psychosis	Delusions, hallucinations, disorganized speech and behavior, and gross distortions of reality *Perceptual distortion*: hearing voices that accuse, blame, or threaten punishment; seeing visions; reporting hallucinations of touch, taste, or odor; or reporting that familiar things and people seem changed *Motor disturbances*: rigid postures; overt signs of tension, inappropriate grins, giggles; repetitive gestures, talking, muttering, or mumbling to oneself; glancing around as if hearing voices
Schizophrenia	Must last for 6+ mo or longer, including at least 1 mo of hallucinations, delusions, disorganized speech, grossly disorganized or catatonic behavior or negative symptoms **Delusions:** misinterpretation of perceptions or experiences (persecutory, referential, somatic, religious, grandiose) **Hallucinations:** any sensory modality (auditory, visual, olfactory, gustatory, tactile), but auditory most common

Positive Symptoms	Negative Symptoms	Cognitive Symptoms	Aggressive and Hostile Symptoms	Depressive and Anxious Symptoms
• Delusions • Hallucinations • Disorganized speech • Disorganized/catatonic or agitated behavior Drugs or diseases that enhance or increase dopamine, enhance/produce positive symptoms: amphetamine, cocaine Drugs that decrease dopamine will decrease/stop positive symptoms	At least 5, start with A: Affective flatting Alogia Avolition Anhedonia Attentional impairment • Considered a deficit in normal function: blunted affect, emotional withdrawal, poor rapport, passivity, apathetic social withdrawal; difficulty in abstract thinking, stereotyped thinking, lack of spontaneity with long periods of hospitalization and poor social function • Can be secondary to EPS, depression, or environmental deprivation	Odd use of language: incoherence, loose associations, neologisms, impaired attention, and information processing Most common/severe: impaired verbal fluency (ability to produce spontaneous speech), problems with serial learning (of a list of items/sequence of events), impairment in vigilance for executive functioning (sustaining/focusing attention, concentrating, prioritizing, and modulating behavior based on social cues)	Emphasize problems in impulse control: overt hostility (verbal or physical abuse/assault), self-injury (suicide, arson, property damage), sexual acting out	Depressed mood, anxious mood, guilt, tension, irritability
*Overactivity of meso-**limbic** dopamine pathway*–caused by ↑ dopamine Treat with D2 receptor dopamine blockers	***Mesocortical** dopamine pathway*–caused by ↓ dopamine Could be due to overactivity of glutamate systems or deficit of dopamine–increase would worsen positive symptoms (*neuroleptic induced deficit syndrome*)		Tuberoinfundibular pathway	

(continued)

(continued)

	*Nigro***striatal** *dopamine pathway*: caused by ↓ dopamine Deficiencies in dopamine cause movement disorders: Parkinson disease (rigidity, akinesia, bradykinesia) and tremors DA deficiencies in the basal ganglia can produce akathisia (restlessness) and dystonia (twisting movements, especially of the face and neck) Replicated by drugs that block D2 receptors—chronic blockade of D2 receptors leads to *neuroleptic-induced tardive dyskinesia* (constant chewing, tongue protrusions, facial grimacing, limb movements that are quick, jerky, and choreiform) Chorea, dyskinesias, tics—caused by ↑ dopamine		

- **Affective flattening:** restriction in range and intensity of emotional expression
- **Alogia:** restriction in the fluency and productivity of thought and speech
- **Avolition:** restrictions in initiation of goal-directed behavior

- **Anhedonia:** lack of pleasure
- **Attentional impairment**

ANTIDEPRESSANTS

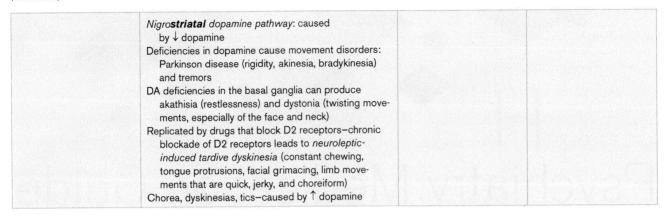

Antidepressants	MOA	Contraindications/ Interactions ± Pregnancy Category and Boxed Warnings	Adverse Effects	Monitoring	Clinical Pearls and Miscellaneous
Monoamine Oxidase Inhibitors (MAOIs)					
Phenelzine (Nardil) HL = 4-5 h Selegiline (EmSam) Selective MAO-B (low dose) Patch HL = 2.5 h	Irreversibly inhibit the monoamine oxidase enzyme, both A and B, resulting in ↑ amounts of: **5HT, NE, DA** Not used very often anymore d/t many interactions and adverse effects of toxicities Indications: Atypical depression (hyperphagia, hypersomnia)	Interactions: • *Stimulants* • *Levodopa* • **A**ntidepressants: SSRIs, TCAs, SNRIs • *Pseudoephedrine* • *Phenylephrine* • *Ephedrine* • **D**extromethorphan • *Tyramine-containing foods* (beer, red wine, aged cheese, dry sausage, smoked fish, liver) • Serotonin agonists, cocaine, MDMA • Meperidine, Tramadol, Fentanyl, Methadone	• **S**edation (greater with phenelzine) • **L**eukopenia, ↑**L**FTs • *Orthostatic hypotension* • *Weight gain* • *Edema* • *Sexual dysfunction* • Tremor • Anxiety • CNS stimulation (greater with tranylcypromine and EmSam) • Nausea and Headache (common with EmSam)	CBC (leukopenia) LFTs	<u>Hypertensive crisis:</u> Sharply elevated BP (diastolic BP >120 mmHg) Occipital headache Stiff or sore neck Nausea, vomiting Sweating (± fever) Palpitations →**end organ damage** <u>Serotonin syndrome:</u> Sweaty **C**lonus, **A**gitation **T**remor, hyperreflexia, Hypertonicity, Hyperpyrexia (fever)

Antidepressants	MOA	Contraindications/ Interactions ± Pregnancy Category and Boxed Warnings	Adverse Effects	Monitoring	Clinical Pearls and Miscellaneous
Tricyclic (TCA) Antidepressants					
Tertiary: • Amitriptyline (Elavil) • Clomipramine (Clofranil) • Imipramine (Tofranil) • Doxepin (Zonalon) • Trimipramine (Surmontil) Secondary: • Amoxapine • Nortriptyline • Desipramine • Protriptyline • Secondary have 1/3 the side effect burden as the tertiary • Okay for use in lactation	• Inhibit the reuptake of **5HT, NE** • Also block **α-1, H1**, and muscarinic **cholinergic** receptors to varying degrees Indications: MDD, depressive disorder *Not used as often for depression d/t toxicity … more commonly prescribed for migraines/ sleep disturbances*	CI: prior hx of *seizure* disorder; concomitant use with MAOIs ↑ TCA levels: • Cimetidine • SSRIs • Quinine (↑ QT interval) ↓ TCA levels: • PHB, phenytoin • CBZ • Barbiturates • **Tobacco** • Terbinafine TCA + MAOI = HTN crisis/serotonin syndrome! Other: phenytoin, warfarin, St. John's Wort, QTc prolonging meds	• **Cardiac toxicity** • **Sexual dysfunction** (~50%) • **Seizures** (lowers threshold) • H1: *sedation, weight gain* (5-25 kg) • α-1: orthostatic hypotension, dizziness Muscarinic (anticholinergic): Dry mouth, constipation, urinary retention, blurred vision, tachycardia	• Blood levels—difficult to measure (low) • Acute doses of >1 g are often toxic and may be fatal • Serum levels >1000 ng/ mL = serious overdose **EKG** (cardiac tox) on initiation • **Death** may result from cardiac arrhythmias, hypotension, or uncontrollable seizures SX of toxicity: • Almost all symptoms develop within 12 h of the overdose • Antimuscarinic effects = dry mucous membranes, warm dry skin, mydriasis, decreased bowel motility • CNS depression or agitated delirium Cardiovascular toxicity = hypotension, arrhythmias (supraventricular tachycardia, ventricular tachycardia or fibrillation, and varying degrees of heart block)	• First pass liver: tertiary broken into secondary (still active) • Taper off: 1-2 wk (GI distress, dizziness, chills, muscle aches) • OCD: responds to clomipramine

(continued)

(continued)

Antidepressants	MOA	Contraindications/ Interactions ± Pregnancy Category and Boxed Warnings	Adverse Effects	Monitoring	Clinical Pearls and Miscellaneous
Serotonin Selective Reuptake Inhibitors (SSRIs)					
Fluoxetine (Prozac)– $5HT_{2C}$ antagonist ($\uparrow$NE and DA) to improve concentration and attention; activating, energizing	<u>MOA</u>: • Selectively inhibit the reuptake of **5HT** by SERT • $5HT_{1A}$ autoreceptors desensitize or downregulate • No M, H1, or A1 blockade • QD: AM or HS • Increased risk of suicidality in patients <25	<u>Adverse effects</u>: • C<u>NS</u>: anxiety, **irritability**, *insomnia*, **headache**, tremor, nervousness • **Sexual dysfunction**: decreased libido, anorgasmia, impotence • **Stomach upset**: *nausea*, diarrhea, anorexia • REM suppression: bizarre, abnormal dreams Thymoanesthesia (emotional blunting, apathy) Headache	• NSAIDs: SSRIs may enhance the antiplatelet effect of NSAIDs (rating: major)–to minimize risk of bleeding, addition of a *gastroprotective agent* (such as a **PPI) should be added** • Clopidogrel: SSRIs may decrease the serum concentration of the active metabolite (s) of clopidogrel–increase monitoring for signs/symptoms of bleeding	Pregnancy: C (avoid in the first trimester) Mildly sedating, high probability of insomnia Not for lactation Longest HL of all antidepressants (no discontinuation syndrome): 1-3 d
		<u>Interactions: CYP 2D6 inhibitor</u> (Prozac > Lexapro > Zoloft)			
			Isoenzyme	Inhibitor (mod-high)	Drugs metabolized
Escitalopram (Lexapro)–pure S-enantiomer; not beneficial until 60 mg for MDD Antihistamine		CYP450 1A2	Fluvoxamine	Theophylline, R-warfarin, TCAs (demethylation), clozapine, tizanidine, pimozide, ramelteon	• Herbal products: (Alfalfa, anise, bilberry)–SSRIs may enhance the adverse/toxic effect of antiplatelet agents. Bleeding may occur	QTc prolongation (>40 mg) HL = 27-30 h
Citalopram (Celexa) Active metabolite of escitalopram (Lexapro)		CYP450 2C9/19	Fluoxetine Fluvoxamine Sertraline Vilazodone	Phenytoin, S-warfarin, TCAs (demethylation), tolbutamide, diazepam, methadone	• Metoclopramide: may enhance adverse/ toxic effects of antidepressants **SSRI/SNRI withdrawal**: mimics depression or	QTc prolongation Pregnancy: C (avoid in the first trimester) HL: 35 h Not for lactation
Paroxetine (Paxil)– mild anticholinergic (calming, sedating) Inhibits NO (*worst* sexual dysfunction)		CYP450 2D6	Fluoxetine Paroxetine Vilazodone	Codeine, 1 C antiarrhythmics, TCAs (hydroxylation), antipsychotics, β-blockers	mania F: flu-like symptoms L: light-headedness U: uneasiness (depression, anxiety) S: sleep disturbance H: headache	*Worst* **sexual dysfunction**, sedation Pregnancy category: D (avoid in the first trimester) Anticholinergic HL = 24 h
Fluvoxamine (Luvox)–Ω-1 (anxiolytic, improves psychosis and delusional depression)		CYP450 3A4	Fluvoxamine Fluoxetine Sertraline Vilazodone	BZD (triazolo-), CBZ, TCAs (demethylation), pimozide, ramelteon, methadone	RF of withdrawal: time on drug, potency, $t_{1/2}$ (shorter = more likely)	Mild insomnia

Antidepressants	MOA	Contraindications/ Interactions ± Pregnancy Category and Boxed Warnings	Adverse Effects	Monitoring	Clinical Pearls and Miscellaneous
Serotonin Partial Agonist/Reuptake Inhibitor (SPARI)					
Vilazodone (Viibryd)	• 5-HT$_{1A}$ receptor partial ago- nist, SERT inhibition (↑DA) • T$_{1/2}$ = ~25 h • Take with food	CYP3A4 (major)—reduce dose with inhibitors (fluoxetine, fluvoxam- ine, sertraline) CYP 2C19, 2C8, and 2D6 (minor) Interactions: Anticoagulants Carbamazepine Clozapine Dextromethorphan Herbals (alfalfa, anise, bilberry) Linezolid Metoclopramide NSAIDs Pimozide Serotonin modulators	• Stomach upset: diarrhea, nausea, vomiting (23%-28%) • Somnolence • Sexual dysfunction: decreased libido, anorgas- mia (4%) • Dry mouth (xerostomia) (8%) • Insomnia (6%)		

	MOA	Contra/ Interactions	Adverse Effects	Monitoring	Toxicity Symptoms and Treatment
Serotonin Norepinephrine Reuptake Inhibitors (SNRIs)					
Venlafaxine (Effexor) • Only affects 5-HT at levels <150	• Potent inhibitor of **5-HT** and **NE** reuptake and a weak inhibitor of **DA** reuptake • Virtually no affinity for cholinergic, H1, or A-1 • Take with food • Indications: GAD and social anxiety	• Reduce dose by 25% for renal dysfunction • Reduce dose by 50% for hemodialysis	• CNS (5HT-2): anxiety, agitation, *insomnia*, headache, tremor, nervousness • **Sexual dysfunction** (5HT-2): decreased libido, anorgasmia, impotence • GI (5HT-3): *nausea, vomiting*, diarrhea, anorexia • **Sustained elevation in dia- stolic blood pressure**	Monitor blood pressure	Pregnancy category: C HL = 3.5 h
Duloxetine (Cymbalta)	• Potent inhibitor of neuronal **5-HT** and **NE** reuptake and weak inhibitor of **DA** reuptake • No significant activity musca- rinic, cholinergic, H1, or A-1 • Indications: GAD and painful dia- betic peripherally neuropathy		• Common: **xerostomia** • CNS: *insomnia, headache* • GI: **nausea, vomiting, constipation** • Others: dizziness, decreased libido, orgasm abnormality, erectile dysfunction, diarrhea, appetite decreased, **sweating, increased LFTs**, orthostasis, increase in B/P	LFTs Monitor blood pressure	Pregnancy category: C HL = 12 h
Desvenlafaxine (Pristiq)	Potent and selec- tive **5-HT** and **NE** reuptake inhibitor	Renal adjust- ment: CrCl <50	• Common: **xerostomia, diaphoresis** • CNS: **dizziness,** *insomnia* • GI: *nausea,* **diarrhea, constipation** • Others: fatigue, abnormal dreams, decreased libido, pro- teinuria, increases cholesterol (dose-related), increased B/P	Monitor U/A– proteinuria Monitor cholesterol Monitor blood pressure	

(continued)

(continued)

	MOA	Contra/ Interactions	Adverse Effects	Monitoring	Toxicity Symptoms and Treatment
Others					
Mirtazapine (Remeron) **α-2-Adrenergic antagonist (AAA)** HL = 20-40 h	• Blocks presynaptic α-2 *autoreceptors* and *heteroreceptors* = increases in both **NE** and **5-HT** (like SNRI) • Potent **5-HT-2** and **5-HT-3** receptor blockade • Blocks **muscarinic cholinergic**, **histamine**-1, and α-1-adrenergic receptors		<u>Common:</u> • **H1: sedation**, *weight gain* • **Muscarinic: constipation**, dizziness, dry mouth • **A-1**: orthostasis • Rare: elevated **LFTs** and elevated **cholesterol/** triglycerides • Serious: agranulocytosis and neutropenia	LFTs Lipid panel CBC	**No sexual interference; no nausea or diarrhea**
Bupropion (Wellbutrin) **Norepinephrine/ dopamine reuptake inhibitor (NDRI)**	No effect on the reuptake of **5-HT** (almost none) or **NE** (very little); weak blockade of **DA** reuptake (*most potent action*) No blockade of cholinergic, histaminergic, and alpha-1 adrenergic receptors	**Seizures**–history of head trauma or seizures History of **bulimia** or **anorexia** due to increased incidence of seizures Abrupt discontinuation of ETOH or Benzos **Panic disorders/ anxiety**	CNS: insomnia, agitation, restlessness, nightmares, psychosis, **headache** (25%-34%) **GI: *upset*** (nausea, anorexia) Muscarinic: constipation, **dry mouth** (17%-26%) **Weight loss** (14%-23%)		
Trazodone (Desyrel) Triazolopyridine Serotonin- antagonist/ reuptake inhibitors (**SARIs**) (Oleptro = ER)	• Inhibits reuptake of **5HT** and blocks **5HT**$_{2A/2C}$ • Blocks **H**$_1$ and **A**$_1$ receptors	Liver failure (Nef) = CYP 3A4 inhibitor	Common: • **CNS**: headache, agitation, fatigue • **GI**: nausea (5HT-3) • **H1**: sedation (Traz > Nefaz), seight gain • **A1**: orthostasis (Traz>Nefaz), Dizziness • **Muscarinic**: constipation, dry mouth • **Priapism** (trazodone only)		Pregnancy category: C Low doses used for sleep, avoid with MAOI

Antidepressant Syndrome Response

Desensitization or downregulation of neurotransmitters is delayed and changes in neurotransmitter receptor sensitivity may mediate clinical effects and side effects.

Days After Starting Therapy	Response
2-3 d	Improved sleep and appetite
1-2 wk	Improved energy
2-4 wk	Improvement in mood
Up to 8 wk	Full antidepressant benefits

MOOD STABILIZERS

	Indications/MOA/Half-Life	Side Effects	Monitoring	Clinical Pearls
Lithium (Lithobid)	• FDA approved for *bipolar disorder* (mania and maintenance) • *Acute mania*–80% effective • Acute *depression*–most patients respond, may take up to 6-8 wk of therapy • *Maintenance*–markedly reduces frequency, duration, and severity of future episodes MOA: inhibits adenylate cyclase enzyme $T_{1/2} = 24 \pm 6$ h Dosing: • Start at 300 mg BID or TID (smaller dose in the elderly) • Increase by 300-600 mg every 1-5 d depending on response, tolerability, and BMI • Goal: therapeutic serum level at 900-1800 mg/d • Target serum level: 0.8-1.2 mEq/L	Acute effects: 1. Nephrogenic diabetes insipidus: ***weight gain***, acne, ***polyuria, polydipsia***: use diuretic (amiloride) 2. ***Tremor***: use β-blocker (propranolol) 3. **Cognitive impairment** 4. GI: ***nausea***, vomiting, ***diarrhea*** 5. Acute renal failure 6. *Hyper*kalemia Late effects: • **Skin** effects • **Kidney** damage • **Ebstein** anomaly • **Thyroid** (hypothyroid) • **Cardiac** effects–in patients with preexisting heart disease • **Hematologic:** leukocytosis	Remember: Pee-THe-BEER: 1. Pregnancy test–before treatment, then annually 2. Thyroid (hypothyroid) 3. Blood (↑ WBC → 13K) 4. EKG (arrhythmias, flattened T-waves)–before treatment and annually 5. Electrolytes (↓ Na, ↑ lithium) 6. Renal (excreted renally): urine specific gravity, BUN/SCr • Measure serum levels every 5-7 d after each dose increase (trough levels) • Monitor lithium serum levels every 3 mo–especially with diuretics, HTN meds, or NSAIDs • Long-term: monitor TSH and SCr every 6-12 mo • Lithium toxicity with increased sodium: *confusion, vertigo, ataxia, hyperreflexia, rigidity*, seizures, coma, *muscle weakness, vomiting, diarrhea, tremor*	• May reduce the risk of suicide attempts and deaths • More effective–in mild, uncomplicated, fewer previous episodes • Take with food • K⁺-sparing diuretics–increase lithium levels • Loop diuretics–do not affect lithium levels • CCB–may cause fatal neurotoxicity

Drugs that ↑ Lithium	Mechanism	Outcome	Management	Drugs that ↑ Lithium	Mechanism	Outcome	Management
Thiazide diuretics and **K⁺-sparing diuretics**	Na⁺ depletion resulting in increased proximal tubular reabsorption of Na⁺ and lithium	Increases lithium levels by 40%	1. Monitor lithium levels *biweekly* 2. Empirically decrease dose by 50% 3. Avoid TDZ and use alternative	ACE/ARBS	Volume depletion and reduction in GFR → less lithium eliminated	Increases lithium levels by 50%-75%	Monitor lithium levels *weekly* for first 3 mo
NSAIDs	Enhanced reabsorption of Na⁺ and lithium due to inhibition of prostaglandin synthesis	Increases lithium levels by 50%	1. Avoid NSAIDs 3+ d 2. Use ASA or sulindac 3. Monitor lithium levels *biweekly*				

ANTICONVULSANTS

	Indications/MOA/Half-Life	Interactions	Adverse Effects	Monitoring	Clinical Pearls
Valproic acid/ valproate/ sodium divalproex (Depakote, Depakene)	• FDA approved for acute mania • Acute or mixed episodes with or without psychotic features $T_{1/2}$ = 8-17 h MOA: opens chloride channels Dosing: 1. Start at 250 mg BID or TID 2. Increase by 250-500 mg every 1-3 d as tolerated 3. Therapeutic levels at 1500-2500 mg/d 4. Target serum level: 50-125 µg/mL	1. HIV medications 2. VPA is an inhibitor of CYP 450 2C9, 2D6 and 3A3/4 (weak) 3. VPA is highly protein bound and may displace other drugs that are highly protein bound (warfarin)	1. Hepatotoxicity 2. Acute pancreatitis (rare) 3. Polycystic ovarian syndrome (PCOS) Dose related (**CHANGE**): 1. <u>C</u>NS: *tremor*, ataxia, cognitive impairment 2. <u>H</u>1: sedation, *weight gain* 3. **Alopecia**: hair loss 4. N 5. <u>G</u>I Upset: **nausea, vomiting,** diarrhea 6. <u>E</u>asy bruising: thrombocytopenia (**easy bruising**), leukopenia	1. CBC (platelets) and LFTs every 6-12 mo and prior to start 2. Serum hCG 3. Pancreatic enzyme levels if abdominal pain/ vomiting • Draw trough levels 2-5 d after each dose increase	1. Pregnancy category: ×(neural tube defects) 2. Less GI upset with sodium divalproex 3. Low risk of hepatic failure and thrombocytopenia
	Drugs that VPA ↑	**Drugs that ↑ VPA**			
	Benzodiazepines	Chlorpromazine			
	Phenobarbital	Cimetidine			
	TCAs	Erythromycin			
	Salicylates	Felbamate			
		Fluoxetine			
Lamotrigine (Lamictal)	• FDA approved for long-term maintenance treatment for bipolar I disorder • First line for maintenance therapy in pregnancy Dosing: 1. 25 mg/d × 2 wk, then 50 mg/d × 2 wk in 2 doses 2. Increase by 25-50 mg/d each wk 3. Goal: 50-200 mg/d up to 400 mg $t_{1/2}$ = 15 h	1. Valproic acid—increases LTG levels 2. Carbamazepine—decreases LTG levels **Black box**: Stevens-Johnson syndrome with abrupt D/C	1. **Rash:** • SJS with starting dose and rapid rate of increase • Occurs in first 8 wk of starting 2. Leukopenia 3. Hepatic failure 4. <u>C</u>NS: headache, lethargy, diplopia or blurred vision, ataxia, somnolence, dizziness 5. <u>G</u>I: **nausea, vomiting, diarrhea. dyspepsia** 6. **Insomnia**	1. Urine pregnancy test before starting 2. CBC with platelet count every 6-12 mo	1. Pregnancy category: C 2. "No rush, no rash," SJS most common in patients with HLA-B*1502 allele (5% incidence, South Asian Indians), the FDA recommends screening in these ethnic groups before starting 3. Estrogen (contraceptives) may reduce the effectiveness

	Indications/MOA/Half-Life	Interactions	Adverse Effects	Monitoring	Clinical Pearls
Carbamazepine (Tegretol)	1. XR: FDA approved for **acute mania** and mixed episodes 2. Acute mania • Comparable to lithium • Onset faster than lithium • More effective in mixed mania, rapid cycling, and organic mania <u>MOA:</u> Inhibits kindling and repetitive firing of action potentials by inactivating sodium channels $t_{1/2}$ = 25-60 h, but decreases to 12-20 h due to autoinduction <u>Dosing:</u> 1. 100-200 mg 1-2×/d 2. Increase by 200 mg/d every 1-4 d, final dose of 800-1000 mg/d 3. No therapeutic serum levels established (4-12 µg/mL recommended)	1. Induces liver enzymes and frequently causes drug-drug interactions 2. Liver enzymes often decrease levels of CBZ	1. **Rash:** • SJS with starting dose and rapid rate of increase • Occurs in first 8 wk of starting • Exfoliative dermatitis • **Toxic epidermal necrolysis** 2. **Leukopenia, agranulocytosis** 3. Hepatic failure 4. <u>CNS:</u> headache, lethargy, diplopia or blurred vision, ataxia, somnolence, dizziness 5. <u>GI:</u> **nausea, vomiting, diarrhea** 6. **Hyponatremia** 7. **Pruritus** 8. **Fluid retention**	1. Na⁺ level, CBC with platelet count, and serum CBZ levels every 6-12 mo 2. Baseline: CBC, platelet, reticulocyte, serum iron, serum electrolytes, and EKG 3. CBC (biweekly first 2 mo, then once every 3 mo) 4. Platelet, reticulocyte, serum iron (annually) 5. LFT (every month first 2 mo, then every 3 mo) 6. CBZ levels, serum electrolytes and EKG (annually)	1. Pregnancy category: X • Teratogenic: craniofacial defects 2. "No rush, no rash," SJS most common in patients with HLA-B*1502 allele (5% incidence, South Asian Indians), the FDA recommends screening in these ethnic groups before starting 3. Reduces effectiveness of oral contraceptives

Drugs that ↓ CBZ	Drugs that ↑ CBZ	Drugs that CBZ↓
Phenytoin Phenobarbital	Cimetidine Diltiazem Verapamil Fluoxetine Fluvoxamine Valproate Erythromycin Danazol INH Propoxyphene Nefazodone	Doxycycline Valproate Clonazepam Theophylline Haloperidol Warfarin Dexamethasone TCA BCP Synthroid

	Indications/MOA/Half-Life		Adverse Effects	Monitoring	
Gabapentin (Neurontin)	$t_{1/2}$ = 5-9 h		• CNS: somnolence, dizziness, ataxia, fatigue • Leukopenia • Weight gain • Rash: can be fatal	**Monitor for rash**	

FIRST-GENERATION ANTIPSYCHOTICS

Typicals (First-Generation Antipsychotics)

Antipsychotics	Class/MOA/Indications	Contraindications/Interactions	Adverse Effects	Monitoring and Toxicity	Clinical Pearls
Chlorpromazine (Thorazine) Haloperidol (Haldol) Fluphenazine (Prolixin) Loxapine Perphenazine Thiothixene Trifluoperazine	1. **D2** antagonists • Differ in potency, not efficacy Indications: 1. *Positive* symptoms 2. Acute agitation (**acute psychosis**) 3. Psychosis in pregnancy—Haldol (gold standard) 4. Mania—preferred MOA: 1. Varying cholinergic, H1 and A1 blockade Dosing: 1. Haloperidol 5-15 mg/d once/d or divided BID	Interactions: 1. Avoid use with *alcohol* and other *CNS depressants* 2. Monitor closely with other QTc prolonging agents • *Chlorpromazine* • *Thioridazine* • *IV haloperidol* 3. ± decreased therapeutic effect with Parkinson's medications 4. Liver: CYP2D6 and CYP3A4 inhibitors and inducers **Black box warning**: • Use in dementia patients→ ↑ risk of death due to CV and infectious causes	1. **H1**: sedation, weight gain 2. **A1**: orthostasis (orthostatic hypotension) 3. **Anticholinergic effects**: Dry mouth, urinary retention, constipation 4. Hyperprolactinemia 5. QT prolongation	1. ↑ CPK: rhabdomyolysis 2. CBC: leukocytosis, thrombocytosis 3. LFTs: ↑ 4. LP: ↑ protein Monitoring for side effects is KEY: 1. EPS: (extrapyramidal symptoms) acute dyskinesias (early) • **Dystonia**: *painful muscle contractions* of the neck, jaw, face, tongue, eyes, limbs • **A**kathisia: motor restlessness (thighs or abdomen), insomnia, refusing to sit down, pacing, anxious • **P**arkinsonism effects: tremor, rigidity, bradykinesia, shuffling gait, stooped posture • **Tardive dyskinesia** (late): • Oral/buccal/lingual: Tongue darting, lip smacking, puckering, chewing • Limb: finger movements, foot movements, hand clenching • Trunk twisting 2. **NMS: (neuroleptic malignant syndrome)**—Potentially fatal idiosyncratic reaction • Fever: hyperpyrexia • Catatonia • Muscle (lead pipe) rigidity, dysarthria • Autonomic dysfunction: blood pressure changes, cardiovascular instability, pulmonary congestion, diaphoresis • Delirium: altered consciousness, confusion	1. Haldol = **gold standard for tx of psychosis in pregnancy** 2. Haldol—preferred for manic episodes because widely studied, less orthostatic hypotension 3. Better bioavailability with *IM preparations* = Depot formulations (also have to give PO to cover until steady state reached in 2-4 mo) 4. Treatment of NMS: supportive (fluids, antipyretics), Dantrolene (Dantrium) and bromocriptine (Parlodel) • **May take weeks to see full improvement in NMS symptoms** 5. Management of EPS • Lower antipsychotic or add anticholinergic drug • Treatment of dystonia: Benztropine 1-2 mg BID-QID, Cogentin, Benadryl, diazepam • Treatment of Tardive dyskinesia: Reserpine • EPS due to ↓ dopamine in nigrostriatal pathway

What is the main difference in mechanism of action between typical and atypical antipsychotic agents?

Answer: **Atypical** antipsychotics typically have **higher affinity for 5HT$_{2A}$** receptors than D$_2$ receptors.

- *Key*: fluphenazine and Haloperidol = high affinity for dopamine receptor, bind less tightly to others = more EPS
- Low-potency agents: bind to other receptors more than dopamine = lots of other side effects

SECOND-GENERATION ANTIPSYCHOTICS

Atypicals (**second-generation**): All block D2 receptors in the brain, except aripiprazole. Overall, less specificity for D2 receptor than typical antipsychotics. All block 5HT2A receptors with more affinity than D2 receptors→ decreased side effects
RICH Queens **ARE CL**UMSY **OL**D Zillionaires
More Effective for negative symptoms than first-generation antipsychotics, treats (+) symptoms as well; monitor FBS for all for development of diabetes (quarterly or semiannual)

	Class/MOA/Indications	Interactions	Adverse Effects	Monitoring	Clinical Pearls
Risperidone (Risperdal)	Class: **5HT$_{2A}$/D$_2$** antagonist MOA: Blocks α$_2$ and α$_1$ (high affinity) Indications: • Acute psychosis (first line) Dosing: 1. 1-2 mg once/d in 1-2 doses $t_{1/2}$ = 23 h		1. Sexual dysfunction (Erectile dysfunction, orgasm dysfunction) 2. Increased pigmentation 3. Rhinitis 4. ***Hyperprolactinemia*** 5. A1: orthostasis and reflex tachycardia, anxiety 6. **Weight gain** 7. GI: **nausea**, vomiting, **dyspepsia** 8. EPS with doses >6 mg/d • ***Akathisia*** 9. **Sedation**	1. Weight, waist circumference, BP, serum glucose, lipids	1. Long-acting IM given q 2 wk 2. Oral dissolvable tablet formulation available
Quetiapine (Seroquel)	Class: **5HT$_{2A}$/D$_2$** antagonist MOA: Blocks **H$_1$** and α$_1$ receptors Dosing: 1. Mania: 100-200 mg/d in 1-2 doses *biweekly* 2. Depression: 50 mg QHS daily, then increased by 50-100 mg daily (goal: 300-600 mg/d) $t_{1/2}$ = 6 h		1. A1: ***orthostatic hypotension***, dry mouth 2. H1: ***weight gain, sedation***, dizziness 3. **Headache** 4. GI: **constipation**	1. Eye examinations–check for **cataracts** 2. Weight, waist circumference, BP, serum glucose, lipids	1. Tablet only
Aripiprazole (Abilify)	Indications: 1. Mania (monotherapy) Class: D$_2$ ***partial*** agonist, **5HT$_{2A}$** antagonist MOA: Blocks **H$_1$** and α$_1$ receptors (moderate), no affinity for M1 receptors Dosing: 10-30 mg/d $t_{1/2}$ = 75 h, active metabolite 94 h; tablet only	1. Beware with anxious pts–can make them worse 2. CYP3A4 interaction	1. **Headache** 2. *A*kathisia (agitation, *restlessness*) 3. **GI: nausea/vomiting, constipation** 4. **Insomnia**		1. Long-acting injectable (depot) 1/mo available for maintenance therapy 2. Comes in oral dissolvable tablet (ODT) formulation

(continued)

(continued)

	Class/MOA/ Indications	Interactions	Adverse Effects	Monitoring	Clinical Pearls
Clozapine (Clozaril)	1. $5HT_{2A}/D_2$ antagonist 2. Blocks **M1, H₁** and α₁ with high affinity 3. Binds to many other receptors Indications: 1. Treats *refractory schizophrenia* 2. **Can improve Tardive dyskinesia** $t_{1/2} = 12$ h	1. Many drug interactions due to metabolism via multiple CYP enzyme pathways 2. Contraindicated: ***uncontrolled epilepsy*** 3. **Black box:** myocarditis, *agranulocytosis*	• High metabolic risk: "metabolic syndrome" (cl > ol > qu = ri > ar = zi) • Anticholinergic (**constipation**) • **A1:** orthostasis (*fatal hypotension*) • **Sedation** • **S**eizures (highest risk) • **S**alivation (drooling)	1. **Baseline CBC:** 2. Requires frequent CBC monitoring • Weekly blood monitoring first 6 mo, then biweekly for next 6 mo, then monthly after 1 y	1. Pregnancy category B (safe)—although not recommended 2. Very effective but associated with many side effects 3. The patient and prescriber *must be registered* with the manufacturer 4. Has been shown to reduce suicide attempts in patients with schizophrenia who are at high risk
Olanzapine (Zyprexa)	Class: $5HT_{2A}/D_2$ antagonist MOA: Blocks **M1, H₁** and α₁ with high affinity Dosing: 1. 10-15 mg/d in 1-2 doses $t_{1/2} = 30$ h		1. H1: **sedation** 2. Anticholinergic effects: **dry mouth, orthostatic hypotension** 3. Metabolic: glucose intolerance, diabetes, hyperlipidemia, **weight gain** 4. GI: constipation 5. **Increased appetite**	1. **LFT**—can be elevated 2. Weight, waist circumference, BP, serum glucose, lipids	1. Pharmacologically and structurally similar to clozapine (sister drug) 2. Relprevv = long-acting version, given every 2-4 wk 3. Oral dissolvable tablet (ODT) formulation available

Ziprasidone (Geodon)	MOA:
	$5HT_{2A}/D_2$ and α₁ antagonist (no H1)
	Dosing:
	1. Mania: start at 40 mg BID
	2. Depression: 5 mg daily QHS, then 5 mg/d each wk, max: 15-20 mg/d
		1. $t_{1/2} = 3.2$-10 h (shorter than other agents = give 2×/d)	1. **QTc prolongation**
			2. **Sedation**, light-headedness, **dizziness**
			3. **A1:** orthostasis, dry mouth
			4. Nausea
			5. **Headache**
			6. EPS
			  • **Akathisia**
			7. Weight gain, increased appetite
				1. EKG	1. Consider if the patient eats frequently before giving this agent
					2. Increased in presence of food (50%)
					  • Must give with food (at least 350 calories) to improve absorption
					3. Highly protein bound

Lurasidone (Latuda)	Indications: 1. Approved in October 2010 for the treatment of **schizophrenia** 2. Bipolar depression (first line) MOA: *Partial* agonist for **5-HT₁A** receptors, blocks α₁ (moderate), little to no muscarinic or histaminic blockade Dosing: 20 mg daily QHS, taken with food, increased every 2-7 d by 20 mg/d (goal: 20-120 mg/d)	1. CYP3A4 metabolism: use with strong inhibitors/inducers	1. **S**edation (23%) 2. **N**ausea (12%) 3. **A**kathisia (15%)—EPS (26%) 4. **P**arkinsonian Symptoms 5. Hyperprolactinemia (8%) 6. Hyperglycemia (14%) 7. Headache		1. Pregnancy category B (safe)—although not recommended 2. ***Must be taken with food >350 calories*** 3. High affinity for $5HT_{2A}/D_2$ and **5HT₇** receptors

MONITORING FOR ANTIPSYCHOTICS

Weight (BMI)	Baseline, then every month for 3 mo, then every 3 mo
Waist circumference	Baseline, then annually
Blood pressure	Baseline, then every 12 wk, then annually
Fasting plasma glucose	Baseline, then every 12 wk, then annually
Fasting lipid panel	Baseline, then every 12 wk, then annually

DOSE ADJUSTMENTS

Renal Impairment	Hepatic Impairment
• Risperidone • Lurasidone	• Risperidone and lurasidone (moderate-severe) • Quetiapine

TIME COURSE TO RESPONSE (FIRST GENERATION)

	Inhibitor	Inducer	Substrate	1-3 d	1-2 wk	3-6 wk	Persistent Symptoms
CYP3A4	Ketoconazole Clarithromycin Erythromycin Fluconazole Protease Inhibitors	Rifampin Phenytoin Carbamazepine Phenobarbital	Haloperidol Clozapine Olanzapine Paliperidone Quetiapine Ziprasidone Aripiprazole	Decreased agitation, hostility, aggression, combativeness, anxiety, normalization of sleep and eating patterns	Improvement in socialization self-care habits and mood	Improvement in thought disorder, delusions, hallucinations, conversations	Impaired insight, inappropriate affect, fixed delusions/hallucinations
CYP2D6	Fluoxetine Paroxetine Bupropion Ritonavir	Rifampin	Haloperidol Chlorpromazine Thioridazine Perphenazine Fluphenazine Risperidone Paliperidone Aripiprazole				
CYP1A2	Fluvoxamine Fluoroquinolones	Smoking	Thiothixene Clozapine Olanzapine				

SMOKING CESSATION THERAPIES

	Class/MOA/Indications	Precautions/Contraindications	Adverse Effects	Dose	Duration
Bupropion SR (Zyban)	First line (FDA approved) for smoking cessation	History of seizure disorder History of eating disorder	1. Insomnia 2. Dry mouth	150 mg every morning for 3 d, then 150 mg BID (treatment starts 1-2 wk pre-quit)	Maintenance: 7-12 wk for up to 6 mo

Nicotine gum (Nicorette)	First line (FDA approved) for smoking cessation	None	1. Mouth soreness
			2. Dyspepsia
				1-24 cigarettes/d:
				  2 mg gum (up to 24 pieces/d)
				25+ cigarettes/d:
				  4-mg gum (up to 24 pieces/d)
					Up to 12 wk

Nicotine patch (NicoDerm CQ, Nicotrol)	First line (FDA approved) for smoking cessation	None	1. Local skin irritation 2. Insomnia	1. 21 mg × 24 h→ 2. 14 mg × 24 h→ 3. 7 mg × 24 h→ 4. 15 mg × 16 h→	4 wk then 2 wk then 2 wk 8 wk

(continued)

(continued)

	Class/MOA/ Indications	Precautions/ Contraindications	Adverse Effects	Dose	Duration
Varenicline (Chantix)	First line (FDA approved) for smoking cessation	Renal impairment	1. Nausea 2. Abnormal dreams	1. 0.5 mg/d for 3 d, then 2. 0.5 mg BID for 4 d, then 3. 0.1 mg BID	1. 12 wk or 24 wk based on response
Clonidine (Catapres)	Second line for smoking cessation (not FDA approved)	Rebound hypertension	1. Dry mouth 2. Drowsiness 3. Dizziness 4. Sedation	0.15-0.75 mg/d	3-10 wk
Nortriptyline	Second line for smoking cessation (not FDA approved)	Risk of cardiac arrhythmias	1. Sedation 2. Dry mouth	75-100 mg/d	12 wk

U.S. Public Health Service.

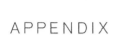
Guide to Contraindications and Precautions for Vaccinations

KEY TAKEAWAYS

Vaccine	Contraindications	Precautions
Hepatitis B	• Severe allergic reaction to vaccine component or previous dose	• Moderate-severe illness ± fever • Infant <2000 g
Rotavirus	• Severe allergic reaction to vaccine component or previous dose • Severe combined immunodeficiency (SCID) • **History of intussusception**	• Moderate-severe illness ± fever • Immunocompetent other than SCID • Chronic GI disease • Spina bifida, bladder exstrophy
DTaP, Tdap, or DT/Td	• Severe allergic reaction to vaccine component or previous dose • If containing pertussis: encephalopathy (coma, decreased consciousness, prolonged seizures)	• Moderate-severe illness ± fever • **Guillain-Barre syndrome** within 6 wk after previous dose of tetanus toxoid–containing vaccine • See link for more
Haemophilus influenzae type b (Hib)	• Severe allergic reaction to vaccine component or previous dose • **Age <6 y**	• Moderate-severe illness ± fever
Inactivated poliovirus (IPV)	• Severe allergic reaction to vaccine component or previous dose	• Moderate-severe illness ± fever
Pneumococcal (PCV13, PPSV23)	• Severe allergic reaction to vaccine component or previous dose	• Moderate-severe illness ± fever
MMR	• Severe allergic reaction to vaccine component or previous dose • Known severe immunodeficiency • **Pregnancy**	• Moderate-severe illness ± fever • Recipient (within 11 mo) of Ab-containing blood product • **History of thrombocytopenia or purpura** • **Need for tuberculin skin testing**
Varicella	• Severe allergic reaction to vaccine component or previous dose • Known severe immunodeficiency • **Pregnancy**	• Moderate-severe illness ± fever • Recipient (within 11 mo) of Ab-containing blood product • **Recipient of antivirals 24 h before vaccine**

(continued)

(continued)

Vaccine	Contraindications	Precautions
Hepatitis A	• Severe allergic reaction to vaccine component or previous dose	• Moderate-severe illness ± fever
Influenza, live attenuated	• Severe allergic reaction to vaccine component or previous dose • **Children aged <2 or adults aged >49 y** • **Concurrent use with aspirin or aspirin-containing meds in children or adolescents up to 17 y old** • **Pregnancy,** immunocompromised, egg allergy, children aged 2-4 y with asthma, people who have taken antivirals for flu treatment in last 48 h	• Moderate-severe illness ± fever • **History of Guillain-Barre Syndrome within 6 wk or prior flu vaccine** • **Asthma in persons aged 5+ y** • **Other chronic medical conditions**
Human papillomavirus (HPV)	• Severe allergic reaction to vaccine component or previous dose	• Moderate-severe illness ± fever • **Pregnancy**
Meningococcal conjugate, polysaccharide (MPSV4)	• Severe allergic reaction to vaccine component or previous dose	• Moderate-severe illness ± fever
Zoster (HZV)	• Severe allergic reaction to vaccine component • Known severe immunodeficiency • **Pregnancy**	• Moderate-severe illness ± fever • **Recipient of antivirals 24 h before vaccine**

A complete source can be found at http://www.immunize.org/catg.d/p3072a.pdf.

Index

Note: Page numbers followed by "f" indicate figures and "t" indicate tables.

A

Abdomen, acute, 257
Abdominal aortic aneurysm, 374t
Abdominal pain, 398–399, 625t
ABG analysis, 686–687, 686t
Abnormal uterine bleeding, 463, 496, 496t
Abortion, 472, 473t–475t
Abruptio placentae, urgent care, 189t–190t
Acanthosis nigricans, 158f, 158t–159t
Achilles tendon rupture, 733
Achondroplasia, 348t, 351f
Acid-base disorders
    arterial blood gases
        acidosis, 683
        alkalosis, 683
        anion gap, 686, 686t
        base deficit/excess, 683
        bicarbonate buffering system, 683
        HCO_3^-, 683
        nonanion gap metabolic acidosis, 686
        $PaCO_2$, 683
        PaO_2, 683
        pH compensation, 684–685, 684f, 685t
        serum chemistry normal ranges, 685, 685t
    metabolic alkalosis, 686–687, 686t
Acidosis homeostasis, 683–684, 684f
Acne vulgaris, 141, 142f, 143, 143t, 144f
Acoustic neuroma, 419t
Acquired hemolytic anemia, 441, 442t
Acromegaly, 233t–234t, 632
Actinic keratosis, 138, 138f, 138t
Acute arterial occlusion, 374, 375f, 375t–376t
Acute coronary syndrome, 562
Acute interstitial nephritis, 239t
Acute lymphoblastic leukemia, 280t
Acute myeloid leukemia, 280t
Acute renal injury, 235–237, 236t
Acute respiratory distress/failure, 392–393, 392, 395t

Addison's disease, 228t–229t
Adjustment disorder, 537, 538t
Adolescent growth, 347
Adrenal carcinoma, 632, 632t
Adrenal insufficiency, 632, 632t
Affective flattening, 740
Agoraphobia, 546
Alcoholic hallucinosis, 552
Alcohol intoxication, 408, 408t–409t
Alcohol-related disorders, 552, 553t–555t, 555
Alkalosis homeostasis, 683–684, 684f
Allergic rhinitis/nasal congestion, 97t
Allergies, 187t–188t
Alogia, 740
Alopecia
    androgenic alopecia hair loss patterns, 148f, 150t
    areata, 147f, 150t
    Norwood-Hamilton classification, 149f, 150t
    telogen effluvium, 148f, 150t
Alzheimer's disease, 117, 117t
Amenorrhea, 463
    primary, 465, 465t–468t
    secondary, 466t–468t
    tanner staging, breast development, 466f
American Burn Association criteria, 189
American College of Chest Physicians (ACCP) Risk Stratification, 604t
American Society of Anesthesiologists (ASA) Classification System, 607, 607t
Amphetamines, 558
Anal fissure and fistula, 35f, 35t, 37f
Analgesia, 639
Anemia, 276t, 652t
Aneuploidy, fetal, 452, 452t
Aneurysm, definition, 373
Angina pectoris, 12, 12t–15t
Anhedonia, 740
Anion gap metabolic acidosis, 686, 686t

Ankle
    dislocations, 727f–728f, 728t
    fractures, 722t–723t, 724f–725f
Ankylosing spondylitis, 734, 735t
Anorectal abscess, 401, 401t
Anorexia nervosa, 399, 588, 589t–590t, 592t
    medical complications, 590, 590t–592t
Anterior cord syndrome, 415, 416t
Anterior drawer test, 733
Antibiotics, preoperative care, 607t
Anticoagulation, 620t
Anticonvulsants, 746t–747t
Antidepressants, 740t–744t
    depressive disorders, 536
Antipsychotics
    atypical, 749
    first-generation, 748t
    second-generation, 749t–750t
Anxiety disorders
    generalized anxiety disorder, 544, 545t
    panic disorder, 546, 546t
    phobic disorders, 548, 549t–550t
    post-traumatic stress disorder (PTSD), 547–548, 547t–548t
Anxiolytic related disorders, 559, 559t–560t
Aortic aneurysm/dissection, 373, 373f, 373t–374t
Aortic stenosis, 669
Apgar scoring, 461, 461t
Aphthous ulcers, 100f, 100t
Apley test, 733
Apnea, 397
Appendicitis, 47t, 321, 322t, 483
Arrhythmia, chronic, 659
Arterial embolism/thrombosis, 374, 374t
Arterial/venous ulcer disease, 208t–209t, 209, 210f
Arteritis, giant cell, 408t
Arthritis. *See under type of arthritis*
Aseptic technique, 612